COMPREHENSIVE FAMILY AND COMMUNITY HEALTH NURSING

Susan Clemen-Stone, RN, MPH
Associate Professor
Community Health Nursing
School of Nursing, University of Michigan

Diane Gerber Eigsti, RN, MS
Project Coordinator, Kellogg Grant
Community Health Accreditation Program (CHAP)
National League for Nursing
New York, NY

Sandra L. McGuire, RN, EdD
Associate Professor
College of Nursing, University of Tennessee-Knoxville

Third Edition

With 128 illustrations

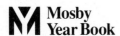

Mosby
Year Book

St. Louis   Baltimore   Boston   Chicago   London   Philadelphia   Sydney   Toronto

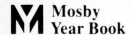

**Mosby
Year Book**

Dedicated to Publishing Excellence

Editor: N. Darlene Como
Developmental Editor: Laurie Sparks
Project Supervisor: Lilliane Anstee
Design: Laura Steube

Printed in the United States of America.

Mosby–Year Book, Inc.
11830 Westline Industrial Drive
St. Louis, MO 63146

Part One opening photo: Visiting Nursing Service of New York City.
Part Three opening photo (*bottom left*): American Society on Aging, San Francisco, photograph by Patricia Lee Chorazy.

Library of Congress Cataloging-in-Publication Data

Clemen-Stone, Susan.
    Comprehensive family and community health nursing / Susan Clemen
-Stone, Diane Gerber Eigsti, Sandra L. McGuire. — 3rd ed.
        p.   cm
    Includes bibliographical references and index.
    ISBN 0-8016-6068-8
    1. Community health nursing.   2. Family—Health and hygiene.
3. Community health nursing—United States.   I. Eigsti, Diane
Gerber.   II. McGuire, Sandra L.   III. Title
    [DNLM: 1. Community Health Nursing.   2. Family.   WY 106 C625c]
RT98.C56   1991
362.1′73—dc20
DNLM/DLC
for Library of Congress   90-13416
                                                                      CIP

UG/DC/DC   9 8 7 6 5 4 3 2 1

PREFACE

When the first edition of this book was published a decade ago, it was obvious that health care trends, one of the most notable being the emphasis on cost containment, would significantly impact community health nursing practice. The 1980s for community health nursing were indeed characterized by major changes such as the shifting of health care delivery to the home and other community-based settings, more active consumer involvement in health care decision making, the development of different models for providing community health nursing services, and the disturbing emergence of health problems which are posing a threat to the health of our society. As we enter the 1990s, community health nursing will continue to face major challenges. It is apparent that our society is no longer willing to pay for escalating health care costs. It is also apparent that changes must occur in all components of the health care delivery system in order to deal with emerging health care crises. Community health nursing is ready to make the needed changes; the struggles experienced during the 1980s were maturing ones. Much rethinking about the goals and values of community health nursing has taken place.

Although *Comprehensive Family and Community Health Nursing* adheres to the original purposes of its other editions, a substantial attempt has been made to reflect the changes and innovations that have occurred within the field since its inception. As originally designed, this text is presented to assist students and practitioners to gain an understanding of the unique role of the community health nurse and the exciting, challenging nature of a specialty field which integrates the knowledge and skills of professional nursing and the philosophy, content, and methods of public health. The third edition, however, places increased emphasis on examining how unprecedented changes in the health care delivery system have expanded the nature and scope of community health nursing practice. The role of the community health nurse in providing health promotion and disease prevention services as well as long-term care is stressed. The importance of achieving our nation's public health goals, as described in major policy documents, is examined carefully. Both the health promotion needs of groups across the life span and strategies to meet these needs are addressed. Neglected public health mandates and growing challenges in community health nursing practice—such as infant mortality, communicable disease control, pediatric AIDS, complex home care demands, homelessness, elder abuse, and nurse shortages—have been expanded on to increase the comprehensiveness of the text. A more thoroughly developed discussion on the role of the community health nurse in addressing these mandates and challenges enhances the usefulness of this book.

In recent years, significant philosophical, economic, social, political, and technological trends have dramatically influenced community health nursing practice. Revisions have been made throughout the text to reflect these trends and the most current data related to major health care legislation, demographic characteristics of the population, health problems of at risk populations, and advancements in nursing. Trends are well documented by recent literature. Extensive information about where the community health nurse can obtain up-to-date statistical data related to the health needs of at risk populations and resources available to assist in meeting community health needs has been added. The appendices provide valuable assessment tools, legislative information, and data that can facilitate the use of the nursing process with various client groups. A significant addition for educators is an instructor's manual with learning objectives, lecture outlines, suggestions for didactic and clinical learning activities, instructor resource materials, and sample test questions.

The organization of this text stems from the philosophy of community and public health nursing practice delineated in the American Nurses' Association and the American Public Health Association definitions of this specialty area. Flowing from these definitions, the authors explore the unique aspects of community health nursing practice throughout the text. The reader is helped to examine the multiple factors that affect the health status of individuals, families, groups at risk, and communities and is encouraged to seek improved ways for providing preventive health care services in an effective and efficient manner. Emphasis continues to be placed on how the community health nurse can provide *quality* nursing care for multiple client groups within the community.

The unique perspective that community health nurses bring to any health care team is a holistic philosophy derived from a synthesis of nursing and public health knowledge. Preventive activities at all three levels—primary, secondary, and tertiary—are implemented by community health nurses to enhance the state of wellness in a community. Community health nurses respect cultural differences and varying life-styles and analyze sociocultural, political, economic, and environmental forces that influence consumer interests, needs, beliefs, and values. This text has addressed the unique role of the community health nurse by:

- Analyzing the scope of community health nursing practice
- Integrating nursing and public health knowledge throughout the text
- Presenting the family-centered approach to nursing care with emphasis on examining significant structural and process parameters of family functioning
- Describing the health care planning process as a problem-solving approach for communities
- Utilizing a developmental approach to address the health needs of populations across the life span and to plan appropriate preventive health services for populations at risk

- Discussing in-depth health, welfare, and environmental services systems and how the community health nurse can facilitate client utilization of these resources
- Presenting specific federal legislation that provides funding for health care services and affects the delivery of nursing services
- Discussing the emerging importance of home health and long-term care and the impact of this trend for community health nurses
- Including the principles of management and quality assurance utilized by community health nurses to manage and evaluate the multiple responsibilities assigned to them
- Integrating theoretical concepts and clinical data in case situations to illustrate the application of nursing and public health theory in the practice setting
- Presenting tools currently being used by practitioners that assist them in delivering quality nursing services to clients
- Including selected bibliographies that expand on the theoretical concepts presented in the text and that describe the multiple situations encountered by the community health nurse

The overall acceptance of the other editions of this book has prompted the authors to retain the basic organization of the original text. The three major parts of this textbook explore how community health nurses utilize concepts from nursing and public health to provide comprehensive, continuous preventive health services for groups (families, populations at risk, and communities). Part One presents a philosophical foundation for nursing practice in the community. It analyzes the origin, scope, and changing nature of current community health nursing practice and examines community dynamics and social, cultural, political, and economic factors that influence the delivery of health and welfare services. Part Two focuses on the direct service functions of the staff community health nurse. It discusses why the family is viewed as the unit of service in community health and outlines relevant theoretical concepts essential for understanding family dynamics. Special emphasis is placed on analyzing how the community health nurse utilizes the nursing process to implement and evaluate intervention strategies with families. Part Three stresses the value of working with populations at risk in the community. Population groups, delineated by age, are examined in terms of developmental characteristics, health needs, health and welfare services, barriers to the utilization of health and welfare services, and the role of the community health nurse in meeting the needs of high-risk groups. Long-term care, which has particular relevance for this specialty area, is discussed. The epidemiological process and the principles of health planning are presented as the tools for studying the determinants of health and disease frequencies in populations and for planning health promotion and disease control programs. The need for health care providers to address the ethical dimension of practice and to become politically active during the health planning process is stressed. Management concepts and information systems are also included because they help community health nurses to integrate and handle their multiple professional commitments in a meaningful way.

The logo for the book, interconnecting systems and subsystems on a continuum, emphasizes a major focus in community health nursing practice—helping clients to effectively fit together community systems and subsystems in their environment to maximize growth—and is stressed throughout the book. One will frequently find, when working in the community setting, that clients (individuals, families, populations at risk, and communities) have not reached their maximum potential because the environment they are functioning in does not enhance the growth process. Community health nurses can and frequently do alter this occurrence. They have unique skills which assist them in bringing together in a meaningful way all the systems encountered by their clients.

Acknowledgments

The authors are greatly indebted to family, friends, colleagues, students, and former faculty and associates for their support, guidance, and assistance as we revised this book. Special appreciation is extended to the following individuals:

- Beverly Smith, our administrative secretary and a special friend, whose painstaking efforts, patience, and dedication to our project made it a reality. This book could never have been published without her help.
- Bill Smith, whose "it only takes a little more to do it right" encouragement, as we began this process a decade ago, provided the impetus to move forward. His willingness to share his wife's time will never be forgotten.
- Nancy Watson, assistant professor, The University of Rochester, who readily shared her ideas and materials related to the population-based health planning process.
- Leslie Davis, Ike Eigsti, and Henry Parks for helping us with our artwork and photography.
- Marilyn Franecki for her assistance in researching current literature in the field.
- Denver Stone, who willingly devoted considerable time to the tedious aspects of the manuscript preparation process.
- Colleagues from the University of Michigan and University of Tennessee Schools of Nursing for their encouragement and support.
- Colleagues from the service setting who have shared with us materials their staff developed to facilitate the delivery of quality client services.
- Publishers and authors who graciously granted us permission to use information from their writings.
- The Mosby–Year Book staff, especially Darlene Como, Laurie Sparks, and Lilliane Anstee, for their support, understanding, and concrete assistance.
- All our friends and family members who "understood" and allowed us to postpone events and activities.

Susan Clemen-Stone
Diane Gerber Eigsti
Sandra L. McGuire

TO OUR SIGNIFICANT OTHERS:

Verna and Al J. Clemen, for their special love that promoted growth and family cohesiveness, and for encouraging and supporting independent thinking even when this was not the norm.

John and Sharon Clemen and **Sara and Henry Parks,** for their caring, friendship, and encouragement.

Denver Stone, for his love, unfailing support, and knowing just the right time to assist.

Teresa and Rick Stone, for their patience and understanding.

Holly Marie Huling, for bringing the joys of childhood into our life and for her loving ways.

To the memory of **Ike**

Heiki-Lara and Inge-Marie Eigsti, for their patience and loving.

Joseph, Matthew, Kelly, and Kerry McGuire, for their love and support.

Donald and Mary Lue Johnson, for their pride in this publication, their continued encouragement, and their love and interest.

Arthur and Sally Johnson, for the belief they instilled in the value of education, the role modeling they provided, and their constant love.

Judy Simpson, for her continued faith in and support of the nursing profession.

Alma Weale, for recognizing the importance of this publication and her unfailing encouragement.

CONTENTS

Part Three: Planning Health Services for Populations at Risk

Unit Four: Foundations for Community Assessment, Diagnosis, and Health-Planning Activities

Unit Five: Meeting the Needs of Populations at Risk across the Life Span

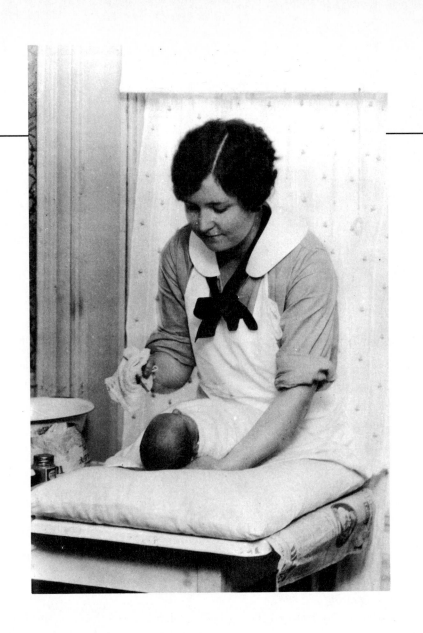

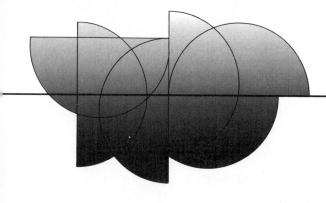

PART ONE

A Foundation for Community Health Nursing Practice

Public health nurses have been leaders in improving the quality of health care for people since the late 1800s. They have been the vanguard of change for both the nursing profession and society as a whole. They stressed the importance of establishing standards for nursing practice, nursing education at the university level, and social reform to improve the quality of life for all individuals. They quickly recognized the need to deal with community dynamics and to influence legislative processes and the direction of our health and welfare systems at the local, state, and national level.

In order for community health nurses to continue the progress made by their early leaders, they must understand where and how they began, the nature of current community health nursing practice, and how community forces contribute to, or distract from, the health of families and populations at risk. Examining how the health-care delivery system is organized and what it provides and does not provide is particularly important because community health nurses focus attention on health planning activities aimed at correcting deficiencies in this system. Part 1 looks at these aspects of community health nursing practice.

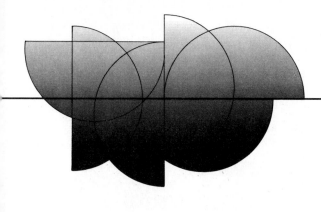

UNIT ONE

Introduction to the Historical and Current Perspectives on Community Health Nursing Practice

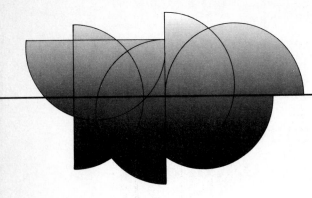

Histories make women wise.

FRANCIS BACON

1

A Historical Overview of Community Health Nursing

_____ OBJECTIVES _____

Upon completion of this chapter, the reader will be able to:

1. Identify how early feminists shaped the development of public health nursing.
2. Relate how societal beliefs about women influenced the development and image of nursing.
3. Discuss how historical events have shaped the development of community health nursing practice.

4. Analyze the contributions of Lillian Wald and Florence Nightingale to nursing and public health.
5. Summarize historical events which influenced beliefs about educational preparation for community health nursing practice.

Today's nurse should be proud of the founders of public health nursing! They are heroines who are role models for persons committed to nursing and to working for the improvement of health care services. Lavinia Lloyd Dock, one early public health nurse pioneer, was picketing, parading, and protesting 70 years ago. Dock, a feminist, scholar, and accomplished musician, devoted 20 years of her life to helping women gain the right to vote (Christy, 1969).

To understand the role the legendary Lavinia Dock and her peers played in establishing public health nursing, we must go farther back into the history of nursing. Looking at significant public health nursing pioneers and events helps us to understand how public health nursing was shaped and how areas of concern within public health nursing developed.

IN THE BEGINNING

Nursing began when humanity began.

The word nurse is a reduced form of the Middle English *nurice,* which was derived, through the old French norrice, from the Latin *nutricius* (nourishing). In Roman mythology, the Goddess Fortuna, in addition to her usual function as Goddess of Fate, was also worshipped as Jupiter's nurse (Fortuna Praeneste) and prayed to for hygiene in the public baths (Fortuna Balnearis). From the dawn of civilization, mankind has sought to acquire a knowledge of pain-relieving remedies and to discover additional means of preventing disease. To alleviate human suffering, man has also developed nursing roles. (Kalisch and Kalisch, 1986, p. 1)

In 1916, Mary Sewall Gardner, another public health nurse pioneer, published the "first really comprehensive and authoritative presentation on the subject of public health nursing" (Nelson, 1954, p. 38). Gardner wrote that "the true ancestors of the modern nurse are the noble abbesses and early Christian women who were trying to do for their day what the nurse of today is trying to do for her's" (Gardner, 1919, p. 3).

Visiting nursing, or the care of ill people at home by a specialized group, has probably existed down through the ages. The New Testament is replete with stories of how the sick were visited. The Apostle Paul wrote of Phoebe in Rom. 16:1–2, "I commend to you our sister Phoebe, a deaconess of the church at Cenchreae, . . . help her in whatever she may require from you, for she has been a helper of many and of myself as well." Phoebe is probably the first visiting nurse we know by name.

The Middle Ages, with the subsequent rise of monasteries and convents, contributed to nursing a specialized effort to care for the ill. Specific convents had as their stated reason for existing the nursing care of sick people. To perform acts of mercy for the well-being of one's eternal soul was, during this time, a common and accepted reason for entering nursing convents. These early nurses included among their numbers males who were drawn into military nursing orders as a result of the Crusades (1091-1291). The Crusades were religious wars between the Turks and the Christians which encouraged both the spread of disease and the exchange of ideas between East and West. It has been well documented that nurses of high intellectual capacity responded to the needs of society in times of war and persecution (Dolan, 1978).

The Renaissance (about 1500-1700) brought about great political, social, and economic expansion. Two names of this period that are important to public health nursing are St. Vincent de Paul and Mademoiselle Le Gras. Gardner says of de Paul that "there is no more prominent figure in the history of nursing and social welfare" (Gardner, 1919, p. 9).

In 1617, de Paul organized the Sisterhood of the Dames de Charité. The ladies went from home to home, visiting the sick. As the movement spread and its numbers increased, difficulties arose because of the lack of supervision of work done by them. St. Vincent reorganized this group by appointing Mademoiselle Le Gras as a supervisor. Together, their greatest contribution to the development of public health nursing was the idea of providing education for those persons helping the poor and the sick, as well as recognizing the need for professional supervision of caregivers. Taking care of ill people at home could not be accomplished simply with intuition; nursing practice must be based on principles somewhat akin to social work as we know it today. They felt that people could best be helped by "helping them to help themselves." De Paul and Le Gras also believed that one must find out the needs of the poor, investigate the causes, and then help supply possible solutions. Taken for granted by people today, these were entirely new concepts of charity for this time (Maynard, 1939).

The Era of Sairy Gamp

It is difficult to imagine how nursing could have sunk to the low levels it did during the time from the end of the seventeenth century to the middle of the nineteenth century. The change from nursing care given by devoted deaconesses to nursing care given by drunks and prostitutes is a change that is baffling. In *Martin Chuzzlewit*, originally published in 1844, Charles Dickens (1910) immortalized the prototype of the nurse of this era by describing a drunk, untrained servant, Sairy Gamp, as a nurse. In order to understand what persons such as Florence Nightingale and her peers accomplished, the reader must know the nursing conditions that were in existence when they began their efforts to professionalize nursing.

The basis for the nursing care given by Phoebe and her contemporaries was charity. Thus the care was only as good as the church organization that supported it. During the time of the Reformation (the 1500s), nursing care degenerated to the greatest extent in countries where Catholic organizations were overthrown. In England, for instance, 100 hospitals were closed, and for a period of time there was no provision for the institutional care of ill people who were poor (Deloughery, 1977, p. 23). When nursing lost the importance once lent it by the church, it also lost its social standing. Thus, it was necessary to recruit nurses from distinctly lower classes, because "respectable" people would no longer do the work.

The status of women also greatly affected the change in the status of nursing. The church had given women an opportunity for a career in nursing. Love for others was the basis of the Gospel, and women were considered to be persons of worth. The Reformation and subsequent Protestant church movement changed this attitude. The general social position of women reached its lowest level in the eighteenth century.

The accompanying conditions in society during the 1600s were also dismal. The slums of European cities were huge and bred disease. Life expectancy was short and mortality rates were high. Before the Industrial Revolution (about 1750-1850) the social and economic structure of the Western world was quite simple: there were only a few large cities and work was largely agrarian. Social classes were rigidly stratified. During this time medicine was at a low level, largely because the scientific basis for it was unknown. Thus, health care was based on folklore and superstition.

Nursing existed in a low and dismal state indeed. It existed without organization and without social standing. No one who could possibly earn a living in some other way performed this service. Those who did so lost caste thereby, for as one is judged partly by the company one keeps, a woman who began to practice nursing was almost certain to become corrupted if she were not so already. (Deloughery, 1977, p. 24)

With this background, the contributions of Florence Nightingale to nursing, to public health, and to women are inestimable.

Florence Nightingale's Legacy

The family of this pioneer nurse leader was a wealthy one, and the environment into which she was born in 1820 became instrumental in her life's work. Nightingale was well educated by her father and, to her family's chagrin, longed to be a nurse. After a delay of many years, in deference to her family's wishes, she entered nurses' training with Pastor Fliedner, at Kaiserswerth on the Rhine, Germany. Her subsequent work in the Crimean War at Scutari has been chronicled by many, among them Longfellow, in his "Santa Filomena." It was there that she demonstrated that thousands of lives could be saved by intelligent nursing care and that capable nurses were needed in military hospitals. This was accomplished in the face of overwhelming obstacles. The hospital at Scutari was built for 1700 patients. When Nightingale arrived, there were 3000 to 4000 wounded men in it, lying naked with no beds, no blankets, and no eating or laundry facilities. Within days of her appearance at Scutari, she had a food kitchen operating as well as a laundry.

When Florence Nightingale began her career, it was a very dreadful thing to be a nurse. By helping establish the first modernly planned training school for nurses at St. Thomas Hospital in 1850, Nightingale set the example for Bellevue Hospital in New York City to follow in 1873. She also began the movement which led to the University Schools of Nursing at Western Reserve and Yale (Winslow, 1946, p. 331). Nightingale was the originator of the concept of the nursing process. She insisted that educated nurses were essential to perform the nurse's role. In this role she included assessment and intervention, followed by evaluation. In her famous *Notes on Nursing,* she defined nursing as that care that puts a person in the best possible condition for nature to either restore or preserve health, to prevent or cure disease or injury (Nightingale, 1859). Furthermore, from the very beginning of her career, she visualized the nurse as not merely an attendant for the sick but also a teacher of hygiene. She described the nurse as a "health missioner," a guide and teacher of health to the individual in the home. She recognized that "from the very nature of the case, compulsion can under no conditions work the changes we want to see wrought by the obedience of consent" (Winslow, p. 331). This was a very early affirmation of the principle that individuals are responsible for their own health.

THE ESTABLISHMENT OF VISITING NURSING

Visiting nursing, or district nursing, was the forerunner of public health nursing. The modern concept of a nurse who provides care to families in the home was visualized and established in 1859 by William Rathbone of Liverpool, England. "It is to Mr. Rathbone that we owe the first definitely formulated district nursing association and in that sense he may be called the father of the present movement" (Gardner, 1919, p. 14). Rathbone

was a wealthy businessman and philanthropist. His wife died after a long illness, and he had been impressed and comforted by the skilled nursing care that was given her in the months before she died. Rathbone had long been interested in helping the many poor people of Liverpool. If nursing care could help his wife who had everything that money could buy, how much more might it do for poor people whose physical illnesses were made increasingly burdensome by their poverty. To test his idea, he employed Mrs. Mary Robinson, the nurse who had cared for his wife, to visit the "sick poor" in their homes. She was to give care, instruct both the patient and the family in the care of the sick, and teach hygienic practices to prevent illnesses. The experiment was so successful that Rathbone decided to establish a permanent system of district or visiting nursing in Liverpool (McNeil, 1967, p. 1).

Rathbone's first problem was that there were no nurses in Liverpool to do this difficult work. So, with the help and advice of Florence Nightingale, he founded a school in 1859 for the training of visiting nurses on the grounds of the Liverpool Infirmary. Within 4 years, 18 nurses were working in this same city, demonstrating dramatically the organization and success of the venture. Even at this early date, these visiting nurses were visualized not only as people who cared for the sick but also as social reformers.

Visiting Nurses in the United States

As is already evident from this historical overview, trends within nursing are directly influenced by trends in society. The development of visiting nursing in the United States was no exception.

By the later 1800s, organized nursing care in hospitals had been demonstrated to be effective. Germ theory was used as the basis for communicable disease control. Poverty was beginning to be seen as the result and cause of multiple social problems.

Florence Nightingale's work and the establishment of her school of nursing in England were well known. Her concept that better nursing care could be given if nurses were educated for the position became more clearly understood.

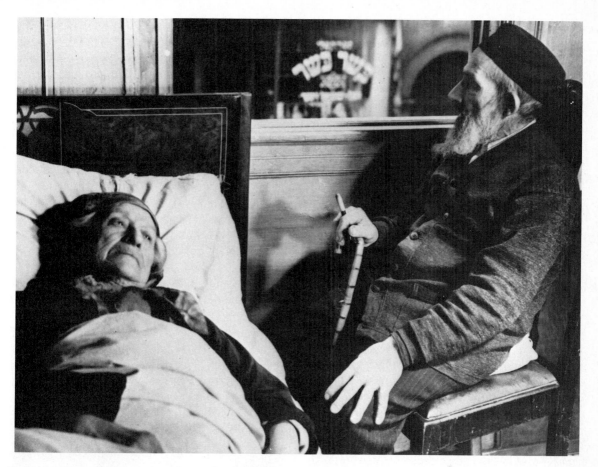

Figure 1-1 It was the year of the great blizzard, 1888, when this Russian blacksmith and his bride emigrated to the New World to build a life. Fifty years later, in sickness and in health, they were still together—thanks to a visiting nurse. (Visiting Nurse Service of New York City.)

The growth of our nation's cities as well as the waves of immigrants to America, the "land of opportunity," were two underlying reasons for the development of visiting nursing. Although every city had its rich people, the poor greatly outnumbered them (Kalisch and Kalisch, 1986, p. 262).

New York had the largest settlement of immigrants and thus faced the most problems concerning them (refer to Figure 1-1). Dismal tenement houses were built for this huge influx of people, and living conditions were horrible. Very young children were expected to work 12 to 14 hours a day in dark, airless factories.

Visiting nursing in the United States, just as in England, was begun by groups of people who were greatly distressed by the conditions in which many poor people lived. Then, as now, the most serious public health problems were in slum areas, and visiting nurse agencies were often located in buildings in low-income areas. Nurses from these organizations provided care to the sick in their homes and gave instruction to families as well. Buffalo, Boston, and Philadelphia developed such services during 1885 and 1886, about 25 years after Rathbone's experiment. The Philadelphia Visiting Nurse Society cared for the sick as well as for the poor and, at a very early date, established a fee for services given.

Visiting nursing in this country did not follow the English system established by Rathbone

(Gardner, 1919, p. 29). In England, Queen Victoria's Jubilee Institute for Nurses was founded in 1889, and it set standards for the preparation of visiting nurses as well as for the care given by them. In 1890 in the United States, there were 21 separate organizations engaged in visiting nursing. These organizations had no connection with each other and also had no common standards of educational preparation for the caregivers. Each city and town established its own visiting nurse service so that there was great diversity in the quality of organization and care given.

In 1896, the Nurses' Associated Alumni (now the American Nurses' Association) was formed and helped to organize the nurses of the country into a professional group. This was the beginning of "group consciousness" among the visiting nurses of the United States.

Enter Lillian Wald

The person who coined the expression *public health nursing* was Lillian Wald. Nightingale had originated the idea of "health nursing"; it was Wald who placed the word *public* in front of it so that all people would know that this type of service was available to them (Haupt, 1953, p. 81). Wald was the "predecessor of the modern public health nurse in the United States" (Christy, 1970, p. 50). *The House on Henry Street* is her story of the work she did as director of the Henry Street Settlement House. Lillian Wald's accomplishments are legendary and involve numerous "firsts" in nursing. She originated the idea of family-focused nursing and stressed the importance of health teaching in preventing disease and promoting health. She saw the value of, and helped to establish, school nursing as well as rural nursing in the Red Cross Town and Country Nursing Service. Wald truly promoted the philosophy of professional nursing. She encouraged the teaching of courses for public health nursing at Teachers College of Columbia University and was founder and first president of the National Organization for Public Health Nursing (Kaufman, Hawkins, Higgins, and Friedman, 1988).

Lillian Wald has been honored for her social reform activities as well as her nursing achieve-

ments. She originated the idea and then helped to establish the U.S. Children's Bureau. She was also instrumental in securing changes in child labor laws, better housing conditions in tenement districts, city recreation centers, more and better parks, pure food laws, graded classes for mentally handicapped children, and humanistic provisions for immigrants to the United States. What a role model for public health nurses today! And how appropriate the title, "predecessor of modern public health nursing"! (Refer to Figure 1-2.)

Lillian Wald was born in 1867 and spent her growing years in Rochester, New York. Though her family was not wealthy, her father, an optical goods dealer, provided a comfortable living for them. She studied at a private school and was an excellent student. Wald chanced to meet a graduate of the Bellevue Hospital Training School for

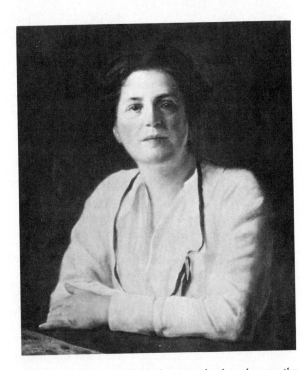

Figure 1-2   Lillian D. Wald, the nurse leader who was the "predecessor of modern public health nursing," was far ahead of her time. She promoted social reform at a time when it was not the norm for women to engage in such activity. Her accomplishments truly reflect the "mark" of a professional nurse. (Visiting Nurse Service of New York City.)

Nurses who had assisted her sister during pregnancy. In this manner, Wald became interested in nursing and entered training at New York Hospital in 1891, where she spent 2 years.

After graduating, she supplemented her nursing instruction with a period of study at a medical college. During this time of study, she was asked to give classes in home nursing and bedside care to a group of women in the Lower East Side tenement district. This was a turning point of Wald's career:

From the schoolroom where I had been giving a lesson in bed-making, a little girl led me one drizzling March morning. She had told me of her sick mother, and gathering from her incoherent account that a child had been born, I caught up the paraphernalia of the bed-making lesson and carried it with me.

The child led me over broken roadways,—there was no asphalt, although its use was well established in other parts of the city,—over dirty mattresses and heaps of refuse,—it was before Colonel Waring had shown the possibility of clean streets even in that quarter,—between tall, reeking houses whose laden fire escapes, useless for their appointed purpose, bulged with household goods of every description. The rain added to the dismal appearance of the streets and to the discomfort of the crowds which thronged them, intensifying the odors which assailed me from every side. Through Hester and Division Streets we went to the end of Ludlow; past odorus fish-stands, for the streets were a marketplace, unregulated, unsupervised, unclean; past evil-smelling, uncovered garbage-cans; and—perhaps worst of all, where so many little children played—past the trucks brought down from more fastidious quarters and stalled on these already over-crowded streets, lending themselves inevitably to many forms of indecency.

The child led me on through a tenement hallway, across a court where open and unscreened closets were promiscuously used by men and women, up into a rear tenement, by slimy steps whose accumulated dirt was augmented that day by the mud of the streets, and finally into the sickroom.

All of the maladjustments of our social and economic relations seemed epitomized in this brief journey and what was found at the end of it. The family to which the child led me was neither criminal nor vicious. Although the husband was a cripple, one of those who stand on street corners exhibiting deformities to enlist compassion, and masking the begging of alms by a pre-

tense at selling; although the family of seven shared their two rooms with boarders,—who were literally boarders, since a piece of timber was placed over the floor for them to sleep on,—and although the sick woman lay on a wretched, unclean bed, soiled with a hemorrhage two days old, they were not degraded human beings, judged by any measure of moral values.

In fact, it was very plain that they were sensitive to their condition, and when, at the end of my ministrations, they kissed my hands (those who have undergone similar experiences will, I am sure, understand), it would have been some solace if by any conviction of the moral unworthiness of the family I could have defended myself as a part of a society which permitted such conditions to exist. Indeed, my subsequent acquaintance with them revealed the fact that, miserable as their state was, they were not without ideals for the family life, and for society, of which they were so unloved and unlovely a part.

That morning's experience was a baptism of fire. Deserted were the laboratory and the academic work of the college—I never returned to them. On my way from the sickroom to my comfortable student quarters my mind was intent on my own responsibility. To my inexperience, it seemed certain that conditions such as these were allowed because people did not know, and for me there was a challenge to know and to tell. When early morning found me still awake, my naive conviction remained that, if people knew things,—and "things" meant everything implied in the condition of this family,—such horrors would cease to exist, and I rejoiced that I had had a training in the care of the sick that in itself would give me an organic relationship to the neighborhood in which this awakening had come. (Wald, 1915, pp. 4-8)

This experience was the cause for the creation of the Henry Street Settlement House in 1893. Along with Mary Brewster, another New York Hospital graduate, Wald elicited funds from wealthy people and founded a place where care was offered to needy people.

Wald's settlement house changed the focus of nursing service: the only other visiting nurses during this period were those associated with sectarian organizations or free dispensaries. Wald felt that a nurse could be most effective if she were independent of any religious agency and not associated exclusively with one doctor. She insisted that nurses should be available to anyone who needed them, without the intervention of a doctor, establishing early in the history of nursing that the profession should be an independent one. She also believed that nurses should live in the neighborhood where they practiced so that they could identify with the needs of the family served, as Wald herself did.

School Nursing Develops

The nursing care of children in public schools began with an idea by Lillian Wald. In 1902 health conditions of school children in New York City were appalling. Thousands of students were sent home from school with diseases such as trachoma (an infectious eye disease), pediculosis, ringworm, scabies, and impetigo. They then played outside with the children from whom they had previously been excluded in the classroom (Wald, 1915, p. 51). Wald offered to show school officials in New York that with the assistance of a well-prepared nurse fewer children would lose valuable school time. It would also be possible to bring under treatment those who needed it. The experiment was to be paid for with public funds.

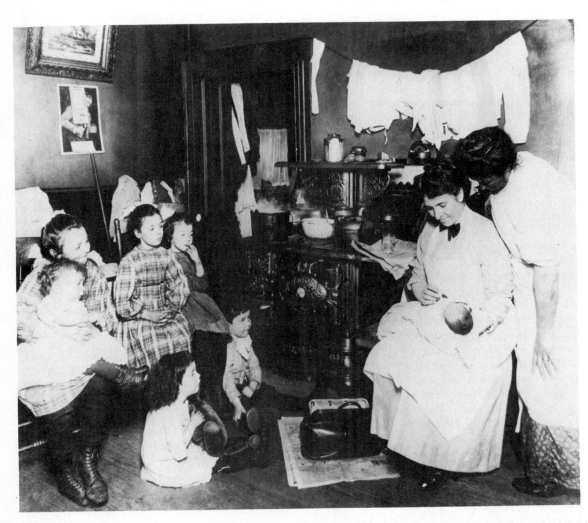

Figure 1-3   Involving the family in baby care, Boston, 1912. (The Metropolitan Life Insurance Company of New York. Used with their permission.)

One month's trial with Lina Rogers, a nurse from Henry Street, proved to be immensely successful. Thirty thousand dollars was approved by the Board of Estimate and Apportionment for the employment of trained nurses, the first municipalized school nurses in the world (Wald, p. 53).

Maternal-Infant Care Becomes a Concern

An appreciation of the needs of children, demonstrated in part by the rise of settlement houses like Henry Street, was a part of the social consciousness of the early 1900s. There were spasmodic efforts to help children to better health, and in 1909 these were united into action at a Conference on Infant Mortality called by the American Academy of Medicine. Finally in 1912, the Children's Bureau was created by Congress to draw the attention of the highest levels of government to the needs of children. Though many nurses and lay associations contributed to its formation, Lillian Wald's activities, initiative, and remarkable skill in securing support for new ideas was fundamental to the establishment of the Children's Bureau (Stewart and Austin, 1938, p. 197).

The passage of the *Shepherd-Towner Act* of 1921 was a historic milestone in the evolution of public health and public health nursing. Studies by the Children's Bureau at the federal level showed that the United States had a higher maternal death rate than most other developed countries. This act, administered by the Children's Bureau, gave grants to states to develop programs that provided care to that at-risk population group.

Marie Phelan was appointed in 1923 as the first nurse consultant to the federal government in peacetime. At the request of state health departments she helped to develop programs that promoted the health of mothers and children. Her work had the effect of creating a demand for nurses to work with established county or official agencies to begin demonstration programs with mothers and infants (refer to Figure 1-3). The results of these nurses' work are difficult to measure, but the maternal death rate was reduced from 7.1 per 1000 live births in 1915 to 6.7 for the years between 1925 and 1929. In a final report on the program, the chief of the Children's Bureau noted that "a nurse working alone had frequently afforded a starting point for the development of full-time health departments" (Roberts, 1954, p. 196). As a result of strong political conservatism, the Shepherd-Towner Act was permitted to lapse in 1929 and was not renewed.

The original Shepherd-Towner Act was subsequently amended and broadened to include under its auspices a network of maternity and infant care programs, as well as children and youth programs, throughout the United States. Nurse-midwives, pediatric nurse practitioners, and family planning nurse practitioners were responsible for providing primary health care in many of these programs.

Metropolitan Employs PHN

In 1909 the first public health nursing program for policyholders of an insurance company was initiated (Haupt, 1953, p. 81). Lillian Wald and Lee Frankel, founder of the Metropolitan Life Insurance Company Welfare Division, convinced the board of directors at Metropolitan that healthier workers live longer and thus profit the company by purchasing insurance longer. Wald felt that nurses supplied by agencies such as Henry Street could provide skilled service needed to produce healthy workers. Increased efficiency on the workers' part could favorably influence the output of industry, which, in turn, would pay for the health services in cash and improve morale.

The two principles underlying this concept were that the company should utilize existing public health nursing services rather than employing their own nurses and that services should be available to anyone, with fees based on the ability to pay. Both of these ideas are utilized today in health agencies.

The Metropolitan project was terminated in 1953 after 44 successful years. The shifting of the voluntary responsibility for health care to professional community organizations was the basis for the change.

There were numerous contributions to public health nursing as a result of this project (Haupt, 1953). Among them, the following:

1. The extension of bedside nursing care on a fee-for-service basis.
2. The establishment of a cost-accounting system for visiting nurses, which is used to this day.
3. The recruitment of nurses, aides, and home nursing programs under the Red Cross by the use of advertisements in paper and radio. This was a new concept of recruitment.
4. The reduction of mortality rates from infectious diseases. Mortality rates were reduced by half in the 44 years of the program among the Metropolitan Life Insurance policyholders.
5. The demonstration of how nursing and a business organization can work together, despite each having an interest in the promotion of its *own* goals.

Public Health Nursing in Rural Areas

While public health nursing in cities and towns was developing at a rapid rate, work in rural areas was progressing slowly. In 1912, the same year the Children's Bureau was formed, Lillian Wald asked her wealthy friend, Jacob Shiff, to donate money to the Red Cross so that a system of rural nursing could be developed (Gardner, 1919, p. 37).

Wald had been a Red Cross member in 1904 and 1905. She expressed strong dissatisfaction at seeing so potent an organization as the Red Cross limited to the uncertainty and irregularity of service in war or calamity; she felt it simply wasteful to have a national organization inactive. Wald believed that the Red Cross was a logical facility to employ in promoting public health nursing in rural areas and scattered towns on a regular national scale (Dock, Pickett, Noyes, Clement, Fox, and Van Meter, 1922, p. 1212).

And so it happened that the Red Cross began a new department, the Town and Country Nursing Service, which was later to be named the Bureau of Public Health Nursing. The purpose of the department was to supply rural areas and small towns with trained public health nurses and to supervise their work. The Red Cross, however, did not assume the local financial responsibility for this work. Voluntary and charitable organizations as well as fees for service financed nursing care given.

PUBLIC HEALTH NURSING BECOMES A GOVERNMENTAL CONCERN

Public health nursing grew out of the need recognized by groups of citizens to help poor people who suffered not only physically but in all other areas of life as well. Thus, public health nurses were financed by voluntary agencies, depending upon contributions and small service charges for financial support. The state of our nation's health forced a change.

In the nineteenth century, threats to the public's health and welfare were increasing due to diseases such as smallpox, yellow fever, cholera, typhoid, tuberculosis, and malaria (refer to Figure 1-4). In Massachusetts in 1850, for example, the tuberculosis death rate was 300 per 100,000 population. The infant mortality rate was 200 per 1000 live births, and smallpox, scarlet fever, and typhoid were the leading causes of death (Pickett and Hanlon, 1990, p. 30).

In response to these problems, some larger cities such as Philadelphia and New York established city health departments. In 1855 Louisiana set up what is called by some historians the first state health department. Its function was to deal with repeated outbreaks of yellow fever and other epidemic diseases. In terms of the more usual concept of the general functions of a state health department, Massachusetts is usually credited with the first state health department, founded in 1869 (Pickett and Hanlon, 1990, p. 33).

An early public health pioneer of this period was Lemuel Shattuck. In 1842, he helped to achieve passage of a law in Massachusetts which resulted in the statewide registration of health-related statistics. In the next few years, Shattuck compiled shocking statistics about unbelievably high infant and maternal mortality rates. The *Shattuck Report,* one of the first public health documents in the United States, was published in 1850. It recommended the establishment of state and local health departments as well as pointing

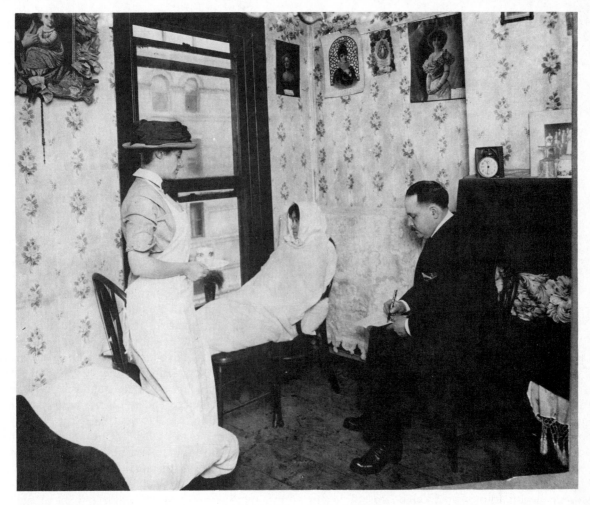

Figure 1-4   Convalescing from typhoid fever, New York City, 1912. (The Metropolitan Life Insurance Company of New York. Used with their permission.)

out the need for sanitary surveys. It unfortunately lay unnoticed for 25 years, although much of it is relevant for today (Pickett and Hanlon, 1990, pp. 31–32).

Thus the concept of the public's health developed near the turn of the century. Personal health services played an increasingly important role in community health programs. A new era was reached when, in Los Angeles in 1889, a nurse was employed by the city's health department to provide home nursing care to the sick poor (Rosen, 1958, p. 380). At this point, public health nursing began to be officially recognized and tax supported. However, it was not until 1913 that the Los Angeles Health Department established a bureau of nursing.

In 1902 Lillian Wald had loaned a nurse to the New York City Health Department to ascertain whether or not pupil absence from the schools could be reduced with nursing care. The reader may recall that this experiment was extremely successful and that a group of nurses was then employed to work in the schools. This was the first use of trained nurses in any large number in health departments. In 1903, this same health department appointed three nurses (annual salary

TABLE 1-1   Distribution of public health nurses in 1912

Visiting nurse associations	205
City and state boards of health and education	156
Private clubs and societies	108
Tuberculosis leagues	107
Hospitals and dispensaries	87
Business concerns	38
Settlements and day nurses	35
Churches	28
Charity organizations	27
Other organizations	19

NOTE: This list, used by the author in 1912, as secretary of a joint committee of the American Nurses' Association and the Society of Superintendents of Training Schools, to circulate names of the agencies then known to be engaged in public health nursing, probably gives a reasonably true picture of the general distribution of nursing work among the different types of agencies. There were 78 letters sent to nurses working in that number of counties in Pennsylvania and 204 to nurses independently employed by the Metropolitan Life Insurance Company.

From Gardner MS, Public health nursing, ed 3, New York, 1936, Macmillan, p 40.

$900) to visit tuberculosis patients at home. The nurses were to teach the patients about sputum disposal and other aspects of care. In 1905 the number of nurses serving tuberculosis patients was increased to 14. Alabama, in 1907, was the first state to legally approve the employment of public health nurses by local boards of health (Rosen, 1958, p. 380).

By 1912 public health nurses were supported by both private and public funds. The need for the skills and knowledge of this kind of professional was generally well recognized. They could be found in many kinds of agencies as well as in both rural and urban settings. Table 1-1, compiled by public health nurse pioneer Mary Gardner, illustrates this distribution well.

ORGANIZING PUBLIC HEALTH NURSES

Leaders among public health nurses, including Lillian Wald, Mary Beard, Ellen Phillips Crandall, Jane Delano, and Mary Gardner, soon realized the need to develop professional standards for this expanding professional group. Although most agencies employing nurses were attempting to do conscientious work, there were no overall professional and ethical guidelines. These same leaders felt clearly that only a new organization "whose sole object should be public health nursing would adequately meet the need" (Gardner, 1919, p. 41).

June 7, 1912, was a momentous day in the history of American public health nursing: at the annual meeting of the American Nurses' Association and the Society of Superintendents of Training Schools, the *National Organization for Public Health Nursing* (now the National League for Nursing) was voted into existence with Lillian Wald as president. The two purposes of the National Organization for Public Health Nursing (NOPHN) were the stimulation and standardization of public health nursing and the furthering of relationships among all people interested in the public's health. It was the *first* national nursing organization to have a headquarters and paid staff. For a long period in the development of nursing, it grew in power, set standards for practice, and influenced education by requiring certain curriculum content as a basis for employment (Fagin, 1978, p. 752). One of the unique features of the NOPHN was that membership was open to public health nursing agencies and other interested people, as well as to nurses. Collaborative relationships among health and social agencies has always been a strength among those who work in public health nursing.

Education for Public Health Nurses

The education of public health nurses presented special problems because, traditionally, all nurses were prepared in apprentice-type programs in hospitals. Their curriculum was determined by the needs of the hospital and was controlled by the physicians whose primary responsibility was service to patients rather than the education of nurses. The education was illness- and individual-oriented and did not adequately prepare (or even claim to prepare) a person to work in the community setting, where the care delivered differed from hospital care. In the community setting, nurses had a greater degree of independence; they did health teaching, carried out case finding, and made referrals; and their responsibility was to population groups.

The first course in public health nursing was offered by the Boston Instructive Nursing Association in 1906 (McNeil, 1967, p. 4). However, considering the broad scope of a public health nurse's work, it soon became apparent that education for this group was a function of the university. Because of the nurse's concern with social and educational problems, most of the early university public health nursing programs were in teacher's colleges or university departments of sociology or social work. By 1921, courses in public health nursing, which met standards developed by the NOPHN, were offered by 15 colleges and universities. These courses taught "preventive medicine," covering topics such as how to examine a class of children, how to find those who were developing measles, and how to visit in a home and evaluate tuberculosis contacts (Jensen, 1959, p. 236).

Public Health Nursing Magazine

On the very day that the NOPHN was formed, the Cleveland Visiting Nurses' Association presented its magazine, *The Quarterly,* to the group as a gift. *The Quarterly* later became *Public Health Nursing* and, still later, *Nursing Outlook.* It was an essential element to the development and dissemination of the public health nursing movement in the United States.

The Goldmark Report

In 1919, under the auspices of the Rockefeller Foundation and at the urging of concerned nursing leaders, the Committee for the Study of Public Health Nursing Education, with C.-E. A. Winslow as chairman, began a 2-year investigation. Josephine Goldmark was secretary of the committee and the study was later to bear her name.

The purpose of the committee was to look at typical examples of public health nursing education and service and to study the education of these workers afforded by hospital training schools, graduate courses for public health nurses,

and special schools of a non-nursing type (Committee for the Study of Nursing Education, 1923, p. 2). The study was expanded the following year to look at the entire field of nursing education.

Ten conclusions were reached that have profoundly affected the course of public health nursing, as well as of all nursing (Committee for the Study of Nursing Education, 1923):

Conclusion 1. That, since constructive health work and health teaching in families is best done by persons:

(a) capable of giving general health instruction, as distinguished from instruction in any one specialty; and

(b) capable of rendering bedside care at need; the agent responsible for such constructive health work and health teaching in families should have completed the nurses' training. There will, of course, be need for the employment, in addition to the public health nurse, of other types of experts such as nutrition workers, social workers, occupational therapists, and the like.

That as soon as may be practicable all agencies, public or private, employing public health nurses, should require as a prerequisite for employment the basic hospital training, followed by a postgraduate course, including both class work and field work, in public health nursing.

Conclusion 2. That the career open to young women of high capacity, in public health nursing or in hospital supervision and nursing education, is one of the most attractive fields now open, in its promise of professional success and of rewarding public service; and that every effort should be made to attract such women into this field.

Conclusion 3. That for the care of persons suffering from serious and acute disease, the safety of the patient, and the responsibility of the medical and nursing professions, demand the maintenance of the standards of educational attainment now generally accepted by the best sentiment of both professions and embodied in the legislation of the more progressive states; and that any attempt to lower these standards would be fraught with real danger to the public.

Conclusion 4. That steps should be taken through state legislation for the definition and licensure of a subsidiary grade of nursing service, the subsidiary type of worker to serve under practicing physicians in the care of mild and chronic illness, and convalescence, and possibly to assist under the direction of the trained nurse in certain phases of hospital and visiting nursing.

Conclusion 5. That, while training schools for nurses have made remarkable progress, and while the best schools of today in many respects reach a high level of educational attainment, the average hospital training school is not organized on such a basis as to conform to the standards accepted in other educational fields; that the instruction in such schools is frequently casual and uncorrelated; that the educational needs and the health and strength of students are frequently sacrificed to practical hospital exigencies; that such shortcomings are primarily due to the lack of independent endowments for nursing education; that existing educational facilities are on the whole, in the majority of schools, inadequate for the preparation of the high-grade of nurses required for the care of serious illness, and for service in the fields of public health nursing and nursing education; and that one of the chief reasons for the lack of sufficient recruits, of a high type, to meet such needs lies precisely in the fact that the average hospital training school does not offer a sufficiently attractive avenue of entrance to this field.

Conclusion 6. That, with the necessary financial support and under a separate board or training school committee, organized primarily for educational purposes, it is possible, with completion of a high school course or its equivalent as a prerequisite, to reduce the fundamental period of hospital training to 28 months, and at the same time, by eliminating unessential, non-educational routine, and adopting the principles laid down in Miss Goldmark's report, to organize the course along intensive and coordinated lines with such modifications as may be necessary for practical application; and that courses of this standard would be reasonably certain to attract students of high quality in increasing numbers.

Conclusion 7. Superintendents, supervisors, instructors, and public health nurses should in all cases receive special additional training beyond the basic nursing course.

Conclusion 8. That the development and strengthening of University Schools of Nursing of a high grade for the training of leaders is of fundamental importance in the furtherance of nursing education.

Conclusion 9. That when the licensure of a subsidiary grade of nursing service is provided for, the establishment of training courses in preparation for such service is highly desirable; that such courses should be conducted in special hospitals, in small unaffiliated general hospitals, or in separate sections of hospitals where nurses are also trained; and that the course should be of 8 or 9 months' duration; provided the standards of such schools be approved by the same educational board which governs nursing training schools.

Conclusion 10. That the development of nursing service adequate for the care of the sick and for the conduct of the modern public health campaign demands as an absolute prerequisite the securing of funds for the endowment of nursing education of all types; and that it is of primary importance, in this connection, to provide reasonably generous endowment for university schools of nursing.

The significance of this very early study is, even today, not fully understood and implemented. However, some positive changes were slowly made: poor schools were closed, qualified faculty members were hired, and the money allotted to education programs was increased.

Changes in Nursing Education

Until World War II it was believed that nurses could be prepared for public health only after they graduated from a hospital (diploma) school of nursing. It became evident, however, that graduates of collegiate schools of nursing did not need the same additional content in public health nursing as did graduates of diploma schools, because the broader background of a liberal arts education helped prepare one for this area of nursing. Content in public health became increasingly evident in collegiate schools of nursing. Finally, in 1944 the first basic collegiate program in nursing was accredited as including adequate preparation for public health nursing, so that graduates did not need additional study to practice public health nursing after graduation from the basic nursing program (National Organization for Public Health Nursing, 1944, p. 371).

During the next 30 years there were drastic changes in nursing education. Like most major changes, they were met with resistance from many sources and caused severe distress for some individuals. These changes included the following:

1. One-year practical nursing programs were established and the numbers of schools and graduates increased rapidly. More than half of these programs were offered under vocational education.
2. Two-year programs in nursing were established (1952), most of them in junior col-

leges. These graduates were qualified to take the examination to become registered nurses.

3. After 1963 no specialized baccalaureate program was accredited unless it prepared its graduates for public health nursing. Emphasis on comprehensive nursing care in both public health and hospital nursing revealed that all baccalaureate graduates should be prepared for staff-level positions in both hospitals and public health nursing agencies. Only three graduate schools of public health had undergraduate programs in public health nursing, and these were discontinued when the content was included in baccalaureate nursing curriculums.

4. Universities assumed more responsibility for clinical field instruction, which enriched both field and classroom teaching.

5. Members of the American Nurses' Association, in 1965, approved a position paper on the educational preparation for nurse practitioners, which stated that education for all those licensed to practice nursing should take place in institutions of higher education.

6. In 1978, the American Nurses' Association, after years of debate, resolved again that the baccalaureate degree should be the minimum preparation for entry into professional nursing practice.

The Effects of World War I on Public Health Nursing

By 1915 the role of the public health nurse was well established and the pioneer stage of this specialized area was drawing to a close. However, with the advent of World War I in 1917 and the involvement of thousands of nurses in military service, public health nursing services were threatened. The American Red Cross (which had been founded in 1882 by Clara Barton to supply nurses for war service) along with a committee chaired by Adelaide Nutting, the "far-seeing dean of American nurses," investigated methods to deal with the situation (Roberts, 1954, p. 131).

The efficient use of the limited supply of public health nurses was ensured by the Red Cross, which set up a roster of nurses who could be called upon to coordinate and supplement health resources. Emphasis was placed upon educational programs for the community as well as the control of communicable diseases.

During World War I, a nurse was loaned to the U.S. Public Health Service from the National Organization of Public Health Nursing, to develop a public health nursing program for the military outposts. This was the first public health nursing service to be established within the federal government (Gardner, 1919, p. 44).

The committee was convinced that the standards for preparing nurses must be maintained and that quick "short courses" to prepare nurses would have a disastrous effect on war and postwar health programs. To alleviate the nursing shortage and to ensure standards of care, they encouraged the development of a quality shortened program.

The Vassar Training Camp for Nurses

A unique experience in the annals of nursing education was the Vassar Camp School of Nursing. Begun in 1918 and supported by the American Red Cross and the Council of National Defense, the program was based on the principle that the 3-year nursing course could be shortened to 2 years for students who had graduated from college majoring in other subjects. It was modeled on the Plattsburg Military Camp at Plattsburg, New York, where college men were given intensive training to become army reserve officers. The purpose was to more rapidly fill the desperate need for women in nursing in wartime. Applicants to the program chose a college and were admitted into selected nursing schools across the country. Graduates of this program numbered 435; the program ended with the Armistice.

This patriotic opportunity attracted high-level faculty and students. The program produced distinguished nursing leaders of the next several decades, including people like Katherine Densford Dreves, who became dean of the University of Minnesota School of Nursing, president of the American Nurses' Association, and second vice-president of the International Council of Nurses.

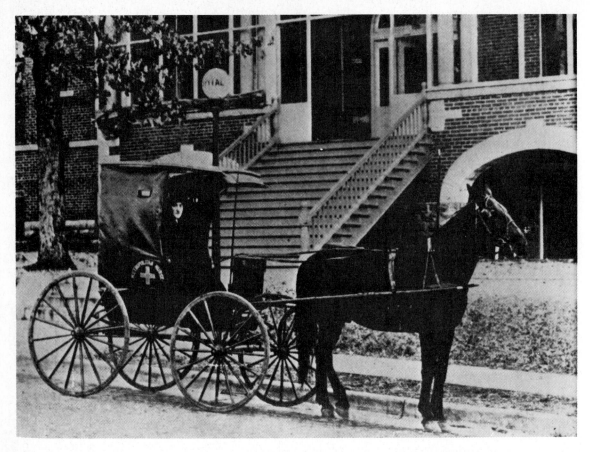

Figure 1-5   Public health nurse utilizing horse and buggy before the advent of the automobile. (The Metropolitan Life Insurance Company of New York. Used with their permission.)

After World War I

Rapid changes came with peace. Economic prosperity, reaction to prohibition, and the increasing use of the automobile created radical changes in the way people lived. These changes brought subsequent changes in public health nursing. The use of the automobile, for instance, permitted nurses to have easy access to rural areas and made once-closed areas accessible (refer to Figures 1-5, 1-6, and 1-7).

The poor physical condition of the nation's males, made evident in wartime, shocked the nation. About 29 percent of those called for service were unfit for military duty because of problems that in many cases were preventable (Roberts, 1954, p. 164). Health programs of both official and nonofficial agencies grew as a result.

Smillie says that "beginning in 1925 and extending through the present time (1952) is the extraordinary phenomenon of the nationalization of the public health. The public health was, for generations, a community affair administered under local self-government with some slight degree of state government supervision. Public health has now become a subject of nationwide interest and importance" (Smillie, 1952, p. 10).

By 1920 there were 28 states that had a statewide public health nursing program. However, only five had divisions of public health nursing within state health departments (Roberts, 1954, p. 168).

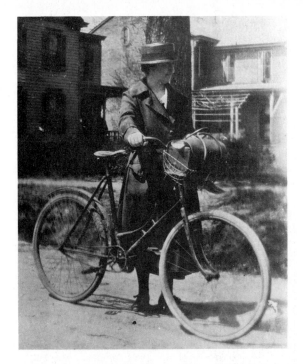

Figure 1-6 Public health nurse utilizing a bicycle before the advent of the automobile. (The Metropolitan Life Insurance Company of New York. Used with their permission.)

Two voluntary (non-tax-supported) agencies were very active during this time: the National Tuberculosis Association and the American Red Cross. The Red Cross supplemented but did not supplant the work of legitimate health agencies. Its goal was that public health nursing would be conducted as a public service by municipalities, counties, or states. In some states the public health nursing supervisors in state health departments also functioned as Red Cross supervisors. In 1921, state tuberculosis associations had supervising nurses in 28 states, the Red Cross in 31. In 29 states, the state board of health had a director of public health nursing or a division of child hygiene (Fox, 1920, p. 180). (Refer to Figure 1-8.)

The Effects of World War II on Public Health Nursing

The Depression of 1929, which preceded World War II, forced many hospitals and schools of nursing to close. The supply of nurses far exceeded the demand. In the health field as a whole, the financial crisis resulted in the wider use of national, state, and local tax funds for health and

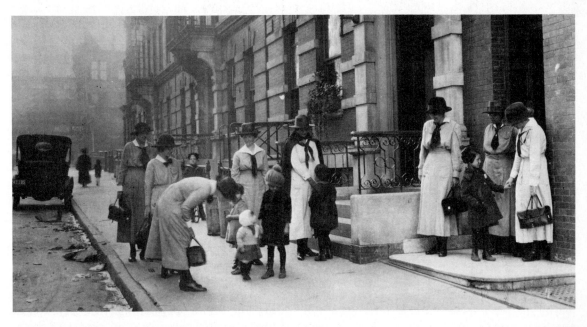

Figure 1-7 To these nurses of the 30s, the city's streets were hospital corridors, and family bedrooms their wards. They carried a cake of soap to protect themselves from germs and a whistle to guard themselves from danger. (Visiting Nurse Service of New York City.)

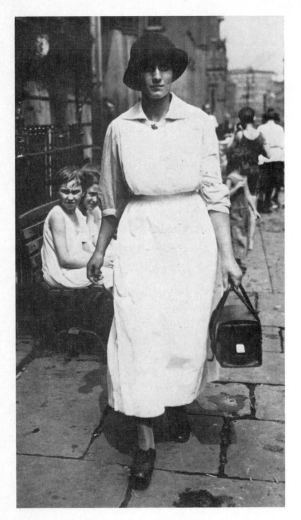

Figure 1-8 From the turn of the century on, the visiting nurse served as the first line of defense in the fight against diphtheria and other "killer" contagions of the era. (Visiting Nurse Service of New York City.)

welfare services. An important aspect of this program on the national level was the passage of the Social Security Act in 1935, which introduced governmental involvement in health care on a larger scale. This meant that the federal government was taking on a new role in assuming responsibility for the health of people. The individualism that was important to the founding of this country was no longer sufficient to solve all problems. The Depression also led to the rapid growth

of voluntary insurance plans for financing hospital and medical care (Stewart and Austin, 1938, p. 219).

In 1933 Pearl McIver, a well-qualified public health nurse in the U.S. Public Health Service, was assigned as a consultant for the placement of nurses on federal relief projects. Many of these nurses were formerly hospital nurses now assigned to public health agencies and clinics, and they became interested in this new field. Thus, when the Social Security Act of 1935 made money available for the education and employment of public health nurses, many of those working on relief projects seized the opportunity to study. Other educational funds followed which made it possible for nurses to complete their education in a shorter time. These included Training for Nurses for National Defense, the GI bill, the Nurse Training Act of 1943, and Public Health and Professional Nurse traineeships. Funds were also available to help prepare nurses at the graduate level for specialities such as tuberculosis, cancer, mental health, maternal and child health, and research (McNeil, 1967, p. 6).

After the war began in 1941, the nurse shortage became acute. The problem was more serious than in World War I because of the duration and scope of the war effort. The National Nursing Council, composed of six national nursing organizations, along with the aid of the U.S. Department of Education, requested $1 million to enlarge facilities for nursing education. The administration of this money was assigned to the U.S. Public Health Service.

In 1943, the Cadet Nurse Corps was authorized by the Bolton Act. Sixty million dollars was appropriated to recruit and educate 70,000 cadets in 1125 schools between 1944 and 1946. These nurses comprised 90 percent of the total enrollment of basic nursing programs for this time. Lucille Petry, chief nurse officer, directed this remarkable program at a difficult time in our nation's history.

World War II, like World War I and the Depression, had a major impact on public health nursing. Specifically, the war influenced the following trends:

1. The importance of public health nursing service was recognized when public health nurses were declared essential for civilian work, although many of them entered military service.
2. Maximum utilization of personnel was essential and official tax-supported public health nursing agencies combined with voluntary non-tax-supported agencies, to avoid duplication.
3. Practical nurses were accepted as an important resource for nursing service.
4. The establishment of priorities for health care became more than a topic for discussion.
5. Additional funds for nursing education became available and the fear of governmental control of education decreased. After the war, the enrollment of nurses who were veterans or widows of veterans strained the resources of universities and agencies providing field experience.

FROM WORLD WAR II TO THE DECADE OF THE 1970s

The depressions before and after World War II, as well as the war itself, provided the milieu for the development of numerous programs designed to help the country renew itself. Chronic disease and accidents replaced infectious disease as the leading causes of death, a result of the effectiveness of new drugs and vaccines. Consequently, life expectancy increased.

The years between 1935 and 1965 produced much legislation that was aimed at improving the health, education, and housing of people, ending discrimination against minorities, and providing proper working conditions for wage earners. This legislation began with the Social Security Act of 1935; it provided monies for old-age benefits, state grants for aid to the blind and disabled, aid for dependent and crippled children, vocational rehabilitation programs, and unemployment compensation programs.

Title VI of the act focused on public health programs, and its overall purpose was to elicit a public health program that would protect and promote the nation's health. One part of title VI provided money to states and counties to establish and maintain health services. Allocations in this part of the act provided money for nurses to study public health nursing. Prior to 1935, only one-third of the states had a public health nursing section within the state health department, and only 7 percent of the public health nurses employed had taken an accredited course in public health nursing. During 1936, the first year that money became available through the Social Security Act, over 1000 nurses received money to study in a program accredited by the National Organization for Public Health Nursing.

Another part of title VI provided money for research and the investigation of diseases and problems with environmental health. Title VI was directly responsible for expanding public health nursing programs and developing new ones. As a result of this legislation, the public health nurse became an integral part of local health departments: the maternal and child health programs of the Social Security Act made the nurse's work with families essential. By 1940, 3000 nurses had received public health training in accredited schools, 970 counties had developed full-time public health services, and 1150 clinics had been added to those already working on the problems of venereal diseases (Williams, 1951, p. 156).

Later, President Kennedy's New Frontier and President Johnson's Great Society epitomized the era in our nation's history when the government took on even more aggressively the role of guardian of the nation's health. The rugged individualism of the early 1900s had disappeared. John Kennedy's inaugural address in 1961 is remembered for the words, "Ask not what your country can do for you—ask what you can do for your country." A new social consciousness swept the country, and the differences between black and white, poor and rich became topics for scrutiny, worth dying for.

Citizens began to see health as a right rather than a privilege, a significant change from the beginning of the century when families with large numbers of children were the norm so that at least some could be expected to live to adulthood. Parents realized that health should be the birthright of every child, not the privilege of a few.

The Constitution of the World Health Organization defined health as "complete physical, mental and social well-being and not just the absence of disease." This definition reflected inclusion of the mental and social aspects of health as well as its physical aspects.

The demand for health care services on the part of an increasingly sophisticated and informed public came about in part as the result of ideas generated through television, magazines, newspapers, and radio. The ability to pay for these services led to the quest for a national compulsory health insurance.

When the war was over in 1945, President Harry Truman presented to Congress a health message with the following proposals for a health care system (Kalisch and Kalisch, 1982, p. 21):

1. Prepayment of medical costs with compulsory insurance and general revenues.
2. Protection from loss of wages as a result of sickness.
3. Expansion of services related to the public's health and including maternal and child health services.
4. Governmental aid to medical schools for research.
5. Increased construction of hospitals, clinics, and medical institutions.

Charges of socialism from the American Medical Association ended the quest for national health insurance in 1949 and 1950 (Kalisch and Kalisch, 1986, pp. 568-573). Much later, in 1965, a health insurance program for people 65 and older, Medicare, financed under the Social Security Act, was enacted by President Johnson.

Hospital Survey and Construction Act, 1946

Only the last of Truman's proposals was enacted. The Hospital Survey and Construction Act, also called the Hill-Burton bill, provided a 5-year program to states for the purpose of assessing needs, and then planning and constructing needed hospitals and public health centers.

The federal government provided one-third of the funds needed for the program, and each state provided the remaining two-thirds of the money. This act gave some nurses an opportunity to help plan the areas where they worked.

Organizing Public Health Nursing Services

It was at this point in our nation's history, after the war, when public health nursing seemed to become more concerned with how services were organized than with responding to health needs. The leadership among public health nurses, demonstrated by Wald and Gardner, appeared to diminish, and this specialty area entered a period in which it took a defensive stance regarding its contributions to health care and to nursing (Tinkham and Voorhies, 1977, p. 88).

In 1946, a committee of representatives from numerous agencies interested in public health nursing published guidelines upon which this area of nursing should be organized (Desirable organization, 1946, p. 387). The reason for the publication of these guidelines lies in the history of public health nursing. Public health nursing began with visits to the sick poor by voluntary agencies. Usually this was the only kind of care given by an agency and was the only organized program of home nursing. As the concept of public health grew, both voluntary and governmental services developed to provide public health nursing for special programs such as tuberculosis or child health. This resulted in duplication of services and unnecessary costs. Although the principal purpose of home nursing agencies was to give home care to the sick, nurses very quickly assumed the role of teaching a family to take responsibility for its own health. Thus, visiting nurses played a big part in helping to prevent and control sickness and epidemics. Gradually, city health departments became aware of the value of nursing and added nurses to their staffs to give health protection to the community as mandated by law. Nursing care of the sick was not accepted by health departments as a public health problem, so this activity remained the focus of voluntary agencies. This meant that in many communities public health nurses from two agencies (as well as an additional nurse from the school setting) might visit the same home, a problem that can still exist today in some communities.

The guidelines adopted by the committee addressed this history and resulting problems. It was agreed that a population of 50,000 was needed to support an adequate health program and that there should be one public health nurse for every 2000 people. Other principles included:

1. That each public health nurse should combine the functions of health teaching, control of disease, and care of the sick
2. That the community should adopt one of three patterns of organization that would best serve that community:
   a. All public health nursing service, including care of the sick at home, administered by the local health department
   b. Preventive services carried on by the health department with one voluntary agency, in close coordination with the health department, carrying responsibility for bedside nursing care
   c. A combination service jointly administered and financed by official and voluntary agencies with all service given by a single group of public health nurses

The Nurse Shortage

Right after World War II a serious undersupply of nurses created critical situations in hospitals and health centers. This was a result of factors including the increase in the population, the increase in insurance plans such as Blue Cross, an increase in the sophistication of surgery and medicine, which kept people alive longer, and the different situations in which nurses were increasingly employed, such as industry and schools.

Also, during the 1940s and the 1950s the place for women to be was in the home with husband and children. Married nurses were affected by this philosophy, and careers came second. It was not until the late 1960s that nurses began to develop a consciousness about their possible role in shaping the health care policies of the country, as well as their role in the political arena. Nurses were finally beginning to see themselves as the very obvious answer to the health care problems in the United States (Grissum and Spengler, 1976). This rise in activism among nurses paralleled the feminist movement among women in general.

In 1972, Nurses for Political Action was organized with headquarters in Washington, D.C. It became affiliated with the American Nurses' Association and later changed its name to N-CAP, Nurses Coalition for Action in Politics. Its purpose as a nonpartisan, nonprofit association was to obtain support for nursing from legislators, governmental officials, and the general public. At a time when a new national health care system was being developed and the present health care system was fragmented and dominated by the medical profession, nurses sought a place where they could make known their thoughts and ideas and help plan a system that comprehensively met people's health care needs.

The Federal Government Prepares Nurses

The government became involved in preparing new nurses with the passage of the Health Amendments Act of 1956. Title II authorized monies to aid registered nurses in the full-time study of either administration, supervision, or teaching.

However, in 1963 the Surgeon General's Consultant Group on Nursing reported that there were still too few nursing schools and not enough capable people being recruited into nursing. Additional problems were that nursing personnel were not well utilized and that only limited research was being done in nursing (U.S. Public Health Service, 1963).

Based upon these conclusions, the Nurse Training Act of 1964 was passed. This act provided money for loans and scholarships as well as for nursing school construction. With this act the federal government greatly helped to improve the quality of nursing in America.

The Expanding Role of the Nurse

By the 1960s the nursing profession began to look at new methods of meeting the health care needs of people, utilizing advanced nursing practice and extending the nursing role to take over some medical functions. The term *nurse practitioner* was first used at the University of Colorado in 1965 in a program that prepared nurses to provide comprehensive well-child care in ambulatory settings.

The concept of primary care nursing also became an important one. Primary care involves three important elements: first contact with the patient, continuity of care, and coordination of care. It is ambulatory care that views a person in relation to family and environment and emphasizes cure as well as prevention. Primary care can prevent both gaps and overlapping in health care services.

Public health nursing evolved from concern for the individual, the family, and the community. In fact, the early public health movement was the historical forerunner of today's primary care movement (Fagin, 1978, p. 752). Though presently other nursing specialties besides public health nursing work outside the hospital setting, and work with a person in terms of the family and the environment, public health nurses first used the concept that nursing could best meet the total health needs of people. The major difference between public health nursing and other areas of primary nursing is that public health nursing deals with the personal and environmental health of populations rather than only individuals and families. Public health practice must deal in concepts such as caseloads, clinics, counties, or census tracts to locate subgroups who have problems and are at risk.

In 1971, a bronze bust of Lillian Wald was placed in the Hall of Fame for Great Americans. An editorial about this event stated:

The kind of health care Lillian Wald began preaching and practicing in 1893 is the kind the people of this country are still crying for. She demonstrated with no need to rest on formal research that nursing could serve as the entry point—not only for health care, but for dealing with many other social ills of which sickness is only a part. She felt that nurses should go to the sick, instead of expecting the sick to come to them (and waiting for physicians to refer them); that care of persons in the home, especially of children, was far more effective

and much less expensive except perhaps for those needing, to use her own word, "intensive" care. (A prophet honored, 1971, p. 53)

There is still not total agreement in nursing on the definition of and preparation for the expanded role of the nurse. However, increasing numbers of people are viewing primary care as the major focus of nursing (Fagin, 1978, p. 753). Attractive federal funding has encouraged the growth of practitioner programs.

THE DECADE OF THE 1970s

Public health nursing, as well as all of professional nursing, was in a state of transition. The contribution of this specialty area to the health needs of people was less clear than it was in Lillian Wald's time. She and her peers had no doubt about their mission and the goals of public health nursing. Through the 1920s and 1930s the public health nursing movement grew in power, set standards for practice, and influenced education by requiring certain content as a condition for employment.

In the 1970s, all areas of nursing, including parent and child nursing, psychiatric nursing, and medical and surgical nursing, began discovering the community. These areas also began to emphasize the importance of the family to the patient, and the clear lines of distinction for what constituted public health nursing started to blur. Now, not even public health nurses agreed on the nature, standards, and scope of public health nursing practice (Ruth and Partridge, 1978, p. 625). However, it must be reemphasized that public health nursing was seen as a generalized area within nursing. Each of the other areas, medical-surgical nursing, psychiatric nursing, and parent and child nursing, had a specialized focus. Public health nursing had always been broad and comprehensive. Efforts were at last made to define the nature, standards, and scope of public health nursing practice.

Further, more and more professionals and semiprofessionals began to work in the community. Social workers, physical therapists, occupational therapists, as well as physicians' assistants and home health aides, were seen in public health settings. To complicate the situation, there were numerous ways to become a "nurse"; associate degree programs, diploma programs, and baccalaureate programs all claimed to prepare a different level of nurse. How these levels functioned in the community setting varied from agency to agency.

Voluntary agencies and health facilities multiplied, and many of them were not coordinated or designed with comprehensive health care plans in mind. Strong, effective official planning often was not evident on the state and local level. Health maintenance organizations, neighborhood health centers, free clinics, and numerous home health care programs based in hospitals and "for-profit agencies" represented the conglomeration of facilities that could spring up in any one community.

The rapid development of health services and specialties created even more confusion for people who found the existing health care system difficult to negotiate. People desperately needed someone to help them, and public health nurses offered hope.

COMMUNITY HEALTH NURSING IN THE 1980s

The concerns of the 1970s in the field of community health nursing (CHN) continued to be the concerns of this decade. Public health, as a specialty area, was undergoing an identity crisis. This crisis had three contributing factors (Chavigny and Kroske, 1983, p. 312):

1. Fragmentation of services whereby CHN roles and responsibilities were shared or delegated to others. For example, health education, once the hallmark of a community health nurse (CHN), was a role now claimed by health educators as well as all others involved in specialty nursing areas.
2. Problems in educational preparation when integrated curriculums combine specialized roles, such as community health nursing,

into a curriculum and virtually eliminate the specialty area. For example, continuity of care was a thread in many integrated curriculums. As a result, home visits were considered the function of the operating room nurse who prepared a client for surgery and of the pediatric nurse who followed up on a child at home while carrying out comprehensive care. These types of visits did not have the same focus as do the visits made by a CHN (refer to Chapter 2).

3. Role confusion that occurs when responsibilities of the CHN were well defined. Home visits were considered the cornerstone of community health nursing in some agencies; in others, most of the care to clients was delivered via clinic visits. Community health nursing professionals are currently debating why it is that a home visit is essential for nursing care in some geographic areas and not in others.

The Cyclical Nature of Issues in Community Health Nursing

The issues that faced CHNs relating to common practices and education in the 1980s were amazingly like those faced by Lillian Wald and her contemporaries. Babies were born to destitute parents; growing numbers of the elderly suffered from neglect, isolation, and lack of adequate care; and clients desired to die at home surrounded by family and familiar circumstances rather than in a hospital. Human needs do not change or diminish—only perhaps our methods of dealing with them.

The current economic crisis, with resulting cuts in the budgets of almost every agency, has meant decreases in services provided as well as reorganization of some of those services and agencies. Community health nursing agencies have had to examine critically each program that they offered. Often programs have lacked adequate documentation of the effectiveness of community health nursing intervention. Preventive efforts and those that are long-term in nature are difficult to evaluate; thus, CHNs must make such research a priority.

THE DECADE OF THE 1990s

As the decade of the 1980s came to an end, a number of trends in nursing's development became apparent (Lynaugh and Fagin, 1988): the acute care model of care delivery and disease-focused insurance systems do not meet the needs of children, the old, the chemically dependent, and the dying. The profession of nursing must address the fact that the age of "delayed degenerative disease" means that aging citizens survive pneumonia to face a life in which they need help with the activities of daily living. Other vulnerable groups such as handicapped children and adults and minorities face this challenge at the same time that they strive to obtain access to health care. "Health Care for All"—a goal being promoted worldwide and discussed throughout this chapter—is not a reality for many people in our society.

Further, the United States is seeing a "Third Revolution in Medical Care," that of assessment and accountability (Relman, 1988, p. 1220). Rapid expansion of the entire health care system took place in the decades of the 1940s through the 1960s, followed by the era of cost containment of health care spending. Presently health care planners agree that we need to know more about the costs, effectiveness, quality, and safety of the methods we use for the prevention, diagnosis, and treatment of disease. Outcome management or methods to link health care management decisions to systematic information about outcomes of practice will improve the effectiveness of care and provide a firm basis for economic decision making.

Challenges for the Future

The key issue that faced CHNs in the 1980s and that will continue to challenge the profession throughout the next decade is the spiralling cost of health care. In 1983, the major payor for health care, the federal government through Medicare, changed its method of payment; hospitalizations are now paid for prospectively, based on established rates for 467 diagnostic related groups (DRGs). Thus, a client's length of stay in a hospital has nothing to do with how much money the hospital receives. Rather, the client's diagnosis is the determining factor; a normal length of hospital stay has been established for each of the DRGs and health care professionals must document unusual circumstances for Medicare to reimburse for hospitalization beyond the average. Consequently, nurses must help clients back to health in the most efficient and effective way possible. Clients have been discharged back into the community "quicker and sicker." CHNs are increasingly called upon to be skilled in acute care. It is not uncommon to find that a year's experience in a hospital setting is a prerequisite for a CHN staff position.

Medicare's influence on the delivery of community-based and institutional services has not always been positive. Medicare's strict eligibility and reimbursement criteria and rigid definition of skilled care have promoted an acute-focused individual model of service. This limits ongoing reassessment and nursing intervention that could *prevent* institutionalization and caregiver/family burnout. Chapter 19 discusses extensively the consequences of acute-focused health care reimbursement mechanisms.

The challenges that need to be addressed in the 1990s are not insurmountable. The early public health nurse pioneers set the standards for the development of the nursing profession and reform in health care delivery. They were on the cutting edge of the suffragette movement, the birth control movement, and the social reform movement that brought health care and civil rights to women, children, immigrants, prisoners, and the mentally ill. They were not infrequently jailed for their beliefs. Their names are seen in the books that tell the story of our nation's history. Further, they worked independently in their profession and set standards for both nursing education and practice. Appendix 1-2 presents an overview of early nurse leaders whose lives we can continue to celebrate today. We can continue to use them as models for our own professional and personal growth.

In the first years of the 1990s there continue to be nurses at the cutting edge of nursing research, education, and practice and in local, state, and national politics. The following chapters tell some of their stories.

SUMMARY

The beginnings of nursing can be traced to the beginnings of humankind since there has always been a need for reducing pain with comfort measures. The early Christian church's contributions to nursing were significant, as were the organizational contributions of St. Vincent de Paul and Mademoiselle Le Gras to public health nursing. The influence of the status of women on nursing can be demonstrated by Sairy Gamp, a prostitute-nurse who cared for people in the 1700s when no "respectable" woman could take this position. Florence Nightingale's legacy to professional nursing and to public health, along with the contributions of William Rathbone, the founder of public health nursing in England, provided the basis for public health nursing in the United States. Events in society at large have shaped nursing as a whole and the development of public health nursing. The life and work of Lillian Wald, predecessor of the modern public health nurse, was powerfully influenced by the waves of immigrants to New York City and the desperate conditions in which they lived. How public health nurses organized themselves along with methods of education for this area of nursing shaped not only the development of this specialty area but the entire field of nursing. Gradually, the nation developed a consciousness about its collective health status, and this was demonstrated by the formation of health services on the national, state, and local level. Both world wars and the Depression forced negative as well as positive changes in public health nursing. Emphases in public health nursing as well as nursing in general are changing; the health scene is chaotic because there is no overall health plan. Public health nursing, with its focus on the health of groups, can involve nurses in health planning and in the necessary task of bringing order out of chaos.

Appendix 1-1 presents some beginnings and developments of significance to public health nursing in a chronological chart form. It is especially important to note other contemporary social events when reviewing the historical transition of public health nursing. Societal changes tremendously influence changes that occur in a profession.

APPENDIX 1-1

Some Beginnings in and Developments of Significance to Public Health Nursing*

Nursing and public health nursing	Other significant events
	1765 First school of medicine (Philadelphia)
	1798 Marine Hospital Service (became USPHS 1912) U.S. Treasury Department established and Act for the Relief of Sick and Disabled Seaman imposed a 20 cent tax on seaman's wages to provide funds for their health care
1813 Ladies Benevolent Society, Charleston, South Carolina	1813 Act to Encourage Vaccination
	1839 First dental school (Baltimore)
	1848 Imports Drug Act becomes the first federal statute to ensure the quality of drugs
1851 Florence Nightingale (1820-1910) went to Kaiserswerth	
1859 First District Nursing Association, Liverpool (William Rathbone and Mrs. Mary Robinson)	
1860 Nightingale Training School established, London	
	1861-1865 Civil War
	1864 International Red Cross (Henri Durant)
	1869 Massachusetts State Department of Health
1872 First schools of nursing in United States (New England Hospital for Women and Children, Boston, and Women's Hospital, Philadelphia)	1872 American Public Health Association founded by Stephen Smith
1873 Linda Richards, first nurse graduated in United States	1878 Act to Enforce Quarantine on Vessels and Vehicles
1877 New York City Mission sent trained nurses into homes of sick poor	1879 Act to Establish a National Board of Health for a 4-year period to cooperate with states on matters of public health
	1880 National Death Registration established by U.S. Bureau of the Census
	1882 American Red Cross (Clara Barton)
	1882-1884 Discovery of bacteria causing tuberculosis, diphtheria, and typhoid
1885 Buffalo District Nursing Association	
1886 Boston Instructive District Nursing Association and Philadelphia Visiting Nurse Association (VNA)	
1889 Chicago Visiting Nurse Association	
	1890-1910 "Golden Age of Bacteriology"
	1890 Pasteurization of milk developed
	Act to Prevent Interstate Spread of Disease passed
1892 School nursing, London (Amy Hughes)	

*Some dates may be disputed.

APPENDIX 1-1

Some Beginnings in and Developments of Significance to Public Health Nursing—cont'd

Nursing and public health nursing	*Other significant events*
1893 Henry Street Visiting Nurse Service, New York (Lillian D. Wald and Mary Brewster); first milk station, New York City; American Society of Superintendents of Training Schools for Nurses (became National League for Nursing Education, 1912)	
	1894 School medical inspection, Boston
1895 Industrial Nursing, Vermont Marble Works (Ada Mayo Stewart)	
1897 Nurses' Associated Alumnae of United States and Canada (became American Nurses' Association 1911)	1897 University of Michigan granted Master of Science degree in Hygiene and Public Health
1898 Los Angeles Health Department paid public health nurses; Detroit Visiting Nurse Association	1898 Course in social work, New York Charity Organization Society
1899 International Council of Nurses; University education for nurses, Teachers College, Columbia University (course in hospital economics)	1899 Association of Hospital Superintendents (became American Hospital Association 1907)
1900 *American Journal of Nursing*	1900-1925 Expansion of voluntary agencies
1901 58 public health nursing associations; 130 public health nurses in United States	
1902 School nursing, New York City (Lina Rogers)	1902 Biologics Control Act
1903 Tuberculosis nursing, Baltimore; First Nurse Practice Acts	
1904 Visiting nurses have program at Conference of Charities and Correction	1904 National Organization for the Study and Prevention of Tuberculosis (became National Tuberculosis Association)
1905 200 public health agencies; 440 public health nurses in United States	1905 Medical social work, Massachusetts General Hospital
1906 Course in district nursing offered by Boston Instructive District Nursing Association	1906 Food and Drug Act
1907 Alabama law permitting employment of public health nurses	1907 Visiting teacher, Boston
1908 English health visitor; Detroit Health Department employed public health nurses	
1909 University of Minnesota School of Nursing	1909 National Committee for Mental Hygiene
Metropolitan Life Insurance Company contracts for visiting nursing service; The *Visiting Nurse Quarterly* published by Cleveland Visiting Nurse Association (later presented to NOPHN and became *Public Health Nursing* monthly until 1953)	First White House Conference; American Association for the Study and Prevention of Infant Mortality
1910 Public health nursing program, Teachers College, Columbia University	1910 *Medical Education in the United States and Canada,* Abraham Flexner
	1911 Boston Instructive Visiting Nurse Association added nutritional service
	Joint Committee on Health Problems in Education, American Medical Association and National Education Association; county health departments in Guilford County, North Carolina, and Yakima County, Washington

Continued.

APPENDIX 1-1

Some Beginnings in and Developments of Significance to Public Health Nursing—cont'd

Nursing and public health nursing	*Other significant events*
1912 American Red Cross Rural Nursing Service (1200 services in 1922); National Organization for Public Health Nursing (NOPHN); U.S. Children's Bureau, Department of Labor	1912 Act to Establish a Children's Bureau (PL 62-116) established maternal and child health services on the federal level
1913 Division of Public Health Nursing, New York State Department of Health	1913 Harvard School of Public Health
1914 NOPHN suggested 4-month course in a visiting nurse association as essential preparation for public health nursing	1914 Harrison Narcotics Act (PL 62-223) established federal controls over narcotics
	1915 National Birth Registration Area established
	1915-1925 Wave of legislation of physical education and hygiene
1916 1922 public health nursing agencies; 5152 public health nurses: University of Cincinnati School of Nursing 5-year program leading to bachelor's degree	
	1917-1918 World War I
	1917 American Dietetic Association; Massachusetts and New York employed public health nutritionists
1918 USPHS organized a division of public health nursing to work in extracantonment zones	Community chests and councils emerged
1918-1923 Increased interest in combining local public health nursing agencies	1918 Compulsory education in all states; American Association of Medical Social Workers
1918 Maternity Center Association, New York	
1919 *Public Health Nursing,* Mary S. Gardner; increase in public health nurses and public health nursing education; public health nursing program, University of Michigan	1919-1929 Demonstrations of child health and public health services
1920 NOPHN-approved university programs in public health nursing	
1921 Industrial and school nursing sections of NOPHN; NOPHN set 1 academic year as minimum for public health nursing certificate	1921 First university program in public health education, Massachusetts Institute of Technology, Harvard; National Health Council; American Association of Social Workers
	1921-1929 Shepherd-Towner Act—federal aid for maternal and child health
1922 4040 public health agencies; 11,548 nurses	1922-1935 American Child Health Association
1923 Public health nursing section, APHA; Nursing and Nursing Education in the United States ("The Winslow-Goldmark Report"); Yale and Western Reserve Universities established collegiate schools of nursing	
1924 U.S. Indian Bureau Nursing Service (Eleanor Gregg)	1924 Oil Pollution Act (PL 68-238) prohibited the dumping of oil in navigable waters

APPENDIX 1-1

Some Beginnings in and Developments of Significance to Public Health Nursing—cont'd

Nursing and public health nursing	*Other significant events*
1925 Frontier Nursing Service—nurse-midwives (Mary Breckenridge); first NOPHN statement of qualifications for public health nurses; John Hancock Mutual Life Insurance Company Visiting Nurse Service	
1925-1926 Chicago Infant Welfare Society and Boston and East Harlem public health nursing agencies employ psychiatric social workers	
1926 Committee on Grading of Nursing Schools began studies	
	1927-1931 Research by Committee on the Cost of Medical Care
	1929 Beginning of the Depression
1930 Unemployment of nurses	1930 Study of maternal mortality in New York City
	Act to Establish a National Institute of Health (PL 71-251)
1931 4355 public health agencies; 15,865 nurses	
1932 Final report of Commission on Medical Education; Association of Collegiate Schools of Nursing; Lobenstine Midwifery Clinic and School (Maternity Center responsible for school 1934); 7% of nurses employed in public health nursing had completed a 1-year program	
1933 Pearl McIver appointed to USPHS as a public health nursing analyst	1933 U.S. Birth and Death Registration Areas complete
1934 *Survey of Public Health Nursing,* NOPHN, published	
1935 *Facts about Nursing,* American Nursing Association (ANA)	1935 Social Security Act (PL 74-721) was designed to provide for the general welfare by establishing a system of federal old-age benefits, and by enabling the states to make provision for aged persons, blind individuals, dependent and crippled children, maternal and child welfare and the unemployed
	1935-1936 National Health Survey
	1937-1947 Beginning of federal appropriations for cancer, venereal diseases, tuberculosis, mental health, heart disease, etc.
	1938 Federal Food, Drug and Cosmetic Act (PL 75-717)
	1939 Reorganization of federal agencies; USPHS transferred from Treasury Department to Federal Security Agency
	1939-1945 World War II
1940 20,434 nurses employed in public health nursing; 22% had completed 1 or more years in an approved public health nursing program	
1941 Nurse Training Act (PL 77-146)	
1942 American Association of Industrial Nurses	*Continued.*

APPENDIX 1-1

Some Beginnings in and Developments of Significance to Public Health Nursing—cont'd

Nursing and public health nursing	Other significant events
1943 Bolton-Bailey Act (PL 77-146) for nursing education and Cadet Nurse Program; Division of Nursing Education, formed in USPHS [Lucile Petry (Leone)—Director]	1943-1947 Emergency Maternity and Infant Care Program
1944 Division of Nursing, USPHS [Lucile Petry (Leone)]; commissioned rank for nurses; NOPHN accredits only public health nursing programs with professional content of at least 1 year, which is part of program leading to a degree; Skidmore College basic nursing program approved for preparation of public health nurses	1944 Public Health Service Act (PL 78-410) consolidated all existing public health legislation into a single statute
	1945 End World War II; educational privileges provided for nurse veterans by GI Bill of Rights; publication of *Local Health Units for the Nation;* APHA accreditation of schools of public health
1946 Nurses classified as professional by U.S. Civil Service Commission	1946 Hospital Survey and Construction Act [Hill Burton](PL 79-725)
1947 Women's Medical Specialist corps (PL 80-36) established a permanent nursing corps in the army and navy	
1948 Publication of *Nurses for the Future* (Esther Lucile Brown)	1948 World Health Organization permanently established and meeting of World Health Assembly
	National Heart Act (PL 80-655) authorized aid for research and training, and established the National Heart Institute at NIH; National Dental Research Act (PL 80-755) established the National Institute of Dental Research in NIH; and Water Pollution Control Act (PL 80-845) to help ensure clean water in the U.S.
1949 National Federation of Licensed Practical Nurses; national nursing organizations support legislation for federal financial aid for practical nursing education	
1950 25,081 nurses employed for public health work in the United States and territories; 34% had completed 1 or more years in an approved public health nursing program	1950 National Research Institutes Act (PL 81-692) expanded NIH to include research and training related to arthritis, rheumatism, multiple sclerosis, cerebral palsy, blindness, and leprosy
1951 National League for Nursing recommendation that collegiate basic nursing education programs include preparation for public health nursing; National Association of Colored Graduate Nurses integrated with ANA	
1952 Reorganization of national nursing organizations, major functions transferred to American Nurses' Association and National League for Nursing	
Boston University program with a major in general nursing approved for preparation of public health nurses	

APPENDIX 1-1

Some Beginnings in and Developments of Significance to Public Health Nursing—cont'd

Nursing and public health nursing	*Other significant events*
1952-1953 American Red Cross, Metropolitan Life Insurance Company, and John Hancock Mutual Life Insurance Company discontinue public health nursing services; *Public Health Nursing,* December 1952, last issue	
1953 *Nursing Outlook* published in January	1953 Department of Health, Education, and Welfare established with cabinet status
1955 27,112 nurses employed in public health work in the United States and territories; 37% had completed at least 1 year of approved public health nursing program; nursing programs preparing for public health nursing:	1955 National Association of Social Workers (seven associations combined)
Major in public health nursing 33	Air Pollution Control Act (PL 84-159); Mental Health Study Act (PL 84-182); and Polio Vaccination Assistance Act (PL 84-377)
Baccalaureate basic 25	
Major in general nursing 9	
	1956 National Health Survey Act (PL 84-652) provided for a continuing survey and special studies of sickness and disability in the U.S.
1959 NLN voted that no new specialized baccalaureate program be accredited and that after 1963 only baccalaureate programs that include public health nursing be accredited	
1960 *NLN Criteria for the Evaluation of Educational Programs in Nursing that Lead to Baccalaureate and Master's Degrees*	1960 International Health Research Act (PL 86-610) and Federal Hazardous Substance Labeling Act (PL 86-813)
	1961 First White House Conference on Aging
	1962 11 accredited schools of public health in United States, 2 in Canada
	National Institute of Child Health and Human Development (PL 87-838) and Vaccination Assistance Act (PL 87-868) aided programs to combat polio, diphtheria, whooping cough, and tetanus
1963 Report of Surgeon General's Consultant Group on Nursing	1963 Health Professional Educational Assistance Act (PL 88-129) and Clean Air Act (PL 88-206)
1964 *NLN Statement of Beliefs and Recommendations Regarding Baccalaureate Programs Admitting Registered Nurse Student*	1964 Economic Opportunity Act of 1964 (PL 88-452) was enacted to mobilize the human and financial resources of the nation to combat poverty, it established the Office of Economic Opportunity, authorized Volunteers in Service to America (VISTA), the Job Corps, Upward Bound, Neighborhood Youth Corps, Head Start, neighborhood health centers, commmunity action programs, assisted small businesses, and was an impetus to antipoverty programs; Civil Rights Act of 1964 (PL 88-352) forbade discrimination based on race or sex in public accommodations, facilities, and educational settings; and Food Stamp Act (PL 88-525)

Continued.

APPENDIX 1-1

Some Beginnings in and Developments of Significance to Public Health Nursing—cont'd

Nursing and public health nursing	*Other significant events*

1964   Agencies and nurses employed for public health nursing:

	Agencies	*Nurses*
Local	9,094	35,209
Board of Education	5,412	13,257
Official	2,712	14,738
VNA	682	3,826
Combination	51	1,478

Population per public health nurse in United States 5586, 43.4% of full-time nurses had completed 30 or more hours in an approved public health nursing program; 39.7% had college degrees

Nurse Training Act of 1964 (PL 88-581)

1965   Social Security Amendment of 1965 (PL 89-97) established Medicare and Medicaid; Federal Cigarette Labeling and Advertising Act (PL89-92) designed to inform the public of the hazards of cigarette smoking; Heart Disease, Cancer and Stroke Amendments (PL 89-239); and Solid Waste Disposal Act (PL 89-272)

1966   NLN programs accredited for public health nursing—June 1966:

Masters	42
Baccalaureate basic (students with no previous nursing preparation and registered nurses)	151
Baccalaureate basic (students with no previous nursing preparation)	91
Baccalaureate basic (registered nurses only)	6

1966   Child Nutrition Act (PL 89-642) established a federal program of research and support for child nutrition, and Comprehensive Health Planning and Public Health Service Amendments (PL 89-749)

1967   Air Quality Act (PL 90-148)

1968   Health Manpower Act (PL 90-490) extended Nurse Training Act of 1964

1969   Federal Coal Mine Health and Safety Act (PL 91-173) and National Environmental Policy Act (PL 91-190)

1970   National Commission on Nursing and Nursing Education—Abstract for Action published

1970   Family Planning Services and Population Research Act (PL 91-572); Occupational Safety and Health Act (PL 91-596); Comprehensive Alcohol Abuse and Alcoholism Prevention Treatment and Rehabilitation (PL 91-616); the

APPENDIX 1-1

Some Beginnings in and Developments of Significance to Public Health Nursing—cont'd

Nursing and public health nursing	*Other significant events*
	Environmental Education Act (PL 91-516) Comprehensive Drug Abuse Prevention and Control Act (PL 91-513); Resource Recovery Act (PL 91-512); Health Training Improvement Act (PL 91-519); Emergency Health Personnel Act (PL 91-623); and Public Health Cigarette Smoking Act (PL 91-222)
1971 "Extending the Scope of Nursing Practice" report was published	1971 Comprehensive Health Manpower Training Act (PL 92-218); National Cancer Act (PL 92-218); and Lead Based Poisoning Prevention Act (PL 91-695)
Nurse Training Act of 1971 (PL 92-158) expanded and continued nurse training provisions of the 1964 and 1968 acts	
	1972 National Sickle Cell Anemia Control Act (PL 92-294); National Cooley's Anemia Control Act (PL 92-414); Federal Environmental Pesticide Control Act (PL 92-516); National Heart, Blood Vessel, Lung, and Blood Act (PL 92-423); National School Lunch and Child Nutrition Amendments (PL 92-433); Federal Environmental Pesticide Control Act (PL 92-516); Consumer Product Safety Act (PL 92-573); Noise Control Act (PL 92-574); Marine Mammal Protection Act (PL 92-522)
	1973 The Health Maintenance Organization (HMO) Act (PL 93-222) and Endangered Species Act (PL 93-205)
1974 Formation of Nurses Coalition for Action in Politics, N-CAP; first certification examinations by the ANA for excellence in practice	1974 Child Abuse Prevention and Treatment Act (PL 93-247); Sudden Infant Death Syndrome Act (PL 93-270); Narcotic Addict Treatment Act (PL 93-281); Research on Aging Act (PL 93-286); National Research Act (PL 93-348); National Diabetes Mellitus Research and Eduction Act (PL 93-354); Safe Drinking Water Act (PL 93-523); National Arthritis Act (93-640)
	1975 National Health Planning and Resources Development Act (PL 93-641); Disabled Assistance and Bill of Rights Act (PL 94-103); and Health Services, Health Revenue, and Nurse Training Act [NTA] (PL 94-63)
	1976 Costs for health care in the United States rose 14% over 1975
	Toxic Substances Control Act (PL 94-469)
1977-1978 Designated the "Year of the Nurse" by ANA to help the public better understand nursing	1977 Passage of the Rural Health Clinic Services bill (PL 95-210)
1978 Massachusetts becomes the seventh state to mandate continuing education as a requirement for relicensure of both registered and practical nurses	1978 President Carter vetoes the Nursing Training Act

Continued.

APPENDIX 1-1

Some Beginnings in and Developments of Significance to Public Health Nursing—cont'd

Nursing and public health nursing	*Other significant events*
1978 Robert Wood Johnson Foundation finances $5 million program to train nurses as school nurse practitioners and place them in areas where children now receive inadequate care	
1979 ANA board determines that future ANA conventions and conferences will be held only in states that have ratified the Equal Rights Amendment; Maryland passes law which requires insurance companies to provide reimbursement "for any service which is within the lawful scope of a duly licensed health care provider"; ANA sponsors a Study of Credentialing in Nursing, which spurs nationwide discussion and debate; N-CAP survey shows that nurses act on their political convictions and back candidates on the basis of issues, not party philosophy (they also vote and let officials know what they think)	1979 Due to antirecession lobbying by nurses and others, NTA funds were cut $15.75 million rather than Carter's $84 million; President Carter's fiscal 1980 budget cut nursing education funds to $15 million in contrast to current levels of $122 million (only nurse practitioner programs fared well); President Carter sent to Congress a national health insurance bill which would require minimum benefits for employed people and upgrade coverage for the poor, aged, and disabled; he became the first president to formally back a plan with the underlying concept that health care is a basic human right President Carter's cost containment bill designed to limit annual revenue for the nation's hospitals ran into many snags and has slim chance of passing
1980 "A Classification Scheme for Client Problems in Community Health Nursing," written by D. Simmons, provided the potential for systematically describing client needs in the community setting Jo Eleanor Elliott was named Director of the Division of Nursing, USPHS, replacing Jessie Scott Colorado passed a new nurse practice act that made it possible for nurses to practice independently in private settings The Supreme Court declined to review the discrimination suit brought by NURSE (Nurses Underrepresented in Social Equality) which charged that the city of Denver paid women less than it did men who performed work of equal value Maryland was the first state to pass the law that mandates reimbursement in all health insurance for services of nurses and other licensed providers	1980 Enrollments in higher education programs, including nursing, declined. The decline was expected to continue through the end of the century Civil Rights of Institutionalized Persons Act (PL 96-247)
1981 In a $5 million project to up-grade long-term care, the Robert Wood Johnson Foundation joined with the ANA to develop "teaching nursing homes" Carolyn Davis became the first nurse to head the Health Care Financing Administration (HCFA) "The more an occupation is dominated by women, the less it pays" stated a new report of the Equal Opportunity Employment Commission	1981 Ronald Reagan was elected president and began a period of retrenchment in numerous health and social programs California legislature passed a vote mandating that women in female-dominated jobs be paid in accordance with their ability to produce the same level or quality of work as men

APPENDIX 1-1

Some Beginnings in and Developments of Significance to Public Health Nursing—cont'd

Nursing and public health nursing	Other significant events
	Omnibus Budget Reconciliation Act (PL 97-35) [refer to Tables 4-1 and 4-3.]; and Migrant and Seasonal Agricultural Worker Protection Act (PL 97-410)
1982 The nation's first directly elected board of nursing met in Raleigh, N.C., for a swearing-in ceremony. North Carolina was the only state where RNs and LPNs nominated and voted for members of their own board of nursing	1982 *Playboy* magazine abandoned a plan to publish a pictorial feature on women in nursing when it was met with widespread protest by nurses across the country
To be licensed as RNs, students of nursing began taking a new comprehensive test developed by the National Council of State Boards of Nursing over the past several years	The USPHS released a report stating that exposure to other people's smoking may increase cancer risks to nonsmokers
The ANA convention adopted a radically new organizational plan for the organization that was designed to make decisions more representative of the total membership	With the nation's cities hard hit by the recession, major cities projected the most declines in expenditures in the areas of health care
Federal support for nursing education took a massive blow from "Reaganomics"; hundreds of nurses and nursing students traveled to Capitol Hill to protest the cutbacks	A 2-year drive by conservatives to ban voluntary abortions was blocked when the Senate voted to table a bill introduced by Senator Jessie Helms
Faye Abdellah became the first nurse and the first woman to be promoted to rank of deputy surgeon general of the USPHS	During a 1-year period, over 600 cases of Kaposi's sarcoma were reported to the Centers for Disease Control. The mortality rate was 40 percent; the disease was considered to be a manifestation of acquired immunodeficiency syndrome (AIDS)
May 6, was voted National Recognition Day for Nurses by Congress	The first annual meeting of the National Association of Home Care was held in Atlanta, Ga. Its goal was to unite the rapidly growing ranks of home care providers in a single, national organization. Elsie Griffith, a nurse, was the founder of the association
The longest nurses' strike in the nation's history (2 years) ended February 8 when nurses at Ashtabula General Hospital voted to accept a 2-year contract	The third White House Conference on the Aging (held every 10 years) stressed the importance of nursing in the care of this population group
Classification of Nursing Diagnoses, the proceedings of the third and fourth national conferences for classification of nursing diagnoses, was published	Members attending the American Public Health Association convention vigorously opposed the Reagan administration's sizable increases in military defense which led to reduced spending in social and health programs
Nurses across the country worked to ensure that the Equal Rights Amendment would be ratified by the necessary 38 states by June 30. The goal was not reached, and on July 14 the ERA amendment was reintroduced into the House and the Senate	November elections revealed that 83% of the political candidates endorsed by N-CAP were winners
	Tax Equity and Fiscal Responsibility Act of 1982 (PL 97-248) [refer to Tables 4-1 and 4-3]; and Nuclear Waste Policy Act (PL 97-425)

Continued.

APPENDIX 1-1

Some Beginnings in and Developments of Significance to Public Health Nursing—cont'd

Nursing and public health nursing	*Other significant events*
1983 Ruth Freeman, a leader in the field of public health nursing, died at the age of 76. For several decades, her writings helped to prepare nurses for CHN practice	**1983** Dr. Barney Clark became the first recipient of an artificial heart
The state of Maine legislated a prospective reimbursement system that called for regular reporting of nursing service data and the nursing costs of treating patients in similar classifications. For the first time anywhere, hospitals were compelled to break down nursing costs as a separate item in their accounting systems	The Reagan administration issued a regulation that would force 5000 family planning centers to inform parents when a teenager under 17 sought birth control prescriptions or devices
The final report of the National Commission on Nursing, sponsored by the American Hospital Association, stated that future progress in the profession would mandate better-educated and more highly qualified nurses	Health and Human Services (HHS), Division of Maternal and Child Health, developed projects to study the prevalence of ventilator-dependent children and to establish guidelines for a regional system for their care
The Department of Public Health Nursing at the University of North Carolina's School of Public Health, a longtime leader in the field, was threatened with closure by the university. Nursing and public health leaders around the country moved to block the plan	AIDS was declared the number one priority of the USPHS
Salaries for nurses in home and community health agencies increased 13.8% in the past year, to a median of $19,148 for official agencies and $17,480 for nonofficial agencies	Seven years into the study, over 100,000 nurses continue to participate in a Harvard project that examines health risks that pose special threats to women
Institute of Medicine completed *Nursing and Nursing Education: Public and Private Action,* which concluded that the shortage of nurses had been eliminated and that funding for nursing education should be targeted for specialty groups	President Reagan supported reductions in nursing education funding totaling $1.2 billion. His FY 84 budget represented an overall funding reduction of 75% for nursing programs
	Deciding to For-go Life-Sustaining Treatment was the report submitted by the President's Commission for the Study of Ethical Problems in Medicine and Biomedical Research
	Health Care Financing Administration (HCFA) set very low Medicare reimbursement rates for hospice care; critics argue that few agencies would be willing to sponsor hospices as a result
	April 20, President Reagan signed Public Law 98-28, which changed payment for Medicare hospital stays. Hospital stays are now reimbursed by Medicare, based on prospectively established rates for 467 diagnosis related groups (DRGs); and International Environmental Protection Act (PL 98-164)
1984 The Diamond Jubilee of the first school of nursing in the world to be located on a university campus where faculty held university appointments was celebrated. The University of Minnesota School of Nursing was founded in 1909	**1984** That the risk of congestive heart disease (CHD) can be reduced by lowering serum cholesterol levels was conclusively demonstrated in a study by the National Heart, Lung, and Blood Institute

APPENDIX 1-1

Some Beginnings in and Developments of Significance to Public Health Nursing—cont'd

Nursing and public health nursing	*Other significant events*
	The Senate debated a bill that would create a National Institute of Nursing within the National Institutes of Health. The Institute would assume research responsibilities now assumed by the Division of Nursing, PHS
	"People Match" in Bristol, N.H., kept people out of nursing homes by matching them with appropriate roommates
	President Reagan signed a bill authorizing the third Monday in January as Martin Luther King Day
	The Missouri Supreme Court vindicated two obstetric/gynecologic nurse practitioners charged with unauthorized practice of medicine. They gave routine care under physician backup with written protocols to 5000 patients a year in a Title X neighborhood agency
	Deficit Reduction Act of 1984 (PL 98-369) [see Table 4-1]; National Organ Transplant Act (PL 98-460)
1985 *Consensus Conference on the Essentials of Public Health Nursing Practice and Education: Report of the Conference, September 5–7, 1984* examines the critical issues confronting PHN; educational preparation needed to practice as a generalist and as a specialist; and collective goals for PHN in the future	1985 Food Security Act of 1985 (PL 99-198)
	"Live-Aid," a 17-hour rock concert broadcast on radio and TV from Philadelphia to London to 152 countries, raised $70 million for starving people in Africa
Patients are discharged "quicker and sicker" from hospitals under Medicare's DRG system	
NLN wages a fight to keep RN licensure for ADN graduates while the ANA strives to make the BSN the legal requirement for practice	
LPNs disappear from acute care settings with the shift to all RN staffs across the country	
1986 American Nurses' Association revises the *Standards for Community Health Nursing Practice* and develops standards for *Home Health Nursing Practice*	1986 Comprehensive Smokeless Tobacco Health Education Act of 1986 (PL 99-252); Consolidated Omnibus Budget Reconciliation Act of 1986 (PL 99-272) [see Table 4-1]; Protection and Advocacy for Mentally Ill Individuals Act of 1986 (PL 99-319); Education of the Deaf Act (PL 99-371); Handicapped Children's Protection Act (PL 99-372); Comprehensive Anti-Apartheid Act of 1986 (PL 99-440); Radon Gas and Indoor air Quality Research Act of 1986 (PL 99-499); Asbestos Hazard Emergency Response Act of 1986 (PL 99-519); Anti-Drug Abuse Act of 1986 (PL 99-570); Child Sexual Abuse and

Continued.

APPENDIX 1-1

Some Beginnings in and Developments of Significance to Public Health Nursing—cont'd

Nursing and public health nursing	Other significant events
	Pornography Act of 1986 (PL 99-628); Employment Opportunities for Disabled American Act (PL 99-643); Health Programs (PL 99-660)
The National Center for Nursing Research is established at NIH	In Chernobyl, Ukraine, there was a major accident at a nuclear power plant that killed 23; 40,000 were evacuated
North Dakota becomes the first state to require the BSN for RN licensure and the ADN for LPN licensure	The Gramm-Rudman Landmark Law cut over $1 billion in the fiscal 1986 budget
The NLN switches positions and backs two levels of nursing practice—professional and associate	
Certified nurse midwives formed an independent mutual insurance firm to solve the malpractice insurance dilemma that threatened to shut down the profession	AZT (aziodothymidine), an antiviral drug and now known as ZDV (zidovudine), was found to improve the health of some AIDS patients but was not a cure. Government officials predicted a tenfold increase in AIDS-related deaths in the next 5 years
Major study in Institute of Medicine says that nursing homes need more RNs to upgrade care	Mounting use of illegal drugs (cocaine as "crack") caused passage of stiff antidrug laws
1987 Public Health Nursing Education and Practice document was published by the USDHHS and addresses the congruence of public health baccalaureate education for practice in public health agencies	1987 Stewart B. McKinney Homeless Assistance Act (PL 100-77); Wilbur J. Cohen Federal Building (PL 100-99); Developmental Disabilities Assistance and Bill of Rights Act Amendments of 1987 (PL 100-146); and Civil Rights Restoration Act of 1987 (PL 100-259)
OSHA changed its rules, and allowed OH nurses to have access to trade secrets in nonemergency situations	Condom ads become prominent in U.S. media, reflecting a concern for "safe sex" to prevent AIDS
UCLA's study of entering students finds sharp drop in number planning nursing careers	Biological father William Stern won custody of Baby M, with parental rights terminated for Mary Beth Whitehead, who had contracted to bear Stern's child for $10,000
The largest pay equity award in the history of nursing was won by the Pennsylvania Nurses' Association against that state	
Secretary's Commission on Nursing report confirms that the reported shortage of RNs is real, widespread, and of significant magnitude	1988 The Institute of Medicine's report, The Future of Public Health examines America's public health system in detail—its mission, its current state, and the barriers to improvement—and makes recommendations for dealing with future public health challenges
Candidates for nursing licensure took the first past/fail test that replaced numerical scores	Medicare Catastrophic Coverage Act of 1988 (PL 100-360); School Asbestos Management (PL 100-368); Hearing Aid Compatibility Act of 1988 (PL 100-394); Technology-Related Assistance for Individuals with Disabilities Act of 1988 (PL 100-407); Hunger Prevention Act of 1988 (PL 100-435); Family Support Act of 1988 (PL 100-485) [refer to Table 4-1]; Health

APPENDIX 1-1

Some Beginnings in and Developments of Significance to Public Health Nursing—cont'd

Nursing and public health nursing	*Other significant events*
	Maintenance Organization Amendments of 1988 (PL 100-517); Forest Ecosystems and Atmospheric Pollution Research Act of 1988 (PL 100-521); Radon Program Development Act (PL 100-551); Lead Contamination Control Act of 1988 (PL 100-572); Native Hawaiian Health Care Act of 1988 (PL 100-579); Medical Waste Tracking Act of 1988 (PL 100-582); Health Omnibus Programs Extension of 1988 (PL 100-607) [refer to Table 4-3]; Water Resources Development Act of 1988 (PL 100-676); Ocean Dumping Ban Act of 1988 (PL 100-688); Anti-drug Abuse Act of 1988 (PL 100-690); Federal Cave Resources Protection Act of 1988 (PL 100-691)
BSN programs saw a 7.8 percent decline in undergraduate enrollments	
Sigma Theta Tau began building a $4 million center for Nursing Scholarship in Indianapolis	
	A 3-year drive to boost a "thoroughly experienced" staff nurse salary to $50,000 was started by The Pennsylvania Nurses' Association
	Nursing: Sixth Report to the President and Congress on the Status of Health Personnel in the United States addresses current developments in various health care practice settings; the increased movement of patients to the community; and future requirements for nursing personnel
	Reagan Administration temporarily halts efforts to enforce new HHS regulations that would prohibit federally funded family-planning clinics from providing abortions
	The AMA approves a proposal to train "registered care technologists" to assume a new role at the bedside, designed to carry out medical protocols, with special emphasis on technical skills
	The term "ecophobia" is coined to illustrate the nation's concern about polluted beaches and water, persistent drought, immense forest fires, and the worst air quality in decades
1989 *Strategies for a Collaborative Future: The Consensus Report from the National Consensus Conference on the Educational Preparation of Home Care Administrators* addresses the educational needs of practitioners preparing for leadership positions in home health care	1989 Whistleblower Protection Act of 1989 (PL 101-12)

Continued.

APPENDIX 1-1

Some Beginnings in and Developments of Significance to Public Health Nursing—cont'd

Nursing and public health nursing		*Other significant events*	
1989	Nineteen hundred nurses are named in liability and malpractice suits yearly; 50% of those claims are upheld. The average claim against a nurse that results in payment is $145,397	1989	A draft of *Promoting Health/Preventing Disease: Year 2000 Objectives for the Nation* is distributed for public review and comment
	The majority of nurses had economic gains of 7-10% in 1988. The average pay for nurses rose 10.6 percent to $32,160, the largest maximum increase on record		The revolutionary abortion pill, RU 486, is increasingly popular in France. Given anti-abortion pressures, it could take years before it becomes popular in other countries
			George Bush is inaugurated President; he urges the nation to "use power to help people."

Used by permission of Ella McNeil, Professor Emeritus of Public Health Nursing, School of Public Health, University of Michigan, Ann Arbor, Michigan. Original compilation of important beginnings was updated to reflect significant changes in the '70s and '80s.

APPENDIX 1-2

Selected Significant CHN/PHN Leaders

Leader	*Contributions*
Clarissa Barton (1821-1921)	The first woman to take to the battlefield as a volunteer nurse and relief worker during the Civil War; founder of the American Red Cross
Mary Beard (1876-1946)	One of the founders of the National Organization for Public Health Nursing; an advocate of preventive health services and a worker for the Rockefeller Foundation
Mary Breckinridge (1877-1965)	Founder of the Frontier Nursing Service, public pioneer in nurse-midwifery and in bringing modern nursing to rural America
Ada M. Carr (1800-1951)	Editor of the *Public Health Nurse* and the first nurse to conduct postgraduate studies in public health nursing
Charity Collins (1882-1900)	The first black public health school nurse in the country
Ella Phillips Crandall (1871-1938)	One of the founders of the National Organization for Public Health Nursing and the Red Cross Rural Nursing Service
Annie Damier (1800-1916)	Instrumental in establishing tuberculosis nursing in New York City
Dorothy Deming (1893-1972)	Directed the National Organization for Public Health Nursing beginning in 1927 and a prolific author, among her books the *Penny Marsh* series for teenagers
Dorothea Dix (1802-1887)	Crusader for the mentally ill and imprisoned, teacher and writer
Lavinia Lloyd Dock (1858-1956)	Helped develop the American Nurses Association; prolific author and educator; historian, advocate of social reform and women's rights
Margaret Dolan (1914-1974)	President of the ANA from 1962-1964 and the second nurse to be President of the American Public Health Association

APPENDIX 1-2

Selected Significant CHN/PHN Leaders—cont'd

Leader	Contributions
Ruth Freeman (1906-1982)	Nurse, educator, and author, using an interdisciplinary outlook which related academic work to the real world, prolific author; worked to persuade personnel in public health to view nurses as team members
Mary Sewall Gardner (1871-1961)	Author of the first public health nursing text; founder of the National Organization for Public Health Nursing
Emma Goldman (1869-1940)	Used nursing as point from which to attack the problems in society, leader of the birth control movement; editor of *Mother Earth,* a radical journal; called the "mother of anarchy in America"; spent time in jail for birth control lectures in America; one of the most significant women in America in the years before WWI
Alma Haupt (1893-1956)	Graduate of the first class at the University of Minnesota in public health nursing; directed the Nursing Bureau of the Metropolitan Life Insurance company where she established a model home nursing program
Clara Maass (1876-1901)	A heroine in the war against yellow fever; volunteered to take part in the experiments in Cuba which proved that yellow fever was transmitted by mosquitoes; died from the disease
Pearl McIver (1893-1976)	The first nurse on the staff of the U.S. Public Health Service which she expanded into a modern and extensive agency to serve the needs of the U.S. public
Mary Adelaide Nutting (1858-1948)	First professor of nursing in an American university, occupying the first endowed chair in nursing; a reformer of nursing education
Linda Richards (1841-1930)	America's first trained nurse; teacher
Margaret Sanger (1879-1966)	Pioneer in the birth control movement, launching the American Birth Control League which became the Planned Parenthood Federation of America
Emilie Sargent (1894-1977)	Directed the Visiting Nurse Association of Detroit for 40 years, improving and diversifying its services. Was the first woman and public health professional to receive the University of Michigan Outstanding Achievement Award
Isabel Maitland Stewart (1878-1963)	Leader in the NLN and curriculum development; author of nursing history; avid supporter of the suffrage movement
Lina Rogers Struthers (1870-1928)	First school nurse in the U.S., chosen by Lillian Wald while a nurse at the Henry Street Settlement House
Stella Boothe Vail (1890-1926)	Implemented unique method for teaching health promotion and disease prevention. Used entertainment techniques at county fairs to emphasize hygiene and public health
Lillian Wald (1867-1940)	Leader of the public health nursing movement in the U.S.; developed the Henry Street Settlement House in New York and improved the lot of immigrants on the Lower East Side; established playgrounds for children who had none; placed the first nurse in a public school setting; developed innovative financing for nursing services; helped to found the National Child Labor Committee; formed the New York State Bureau of Industries and Immigrations and the Joint Board of Sanitary Control to enforce basic sanitary rules; helped develop the forerunner of the ACLU; prolific writer and teacher

Adapted from Kaufman M, Hawkins WJ, Higgins LP, and Friedman AH: Dictionary of American Nursing Biography, Westport, Conn, 1988, Greenwood Press; and Kalisch P and Kalisch BJ: The advancements of American nursing, ed 2, Boston, 1986, Little, Brown.

REFERENCES

Archer SE: Marketing public health nursing services, Nurs Outlook 31:305-309, 1983.

Barkauskas V: Public health nursing practice—an educator's view, Nurs Outlook 30:384-389, 1982.

Chavigny K and Kroske M: Public health nursing in crisis, Nurs Outlook 31:312-316, 1983.

Christy TE: Portrait of a leader: Lavinia Lloyd Dock, Nurs Outlook 17:72-75, 1969.

Christy TE: Portrait of a leader: Lillian Wald, Nurs Outlook 18:50-54, 1970.

Committee for the Study of Nursing Education: Nursing and nursing education in the United States, New York, 1923, Macmillan.

Davis C: Nursing and the health care debate, Image: J Nurs Scholarship 15:67, 1983 (editorial).

Deloughery GL: History and trends of professional nursing, ed 8, St Louis, 1977, The CV Mosby Co.

Desirable organization of public health nursing for family service, Public Health Nurs 38:387-389, 1946.

Dickens C: Martin Chuzzlewit, New York, 1910, Macmillan.

Dock L, Pickett SE, Noyes CD, Clement FE, Fox EE, and VanMeter AR: History of American Red Cross nursing, New York, 1922, Macmillan.

Dolan JA: Nursing in society. A historical perspective, Philadelphia, 1978, Saunders.

Fagin CM: Primary care as an academic discipline, Nurs Outlook 26:750-753, 1978.

Fox EG, ed: Red Cross public health nursing, Public Health Nursing 12:175–181, 1920.

Gardner MS: Public health nursing, ed 1, revised, New York, 1919 Macmillan.

Gardner MS: Public health nursing, ed 3, New York, 1936 Macmillan.

Grissum M and Spengler C: Woman power and health care, Boston, 1976, Little, Brown.

Haupt AC: Forty years of teamwork in public health nursing, Am J Nurs 53:81-84, 1953.

Jensen DM: History and trends of professional nursing, ed 4, St Louis, 1959, The CV Mosby Co.

Kalisch P and Kalisch BJ: Politics of nursing, Philadelphia, 1982, Lippincott.

Kalisch P and Kalisch BJ: The advancement of American nursing, ed 2, Boston, 1986, Little, Brown.

Kaufman M, Hawkins JW, Higgins LP, and Friedman AH, eds: Dictionary of American nursing biography, Westport, Conn, 1988, Greenwood Press.

Lynaugh JE and Fagin LM: Nursing comes of age, Image: J Nurs Scholarship 20:1184, 1988.

Maynard T: The apostle of charity: the life of St. Vincent de Paul, New York, 1939, Dial Press.

McNeil EE: Transition in public health nursing, John Sundwall Lecture, University of Michigan, 1967.

National Organization for Public Health Nursing: Approval of Skidmore College of Nursing as preparing students for public health nursing, Public Health Nurs 36:371, 1944.

Nelson SC: Mary Sewall Gardner, Nurs Outlook 2:37-39, 1954.

Nightingale F: Notes on nursing, London, 1859, Harris and Sons; Philadelphia, 1944, Lippincott.

Pickett G and Hanlon JJ: Public health adminstration and practice, ed 9, St Louis, 1990, Times Mirror/Mosby.

A prophet honored, Am J Nurs 71:53, 1971 (editorial).

Relman A: Assessment and accountability. The third revolution in medical care, N Engl J Med 319:1220, 1988.

Roberts MM: American nursing, history and interpretation, New York, 1954, Macmillan.

Rosen G: A history of public health, New York, 1958, MD Publications.

Ruth MV and Partridge KB: Differences in perception of education and practice, Nurs Outlook 26:622-628, 1978.

Smillie WG: Preventive medicine and public health, ed 2, New York, 1952, Macmillan.

Stewart IM and Austin AL: A history of nursing, ed 5, New York, 1938, Putnam.

Tinkham CW and Voorhies EF: Community health nursing. Evolution and process, ed 2, New York, 1977, Appleton-Century-Crofts.

US Public Health Service: Toward quality in nursing: Needs and goals. Report of the Surgeon General's consultant group on nursing, Washington, DC, 1963, US Government Printing Office.

Wald L: The house on Henry Street, New York, 1915, Holt.

Williams R: The United States public health service, Bethesda, Md, 1951, Commissioned Officers Association of the US Public Health Service.

Winslow C-EA: Florence Nightingale and public health nursing, Public Health Nurs 38:330-332, 1946.

SELECTED BIBLIOGRAPHY

Bigbee JL and Crowder ELM: The Red Cross Rural Nursing Service: an innovative model of public health nursing delivery, Public Health Nurs 2:109-121, 1985.

Brainard AM: The evolution of public health nursing, Philadelphia, 1922, Saunders.

Carr AM: Development of public health nursing literature, Public Health Nurs 5:81-85, 1988.

Dock LL and Stewart IM: A short history of nursing, New York, 1931, Putnam.

Fiedler LA: Images of the nurse in fiction and popular culture, literature and medicine, Albany, NY, 1983, Albany State University of New York Press.

Frachel RR: A new profession: the evolution of public health nursing, Public Health Nurs 5:86-90, 1988.

Gardner MS: The National Organization for Public Health Nursing, Visiting Nurse Quart 4:13-18, 1912.

Hamilton D: Clinical excellence, but too high a cost: The Metropolitan Life Insurance Company Visiting Nurse Service (1909-1953), Public Health Nurs 5:235-240, 1988.

Hamilton D: Faith and finance, Image: J Nurs Scholarship 20:124, 1988.

Herrmann EK: Clara Louise Maass: heroine or martyr of public health? Public Health Nurs 2:51-57, 1985.

Kalisch PA and Kalisch BJ: The advance of American nursing, Boston, 1986, Little, Brown.

Rathbone W: History and progress of district nursing, New York, 1890, Macmillan.

Watson J: The evolution of nursing education in the United States: one hundred years of a profession for women, J Nurs Educ 16:31-37, 1977.

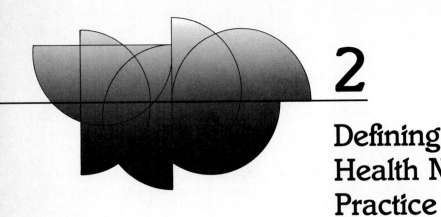

2

Defining Community Health Nursing Practice

───────────────── OBJECTIVES ─────────────────

Upon completion of this chapter, the reader will be able to:

1. *Discuss how community health nursing differs from other specialty areas within nursing.*
2. *Formulate a personal definition of community health nursing practice, incorporating key concepts delineated by professional organizations.*
3. *Describe White's Conceptual Model for Public Health Nursing Practice and discuss terms specific to this model.*
4. *Discuss the mission of public health and how the concept of "Health for All" relates to this mission.*
5. *Identify the client groups in community health nursing practice and the roles nurses can assume when working with these groups.*
6. *Describe how community health nurses provide population-based nursing care.*

When public health nursing began in the early 1900s, it was a simple matter to define it as a specialty area within nursing. Public health nursing took place outside the hospital setting; it was "nursing without walls," nursing that was community-focused and family- and group-oriented. Early public health nurses functioned relatively independently and worked to maintain and improve the health of the entire community. Thus, public health nursing was "*nursing for the public health*" (Brainard, 1921, p. 5).

Today, as the focus of health care continues to move outside the hospital setting and as more and more nurses assume expanded roles, defining community health nursing as a specialty area is less easily done. The definition becomes sharper and clearer, however, when it is understood that it is the *nature of the practice* and not the *setting* that defines community health nursing as a specialty area. Now, nursing outside walls is not necessarily community health nursing: pediatric nurses who do assessments of newborns in physicians' offices and nurses who counsel clients in mental health centers may not be practicing community health nursing. These nurses are probably specialty-focused nurse *practitioners;* nurse practitioners have advanced physical assessment skills and have been prepared to exercise independent and collaborative judgment in the health care management of patients (Secretary of Health and Human Services, 1988). The holistic *community* focus characteristic of community health nursing practice is not a major emphasis of nurse practitioners in many ambulatory care and other community-based health care settings. Many of these practitioners place emphasis on delivering care to individuals and are not necessarily oriented to the community (Goeppinger, 1984).

Community health nursing is "nursing for the community's health." Its uniqueness lies in its emphasis on the health of the population as a whole. Community health nurses address both the personal and the environmental aspects of health and deal with community factors which either inhibit or facilitate healthy living. Personal health involves the biopsychosocial and spiritual aspects of individual, family, and group functioning, whereas environmental health deals with people's surroundings, settings such as homes, schools, workplaces, or recreational facilities. In community health nursing, nurses enter the environment in which people live, and they practice within this environment, in sharp contrast to the situation where the client enters the nurse's environment in a hospital or clinic. In addition to the one-to-one or single-family approach to health care, the community health nurse thinks in terms of populations such as caseloads, clinics, districts, census tracts, and cities. Groups at risk within these populations, including families at risk, are identified so that preventive measures and resources can be targeted for them. In this manner, available resources can be wisely utilized (Ruth and Partridge, 1978, p. 625). Effective resource management is discussed in Chapters 9 through 18.

An example can best illustrate how the community health nurse expands the nurse practitioner role by focusing on groups at risk and the community:

Julie Cherry, a community health nurse working for an official health department, was assigned a census tract as her population to be served. This census tract was located in a decaying area of town with substandard housing and no transportation, playgrounds, or parks. A large industrial complex lay in the census tract, and consequently large numbers of young laborers and their families lived there. There was no hospital located in the area and only one physician. The community health nurse received numerous referrals from the physician and outlying hospitals to visit young mothers with newborns who needed support with parenting their children. The nurse assessed the need for a parenting group by talking with the families whom she served as well as with her supervisors. She and the families she visited planned a weekly sharing and support group that met in a neighborhood church. The group was well attended and continued to function after the nurse left.

The nurse in this situation demonstrated the focus in community health, planning preventive health measures for groups at risk, which is a step beyond providing primary health care to families who need it.

The World Health Organization has defined three necessary components of community health nursing practice that further delineate the uniqueness of this specialty area (WHO, 1974):

1. A sense of responsibility for coverage of needed health services in a community. It is not necessary that community health nursing provide these services. The sense of responsibility for their provision, however, must be present.
2. The care of vulnerable groups in a community is a priority. The basis for involvement in the health care of groups is based upon their vulnerability. The long involvement of community health nursing in maternal-child health is based upon this component.
3. The client (individual, family, group, community) must be a partner in planning and evaluating health care.

The unique aspects of community health nursing practice do not negate direct individual client care or practitioner-focused nursing. One-to-one clinical practice, illustrated by pediatric nurse practitioners and geriatric nurse specialists, certainly has a place in community health nursing when it is performed for the explicit purpose of improving the level of health in a community. Nurses in these roles can have the expertise needed to plan for populations at risk and are also very valuable consultants for other community health nurses. One official health department has, for example, a pediatric nurse practitioner who holds well-child conferences weekly in impoverished rural areas where there are almost no other health care resources available. This nurse is serving the high-risk population of children, from birth through 5 years of age, in that county. Other staff nurses in the agency use her as a resource person when they have questions about the growth and development of the children they serve.

TITLE EVOLVES OVER TIME

Historically, varying titles have been used to describe the type of nursing provided in the community setting, including district nursing, health nursing, visiting nursing, public health nursing, and community health nursing (McNeil, 1967). *District nursing,* which was the origin of our present concept of public health–community health nursing, was the title used by Rathbone when he hired nurses in England to care for the sick poor in their homes (refer to Chapter 1). When home nursing services were started in the United States, the term *visiting nursing* was used to identify the specialty area of practice which emphasized home-based nursing care. *Public health nursing* has its historical roots in Florence Nightingale's *health nurse* and Lillian Wald's *public health nurse.* Wald thought the word *public* denoted a service that was available to *all* people and, thus, coined the term *public health nursing* when she was director of the Henry Street Settlement in New York City. She hoped by doing so that the public would realize that the nursing services provided by the Henry Street Settlement were available to all individuals in the community. However, as federal, state, and local governments increased their involvement in the delivery of health services, the term *public health nursing* became associated with "public," or official, agencies and in turn with the care of poor people.

The phrase, *community health nursing,* recently emerged out of an interest to reaffirm the original major thrust of public health nursing or community-based practice: nursing for the health of the entire public/community versus nursing only for the public who are poor. Some people use the terms community health nursing and public health nursing interchangeably. It must be remembered, however, that not every nurse who works in the community setting is a public health–community health nurse. Public, or community, health nurses have a definitive philosophy of practice which is described in the next section of this chapter.

In this text, the authors have chosen to use the terms *community health nurse* and *community health nursing,* believing that these terms help to emphasize the major focus of the nurse's work— the community—as well as the services provided and the underlying philosophy. It is recognized that, in addition to these terms, other titles (visiting nursing and public health nursing) are still being used in the practice setting.

DEFINING COMMUNITY HEALTH NURSING: PURPOSES AND GOALS

Throughout the history of public/community health nursing, leaders in the field have stressed the importance of defining beliefs about nursing practice and developing standards for practice which reflect these beliefs. The National Organization for Public Health Nursing (NOPHN) grew out of a concern for the rights and safety of clients. Public/community health nursing professionals were finding that as their specialty-based practice was rapidly expanding, "there were no generally accepted standards for anything" (Gardner, 1948). Gardner, a noted public health leader and an early president of the NOPHN, stated, when reminiscing about the development of the NOPHN, that "we realized that a body of poorly prepared and unsupervised nurses, some of whom might be without an ethical background for this work, were a dangerous element to let loose in the homes of the people and might easily jeopardize, in a short time, all the confidence we had been building throughout the country" (Gardner, 1948).

One of the major purposes of the NOPHN was to promote standardization of public health nursing practice. The first comprehensive statement of public health nursing objectives and functions was prepared by the NOPHN in 1931 (McIver, 1949, p. 65). Since that time, public/community health nursing professionals have periodically reexamined their basic beliefs about public/community health nursing practice and have disseminated these beliefs to nurses across the country. Most recently, the ANA and APHA, the two professional organizations which represent community health nurses on the national level, have each published documents which delineate their concept of community and public health nursing practice.

In its document, *Standards of Community Health Nursing Practice,* the American Nurses'

Association (ANA) defines community health nursing practice as follows (ANA, 1986, pp 1-2)*:

Community health nursing practice promotes and preserves the health of populations by integrating the skills and knowledge relevant to both nursing and public health. The practice is comprehensive and general, and is not limited to a particular age or diagnostic group; it is continual, and is not limited to episodic care. In the *Standards of Community Health Nursing Practice* document, the terms community health nursing and public health nursing are synonymous.

Community health nursing practice promotes the public's health. The programs, services, and institutions involved in public health emphasize promotion and maintenance of the population's health, and the prevention and limitation of disease. Public health activities change with changing technology and social values, but the goals remain the same: to reduce the amount of disease, premature death, discomfort, and disability (Milbank Memorial Fund Commission, 1976, 3).

While community health nursing practice includes nursing directed to individuals, families, and groups, the dominant responsibility is to the population as a whole. Nurses' efforts to promote and maintain the population's health entail the understanding and application of (a) concepts of public health and community; (b) skills of community organization and development; and (c) nursing care of selected individuals, families, and groups for health promotion, health maintenance, health education, and coordination of care.

The World Health Organization defines a community as a social group determined by geographical boundaries and/or common values and interests. Its members interact with each other. It functions within a particular social structure, exhibits and creates norms and values, and establishes social institutions (World Health Organization, 1978).

The nurse's actions reflect awareness of the need for comprehensive health planning in partnership with communities; the influence of social, economic, ecological, and political issues; the needs of populations at risk; and the dynamic forces that stimulate change. Because the nurse's primary responsibility is to a population, some practice occurs through organization and coordination of the actions of others in response to health needs. When care is given to individuals, families, or

---

*Reprinted with permission from Standards of Community Health Nursing Practice, © 1986, American Nurses' Association, Kansas City, Mo.

groups, this responsibility dictates that the nurse's priorities concerning which clients to serve are determined by the needs of the population.

Professional community health nurses recognize that many local health issues are directly and profoundly affected by larger policy issues. Consequently, their practice reflects awareness of and responsiveness to legislative action and other means by which health and social policies are set at all levels within the health care system and the government.

The theoretical and factual context within which the community health nurse understands phenomena and their interrelationships derives from an interdisciplinary base including public health, the humanities, the social and behavioral sciences, epidemiology, and nursing science.

Community health nursing practice should be consistent with the World Health Organization's concept of primary health care as "essential health care made universally accessible to individuals and families in the community by means acceptable to them, through their full participation, and at a cost that the community and country can afford. Primary health care forms an integral part both of the country's health system (of which it is the nucleus) and of the overall social and economic development of the community" (World Health Organization, 1978).

Imbedded in this definition is the assumption that health care is a right and not a privilege.

The American Public Health Associations' (APHA) position paper, *The Definition and Role of Public Health Nursing in the Delivery of Health Care,* was designed "to elucidate the essence of public health nursing practice and to clarify the role of public health nursing in the delivery of health care" (APHA, 1981, p. 3). This association's definition, emanating from the Public Health Nursing Section, is identified below (APHA, 1981, p. 4):

Public health nursing synthesizes the body of knowledge from the public health sciences and professional nursing theories for the purpose of improving the health of the entire community. This goal lies at the heart of primary prevention and health promotion and is the foundation for public health nursing practice. To accomplish this goal, public health nurses work with groups, families, and individuals as well as in multidisciplinary teams and programs. Identifying subgroups (aggregates) within the population which are at high risk of illness, disability, or premature death and directing resources toward these groups, is the most effective approach for accomplishing the goal of PHN. Success in reducing the risks and in improving the health of the community depends on the involvement of consumers, especially groups experiencing health risks, and others in the community, in health planning, and in self-help activities.

The major concern of public/community health nurses, the health of the community, has not changed over time. In both the ANA and APHA definitions, emphasis is placed on "improving the health of the entire community' (APHA) or "the population as a whole" (ANA). In 1912, the NOPHN stated in its constitution that "the object of this organization shall be to stimulate responsibility for the health of the community" (NOPHN, 1912, p. 27).

A MODEL FOR COMMUNITY HEALTH NURSING PRACTICE

"While community health nursing practice includes nursing directed to individuals, families, and groups the dominant responsibility is to the population as a whole" (ANA, 1986, p. 2). Community health nurses, like all nurses, utilize the nursing process to ensure that the needs of clients are met. They use content and methods from nursing and public health in delivering *preventive* community health nursing services to populations and to establish priorities for care. The goal of community health nursing practice is health—that is, helping clients to obtain their maximum level of physical, mental, social, and spiritual functioning. The term *health* reflects the wellness orientation of the practice: A health orientation assumes that people always have the potential for higher levels of functioning and that people in all stages of living, including those who are dying, are growing and developing. The concept of health is further elaborated in Chapters 3, 7, and 8.

Multiple determinants in the environment influence how well clients function. *Environmental forces* encompass all internal and external factors which affect aggregate and individual functioning. Because people and their environments are dynamic and constantly changing, community health nurses must analyze interactions and mutual influences between humans and their environments. The concept of the environment is very broad and includes biologic, sociocultural, ecological, and technological dimensions—all of which affect healthy functioning. These dimensions are discussed further in Chapter 10.

White's (1982) Conceptual Model for Public Health Nursing Practice depicts the relationships between the determinants of healthy functioning and the dynamics of public health nursing practice (refer to Figure 2-1). This model illustrates that the scope of public health nursing practice is very broad, extending from "one-to-one nursing intervention to a global perspective of world health. The overall focus of public health nursing is achieving and maintaining the public's health-

at-all times" (White, 1982, pp. 527, 528). To accomplish this goal, preventive strategies ranging from health promotion to rehabilitation are used by the nurse in the public/community health setting. Knowledge of what factors impact on health (health determinants), either positively or negatively, assists the public/community health nurse to plan appropriate prevention strategies. Intervention strategies are based on sound data and are planned in collaboration with the client. They include, but are not limited to, health education with individuals and aggregates, political action to promote effective public policy, and safety investigations to ensure a healthy environment.

The essential dynamics of this model consist of the nursing process and the valuing process (White, 1982, p. 529). The *nursing process* is a

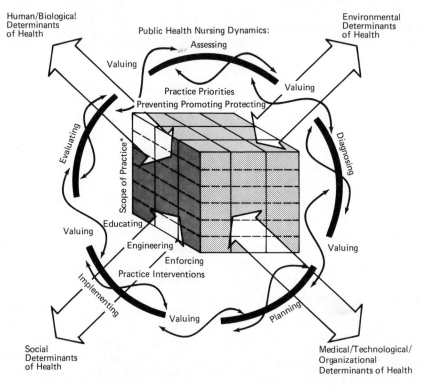

*The scope of practice is an open-ended continuum extending from individuals through such aggregates as groups, communities, entire populations to include the entire globe.

Figure 2-1 A public health nursing conceptual model. The determinants of the health framework presented are modified from those in Healthy People, The Surgeon General's Report on Health Promotion and Disease Prevention, DHEW (PHS) Pub No 79-55071, 1979. (From White MS: Construct for public health nursing, Nurs Outlook 30:529, November/December 1982. Copyright 1982, American Journal of Nursing Company. All rights reserved.)

systematic approach to scientific problem solving, involving a series of circular dynamic actions—assessing, analyzing (diagnosing), planning, implementing, and evaluating (refer to Chapter 8). It is used to assess and diagnose client needs and to plan, implement, and evaluate effective nursing interventions.

According to White (1982), community health nursing interventions fall into three major categories: education, engineering, and enforcement. *Educative* nursing actions help clients to voluntarily acquire knowledge essential for understanding healthy functioning, to develop attitudes that foster preventive health behaviors, and to establish practices conducive to effective living. Educative strategies are commonly used in community health nursing practice. Community health nurses help families, for example, to learn about normal growth and development and child care, conduct discussions related to sexuality issues in the school setting, and distribute health education materials in clinics, industrial plants, and other community health settings. *Engineering* strategies focus on environmental modification for the purpose of eliminating or managing environmental risk factors which affect healthy living. Campaigning against television advertisements which promote alcohol and cigarette usage, conducting clinics for the treatment of sexually transmitted diseases, and promoting actions to eliminate safety hazards in a schoolyard are examples of engineering nursing actions. *Enforcement* interventions are actions which impose regulatory controls and are designed to prevent disease, promote health and protect society from harmful substances and conditions. Enforcement actions encourage the passage of regulations and legislation, such as seat belt and drug abuse laws, which mandate health promoting behaviors.

To intervene effectively in the public/community health setting, the nurse must engage in political activity. The political arena is where health care decisions are made for the public as a whole. Sound public policy is needed to eliminate or manage environmental risk factors, prevent disease, and promote public health. Political activism is emphasized in Chapters 12 and 23.

Valuing, the second dynamic process in White's model, guides nursing interventions and decision making and influences the development of goals and priorities for care. Valuing is "the process of assigning or determining the worth or merit of something" (White, 1982, p. 529). The influence that valuing has on decision making becomes particularly evident during times of scarce resources. When resources are limited, professionals must critically examine their beliefs about practice and target resources so that they are used effectively and efficiently. Community health professionals place a high priority on targeting resources for at-risk groups in the community (APHA, 1981, p. 3). Their overall focus is "nursing for the health of the community." Identifying groups at risk and planning services to meet their needs, benefits the community as a whole. *Groups at risk are those who engage in certain activities or who have certain characteristics that increase their potential for contracting an illness, injury, or a health problem.* Individuals who smoke, for example, constitute a group at high risk for developing cancer. The at-risk concept is a basic concept of public health practice which guides epidemiological study, and thus, is discussed further in Chapter 10.

Prevention, another basic concept valued by community health professionals, is a primary focus of community health nursing intervention and identified as "practice priorities" in White's model. This focus entails a continuum of activities essential for preventing disease, prolonging life, and promoting health. These activities can be grouped under the three classic levels of prevention: primary, secondary, and tertiary (Leavell and Clark, 1965, p. 21). *Primary prevention* deals with health promotion and specific protection from health problems. "*Health promotion* begins with people who are basically healthy and seeks the development of community and individual measures which can help them to develop lifestyles that can maintain and enhance the state of well-being. *Disease prevention* or specific protection begins with a threat to health—a disease or environmental hazard—and seeks to protect as many people as possible from the harmful consequences of that threat" (Surgeon General, 1979, p. 119).

The significance of implementing health promotion activities is recognized worldwide. In 1986, the World Health Organization (WHO) institutionalized this concept through the development of *The Charter for Health Promotion*. WHO views health promotion as "a process of advocacy for health, encouraging a healthy lifestyle and mediating between different interests in society in the pursuit of health. Health promotion means building healthy public policy, creating supportive personal skills, and reorienting health services" (Turner, 1986).

Encouraging a healthy lifestyle is currently being stressed because personal lifestyles play a critical role in the development of many serious diseases, injuries, and health conditions. It is believed that if personal habits (e.g., regular exercise, adequate diet, no smoking, and appropriate use of alcohol and antihypertensive drugs) were changed, the mortality or death rate for seven of the ten leading causes of death could be substantially reduced (Surgeon General, 1979, p. 14). Immunizations, family planning services, antepartal care, classes for retirement preparation, smoking cessation, teaching, anticipatory guidance in family health and child care, and counseling on accident prevention are all examples of activities which focus on primary prevention. Health promotion activities such as regular exercise and adequate diet, and strategies for encouraging health promotion are discussed throughout the text and in Pender's (1987) book, *Health Promotion in Nursing Practice*.

Secondary prevention or health maintenance involves activities aimed at early diagnosis, prompt treatment, and disability limitation. Identification of health needs, health problems, and clients at risk is inherent in secondary prevention. The community health nurse who conducts a health risk appraisal, observes for poor maternal-infant bonding, assesses for developmental delays in the young child, and reinforces the need to do self-examination of the breasts illustrates the concept of secondary prevention. The types of health needs a community health nurse should focus on when doing a health risk appraisal with individuals across the life span are discussed in Chapters 12 through 19.

Health risk appraisal is a process whereby a health history (refer to Chapter 8) is collected, data obtained from this history are analyzed to identify characteristics which might make clients vulnerable to illness or premature death (e.g., personal and/or family history of hypertension and smoking), and educational nursing actions are instituted for the purpose of helping clients to acquire knowledge about ways to reduce health risks. When conducting a health risk appraisal, community health nurses focus on collecting data about health problems which are likely to occur in a particular age group such as inappropriate use of medication among the elderly, heart disease and cancer among well adults, and developmental delays among infants and children. Assessment tools and screening tests which facilitate risk appraisal are discussed in Chapters 13, 15, and 18. The ultimate goal of a health-risk appraisal is to increase a client's self-care capabilities. *Self-care* is defined by Orem (1980), as "the practice of activities that individuals initiate and perform on their own behalf in maintaining life, health, and well-being."

Community health nurses focus on identifying at-risk populations as well as individuals at risk. Using the epidemiological process (refer to Chapter 10), they collect and analyze community assessment data to identify which groups in the community are at risk for developing significant health problems. Pregnant women in a specific area of a community might, for example, be at risk for developing complications of pregnancy due to poor living conditions and inadequate health care resources. If this were found to be the case, the community health nurse would use the health planning process (Chapter 12) to educate these women about their potential health risks and to develop health programs which better meet their needs.

Tertiary prevention has rehabilitation as the major focus. Rehabilitation activities assist clients to reach their maximum potential. The nurse who teaches an arthritic client how to rest at intervals throughout the day provides an example of tertiary prevention. Assisting the postcerebrovascular accident client to continue with a physical and speech therapy regimen is also carrying out aspects of tertiary prevention. Chapter 17 discusses in depth the role of the community health nurse in rehabilitation.

To achieve the goal of community health nursing—*optimal health*—all three levels of prevention—primary, secondary, and tertiary—must be implemented. Populations must develop behaviors that promote health as well as prevent disease to achieve an optimal level of functioning.

The dynamics and dimensions in White's model (Figure 2-1) stress the value of preventive activities. According to White (1982) preventing, promoting, and protecting are practice priorities. This model illustrates that the community health nurse utilizes the nursing process, on the individual and aggregate level, to provide preventive

health services and that multiple dimensions or determinants of health must be addressed in order to successfully enhance individual and group health. It also illustrates that a range of intervention strategies, including political activism, is used to dilute or eliminate negative health determinants in the environment.

UNIQUENESS OF COMMUNITY HEALTH NURSING PRACTICE

Community health nursing's philosophy and scope of practice distinguish this practice field from other specialty areas in nursing. Community health nurses focus on providing *preventive* health services, versus curative care, to enhance the

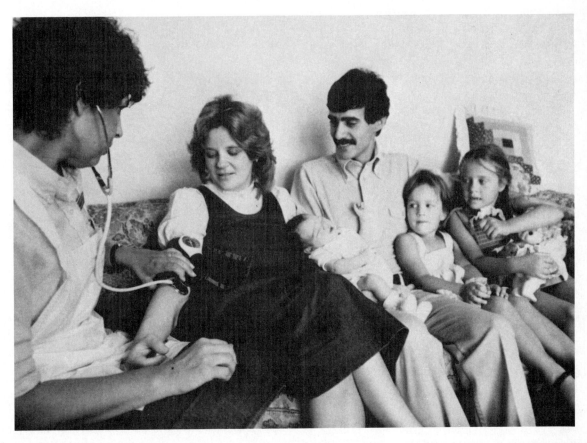

Figure 2-2 The family is seen as the natural unit of service in community health nursing practice. During a home visit, the community health nurse determines the health status of all family members and assesses family dynamics as well. (Genesee Region Home Care Association, Rochester, New York,)

health of individuals, families, and groups within the community. Nursing service to individuals is viewed within the context of the family. It is recognized that the health of individuals can affect the health of all family members and that the family provides an environment which influences the health of its members. The family is seen as a natural unit of service (refer to Figure 2-2). It is also seen as a significant entry point from which to identify community strengths, needs, and resources related to the provision of health care services.

Community health nursing practice is general and comprehensive, not limited to a particular age group or diagnosis (ANA, 1980, p. 2). Community health nurses work with clients (individuals, families, and groups) across the life span. They are committed to improving *the health of the community* by identifying subgroups (refer to Figure 2-3) which are at high risk of illness, disability, or premature death and directing resources toward these groups (APHA, 1981, p. 4). Determining specific populations at risk facilitates the identification of individuals and families at risk.

The words *client* or *consumer* rather than *patient* are used in community health nursing because they reflect a *wellness* orientation. In addition, they denote an active, independent relationship, in contrast to the passivity denoted in the word *patient.* The client asks questions and is a participant in assessing needs and in planning and implementing preventive health care. Care is not given to clients; rather, clients have a full part in their care. "Success in reducing the risks and in improving the health of the community depends on the involvement of consumers, especially groups experiencing health risks, and others in the community, in health planning and in self-help activities" (APHA, 1981, p. 4).

In order to assess needs and plan health services for individuals, groups, and the community

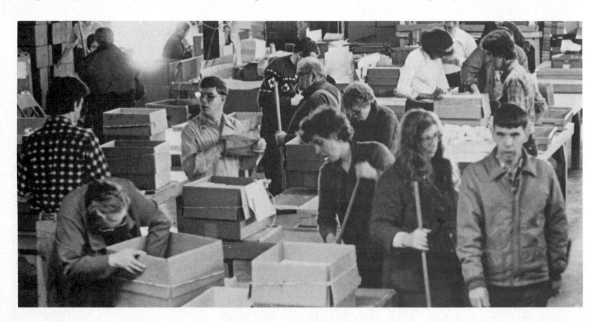

Figure 2-3 Aggregates as well as individuals are *clients* in community health nursing practice. An aggregate is a group of individuals who have in common one or more personal or environmental characteristics (Williams, 1977). Community health nurses focus on identifying at-risk aggregates in the community in order to target resources more effectively. Individuals who are retarded, for example, make up a high-risk aggregate, because often persons in this population group need an array of community services in order to strengthen their self-care capabilities. (Courtesy of Sunshine Workshop, a nonprofit voluntary agency sponsored by the Association of Retarded Citizens in Knox County, Tennessee. Photographer, Mary Louise Peacock.)

as a whole, a public health knowledge base is mandatory. Community health nursing is a *synthesis of nursing and public health* practice. Community health nurses use the knowledge and skills of professional nursing and the philosophy, content, and methods of public health when delivering services in the community. The ANA, in its recent Social Policy Statement, defines nursing as "the diagnosis and treatment of human responses to actual or potential health problems" (ANA, 1980, p. 9). Nursing emphasizes assisting *individual* clients in dealing with responses to health problems. In contrast, public health focuses on the health of the *community.*

Public health was described by Winslow (1952, p. 30) as follows: [The] science and art of preventing disease, prolonging life, and promoting physical and mental health and efficiency through organized community efforts focused toward

1. maintaining a sanitary environment;
2. controlling communicable diseases;
3. providing education regarding principles of personal hygiene;
4. organizing medical and nursing services for early diagnosis and treatment of disease; and
5. developing social machinery to ensure everyone a standard of living adequate for health maintenance, so organizing these benefits as to enable every citizen to realize his birthright of health and longevity.*

The values held by public health professionals when Winslow proposed this classic description of public health continue to guide the direction of practice in the field. A recent report prepared by the Institute of Medicine's Committee for the Study of Public Health reaffirms "the mission of public health as fulfilling society's interest in assuring conditions in which people can be healthy. Its aim is to generate organized community effort to address the public interest in health by applying scientific and technical knowledge to prevent disease and promote health" (Committee for the Study of the Future of Public Health, 1988, p. 7).

This report, entitled *The Future of Public Health* and known as the "IOM Report," addresses the need to deal with environmental health concerns, to control communicable disease, to provide personal health care services, and to encourage healthful behaviors through education and through modification in the social environment.

HEALTH FOR ALL

"What unites people around public(community) health is the focus on society as a whole, the community, and the aim of optimal health status" (Committee for the Study of the Future of Public Health, 1988, p. 39). This is the theme that guides public/community health action at all levels of national and international government. In 1978, 158 countries attending the International Conference on Primary Health Care, held in Alma-Ata, USSR, set for themselves a common goal, "Health for All by the Year 2000" (WHO, 1978). In committing themselves to this goal, countries did not mean that by the year 2000 disease and disability would no longer exist. The focus was placed on all people having access to health services which would assist them to lead socially and economically productive lives (Mahler, 1979). "The goal of Health for All by the Year 2000 is a vision founded on social equity; on the urgent need to reduce the gross inequality in the health status of people in the world, in developed and developing countries, and within countries" (Maglacas, 1988).

The Declaration of Alma-Ata specifies that primary health care is the key vehicle for attaining the "health for all" goal. Primary health care is a blend of essential health services, personal responsibility for one's own health, and health-promoting action taken by the community. It must include at least the following eight components (WHO, 1988, p. 23):

• Education concerning prevailing health problems and the methods of preventing and controlling them
• Promoting of food supply and proper nutrition

---

*Reprinted by permission of Princeton University Press.

- An adequate supply of safe water and basic sanitation
- Maternal and child health care, including family planning
- Immunization against the major infectious diseases
- Prevention and control of locally endemic diseases
- Appropriate treatment of common diseases and injuries
- Provision of essential drugs

Primary health care facilitates client entry into the health care system, promotes integrated and co-ordinated services, requires client participation in the program planning and evaluation process and in policy making, and promotes self-reliance and self-determination (WHO, 1978). Community health nurses promote these types of services, activities, and values.

A recent development in the United States has been the effort of the American Public Health Association (APHA) to establish a program of national health care. APHA is promoting a "Health Care for All" Sense of the Congress resolution outlining APHA's broad policy goals for a system of national health care (APHA, 1989, Action alert). The current resolution states that the United States should enact a national health program that will remove economic and other major barriers to health care while encouraging efficient delivery of effective, high-quality services (Health Care, 1990, p. 3). The APHA plan envisions universal, nondiscriminatory coverage; financing based on ability to pay; disease prevention and health promotion emphasis; education and training for health workers; consumer health education; quality assurance; and ongoing program evaluation (APHA, 1989, For national health care and APHA, 1989, A national health program). APHA is urging Americans to tell their members of Congress that they want tax money spent on a national health program for everyone that responds to community needs, is preventive in nature, and does not discriminate (APHA, 1989, A national health plan).

Basic public health knowledge is needed to practice effectively in community health nursing.

This includes the philosophy, content, and methods of epidemiology, biostatistics, social policy, health planning, public health organization and administration, and public health law. These topics are explored more fully in later sections of this text.

No one discipline can address all of the health needs in the community. That is why community health nurses stress the importance of multidisciplinary planning. Multidisciplinary planning and cooperation can facilitate community diagnosis (Chapter 11) and health planning (Chapter 12). It also promotes effective and efficient utlization of resources.

SETTINGS, WORK FORCE, ROLES, AND SERVICES

Community health nurses implement a variety of roles in the practice setting and provide a broad range of services aimed at promoting individual and aggregate health. They work in diverse health and health-related organizations. Changing health care delivery trends have resulted in a need for increased numbers of nurses who can function in the community setting: Deinstitutionalization is being stressed and community-based care is being advocated.

Settings in Which Community Health Nurses Function

Community health nurses have traditionally been employed by health departments or other tax-supported agencies, visiting nurse associations or other non-tax-supported agencies, schools, and occupational health programs.

State and local health departments are mandated to protect the health of the community and, as such, provide a broad range of services which address the needs of groups across the life span. Visiting nurse associations primarily emphasize the delivery of home health care or bedside nursing services. Health programs in schools and occupational settings mainly serve a specific segment of the community. School-age children are the focus in school health programs, whereas the well adult is the target of service in the occupational health setting. Migrant health clinics and senior citizen centers are other settings in which the community health nurse works and where services are targeted for specific aggregates.

Community health nurses have always functioned rather independently in a way that corresponds to the current definition of the expanded or extended role of the nurse (refer to Figure 2-4). In addition to the above settings, health maintenance organizations, neighborhood health centers, and home health care agencies have also used community health nurses in an expanded role as the source of primary health care.

Size of the Work Force in Community Health Nursing

The number of nurses working in community health has increased dramatically. Some of these changes have been brought about by legislation such as the Social Security Amendments of 1965, Medicare, and Medicaid.

The earliest-known count of public health nurses in the United States was reported by Harriett Fulmer at the International Congress of Nurses in Buffalo, N.Y., in 1901. At that time, there were 58 public health nursing organizations, employing about 130 nurses. In 1912 Mary Gardner found that approximately 3000 nurses were engaged in community health nursing services. From 1916 to 1931, periodic enumerations of public health nursing agencies and the nurses they employed were recorded by the Statistical Department of the National Organization for Public Health Nursing. Since 1937, the state directors of public health nursing and the Division of Nursing, U.S. Public Health Service, have systematically collected and compiled data about numbers and educational preparation of nurses employed in public health work in the United States. State and local official and nonofficial (voluntary) public health agencies, boards of education, national agencies, universities, and, in some years, industries, have supplied the information (Source Book, 1975, p. 187). Table 2-1 shows the number and distribution of active registered nurses by employment setting in 1972 and 1984. In 1984, the latest year in which a national survey of registered

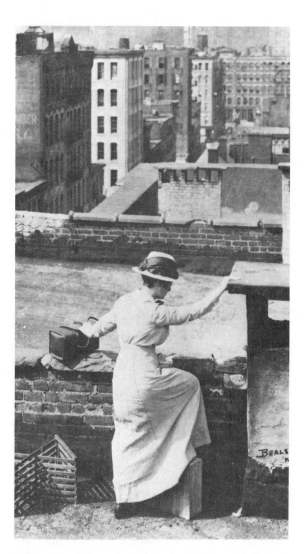

Figure 2-4 Community health nurses have traditionally gone into a variety of community settings to serve individuals, families, and groups. In this picture, a Henry Street nurse is climbing over a tenement roof on New York's Lower East Side to visit her clients in the home. Today, community health nurses usually do not need to climb over rooftops. They do, however, reach out to clients in all types of settings (e.g., homes, schools, rural clinics, neighborhood health centers, and sheltered workshops). (Visiting Nurse Service of New York City.)

TABLE 2-1 Number and distribution of active registered nurses by employment setting, 1972 and 1984*

Employment setting	1972†		1984‡	
	Number of active RNs	Percent of RNs	Number of active RNs	Percent of RNs
Hospitals	449,594	64.2	1,011,955	68.1
Nursing homes	53,988	6.9	115,077	7.8
Nursing education	28,820	3.7	40,311	2.7
Public, community, and school health	68,945	8.9	144,574	9.7
Private duty	38,923	5.0	22,675	1.5
Occupational health	19,403	2.5	22,890	1.6
Offices	52,390	6.7	97,374	6.6
Other and not reported	16,407	2.1	30,871	2.0
TOTALS	778,407	100.0	1,485,725	100.0

*For 1972, at license renewal time; for 1984, November data.

†1972 data from Division of Nursing: Source book of nursing personnel, 1974, UDHEW Pub No HRA 75-43, Washington, DC, 1975, US Government Printing Office.

‡1984 data from Moses E: The registered nurse population: findings from the National Sample Survey of Registered Nurses, November 1984, NTIS Accession No HRP-0906938, Springfield, Va, 1986, National Technical Information Service.

nurses was conducted, 75,629 more nurses were working in community health settings than in 1972. The overall demand for community health nurses, especially for those functioning in the home health subsector, has increased substantially in the 1980s (Secretary's Commission on Nursing, 1988). It is projected that in the years 2000 and 2020 the requirements for full-time-equivalent registered nurses will increase significantly in many health care settings, but that the highest percentage increase will occur in the community health setting. The RN community-health requirements represent increases of 75 percent and 205 percent in the years 2000 and 2020, respectively, over the 1985 requirements (Secretary of Health and Human Services, 1988).

Roles of Community Health Nurses

A variety of roles can be assumed by nurses in providing community health nursing services (Green and Driggers, 1989; Gulino and La-Monica, 1986). Other chapters in this text discuss these roles in depth. Below is a partial listing of the types of roles community health nurses implement:

1. *Advocate.* Clients in the CHN setting frequently are unable to obtain needed health care services or to negotiate for change in the health care system. Community health nurses seek to promote an understanding of health problems, lobby for beneficial public policy, and stimulate supportive community action for health. This role is discussed in more detail throughout the text.
2. *Care manager.* Helping clients to make decisions about appropriate health care services and to achieve service delivery integration and coordination is a major role of the community health nurse. Chapter 9 focuses on this care manager role.
3. *Case finder.* Community health nurses look for clients at risk among the popula-

tion being served. Chapters 8, 9, and 12 through 20 discuss ways in which nurses serve as case finders.

4. *Counselor.* Clients in the community health setting frequently face difficult and complex health concerns and desire supportive and problem-solving assistance. Community health nurses are often in a unique position to help clients deal with stress related to health concerns. The counselor role of the CHN is highlighted in Chapter 7.

5. *Clinic nurse.* Chapter 20 expands on the role of the nurse in the ambulatory care setting. Clinic services are increasingly being expanded to meet the needs of populations at risk (e.g., noninsured groups of individuals).

6. *Epidemiologist.* The community health nurse uses the epidemiological method to study disease and health among population groups and to deal with community-wide health problems. Chapter 10 explains this role.

7. *Group leader.* Chapter 20 also discusses the role of the nurse who works with groups in practice.

8. *Health planner.* Providing health programs for populations at risk is described in Chapters 11 through 19.

9. *Home visitor.* Perhaps the most unusual aspect of this specialty is that the community health nurse enters the client's setting. The nurse not only assesses the environment but also works within it. Home visitors are able to gather environmental information as well as data about how a family system functions within its own setting. They also are able to provide direct care services in a situation familiar to the client.

10. *Occupational health nurse.* Chapter 16 presents this expanding and changing area of community health nursing.

11. *Researcher.* The goals for community health nursing practice are far from being realized. The critical need for research to assist health care professionals in reaching their goals is addressed throughout the text.

12. *School nurse.* Chapter 14 presents the role of the nurse with this vital population group.

13. *Teacher.* Application of teaching-learning principles to facilitate behavioral change among clients is a basic intervention strategy in community health. Chapter 7 presents the educative approach with families. Chapter 20 discusses the group educative approach.

Many of the above roles are carried out with all populations and within all community health nursing service delivery settings. For example, advocacy, case finding, and teaching are essential components of the community health nurse's activity whether in a clinic, home, school, workplace, or senior citizen center.

Many other roles are assumed by the community health nurse; those described above are by no means all-inclusive. The excitement of this specialty area lies in its diversity.

SERVICES PROVIDED BY COMMUNITY HEALTH NURSES

In order to accomplish their goals, community health nurses provide multiple and diverse direct and indirect client services. Direct client services usually involve a personal relationship between the nurse and client (which can be a person, a family, a group, or the community). Teaching, hands-on bedside care, health risk appraisal, counseling, health planning with consumers, and the delivery of clinic services are examples of direct client services. Indirect client services include such things as record keeping, talking to a community agency about available resources to meet client needs, and supervising the care provided by a home health aide.

The following typical day in the life of a community health nurse vividly illustrates the range of services provided by the nurse in the community health setting (Haradine, 1978):

—————————————— A Day in the Life of a Community Health Nurse ——————————————

Her first stop by 8 a.m. each day is at her desk in the health department to pick up messages from the day before, make phone calls, and plan her day's schedule.

After morning coffee with the other nurses, which offers time for comparisons, she starts her calls.

"Sometimes you've had a dark day and you need input, you need to talk to someone," she explains. "I could get depressed if I allowed myself, but I realize whose problem it is. It's not my problem. It's only my place to help when I'm accepted."

Many calls start with a request from a school or another public health nurse, or Charlene's own case finding.

Her first stop on a gray, cheerless day recently was a happy one, to visit a new baby. Paul Daniel Conner had spent 2 months in a hospital nursery after being born prematurely, weighing only 3 pounds, 7 ounces. Now 2½ months old, he had adjusted easily to his mother's style in the 2 weeks he has been home.

"He's a perfect baby," says his mother, Julie. "He doesn't ever cry." But she does have a few questions, written on a scrap of paper.

"I was surprised how easy it has been. I've been just really relaxed with him," she tells Charlene.

The routine on a visit to a new baby includes leaving a sheaf of pamphlets for the mother's spare-time reading. Topics include first aid, exercises for the mother, feeding, birth control, and descriptions of the free services offered by the health department.

Charlene advises Mrs. Conner not to put Paul Daniel to bed with a bottle.

"A baby will get a pool of milk, juice or Kool-Aid in its mouth that causes tooth decay. I see children with nothing but little brown stubs left of their teeth," she explains.

"You can use your blender to make baby food from table food, then freeze it in an ice cube tray and put it in a bag. But be sure to freeze it."

The telephone number for the Western Michigan Poison Center and instructions on taking a baby's temperature are all part of the routine which ends with a full examination of the baby and measuring its height and weight.

Charlene tells Mrs. Conner she can take her baby to the health department's well-baby clinic, in the Belmont area, for children from birth to school age.

"It's one of your benefits as a taxpayer. You can take the baby in for his shots, but continue to see the doctor."

The idea appeals to Mrs. Conner. She takes the information, the telephone number she would use for an appointment.

"You can call me anytime," Charlene says as she leaves. "I'm usually in early in the morning."

Few newborns in Kent County are seen by a public health nurse. Many don't need it; more probably do. All it would take is a call—from the hospital, from the mother, or even from a relative.

"There are many out there I'm not getting, mothers who are having problems adjusting to a new baby, who didn't like children or babies before and now overcompensate," Charlene explains.

A stop at West Oakview School is squeezed in before the students' lunch break to check a girl with bites on her arms and legs (probably flea bites from a cat, Charlene thinks) and a progress report from a class for emotionally impaired youngsters.

At North Oakview School, after lunch, Charlene calls in to her office for messages. Then she visits a "readiness room" for 5- to 7-year-olds taught by Ann Westerhof.

"If Charlene didn't come in once a week, I don't know what I'd do," Mrs. Westerhof exclaims. "She's the go-between for me and the families. She helps me know what I can and can't do."

The "star" of this visit is Jim Fragale, 6, who is sporting a new brace, an unusual contraption with a tripod base and straps that keep his legs bent to aid healing of the hip joints.

The cause of Jim's hip problem is unknown, Charlene explains. "The ball joint of the hip softens, then starts coming back. But the regeneration is dependent on rest and nutrition."

Jim had a little trouble balancing when he was first fitted with the brace, and even fell backwards, Mrs. Westerhof explains. "And he was a little embarrassed by it at first. But now he can show the other students tricks they can't do."

Charlene's link was knowing what agency to contact to make the brace a reality. "So many times, parents can't afford the treatment needed, and Char knows how to get it," Mrs. Westerhof adds.

From the young to the old—that switch in thinking is typical for public health nurses.

Twice a month, Charlene is in charge of the well-baby clinic in Belmont. She sees humanity at its beginnings there, in the tots brought in for free care—routine physical examinations by a doctor, immunizations, and advice for parents.

Although the wait can be long, the time can be used to ask a public health nurse about the little doubts, those questions that seem too insignificant for the doctor.

"I thought he'd outgrow it by this time. I guess he won't," one mother was overheard commenting to one of the three nurses staffing the clinic.

These chats, informal and friendly, offer help on parenting to start the young out right.

When the young, at 14 or 15, stumble along the way, Charlene and the other public health nurses are there, just a telephone call away.

Sometimes it's the child's problem, and sometimes it's the parent's, spreading over to the child. "Rare is the teenager who will say, 'Hey, I've got a problem,'" Charlene notes. "Some social workers do refer kids to me.

"We see some child abuse cases and we see neglect, which is so hard to prove. It's insidious and camouflaged. Sometimes the parents are too wrapped up in themselves, or it might be a lack of resources, of money.

"We have to know what help is available from the different agencies."

The old pose a different problem, when loneliness and loss have taken their toll. Charlene pulls into a driveway along the Grand River, next to a small house with a tidy yard at 4566 Abrigador Trail NE. It's a call to the other end of life.

"They say I'll live to be 90, but I don't care to," says Josephine Robbins as Charlene takes her blood pressure.

"I know that," Charlene replies, acceptingly, as she removes the blood pressure cuff from the arm of the woman, who is 80.

The youngest of seven, Josephine says, "The others, they're all gone. My sister was 92."

Her husband, Lloyd, died in March. "What do I have to live for?" she asks.

In answer to Charlene's questions on her health, she reports only "a catch in my side" now and then. But she takes "just a little Lydia Pinkham's and it goes away."

An active woman now very lonely and anxious, Josephine looks forward to the weekly nurse visit. "You're not taking any of those pills, are you?" Charlene asks in a warning tone.

"No, I threw them out." A neighbor had given Josephine two drugs, Librium (a tranquilizer) and nitroglycerine (a heart drug), saying, "They always helped me. Maybe they'll help you."

Charlene had become aware of them on her last visit when she had asked what medications Josephine was taking.

Josephine worries about getting her things in order, her will, her records and being able to pledge her eyes and kidneys before she dies. "They said I had to come down and sign in front of two witnesses, but I can't get down there," she tells the nurse. Charlene explains, "Not necessary; just witnesses, here in your home."

Besides the decisions for her will, on the who and what of all she owns, Josephine must finish the mural she is painting on one wall, then paint a scene in a window and refinish some furniture. And then. . . .

"There's just an awful lot of red tape," the gray-haired woman comments sadly. "I'm never going to be through."

The public health nurse visits often when the need is great, then as the crisis eases, the visits taper off, to make time and room for someone else with other pressing needs.

Days are filled with joy and sadness. Charlene believes she gets as much as she gives in her 8-5 job. "I need people. I see myself as a helping person and they are fulfilling to me."

But in public health the rewards are seldom quick in coming. "You see something grow. You see a person who has never had any self-confidence make strides.

"I'm really in preventive medicine," Charlene says. "By educating others and by my intervention, I believe I'll make a difference."

The community health nurse in the above story illustrates several important concepts in community health nursing. The community health nurse is a generalist and serves all population groups. She or he works in the client's setting, utilizing principles of primary, secondary, and tertiary prevention. The community health nurse also serves population groups in clinics and schools; concepts from the public health sciences of biostatistics, epidemiology, and administration help the nurse to identify needs of these groups.

SUMMARY

Community health nursing is a synthesis of nursing and public health practice applied to promoting and preserving the health of populations (ANA, 1980). The community health nurse's philosophy and scope of practice distinguishes her or him from other nurses in the practice setting. Community health nurses serve individuals and aggregates (groups of people) across the lifespan on a continuing basis. Their major goal is to protect and promote the health of the community. Prevention is their primary focus in nursing practice. Identifying at-risk populations within the community assists community health nurses to effectively and efficiently provide preventive health care services.

Community health nurses work in a variety of settings and implement multiple roles such as case finder, teacher, group worker, and health planner. Changing health care delivery trends have increased the demand for community-based services and, in turn, the number of qualified community health nurses. The excitement of this specialty area lies in its diversity.

REFERENCES

American Nurses' Association, Community Health Nursing Division: Standards of community health nursing practice, Pub No CH-10, Kansas City, Mo, 1986, The Association.

American Nurses' Association: Nursing: a social policy statement, Pub No NP-63, Kansas City, Mo, 1980, The Association.

American Public Health Association, Public Health Nursing Section: The definition and role of public health nursing in the delivery of health care, Washington, DC, 1981, The Association.

American Public Health Association: For national health care principles: APHA to push for support of 'Sense of Congress' on care, Nation's Health XIX(9): 1, 10, Washington, DC, 1989, The Association.

American Public Health Association: Action alert, Washington, DC, 1989, The Association.

American Public Health Association: A national health program for all of us, Washington, DC, 1989, The Association.

Brainard, A. Organization of public health nursing, New York, 1921, Macmillan.

Committee for the Study of the Future of Public Health, Institute of Medicine: The future of public health, Washington, DC, 1988, National Academy Press.

Fry ST: Dilemma in community health ethics, Nurs Outlook 31:176-179, 1983.

Gardner MS: Typewritten Reminiscences, Feb. 5, 1948, NOPHN Archive Microfilm H25. In Fitzpatrick ML, ed: The national organization for public health nursing, 1912-1952: development of a practice field, New York, 1975, National League for Nursing, p 17.

Goeppinger J: Primary health care: an answer to the dilemmas of community nursing? Public Health Nurs 1:129-140, 1984.

Green JL and Driggers B: All visiting nurses are not alike: home health and community health nursing, J Community Health Nurs 6:83-93, 1989.

Gulino C and LaMonica G: Public health nursing: a study of role implementation, Public Health Nurs 3:80-91, 1986.

Haradine J: Public health nurse makes a difference, Grand Rapids Press, pp 29-33, December 3, 1978.

Health Care for All Sense of the Congress Proposed Resolution, Nations Health XX(2):3, 1990.

Leavell HR and Clark EG: Preventive medicine for the doctor in his community. An epidemiological approach, ed 3, New York, 1965, McGraw-Hill.

Maglacas AM: Health for all. Paper presented at a conference on international health, Ann Arbor, September 1988.

Mahler H: What is health for all? World Health, pp 3-5, November 1979.

McIver P: Public health nursing responsibilities, Public Health Nurs 41:65-66, 1949.

McNeil E: Transition in public health nursing, U Michigan Medical Center J 33:286-291, 1967.

Milbank Memorial Fund Commission: Higher education for public health: a report, Nantucket, Mass, 1976, Prodist.

Moses E: The registered nurse population: findings from the National Sample Survey of Registered Nurses, November 1984, NTIS Accession No HRP-0906938, Springfield, Va, 1986, National Technical Information Service.

National Organization for Public Health Nursing: Constitution of the National Organization for Public Health Nursing, Article 2, 1912. Wald: New York Public Library folder: NOPHN No 1. In Fitzpatrick ML, ed: The national organization for public health nursing, 1912-1952: development of a practice field, New York, 1975, National League for Nursing, p 27.

Orem D: Nursing: concepts of practice, ed 2, New York, 1980, McGraw-Hill.

Parker EW: Normative approach to the definition of primary health care, Milbank Mem Fund Q 54:415-438, 1976.

Pender NJ: Health promotion in nursing practice, ed 2, Norwalk, Ct, 1987, Appleton-Lange.

Ruth MV and Partridge KB: Differences in perception of education and practice, Nurs Outlook, 26:622-628, 1978.

Secretary's Commission on Nursing (1988). Secretary's Commission on Nursing, final report, vol 1, Washington, DC, 1988, US Government Printing Office.

Secretary of Health and Human Services: Nursing, sixth report to the President and the Congress on the status of health personnel in the United States, June, 1988, NTIS Accession No HRP-0907204, Springfield, Va, 1988, National Technical Information Service.

Source Book, Nursing Personnel, December 1974, DHEW Publication No HRA 75-43, Bethesda, Md, 1975, US Government Printing Office.

Surgeon General: Healthy people: the Surgeon General's report on health promotion and disease prevention, DHEW [PHS] Pub No 79-55071, Washington, DC, 1979, US Government Printing Office.

Turner J: Charter for health promotion, Lancet 2:1407, 1986.

White MS: Construct for public health nursing, Nurs Outlook 30:527-530, 1982.

Williams CA: Community health nursing—what is it? Nurs Outlook 25:250-254, 1977.

Winslow C-EA: Man and epidemics, Princeton, 1952, Princeton University Press.

World Health Organization: Community health nursing, 1974. WHO Expert Committee Report 558, Geneva, 1974, The Organization.

World Health Organization: Alma-Ata 1978: primary health care: report of the International Conference on Primary Health Care, Alma-Ata, USSR, Geneva, 1978, The Organization.

World Health Organization: Four decades of achievement: highlights of the work of WHO, Geneva, 1988, The Organization.

SELECTED BIBLIOGRAPHY

Allen RJ and Allen J: A sense of community, a shared vision and a positive culture: care enabling factors in successful culture based health promotion, Am J Health Prom 1(3):40-47, 1987.

Archer SE: Synthesis of public health science and nursing science, Nurs Outlook 30:442-446, 1982.

Becker M: The tyranny of health promotion, Public Health Rev 14:15-25, 1986.

Bernal B: Levels of practice in a community health agency, Nurs Outlook 26:364-369, 1978.

Consensus conference on the essentials of public health nursing practice and education, HRSA 84-564 (POLP), Rockville, Md, 1985, Health Resources and Services Administration.

Cross J, Northrop C, and Strasser J: How community health nurses spend their time, Nurs Health Care 4:314-317, 1983.

Duffy M and Pender N, eds: Conceptual issues in health promotion: report of proceedings of a Wingspread Conference, Racine, Wi, 1987, Sigma Theta Tau.

Goodstadt M, Simpson R, and Loranger P: Health promotion: a conceptual integration, Am J Health Prom 1(3):58-63, 1987.

Hanchett E: Nursing frameworks and community as client: bridging the gap, Norwalk, Ct, 1988, Appleton and Lange.

Hollen P: A holistic model of individual and family based on a continuum of choice, Adv Nurs Sci 3(3):27-42, 1981.

Maglacas AM: Health for all: nursing's role, Nurs Outlook 36:66-71, 1988.

McKay R and Segall M: Methods and models for the aggregate, Nurs Outlook 31:328-334, 1983.

McLaughlin JS: Toward a theoretical model for community health programs, Adv Nurs Sci 4(2):7-28, 1982.

Shamansky SL and Clausen CL: Levels of prevention: examination of the concept, Nurs Outlook 28:104-108, 1980.

Sills G and Goeppinger J: The community as a field of inquiry in nursing. In Werley H and Fitzpatrick JJ, eds: Annual Review of Nursing Research, 3, New York, 1985, Springer, pp. 4–23.

Smith JA: The idea of health: a philosophical inquiry, Adv Nurs Sci 3(3):43-51, 1981.

Smith JB: Levels of public health, Public Health Nurs 2:138-144, 1985.

Walker B: The future of public health: the Institute of Medicine's 1988 report, J Public Health Policy 10:19-31, 1989.

Whall AL: The family as the unit of care in nursing: a historical review, Public Health Nurs 3:240-249, 1986.

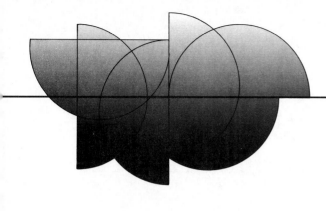

UNIT TWO

The Community and Its Health, Welfare, and Environmental Resources

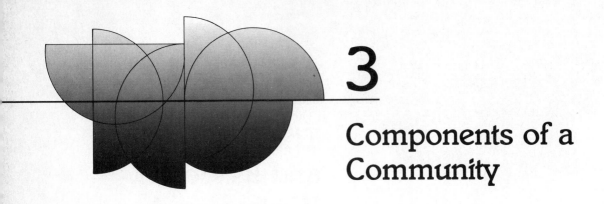

3

Components of a
Community

OBJECTIVES

Upon completion of this chapter, the reader will be able to:

1. *Discuss several interpretations of the term community and identify concepts which are common to most definitions of community.*
2. *Describe the common components of a community.*
3. *Discuss the functions of a community.*
4. *Analyze how community dynamics impact on the functional level of a community.*
5. *Differentiate between a community's normal line of defense and its flexible line of defense.*
6. *Explain the concept of "community as client."*
7. *Discuss the relevance of community assessment to community health nursing practice.*

Community health nurses have recognized since their early beginnings the importance of viewing the community-as-client. Lillian Wald and other historical leaders in the field realized that health problems, and their solutions, were deeply embedded in the structure of the community. These leaders promoted the idea that the dominant responsibility of the public/community health nurse was to the population as a whole—the community (ANA, 1980; NOPHN, 1912).

The concept of community-as-client implies that the focus of practice is on promoting and preserving the health of the community for the common good, and that the community becomes the target of practice (Sills and Goeppinger, 1985, p. 6). Within this target of practice direct care services are provided to individuals, families, and aggregates. Community health nurses become involved in activities such as community outreach and advocacy, community health planning and intervention, and community-wide health education. Two nursing research studies (Anderson, 1983; Cruise and Storfjell, 1980) elaborate on the community-focused activities of the community health nurse. Community-oriented nurses recognize that communities influence nursing practice (Hamilton, 1983), and learn to work in collaboration with community leaders to achieve their goals.

The concept of community-as-client provides a broad and comprehensive approach to the study of contemporary community health problems (Rodgers, 1984, p. 211). A community-wide approach to health problems is merited when risk factors are widespread throughout the community (Chamberlin, 1988, p. 301). Community-wide services are frequently implemented in areas such as communicable disease control, services to handicapped people, services to aged people, services to children, environmental health, domestic violence, and personal health services.

The transition to community-as-client can be difficult for the nurse, since nurses often provide services to individuals and families but not as often to aggregates or communities. While providing direct services to individuals, families, and aggregates it is important for the nurse to realize that the community may contribute to or detract from the health of these client groups. When this is recognized the value of community-oriented practice becomes evident.

In order to work effectively in the community the nurse needs to understand the concept of community. The purpose of this chapter is to promote this understanding, as well as to introduce the concept of community-as-client. Chapters 11 and 12 expand upon this understanding. They discuss how community diagnosis and health planning influence nursing practice and help community health nurses to achieve population-focused goals.

DEFINING COMMUNITY

The word *community* has been in common usage since its Latin origin as *communitas,* and there are no less than 100 definitions for the word *communis* from which *community* was derived (Shamansky and Pesznecker, 1981, p. 182). Health, social, and political scientists have defined *community* from several different perspectives, and each perspective has merit and relevant applications (Lyons, 1988, p. 93). Nursing literature also reveals a diverse use of the term *community* (Sills and Goeppinger, 1985; Goeppinger, Lassiter, and Wilcox, 1982; Shamansky and Pesznecker, 1981; Williams, 1977).

The American community has been studied extensively since the early 1900s and many early studies have become classics in the field. Early researchers on the community such as MacIver (1917), Hillery (1955), Sanders (1963), and Warren (1966) are frequently cited in today's social science and nursing literature.

Communities are frequently defined within one of two frameworks: (1) geographic area or (2) relational (McMillan and Chavis, 1986, p. 6). Geographic definitions usually look at communities in terms of legal or geopolitical jurisdictions such as cities, towns, municipalities, or census tracts. Relational definitions are more abstract and examine how a group of people is organized and interacts to achieve common goals and needs.

Urban sociologists have moved from research

in the 1920s and 1930s, which placed community into a conceptual framework focusing on *natural area,* to a contemporary view of community, which follows a *natural network* approach (Hunter and Riger, 1986, p. 56). The natural network approach takes into account the widening scope of service and support areas necessary to maintain a community; the necessity of interactions not only among community residents, but between community residents and those outside the community; the increased mobility of community members; and the increased population base of contemporary communities.

Community is a somewhat nebulous term. Sanders (1975, pp. 26-33; 1979, pp. 412-441) has described a community as a place to live, a collection of people, and a social system. Warren (1988, p. 84) has described the community as a social system including people, spatial arrangements, shared institutions, interaction, and power structure. Heller (1989, p. 3) views the community as being a locality, a relational community, and as a collective political power. The American Public Health Association (1985, p. 5) has said that the term community implies an entity from which the nature and scope of a public health problem, as well as the capacity to respond to that problem, can be defined; and that depending on the problem area and response capacity the definition of community may vary. According to the Association, for most instances of public health the community is defined as a geopolitical unit, such as a town, city, or county (APHA, 1985, p. 5).

The World Health Organization (1974) has defined a community as being a social group determined by geographic boundaries and/or common values and interests. Its definition states that community members know and interact with one another, that the community functions within a particular social structure, and that the community creates norms, values, and social institutions. This World Health Organization definition is incorporated into the latest American Nurses' Association *Standards of Community Health Nursing Practice.*

While definitions of the term community vary, there are some common elements in all these definitions. Specifically, four major elements are seen as being essential to the definition: (1) people, (2) social interaction, (3) area, and (4) common ties (Hillery, 1955, pp. 118-119; Wellman and Leighton, 1988, p. 58).

A community is defined in its broadest sense as a group of people living in an environment that has the ability to meet their life goals and needs. Communities are social units that have characteristics similar to those of an individual, a family, or an aggregate but exist within a larger social environment or system (Higgs and Gustafson, 1985, p. 11). In a community, people live together in such a way that they share not just a particular interest but the elements of a common life (MacIver and Page, 1949, pp. 8-10). A community is differentiated from other social organizations in that one's life can be lived within its bounds (MacIver and Page, 1949, pp. 8-10; Arensburg and Kimball, 1972, p. 17; Warren, 1978, p. 6). Community organization and function serve to meet the goals and needs of community members (Higgs and Gustafson, 1985, p. 11).

A community is part of, and has ties to, larger societies such as a county, a state, a region, a nation. A community has patterns of communication, leadership, and decision making. It is a setting for action (Sanders, 1963, p. 642; 1975, p. 43). It is a place where people maintain their homes, earn their livings, rear their children, and carry on most of their life activities (Poplin, 1979, p. 8). It appears to be the basic unit of organization which transmits cultural values, beliefs, and attitudes to its members (Arensburg and Kimball, 1972, p. 15).

Some communities will have greater autonomy than others. People will have varying degrees of loyalty to different communities. In some communities, a sense of community will exist, and in others, it will not. The movement in the American community from natural area to natural network is fertile for the loss of a "sense of community" within its membership. Research has shown that a population base of 10,000 to 20,000 is preferred for maintaining a sense of community, that larger cities of up to 100,000 can still maintain this sense, and that cities or geographic areas larger than 100,000 often need to be broken down into target areas to maintain this sense of community (Chamberlin, 1988, p. 302). In order for these target areas to be effective modes for health care delivery they need to be able to function like a community in terms of residents sharing some common goals, and having an established pattern of shopping, employment, and political representation (Chamberlin, 1988, p. 303).

A community must be organized to achieve its goals. It must contain a set of institutions—industry, stores, churches, organizations, schools, and government—so its residents can carry on life within its bounds. A community encompasses a variety of health care resources which provide both inpatient and outpatient health care services.

COMPONENTS OF A COMMUNITY

Communities have the common components of *people, goals, needs, environment, service systems,* and *boundaries.* The characteristics of these components will vary from one community to another.

People

People are a community's most important resource: they are the core of the community. People in the community often will have shared values. Shared values are an integrative force for cohesive, functional communities (McMillan and Chavis, 1986, p. 13).

Within communities, people will cluster or separate based on a variety of individual, demographic, health, psychosocial, socioeconomic, and cultural characteristics. These characteristics can either positively or adversely influence the community's health status. For example, when analyzing health status measures (mortality, morbidity, sociodemographic statistics, and health care utilization patterns), it becomes evident that persons disadvantaged by virtue of their income, educational level, age, residence, and membership in racial or minority groups, are characterized by lower levels of health than are the advantaged (USDHHS, 1986).

People in the community will take part in varying levels of social interaction with one another. The community itself exerts an effect on the social status, roles, and social mobility of its members (Reiss, 1959). However, community positions, roles, and status may not be commensurate with the ones the person assumes in the larger society.

Goals and Needs

The people, family, and aggregates of the community have mutual as well as independent goals and needs. These are reflected in, and determine, community goals and needs. Community goals and needs follow Maslow's hierarchical order of physiology, safety, social affiliation, esteem, and self-actualization (Meneshian, 1988, p. 116). People are often attracted to others whose skills or competence can help them to meet these goals and needs (McMillan and Chavis, 1986, p. 13).

Community Environment

The community's environment includes (1) *physical characteristics* such as geography, climate, terrain, natural resources, and structural entities (buildings such as schools, workplaces, and homes); (2) *biologic and chemical characteristics* such as flora, animal reservoirs, vectors, bacteria, agents, toxic substances, and food and water supplies; (3) *social characteristics* such as economics, education, health and welfare services, leadership, recreation, and religion. These characteristics combine to make each community unique; they have a major impact on the health and welfare resources a community can provide, and have a major impact on the health status of the community. Take, for example, rural communities where well water is the only source of fresh water. If children in these communities do not have regular, preventive dental fluoride treatments, these children may develop serious dental problems.

Often the social environment of the community is overlooked. However, the social environment involves significant networks which influence well-being and health care decision-making (Dean, 1986, p. 545). The social environment provides the mechanisms for passing on the culture and values of the community. Communities can lose their cultural heritage if they become too large. The defined geographic area of a community should be large enough to provide an adequate population base for comprehensive, efficient services, but remain small enough to maintain a sense of community (Chamberlin, 1988, p. 302).

Service Systems

In order for its residents to carry on life within its bounds, a community must be of sufficient size to contain a set of service systems. The community must organize these systems so that the goals and needs of its populace are met. The service systems of a community help its citizenry to meet basic needs of daily living as well as special health and welfare needs. These service systems are represented by a multiplicity of agencies and organizations aimed at meeting some community need (Cottrell, 1977, p. 546). If there is a gap within a community service system, mechanisms should exist within the community to assist its members in finding the service elsewhere. In this way a "community of solution" is developed.

Sanders (1966, p. 170) viewed the major service systems of the community as (1) health, (2) social welfare, (3) education, (4) economic, (5) government, (6) recreational, and (7) religious. Community service systems have the following identifiable characteristics (Sanders, 1966, pp. 175-180):

- A structure comprising a network of agencies, organizations, and establishments which frequently can be viewed as subsystems
- A set of functions, both manifest and latent
- Ideology or rationale, which provides the justification for the continuation of the system
- Norms and standardized procedures (standards of right and wrong)
- Functionaries, people charged with the responsibility of watching out for the interest of the system
- Paraphernalia, or the materials, resources, and artifacts required for system operation

These characteristics help community systems to form a network of resources that deliver services to community members. This network of resources has linkages within and outside the community.

Each system is important and will in some way affect health. Not all systems have equal importance within the community, and they can become out of balance with one another. An example of this occurs when local government becomes so powerful that it uses a disproportionate amount of the tax dollars—tax dollars needed by other community systems such as education or health (Poplin, 1979, p. 167). Once this system equilibrium has been disturbed, it may never be restored, or it may take years to recover.

Community systems are extremely important to the community health nurse, because it is through them that services are provided to individuals, families, and population groups. The nurse should assess all community systems, identify their services and linkages, discover how each fits into the overall structure of the community, and then know how to utilize them effectively. All community systems are essential for maintaining and promoting community wellness.

The health system is the central focus for the community health nurse. However, the economic system (economic sufficiency) has long been recognized as the usual focus for the citizenry and leadership of the community (National Commission on Community Health Services, 1966, p. 7). Until a community's basic economic needs are met, it is not likely that people will work diligently on other needs, such as health.

Boundaries

A community has *boundaries*. These boundaries serve to regulate the exchange of energies between a community and its external environment. They define the community's area. In general, boundaries may be concrete (definite, spatial) or conceptual (elusive, nonspatial). Concrete boundaries are more absolute and easier to see and to define. They include *geographic* boundaries (mountains, valleys, and deserts), *political* boundaries (cities, towns, counties, states, and nations), and *situational* boundaries (home, school, and work). Conceptual boundaries are less definite and do not necessarily fit into a neatly defined space. They can be such factors as interest-area, problem-solving, or service-area boundaries, social ties, or social interactions.

The service area boundaries of the community are flexible, dynamic, and ever-changing. Communities may overlap and intermingle and will not always conform to the boundaries of a local political jurisdiction, such as a town or city. Many local health departments serve counties or districts.

Community health nurses are frequently assigned to work within specific geographic areas such as cities and counties. The community for them will be centered around these geographic areas no matter how arbitrary that may be. Nurses must remember that even though their service area may be a specified geographic region, that area may not reflect "the community" for the populace. The community health nurse should be aware of this when doing a community assessment. For example, it is not uncommon for community health nurses to discover multiple problem-solving boundaries when working in a rural setting. If the geographic rural area is surrounded by several large cities, clients in this rural community will probably be using health resources in several of the larger cities close to them.

Population Groups in the Community

A community is made up of various population groups. *Population groups are aggregates of persons who have one or more shared personal or environmental characteristics.* They can be identified in an infinite number of ways, based on such variables as health conditions, place of location (geography), climate, age, sex, race, marital status, religion, and sociocultural and recreational characteristics. The environmental characteristics of a population should not be overlooked, since people are identified according to the characteristics

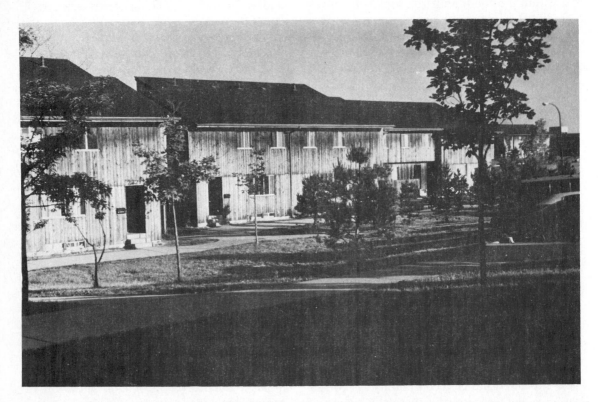

Figure 3-1   Students in a university married housing project form an aggregate of persons who have shared personal and environmental characteristics.

they share by living in a particular geographic area. An example of this is students living in a "married housing" area provided by a university (refer to Figure 3-1), which forms a population group. Students in married housing are frequently seen as a population at risk, because they can experience multiple stresses such as crowded living conditions, financial difficulties, and educational pressures.

The community health nurse's role in providing services to population groups, based on age-related developmental tasks and at-risk characteristics, is discussed throughout this text (refer to Chapters 13 to 20). By using the developmental approach, the community health nurse can assess the health needs of all individuals and groups within the community and can identify health promotion activities needed for age-correlated groups across the life span.

The developmental approach views human life as a process of continued development. Eric Erikson, Sigmund Freud, Jean Piaget, Evelyn Duvall, and others have written about the process of human development. Erikson's eight stages of the life cycle (infancy, early childhood, play age, school age, adolescence, young adulthood, adulthood, and senescence) have been used widely in nursing (Erikson, 1978). Duvall (1977) continues to be a source for the study of developmental tasks to be accomplished by individuals and families. Reviewing the writings of these authors gives the reader an in-depth perspective on individual development throughout the lifespan as well as family development across the family life cycle.

The developmental approach is based on the theory that individuals develop in their own way, yet in conformity with a common developmental pattern. It postulates that failure to accomplish developmental tasks at the appropriate time makes subsequent development more difficult. Community health nurses can use the developmental framework as a foundation for identifying problems that exist or have the potential to exist and for determining health programs needed in a community for a particular developmental population group. For example, a major developmental task of aging is to make an adjustment to changing sensory perceptions and strengths. These changes may increase the aging person's need for medical care and decrease that person's ability to handle activities of daily living. If health statistics reflect an increased number of senior citizens living in the community, services that are frequently used by seniors such as geriatric screening clinics, meals on wheels, and dial-a-ride should be assessed to determine if they are adequate. A community with a large preschool population, on the other hand, would likely benefit from services such as child health conferences, immunization clinics, and family planning. Community health nurses focus their thinking on various population groups and what type of services each group needs.

The community health nurse works extensively with individuals, families, and groups in the neighborhoods in which they live. Therefore, a population group that has special significance to this chapter is that cluster of people who make up a neighborhood.

Neighborhoods

Neighborhoods have a specific population and boundaries and may provide resources to meet the needs of residents, such as recreational facilities, schools, and shops. A neighborhood is usually unable to meet all the health and welfare needs of its population and must have ties with the larger community. People may identify more closely with their neighborhood than with the community as a whole. Neighborhoods can be looked at in terms of *interaction* in the neighborhood, *identification* with the neighborhood, and *connections* outside the neighborhood (Warren and Warren, 1975, pp. 72-76). Neighborhoods vary greatly in leadership, cohesiveness, self-sufficiency, and ties with the larger community. These neighborhood variances play a significant role in relation to the health services the community health nurse is able to provide residents. Warren (1977, pp. 224-229) has elaborated on the varying characteristics in neighborhoods by using the following classifications to identify differences between them: Descriptions of these neighborhoods are given in the box on p. 78.

Classifications of Neighborhoods

INTEGRAL

The individuals in this setting have frequent face-to-face contacts. The norms, values, and attitudes of the neighborhood support those of the larger community. People are cohesive within the neighborhood but belong to other groups outside their area of residence. There is a form of power, authority, and leadership within this type of neighborhood which aids its members to reach out to the larger society for assistance when a problem arises that cannot be handled internally.

PAROCHIAL

People in this setting also have face-to-face contacts, but there is an absence of ties to the larger community. These neighborhoods tend to be protective of their status, to screen out values that do not conform to their own, and to enforce their own beliefs within the neighborhood. The power, authority, and leadership structure within this type of neighborhood encourages isolation from the larger community.

DIFFUSE

Neighbors within this type of environment interact infrequently with each other and have few ties with the larger community. There is often a lack of shared norms, values, and attitudes. A primary tie between these neighbors is geographic proximity to one another. There may be little or no leadership in these areas. When leadership exists, it is often not representative of the entire neighborhood, but is composed of an "elitist" leadership that ignores or subverts the values of most residents. Groups of residents, such as those living in a public housing unit, may be categorized and separated from the mainstream of the neighborhood.

STEPPING-STONE

This type of neighborhood is characterized by a rapid membership turnover and families who have a weak sense of identity with the neighborhood. Members are willing to give up the ties established in the neighborhood if other commitments arise; they strive to attain a higher social status. Residents of these areas do, however, have close ties to the larger community and do interact regularly with neighbors. Leadership is usually not effective because of the high rate of mobility; conflicts arise between the needs of the local neighborhood and the values of social mobility.

TRANSITORY

Members of this kind of neighborhood fail to participate in or identify with the local community. There is an emphasis on people keeping to themselves, because links with others may interfere with the goals of the individual and the family. There may be a widespread feeling of mistrust in this type of neighborhood.

ANOMIC

Such a neighborhood is completely disorganized; its residents lack participation in and a common identification with the neighborhood or the larger community. This neighborhood reflects mass apathy and is not likely to influence or alter the values of its residents through any form of socialization. There is little interaction between people within the neighborhood or between the neighborhood and the larger community, and leadership activity is largely lacking.

Warren DI: Neighborhoods in urban areas. In Warren RL, ed: New perspectives on the American community, ed. 3, Chicago, 1977, Rand McNally, pp 224-237.

Identifying the type of neighborhood in which one is working helps the community health nurse to assess and plan for meeting health needs. For example, if a community health nurse is working in a parochial neighborhood, it would be imperative for her or him to work closely with neighborhood leaders in the delivery of health care services. The nurse may find that the parochial neighborhood readily becomes involved in providing services for its residents. However, there also may be more resistance in this neighborhood to health services proposed by the larger community which do not coincide with neighborhood values and beliefs. In an anomic neighborhood, on the other hand, the community health nurse may find little neighborhood leadership and may want to invest effort in developing this leadership to facilitate implementation of health care services. In addition, the nurse may find that the anomic neighborhood offers few services to its residents and that services need to be sought extensively from outside the neighborhood.

Whatever the type of neighborhood, its structure has implications for the activities of the community health nurse. Neighborhoods, as part of the community, play an important role in providing for the needs of the population. Communities meet these population needs by carrying out specific functions.

COMMUNITY FUNCTIONS

In order to provide for the life goals and needs of its population, the community carries out a number of functions. Warren (1978, pp. 171-12) gives the following functions of a community:

1. *Production-distribution-consumption.* The community produces, distributes, and utilizes goods and services that are essential for meeting the health and welfare needs of its residents. This triad of activities provides opportunities which help community residents to carry out activities of daily living, and it involves extensive resource coordination. Establishing and supporting local companies and businesses are an integral part of this function, because community residents need employment to meet their basic needs (food, clothing, and shelter) and the community needs funds from taxes to maintain its systems. Tax funds from industry and business significantly contribute to the economic stability of a community.
2. *Socialization.* This is the process by which prevailing knowledge, values, beliefs, customs, and behavior are transmitted to a community's members. It is a lifelong process which helps persons to learn how to effectively relate in a social environment and to develop a philosophy of life. Educational services for the populace are included here.
3. *Social control.* The community influences the behavior of its members through norms and rules of social control. Social control has a legal component that is often enforced through law agencies, courts, and the government. It also has a "social sanction" component that is enforced by the family, neighborhood residents, friends, and the educational, religious, and recreational systems. Social control helps to safeguard and protect the community by providing mechanisms for safety and order.
4. *Social participation.* People have basic needs for self-expression and self-fulfillment. These needs are largely met through interaction with others. Social participation is primarily carried out through the community's private sector. This function provides opportunity for members of the community to achieve psychosocial wellness, communication, social interaction, and support. Social networks evolve through social participation.
5. *Mutual support.* This involves people lending help and assistance to one another. It is frequently offered through family, friends, neighbors, and religious groups, as well as official health departments and departments of social service within the community.

The ability to carry out these functions is a major determinant of whether or not a community really exists. These functions provide for the services and activities necessary for community life. The community health nurse must be aware of these functions and how a community implements them in order to effectively assess and plan for essential nursing services in the community.

The way in which a community carries out all its functions makes an impact on how well the community health nurse will be able to meet the needs of the population. For example, if there is a gap in production-distribution-consumption, the community may not have the health resources to meet the health needs of its population. If people have not been socialized to value preventive health care, or if they have customs (such as religious fasting) that affect the delivery of health care services, the nurse's ability to implement preventive health care services can be hindered. If community health policy is inadequate, or if the health policy is not enforced, the health of the community may be in jeopardy. If the members of the community do not value social interaction and participation, the community's response to clinics, classes, and group activities may not be maximized. If a community does not support its residents, there may be few health and welfare assistance programs that provide community services.

COMMUNITY DYNAMICS

Community dynamics occur as a result of interactions within the community and between the community and the larger society. Critical to the dynamics of the community are its patterns of communication, leadership, and decision making.

Communities have both horizontal and vertical patterns of communication (Warren, 1978, pp. 163-164). *Vertical patterns* of communication link the community to the larger society (state, national, and international); *horizontal patterns* of communication link the community to itself, its people, environment, and systems. The strength, cohesiveness, and ease with which these patterns operate will largely determine the extent to which the community is able to be self-sufficient and provide for the needs of its membership. The horizontal patterns of communication are especially important, because they influence the internal dynamics of the community.

The *leadership* and *decision-making* processes within a community critically influence how well a community will function. The community usually has elected, appointed, and legal (official, manifest) leadership, such as a mayor or city council. However, much of a community's leadership is less obvious and takes more effort to decipher and detect. A community may have the obvious political leadership of a mayor but also many other leaders who are unofficial. This nonofficial leadership includes the "heroes" of the community, those whom the people in the community revere and respect, plus people of power and authority. The local community religious leader whom people often go to for advice and guidance and the wealthy philanthropist who heavily subsidizes community activities are examples of nonofficial leaders. These people may have more influence, power, and control over community decision making and action than the elected government leaders. They are also more diverse and numerous.

Table 3-1 presents a summary of the types of leadership in a community. The community health nurse will find it useful to identify individuals under each of these categories when doing an assessment of the community. The leadership in the community needs to be assessed by the community health nurse, because community leaders greatly influence what type of services will be available for community residents. The nurse should be aware of official leaders and their health and welfare responsibilities within a community,

TABLE 3-1 Types of community leaders

Type	Basis for leadership	Area of authority	Examples
Institutional	Occupies a formal leadership position in the community and is elected or appointed to his or her post	Confined to routinized community actions	Mayor, city council, school principal, ministers, and labor union officials
Grassroots	Has personal influence and the ability to get other people interested in a "cause"	Confined to community actions of a spontaneous and/or initiated nature	Opponent of school desegregation, or a leader of a campaign against water fluoridation
Power elite	Has wealth, economic power, and/or personal influence	Makes his or her influence felt in all areas of community action and decision making	Wealthy business person, or a top-echelon employee of a commercial, banking, or industrial firm

From Poplin DE: Communities, New York, 1979, Macmillan, p 216.

as well as the nonofficial leaders. Knowing these leaders and their patterns of functioning can facilitate the implementation of health care services in the community.

One major community system may have a form of leadership or authority over another. The religious system is a good example, because it influences the health practices of its members. The religious practices of fasting, eating or not eating certain foods, and prohibiting the use of certain health care services, such as general medical care, blood transfusions, and family planning methods, are examples of how religious beliefs make an impact on the health care delivery system.

Many aspects of community life are in part controlled by decisions made outside the community. These decisions frequently result from the enactment of state and federal laws. The community must adhere to these decisions, although they may be in conflict with community ideology.

The dynamics of a community result in community action, change, and development. They will determine the community's ability to promote health (Turner and Chavigny, 1988, p. 117). Figure 3-2 summarizes these dynamics.

This figure illustrates that many forces interact to establish a functional, healthy community. According to Warren (1988, pp. 413-418) a functional community is one in which people interact (primary group relationships), participate, and have a degree of commitment to the community; the community has some autonomy from the larger society; people can confront their problems through concerted action (viability); decision making is relatively equally distributed throughout the population and not concentrated (power distribution); there is a balance of differences (degree of heterogeneity); and the degree of conflict is manageable.

Cottrell (1977, pp. 549, 554) has cited the variables of commitment and participation as necessities for a competent, functional community. Cottrell (1977, pp. 551-556) further discussed the need of each segment of the community to be aware of its own interests and of how these relate to the interests of other elements (self-other awareness); the ability of each segment of the community to articulate its views, attitudes, needs, and intentions in relation to itself and the community at large (articulateness); the ability of the community to communicate with itself and the larger society (communication); the ability of the community to manage its relations with the larger society; and the ability of a community to utilize appropriate decision-making and leadership approaches so as to be representative of its membership. Communities with these characteristics can more successfully deal with stressors in the environment.

Community stressors are tension-producing stimuli that have the potential of causing disequilibrium and can result in disruption in the community (Anderson, McFarlane, and Helton, 1986, p. 221). Stressors often arise when service

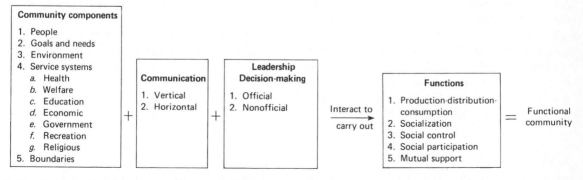

Figure 3-2   Community dynamics. (Service systems data from Sanders IT: The community: an introduction to a social system, ed 2, New York, 1966, Ronald Press. Communication and function data from Warren RI: The community in America, ed 2, Chicago, 1972, Rand-McNally, pp 167, 237.)

systems are unable to provide the necessary services for effective community functioning. An example of this is the inability of a community to maintain a sufficient tax base to adequately operate the local health department, or an absence of health care services to senior citizens. The reaction to these stressors may be reflected in community health statistics such as morbidity and mortality rates (Anderson, McFarlane, and Helton, 1986, p. 221).

A functional community can identify, prioritize, and address community needs and stressors. It provides health interventions at all three levels of prevention: primary, secondary, and tertiary. It is a community that is capable of problem solving and crisis resolution (Turner and Chavigny, 1988, p. 117). A functional community maintains a high degree of system equilibrium while promoting growth and development.

Rural and Urban Communities

An awareness of the general characteristics of urban and rural communities will assist the nurse in community assessment, diagnosis, and planning. Several authors have written about the differences between urban and rural communities and how these differences influence community dynamics and ultimately the community's health. A group of community health nurses learned this dramatically when they carried out a community diagnosis of a rural county, which included some 760,000 people, or 578 persons in each of its 1313 square miles. By contrast, an adjacent county included 10,404 people in each of its 675 square miles and a major industrial city. The results of both community assessments surprised the community health nurses. The major health problem of the rural county was traffic deaths among males 16 to 24 years of age; the death rates for this age group were significantly higher than the death rates for the same age group in the urban community. After data analysis, the reasons given for this were narrow, winding, two-lane roads with no shoulders; an image among the young males that fast cars were "macho"; no recreational facilities except bars; and the necessity of driving very long distances to employment sites.

Rural communities are more sparsely populated than urban communities and often contain fewer health and welfare resources within their geographic boundaries. Rural communities often have restricted access to emergency and specialized health care services. The number of rural hospitals has declined 12% in the last decade (AHA study, 1990, p. 3). This can increase levels of morbidity and mortality. For example, in the above situation residents had to travel 35 miles to obtain emergency care services. If the young males in this community had easy access to a trauma center designed to treat injuries suffered during a major accident, the mortality rate for automobile injuries might be significantly reduced.

When resources are not available in rural areas, residents are forced to recruit these services from other communities, which then become areas of trade. Rural communities often have extensive trade areas, to which their residents go for necessary health and welfare services.

Rural communities are often more closely knit than urban communities, with many people knowing each other on a first name basis and having a higher frequency of contact with community members. This means that individual anonymity is more difficult to maintain in the rural community than in the urban. Conversely, urban communities are known for the isolation that is produced when people living next to each other do not know each other's names.

Rural communities are often classified on the basis of their dominant economic activity—farming, mining, or resort area (Poplin, 1979, p. 42). This activity tends to dominate community dynamics and function. For example, coal mining communities in the south have high concentrations of men with "black lung" disease, who have had to retire early.

Both urban and rural communities have populations at risk, but until recently, very little attention has been given to the needs of at-risk groups in rural communities. In some rural areas, the tranquility of the environment (refer to Figure 3-3) can be deceiving; it makes health hazards less obvious. However, statistics reveal that farm settings are not as safe as they appear. Agricultural

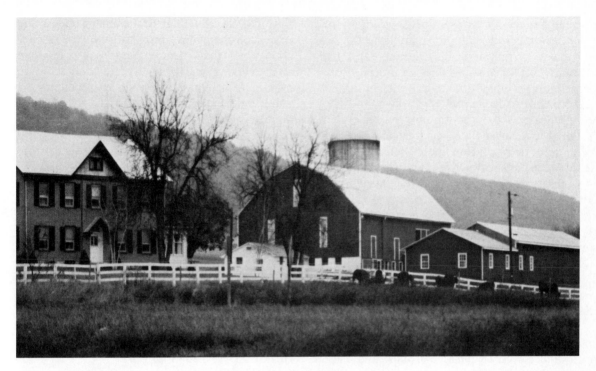

Figure 3-3 Some 60 million Americans, or 26.3% of the U.S. resident population, live in rural communities. Public health efforts need to be strengthened in these communities. Residents in rural settings are regularly exposed to environmental hazards such as chemical pollutants and diseases transmitted by animals, yet often lack adequate health care resources to meet emergency as well as basic health care needs. The shortage of health care in rural communities presents serious problems for many rural Americans. (Courtesy of photographer, Henry Parks.)

workers have some of the highest rates of occupational illness, injury, disability, and death in the nation.

It is increasingly being recognized that many of our nation's rural areas have serious health problems, because of the lack of needed health care resources and environmental surveillance, which are not being resolved. The rural population groups most often in need of health services—farm workers, the poor, elderly, persons with chronic illnesses, and migrant families—are the ones which are least capable of obtaining them. The needs of these at-risk populations are discussed in Unit 5 of this text.

THE HEALTH SYSTEM AND THE COMMUNITY

The health system is a major community system. It consists of facilities, organizations, a work force, and funding to implement health care services. The health of a community depends upon its ability to work toward common health goals and upon adequate distribution of health resources to all members (Hanchett, 1979, p. 46). Organized community effort to prevent disease and promote health is both valuable and effective (Committee for the Study of the Future of Public Health, 1988, p. 159).

The priority a community places on health varies and will affect health care resources and their distribution. Health care resources include individuals and groups or agencies, such as private health practitioners, volunteers, hospitals, clinics, pharmacies, nursing homes, health departments, and departments of social services.

Health resources are both governmental and private. Private-sector provision of health care services in the community is based on supply and demand and fee-for-service. The government (official) sector provides traditional public health services, such as communicable disease control, and preventive health services through official health departments at no or little cost to the consumer.

According to Anderson, McFarlane, and Helton (1986, p. 220), a community has a level of health reached over time which is called its *normal line of defense.* This line of defense can include characteristics such as high immunity and low infant mortality. They contrast this with the community's *flexible line of defense,* which represents a state of health that is more dynamic or in flux owing to temporary stressors such as environmental disasters and epidemics. It is important for the nurse to be aware of these normal and flexible lines of defense for community health, and to use the information for effective health planning, implementation, and evaluation.

The health service area for a community is the area within which a problem can be defined, dealt with, and solved (Ruybal, Bauwens, and Fasla, 1975, p. 365). Within this health service area, the nurse must be familiar with the health needs of the people and available health resources and services. In order to meet client needs, the community health nurse often utilizes health resources outside the confines of a political jurisdiction. For instance, she or he may refer families to a medical center in another area, because the medical care needs of these persons cannot be met by local community resources.

Difficulties in the Community Health System

When the nurse analyzes the community's health system, there are several concerns that may become apparent. Communication between the health care system and the other community systems has historically been weak (refer to Chapter 5). In many communities, official local health departments have little contact with private health care resources and other official health and welfare resources. The health system of the community also may have little direct communication with the people of the community.

No one agency has statutory (legal) responsibility for coordinating the health resources and services in the community, and thus the responsibility for management of these resources is often vague. Having one agency whose major role is to coordinate health services and to function as a health information center for the community would facilitate more effective delivery and utilization of community health resources. Local health departments are an excellent source of information on the health resources of a community.

Not only is the overall management of the health system weak, but the management skills of individual health practitioners are also weak. Health practitioners frequently have not had educational experiences which prepare them to manage health care resources (refer to Chapter 21). Health care professionals must understand the principles of management if the health care system is to exist effectively and carry out its functions (National Commission on Community Health Services, 1966, p. 134).

Another problem community health nurses frequently experience is the community's adherence to traditional stands on health. American communities have historically reacted better to disaster and catastrophic health events than to providing ongoing, preventive community health services. There is usually general indifference to a health problem as long as no serious or long-term effects are apparent (Smolensky, 1982, p. 68). The feeling within the community that the responsibility for health concerns rests with official health departments, private health care practitioners, and health care facilities deters community involvement in health. This is unfortunate, because "health is a community affair" (National Commission on Community Health Services, 1966).

The community may not actively support health activities. This can occur for a variety of reasons, including other community priorities, a lack of information on health issues and resources, and a lack of understanding about the role the community can play in establishing and promoting positive health practices for its membership. The health system often does not include the community in health planning, implementation, and evaluation. There is a need for increased cooperation and collaboration between the community and the health care delivery system; an appreciation of all aspects of health, as well as a plan to meet future health needs, could evolve from such efforts.

The National Commission on Community Health Services (1966) issued the following goals for community health systems that are still to be fulfilled:

All communities of this nation must take the action necessary to provide comprehensive personal health services of high quality to all people in the community. These services should embrace those directed toward promotion of positive good health, application of established preventive measures, early detection of disease, prompt and effective treatment, and physical, social, and vocational rehabilitation of those with residual disabilities. This broad range of personal health services must be patterned so as to assure full and intelligent use by all groups in the community.

Success in this endeavor will mean change. It will require removal of racial, economic, organizational, residential, and geographic barriers to the use of health services. It will require strengthened and expanded licensure and accreditation of services, manpower, and facilities. It will require maximum coverage through health insurance and other prepayment plans, and extension of such insurance to cover the broad range of services both in and out of hospitals. Finally, success will require citizenry that is sufficiently well informed and motivated to follow established principles conducive to good health services in all phases of prevention and treatment of illness and disability.

COMMUNITY CONCEPTS: IMPLICATIONS FOR THE COMMUNITY HEALTH NURSE

The community health nurse is in the unique position of being able to see the community carry out its functions and activities on a day-to-day basis. Unlike many other health practitioners, the community health nurse is out in the community on a regular basis, working with its people and systems. She or he provides services in homes, schools, clinics, industry, and other settings and thus has multiple opportunities to collect data about community dynamics and to comprehen-

sively assess the community. Through the knowledge gained from these opportunities, the community health nurse has a base for analyzing strengths and deficiencies in the health care delivery system. Community data need to be gathered systematically and community diagnoses must be made (refer to Chapter 11).

Community Assessment

The nursing process can be applied to community assessment (Martin, 1988; Meneshian, 1988; Selvy and Tuttle, 1987). Community information gathering and awareness of community needs and problems are a major dimension of community-focused nursing (Cruise and Storfjell, 1980, p. 10). Community data are needed to work with the community-as-client.

The Committee for the Study of the Future of Public Health (1988, p. 7) recommended that every public health agency regularly and systematically collect, assemble, analyze, and make available information on the health of the community. The responsibility of community assessment is often delegated to the nursing staff.

A community assessment provides a "window" through which to view the community. It provides the means for looking at community strengths, problems, and potential problems. It can identify populations at risk and gaps in community resources. It is the basis for health planning.

Various methods can be used to assess a community. It can be difficult for both neophytes and professionals to handle all of the information that must be obtained when doing a community assessment. It is important to have assessment tools which help professionals to collect and organize community data. Included in Appendix 3-1 is such a tool. This tool is based on a set of master categories that characterize community data (Stein and Eigsti, 1982). It quickly helps the beginning practitioner to complete a "windshield" survey of a community. A windshield survey is a process that provides observational information about a community's environment, mode of functioning, and social and health resources. A community health nurse collects these data while driving through or walking around in a community. A windshield assessment of a community provides a beginning data base about a community's lifestyle.

An assessment tool which assists health agencies to obtain a comprehensive profile of a community is presented in the appendix to Chapter 11. Other community assessment tools and frameworks for nurses can be found in Meneshian (1988), Martin (1988), Ruffing-Rahal (1987), Rodgers (1984), Allor (1983), Rauckhorst, Stokes, and Mezey (1980), and Hanchett (1979). Chapter 11 also discusses pertinent sources of data when using these tools.

Through the knowledge gained from a community assessment, the community health nurse has a data base for analyzing strengths and deficiencies in the health care delivery system. The community health nurse through the health planning process uses this knowledge base to correct deficiencies in the health care system (refer to Chapter 12).

Another useful nursing outcome of community assessment is in the area of marketing. After a community assessment is done, decisions can be made as to what nursing services should be of-fered to a community, what nursing services would fit into the health care market of the community, and the scope and depth at which services should be offered (Archer, 1983; Martin, 1988).

SUMMARY

The community is not an easily or consistently defined entity. It is a nebulous, complex concept. However, it is within the confines of the community that nurses diagnose and solve health problems. Developing a conceptual understanding of the word *community* and how health problems are assessed and solved within the community is the first step in carrying out the unique responsibilities of the community health nurse.

Working with clients (individuals, families, populations at risk, and communities) becomes far more exciting when the community health nurse understands community concepts. This knowledge, coupled with flexibility in meeting the changing and diverse health needs of the community, facilitates the achievement of a high-level of community wellness. Understanding the concept, community-as-client, helps the nurse to recognize the value of community-focused practice.

APPENDIX 3-1

University of Rochester School of Nursing: Categories for Recording Descriptive Community Data*

Find a place to eat in the community in which your caseload exists. After lunch, drive around or walk in the community in pairs, essentially observing on as many streets as possible for the following assessment categories, which are grouped according to community systems. Do not be concerned if all categories are not covered.

I. Physical environment

    A. Land use
- 1. Open spaces (look for play areas, parks)
- 2. Undeveloped space (vacant lots, fields)
- 3. Residential space
  - a. Single-family housing (note better or poorer housing)
  - b. Multiple-family housing
- 4. Commercial space
  - a. Go into stores; note prices, atmosphere, selection
  - b. Visit gas stations; find out where you could go for car repairs and gas, and what the costs are
- 5. Industrial space
  - a. Note location and condition
  - b. Determine type of industry
- 6. Water in area
  - a. Note open ditches
  - b. Stagnant water
  - c. Bodies of water (lakes, rivers, or streams)
- 7. Roads
  - a. Note paved streets, condition
  - b. Dirt roads, condition
- 8. Boundaries
  - a. Note any geographical boundaries which tend to separate communities, such as "the other side of the tracks"
- 9. Agriculture
  - a. Note types of crops
  - b. Note types of animals kept

    B. Environmental status
- 1. Sanitation
  - a. Note debris, location
  - b. Note garbage cans in area
  - c. Waste disposal systems
- 2. Air
  - a. Note smell, color
  - b. Note location of unusual odors
- 3. Note utilities—note availability of water, gas, public telephones, telephone lines, and electricity
- 4. Household pets—where kept, what type?
- 5. Topography and geology
  - a. Note general topography of land
  - b. Obstacles to travel and hazards (such as rock slides)

II. Social and behavioral environment

    A. Education
- 1. Note church or synagogue schools: how many are there, what condition are they in? Types?
- 2. Alternative education systems: e.g., Montessori schools, encounter workshops, martial arts

---

*Areas currently found to be "essential" sources of data about communities. These areas are broad to allow you to add to or delete from categories, since some areas of community life may be of more concern than others in health assessment.

Continued.

APPENDIX 3-1

University of Rochester School of Nursing: Categories for Recording Descriptive Community Data—cont'd

---

   B. Religion
     1. Locate churches, synagogues: How many are there, what condition are they in? Types?

   C. Recreation and entertainment
     1. Movie house, auditoriums
     2. Bars—how many are there?
     3. Recreational centers

   D. Health
     1. Services (clinics, hospitals, physicians)
     2. Status—do you get an overall impression of a "healthy" or "unhealthy" community? State rationale

   E. Communications
     1. Public (radio, television)
     2. Informal: note "hangouts" and which groups congregate

   F. Transportation and travel
     1. Availability and type of transportation

III. Government

   A. Note police protection: How are police transported?

Adapted from Christianson, JZ: A community data base record (unpublished master's thesis), Houston, Tx, 1977, The University of Texas Health Science Center. In Stein KZ and Eigsti DG: Utilizing a community data base system with community health nursing students, J Nurs Educ 21: 26–32 March 1982.

REFERENCES

AHA study reports changes, trends in 1980s, Reflects 16(2):3, 1990.

Allor MT: The "community profile," J Nurs Educ 22:12-17, 1983.

American Nurses' Association, Community Health Nursing Division: Conceptual model of community health nursing, Pub No CH-10, Kansas City, Mo, 1980, The Association.

American Public Health Association: Model standards: a guide for community preventive health services, ed 2, Washington, DC, 1985, The Association.

Anderson ET: Community focus in public health nursing: whose responsibility? Nurs Outlook 31:44-48, 1983.

Anderson ET, McFarlane J, and Helton A: Community-as-client: a model for practice, Nurs Outlook 34:220-224, 1986.

Archer SA: Marketing public health nursing services, Nurs Outlook 31:304-306, 1983.

Arensburg CM and Kimball ST: Culture and community, Gloucester, Ma, 1972, Peter Smith.

Chamberlin RW: Beyond individual risk assessment: community wide approaches to promoting the health and development of families and children—conference proceedings, Washington, DC, 1988, National Center for Education in Maternal and Child Health.

Christianson JZ: A community data base record, Houston, Tx, 1977, unpublished Master of Public Health thesis, University of Texas Health Science Center.

Committee for the Study of the Future of Public Health–Institute of Medicine: The future of public health, Washington, DC, 1988, National Academy Press.

Cottrell LS: The competent community. In Warren, RL, ed: New perspectives on the American community, ed 3, Chicago, 1977, Rand McNally, pp 546-560.

Cruise P and Storfjell J: The Storfjell-Cruise community focused model of community health nursing, unpublished master's thesis, Ann Arbor, 1980, University of Michigan.

Dean PD: Expanding our sights to include social networks, Nurs Health Care 7:545-550, 1986.

Duvall EM: Marriage and family development, ed 5, Philadelphia, 1977, Lippincott.

Erikson EH: Childhood and society, ed 2, New York, 1978, Norton.

Goeppinger J, Lassiter PG, and Wilcox B: Community health is community competence, Nurs Outlook 30:464-467, 1982.

Hamilton P: Community nursing diagnosis, Adv Nurs Sci 5(3):21-36, 1983.

Hanchett ES: Community health assessment, New York, 1979, Wiley.

Heller K: The return to community, Am J Community Psychol 17:1-15, 1989.

Higgs ZR and Gustafson DD: Community as a client: assessment and diagnosis, Philadelphia, 1985, FA Davis.

Hillery GA Jr: Definitions of community: areas of agreement, Rural Sociol 20(2):118-120, 1955.

Hunter A and Riger S: The meaning of community in community mental health, J Community Psychol 14:55-71, 1986.

Lyons L: Choosing the best approach to the community. In Warren RL and Lyon L, eds.: New perspectives on the American community, ed 5, Chicago, 1988, Dorsey Press, pp 87-96.

MacIver RM: Community, London, 1917, Macmillan.

MacIver RM and Page CH: Society: an introductory analysis, New York, 1949, Rinehart.

Martin A: Community assessment: the cornerstone of effective marketing, Pediatr Nurs 14:50-53, 1988.

McMillan DW and Chavis DM: Sense of community: a definition and theory, J Community Psychol 14:6-23, 1986.

Meneshian S: Nursing assessment of a community. In Caliandro G and Judkins B, eds: Primary nursing practice, Glenview, Il, 1988, Scott, Foresman, pp 111-118.

National Commission on Community Health Services: Health is a community affair, Cambridge, Ma, 1966, Harvard University Press.

National Organization for Public Health Nursing (NOPHN): Constitution of the National Organization for Public Health Nursing, Article 2, 1912, Wald: New York Public Library folder: NOPHN No. 1. In Fitzpatrick ML, ed: The National Organization for Public Health Nursing, 1912-1952: development of a practice field, New York, 1975, National League for Nursing.

Poplin DC: Communities: a survey of theories and methods of research, ed 2, New York, 1979, Macmillan.

Rauckhorst LM, Stokes SA, and Mezey MD: Community and home assessment, J Gerontol Nurs 6:319-327, 1980.

Reiss AJ: The sociological study of communities, Rural Soc, 24:118-127, 1959.

Rodgers SS: Community as client—a multivariate model for analysis of community and aggregate health risk, Public Health Nurs 1:210-222, 1984.

Ruffing-Rahal MA: Qualitative methods in community analysis, Public Health Nurs 2:130-137, 1985.

Ruffing-Rahal MA: Resident/provider contrasts in community health priorities, Public Health Nurs 4:242-246, 1987.

Ruybal SE, Bauwens E, and Fasla MJ: Community assessment: an epidemiological approach, Nurs Outlook 23:365-368, 1975.

Sanders IT: The community: an introduction to a social system, New York, 1958, Ronald Press.

Sanders IT: The community: structure and function, Nurs Outlook 11:642-645, 1963.

Sanders IT: The community: an introduction to a social system, ed 2, New York, 1966, Ronald Press.

Sanders IT: Public health in the community. In Freeman HE, Levine S, and Reeder LG, eds: Handbook of medical sociology, ed 2, Englewood Cliffs, NJ, 1972, Prentice Hall, pp 407–434.

Sanders IT: The community: an introduction to a social system, ed 3, New York, 1975, Ronald Press.

Sanders IT: Health in the community. In Freeman HE, Levine S, and Reeder LG, eds: Handbook of medical sociology, ed 3, Englewood Cliffs, NJ, 1979, Prentice Hall, pp. 412–433.

Selvy ML and Tuttle DM: Community health assessment and program planning in the nurse practitioner curriculum: evaluation of a guided design learning module, Public Health Nurs 4:160-165, 1987.

Shamansky SL and Pesznecker B: A community is . . . , Nurs Outlook 29:182-185, 1981.

Sills GM and Goeppinger J: The community as a field of inquiry in nursing. In Werly HH and Fitzpatrick JJ, eds: Annual Review of Nursing Research 3, New York, 1985, Springer, pp 4-23.

Smolensky J: Principles of community health, ed 6, Philadelphia, 1982, Saunders.

Stein KZ and Eigsti DG: Utilizing a community data base system with community health nursing students, J Nurs Educ 21:26-32, 1982.

Stein M: The eclipse of community. In Warren RL and Lyons L, eds: New perspectives on the American community, ed 5, Chicago, 1988, Dorsey Press, pp 120-127.

Turner JG and Chavigny KH: Community health nursing: an epidemiologic perspective through the nursing process, Philadelphia, 1988, Lippincott.

USDHHS: Health status of the disadvantaged chartbook, 1986, Washington, DC, 1986, US Government Printing Office.

Warren DI: Neighborhoods in urban areas. In Warren RL, ed: New perspectives on the Americam community, ed 3, Chicago, 1977, Rand McNally, pp 224–237.

Warren RL: Perspectives of the American community, Chicago, 1966, Rand McNally.

Warren RL: Toward a non-utopian normative model of community, Am Sociol Rev 35:219-228, 1970.

Warren RL, ed: New perspectives on the American community, ed 3, Chicago, 1977, Rand McNally.

Warren RL: The community in America, ed 3, Chicago, 1978, Rand McNally.

Warren RL: Observations on the state of community theory. In Warren RL and Lyon L, eds: New perspectives on the American community, ed 5, Chicago, 1988, Dorsey Press, pp 84-86.

Warren RL: The community in America, In Warren RL and Lyon L, eds: New perspectives on the American community, ed 5, Chicago, 1988, Dorsey Press, pp 152-157.

Warren RL: The good community—what would it be? In Warren RL and Lyon L, eds: New perspectives on the American community, ed 5, Chicago, 1988, Dorsey Press, pp 412-419.

Warren RL and Warren RB: Six kinds of neighborhoods, Psychol Today June:72-76, 1975.

Wellman B and Leighton B: Networks, neighborhoods, and communities: approaches to the study of the community question. In Warren RL and Lyon L, eds: New perspectives on the American community, Chicago, 1988, Dorsey Press, pp 57-72.

Williams CA: Community health nursing: what is it? Nurs Outlook 24:250-254, 1977.

World Health Organization: Community health nursing: report of a WHO expert committee, Technical Report Series No 558, Geneva, 1974, The Organization.

SELECTED BIBLIOGRAPHY

American Nurses' Association: A guide for community-based nursing services, Kansas City, 1985, The Association.

Archer SE and Fleshman RP: Community health nursing: a typology of practice, Nurs Outlook 23:358-364, 1975.

Buhler-Wilkerson K: Public health nursing: in sickness or in health? Am J Public Health 75:1155-1161, 1985.

Burbach CA and Brown BE: Community health and home health nursing: keeping the concepts clear, Nurs Health Care 9:97-100, 1988.

Colcord JC: Your community, New York, 1947, Russell Sage.

Eigsti DG, Stein KZ, and Fortune M: The community as client for continuity of care, Nurs Health Care 3:251, 1982.

Frost H: Nursing in sickness and in health: the social aspects of nursing, New York: 1939, Macmillan.

Goeppinger JE and Baglioni AJ Jr: Community competence: a positive approach to needs assessment, Am J Community Psychol 13:507-523, 1986.

McLaughlin JS: Toward a theoretical model for community health programs, Adv Nurs Sci 5(1):7-28, 1982.

Nisbet RA: The quest for community, New York, 1953, Oxford.

Steward M and White L: Nursing the community, Canad Nurse 77:32-33, 1981.

Storfjell JL and Cruise PA: A model of community-focused nursing, Public Health Nurs 1:85-96, 1984.

Vernon CL and D'Augelli AR: Community involvement in preventions: the use of a telephone survey for program development, Am J Community Psychol 15:23-28, 1987.

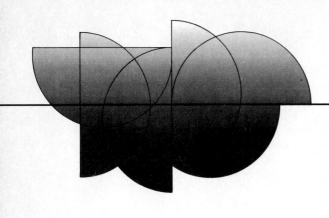

4

United States Health, Welfare, and Environmental Legislation and Services

OBJECTIVES

Upon completion of this chapter, the reader will be able to:

1. Summarize the development of health, welfare, and environmental policy and legislation in the United States.
2. Discuss the purpose and mandates of significant health, welfare, and environmental legislation in the United States.
3. Explain how the Social Security Act and the Public Health Service Act and their amendments have influenced health and welfare practices for a half of a century.
4. Discuss how health, welfare, and environmental legislation impacts on community health nursing practice.
5. Differentiate between voluntary and governmental health and welfare agencies.
6. Explain resources for health care financing in the United States.
7. Give an overview of the welfare system in the United States.

Health and welfare practices have evolved over the ages. It is known that as early as 1500 B.C. the Hebrews had a written hygienic code in Leviticus that dealt with personal and community hygiene (Pickett and Hanlon, 1990, p. 21). The Egyptians and Romans of 1000 B.C. had elaborate sewage, drainage, and water supply systems, provisions for keeping public streets clean, pharmaceutical preparations, surgical treatments, and rigorous personal hygiene measures.

Health, welfare, and environmental policies have continually changed to meet the demands and societal attitudes of the time. Throughout the history of public health, two major factors have determined how problems were solved: the level of scientific and technical knowledge, and the content of public values and popular opinions (Institute of Medicine, 1988, p. 1). Many of the major improvements in the health of the American people have been accomplished through public health measures such as the control of epidemic diseases, ensuring safe food and water, and maternal and child health services. These measures have prevented countless deaths and improved the quality of American life. Unfortunately, public health in the United States is often taken for granted, and areas where in the past we had made strides, such as infant mortality, are beginning to slip backward.

This chapter is designed to create an awareness of the historical evolution of the health and welfare systems and practices in the United States, as well as an understanding of current legislation, legislative trends, and existing health, welfare and environmental services and resources. The services discussed in this chapter are designed to assure Americans access to health care, provide an adequate standard of living and quality of life,

and protect them from the possibility of income loss as a result of old age, unemployment, illness, or disability. Nurses need to be familiar with these programs when they work with clients in the community.

Application of this information to community health nursing practice is discussed throughout the text; the organization of these services is discussed in Chapter 5.

An examination of the historical evolution of health, welfare, and environmental programs in the United States demonstrates that the development of these programs has largely been in response to specific problems rather than a preventive or national approach. Health, welfare, and environmental programs remain decentralized, operating at all levels of government and in the private sector.

EUROPEAN INFLUENCE ON UNITED STATES HEALTH, WELFARE, AND ENVIRONMENTAL POLICY

European influence has been singled out because of the significant impact it had on the development of United States health and welfare policy. Health and welfare policies in the United States reflect a background that is European, primarily English.

Europe was not always a pacesetter in health practices. Europeans of the Middle Ages chose to ignore many of the health practices of previous times and cultures. They allowed refuse to accumulate in streets and dwellings, dumped human waste into public water supplies, improperly stored and prepared foods, and often ignored personal hygiene. These practices did little to promote health, but did much to establish European trade routes as the demand for perfumes and spices rose.

During this time, epidemics of cholera, smallpox, typhoid, plague, and diphtheria raged. In the 1300s, bubonic plague came close to exterminating the human race, killing nearly one half of the world's population. Epidemics have never been seen since at such magnitude. There was little government intervention in matters of public

The authors are indebted to Professor Dorothy Donabedian, colleague and friend, whose efforts have stimulated both student and faculty awareness of the health and welfare systems, as they apply to community health nursing practice. Her enthusiasm, encouragement, and suggestions in this work have been greatly appreciated.

health, and the major impetus to the development of public health practices was the control of communicable disease.

During the Middle Ages (500-1350 A.D.) the belief in divine causation, that conditions reflect the will and judgment of God, flourished and greatly influenced the direction of health and welfare policies. Conditions such as poverty, illness, and disability were viewed as originating in divine causation rather than societal causation. The sick, disabled, and poor were largely ignored as a public responsibility. Self-help, the responsibility of individuals to care for themselves, was the prevailing policy, and poverty was often equated with crime. Beggars and vagrants could be physically punished or imprisoned. Welfare assistance was usually church sponsored rather than government sponsored. When assistance was given it was usually in the form of food, shelter, or both, rather than money. Government involvement in issues of health and welfare was more forced than voluntary, and usually came about as a corrective response to a problem rather than as a primary preventive approach. Economic depressions, wars, natural disasters, epidemics, threat of government overthrow, and mass public indignation have played an important role in shaping public policy making. It was an economic depression that brought about the Elizabethan Poor Law of 1601.

The Elizabethan Poor Law of 1601

A severe economic depression spurred the enactment of the Elizabethan Poor Law of 1601. Large-scale, involuntary unemployment and the fear of insurrection stimulated the government to provide welfare aid for select persons (Coll, 1969, p. 5). This law granted the right to assistance through taxation, and established three major categories of dependent people: the vagrant, the involuntarily unemployed, and the helpless (Coll, 1971, p. 5). The helpless included widows, the disabled, and dependent children. The last two categories were deemed as the "worthy" poor. Poor law concepts included:

1. *Local administration.* It was the responsibility of local government to aid and support those in need. The locality decided on the amount and type of aid to be given and who would receive it. Aid was often administered through the church.
2. *General aid.* Aid was usually available to the worthy poor, and others could be jailed or physically punished.
3. *Responsible relative.* Relatives could be held responsible for the financial support of each other.
4. *Restrictive residence.* The locality of the individual's origin was responsible for the financial support of the individual. An indigent who migrated from his or her locality of origin could be returned to it.
5. *Individual means test.* Aid was administered on an individual basis through determination of means and needs. Local jurisdictions exercised the right to use moral qualifications to determine who was worthy of assistance.
6. *Minimal subsistence.* A recipient was to receive no more assistance than what was necessary to exist.
7. *Compulsory work or service.* Work or service by the recipient was often compulsory to obtain assistance, and refusal to work could be a punishable crime. Workhouses for the indigent were commonplace.
8. *Funding through taxation.* Funds to administer the poor law were raised through local taxes.

The Elizabethan Poor Law was a forerunner of United States welfare policy, and all of the original 13 colonies adopted it in some form. Following poor law tradition, the United States left administration of assistance programs largely under local control, implemented responsible relative clauses, administered means tests, provided only minimal subsistence, encouraged or mandated work or service, imposed restrictive residency, and derived welfare revenues through taxation. Restrictive residency laws are now unconstitutional in the United States. However, most original poor law concepts are still evident in our health and welfare policy.

THE DEVELOPMENT OF UNITED STATES HEALTH, WELFARE, AND ENVIRONMENTAL POLICY

The concepts of divine causation, self-help, minimal government intervention, and control of communicable disease prevailed in the United States. The word *health* was left out of the United States constitution, and each state was made responsible for legislating its own health law. Federal intervention in public health and welfare assistance programs was almost nonexistent in early U.S. history. When government health, welfare and environmental programs existed, they were largely administered by the individual states.

A forerunner to U.S. health, welfare, and environment policy was a report written in England in the seventeenth century. In 1832, the British Parliament appointed a royal commission to revise the poor law, and in 1834 the revisions were implemented. Edwin Chadwick was a member of this commission and later, in 1842, he published the *Report of the Labouring Population and on the Means of Its Improvement.* It detailed the unsanitary conditions under which the laborers lived, the lack of proper refuse disposal, contaminated water supplies, and generally poor living conditions. He cited these conditions as the primary reasons for public health problems, such as high morbidity and mortality rates, rather than divine causation. Chadwick's report helped to bring about the passage of the English Public Health Act of 1848.

The *Shattuck Report*

A major impetus to developing United States public health policy was the *Shattuck Report,* written in 1850 by Lemuel Shattuck, a teacher, statistician, and legislator. This report recommended such measures as the creation of state and local boards of health; collection of vital statistics; supervision of housing, factories, sanitation, and foods; procurement of immunizations; community health control measures; and school health and health education (Pickett and Hanlon, 1990, p. 31). The majority of Shattuck's recom-

mendations are accepted today as sound public health practice.

Before the *Shattuck Report,* local boards of health had begun to emerge in the United States. Some of the earliest of these were in Baltimore, Maryland (1798); Charleston, South Carolina (1815); Philadelphia, Pennsylvania (1818); and Providence, Rhode Island (1832). Following the Shattuck Report, the number of boards of health expanded. In 1869 Massachusetts established the first state board of health in line with Shattuck's recommendations (Pickett and Hanlon, 1990, p. 32). These local boards of health were the forerunners of today's health departments.

At the time of Shattuck's report, institutions and almshouses (poorhouses) were the major form of welfare assistance in this country. These residential placements served to separate the poor, disabled, frail elderly, and ill from the mainstream of the population. Many people who were mentally ill or mentally retarded were placed in institutions. These institutions are still a part of our country's health and welfare tradition. The constitutionality of institutional placements for individuals, such as people who are mentally retarded, is being challenged in the U.S. court system.

The years following Shattuck's report saw significant strides worldwide in health theory and practice: Disease conditions were recognized and differentiated; the sciences of bacteriology, virology, immunology, and pharmacology emerged; antibiotics and sterile techniques were developed; the importance of vectors in disease transmission and control became known; and advanced training for health professionals was expanded.

Development of Voluntary Agencies

When the term *voluntary* is used in relation to health, welfare, and environmental services it can be somewhat confusing. *Voluntary* refers to private, nonprofit resources that are not under the auspices of federal, state, or local government; are not tax supported; have no legal powers; and rely heavily on donations, endowments, grants, and fee-for-service as funding mechanisms. Voluntary resources traditionally represent people doing for people and a willingness to share with others. These resources usually have a large volunteer staff.

Voluntary agencies have a long history. By the 1870s voluntary agencies were beginning to emerge and to work with America's health and welfare and environmental problems. In 1872, the American Public Health Association (APHA) was founded by Dr. Stephen Smith. This voluntary health association was and is concerned with protecting and promoting the health of the nation.

In 1882, one of our country's best known voluntary organizations, the American Red Cross, was founded by Clara Barton. In 1892 the Anti-Tuberculosis Society of Philadelphia, a forerunner of today's American Lung Association, was established. Other voluntary organizations continued to develop.

In 1877, the first charity organization society was founded in Buffalo, New York, to coordinate private, voluntary (nonprofit) welfare assistance activities. Similar organizations began to develop in other cities. By the early twentieth century, groups such as the Rockefeller Foundation, the Commonwealth Foundation, and the Kellogg Foundation were established as private, voluntary health and welfare organizations. At the time of this writing, private profit-making health insurance programs were emerging as well (refer to Figure 4-1). Today there are more than 165,000 voluntary health, welfare, and environmental organizations in the United States, and estimates have gone as high as 785,000 (Tropman and Tropman, 1987, p. 829).

Voluntary organizations and individuals are an integral part of our health and welfare services. This voluntary tradition is to be applauded. Voluntary resources are discussed in Chapter 5.

The Volunteer Tradition

The American volunteer tradition has very early roots. Many of the founding fathers of America were trying to break from the traditional and sometimes oppressive influences of church and

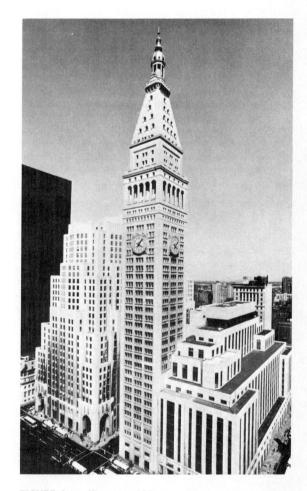

FIGURE 4-1 "For over 100 years, Metropolitan Life has been unique in performing a public health service in an insurance company setting. Its efforts have included the promotion of health and safety through publications, films, filmstrips, TV and radio, as well as demonstration projects, research and consultation and cooperation with local, state and national health organizations, both voluntary and governmental. Through the years, as various public health problems were brought under control and others arose, the Company's programs changed to meet the current health challenge." (Metropolitan Life Insurance Company: Brief History of Metropolitan Life's Health and Safety Activities 1871-1983, New York, 1983 Metropolitan Life Insurance. Photo courtesy of Metropolitan Life Insurance.)

state from which they came. They were often mistrustful of governmental intervention into matters of personal health and welfare. Even had they wanted governmental help, there was little to be had in the new and expanding nation. People helped each other, charities developed, and voluntary organizations began to emerge. The United States went through what is termed by some the "voluntaristic period," which fit into the time between the Civil War and 1935. It was during this time period that many voluntary resources were founded. The passage of the Social Security Act of 1935 signaled governmental involvement in the provision of health and welfare services, and eliminated some of the need for voluntary programs (Tropman and Tropman, 1987, p. 827).

The volunteer tradition has existed since the beginnings of our country and is very important to American voluntary service agencies. Voluntary agencies typically have an active volunteer staff. However, governmental and proprietary agencies all across the country also utilize volunteers.

Volunteers are frequently the backbone of a voluntary agency. They provide direct services, promote change, act as advocates, serve on boards of directors, and assist administration. They are involved in many activities including telephone services, newsletters, transportation, public relations, fund-raising, and recruiting. It is estimated that over 92 million American adults are involved in volunteering each year (Manser, 1987, pp. 842-846).

Unfortunately, negative relationships between volunteers and professionals are often the greatest barrier to the effective use of volunteers (Manser, 1987, p. 846). Nurses should be aware of this when they utilize volunteer services, and should promote an environment which fosters positive professional relationships with these workers. Volunteers provide many important services that could not be provided otherwise, or could only be provided otherwise at great time and expense. There is a great need to keep this volunteer tradition alive in the United States.

Establishing Government Involvement in the Delivery of Health, Welfare, and Environmental Services

Under the U.S. Constitution issues of health and welfare were left primarily to the states. Federal involvement in these issues emerged slowly and cautiously. Major federal legislation began to emerge in the early 1900s.

The U.S. Public Health Service was established in 1798. In 1879, the National Board of Health, forerunner of the Department of Health, Education, and Welfare, was established. In 1912, the United States enacted a Public Health Act. Still, involvement by the federal government in public health and welfare was minimal, and health and welfare services were largely left to the states. The system of federal grant-in-aid to states originated in 1919 and supplied revenue to states for health and welfare programs.

By 1919, all states had a government branch dealing with health, often known as the state department of public health (Smolensky, 1977, p. 168). State public health programs focused on the control of communicable disease and maternal-child health problems. Also by this time, many states had a government branch dealing with welfare, often a state department of social services. State welfare assistance programs largely focused on providing services to widows, dependent children, and the indigent elderly. State welfare insurance programs, in the form of workers' compensation, began to evolve in 1911. State and local taxes comprised the major source of revenue for health and welfare assistance programs.

The Great Depression

The Great Depression started with the stock market crash of 1929 and reached a peak in 1933 when 13 million persons, 25 percent of the work force, were unemployed, and 19 million persons were on state relief rolls. Neither privately nor government-funded health and welfare programs could handle the health and welfare demands created by this event, and possibly no other single event has had such an impact on U.S. health and welfare policy. The Depression showed the general public that anyone could become poor. It dealt a mortal blow to the belief of divine causation, because many people whom the general public believed were not deserving of poverty became impoverished. There was considerable public pressure for the federal government to assist those in need.

A major concern that developed as a result of the Depression was the large, young, unemployed labor force. New jobs were hard to generate, and many jobs were held by older workers with seniority. There was no mandatory retirement age, and there were few retirement pension plans. The idea of mandatory retirement of workers with the retiree being eligible for a government pension emerged. The federal government needed to assist the states in meeting these needs.

The Social Security Act of 1935

Out of the Depression, and under the presidency of Franklin D. Roosevelt, came the federal Social Security Act of 1935. For the first time, major welfare programs were consolidated under one law (Donabedian, 1990). The passage of the Social Security Act gave the United States the dubious distinction of being the last of the major industrial nations to develop a federal welfare program (Institute of Gerontology, 1970, p. 2).

The Social Security Act established insurance programs (contributory) and assistance programs (noncontributory). Contributory programs are financed through both taxation and individual contributions, whereas assistance programs are financed only through taxation. It is a landmark piece of legislation, possibly the most important one of our time. Since 1935, the Social Security Act has been amended numerous times to incorporate other health and welfare programs.

Environmental Health

Although the *Shattuck Report* identified in 1850 a need for improved sanitation, the federal, state and local governments were slow to become involved in environmental health issues. When legislation was enacted it was usually remedial instead of preventive in nature. Early federal laws included the Water Pollution Control Act (Public Law 80-845) in 1948, the Air Pollution Control Act (Public Law 84-159) in 1955, the Clean Air Act (Public Law 88-206) in 1963, the Solid Waste Disposal Act (Public Law 89-272) in 1965, and the National Environmental Policy Act (Public Law 91-190) in 1969. The recency of these early laws clearly illustrates how long it took for our country to become actively involved in environmental health issues.

UNITED STATES HEALTH, WELFARE, AND ENVIRONMENTAL LEGISLATION

Each year many laws with health, welfare, and environmental implications are enacted, and many existing laws are amended. Health and welfare legislation should be examined and understood in terms of its administration, funding, services offered, clients served, service delivery, and quality control. An in-depth perspective on laws can be obtained by reading materials specific to each piece of legislation in the *United States Code— Congressional and Administrative News* and the *United States Statutes at Large.* This type of information is needed in order for the community health nurse to effectively help clients to obtain services available to them, as well as to identify gaps in the delivery of health and welfare services. When gaps or deficiencies are identified, the community health nurse utilizes the principles of health planning to correct these problems (refer to Chapter 12).

Administration of Health, Welfare, and Environmental Legislation

The organization of health, welfare, and environmental resources and services is discussed in depth in Chapter 5. It is a complicated system, but one with which the community health nurse should be familiar in order to facilitate the utilization of services by clients.

Health, welfare, and environmental legislation is administered through many offices, staffs, agencies, and departments of government. The responsibility to carry out this legislation is often as much a matter of historical development and organizational relationships as it is of rational decision making (Wilner, Walkley, and O'Neill, 1978, p. 34). Most federal health and welfare legislation is administered by the U.S. Department of Health and Human Services (USDHHS), formerly the Department of Health, Education, and Welfare. Most federal environmental health legislation is administered by the Environmental Protection Agency.

Health, welfare, and environmental administration varies in each state; it is not always identical to the federal system of administration. Some states have "super agencies," much like the Department of Health and Human Services, that incorporate a variety of health and welfare programs. Other states separate health and welfare components and administer them through separate agencies. State welfare services are often administered by a department of human or social services; health services are often administered by a department of public health. State governments must adhere to federal health, welfare, and environmental law.

Local health and welfare administration, agencies, ordinances, rules, and codes will vary. However, local governments must adhere to state and federal laws. If a locality is unable or refuses to enforce health and welfare law, the state can assist the locality in enforcement or assume control itself.

Major United States Health, Welfare, and Environmental Legislation

Several acts of legislation had a major impact on the development of health, welfare, and environmental policy and practices in the United States. The nurse needs to be aware of this legislation because it has significant impact on the resources and services in this country.

The Social Security Act of 1935 and the Public Health Service Act of 1944 are two of the most significant pieces of U.S. legislation enacted. Many newer laws are amendments to these two acts, and a large number of the health and welfare resources that the community health nurse will utilize on behalf of clients relate to them. When examining the legislation presented, please note that federal laws are designated *public law* and are followed by the number of the congressional session and the sequential number of the law.

Social Security Act of 1935 (Public Law 74-721) as Amended

The Social Security Act of 1935 provided for the general welfare by establishing a system of federal old-age benefits, and by enabling the states to make adequate provision for aged persons, blind persons, dependent and crippled children, maternal and child welfare, public health, and the administration of state unemployment compensation laws. This act established a Social Security Board and mechanisms for raising revenue for retirement income and welfare purposes.

The Social Security Act was a giant step toward safeguarding the health and welfare of Americans. When the act was passed in 1935, it included both welfare insurance and welfare assistance programs. Originally its *welfare insurance* programs included the federal program of old age insurance (OAI) and the state-federal program of unemployment insurance. Its categorical *welfare assistance* programs were originally the federal-state programs of Aid to the Blind (AB), Old Age Assistance (OAA), and Aid to Dependent Children (ADC). It also provided funds for services to crippled children and high-risk mothers and children. In 1939, the Act was amended to provide for Survivors Insurance (OASI); in 1950, to provide Aid to the Permanently and Totally Disabled (APTD); and in 1956, to include Disability Insurance (OASDI). Medicare and Medicaid were added to the act in 1965; in 1988 Medicare Catastrophic Health Insurance was added to Medicare coverage; this coverage was repealed in 1989.

Appendix 4-1 chronologically summarizes some of the major amendments to the Social Security Act and the purpose of the amendments. When nurses examine new legislation, they will find that it is often an amendment to an existing law rather than an entirely new law. It is important to note amendments because they can significantly alter a law.

TABLE 4-1 Some major Social Security Act programs and their source of administration

	Type of programs		
Type of benefits	Federal programs*	State-federal programs†	Federal-state programs‡
Welfare insurance (cash benefit)	Old Age, Survivors, and Disability Insurance (OASDI)	Unemployment Insurance [Department of Labor, Department of the Treasury]	None
Welfare assistance (cash benefit)	None	Aid to Families of Dependent Children (AFDC) [Social Security Administration]	Supplemental Security Income (SSI)
Health insurance	1. Medicare A— hospital insurance, prepaid through social security contributions 2. Medicare B— medical insurance, individual premium required	None	None
Health assistance	None	1. Medicaid [Health Care Financing Administration] 2. Miscellaneous maternal and child health programs (i.e., services to crippled children, PRESCAD)	None

*Administered *federally* through the Social Security Administration and/or the Health Care Financing Administration.

†Administered through the *state* government. Federal sharing agency may be indicated in brackets by program.

‡Administered federally through the Social Security Administration. State sharing agency or agencies will vary in each state.

NOTE: Programs such as workers' compensation, general assistance, and food stamps are not provided for under the Social Security Act of 1935 and are discussed later in this chapter.

Today, nearly every American family is involved with the Social Security Act in some form. Employers, employees, and the self-employed pay into the insurance programs of the act, and almost 90 percent of all United States workers contribute to these programs. The social security insurance protection (OASDI) earned by a worker stays with the worker and his or her family even in a new job or residence. The contributions made by a worker determine eligibility and the amount of benefits. When the contributing worker's earnings stop or are substantially reduced because of retirement, disability, or death, insurance benefits can be paid to the worker or qualifying survivors. The worker or survivors must apply for these benefits in order to obtain them.

Table 4-1 summarizes the health and welfare insurance and assistance programs of the Social Security Act. Determination of eligibility for social security assistance programs is handled through a number of federal, state, and local agencies. Determining social security insurance eligibility is handled through local branches of the federal Social Security Administration. Social Security Administration offices are located throughout the country and representatives are sent to communities in which there are no offices. Applications for the insurance programs of Old

Age, Survivors, and Disability Insurance (OASDI) and Medicare, as well as the assistance program of Supplemental Security Income (SSI) can be made at these offices. One should contact the office in advance to determine what information is necessary to complete the application.

Public Health Service Act of 1944 (Public Law 78-410) as Amended

The Public Health Service Act of 1944 consolidated and revised the laws relating to the Public Health Service and has since served to consolidate national public health legislation. It is the major piece of health legislation in the country, but does *not* have administration over the health programs, Medicaid and Medicare, of the Social Security Act.

This act incorporates legislation on health care personnel, health facility construction and modernization, and services to specific population groups. Over the years, this law has been frequently amended (refer to Appendix 4-2) to provide financing for traineeships for health care professionals (nurse training acts and traineeships for graduate students in public health); grants-in-aid to schools of public health; construction of community mental health centers and facilities; national comprehensive health planning and resource development; the development of health maintenance organizations (HMOs); health services for migratory workers; family planning services and communicable disease control; emergency medical services; and research and facilities for the prevention and control of conditions such as heart disease, cancer, stroke, kidney disease, sudden infant death syndrome, arthritis, Cooley's anemia, sickle-cell anemia, and diabetes mellitus. Amendments such as the Heart Disease, Cancer, and Stroke Amendments gave research and service priority to some of the leading causes of death in this country. Recent amendments have dealt with services to AIDS victims.

Areas covered by the Public Health Services Act are broad and comprehensive. Many of them (e.g., chronic disease, communicable disease, and family planning) should be known to community health nurses who work with them extensively.

Civil Rights Act of 1964 (Public Law 88-352)

Most states and many municipalities have enacted civil rights laws that forbid discrimination and ensure constitutional rights. Federal civil rights legislation has existed in the United States since the early civil rights legislation of the Reconstruction era, enacted in 1866, 1870, and 1871. Four major contemporary civil rights acts were enacted in 1957, 1960, 1964, and 1968. In 1980 the Civil Rights of Institutionalized Persons Act (Public Law 96-247) was enacted.

Of all the civil rights legislation, the Civil Rights Act of 1964 is frequently considered to be the most significant; it was designed to ensure fair and equal treatment for all. The act forbade discrimination on the basis of race or sex in public accommodations, public facilities, and public education. It also enforced the constitutional right to vote. In addition, it established a Commission on Equal Employment Opportunity and attempted to ensure fair employment practices. The original act covered private employers but not government employers. The act was amended in 1972 to cover public employees. Since 1972, if a state or local government is found to be practicing discrimination, the federal Attorney General can sue to have that state's revenue-sharing funds cut off. More recently the Civil Rights Restoration Act of 1987 (Public Law 100-259) has attempted to restore, clarify, and enlarge the broad scope of coverage of the Civil Rights Act of 1964 and the other civil rights statutes.

Economic Opportunity Act of 1964 (Public Law 88-452)

The Economic Opportunity Act of 1964 was designed to mobilize the human and financial resources of the nation to combat poverty. It included work training and study programs, established the Office of Economic Opportunity, authorized Volunteers in Service to America (VISTA), the Job Corps, Upward Bound, Neighborhood Youth Corps, Head Start, neighborhood health centers, and community action programs. An impetus to antipoverty programs, it also incorporated urban and rural community action programs and assistance to small businesses and work experience programs. The future of Public Law 88-452 is now questionable.

Older Americans Act of 1965 (Public Law 89-73)

This act was passed to provide assistance in the development of programs to help older Americans. It provided grants to states for community planning and services and for training and research in the field of gerontology and aging. It established the Administration on Aging which is now located in the Department of Health and Human Services. This act gave national attention to the needs of the elderly and facilitated state and area planning on the needs of this population group. It established state and local agencies on aging.

The purpose of the act was to assist older Americans in securing equal opportunity to the full and free enjoyment of the following objectives:

1. An adequate income in retirement in accordance with the American standard of living
2. The best possible physical and mental health which science can make available, and without regard to economic status
3. Suitable housing, independently selected, designed, and located with reference to special needs and available at costs which older citizens can afford
4. Full restorative services for those who require institutional care
5. Opportunity for employment with no discriminatory personnel practices because of age
6. Retirement in health, honor, dignity—after years of contribution to the economy
7. Pursuit of meaningful activity within the widest range of civic, cultural, and recreational opportunities
8. Efficient community services which provide social assistance in a coordinated manner and which are readily available when needed
9. Immediate benefit from proven research knowledge which can sustain and improve health and happiness and
10. Freedom, independence, and the free ex-

ercise of individual initiative in planning and managing their own lives.

Over the years, the act has been amended to include senior work and volunteer programs, senior nutrition and social programs, health education, preventive health, in-home health care and multipurpose senior centers. This act is a major piece of legislation relating to services for seniors in the United States. Appendix 4-3 presents some significant amendments to this act.

Occupational Safety and Health Act of 1970 (Public Law 91-956)

The Occupational Safety and Health Act is the most comprehensive piece of legislation on occupational health and safety in the United States. Championed by organized labor, its intent is to protect the health of the worker, and it made worker health a public concern. The United States was the last major industrial nation to enact such a law; this act is discussed in depth in Chapter 16.

Rehabilitation Act of 1973 (Public Law 93-112)

The Vocational Rehabilitation Act of 1920 (Public Law 66-236) was an outgrowth of the health care needs evidenced by veterans after World War I. A forerunner of the 1973 act, it provided training for the physically handicapped and was one of the first federal-state grant-in-aid programs to be established. The Rehabilitation Act of 1973 replaced the 1920 act but retained its major components. This new act extended and revised the authorization of grants to states for vocational rehabilitation services; emphasized services to those with severe handicaps; expanded federal responsibilities and training programs; defined services necessary for rehabilitation programs; established the National Architectural and Transportation Barriers Board to enforce legislation designed to remove architectural barriers for the handicapped; and began affirmative action programs to facilitate employment of the handicapped. Its ultimate goal is to help persons become productive members of society. The Rehabilitation Act Amendments of 1974 (Public Law 93-516) transferred the Rehabilitation Services Administration to the Department of Health, Education and Welfare, strengthened services for the blind, and authorized a White House Conference on Handicapped Persons. (This act is discussed further in Chapter 17.)

Education for All Handicapped Children Act of 1975 (Public Law 94-142)

This act amended the Education of the Handicapped Act (Public Law 90-247). Through it, the federal government took an active role in ensuring the educational rights of people who are handicapped. The law helps to provide free, public education for handicapped children (refer to Chapters 13 and 14). Before the passage of this law, many children in the United States who were handicapped had been denied access to the public educational system. Recently, the government has tried to deregulate the act and to become less involved in protecting the educational rights of handicapped persons. Active lobbying by parent groups and professionals has prevented this.

Omnibus Budget Reconciliation Act of 1981 (Public Law 97-35)

This was a major cost containment law. It has a great impact on services provided by health, welfare, and environmental programs in the United States. It mandated cost containment in aspects of government including taxation, government operations, health and human services, veterans' affairs, consumer affairs, labor/employment, transportation, communications, energy, environment, agriculture, foreign, and military operations. The massive cutbacks in public spending will need to be monitored in the coming years to ascertain that needs of at-risk groups are not being neglected.

This act also provided for *block grants* and reduced the number of categorical aid programs. Block grants to states give the states increased flexibility in the manner in which money is spent, but they place individual programs and agencies in competition with one another for funding. This act places more responsibility on the states and localities for program provision.

Comprehensive Smokeless Tobacco Health Education Act of 1986 (Public Law 99-252)

This public law established and implemented a program of public education about the dangers to human health resulting from the use of smokeless tobacco products. It legislated the development of educational programs and materials and public service announcements and made these available to states, local governments, schools, media, and interested others; and established grants to state and local governments to assist in program development and implementation. The act supported research on the effects of smokeless tobacco on human health. It provided regulations for the labeling of smokeless tobacco products and for the advertising of such products. This act followed the historic Public Health Cigarette Smoking Act of 1969 (Public Law 91-222), which informed the American public of the hazards of cigarette smoking, required that a health warning be placed on each package of cigarettes sold in the United States, and banned, as of January 1, 1971, advertising of cigarettes by any electronic medium of communication subject to jurisdiction of the Federal Communications Commission. That is why we do not see or hear cigarette ads on American radio or TV today.

Consolidated Omnibus Budget Reconciliation Act of 1985 [COBRA] (Public Law 99-272)

This act contained many Medicaid and Medicare amendments. A significant change in regard to public health is that it makes available Medicaid coverage to low-income pregnant women in two-parent families and thereby increases their opportunities for obtaining appropriate prenatal and postnatal care (refer to Appendix 4-1).

Omnibus Budget Reconciliation Act of 1986 [OBRA] (Public Law 99-509)

This act contained several Medicaid and Medicare amendments. Of significant interest to public health was the change in Medicaid to allow states the option of expanding Medicaid coverage to pregnant women, infants up to age 1, and children up to age 5 whose family incomes were below the federal poverty level. The act also required states to continue Medicaid coverage to disabled individuals who lost their eligibility for SSI as a result of work earnings, and clarified Medicaid coverage for the homeless (refer to Appendix 4-1).

Stewart B. McKinney Homeless Assistance Act (Public Law 100-77)

This important and comprehensive act dealt with the increasing problem of homelessness in American society and provided urgently needed assistance to protect and improve the lives and safety of the homeless, with special emphasis on elderly persons, handicapped persons, and families with children. It established the Interagency Council on the Homeless, Emergency Food and Shelter Program National Board, Emergency Food and Shelter Grants, Supportive Housing Demonstration Program, Primary Health Services and Substance Abuse Services Grant Program, and Food Assistance for the Homeless Food Stamp Program. It authorized emergency food supplies for the homeless, HUD programs for emergency shelter, supportive housing, programs for primary health care, substance abuse services, community mental health care, adult education for the homeless, education for homeless children and youth, job training for the homeless, and studies of youth homeless and native American homeless.

Medicare Catastrophic Coverage Act of 1988 (Public Law 100-360)

This act was a monumental piece of health legislation. In recognition of the rising costs of health care, and the economically devastating impact catastrophic health care can bring, this act attempted to protect the elderly against catastrophic health care expenses under Medicare. It was financed through an increase in the part B premium and an income-related supplemental surtax. From the beginning, the act met with much resistance, even though it had the backing of such major organizations as the American Association of Retired Persons (AARP). This act was *repealed* in 1989 largely as a result of senior citizens objections to the surtax. However, many national organizations still recognize the need to provide cat-

astrophic health care coverage for the elderly. Presently, the provisions of Medicare coverage are in a state of change. Information about changes on Medicare benefits can be obtained by contacting a local Social Security office. Appendix 4-1 presents an overview of the act.

Family Support Act of 1988 (Public Law 100-485)

This act is said to have overhauled and reformed the federal welfare system. It established the first federal requirement that welfare recipients seek employment, and revised the AFDC program to emphasize that requirement. It provided a federal mechanism for enforcement of child support orders (refer to Appendix 4-1).

Health Omnibus Programs Extension of 1988 (Public Law 100-607)

This act extended and revised all major sections of the Public Health Service Act of 1944. Included in the act were the National Institute on Deafness and Other Communication Disorders and Health Resource Extension Act of 1988, Organ Transplant Amendments of 1988, AIDS Amendments of 1988, and the Health Professions Reauthorization Act of 1988. This act created Title XXIV-Health Services with Respect to Acquired Immune Deficiency Syndrome in the Public Health Service Act (refer to Appendix 4-2).

Environmental Health Legislation

Environmental health legislation cannot be classified under *one* specific federal law. Thus, management of environmental health issues becomes very complicated. Appendix 4-4 summarizes the major environmental health legislation.

Environmental health legislation is diverse and encompasses such areas as Superfund funding (the fund created to finance the cleanup of spills of hazardous substances and leaking hazardous wastes), water quality, air quality, toxic substances in the environment, pesticides, soil conservation, solid waste disposal, radiation, ocean dumping, environmental research and program development, noise pollution, endangered species, and nuclear waste.

The National Environmental Policy Act (Public Law 91-190) is one of the most significant and best-known, pieces of U.S. environmental health legislation. From this legislation the Environmental Protection Agency evolved. Unfortunately, even major environmental health legislation contains significant gaps and enforcement problems. For example, the basic purpose of the Clean Air Act of 1970 was to protect and enhance the quality of the Nation's air resources in order to promote public health, welfare, and productive capacity. While long-term emissions of air pollutants have been reduced under this act, over 100 areas, mostly large cities, did not meet the August 31, 1988, deadline to attain ambient air quality standards (Courpas, 1988, MLC-035). There are still many major issues not covered under this act such as acid rain, hazardous air pollutants, indoor air pollution, and ozone depletion (Courpas, 1988, MLC-035). Appendix 4-4 presents an overview of environmental health legislation in the United States, and environmental health is discussed in Chapter 5.

State Workers' Compensation Acts

The state workers' compensation acts are the oldest form of government *health* and *welfare* insurance in this country. The first act was legislated in 1911, and by 1948 all states had such acts.

In 26 states workers' compensation laws are administered by the state labor department or other relevant agencies, in 20 states the law is administered by an independent workers' compensation agency, and court administration exists in 4 states (Nelson, 1989, Social Security, p. 34).

Approximately 87 percent of the U.S. work force—88.4 million employees—is covered by workers' compensation legislation (Nelson, 1989, Workers' compensation, p. 32). Employees most likely to be excluded from coverage are domestic workers, agricultural workers, railroad employees, seamen in the U.S. Merchant Marine, and casual laborers; and coverage is incomplete among workers in small firms, nonprofit organizations, and state and local government (Nelson, 1989, Social Security, p. 28; Nelson, 1989, Workers' compensation, p. 35). Workers' compensation benefits in excess of $25 billion are awarded each year (Nelson, 1989, Workers' compensation, pp. 34-35; Nelson, 1989, Social Security, p. 28).

Workers' compensation provides *cash benefits* and *health care* to workers and cash benefits to their dependents when the worker suffers a work-related injury or disability (permanent or temporary) or dies. There are no mandatory standards for state workers' compensation legislation, and programs vary greatly from one state to another in relation to the amount of cash benefits and health care services provided. All compensation acts require that medical care be furnished to injured workers without delay. There is no limit placed on the amount of medical care that can be received when accidental injuries are involved, but there may be limits placed on the amount of medical services available for occupational disease, dental care, or prostheses. In some states the employee has the right to choose his or her own physician under workers' compensation and in others the employee must choose from a designated list. All workers' compensation programs provide for physical rehabilitation when needed.

Compensation is awarded regardless of who is at fault for the occurrence; this no-fault principle precludes legal suits against employers when the acquired injury, illness, disability, or death is covered under the workers' compensation program. The employer is liable for the cost of the program.

Employers are allowed to self-insure, contract with private insurance providers, or purchase a policy with the state-operated insurance fund (Nelson, 1989, Workers' compensation, p. 36). Private insurance is the popular method of worker's compensation insurance. In 1986, $13.8 billion was paid for workers' compensation through private insurance, $6.4 billion through public funds, and $4.8 billion through self-insurance (Nelson, 1989, Workers' compensation, p. 36).

The amount of the compensation awarded to the worker is related to the degree and permanence of the injury as well as the number of the worker's dependents (Wilner, Walkley, and O' Neill, 1978, p. 152). In some cases, if the worker is injured but suffers no loss of ability to work, such as in the case of certain types of hearing loss, the injury may not be compensated. Loss of ability to work is generally a criterion for awarding a workers' compensation claim. If a worker is able to return to work, the compensation award is usually discontinued or substantially reduced. Workers may receive benefits only for a specified period of time, or for a specific monetary amount even if the disability is permanent. Workers are often subject to waiting periods before the compensation award can begin.

Each state sets a minimum and maximum payment range for workers' compensation benefits. The median maximum weekly benefit amount for temporary total disability was $340 in 1988, with the maximum weekly (excluding dependents' allowances) ranging from $175 to $1094 (Nelson, 1989, Social security, p. 30). Minimum cash benefits are as low as $20 weekly in Arkansas.

The amount a worker receives under workers' compensation is often considerably less than the wage received prior to work disability. Workers' maximum wage replacement under worker's compensation averages about 67 percent of their previous take-home pay before taxes. This reduction in pay can cause financial hardship for a family in addition to all the other adjustments the family is making in relation to the disability. The nurse should be aware that some disabled workers and their families may also be eligible for benefits under other programs, including Old Age, Survivors, and Disability Insurance (OASDI), and Supplemental Security Income (SSI).

THE UNITED STATES HEALTH CARE SYSTEM

Silver (1974) provides what is possibly the best description of health care in America by utilizing the following passage from the *Book of Common Prayer:*

We have left undone those things which we ought to have done and we have done those things which we ought not to have done, and there is no health in us.

In the United States, comprehensive health services exist, but they are unequally distributed, fragmented, expensive, and often of questionable quality. Almost any type of health care service is available in the United States, but often these services are neither accessible nor affordable. Health care resources and services are found in both government (official) and private sectors. There is often little coordination between health care resources, and there is great complexity and diversity in the United States health care delivery system. Although diversity can be advantageous, it also presents major problems when one is attempting to coordinate available services and resources.

For a variety of reasons (discussed in Chapter 9 under barriers to utilization of resources), many people are not making use of available health resources. Free or low-cost immunization clinics are numerous in this country, yet many children and adults are not immunized or are inadequately immunized. Preventive and early health care is available, but many people do not utilize it. Of the approximately one-half million Americans who die of cancer each year, it is estimated that 178,000 could have been saved if they had had early diagnosis and treatment (American Cancer Society, 1989, p. 3). Prevention and early diagnosis are too important to be ignored. Yet, health care is sought and offered in this country largely on a treatment basis rather than on a preventive one. Despite these and other discrepancies in health care theory and practice, Americans are among the healthiest people in the world. The average life expectancy of Americans continues to increase, the death rate is historically low, and the infant mortality rate continues to decline. Sometimes we appear to make advances in spite of ourselves.

Health Care Facilities
and the Health Care Work Force

Health care resources exist autonomously, are fragmented, unequally distributed, and increasingly expensive. Accessibility to these resources is affected by individual and resource variables, such as cost, geographic location, and time factors. Because there is little coordination between health care resources, it is difficult to ensure continuity and quality of care. It is no wonder that the American public is becoming increasingly dissatisfied with the system.

There are some 6035 acute-care hospitals, 542 long-term hospitals, and 16,033 nursing homes in the United States (USDHHS, 1989, pp. 140, 148). Of these hospitals 307 are federally owned, 3338 are nonprofit, 834 are for-profit, and 1556 are run by state and local governments (USDHHS, 1989, p. 139). There is a trend toward increased for-profit ownership and less government ownership. The U.S. government closed its Public Health Service hospitals at the end of fiscal year 1981. Government ownership of hospitals includes armed forces hospitals, prison hospitals, state long-term psychiatric care facilities, mental retardation facilities, state university medical school hospitals, and city and county hospitals for the medically indigent. There are thousands of state and local health departments and departments of social services, as well as many private agencies and individuals who provide health care services.

Hospital care in the United States accounts for over 46 percent of personal health-care money spent each year (USDHHS, 1989, p. 152). Hospitals are becoming increasingly competitive in the services and incentives they offer to clients; many are offering alternative health care services such as home care, occupational health services, rehabilitation services, decentralized services (minihospitals distributed throughout an area providing broad outpatient and emergency facilities), and alternative care programs similar to programs offered by health maintenance organizations.

Nursing homes are increasing in number in the United States, and their ownership is largely in the private profit-making sector. Approximately 5 percent of Americans aged 65 and over occupy a bed in a nursing or related home. Nursing homes are licensed by the state and are usually certified for Medicaid and Medicare funding. The average individual monthly cost for all types of nursing home facilities was $1456 in 1986 (USDHHS, 1989, p. 163), and this cost is continually rising. Some states have put a freeze on nursing home construction in an attempt to limit institutional care for the aged and to expand home-based services. This has resulted in long waiting lists at many nursing homes, with some people who need this type of care being unable to obtain it.

There are more than 8 million people employed in health care occupations in the United States (USDHHS, 1983, p. 160). Health care is the nation's second biggest business. Education, certification, and licensing help to identify and distinguish various health care workers. There has been an increase in federal funding since World War II to train various health professionals, especially in schools of public health. There are approximately 22 physicians, 66 registered nurses, 6 dentists, 6 pharmacists, and 1 optometrist per 10,000 population active today in the United States (USDHHS, 1989, p. 134). Health professions have generally grown in numbers in recent years.

There is, however, a great disparity between the number of health care providers in urban, rural, and inner-city areas. Time after time, studies have shown rural and inner-city areas to have a significantly smaller health work force than suburban areas. Resource distribution is also often related to the affluence of the area. The more affluent the area, the more available the health work force. The federal government is attempting to use financial incentives, to alter the training and distribution of health care personnel by offering fellowships and grants to students who commit themselves to serving in shortage areas. The government also offers financial incentives to universities and colleges that make a commitment to increase their output of health practitioners to areas where there is a shortage of health care personnel.

Health Care Cost

In general, health care in the United States is uneconomical and disproportionately inflationary. Although growing more slowly than in recent years, spending for health continues to account for an increasing share of the Nation's gross national product. In 1987, spending for health cost $500 billion, and amounted to 11.1 percent of the gross national product, and 9.8 percent more than 1986 (NLN, 1989, p. 1). The following statistics highlight the extent of health care spending in the United States in 1986 (USDHHS, 1989, pp. 134, 153, 159, 169; Health Insurance Association of America, 1988, pp. 2, 17):

• Expenditures for health increased by 8.4 percent from 1985 and amounted to six times the $75 billion spent in 1970.
• The federal government's share of personal health expenditures was 30 percent, up from 10 percent in 1965.
• Health expenditures amounted to $1836 per person, $122 more than 1985. Of that amount, $760 came from public funds.
• Hospital care expenditures rose to a level of $179.6 billion—an increase of 7.4 percent from 1985.
• Spending for the services of physicians increased 11.1 percent to $92 billion.
• Public sources provided approximately 40 cents of every dollar spent on health.
• Health insurance premiums cost almost $60 billion, up 67.7 percent from 1981.
• Medical research amounted to less than 4 percent of national health expenditures.
• Government public health activities amounted to only 2.9 percent of all national health expenditures.

Health care expenditures rise each year, and the cost of health care makes it inaccessible to many people. According to predictions made by the Health Care Financing Administration, national health expenditures will reach $756 billion by 1990 (Health Insurance Association of America, 1983, p. 39). It is obvious that cost containment is an important issue and that legislation will be enacted to deal with it. Some cost controls implemented in recent years have been certificate of need before a health facility can be constructed, deductibles and coinsurance as financial deterrents to a client's using unnecessary services, utilization reviews, and rate-setting commissions. The federal government has influenced the financing of health care through tax subsidies and incentives, including provisions for deductions of medical expenses with personal income tax, allowing employer's contributions to health insurance plans to be nontaxable, allowing income tax deductions for contributions made to charitable organizations engaged in health care, and extending tax exempt status to nonprofit health care resources.

Health care is financed through direct individual payment, insurance, and assistance programs. These methods of payment are discussed in this chapter because the health resources and services that an individual will use are largely dependent on the method of payment available.

RESOURCES FOR HEALTH CARE FINANCING IN THE UNITED STATES

The methods for health care financing in the United States are diverse, complicated, and confusing. Health care services often are not utilized because the individual is unable to afford them. Both the government and private sectors are active in health care financing, and both methods of financing are discussed here. To help make this varied system of financing clearer, the following outline is used:

1. Individual payment (direct, out-of-pocket)
2. Health insurance
   a. Government
      (1) Medicare
      (2) Workers' compensation
   b. Private
      (1) Blue Cross-Blue Shield
      (2) Commercial insurance
      (3) Self-insurance
      (4) Health maintenance organizations (HMOs)
   c. National Health Insurance
3. Health assistance
   a. Government
      (1) Medicaid
      (2) Maternal-child health (MCH)
   b. Private
4. Health service programs
   a. Government
   b. Private

Individual Payment (Direct, Out-of-Pocket)

Individual payment for health care services is exactly what it says—the individual pays for the health care directly. For the 15 percent of American people who are not covered under health insurance and assistance programs, individual payment is a hard reality. Data from the 1987 National Medical Expenditure Survey indicate that the uninsured are overrepresented among young adults, blacks and Hispanics, the unmarried, and in families without a working adult. However, in terms of absolute numbers most of the uninsured population under age 65 is composed of workers and their families. About 25 percent of families with working adults lack work-related health insurance through employers or labor unions and many of these families cannot afford to purchase private health insurance. Workers at risk for being uninsured are the low-wage or part-time employee, the self-employed, workers in industries with seasonal or temporary employment, and employees of small firms (Short, Monheit, and Beauregard, 1989).

Even with health insurance, many persons are involved in some form of individual payment due to insurance deductibles, coinsurance, fixed payment amounts, and uncovered services. A *deductible* is a set expense that must be paid by the insured before the insurer will reimburse for services (e.g., $100 deductible). With *coinsurance,* the insured pays a percentage of the covered health care expenses, which is often in addition to a deductible (e.g., 20 percent coinsurance rate). *Fixed payments* are arrangements whereby only a specified amount for a health service is paid by the insurer, regardless of the cost to the client (e.g., $300 for antepartal care). *Uncovered services* are easily understood: they are services that the insurer does not pay for, and payment is left to the insuree (e.g., prescriptions are not covered). The rising costs of health insurance are prompting more employers to institute coinsurance plans or to limit covered services. This presents a real hardship for many wage earners and their families.

Many people are involved in direct payment for health care costs; in 1987, it accounted for almost 28 percent of personal health care expenditures, or $123 million in the United States (Health Insurance Association of America, 1989, p. 54). When direct payment for health care becomes excessive, it can place the individual and family at great financial risk. A form of health care financing that helps to protect the individual and family from the financial risk of health care is health insurance. Unfortunately, the fact that uninsured and underinsured populations are growing has significant implications for all health care providers and persons within these groups. Individuals and families without or with inadequate health insurance coverage often seek only crisis health care. This, in turn, may present serious consequences for their health status in later life.

Health Insurance

Health insurance is a contractual agreement between an insurer and an insuree for the payment of health care costs. The insuree pays a prepaid premium for specified benefits; the benefits under the insurance program are variable. Health insurance is administered by both government and private agencies. Private health insurance programs serve the majority of the American people, whereas government programs are limited largely to serving the aged and disabled.

Most health insurance programs cover hospital and surgical costs for the insuree because these costs are the most predictable and insurable of health care costs. Many insurance plans do not include regular medical, major medical, disability, or dental insurance. Some insurance plans do not cover the cost of prescription medications or health care equipment. Approximately 15.5 percent of the American population, 37 million people, are not covered by any form of health insurance (Short, Monheit and Beaureguard, 1989, p. 4). The following are some forms of health insurance coverages:

> *Hospital.* Insurance covering the cost of inpatient hospital expenses.
> *Surgical.* Insurance that covers physicians' fees for surgical care.
> *Regular medical.* Insurance that pays for physicians' fees for nonsurgical care. There are usually maximum benefit amounts for specified services.
> *Major medical.* Insurance that helps protect

against large, unpredictable medical costs, usually supplements an existing insurance program, frequently has maximum benefit limits, and is subject to deductibles and co-insurance.

Dental. Insurance providing payment for the cost of specified dental care.

Disability. Insurance that protects against wages lost from disability. This insurance may provide long-term or short-term benefits.

Catastrophic. Insurance that protects against the high cost of acute or long-term illness that would otherwise not be covered by insurance.

Most people are vulnerable to the cost of long-term disability health services and catastrophic illness. Chapter 19 examines in-depth the extent of this problem and actions needed to correct it.

Government

Federal government health insurance did not exist in any significant form until 1965, with the passage of Medicare under the Social Security Act. Government health insurance incorporates many of the same types of coverage as private health insurance. There are two major forms of government health insurance: Medicare and workers' compensation programs. Medicare is a federal program, and workers' compensation is a state program.

Medicare is a federally administered health insurance program created by the 1965 amendments to the Social Security Act. It provides health insurance for eligible persons age 65 and over and for qualifying people who are disabled. It covered 32.4 million Americans in 1987 (USDHHS, 1989, p. 4). Medicare expenditures of $80.3 billion comprised approximately 60 percent of total federal outlays for health care in 1987. Total Medicare outlays are projected to reach $131 billion by 1990 (Arnett, Cowell, Davidoff, and Freeland, 1985, p. 11). Two excellent publications by the Health Care Financing Administration dealing with Medicare are *Your Medicare Handbook* and *Medicare and Medicaid Data Book.*

Medicare is a contributory program, paid into during the insured's working years. The program is administered through the Social Security Administration, Bureau of Health Insurance. Clients apply for it at local Social Security Administration offices. Reimbursement for Medicare services is provided through private insurance companies, intermediaries, under contract with the federal government. These intermediaries are often Blue Cross-Blue Shield organizations.

Medicare includes two parts, Medicare A and Medicare B. *Medicare A* is a hospital insurance program, financed through individual social security contributions. In addition to inpatient hospital care, Medicare A covers selected posthospitalization home health care services, such as skilled nursing care, and physical or speech therapy on a qualifying basis. It sets limits on the number of hospital and extended care facility days that will be covered and is subject to yearly changes in services and deductibles.

Medicare B is a voluntary, supplemental medical insurance program. In 1990 the monthly premium was $28.60. It covers physicians' services; limited services by dentists, podiatrists, optometrists, and chiropractors; hospital outpatient services; some home health service visits; outpatient physical therapy and speech therapy; specified equipment; radiation therapy; hospice services; and other services on a qualifying basis. It excludes coverage for prescription drugs, glasses, dentures, hearing aids, yearly physical examinations, dental care, and routine foot care. Because of these exclusions, many persons 65 and older have obtained supplemental private health insurance policies to augment their Medicare benefits.

Workers' compensation was discussed under the legislative section in this chapter. These state programs include health and disability insurance from occupational illness or injury. Workers' compensation health care benefits cost the individual states more than $8.6 billion a year (Nelson, 1989, Worker's Compensation, p. 34).

Private

A forerunner of private health insurance in the United States was the Baylor University Plan of

1929. The monthly premium was 50 cents, and the plan offered 21 days of semiprivate care at Baylor Hospital, Dallas, Texas (Wilner, Walkley, and O'Neill, 1978, pp. 138-139). Out of this plan came the Blue Cross-Blue Shield concept of 1939. In 1940 less than 10 percent of the civilian, non-institutionalized population was covered by any kind of private health insurance (Health Insurance Association of America, 1983, p. 13).

In the 1950s health insurance became a major point in employees' collective bargaining, and United States industry became increasingly involved in prepayment of health care services. Today, health insurance plans are often a part of employee work benefits, and private health insurance is predominantly paid for by industry.

Americans are protected by private health insurance offered through approximately 1100 private insurance companies and 70 Blue Cross-Blue Shield organizations (Wilson and Neuhauser, 1985, pp. 110-111). The most common forms of health insurance in this country are Blue Cross-Blue Shield, commercial insurance, self-insurance, and health maintenance organizations (HMOs). Each of these forms is discussed here.

Blue Cross and Blue Shield are nonprofit (voluntary) organizations. Blue Cross provides protection against the cost of hospital care, and Blue Shield provides protection against the cost of medical and surgical care. They are tax-exempt organizations and exist through state legislation enabling them to provide health insurance. The state insurance commissioner usually has powers of regulation over these programs, with rate increases being approved by the commissioner and subject to public hearings. These organizations are usually the only organizations allowed to contract with providers of service for agreed-upon fees, and payment is made directly to the service provider (Wilson and Neuhauser, 1985, p. 11).

Blue Cross and Blue Shield are legally independent of each other but usually work in close cooperation. Their boards of directors are composed of evenly distributed representation from the public, contracting providers, and their own organizations. These organizations paid more than $77 billion in insurance benefits in 1986 and insured more than 78 million people (Health Insurance Association of America 1988, pp. 4, 9).

Commercial insurance companies are private profitmaking organizations. They provide health insurance for more than 100 million Americans and cover services similar to those offered under Blue Cross-Blue Shield plans. Commercial insurers compete with Blue Cross-Blue Shield and have pioneered several types of health insurance coverage now common to other carriers, including major medical care, prescription drugs, and post-hospitalization home care services. Commercial insurers contract with clients for prepaid premiums and benefits. Clients are expected to pay the service provider and are then reimbursed by the insurer for the agreed-upon cost.

Self-insurance was stimulated by the passage of the Employee Retirement Income Security Act of 1974 (Health Insurance Association of America, 1978, p. 20). Under this act, corporations and organizations can establish self-funded, nonprofit health plans and escape the taxes and regulations of state insurance laws.

Health maintenance organizations (HMOs) provide a wide range of comprehensive health care services for a specified group at a fixed, prepaid cost to the insured. Health maintenance organizations combine the principles of health insurance and group health practice and stress the preventive aspects of health care. The Health Maintenance Organization Act of 1973 (Public Law 93-222), an amendment to the Public Health Service Act of 1944, provided financial and other assistance to aid in HMO development. There are hundreds of HMOs in the United States, serving millions of Americans. These organizations are characterized by:

- Direct service provision to enrollees on a prepayment basis, with each enrollee paying a fixed amount regardless of the volume or expense of the services utilized
- Service provision through physicians, nurses, and other health care providers, who are under contractual agreement with the HMO. Their practice is limited to the HMO, and subscribers to the HMO are limited to usage

of the health workers employed by the plan
- Comprehensive services that include both inpatient and outpatient care and emphasize preventive health practices
- Internal, self-regulatory mechanisms to ensure quality of care and cost control

National Health Insurance

Teddy Roosevelt first tried to have national health insurance enacted in 1912 (Harrington, 1989, p. 214). However, efforts have been unsuccessful and there is still *no* form of national health insurance in this country. Most of the proposed plans have involved employer and employee contributions. Generally, they include provisions that would provide basic health care for the entire population and that would eliminate financial hardship as a result of catastrophic illness. Proposed programs have varied as to whether they will be federally or privately administered, who will be covered, what will be covered, how they will be funded, and what quality control measures will be taken. Possibly the biggest barrier to passage of a national health insurance plan is the proposed cost. (Harrington, 1989, p. 214). Health care professionals must monitor carefully all proposed legislation to ensure that the proposed program actually provides the services needed by the population as a whole. There has been little movement toward national health insurance in this country in the past decade. However, recently the American Public Health Association (APHA) has championed the platform of "Health Care for All" in the United States by the year 2000 (refer to Chapters 2 and 23).

Health Assistance

Health assistance resources provide health services for a qualifying individual without the prepayment of premiums by the individual, and generally without the individual participating in cost sharing for the services rendered. These programs are largely noncontributory ones.

Government

The major government health assistance programs are the federal-state, state-administered program of Medicaid and a number of maternal-child health programs. The private-sector health assistance programs are diverse and belong largely to the private nonprofit (voluntary) sector.

Medicaid was created by the 1965 Social Security Act amendments that created Medicare. It is a noncontributory health assistance program that provides both medical and hospital services for the qualifying medically indigent; however, its services are provided as health insurance to the client. It is designed to provide more adequate medical assistance to people who are eligible to receive assistance under the AFDC and SSI programs. In addition, states may provide Medicaid to the medically needy, people who have enough money to pay for basic living expenses but not medical care.

Medicaid has provided millions of Americans with health services they would not otherwise have. States have great discretion in determining who will be covered by Medicaid, what services will be covered, and financial eligibility criteria. As a result of recent federal legislation, under Medicaid states must now cover:

- Children aged 1 through 6 and pregnant women and children who meet the state's AFDC financial requirements
- Recipients of adoption assistance and foster care under Title IV-E of the Social Security Act
- Pregnant women and infants up to age 1 whose family income is at or below 75 percent of the federal poverty level
- Certain Medicare beneficiaries
- Special protected groups such as persons who lose SSI and AFDC eligibility as a result of work earnings

The client does not pay for medical and hospital services. The federal government contracts with intermediaries, usually Blue Cross-Blue Shield organizations, to insure the client against health costs. It is a health assistance program, operating on a health insurance basis.

Both federal and state funds pay for Medicaid services, with the ratio of federal funding varying from 50 to 78.5 percent of actual state expenditure, depending on the state's economic status (Simon, 1989, p. 50). This program is federally administered through the Medical Services Administration of the Social and Rehabilitation Service, which is under the Social Security Administration. Each state administers its own Medicaid program through various offices of state government.

Medicaid benefits vary from one state to another. Federal law does not mandate that a state operate a Medicaid program. If the state does operate the program, it must meet federal standards. All states participate in Medicaid (Arizona provides medical assistance through a Medicaid demonstration project). There is no residency or age requirement for the program. A person receiving Medicare may also be eligible for Medicaid. Persons who are eligible for both are called "dual eligibles." A state's Medicaid program pays the Medicare premium for such individuals, and then Medicaid supplements the Medicare coverage with services not available under Medicare such as hearing aids, eye glasses, and long-term care (Simon, 1989, p. 50).

Maternal-child health programs (MCH) have traditionally been a major source of funding for activities that are carried out by local health departments to meet the needs of high-risk mothers and children. These activities include the nutrition and health programs of women, infants, and children (WIC), medical or dental care, and comprehensive preventive medical care services through centers such as PRESCAD (Preschool, School-age, and Adolescent). These services are discussed more extensively in Chapter 13. The monies appropriated for these programs now are largely available through federal block grants.

Private

Health assistance in the private sector is primarily voluntary nonprofit in nature. This volunteerism is prevalent, with many people donating time, money, and effort to help procure health services for others. The candy stripers in the local hospital, as well as the readers for the blind, are examples of volunteers who are helping clients to obtain health care services.

Service groups such as the American Cancer Society, American Diabetes Association, American Heart Association, Associations for Retarded Citizens, Lions' Clubs, Rotarians, Goodfellows, Knights of Columbus, church groups, and Visiting Nurse Associations provide cash and service benefits in the health field. A majority of United States hospitals operate on a voluntary, nonprofit basis. The dedicated leadership, financial support, and personal service of volunteers and voluntary agencies (non-tax-supported) has greatly aided the health care delivery system in this country, and an extension of this voluntary tradition is essential to continuing health services.

Health Service Programs

Some government and private health service programs are administered through an organization for the benefit of specified employees or service groups. These programs often encompass a combination of insurance and assistance benefits.

Government

Government programs have been generally established to meet the health care needs of specific population groups. Health service programs for veterans, military personnel, merchant marines, American Indians on reservations, native Hawaiians and federal employees are available in the United States. These programs vary in relation to the type of services and benefits offered by each, and one should check with the resource provider to determine what benefits are available to the client.

Private

Private service programs are often part of a benefit package for employees in the work setting. In addition to payment of employee health insurance premiums, many industries provide on-grounds employee health services. These services are usually preventive and treatment-oriented for work-related disease and disability. In addition, there are some industry-sponsored group health maintenance organization plans such as Kaiser-Permanente (French, 1979, pp. 187-188).

THE UNITED STATES WELFARE SYSTEM

The primary task of the welfare system is to alleviate the hardships of the most disadvantaged. Welfare programs reflect an effort to ensure a basic standard of living and to promote social well-being. Like the health care financing system, the welfare system is complex. In this text, programs are arbitrarily divided into welfare insurance and assistance programs as shown in the following outline:

1. Welfare insurance
    a. Government
        (1) Old Age, Survivors, and Disability Insurance (OASDI)
        (2) Unemployment insurance
        (3) Worker's compensation
    b. Private
2. Welfare assistance
    a. Government
        (1) Aid to Families of Dependent Children (AFDC)
        (2) Supplemental Security Income (SSI)
        (3) Food Stamps
        (4) Supplemental Food Program for Women, Infants, and Children (WIC)
        (5) General assistance
    b. Private

Welfare Insurance

Welfare insurance programs are contributory. The individual or someone on behalf of the individual, such as the employer or the government, pays a premium, and benefits are awarded by virtue of these past premium contributions. Welfare insurance programs are found in both the government and private sectors.

Government

The federal government became extensively involved in welfare insurance programs with the passage of the Social Security Act in 1935. This act and its amendments are the basis for existing federal government welfare insurance programs today. State governments also provide welfare insurance. A discussion of the major government welfare insurance programs follows.

Old Age, Survivors, and Disability Insurance (OASDI) is the largest income maintenance program in the country and is commonly called *Social Security.* It originated in the Social Security Act of 1935. Presently, more than 38.6 million Americans are collecting OASDI benefits amounting to more than $217.2 billion yearly in total payments (Grundmann, 1989, p. 4). In 1986 nearly three out of five OASDI beneficiaries aged 65 and over relied on OASDI benefits for at least half their income (Grundmann, 1989, p. 6).

Cash benefits are awarded on the basis of money paid in, as well as time spent in the program. The old age component of the program is often called retirement insurance. A worker often begins to receive retirement benefits at age 65. If a worker retires before the age of 65, the amount of his or her check is reduced permanently. If a worker delays retirement past age 65, certain financial rewards and incentives accrue. The retirement age under the program is gradually being raised to age 67. If a worker returns to work after beginning retirement benefits, there is a ceiling limit on the amount that the worker can earn and still collect retirement benefits. The average monthly benefit for a retired worker is $537 and $921 for a couple (OASDI and SSI, 1989, p. 27).

The survivors component provides benefits to survivors in the family of a deceased or disabled qualifying worker. Ninety-five percent of American children and their surviving parent are eligible for benefits should the family breadwinner die. Disability benefits are payable to qualifying persons under 65 years of age on the basis of medical evaluations and the person's continued inability to work. After age 65, the disabled worker can apply for the old age component of the insurance program.

Unemployment insurance provides protection against earnings lost as a result of unemployment. It is a federal-state cost-sharing program provided by the Social Security Act of 1935 and is *state* administered. By 1937 all states had enacted unemployment legislation. A worker who becomes unemployed on a job covered by unemployment insurance and who has worked a specified amount of time can apply for these benefits. The worker must remain registered to work and must actively seek employment while collecting benefits. Most states provide a maximum of 26 weeks of benefits each year. A federal-state program of extended benefits for workers who have exhausted state benefits is available during times of high unemployment. The average duration of state benefits is 13.9 weeks (Bretz, 1989, p. 22).

Employers pay into the program on behalf of the employee while the employee is working for them. There is no commercial insurance and no self-insurance by employers. Benefits and contributions are determined primarily by state law, but federal law sets minimum standards. The federal government pays the costs of administration and makes loans to states when their unemployment insurance accounts run low.

All contributions collected under the state laws must be deposited in the Unemployment Trust Fund in the U.S. treasury, in which each state has an interest-drawing account. A state can withdraw funds only to pay benefits.

There is great variation in program benefits from state to state. In 1988, unemployment insurance covered 100 million workers, 97 percent of all wage and salary workers, and had an average weekly benefit amount of $119.39 (Bretz, 1989, p. 20-22). The maximum weekly unemployment benefit for states varies from $96 to $268 (Bretz, 1989, p. 22).

Workers' compensation is discussed under the legislative section on state workers' compensation laws in this chapter. Refer to that section for information.

Private

Private welfare insurance is available through a number of agencies. A major form of private welfare insurance is employer-employee-funded retirement insurance; another form is disability insurance. Many persons are covered by private retirement insurance as well as the government program of OASDI. Retirement and disability insurance can be purchased by individuals who desire to have additional financial protection when they are no longer working. Millions of American workers are covered by private retirement insur-

ance through their place of work. The Retirement Income Security Act of 1974 helped to safeguard the financial integrity of these private retirement programs. Disability insurance was discussed under health insurance in this chapter.

Welfare Assistance Programs

Welfare assistance programs are noncontributory or minimally contributory programs for qualifying indigent individuals, and they provide cash and service benefits (e.g., food, shelter, clothing). They exist largely as a result of state and federal legislation and are locally administered. Once a person's eligibility for a categorical government welfare assistance program has been determined, he or she receives cash benefits, social service benefits, and medical benefits through Medicare or Medicaid (Donabedian, 1990). The individual is generally eligible for food stamps also. Welfare assistance programs include both government and private programs.

Government

Government welfare assistance programs provide subsistence benefits for those without other resources. Applicants often apply for these programs through local departments of social service or through the Social Security Office, depending on the program. An applicant is generally asked to provide the following information when applying for government assistance programs:

- Proof of residence
- Proof of gross income from all sources, for all household members
- Record of all property, including savings accounts, checking accounts, bonds, and land owned
- Record of house payments or rent and also insurance and taxes
- Record of utility bills
- Record of current medical and dental expenses
- Birth dates and social security numbers of household members
- Records of child support and alimony
- Proof of tuition and other required educational expenses

• Records of child care payment for employment or training purposes

Some major categorical government welfare assistance programs include the AFDC and SSI. Other government assistance programs include general or direct assistance and food stamps. These programs are discussed below.

Aid to Families of Dependent Children (AFDC) is the state-federal program provided for under the Social Security Act of 1935 that helps needy families with children by authorizing federal matching grants to states. Families usually apply for AFDC at local branches of the state Department of Human or Social Services. In 1988, over 3.7 million families received $16.6 billion in AFDC payments, amounting to approximately $4500 per family per year or $375 per family per month (Grundmann, 1989, p. 4). This amount of financial assistance puts AFDC families below the poverty level of income. All AFDC families are eligible for food stamps, and most receive them. Payments are usually made directly to AFDC recipients, but individuals who are physically or mentally incapable of managing their own funds can have their payments go to a representative on their behalf.

AFDC furnishes financial and other assistance to encourage the care of dependent children in their own homes, to help parents become capable of self-support, and to maintain family life. In order for a family to qualify for AFDC, there must be children who are deprived of the financial support of one parent because of death, disability, absence from the home, or, in some states, unemployment. The family's income must fall below a "needs standard" set by each state, which is the dollar amount necessary to meet a minimum standard of living in that state. AFDC funds are available to pregnant women, and in most states, a woman can apply for AFDC or for an increase in her present allotment once a physician has verified in writing that she is pregnant. The actual amount of the AFDC payment will depend on the number of persons in the family and the amount of other income.

Any United States citizen or legal alien can apply for AFDC; there is no age requirement. However, aliens sponsored by private individuals or public or private agencies are usually not eligible until 3 years after they enter the United States because they are considered to have the resources of their sponsors.

The Family Support Act of 1988 (Public Law 199-485) made major revisions in the AFDC program to assist AFDC families in obtaining education, training, and employment to avoid long-term welfare dependence. It established the first federal requirement that AFDC recipients seek employment, and it required that each state establish an education, training, and work (NETWork) program, as well as enforce child support efforts (refer to Appendix 4-1 for additional information on this act).

Supplemental Security Income (SSI) is a federal-state assistance program that is *federally* administered through the Social Security Administration. It became effective January 1, 1974, and provides aid to qualifying aged, blind, and disabled people who have limited financial resources. The objective for establishing this program was to develop a uniform national minimum cash income for the indigent aged, blind, and disabled.

In 1989 the federal standard before state supplementation was $368 per month for an individual and $553 per month for a couple (OASDI and SSI, 1989, p. 27). Federal monetary benefits under the program remain constant throughout the nation and are adjusted to reflect Social Security cost-of-living increases. Forty-eight states supplement the program with additional cash benefits. State supplementary benefits vary and may be made directly to the beneficiary or paid through the federal Social Security Administration. Adults are usually the beneficiaries of SSI, but a child may be eligible if he or she suffers from an impairment expected to last a year or longer, such as mental retardation, terminal illness, or blindness. Applications for SSI are made at local branches of the federal Social Security offices. Qualifying United States citizens and legally admitted aliens are eligible.

The *food stamp program* was begun on a pilot

basis in 1961 to improve the nutritional adequacy of low-income individuals and families. It was formally established by the Food Stamp Act of 1964. It is a federal-state program under *state* administration. The federal sharing agency is the Department of Agriculture. Application is made at the local office of the state Department of Human or Social Services. As of October 1988 an eligible family of four persons with no personal income received $300 per month in food stamps (Loeff, Bretz, and Kerns, 1989, p. 69). The average food stamp recipient has approximately 55 cents' worth of food stamps to use for each meal ($50.04 per person per month) for food. In 1988, over 18.7 million Americans took part in this program at a cost to the government of $11.2 billion (Loeff, Bretz, and Kerns, 1989, p. 69). Persons qualify on the basis of financial need. A household receiving food stamps that is intending to move to another area may apply for transfer of certification before moving. Federal law states that the food stamp office must determine eligibility within 30 days after a signed application is submitted. The Hunger Protection Act of 1988 (Public Law 100-435) raised the maximum amount of food stamp allotments.

Food Stamps are available across the nation. Coupons are given to those who are eligible and are used like money at participating stores. Food stamps can be used only to purchase *edible items;* no imported foodstuffs, alcoholic beverages, or tobacco products can be bought with them. They are not transferable to another person and must be used by the person who purchased them. Food stamp regulations apply nationwide and most grocery stores are authorized to accept food stamps.

Supplemental Food Program for Women, Infants and Children (WIC) is a federal nutrition and health assistance program authorized under the Child Nutrition Act of 1966 and administered by the Food and Nutrition Service of the U.S. Department of Agriculture. It is designed to help pregnant and postpartum women, infants, and children up to age 5 years who have been identified by health professionals as being at nutritional risk. The program includes food distribution, health assessment, and a mandatory nutrition education component. More than 30 percent of infants born in the United States participate (Loeff, Bretz and Kerns, 1989, p. 72). Participants receive vouchers that are redeemable at participating grocery stores for items such as infant formula, infant cereal and juices, milk, cereal, and cheese. In 1988, the WIC program included 3.6 million recipients at a cost of $1.8 billion, amounting to $33.40 per person per month (Loeff, Bretz, and Kerns, 1989, p. 72). WIC programs are frequently administered through local health departments and there are approximately 7600 approved WIC service agencies in the United States. If a family is receiving food stamps, participation in WIC does not affect their food stamp eligibility. The WIC program has been very successful in promoting adequate nutrition and nutrition education to qualifying families. Other food programs in which the federal government is involved are school lunch programs, school breakfast programs, school milk programs, needy family commodity foods, and food programs for the elderly.

General assistance is a state and locally funded and administered program which is offered in 32 states. There are no federal monies involved. In approximately one fourth of the states it is financed by local funds (Loeff, Bretz, and Kerns, 1989, p. 74). The program is often administered through the state's department of social services or a comparable department and is frequently referred to as direct assistance.

General assistance is usually made available to indigent persons who do not meet the criteria for other forms of welfare insurance or assistance but are unable to meet their basic survival needs of food, shelter, and clothing. This may be the only form of government assistance available for individuals who are poor but who do not qualify for AFDC, unemployment, OASDI, or SSI. In many states, general assistance is limited to emergency relief (e.g., for a catastrophic event such as a flood), short-term relief, and burial benefits. Any citizen or legally admitted alien may apply. In some states, people receiving general assistance do not receive cash benefits but instead receive vouchers for food, rent, or clothing.

In addition to the cash benefit programs discussed, many state and local governments offer a number of other welfare services. The following list itemizes some of these services:

- Adoption services: accepting and placing children for adoption, recruiting adoptive families, and supporting the adoption placement
- Foster care: funding, licensing, and monitoring
- Day care: locating suitable day-care placements for children during part of the day, licensing and monitoring such placements, and funding services provided by them
- Counseling: counseling individuals, parents, and children with personal or family problems to strengthen family functioning and to prevent family breakdown
- Chore services: paying part or all of the cost for unskilled help with household tasks, personal care, home maintenance, or other activities for qualifying aged and disabled
- Education or training: providing funds and counseling services so that persons can improve their job skills through education and training programs
- Employment: helping people find jobs
- Family planning: providing information and referral to appropriate agencies
- Homemaking: teaching people about home management
- Housing: helping people to find or improve housing and landlord-tenant relations
- Information and referral: helping people to learn about community services
- Mental health treatment and rehabilitation: providing services to persons with mental health problems through community mental health agencies
- Money management: helping people to learn to budget and to use credit
- Placement: helping to place youth and adults in appropriate living facilities with follow-up
- Problem services: investigating reports of abuse and neglect and providing counseling services to prevent recurrence of such problems, counseling services for runaway youth, foster care or housing in emergency situations, and protection of aging clients and children from abuse and neglect (protective services)

Private

The United States is one of the few countries in the world to offer so many private welfare assistance programs and so comprehensive an array of them. Most offer short-term, acute relief, but do not provide long-term assistance for chronic problems. These programs offer services to meet homemaker, health care, counseling, and adoption needs; residential services for the handicapped; day care; recreational activities; Meals-on-Wheels; and so on. The indigent may be helped with temporary food, shelter, clothing, emotional support, or other services through a variety of community groups such as Goodfellows, Lions, Rotarians, Community Self-Help, and the Salvation Army.

Knowledge of private as well as of all other health and welfare resources is essential when one is nursing a community. Though these systems are complex, time and effort spent learning them will equip the community health nurse to more effectively deal with the situations encountered daily in the practice setting. Chapter 12 discusses ways in which the community health nurse can become involved in making these health and welfare systems more efficient and effective.

SUMMARY

Community health nurses must be aware of the major legislation affecting health, welfare, and environmental policy and practices in the United States, and the services provided by this legislation, in order to fulfill their responsibilities to clients. Programs enacted through the Social Security Act of 1935 and the Public Health Service Act of 1944 are extensively used by community health nurses. The Social Security Act provides for the major government health and welfare insurance and assistance programs in the United States today. Legislation in the 1980s has significantly affected the provisions of these acts and the general availability of funding for health, welfare, and environmental programs. It is imperative that community health nurses remain informed about pertinent health, welfare, and environmental legislation and that they become increasingly politically astute.

The health and welfare systems in the United States are complex, diverse, and poorly coordinated. The community health nurse is in a favorable position for explaining the relationship between these system resources and services in a way that few other professionals can. The community health nurse is integrally linked with the health care system, and through community affiliations she or he is in continual contact with the welfare system as well. For many clients, basic welfare needs are a higher priority than health needs; health needs may not be viewed as a priority until the nurse can help the client meet his or her welfare needs.

The nurse should be aware of resources and services in the private sector as well as the government sector. Keeping up with private-sector resources requires diligent effort on the part of the nurse because these resources will vary greatly from locality to locality and are not as obvious as government resources. Contact with local leadership, clients, other nurses, service groups, and professional organizations is helpful to the nurse who desires to remain informed.

APPENDIX 4-1

The Social Security Act of 1935: Major Amendments and Changes

---

1935 *Social Security Act of 1935 (Public Law 74-721)*—An act arising out of the Great Depression and designed to provide for the general welfare by establishing a system of federal old age benefits, and by enabling the states to make more adequate provision for aged persons, blind persons, dependent and crippled children, maternal and child welfare, public health, and the administration of their unemployment compensation laws. It consolidated existing welfare legislation under one law and established both insurance (contributory) and assistance (noncontributory) programs. Its original welfare insurance programs were Old Age Insurance (OAI) and the state-federal program of unemployment insurance. Its original categorical welfare assistance programs included the federal-state programs of Aid to the Blind (AB), Old Age Assistance (OAA), and Aid to Dependent Children (ADC)

1939 *Social Security Amendments (Public Law 74-271)*—Provided for the payment of insurance benefits to qualifying survivors of workers. The insurance program under the act now was Old Age and Survivors Insurance (OASI).

1950 *Social Security Amendments of 1950 (Public Law 81-734)*—Provided for federal aid to states for financial assistance to people who were disabled under Aid to the Permanently and Totally Disabled. Under a new title, Title XIV, Aid to Dependent Children was broadened to include the relative with whom the child was living and became known as: Aid to Families with Dependent Children. The federal-state public assistance programs under the act were now: Old Age Assistance (OAA), Aid to Families with Dependent Children (AFDC), Aid to the Blind (AB), and Aid to the Permanently and Totally Disabled (APTD). Federal matching of state payments to providers of medical services to persons on public assistance (vendor payments) was added.

1956 *Social Security Amendments of 1956 (Public Law 85-880)*—Provided disability insurance benefits for qualifying disabled individuals, reduced to 62 the age at which benefits could be paid to women (The Social Security Amendments of 1961, Public Law 87-64, would make this the age for men also). The insurance portion of the act was Old Age, Survivors and Disability Insurance (OASDI).

1960 *Social Security Amendments of 1960 (Public Law 86-778)*—Established grants to states for medical care for the indigent aged, improved unemployment compensation and disability insurance benefits, eliminated the waiting period for disability insurance, and increased the insurance benefits for children of deceased workers.

1963 *Maternal and Child Health and Mental Retardation Planning Amendments (Public Law 88-156)*—Amended the act to assist the states and communities in preventing mental retardation through expansion and improvement of maternal child health and crippled children's programs. This amendment provided for prenatal, maternity, and infant care for individuals with conditions associated with child bearing which may lead to mental retardation; it also provided funds for planning efforts which would promote comprehensive action to combat mental retardation.

1965 *Social Security Amendments of 1965 (Public Law 89-97)*—Provided for Medicare *(Title XVIII)* and Medicaid *(Title XIX)*. The insurance program (Medicare) under the act became Old Age, Survivors, Disability and Health Insurance (OASDHI). Medicaid was added to the assistance programs under the act. This was a landmark piece of legislation and marked the advent of major federal government involvement in health care delivery. Medicare greatly influenced the expansion of home health care services (refer to Chapter 19).

1967 *Social Security Amendments of 1967 (Public Law 90-248)*—Consolidated all maternal and child health and crippled children programs under one authorization and provided for funding of family planning services. Initiated the Work Incentive Now (WIN) program. Provided for the coverage of outpatient physical therapy and the purchase of durable medical equipment (DME) under Medicare. Established the Early, Periodic, Screening and Development Testing (EPSDT) under Medicaid and allowed Medicaid recipients free choice in the selection of qualified medical facilities and practitioners.

1972 *Social Security Amendments of 1972 (Public Law 92-603)*—Mandated the establishment of Professional Standard Review Organizations (PSROs) in health care. Established the assistance program of Supplemental Security Income to replace the categorical assistance programs of Old Age Assistance, Aid to the Blind, and Aid to the Permanently and Totally Disabled. This change provided for more nationally uniform payment levels to people qualifying for these programs and set a minimum level of payment. States were encouraged to supplement the federal Supplemental Security Income (SSI) payments. The assistance programs under the act were now Supplemental Security Income (SSI) and Aid for Families of Dependent Children (AFDC), along with the medical assistance program of Medicaid. Health insurance coverage for the disabled was made available under Medicare.

1974 *Social Services Amendments of 1974 (Public Law 93-647)*—Consolidated previous federal-state social service programs into a block grant that would incorporate a ceiling on federal matching funds while providing reasonable flexibility to the states in determining the services to be provided. Reduced the federal regulatory role in social service programs. Included child support enforcement provisions and established the Parent Locator System to aid in collecting child support.

Continued.

APPENDIX 4-1

The Social Security Act of 1935: Major Amendments and Changes—cont'd

1977   *Social Security Amendments (Public Law 95-216)*—Strengthened the financing of the Social Security system through increased rates of contribution; provided benefits to young fathers who have in their care qualifying surviving children of deceased mothers; reduced the duration of marriage requirements for benefits to divorced spouses from 20 years to 10 years, and set a limit on retroactive benefits for a period of up to 12 months before the month of filing. A significant attempt of these amendments was to eliminate sex bias from the act. The establishment of fathers' benefits was significant to maintaining the financial stability of a young family. The National Commission on Social Security was also established.

Medicare-Medicaid Antifraud and Abuse Amendments (Public Law 95-142)—Established regulations and procedures to help protect these health care programs from fraud and abuse.

Social Security Act-Rural Health Clinic Amendments (Public Law 95-210)—Provided payment for rural health clinic services and allowed for direct reimbursement for nursing services in these settings. Also allowed the National Institute for Occupational Safety and Health (NIOSH), upon written request, to obtain the mailing address of taxpayers for the purpose of locating individuals who are, or may have been, exposed to occupational hazards, in order to determine the status of their health or to inform them of the possible need for medical treatment.

1978   *Medicare Endstage Renal Disease Amendments (Public Law 95-292)*—Made improvements in the end stage program for clients with renal disease and kidney donors. Authorized experiments and pilot projects for the purchase of new or used durable medical equipment for end stage renal dialysis clients. Encouraged public participation in the donor programs and authorized studies and measures to look at the costs of the program.

1980   *Medicare and Medicaid Amendments of 1980 (Public Law 96-499)*—The 100-visit-a-year limit was removed from both Part A & B home health care service provisions. Alcohol detoxification facility services were added to Part A benefits. These amendments also provided for payment of nurse-midwives services.

1981   *Omnibus Budget Reconciliation Act (Public Law 97-35)*—An act separate from the Social Security Act, but amended it. Made an impact on many matters of health and welfare in the United States. In relation to the Social Security Act, it changed the following:

Medicare and Medicaid Amendments of 1981—Title XXI of the Omnibus Budget Reconciliation Act eliminated payment for alcohol detoxification services and occupational therapy as a basis for home health services. The part B deductible under Medicare was increased to $75, and federal Medicaid payment was decreased by 3 percent in 1982, 4 percent in 1983, and 4.5 percent in 1984, setting the trend for future disengagement from the program on the part of the federal government.

Maternal and Child Health Block Grant Act—Title XXI of the act provided for the consolidation, into one block grant, of seven grant programs from Title V of the Social Security Act and programs from the Public Health Service Act. The consolidated programs include the maternal-child health and crippled children's programs, genetic disease research; adolescent pregnancy services, sudden infant death syndrome research, hemophilia research, SSI payments to crippled children, and lead poisoning research.

Social Service Block Grant—Retained foster care, adoption assistance and child welfare services as categorical programs while incorporating most of the programs administered by the Community Services Administration into a single social services block grant. Categorical funding was continued for immunizations, tuberculosis, venereal disease, family planning, and migrant health programs.

Other—The Omnibus Budget Reconciliation Act phased out benefits for students under the Social Security Act after the age of 18 years (students who were survivors of a deceased, qualifying parent) and eliminated the minimum benefit available under the Social Security Act, except for those eligible before January 1982. In addition, it authorized states to establish community work experience programs for AFDC recipients that could require work on useful public projects in return for benefits.

1982   *Tax Equity and Fiscal Responsibility Act of 1982 (Public Law 97-248)*—An act separate from the Social Security Act, but amended it. The mandates of this act were designed to reduce Medicare and Medicaid payments by the federal government by more than $14 billion between 1983 and 1985. The act set forth a system of prospective payment for Medicare services, called Diagnostic Related Groups (DRGs). The overall intent of the act was to save the federal government money. However, professionals need to look carefully at the benefits and losses that result in relation to client care and then address these issues.

1983   *Social Security Amendments of 1983 (Public Law 98-21)*—Strengthened the financial basis of the program by increasing contributions by employers, employees, and self-employed individuals. Beginning in 1984, a portion of the Social Secu-

APPENDIX 4-1

The Social Security Act of 1935: Major Amendments and Changes—cont'd

rity retirement benefits paid to higher income recipients will be considered taxable income. Effective January 1, 1984, the Social Security system covers all employees of nonprofit organizations and all federal employees hired on or after that date. Prior to this time, these employees had their own retirement program. Under this amendment, state and local governments which have withdrawn from the Social Security system will be permitted to rejoin. This amendment increases the bonus for individuals who delay their retirement. Regular retirement age, at which time individuals can receive Social Security benefits, will be increased in steps from 65 to 67. This amendment also authorized extended interfund borrowing, between the funds making up the Social Security system, and established a prospective payment plan for hospital reimbursement under the Medicare program.

Medicare Hospice Reimbursement (Public Law 98-90)—Amended title XVIII of the Social Security Act to increase the cap amount allowable for the reimbursement of hospice services under the Medicare program to $6500 for accounting years that end after October 1984.

1984 *Deficit Reduction Act of 1984 (Public Law 98-369)*—An act separate from the Social Security Act, but amended it. Directed the Secretary of Health and Human Services to establish a national fee schedule for *all* Medicare laboratory services, except those provided in hospital facilities; for 15 months (beginning July 1, 1984), Medicare-participating physicians *must* accept Medicare payments as payment in full; conducted a study to determine how more physicians can be induced to accept Medicare assignment; limited for a 2-year period (beginning October 1, 1984) the increase in hospital costs eligible for reimbursement under the Medicare program; provided for the operation of *mobile* intensive care units by Medicare-reimbursed hospitals; making for-profit hospitals eligible for research and demonstration grants; permitted Medicare benefit payment to a third party, a health benefits plan, if the physician or supplier accepts the plan's payment as payment in full; terminated the Health Insurance Benefits advisory council; required states to provide Medicaid benefits to first-time pregnant women meeting Aid to Families with Dependent Children (AFDC) requirements; increased the assets ceiling for SSI beneficiaries, the ceiling increasing in steps to $2000 for an individual and $3000 for a married couple in 1989; provided that in cases of SSI overpayment of benefits, not involving fraud, willful misrepresentation, or concealment, recoupment will not exceed 10 percent of the recipient's monthly salary; increased the gross income limitations for AFDC; made an alien basically *ineligible* for AFDC benefits for 3 years, if his entry into the United States had been sponsored by an agency or organization.

Child Support Enforcement Amendments of 1984 (Public Law 98-378)—Amended Title IV of the Act to assure, through *mandatory* income withholding, incentive payments to states, and other improvements in the child support enforcement program, that all children in the United States who are in need of assistance in securing financial support from their parents will receive such assistance. This amendment included provisions for increasing the availability of federal parent locator services to state agencies and provides for collection of past-due support from federal tax refunds. It also provided for the inclusion of medical support in child support orders. In addition, it required that availability of child support enforcement services be publicized, encouraged state guidelines for child support awards, and directed state and local governments to focus on the problems of child custody, support, and related domestic issues.

Social Security Disability Benefits Reform Act of 1984 (Public Law 98-460)—Provided for reform in the social security disability determination process

1985 *Consolidated Omnibus Budget Reconciliation Act of 1985 [COBRA] (Public Law 99-272)*—Amended the Social Security Act under Medicaid to extend Medicaid coverage for prenatal and postnatal care to low-income women in two-parent families where the primary breadwinner is unemployed; expanded the Medicaid services available under home and community-based services waivers; permitted state to offer hospice services to the terminally ill as an optional Medicaid benefit; required states to formulate policies for Medicaid coverage of organ transplants; and enhanced third-party liability connections. Under Medicare it postponed full implementation of the prospective payment system until October 1, 1987; delayed for 1 year the transition from regional DRG rates to uniform national rates; established extra payment of up to 15 percent of the regular DRG rates for hospitals serving a disproportionate number of low-income persons in an effort to compensate for the higher costs of caring for low-income clients—"disproportionate share allowance"; made permanent a temporary provision in the law allowing Medicare reimbursement for hospice care of the terminally ill and increased by $10 per day the rate of hospice payment; restructured the way Medicare paid teaching hospitals for the direct costs of graduate medical education; established an 11-member committee to study ways to improve the system for physician reimbursement under Medicare; extended the fee freeze for nonparticipating physicians; authorized demonstration projects in at least five states to determine cost effectiveness of providing Medicare coverage for preventive services such as immunizations and drug-abuse prevention; and required Medicare patients to receive a second medical opinion before certain elective surgery, denying Medicare reimbursement to those who failed to do so. The "anti-dumping" provisions required hospitals that participated in Medicare to provide emergency services for people with an urgent need for care, including women in labor, regardless of their ability to pay, and prohibited transfers of such patients un-

Continued.

APPENDIX 4-1

The Social Security Act of 1935: Major Amendments and Changes—cont'd

less their condition had been stabilized or a doctor certified that the move would be beneficial. Hospitals that violated the "anti-dumping" provisions could be barred from participating in Medicare and both the hospital and the responsible physician could face civil penalties of up to $25,000 per violation. Also, provided for a study of physician payments; established a Council on Graduate Medical Education to assess long-term physician training issues; and required the Department of Health and Human Services to establish a task force to develop recommendations for insurance policies to offer long-term health care.

1986   *Omnibus Budget Reconciliation Act of 1986 [OBRA](Public Law 99-509)*—Amended the Social Security Act under Medicaid to allow states to have the option of expanding coverage for pregnant women, infants up to age 1, and children up to age 5 who had incomes below the Federal poverty level; required states to continue Medicaid coverage to disabled individuals who lost their eligibility for SSI assistance as a result of work earnings; clarified Medicaid coverage policies with regard to aliens and homeless individuals; and gave states the option of expanding Medicaid coverage for respiratory care services in the home. Under Medicare it established the rate of increase in prospective payment for fiscal years 1987 and 1988; provided for reductions in expenditures for inpatient hospital services; required prompt payment for provider claims; limited the Part A deductible to $520 in 1987; made a number of requirements to protect the quality of patient services; modified payment for physician services; authorized payment for services of physician assistants; authorized direct reimbursement for the services of certified nurse anesthetists; established a new payment system for hospital outpatient services; limited payment for cataract surgery involving a lens implant; and expanded beneficiary appeal rights under the Part B program.

1987   *Medicare and Medicaid Patient and Program Protection Act of 1987 (Public Law 100-93)*—Amended Titles XI, XVII, and XIX of the Social Security Act to protect beneficiaries under the act's health care programs from unfit health care practitioners, and otherwise to improve the antifraud provisions relating to those programs.

Omnibus Budget Reconciliation Act of 1987 (Public Law 100-203)—Under Medicare specified allowable increases in payments for all physician services and provided for reductions in payments for certain overpriced surgical procedures; increased the "disproportionate share allowance" for hospitals caring for a large number of medically indigent and specified the increases in hospital payment rates for fiscal years 1988 and 1989; established a home health toll-free hotline and investigative unit; permitted disabled individuals to renew entitlement to Medicare after gainful employment without a 2-year waiting period; provided incentive payments for physician's services in underserved areas; and allowed for collection of past-due amounts owed by physicians who breached contracts under the National Health Service Corps Scholarship program. It also established the Boarder Babies Demonstration Project for the development of model projects to develop alternative care for infants who do not require hospitalization, but who would otherwise remain in hospital settings owing to parental inability to care for them for such reasons as drug or alcohol addiction. Infants under this program could remain with a parent who resides in community residential setting (e.g., alcohol or drug treatment) or be placed in foster care, the goal being to rehabilitate the parent and eliminate the need for such infant care. In addition, this act authorized the Study of Infants and Children with AIDS in Foster Care to determine the total number of infants and children in the United States diagnosed as having acquired immune deficiency syndrome and placed in foster care, to determine the problems encountered in placing such children, and the potential increase over the next 5 years in the number of such children. Provided a vaccine compensation program to compensate victims of vaccine side effects.

1988   *Family Support Act of 1988 (Public Law 100-485)*—Reformed the federal welfare system. It revised the AFDC program to emphasize work, child support, and family benefits. It amended Title IV of the Social Security Act to encourage and assist needy children and their parents to obtain the education, training, and employment needed to avoid long-term welfare dependence. It established child support and withholding programs, job opportunitiues and basic skills and training programs, and supportive services for families. Established the first federal requirement that welfare recipients seek employment and restored the permanent work incentive. Ended the WIN (Work Incentive Now) Program as of fiscal year 1990. Required that each state establish an education, training, and work (NETWork) program for parents seeking assistance under the family support program, and required parental participation in children age 3 and over (provided child care is guaranteed for children under 6 years of age and that participation is part-time for parents with a child under age 6 years old). Required states to offer a family support supplement to needy two-parent families in which the principal wage earner is unemployed. Required state Medicaid programs to provide 6 months of transitional coverage for families leaving AFDC roles and beginning employment that may not provide health insurance and to offer an additional 6-month extension (for a 12-month total) at the family's option (with the state being allowed to impose a modest premium for the second 6 months and/or allowing the state to fund the family's enrollment in an employer health plan.) Required that states provide Medicaid to two-parent families with an unemployed head that meet AFDC income standards—health insurance for the unemployed. Established rules regarding recipient rights.

APPENDIX 4-1

The Social Security Act of 1935: Major Amendments and Changes—cont'd

Medicare Catastrophic Coverage Act of 1988 (Public Law 100-360)*—A controversial and comprehensive act that amended the Social Security Act to protect Medicare beneficiaries from catastrophic health care expenses related to acute illness. Coverage was financed through increased Medicare Part B monthly premiums and a supplemental premium or "surtax" based on yearly income. In addition to covering catastrophic health care expenses, it provided under *Medicare* the first broad coverage of outpatient prescription drugs, removed the limit on hospice coverage, limited the inpatient hospital deductible to one per year, eliminated the durational limits and coinsurance charges for inpatient hospital services, limited coinsurance charges for posthospital skilled nursing facility (SNF) service to the first 8 days, and provided for 150 days of posthospital SNF benefits each year. It prohibited the misuse of symbols, emblems, or names in reference to Social Security or Medicare. Under *Medicaid* it required states, on a phased-in basis, to pay Medicare premiums, deductibles, and coinsurance for elderly and disabled individuals with incomes below the federal poverty level, and resources at or below twice the SSI standard; by 1990 to provide Medicaid coverage to all pregnant women and infants up to 1 year old with family incomes below poverty level; increased the amount of income and assets that may be retained by one member of a couple when the spouse enters a nursing home; and established uniform standards relating to disposal of resources for less than their fair market value in order to gain Medicaid eligibility.

1989   *Medicare Catastrophic Coverage Repeal Act of 1989 (Public Law 101-234)*—This act repealed the Medicare provisions of the Medicare Catastrophic Coverage Act of 1988 (Public Law 100-360) effective as of January 1, 1990. The Medicaid provisions of the 1988 Catastrophic Act that were left intact were the spousal impoverishment adjustment enabling a spouse of an institutionalized older person to protect up to $60,000 in jointly held liquid assets while receiving Medicaid assistance for nursing home bills; the Medicaid "buy-in" requirement that states buy-in to Medicare, and pay the Medicare premiums, copayments, and deductibles for impoverished individuals; and Medicaid benefits for low-income pregnant women and infants. The act included transitional assistance for those persons already receiving nursing home and hospital benefits under the 1988 Catastrophic Act. The act also provided for reinstatement of MediGap policies held by persons covered previous to the 1988 Act.

Omnibus Budget Reconciliation Act of 1989 (Public Law 101-239)—Increased individual Social Security contributions; established an outreach program to make families of children who are potentially eligible for SSI benefits aware of their eligibility; provided a Medicare buy-in for selected disabled individuals under age 65; and required that state Medicaid programs pay, on a sliding scale, the Medicare Part A premiums for disabled individuals who are eligible to purchase Medicare under Section 6012 of the Act, whose income under the SSI program does not exceed 200 percent of the official poverty line, and whose resources do not exceed twice the SSI limits.

*As of 1-1-90 the *Medicare* provisions of this act were repealed by the Medicare Catastrophic Repeal Act of 1989 (Public Law 101-234). Many of the *Medicaid* provisions were retained.

APPENDIX 4-2

The Public Health Service Act of 1944: Some Major Amendments and Changes

1944   *Public Health Service Act (Public Law 78-410)*—An act to consolidate and revise the laws relating to the Public Health Service.

1946   *Hospital Survey and Construction Act (Public Law 79-725)*—Authorized grants to states for surveying their hospitals and public health centers and for planning and construction grants for facilities. This legislation is commonly referred to as the *Hill-Burton Act;* it was frequently amended over the years and was incorporated into the 1974 PHSA amendments of the National Health Planning and Resources Development Act—Title XVI.

1954   *Medical Facilities Survey and Construction Act (Public Law 83-482)*—Amended the Hill-Burton provisions of the act to provide for assistance to states in surveying the need for diagnostic or treatment centers, hospitals for the chronically ill and impaired, rehabilitation centers, and nursing homes. Provided construction assistance for such facilities through grants to public and nonprofit agencies.

1956   *Health Research Facilities Act (Public Law 84-835)*—Provided for grants-in-aid to nonfederal public and nonprofit agencies for constructing and equipping facilities for research in the health sciences.

   National Health Survey Act (Public Law 84-652)—Provided for a continuing survey and special studies of sickness and disability in the United States and for periodic reports on the results.

   Health Amendments Act (Public Law 84-911)—Improved the health of the people by assisting in increasing the number of adequately trained professional and practical nurses and professional public health personnel and in developing improved methods of care and treatment in the field of mental health.

1958   *Grants-in-Aid to Schools of Public Health (Public Law 85-544)*—Authorized the Surgeon General to make certain grants-in-aid to public and nonprofit accredited schools of public health for training in the fields of public health and public health administration of state and local public health programs.

1960   *Graduate Training in Public Health (Public Law 86-720)*—Amended Title III of the act to authorize project grants for graduate education in public health.

   Health Promoting Sciences-Grants-In-Aid (Public Law 86-798)—Authorized grants-in-aid to universities, hospitals, laboratories, and other public or nonprofit institutions to strengthen their programs of research and training in sciences related to health.

1961   *Community Health Services and Facilities Act (Public Law 87-395)*—Assisted in expanding and improving community facilities and services for the health care of the aged and other persons; provided grants for research, experiments, and demonstration projects. Amended the Hill-Burton portion of the act.

1962   *Migrant Health Act (Public Law 87-692)*—Amended Title III of PHSA to authorize grants for family clinics for domestic, agricultural migratory workers.

1963   *Health Professions Educational Assistance Act (Public Law 88-129)*—Amended Title VIII to increase the opportunities for training physicians, dentists, and professional public health personnel. Provided for grants for construction of medical, dental, pharmaceutical, optometric, podiatric, nursing, osteopathic, and public health teaching facilities. Established the National Advisory Council on Education for Health Professions.

1964   *Nurse Training Act (Public Law 88-581)*—Increased opportunities for training professional nursing personnel and for construction of nursing schools.

   Hospital and Medical Facilities Amendments (Public Law 88-443)—Amended the Hill-Burton portion of the act to include long-term care facilities and rehabilitation facilities.

1965   *Health Profession Educational Assistance Amendments (Public Law 89-190)*—Improved the educational quality of schools of medicine, dentistry, and osteopathy by authorizing grants to such schools for the awarding of scholarships to needy students. It also extended expiring provisions of the act for student loans and for aid in the construction of teaching facilities for such schools.

   Heart Disease, Cancer, and Stroke Amendments (Public Law 89-239)—An act to assist in combating heart disease, cancer, and stroke, and related diseases by providing for education, research, training, and demonstration projects.

1966   *Comprehensive Health Planning and Public Health Service Amendments (Public Law 89-749)*—An act to promote and assist in the extension and improvement of comprehensive health planning and public health services and to provide for a more effective use of available federal funds for such planning and services.

   Allied Health Professions Personnel Training Act (Public Law 89-751)—An act to increase the opportunities for training

APPENDIX 4-2

The Public Health Service Act of 1944: Some Major Amendments and Changes—cont'd

of medical technologists and personnel in other allied health professions; to improve the educational quality of schools training such allied health professions' personnel; and to strengthen and improve the existing student loan programs for medical, dental, podiatry, pharmacy, optometric, and nursing students.

1968   *Public Health Service Amendments (Public Law 90-574)*—Extended and improved provisions of the PHSA relating to Title I regional medical programs. It also extended the authorization for Title II migratory agricultural workers and provided for construction of facilities for alcoholic and narcotic addict rehabilitation. Commonly referred to as the *Alcoholic and Narcotic Addict Rehabilitation Amendments of 1968.*

Health Manpower Act (Public Law 90-490)—A major amendment to the PHSA, it extended and improved programs relating to the training of nursing and other health professions and allied health professions personnel, and the programs relating to student aid for such personnel and research facilities authorization. It authorized the study of school aid and student programs to establish aid levels for the future, along with the adequacy of health care personnel to meet long-term needs. Increased the monies available for nursing training.

1970   *Medical Facilities Construction and Modernization Amendments (Public Law 91-296)*—Revised, extended, and improved the programs previously established by Title VI relating to medical facility construction and modernization, and increased appropriations. It amended the Hill-Burton portion of the act.

Communicable Disease Control Amendments of 1970 (Public Law 91-464)—Authorized grants for communicable disease control, vaccination assistance, and studies to determine community-based communicable disease needs and strategies. Supported communicable disease programs designed to contribute to national protection against tuberculosis, venereal disease, rubella, measles, RH disease, poliomyelitis, diphtheria, tetanus, pertussis, and other communicable diseases transmissible from state to state that are amenable to treatment.

Comprehensive Drug Abuse Prevention and Control (Public Law 91-513)—Provided for increased research into, and prevention of, drug abuse and dependence; provided for treatment and rehabilitation of drug abusers and drug-dependent persons; and strengthened existing law enforcement authority in the field of drug abuse.

Heart Disease, Cancer, Stroke, and Kidney Disease Amendments of 1970 (Public Law 91-515)—Improved and expanded research, education and training, and demonstration programs in these areas.

Health Training Improvement Act (Public Law 91-519)—Established eligibility of new schools of medicine, dentistry, osteopathy, pharmacy, optometry, veterinary medicine, and podiatry for grants; extended the program related to training of personnel in allied health professions.

Family Planning Services and Population Research Act (Public Law 91-572)—Established Title X, Population Research and Voluntary Family Planning Programs, to promote public health and welfare by expanding, improving, and better coordinating the family planning services and population research activities of the federal government.

Emergency Health Personnel Act (Public Law 91-623)—Authorized assignment of commissioned officers of the Public Health Service to areas with critical medical manpower shortages, in order to encourage health personnel to practice in such areas.

1971   *Comprehensive Health Manpower Training Act (Public Law 91-157)*—Provided for increased funding for health personnel through loan guarantees to students, student subsidies, startup assistance to schools, assistance to schools in distress, and health personnel initiative awards. Established the National Advisory Council on Health Professions Education and the National Health Manpower Clearinghouse. Mandated studies to look at the cost of educating health personnel students.

Nurse Training Act (Public Law 92-158)—Provided for training increased numbers of nurses through construction grants and student loan guarantees, advanced training traineeships, scholarships, loan repayment and forgiveness and capitation grants. Prohibited sex discrimination in student selection.

National Cancer Act (Public Law 92-218)—Strengthened the National Cancer Institute and National Institutes of Health in order to more effectively carry out national efforts against cancer.

1972   *National Sickle Cell Anemia Control Act (Public Law 92-294)*—Provided funding to aid in the control of sickle cell anemia.

National Cooley's Anemia Control Act (Public Law 92-414)—Provided funding to aid in the control of Cooley's anemia.

Continued.

APPENDIX 4-2

The Public Health Service Act of 1944: Some Major Amendments and Changes—cont'd

Communicable Disease Control Amendments Act of 1972 (Public Law 92-449)—Extended and revised the program of assistance to states for control and prevention of communicable disease, including grants for vaccinations, venereal disease prevention and control, and family planning services, grants and contracts.

1973 *Emergency Medical Services System Act (Public Law 93-154)*—Provided assistance and encouragement to states for the development of comprehensive area emergency medical services systems.

Health Maintenance Organization Act (Public Law 93-222)—Provided assistance and encouragement for the establishment and expansion of HMOs.

Safe Drinking Water Act (Public Law 93-253)—Significant environmental health legislation to assure safe drinking water in the United States.

1974 *Sudden Infant Death Syndrome Act (Public Law 93-270)*—Provided financial assistance for research, counseling, information, education, and statistical programs related to sudden infant death syndrome (SIDS).

National Cancer Program Improvement (Public Law 93-352)—Improved the national cancer program and reauthorized appropriations. Mandated an information dissemination program for professionals and the general public. Established the President's Biomedical Research Panel.

Health Services Research, Health Statistics and Medical Libraries Act (Public Law 93-353)—Revised programs of health services research and extended assistance for medical libraries. Established the National Center for Health Services Research.

National Diabetes Mellitus Research and Education Act (Public Law 93-354)—Provided for greater and more effective efforts in research and public education on diabetes mellitus. Established the National Commission on Diabetes within the National Institutes of Health and the Diabetes Mellitus Coordinating Committee to oversee federal activities on the subject. Authorized prevention and control programs and research and training centers.

National Arthritis Act (Public Law 93-640)—Expanded the authority of the National Institute of Arthritis, Metabolism, and Digestive Diseases in order to advance a national attack on arthritis.

National Health Planning and Resource Development Act (Public Law 93-641)—Authorized the development of national health policy and effective state and area health planning resources development programs. Established Titles XV and XVI. *Title XV,* National Health Planning and Development, dealt with national health policies and priorities, established health service areas and health systems agencies, and required state health planning and development agencies. *Title XVI,* Health Resources Development, dealt largely with construction and modernization of health care facilities. Existing Hill-Burton legislation was integrated into this act under Title XVI.

1975 *Public Health Service Act Amendments (Public Law 94-63)*—Revised and extended the revenue-sharing programs, family planning programs, community mental health programs, programs for migrant health centers, community health centers, hemophilia programs, the National Health Service Corps, and nurse training assistance. These amendments include: The Special Health Revenue Sharing Act, Family Planning and Population Research Act, and Community Mental Health Centers Amendments and Nurse Training Act of 1975. Established the National Center for the Prevention and Control of Rape.

1976 *National Consumer Health Information and Health Promotion Act (Public Law 94-317)*—Added title XVII, Health Information and Promotion, to the act. Called for the development of consumer and community information programs related to health information, prevention, and promotion activities and health education.

Indian Health Care Improvement Act (Public Law 94-437)—Improved federal Indian health programs and dealt with provision of services, construction and renovation of facilities, insured safe water, promoted construction of sanitary waste disposal sites, promoted access to health care services and these services for urban Indians, and authorized an American Indian School of Medicine feasibility study.

Health Maintenance Organization Amendments of 1976 (Public Law 94-460)—Revised and extended the program for establishment and expansion of HMOs.

Health Professions Educational Assistance Act (Public Law 94-484)—Revised and extended the programs of assistance under Title VII for training in health and in allied health professions. New authorization for special projects for departments of family medicine and programs related to the recruitment and enrollment of disadvantaged students. Also authorized special project grants for schools of public health and graduate programs in health administration for enlarging programs in biostatistics, epidemiology, health administration, health planning, health policy, environmental and occupational health, and nutrition. Traineeships for students in schools of public health were initiated under Title VII.

APPENDIX 4-2

The Public Health Service Act of 1944: Some Major Amendments and Changes—cont'd

Arthritis, Diabetes, and Digestive Diseases Amendments of 1976 (Public Law 94-562)—Established the National Arthritis Advisory Board, National Diabetes Advisory Board, and National Commission on Digestive Diseases.

1977   *Rural Health Clinics Act (Public Law 95-210)*—Established rural health clinics in underserved sections of the country.

Health Services and Extension Act of 1977 (Public Law 95-83)—Mandated the development of standards for community preventive health services ofer a 2-year period.

1978   *Public Health Amendments (Public Law 95-622)*—Biomedical and behavioral research amendments. Established the President's Commission for the Study of Ethical Problems in Medicine and Biomedical and Behavioral Research.

Health Services Research, Health Statistics, and Health Care Technology Act of 1978 (Public Law 95-623)—Established a National Center for Health Care Technology.

1979   *Health Planning and Resources Development Amendments (Public Law 96-79)*—Addressed the rising cost of health care and cost containment by establishing national health priorities and by eliminating inappropriate placement of people in institutions for the mentally ill and mentally retarded and increasing the quality of care in those institutions for people who needed it. This amendment also placed increased emphasis on community mental health centers utilizing outpatient rather than inpatient treatment. In addition, it developed a *certificate of need* program for health care facilities seeking federal funds, in order to minimize duplication of services and unnecessary services.

1980   *Health Planning Amendments (Public Law 96-538)*—Revised and extended the act. Deleted the National Commission on Diabetes and formulated the Diabetes Mellitus Interagency Coordinating Committee. Established the Diabetes, Arthritis, and Digestive Diseases Advisory Boards and the Information and Education Center on Digestive Diseases.

1981   *Omnibus Budget Reconciliation Act (Public Law 97-35)*—Enacted many budget and program cuts under the Public Health Service Act. It revised health planning policy; eliminated Public Health Service Hospitals as of the end of fiscal year 1981; consolidated many categorical programs of the Public Health Service Act into *block grants* to states, but left in place categorical funding for immunization, tuberculosis, venereal disease, family planning, and migrant health programs.

1982   *Tax Equity and Fiscal Responsibility Act of 1982 (Public Law 97-248)*—Authorized massive federal spending cutbacks that have an impact on public health.

1983   *Alcohol and Drug Abuse Amendments (Public Law 98-24)*—Established the National Institute on Alcohol Abuse and Alcoholism and the National Institute on Drug Abuse. Mandated Drug Abuse Strategy Reports on a yearly basis, which represented a continued federal effort to combat the problems of alcoholism and drug abuse. It also represented increased effort to disseminate information and research findings to the states, to provide technical assistance to research and service personnel, and to develop preventive programs designed to reduce alcohol and drug abuse problems. It encouraged the development of effective occupational prevention and treatment programs and private sector programs.

National Organ Transplant Act (Public Law 98-507)—Provided for the establishment of the Task Force on Organ Transplantation and the Organ Procurement and Transplantation Network.

1985   *Nurse Education Amendments of 1985 (Public Law 99-92)*—Extended the programs of assistance for nurse education through fiscal year 1988. Appropriated $9,500,000 yearly for 1986 through 1988.

Health Research Extension Act of 1985 (Public Law 99-158)—Created the National Center for Nursing Research and the National Institute of Arthritis and Musculoskeletal and Skin Diseases.

1986   Health Services Amendments Act of 1986 (Public Law 99-280)—Revised and extended the community and migrant health centers programs for 2 fiscal years and repealed the Primary Care Block Grant authority.

Safe Drinking Water Act Amendments of 1986 (Public Law 99-339)—Amended Title XIV of the Public Health Service Act, the Safe Drinking Water Act, to authorize EPA to establish national drinking water regulations and to determine maximum allowable water contaminant levels. Mandated that public water systems increase their monitoring for unregulated contaminants. Increased fines and sentences for tampering with public water systems, and prohibited the use of lead pipes and solder in public water systems.

Health Programs (Public Law 99-660)—Amended the Public Health Service Act to include the National Commission to Prevent Infant Mortality Act of 1986, National Childhood Vaccine Injury Act of 1986, Health Care Quality Improvement Act of 1986, Health Maintenance Organization Amendments of 1986, and the Alzheimer's Disease and Related Dementias Services Research Act of 1986. Repealed Title XV: Health Planning; revised and extended the health mainte-

Continued.

APPENDIX 4-2

The Public Health Service Act of 1944: Some Major Amendments and Changes—cont'd

nance organization program through 1989; established an authority within the Public Health Service under which states can apply for grants for the development of state comprehensive mental health plans and under which grants may be awarded for the training of health professionals in geriatric medicine; established a National Commission to Prevent Infant Mortality; encouraged professional peer review as a deterrent to malpractice and incompetence in health care; and established a Council on Alzheimer's Disease. The National Vaccine Program was given the responsibility for vaccine research, development, safety, and efficacy testing; licensing of vaccine manufacturers and vaccines; production and procurement of vaccines; evaluating the need for, effectiveness of, and adverse effects of vaccines; and coordinating government and nongovernmental vaccine activities. Established a National Vaccine Injury Compensation Program.

Public Health Service Act Amendments of 1987 (Public Law 100-177)—Amended the Public Health Service Act to extend the authorizations for the National Center for Health Services Research, National Center for Health Statistics, National Health Service Corps, and preventive health programs relating to immunizations and tuberculosis control. Established a Loan Repayment Program for the National Health Service Corps.

1988   *Family Health Services Amendments of 1988 (Public Law 100-386)*—Amended Title III of the Public Health Service Act to revise and extend the community and migrant health centers programs and the program of health services for the homeless.

Grants for Purchase of Drugs Used in the Treatment of AIDS (Public Law 100-471)—Provided for the awarding of grants for the purchase of drugs used in treatment of AIDS. $15,000,000 was appropriated to be used through March 31, 1989.

National Deafness and Other Communication Disorders Act of 1988 (Public Law 100-553)—Amended the Public Health Service Act to establish within the National Institutes of Health a National Institute on Deafness and Other Communication Disorders. The general purpose of the Institute is to conduct and support research and training, disseminate health information, and sponsor other programs with respect to disorders of hearing and other communication processes, including diseases affecting hearing, balance, voice, speech, language, taste, and smell. Established a National Deafness and Other Communication Disorders Data System, and a National Deafness and Other Communication Disorders Information Clearinghouse.

Lead Contamination Control Act of 1988 (Public Law 100-572)—Amended Title XIV of the Public Health Service Act, the Safe Drinking Water Act, to eliminate the use of lead-lined watercoolers.

Clinical Laboratory Improvement Amendments of 1988 (Public Law 100-578)—Amended the Public Health Service Act to revise the authority for the regulation of clinical laboratories. Provided for uniform standards for the certification of clinical laboratories.

Native Hawaiian Health Care Act of 1988 (Public Law 100-579)—Intended to improve the health status of native Hawaiians. Provided for grants and contracts with Papa Ola Lokahi for the purpose of developing native Hawaiian comprehensive health care master plan to promote comprehensive health promotion and disease prevention services, to maintain and improve the health status of native Hawaiians, and to provide for the establishment of Native Hawaiian Health Centers.

Health Omnibus Programs Extension of 1988 (Public Law 100-607)—Amended the Public Health Service Act to include National Institute on Deafness and Other Communication Disorders and Health Research Extension Act of 1988, Organ Transplant Amendments of 1988, AIDS Amendments of 1988, and Health Professions Reauthorization Act of 1988. The amendments extended Public Health Service Act authorities for the Preventive Health Block Grant; sexually transmitted diseases prevention and control grants; health professions education; and nurse training. Established the National Center for Biotechnology Information, the National Commission on Sleep Disorders, and the National Deafness and Other Communication Disorders Program. Created Title XXIV—Health Services with respect to acquired immune deficiency syndrome that provided comprehensive AIDS services including formula grants to states for home and community-based health services for AIDS patients. Required an annual comprehensive report to Congress each year on AIDS expenditures by the Secretary of Health and Human Services, and mandated the Secretary to expedite AIDS grants and research monies. Mandated Clinical Evaluation Units at the National Cancer Institute and the National Institute of Allergy and Infectious Diseases to evaluate AIDS treatment. Mandated support of international AIDS efforts with special emphasis being placed on cooperation with World Health Organization and Panamerican Health Organization AIDS efforts. Established a public information program with respect to AIDS research, treatment, and prevention activities including a toll-free hotline number, data bank on research information, and data bank on clinical trials and treatments. Provided grant monies for the establishment of projects to develop model protocols for the clinical care of individuals infected with the AIDS virus. Established the National Blood Resource Education Program to increase public awareness that giving blood is safe and other aspects of blood donation. Established the Office of AIDS Research within the Na-

APPENDIX 4-2

The Public Health Service Act of 1944: Some Major Amendments and Changes—cont'd

tional Institutes of Health. Provided for ongoing data collection on the national prevalence of AIDS, long-term AIDS research, and social sciences AIDS research. Established fellowships and training programs, to be conducted by the Centers for Disease Control, to train individuals to develop skills in epidemiology, surveillance testing, counseling, education, information, and laboratory analysis relating to AIDS. Established projects to promote cooperation between public and private sector AIDS programs and research.

Indian Health Care Amendments of 1988 (Public Law 100-713)—Reauthorized and amended the Indian Health Care Improvement Act.

Health Maintenance Organization Amendments of 1988 (Public Law 100-715)—Allowed insurance companies and other entities to sponsor HMOs.

APPENDIX 4-3

The Older Americans Act of 1965: Significant Amendments and Changes

1967 *Older Americans Act; Amendments of 1967 (Public Law 90-42)*—Authorized studies to look at the availability and adequacy of training resources in gerontology and to evaluate present and future trends and needs for such personnel and programs. Resulted in increased funding and training in the field of gerontology. Placed new emphasis on providing services to seniors.

1969 *Older Americans Act; Amendments of 1969 (Public Law 91-69)*—Mandated increased state planning for act programs through state agencies on aging. Increased the emphasis on coordination with local programs and program evaluation. Authorized grants to states and communities for model projects on services to the elderly. Established the National Older Americans Volunteer Program (NOAVP). NOAVP's main purpose was to help retired persons avail themselves of opportunities for voluntary service in their communities and helped to subsidize this through provision of transportation, meals, and other necessary services needed for them to participate. Major components of NOAVP were: (1) *Retired Senior Volunteer Program (RSVP)* and (2) *Foster Grandparents.*

1972 *Older Americans Act; Amendments of 1972 (Public Law 92-258)*—Amended the act to provide grants to states for the establishment, maintenance, operation, and expansion of low-cost meal projects, nutrition training, and education, as well as opportunity for social contacts for the elderly. Established the Nutrition Program for the Elderly and brought the nutrition of the elderly into the national limelight. From this legislation sprang many senior nutrition services.

1973 *Older Americans Act; Comprehensive Amendments of 1973 (Public Law 93-29)*—Established the Federal Council on Aging and the National Information and Resources Clearinghouse for the Aging. Required that a sole state agency administer the provisions of the act in conjunction with local agencies on aging. Established Multipurpose Senior Centers and Older Readers Services. These multipurpose centers combined social, recreational, health, and nutrition aspects for seniors into one accessible program. These centers also placed a new and increasing emphasis on the social needs of seniors and attempted to decrease social isolation for seniors through a community-based program.

1974 *Older Americans Act; Amendments of 1974 (Public Law 93-351)*—Provided for increased funding for transportation for the elderly, especially transportation services that facilitated the elderly in utilizing the nutrition programs and multipurpose centers already designated under the act. The transportation needs of the elderly living in rural areas were explored. This same year, a separate presidential proclamation declared *May* to be Older Americans Month, and this tradition has been carried on by a presidential proclamation each year since.

1975 *Older Americans Act; Amendments of 1975 (Public Law 94-135)*—Established social services programs especially for seniors. A significant part of these amendments involved two separate acts: *Age Discrimination Act of 1975* and *Older Americans Community Service Employment Act of 1975.* Both of these acts carry the same public law number as the amendments and are incorporated into the amendments. The Age Discrimination Act prohibited discrimination on the basis of age, largely in relation to employment. The Community Service Employment Act section of the amendments provided for community service employment for seniors where they were eligible to receive a wage. Most employment programs under the act, prior to this time, had involved voluntary employment for seniors. These amendments also attempted to attract more qualified people into the field of gerontology through increased funding for training.

Continued.

APPENDIX 4-3

The Older Americans Act of 1965: Significant Amendments and Changes—cont'd

1978   *Comprehensive Older Americans Act; Amendments of 1978 (Public Law 95-478)*—The Amendments of 1978 were extensive and provided for improved and increased programs for older Americans. These amendments called for a great reduction in the paperwork necessary to run the program; increased planning, coordination, evaluation, and administration efforts; and facilitated the quality of programs. They also established the Advisory Council on Aging; provided for area agencies on aging to contract for legal services and to carry out demonstration projects on the legal services necessary for older Americans; provided for exploring alternative work modes for older Americans such as the Senior Environmental Protection Corps with the Environmental Protection Agency (EPA); provided for grants to Indian tribes for older American services to tribes' members; set up a White House Conference on Aging for 1981 (there had previously been such conferences in 1961 and 1971); provided for a study of racial and ethnic discrimination in programs for older Americans; and outlined the programs of (1) *Congregate Nutrition Services* and (2) *Home Delivered Nutrition Services for the Elderly.* In addition, these amendments mandated development and implementation of national labor policy for the field of aging; discussed the concept of "preretirement" education and planning services; authorized special projects on long-term care and alternatives to institutionalization such as adult day care, supervised living in public or nonprofit housing, family respite, preventive health services, home health and homemaker services, home maintenance programs, and geriatric health maintenance organizations; and authorized demonstration projects for community model programs to improve and expand social services, and nutrition services, and to promote the well-being of older Americans. High priority for placement of these demonstration projects was given to rural areas and rural agencies on aging.

1981   *Older Americans Act; Amendments of 1981 (Public Law 97-115)*—Emphasized the provision of nutritional programs in congregate settings and facilitated access to such programs. These amendments also encouraged the formation of university-affiliated and other multidisciplinary centers on aging as well as long-term-care projects, and brought migrant and seasonal farm workers and organizations more in line with the provisions of the act.

1984   *Older Americans Act Amendments of 1984 (Public Law 98-459)*—Often referred to as the Older Americans Personal Health Education and Training Act. Provided for a comprehensive array of community-based, long-term care services to appropriately sustain older people in their communities and homes. Authorized the designing of a uniform, standardized *program of health education and training* for older Americans with direct involvement of graduate educational institutions of public health in the design of such a program and direct involvement of graduate education institutions of public health, medical sciences, psychology, pharmacology, nursing, social work, health education, nutrition, and gerontology in the implementation of such a program. Planned for such education and training programs to be carried out in multipurpose senior centers as already provided for under the act.

1986   *Older Americans Act Amendments of 1986 (Public Law 99-269)*—Amended the Older Americans Act to increase the federal contribution to senior nutrition programs covered under the act to about 57 cents per meal. Mandated that the Secretary of Agriculture and the Secretary of Health and Human Services jointly disseminate to state agencies, area agencies on aging, and providers of nutrition services covered under the act information concerning the existence of *all* federal commodity processing programs in which they would be eligible to participate, and the procedures necessary to participate in such programs.

1987   *Older American Act Amendments of 1987 (Public Law 100-175)*—Often referred to as the Health Care Services in the Home Act of 1987. Established grants to states for *in-home health care services* for the frail elderly, for periodic *preventive health* services to be provided at senior centers or appropriate alternative sites, and to implement programs with respect to the prevention of abuse, neglect, and exploitation of the elderly. Authorized a 1991 White House Conference on Aging, and reauthorized the Act through fiscal year 1991. Required on direct reporting relationship between the Commissioner on Aging and the Secretary of Health and Human Services; added an outreach program on Supplemental Security Income, food stamps, and Medicaid benefits; increased funds for administration of area agencies on aging and community service employment projects; added a Demonstration Project Authority in areas of health education and promotion, volunteerism, and consumer protection for home care services; and added a program for grants to assist older Hawaiian natives.

APPENDIX 4-4

Major Environmental Health Legislation

1924   *Oil Pollution Act (Public Law 68-238)*—Prohibited the dumping of oil in navigable waters except in dire emergencies.

1946   *Atomic Energy Act of 1946 (Public Law 79-585)*—Legislated the development and control of atomic energy.

1947   *Federal Insecticide, Fungicide and Rodenticide Act (Public Law 80-104)*—Required all pesticides to be registered prior to sale and to be properly labeled as to use.

1948   *Water Pollution Control Act (Public Law 80-845)*—Authorized the Public Health Service to help states develop water pollution control programs and to aid in the planning of sewage treatment plants.

1954   *Atomic Energy Act of 1954 (Public Law 83-703)*—Amended and superseded the 1946 act to include titles on purpose, research, production of nuclear material, byproduct materials, military application of atomic energy; atomic energy licenses, international activities, control of information, patents on inventions, and compensation for private property acquired, and established the *Joint Commission on Atomic Energy.*

1955   *Air Pollution Control Act (Public Law 84-159)*—Provided aid to states, and localities to protect air quality. Forerunner of Clean Air Act of 1963. Emphasized *state* responsibility for abatement of air pollution.

1956   *Federal Water Pollution Control Act (Public Law 84-600)*—Expanded the 1948 law to deal more aggressively with water pollution.

1960   *Federal Hazardous Substances Labeling Act (Public Law 86-613)*—Required that hazardous substances intended or suitable for household use be prominently and distinctly labeled "warning," "danger," or "caution," as necessary. Regulated interstate sale, transportation, and distribution of such substances. Repealed Federal Caustic Poison Act.

1961   *Oil Pollution Act (Public Law 87-167)*—To implement the provisions of the International Convention for the Prevention of the Pollution of the Sea by Oil, 1954; and provided fines and sentences for such pollution.

1963   *Clean Air Act (Public Law 88-206)*—Authorized direct grants to states and localities for air pollution control; *established federal enforcement* of laws regarding interstate air pollution; directed major research efforts into control of motor vehicle exhaust, removal of sulfur from fuel, and the development of air quality criteria.

1964   *Water Resources Research Act (Public Law 88-404)*—Authorized research to protect U.S. water resources.

1965   *Solid Waste Disposal Act (Public Law 89-272)*—Created a new Title II that established a program of grants-in-aid to states for solid waste disposal.

      Land and Water Conservation Act (Public Law 88-578)—Established a land and water conservation fund to assist state and federal agencies in meeting present and future outdoor recreation needs of the American people.

      Water Resources Planning Act (Public Law 89-90)—Attempted to consolidate the efforts of the river basin planning commission authorized to promote pollution control programs.

1967   *Air Quality Act (Public Law 90-148)*—Established a program of criteria and standards development and enforcement to control air pollution; set up air quality regions and basically strengthened the federal role in air quality maintenance.

1968   *Radiation Control for Health and Safety Act (Public Law 90-602)*—Authorized setting of state performance standards for electronic products such as x-ray machines, TV sets, microwave ovens, and similar devices.

1969   *National Environmental Policy Act (Public Law 91-190)*—Established a national policy for the American environment. Created the *Council on Environmental Quality* to advise the President and required environmental impact statements before major federal actions that might have environmental signfiicance. Through this legislation the *Environmental Protection Agency* was created. One of the best-known pieces of environmental health legislation.

1970   *Resource Recovery Act (Public Law 91-512)*—Shifted the emphasis from solid waste disposal to overall problems of control, recovery, and recycling of wastes.

      Environmental Education Act (Public Law 91-516)—Authorized the establishment of education programs to encourage public understanding of policies and support of activities designed to enhance environmental quality and maintain an ecological balance. Established the *Office of Environmental Education.*

      Environmental Quality Act (Public Law 91-224)—An attempt to limit the effects of pollution on the environment by establishing a national policy for the environment that would provide for enhancement of environmental quality. Authorized the Office of Environmental Quality with the Chairman of the Council on Environmental Quality as the director. Included provisions to increase water quality in the United States including Great Lakes demonstration projects and undergraduate scholarships for persons planning to study water treatment and pollution control.

Continued.

APPENDIX 4-4

Major Environmental Health Legislation—cont'd

Lead-Based Paint Poisoning Prevention Act (Public Law 91-695)—Provided federal assistance to help cities and communities combat lead-based paint poisoning. Established demonstration and research projects.

Clean Air Act Amendments (Public Law 91-604)—Strengthened and expanded air pollution control activities; granted broad regulatory responsibilities to the Environmental Protection Agency. Emphasized research, training, and control. Addressed the problem of motor vehicle emissions and aircraft emissions. Established a new Title IV: Noise Pollution.

1972   *Marine Mammal Protection Act (Public Law 92-522)*—Developed to protect marine mammals from extinction. Established a Marine Mammal Commission, an international program, and research grants.

Federal Water Pollution Control Amendments (Public Law 92-500)—Totally revised the Clean Water Act of 1948 and the federal water program; shifted efforts from the preservation of available water to the improvement of water quality through technology; set as a goal the elimination of pollutant discharge from all navigable waters and dealt with sewage treatment.

Federal Environmental Pesticide Control Act of 1972 (Public Law 92-516)—Expanded and strengthened provisions on product registration, labeling, environmental protection, registration of manufacturers, and national monitoring of pesticide residues in water and food.

Noise Control Act (Public Law 92-574)—Authorized a broad federal program to coordinate noise research and control activities, to establish standards, and to improve public information.

1973   *Endangered Species Act (Public Law 93-205)*—Designed to provide for the conservation of endangered and threatened species of fish, wildlife, and plants.

1974   *Safe Drinking Water Act (Public Law 93-523)*—Amended the Public Health Service Act of 1944 to require the Environmental Protection Agency to set national drinking water standards and to aid states and localities in enforcement.

1975   *Hazardous Materials Transport Act (Public Law 93-633)*—Regulated commerce by improving public protections against the risks connected with the transport of hazardous materials

1976   *Toxic Substances Control Act (Public Law 94-469)*—To prevent unreasonable injury to health or the environment associated with the manufacture, processing, distribution in commerce, use, or disposal of hazardous chemical substances. Required EPA to test existing chemicals; prevent future chemical risks by premarket screening and tracking, and gather and disseminate information about such chemicals.

1977   *Soil and Water Resources Conservation Act (Public Law 95-192)*—Provided for furthering the conservation, protection, and enhancement of the nation's soil, water, and related resources to enhance sustained use. Authorized public participation in the program and directed specific present and future mandates to the Department of Agriculture in this area.

Clean Water Act of 1977 (Public Law 95-217)—Amended the Federal Water Pollution Control Act to provide for additional authorizations and to establish a National Clearinghouse for Alternative Treatment Information within EPA. Grants to municipalities for research, demonstration projects, and training.

Clean Air Act Amendments (Public Law 95-95)—A major overhaul to the act. Established a *National Commission on Air Quality* and a *Task Force on Environmental Cancer and Heart and Lung Disease.*

1978   *Water Research and Development Act (Public Law 95-467)*—Endeavored to promote a more adequate and responsive national program of water research and development. Established centers for cataloging scientific research. Mandated interagency coordination and EPA consultation.

National Ocean Pollution Research, Development and Monitoring Planning Act of 1978 (Public Law 95-273)—Established a program of ocean pollution research, development, and monitoring.

1980   *Asbestos School Hazard Detection and Control Act (Public Law 96-270)*—Established a program for the inspection of schools to detect the presence of hazardous asbestos materials; to provide loans to states or local educational agencies to contain or remove hazardous asbestos materials from schools; and to replace such materials with suitable building materials.

Solid Waste Disposal Act Amendments (Public Law 96-482)—Required 5-year action plans for federal resource conservation and recovery activities that were coordinated and nonduplicated. Established the *Interagency Coordinating Committee on Federal Resource Conservation and Recovery Activities.*

APPENDIX 4-4

Major Environmental Health Legislation—cont'd

Comprehensive Environmental Response, Compensation and Liability Act (Public Law 96-510)—Known as the Super-fund, this act provided for liability, compensation, cleanup, and emergency response for hazardous substances released into the environment and cleanup of inactive hazardous waste disposal sites. EPA overseeing programs. Established *Agency for Toxic Substances and Disease Registry* and the *Hazardous Substance Response Trust Fund.* A total of $44 million was appropriated to the fund for the years 1981-1985 with the federal government being liable only up to that amount.

1981 *Consumer-Patient Radiation and Health Safety Act (Public Law 97-35)*—Part of the Omnibus Budget Reconciliation Act. Minimized the risk of unnecessary exposure to potentially hazardous radiation related to medical and dental proce-dures. Encouraged accredited and certified technicians.

1982 *Nuclear Waste Policy Act (Public Law 97-425)*—Provided for the development of repositories for the disposal of high-level radioactive waste and spent nuclear fuel and established a program of research and demonstration projects on the disposal of these products.

1983 *International Environmental Protection Act (Public Law 98-164)*—Title VII of the Department of State Authorization Act. Increased international environmental protection activities, especially in relation to endangered species and wildlife conservation.

1984 *Water Resources Research Act (Public Law 98-242)*—Preceded by an act in 1964. Authorized an ongoing program of water resources and research. Acknowledged the need for a water supply of high quality and quantity. Grant programs established.

1986 *Safe Drinking Water Act Amendments of 1986 (Public Law 99-339)*—The most significant amendments to the Safe Drinking Water Act to date. Authorized EPA to set national drinking water standards and determine maximum allowa-ble water contaminant levels. Set a 3-year deadline for EPA to set these standards for 83 specified contaminants. Re-quired EPA to promulgate requirements for disinfection and filtration of public water and provide technical assistance on these practices. Mandated that public water systems increase their monitoring of unregulated contaminants. Increased fines and sentences for tampering with public water systems and required EPA to take enforcement action in cases in which drinking water was tampered with and the state did not take action. Established grants to state and local authori-ties to develop groundwater protection programs. Prohibited the use of lead pipes and solder in public water systems.

Federal Lands Cleanup Act of 1986 (Public Law 99-402)—Provided for a program of cleanup and maintenance on fed-eral lands. A public lands cleanup day was designated as the first Saturday after Labor Day each year (states may select another day if the designated day is not climatically or otherwise appropriate).

Superfund Amendments and Reauthorization Act of 1986 (Public Law 99-499)—Directed the administrator of EPA to identify and assess locations and levels of radon gas and radon daughters in naturally occurring deposits of uranium col-lecting in residences and structures. Amended and extended the Comprehensive Environmental Response, Compensa-tion, and Liability Act of 1980 through fiscal year 1988.

Asbestos Hazard Emergency Response Act of 1986 (Public Law 99-519)—Amended the Toxic Substances Control Act to require the Environmental Protection Agency to promulgate regulations and issue rules requiring inspection and rein-spection of the nation's schools for asbestos. Required development of asbestos management plans for the nation's schools.

Emergency Wetlands Resources Act of 1986 (Public Law 99-645)—Promoted the conservation of migratory waterfowl and offset or prevented the serious loss of wetlands by the acquisition of wetlands and other essential habitat for migra-tory waterfowl.

Water Resources Development Act of 1986 (Public Law 99-662)—Provided for the conservation and development of water and related resources and the improvement and rehabilitation of the nation's water resources.

1987 *Water Quality Act of 1987 (Public Law 100-4)*—Amended the Federal Water Pollution Control Act to provide for the renewal of the quality of the nation's waters.

Toxic Substances Control Act Amendment—School Asbestos Management (Public Law 100-368)—Amended the provi-sions of the Toxic Substances Control Act relating to asbestos in the nation's schools by providing adequate time for educational agencies to submit asbestos managment plans to state governors and to begin implementation of those plans.

From U.S. Statutes-at-Large (selected years), U.S. Department of Health, Education, and Welfare, Health in America 1776-1976, Washington, DC, 1977, U.S. Government Printing Office.

REFERENCES

American Cancer Society: Cancer facts and figures—1989, New York, 1989, American Cancer Society.

Arnett RH, Cowell CS, Davidoff LM, and Freeland MS: Health spending trends in the 1980's: adjusting to financial incentives, Health Care Financ Rev Spring 6:1-26, 1985.

Bretz J: Social security programs in the United States—unemployment insurance, Social Sec Bull 52(7):19-27, 1989.

Bretz J: Social security programs in the United States—Medicare, Social Soc Bull 52(7):43-48, 1989.

Coll, BD: Perspectives in public welfare: a history, Washington, DC, 1969, US Government Printing Office.

Courpas M: Environmental protection. Air quality issues. Major legislation of the Congress—100th Congress summary issue, December 1988, MLC-035.

Donabedian D: Health and welfare systems, Ann Arbor, University of Michigan School of Nursing, 1979.

Donabedian D: Conversation with author on health and welfare systems as they apply to nursing, Ann Arbor, April 9, 1990.

French, RM: Dynamics of health care, ed 3, New York, 1979, McGraw-Hill.

Georke LS, and Stebbins EL: Mustard's introduction to public health, ed 5, New York, 1968, Macmillan.

Grundmann H: Social Security programs in the United States—introduction, Social Sec Bull 52(7):1-6, 1989.

Harrington C: A national health care program: has its time come? Nurs Outlook 36:214-216, 225, 1989.

Health Care Financing Administration–Office of Public Affairs: Your Medicare handbook, Washington, DC, 1989, US Government Printing Office.

Health Care Financing Administration–Office of Research and Demonstrations: Medicare and Medicaid data book 1989, Washington, DC, 1989, US Government Printing Office.

Health Insurance Association of America: Source book of health insurance data: 1977-78, Washington, DC, 1978, The Association.

Health Insurance Association of America: Source book of health insurance data: 1983-84, Washington, DC, 1983, The Association.

Health Insurance Association of America: Source book of health insurance data: 1988, Update, Washington, DC, 1988, The Association.

Health Insurance Association of America: Source book of health insurance data: 1989, Washington, DC, 1989, The Association.

Institute of Gerontology: Social security the first thirty-five years, Ann Arbor, 1970, University of Michigan Press.

Institute of Medicine–Committee for the Study of the Future of Public Health: The future of public health, Washington, DC, 1988, National Academy Press.

Loeff J, Bretz J and Kerns W: Social security programs in the United States—income-support programs, Social Sec Bull 52(7):62-77, 1989.

Manser G: Volunteers. In Minahan A, ed-in-chief, Encyclopedia of social work, ed 18, Silver Spring, Md, 1987, National Association of Social Workers, pp 842-851.

Metropolitan Life Insurance Company: Brief history of Metropolitan Life's health and safety activities, 1871-1983, New York, 1983, The Company.

National League for Nursing: Position statement on national health insurance, New York, 1981, The League.

National League for Nursing: Building a public policy agenda: constituents are key, Public Policy Bull Summer 1989:1-4, The League.

Nelson WJ: Social Security programs in the United States—workers' compensation, Social Sec Bull 52(7):27-36, 1989.

Nelson WJ: Workers' compensation coverage, benefit, and costs, 1986, Social Sec Bull 52(3):34-41, 1989.

OASDI and SSI cost-of-living increases for 1989, Social Sec Bull 52:(1):27, 1989.

Pickett G and Hanlon JJ: Public health administration and practice, ed 9, St Louis, 1990, The CV Mosby Co.

Schwartz D and Grundmann H: Social Security programs in the United States—Old Age, Survivors, and Disability Insurance, Social Sec Bull 52(7):6-19, 1989.

Short PF, Monheit AC, and Beauregard K: A profile of uninsured Americans, DHHS Pub No (PHS) 89-3443, National Medical Expenditure Survey Research Findings, 1, National Center for Health Services Research and Health Care Technology Assessment, Rockville, Md, 1989, US Government Printing Office.

Silver GA: Family medical care: a design for health maintenance, Cambridge, Ma, 1974, Ballinger.

Simon M: Social security programs in the United States—Medicaid, Social Sec Bull 52(7):48-51, 1989.

Smolensky, J: Principles of community health, ed 4, Philadelphia, 1977, Saunders.

Starr, P. Transformation in defeat: the changing objectives of national health insurance: 1915-1980, Am J Public Health 72:78-88, 1982.

Tropman EJ and Tropman JE: Voluntary agencies. In Minahan A, ed-in-chief, Encyclopedia of social work, ed 18, Silver Spring, Md, 1987, National Association of Social Workers, pp 825-842.

US Department of Health and Human Services: United States 1983, Washington DC, 1983, US Government Printing Office.

US Department of Health and Human Services: United States 1988, Washington, DC, 1989, US Government Printing Office.

United States Statutes-at-Large: selected years.

Wilner DM, Walkley RP, and O'Neill EJ: Introduction to public health, ed 7, New York, 1978, Macmillan.

Wilson FA, and Neuhauser D: Health services in the United States, ed 2, revised, Cambridge, Ma, 1985, Ballinger.

SELECTED BIBLIOGRAPHY

Ballantyne HC: Social security financing in North America, Social Sec Bull 52(4):2-13, 1989.

Bixby AK: Public social welfare expenditures, fiscal year 1986, Social Sec Bull 52(2):29-39, 1989.

Gronbjerg K: Private welfare in the welfare state, Social Serv Rev 56(1):1-26, 1982.

Haanes-Olsen L: Worldwide trends and developments in social security, 1985-1987, Social Sec Bull 52(2): 14-26, 1989.

Hamilton CL and Wilson CN: The new Medicare catastrophic coverage act: will it affect nursing? Nurs Health Care 10:31-34, 1989.

Iams H and Ycas M: Women, marriage, and social security benefits, Social Sec Bull 51(5):3-9, 1988.

Kerns WL and Glanz MP: Private social welfare expenditures, 1972-1985, Social Sec Bull 51(8):3-11, 1988.

Kramer RM: Voluntary agencies in the welfare state, Berkeley, Ca, 1981, University of California Press.

Lake RS and Lamper-Linden C: A subject bibliography on legislative and political action, Nurs Health Care 4:334-337, 1983.

Naylor HH: Volunteers: resource for human services. In Kramer R and Specht H, eds: Readings in community organization practice, ed 3, Englewood Cliffs, NJ, 1983, Prentice-Hall, pp 154-164.

O'Connell, B: America's voluntary spirit: a book of readings, New York, 1981, Foundation Center.

Pearce JL: Leading and following volunteers: implications for a changing society, J Appl Behav Sci 18:385-394, 1982.

Social Security Administration: The social security handbook, Washington, DC, 1988, US Government Printing Office.

Trattner W: From poor law to welfare state, ed 3, New York, 1984, Free Press.

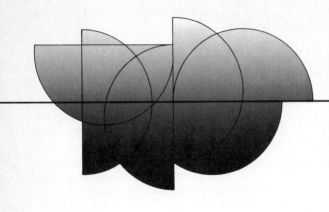

5

Organization of United States Health, Welfare, and Environmental Resources

---

OBJECTIVES

Upon completion of this chapter, the reader will be able to:

1. *Identify the national health objectives for health promotion and protection and disease prevention.*
2. *Explain the basic functions of local, state, and federal governmental health resources.*
3. *Discuss the major divisions of the U.S. Department of Health and Human Services (USDHHS).*
4. *Describe patterns of organizational structure*
   between state health authorities (SHAs) and local health departments (LHDs).
5. *Discuss service functions of SHAs and LHDs.*
6. *Discuss local and state governmental welfare organization.*
7. *Identify voluntary resources on the federal, state, and local level.*

The intent of this chapter is to assist the community health nurse in becoming more familiar with the health, welfare, and environmental resources safeguarding public health in the United States. The mission and organization of these resources are discussed with accompanying model health standards. In 1988, the Institute of Medicine's Committee for the Study of the Future of Public Health published a report that scrutinized public health in the United States: *The Future of Public Health.* As previously discussed in Chapter 3, this report will shape U.S. public health policy for years to come.

The committee broadly defined the mission of public health to be the measures we, as a society, take collectively to provide the conditions that ensure the people's health (Institute of Medicine, 1988, p. 17). The committee stated that "an impossible responsibility has been placed on America's public health resources: to serve the basic health needs of entire populations, while at the same time averting impending disasters, providing personal health care to those rejected by the rest of the health system; and to take on the new public health problems while confronting the old" (Institute of Medicine, 1988, pp. 2, 138). According to the committee, public health in the United States requires that continuing and emerging threats to the public health be successfully countered including *immediate crises* such as the AIDS epidemic and access to health and welfare services for the indigent; *enduring problems* such as injuries, chronic illness, teen pregnancy, control of high blood pressure, smoking, and substance abuse; and *growing challenges,* such as the aging of our population, homelessness, and environmental health (Institute of Medicine, 1988, pp. 19-30). Additionally, the American public has come to take the successes of public health for granted, and has sometimes become lax in public health practices. The committee concluded that it

The authors are indebted to Loraine Black, friend and colleague, who taught both faculty and students the philosophy and practices of health care administration and who stimulated an interest in discovering how the health care system works. We appreciate her efforts in facilitating the writing of this chapter.

was no wonder the American public health system is in trouble and has problems—the wonder is that it has done so much, for so long, with so little (Institute of Medicine, 1988, p. 2).

The United States has a wealth and diversity of health, welfare, and environmental resources, the scope of which is not seen elsewhere in the world. However, these resources are often of questionable quality, fragmented, and poorly coordinated. Resources and responsibilities have become so fragmented that deliberate action is difficult, if not impossible (Institute of Medicine, 1988, p. 17). States have primary responsibility for ensuring the public health, and public health services vary greatly across the nation.

The Health Services Extension Act of 1977 (Public Law 95-83) mandated the development of model standards for community preventive health services in American communities. These standards were to be flexible enough to be utilized across the nation. The American Public Health Association, National Association of County Health Officials, Centers for Disease Control, Association for State and Territorial Health Officials, and United States Conference of Local Health Officers worked collaboratively to formulate these model standards. The result was *Model Standards: A Guide for Community Preventive Health Services,* now in its second edition, which has become a classic in the field and is frequently referred to in community health literature.

The model standards addressed preventive services and some regulatory aspects of prevention. Areas such as health care delivery, financing and licensure; community health planning; and nursing home services were not addressed. For each standard there was a goal statement, process objectives, and outcome objectives. The program areas for these standards are given in the box on p. 141. To date, the federal government has not mandated nationwide implementation of the standards, but encourages state and local official health agencies to utilize them.

Public health resources are found at all levels of government (federal, state, and local), and in both the private nonprofit (voluntary) and for-profit (proprietary) sectors. The United States is

Model Standards for Preventive Health—Program Areas		
Administration and supporting services	Health education	Primary care
Aging and dependent populations	Home health services	Radiological health
Air quality	Housing services	Sanitation facilities
Alcohol and drug abuse and addiction	Injury control	School health
Chronic disease control	Institutional services	Solid waste management
Communicable disease control	Laboratory services (public health)	Tobacco use and addiction
Dental health	Maternal and child health (MCH)	Toxic and hazardous substances
Emergency medical services (EMS)	Mental health	Vector and animal control
Epidemiology and surveillance	Noise control	Violent and abusive behavior
Family planning	Nutrition services	Wastewater management
Food protection	Occupational safety and health	Water (safe drinking)
Genetic disease control		

From American Public Health Association: Model standards: a guide for community preventive health services, ed 2, Washington, DC, 1985, The Association.

notable among the countries of the world for complicated policy relationships among national, state, and local levels of government; and for interweaving of private and public sector activity (Institute of Medicine, 1988, p. 37). Decision making in public health is frequently driven by crises and the concerns of organized interest groups, rather than by comprehensive analysis or the objective of enhancing the quality of life (Institute of Medicine, 1988, p. 5). Barriers to public health problem solving exist such as the lack of consensus on the mission of public health, fragmented decision making, inequities in public health services, problems in relationships among the several levels of government, and the poor public image of public health (Institute of Medicine, 1988, p. 108).

Under the U.S. Constitution the states have primary responsibility for public health. From state to state there are great differences in public health resources, services, and administration. The diversity and fragmentation of the U.S. public health system make it difficult to succinctly discuss, define, or conceptualize it. The following is an overview of the mission and administration of governmental (official) and private (nonofficial)

public health resources in the United States. This material should assist the health care professional in working with clients in the community, and will give community health nurses a better understanding of the public health system in which they work.

THE FEDERAL GOVERNMENT: HEALTH, WELFARE, AND ENVIRONMENTAL ORGANIZATION

The word *health* was left out of the United States Constitution. The federal government bases its involvement in health and welfare activities on the Preamble to the Constitution, which charges it with providing for the general welfare of the people. Public health is the responsibility of the individual states and is provided for through their constitutions, legislation, and public health codes.

In 1979, under the presidency of Jimmy Carter, the Surgeon General of the United States issued a landmark report that has shaped public health policy for the past decade: *Healthy People: The Surgeon General's Report on Health Promotion and Disease Prevention.* This report analyzed the leading causes of death in the United States,

---

Major Documents on United States Public Health Goals, Objectives, Services, and Standards since 1979

United States Public Health Service: Healthy people. The Surgeon General's report on health promotion and disease prevention, Washington, DC, 1979, US Government Printing Office.

United States Public Health Service: Promoting health/preventing disease: objectives for the nation, Washington, DC, 1980, US Government Printing Office.

United States Public Health Service: The 1990 health objectives for the nation: a midcourse review, Washington, DC, 1986, US Government Printing Office.

American Public Health Association: Model standards: a guide for community preventive health services, ed 2, Washington, DC, 1985, The Association.

Public Health Foundation: Status report: state progress on 1990 health objectives for the nation, Washington, DC, 1988, The Foundation.

United States Public Health Service: Year 2000 national health objectives, Washington, DC, 1990 (tentative), US Government Printing Office.

---

and suggested that many of these deaths are preventable. It estimated that approximately one half of all U.S. mortality was due to unhealthful behavior, one fifth to environmental hazards, one fifth to human biological factors, and one tenth to inadequacies in the health care system. *Healthy People* was the first in a series of documents that outlined U.S. public health goals, objectives, services and standards. These documents are discussed in this chapter, and are listed in the box above.

Healthy People established broad national health goals targeted for achievement in 1990, and issued a challenge to the nation to accomplish them. It launched an unprecedented initiative to promote healthful lifestyles and improve the health of Americans, and called on all levels of government, professionals, and lay people to undertake a venture that promised to reduce preventable death and disability across the lifespan (USPHS, 1986 p. v). The goals and subgoals were

listed under the areas of healthy infants, healthy children, healthy adolescents and young adults, healthy adults, and healthy older adults. The box on p. 143 lists the 1990 health goals and subgoals for the nation as outlined in *Healthy People*.

Healthy People established three target areas for health, with five priority subsets in each area: *Preventive health services* (priority areas: family planning, pregnancy and infant care, immunizations, sexually transmissible diseases, and blood pressure control); *Health protection* (priority areas: toxic agent control, occupational safety and health, accidental injury control, fluoridation of community water supplies, and infectious agents control); and *health promotion* (priority areas: smoking cessation, reducing the misuse of alcohol and drugs, improved nutrition, exercise and fitness, and stress control).

In 1980, the federal document *Promoting Health/Preventing Disease: Objectives for the Nation* set forth 226 specific and quantifiable objectives necessary for the attainment of the broad national goals established in *Healthy People*. Objectives were established for each of the 15 priority areas, and became the national health objectives for 1990. When the second edition of *Model Standards* was published, these objectives were cross referenced with the model standards to facilitate implementation of each. Table 5-1 outlines the 1990 objectives cross referenced with model standards.

In 1986, the Public Health Service published *The 1990 Health Objectives for the Nation: A Midcourse Review*. This midcourse review was meant to provide Americans with an assessment of how the nation was doing in its decade-long quest to improve health status. Because of the different data gathering and reporting mechanisms in individual states, it was often difficult to obtain information on the various objectives.

The midcourse review showed that the nation was on its way to achieving nearly half of the 226 objectives, that about one fourth were unlikely to be achieved, and that in eight cases the trend was away from reaching the 1990 targets (USPHS, 1986, p. iii). The midcourse review found reductions in both smoking and per capital alcohol

HEALTHY INFANTS

Goal: Continue to improve infant health, and, by 1990, reduce infant mortality by at least 35 percent to fewer than 9 deaths per 1000 live births.

Subgoals
• Reduce the number of low birth weight infants
• Reduce the number of birth defects

HEALTHY CHILDREN

Goal: Improve child health, foster optimal childhood development, and by 1990 reduce deaths among children ages 1 to 14 years by at least 20 percent to fewer than 34 per 100,000.

Subgoals
• Enhance childhood growth and development
• Reduce childhood accidents and injuries

HEALTHY ADOLESCENTS AND YOUNG ADULTS

Goal: Improve the health and health habits of adolescents and young adults, and by 1990 reduce deaths among people ages 15 to 24 by at least 20 percent to fewer than 93 per 100,000.

Subgoals
• Reduce fatal motor vehicle accidents
• Reduce alcohol and drug misuse

HEALTHY ADULTS

Goal: Improve the health of adults, and by 1990 reduce deaths among people ages 25 to 64 by at least 25 percent to fewer than 400 per 100,000.

Subgoals
• Reduce heart attacks and strokes
• Reduce death from cancer

HEALTHY OLDER ADULTS

Goal: Improve the health and quality of life for older adults, and by 1990 reduce the average annual number of days of restricted activity due to acute and chronic conditions by 20 percent, to fewer than 30 days per year for people aged 65 and older.

Subgoals
• Increase the number of older adults who can function independently
• Reduce premature death from influenza and pneumonia in older adults

From USPHS: Healthy people. The Surgeon General's report on health promotion and disease prevention, Washington, DC, 1979, U.S. Government Printing Office, pp. 21-78.

consumption, an increase in the use of automobile seat belts, and reduced death rates from strokes, cirrhosis, and traffic accidents. The review showed that Americans still need to work on the health areas of weight control, illicit drug use, control of violent behavior, teenage pregnancy, infant health, family planning, physical fitness and exercise, and control of sexually transmitted diseases.

In 1988, the Public Health Foundation published *Status Report: State Progress on 1990 Health Objectives for the Nation.* This report reviewed the individual states' progress toward 29 of the 226 national objectives set forth in *Promoting Health/Preventing Disease: Objectives for the Nation,* and served as a resource for state health planning and evaluation activities for the 1990 objectives. The report found that states did not always have the information necessary to evaluate their progress toward the 1990 objectives. The Public Health Foundation plans to help states in gathering information and reporting on the 1990 objectives, especially for those objectives on which data are not presently available (Public Health Foundation, 1988, p. 6).

The leadership efforts that were started by the federal government in 1979 to set national health objectives and to promote the health of Americans are ongoing. The U.S. Public Health Service plans to finalize *Year 2000 National Health Objectives* in 1990. These health objectives will encompass 21 priority areas. New priority areas are planned to address improving mental health; prevention and control of HIV infection and AIDS; increased prevention, detection, and control of chronic diseases; maintaining the quality of life for older people; improving health education access to preventive health services; and improving public health surveillance and data systems (Public Health Foundation, 1989, Year 2000, p. 2). The Association for State and Territorial Health Officials (ASTHO) is promoting a National Health Objectives Act that would provide a billion-dollar federal grant initiative to states, localities, and others to implement the nation's year 2000 objectives (Harmon, 1988, p. 4).

The following is a discussion of the functions

TABLE 5-1 1990 objectives cross referenced with model standards

1990 objectives	Model standards
Preventive health	
High blood pressure control	Chronic disease control
Family planning	Family planning
Pregnancy and infant health	Maternal and child health Genetic disease control
Immunization	Communicable disease control (immunization)
Sexually transmitted diseases	Communicable disease control (sexually transmitted diseases)
Health protection	
Toxic agent and radiation control	Toxic and hazardous substances Solid waste management Air quality Water (safe drinking) Wastewater management Radiological health
Occupational safety and health	Occupational safety and health
Injury prevention	Injury control
Fluoridation and dental health	Dental health
Surveillance and control of infectious diseases	Epidemiology and surveillance Vector and animal control Communicable disease control Solid waste management Sanitation in facilities Food protection Water (Safe drinking)
Health promotion	
Smoking and health	Tobacco use and addiction
Alcohol and drug misuse prevention	Alcohol and drug abuse and addiction
Nutrition	Nutrition services
Physical fitness and exercise	Chronic disease control
Control of stress and violent behavior	Violent and abusive behavior

From American Public Health Association: Model standards: a guide for community preventive health services, ed 2, Washington, DC, 1985, The Association, p 181.

of the federal government in providing public health services and the federal agencies responsible for administering the health, welfare, and environmental programs essential to maintaining the public health.

Functions

In *The Future of Public Health,* the Committee for the Study of the Future of Public Health (CSFPH) stated that core functions in ensuring public health at all levels of government are assessment, policy development, and assurance (Institute of Medicine, 1988, pp. 7-8, 41-42, 141-142). At *all* levels of government the governmental role in assuring these core functions is the following (Institute of Medicine, 1988, pp. 141-142):

- *Assessment:* Regularly and systematically collect, assemble, analyze, and make available information on the health of the community, including statistics on health status, community health needs, and epidemiologic and other studies of health problems. This is a governmental function that cannot be delegated.
- *Policy development:* Exercise responsibility to serve the public interest in the development of comprehensive public health policies by promoting use of the scientific knowledge base in decision making about public health and by leading in developing public health policy. Agencies must take a strategic approach, developed on the basis of a positive appreciation for the democratic political process.
- *Assurance:* Assure constituents that services necessary to achieve agreed-upon goals are provided, either by encouraging actions by other entities (private or public sector), by requiring such action through regulation, or by providing services directly. Involve the general public and key policymakers in determining a set of high-priority personal and community wide health services that governments will guarantee to every member of the community. This guarantee should include subsi-

dization or direct provision of high-priority personal health services for those unable to afford them.

In addition to these functions the committee assigned *unique* responsibilities to each level of government. The committee recommended the following as additional federal government public health functions (Institute of Medicine, 1988, p. 9):

- Support knowledge development and dissemination through data gathering, research, and information exchange
- Establish nationwide health objectives and priorities, and stimulate debate on interstate and national public health issues
- Provide technical assistance to help states and localities determine their own objectives and

to carry out action on national and regional objectives

- Provide funds to states to strengthen state capacity for services, especially to achieve an adequate minimum capacity, and to achieve national objectives
- Assure actions and services that are in the public interest of the entire nation, such as control of AIDS and similar communicable diseases, interstate environmental actions, and food and drug inspection.

The functions of the federal government in relation to public health can be listed under six major categories. Table 5-2 delineates these categories and presents examples of programs and services under each.

The following is an overview of major federal

TABLE 5-2   Federal government health, welfare, and environmental functions: categories of functions with examples of programs and services

Categories of functions	Examples of programs and services by category
Personal health, welfare, and environmental health	Carries out extensive personal health services under the mandates of the Social Security Act of 1935, Public Health Service Act of 1944, Occupational Safety and Health Act of 1970, and various environmental health legislation. Sets national health objectives and mandates model public health standards. Sponsors services in areas such as research, environmental health, occupational health, disaster relief, civil defense, laboratory, biologics, communicable disease, substance abuse and addiction, physical fitness, stress control, health education, maternal and child health, adult health, chronic diseases, nutrition, and provides services to special population groups (e.g., American Indians, native Hawaiians, and migrant workers).
International health, welfare, and environmental health	Is a member of and supports international health and welfare organizations including the United Nations, WHO, and Peace Corps; and international disaster relief, foreign aid, and international pollution control programs.
Assessment, planning, and assurance	Includes national health assessments, setting national health and welfare goals and objectives, developing intervention strategies, and ensuring certain health, welfare, and environmental services through grants and legislation. An important service is the collection and dissemination of national health, welfare, and environmental statistics.
Policy development	Includes enacting effective and necessary health and welfare legislation and making adequate appropriations for such legislation.
Education and training	Involves promotion of programs preparing health and welfare professionals through such activities as training grants and loans, grants-in-aid to training programs, and continuing education. It also involves federal health education activities and ongoing and significant public health publications. Maintains the U.S. Government Printing Office.
Research	The federal government subsidizes research for the advancement of health, welfare, and environmental sciences and encourages research activities. It has established a number of national clearinghouses for health and welfare research and information, maintains the National Institutes of Health which conducts rigorous research programs and collaborates on international research.

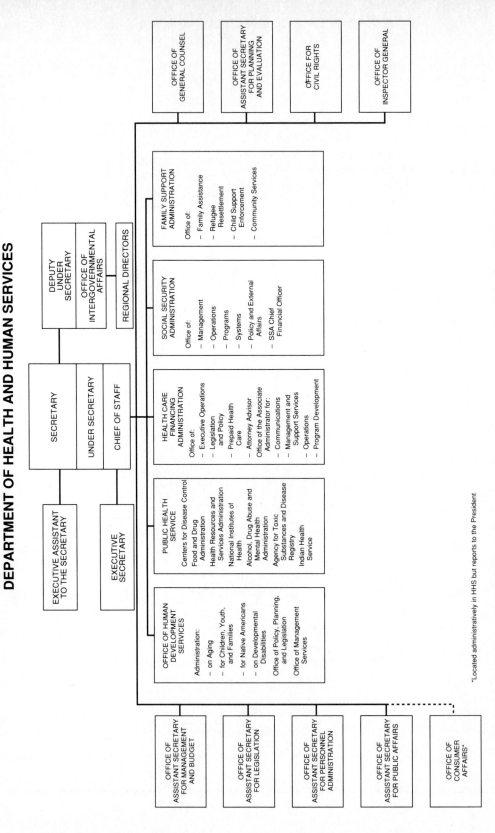

DEPARTMENT OF HEALTH AND HUMAN SERVICES

Figure 5-1 Organization of the U.S. Department of Health and Human Service. (From Office of the Federal Register: The United States government manual 1988/89, Washington, DC, 1989, US Government Printing Office, p 291.)

*Located administratively in HHS but reports to the President involvement in public health. There are *many* federal agencies involved in public health activities concerning health, welfare, and environmental issues. The federal government needs to identify more clearly the specific officials and agencies that are responsible for these public health activities (Institute of Medicine, 1988, p. 12). In the following discussion the Department of Health and Human Services is presented first, since it is the single most important federal agency in this area. Most of the health, welfare, and environmental functions of the federal government are coordinated and administered through this department.

DEPARTMENT OF HEALTH AND HUMAN SERVICES (DHHS)

This department assumed a cabinet-level position on April 11, 1953 as the Department of Health, Education, and Welfare (DHEW), with a charge to safeguard the health and welfare of the nation. In 1980, the DHEW split and became the Department of Health and Human Services (DHHS) and the Department of Education. The DHHS is the department most involved with the nation's human resources and concerns, and touches the lives of more Americans than any other federal agency. The secretary of the department advises the President on health, welfare, and income security issues. Figure 5-1 depicts the organization of the DHHS.

Several important health and welfare programs are administered through this department including Old Age, Survivors and Disability Insurance (OASDI), Medicare, Medicaid, Supplemental Security Income (SSI), Aid to Families of Dependent Children (AFDC), as well as many programs of the Public Health Service Act and Occupational Safety and Health Act. Major components of this department are discussed here, utilizing information from the *U.S. Government Manual* and the *U.S. Budget Report.* Both of these sources are updated yearly and are excellent resources.

Social Security Administration (SSA)

This administration was established on July 16, 1946, when its predecessor, the Social Security Board, was abolished. It guides and directs all of the cash benefit programs of the Social Security Act (SSA) of 1935. Other functions of this agency include research and recommendations on poverty in the United States, the planning and implementation of SSA administrative plans, statistical measurement and evaluation of SSA-administered programs, and development of public information on social security programs. The SSA includes 10 regional offices and over 1300 local offices across the country, and is the major federal agency dealing with social welfare programs for specific population groups (refer to Chapter 4).

Public Health Service (PHS)

This agency is charged with protecting the nation's physical and mental health and is also responsible for developing international health policies. It is the oldest of the department's component agencies, established in 1798, and is under the direction of the Surgeon General. It carries out the mandates of the Public Health Act of 1944 and is the major health agency of the federal government.

The Public Health Service collects and disseminates national health statistics, oversees national health resource planning, coordinates with states to set and implement national health policy, and sponsors programs for the prevention and control of communicable disease. It is actively involved in AIDS research and programs. It operates laboratory services, funds the construction and modernization of health care facilities, conducts and supports health research, provides grants-in-aid to schools of public health, provides funding for the training of health care professionals, coordinates health activities with international governments, and enforces public health laws. The National Center for Health Statistics is housed here. Major components of the Public Health Service are presented in Table 5-3.

Health Care Financing Administration (HCFA)

This agency was created by the DHEW reorganization of March 8, 1977, and oversees the administration of Medicare, Medicaid, and related federal quality control measures designed to improve the delivery of health care services. Chapters 4,

TABLE 5-3   Major components of the U.S. Public Health Service

Agency	Structure and purpose
Centers for Disease Control (CDC)	The centers were established in 1973 and constitute the federal agency charged with protecting the public health of the nation. The centers include nine operating agencies: Epidemiology Program Office, International Health Program Office, Training and Laboratory Program Office, Center for Prevention Services, Center for Environmental Health and Injury Control, Center for Health Promotion and Education, Center for Infectious Disease, The National Institute for Occupational Safety and Health (NIOSH), and the National Center for Health Statistics. Some major program components focus on communicable disease prevention and control, chronic disease prevention, occupational safety and health, public health emergencies, and international health. The centers also coordinate the use of rare therapeutic and immunoprophylactic agents and collect and disseminate health statistics.
Food and Drug Administration (FDA)	The FDA was formally established in 1931. Its activities are directed toward protecting the health of the nation against impure and unsafe drugs, foods, cosmetics, and other hazards. Major divisions include the Center for Drugs Evaluation and Research, Center for Biologics Evaluation and Research and Biologics, Center for Veterinary Medicine, National Center for Devices and Radiological Health, National Center for Toxicological Research, and Center for Food Safety and Applied Nutrition.
Health Resources and Services Administration (HRSA)	The HRSA provides leadership and direction to activities designed to improve U.S. health services, and to develop health care programs which are responsive to the needs of individuals, families, and communities. Funds AIDS demonstration projects and administers the National Organ Transplant Act. Provides leadership to improve the training, and utilization of health care personnel. Major components of the administration include the Bureau of Health Care Delivery and Assistance, Bureau of Health Professions, and Bureau of Maternal and Child Health and Resources Development.
National Institutes of Health (NIH)	The goal of NIH is to improve the health of the nation through biomedical research, training, and dissemination of information. Some of the major components are the National Cancer Institute; National Library of Medicine; National Institute of Arthritis, Musculoskeletal, and Skin Diseases; National Institute of Allergy and Infectious Diseases; National Institute of Dental Research; National Institute of Environmental Health Sciences; National Institute of General Medical Sciences; National Institute of Neurological and Communicative Disorders and Stroke; National Eye Institute; Institute on Aging; Division of Research Resources and the Division of Research Services; Division of Research Grants; Division of Computer Research and Technology; National Heart, Lung, and Blood Institute; National Institute of Diabetes and Kidney Disease; National Institute of Child Health and Human Development; and Fogarty International Center. The National Center for Nursing Research is centered in the National Institutes of Health.
Indian Health Service (IHS)	The IHS is responsible for providing a comprehensive health services system for American Indians, Alaskan natives, and native Hawaiians. The service assists Indian tribes in developing their health programs by providing health management assistance, training, and health planning activities, and serves as the principal federal advocate for Indian health care and Indians in the health care field.
Alcohol, Drug Abuse, and Mental Health Administration (ADAMHA)	The ADAMHA was established to provide a national focus for the federal effort to increase knowledge and promote effective strategies for control of alcohol and drug abuse, and mental illness. The administration conducts and supports research, gathers and analyzes data, and provides public information services. Its major components are the National Institute on Alcohol Abuse and Alcoholism, National Institute on Drug Abuse, and National Institute of Mental Health.
Agency for Toxic Substances and Disease Registry (ATSDR)	The ATSDR was established as an operating agency within the service on April 9, 1983. ATSDR provides leadership and direction to activities designed to protect public and worker health from the adverse effects of hazardous substance exposures and transporting accidents. ATSDR collects and disseminates information relating to serious disease and mortality from human exposure to toxic substances or hazardous substances, and maintains a listing of all areas in the nation closed to the public due to toxicity.

From Office of the Federal Registry, *The United States government manual 1988/89,* Washington, DC, 1988, US Government Printing Office.

12, and 19 address issues handled by this administration.

Family Support Administration (FSA)

This administration consolidated and absorbed the Office of Community Services and the Office of Child Support Enforcement into one administration. It serves America's children and families, especially low-income families; provides leadership and direction in family support programs; and is designated to carry out the Aid to Families with Dependent Children (AFDC) program of the Social Security Act. Its major components are the Office of Child Support Enforcement and the Office of Community Services.

OTHER AREAS OF FEDERAL INVOLVEMENT IN HEALTH, WELFARE, AND ENVIRONMENTAL RESOURCES

All cabinet level departments in the United States have functions which relate to the improvement of health and welfare conditions in our nation or foreign countries. These departments do not have the scope of public health responsibilities that DHHS has, but they provide essential services that enhance the health status and quality of life of Americans. Briefly summarized are some of the health and welfare functions carried out by other federal departments as presented in the *U.S. Government Manual (1988/89).*

Cabinet-Level Involvement

• *Department of Agriculture.* Carries out environmental health activities in the areas of food safety and inspection, sanitation, and assessment of plant and animal disease. It operates programs to protect and develop the nation's natural resources, coordinates rural development programs, and maintains the National Agricultural Library, which houses almost 2 million volumes. It conducts agricultural research, and operates cooperative extension services out of the land grant universities, and also operates international food assistance and information exchange programs. Through its food and nutrition programs the department works to minimize poverty, hunger, and malnutrition in the United States. These programs include food stamps, National School Lunch Program, School Breakfast Program, Special School Milk Program, senior citizen nutrition programs, and Supplemental Food for Women, Infants, and Children program (WIC). WIC is one of the department's largest, most successful, and best-known programs. WIC funding from the department to state health authorities amounted to 57 percent of the funding state health authorities received in 1986 from the federal government (PHF, 1989, USDA provides, p. 1). WIC is discussed more extensively in Chapter 13.

• *Department of Commerce.* Seeks to promote an understanding of the physical environment and oceanic life. Promotes economic development and encourages technological advancements. Its *Bureau of the Census* collects and disseminates data about the economy of the country and the characteristics of population groups; census information is discussed more thoroughly in Chapter 11. Its National Bureau of Standards maintains a national measurement system.

• *Department of Defense.* Provides the military forces necessary to deter war and to protect the national security. Administers the health and medical care services for military forces as well as civilian dependents of service personnel. This department also operates the National Civil Defense Program.

• *Department of Education.* Safeguards the nation's educational system. Oversees bilingual education; educational civil rights; education of the handicapped; vocational and adult education; rehabilitative services; elementary, secondary, and post-secondary education.

• *Department of Housing and Urban Development* (HUD). Is the principal agency concerned with national housing needs, especially for low-income families. It provides assistance for low-income housing, for the development and modernization of impoverished communities, and for the establishment of new communities. It oversees emergency shelter grants.

- *Department of the Interior.* Is the nation's conservation agency and is responsible for most of our national public lands and natural resources, overseeing the use of land and water resources, protecting fish and wildlife, and conducting research and health education programs to improve the ecological conditions in the United States. Its *Bureau of Mines* does research and fact finding on mine safety standards. The *Bureau of Indian Affairs* actively promotes improvement of health and welfare conditions for native Americans. Emphasis is placed on assisting communities in environmental land use, and management. It implements policies for the protection of the environment pursuant to the National Environmental Protection Act of 1969, develops environmental impact statements, and enforces laws on floodplains, wetlands, and endangered species.
- *Department of Justice.* Protects the health of the American public by enforcing federal laws. The department's Bureau of Prisons has a health services divison that maintains a health program in federal prisons to provide medical, psychiatric, dental, and other health support services for prisoners, and is involved in programs to help reduce homicidal deaths, violence, and drug addiction. It is instrumental in protecting civil rights and prosecutes high-level narcotic and dangerous drug offenders. The land and natural resources division represents the United States in litigation involving public lands and natural resources, environmental quality, Indian lands, wildlife resources, hazardous chemical waste, clean air and water laws, and EPA issues.
- *Department of Labor.* Promotes the welfare of workers and strives to improve working conditions. Is responsible for helping disadvantaged segments of the population such as migrant workers, older workers, native Americans, and handicapped workers to obtain employment. Coordinates federal worker compensation programs and enforces safety standards and fair employment practices. *The Occupational Safety and Health Administration* is housed in this department and the department is charged with carrying out many of the mandates of the Oc-

cupational Safety and Health Act of 1970. Provides labor-management services. Sets standards under the Mine Safety Health Administration for mines. Has a Women's Bureau, Job Training Programs, Senior Community Services Employment Program, Apprenticeship Training, and Veterans' Employment Program. This department also compiles extensive labor statistics.
- *Department of State.* Assists the President in formulating foreign policy. Carries out foreign aid and trade agreements, assists in improving the quality of life in underdeveloped countries and is an advocate of international human rights and humanitarian affairs. Responsible for refugee programs, international travel, passports, and representing our country abroad.
- *Department of Transportation.* Protects the environment by implementing portions of the National Environmental Protection Act. Protects the marine environment from damaging pollutants and advocates boating safety. Enforces certain air, land, and water standards in relation to interstate transport. Conducts programs aimed at reducing the increasingly large number of deaths and injuries due to traffic accidents.
- *Department of the Treasury.* Assists other government agencies in preventing illegal drug traffic, illegal possession of firearms, alcoholic beverages, and tobacco products through the U.S. Customs Service and the Bureau of Alcohol, Tobacco, and Firearms.

Besides our federal departments, numerous other agencies on the federal level have significant health and welfare functions. *The Veterans' Administration,* for instance, provides hospital, nursing home, and outpatient medical and dental care to eligible veterans of military service. This agency is also responsible for coordinating compensation, pension, and assistance programs; rehabilitation training for disabled veterans; and life insurance programs and burial services for veterans. In addition, the federal government sponsors the Endangered Species Committee, United States Information Agency, Architectural and Transportation Barriers Compliance Board, Commission on Civil Rights, the Tennessee Valley Authority, National Council on Handicapped, President's Committee on Employment of People with Disabilities, and the Prospective Payment Commission, to name a few.

Two very important governmental agencies that do not have cabinet status are the Environmental Protection Agency and ACTION.

ACTION

ACTION was created as an independent agency in 1971. It is the principal agency in the federal government administering volunteer service programs. Its purpose is to mobilize Americans for voluntary service in the United States through programs which help meet basic needs and support self-help efforts of low-income people and communities. Some of its major programs include Foster Grandparents Program, Retired Senior Volunteer Program, Senior Companion Programs, Volunteers in Service to America (VISTA), and student community service projects.

Environmental Protection Agency (EPA)

The federal government is actively involved in promoting environmental health; however, there is no one umbrella piece of federal environmental health legislation (refer to Chapter 4, Appendix 4-4), and environmental programs are housed in many agencies and departments. Although the federal government spent $3.5 billion on environmental programs in 1986 (Institute of Medicine, 1988, p. 193), many programs remain underfunded. Federal Superfund legislation provides funding for the cleanup of spills and other accidents involving hazardous or toxic materials. The federal government's environmental programs are handled primarily by the Environmental Protection Agency and the Agriculture Department. The Environmental Protection Agency is well known for its efforts to protect the American environment.

The Environmental Protection Agency was created in 1970. It is an agency separate from the Public Health Service, and sometimes coordination between the two agencies is lacking. It is the primary federal agency responsible for protecting and enhancing our environment and serves as the public's advocate for a livable environment. The EPA controls and abates pollution in the areas of air, water, solid waste, noise, radiation, and toxic substances, and it is mandated to mount an integrated, coordinated attack on environmental pollution in cooperation with state and local governments. The EPA coordinates and supports research and antipollution activities and develops and disseminates information. It is actively involved in pesticide programs. It has 10 regional offices. An organizational chart for this agency is presented in Figure 5-2.

International Involvement

Every nation has its own health, welfare, and environmental policies. However, there is international cooperation and coordination on these issues. The United States is involved with a number of agencies, groups, and governments on an international level, to maintain and improve health, welfare, and environmental conditions throughout the world. Several intergovernmental agreements, especially in relation to disease control, trade, immigration, world peace, and respect for basic human rights, have been developed to enhance the well-being of all people.

United Nations (UN)

The United States is extensively involved in international health and welfare issues through the United Nations. This international assembly is dedicated to promoting welfare, peace, and health. Two major United Nations–sponsored groups with which the United States works are the World Health Organization (WHO) and the United Nations' Children's Fund (UNICEF).

World Health Organization (WHO)

Efforts to organize international health activities took place between 1851 and 1909, when a series of meetings known as the International Sanitary Conferences occurred. These meetings were the precursor to the International Office of Public Health in 1909 (Pickett and Hanlon, 1990, p. 74). The primary focus of most international

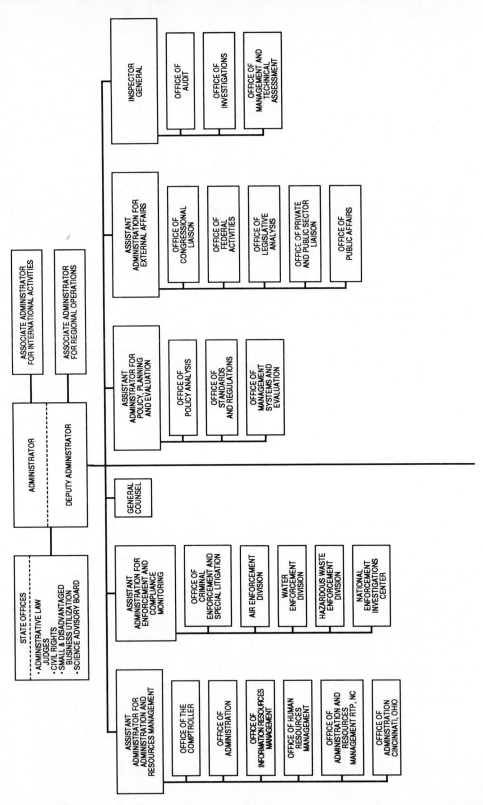

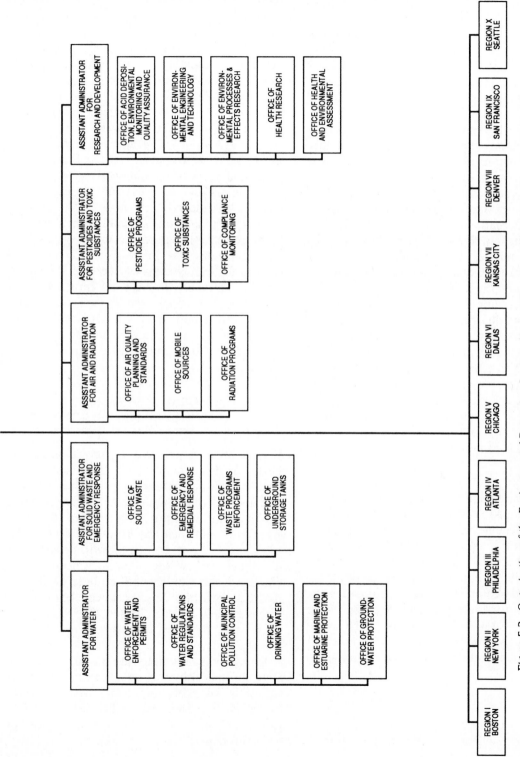

Figure 5-2 Organization of the Environmental Protection Agency. (From Office of the Federal Register: The United States government manual 1988/89, Washington, DC, 1988, US Government Printing Office, p 526.)

health activity is the control of communicable disease.

In 1948, the World Health Organization was created and became a part of the United Nations (WHO, 1988). The World Health Organization is concerned with standardizing international health activities and regulations, providing statistical and health educational services, promoting research, training health workers, promoting maternal-child health, and controlling communicable diseases. Any nation can belong to WHO without being a member of the United Nations.

A major goal of WHO is to prevent the spread of disease from one continent to another and to achieve international cooperation for better health throughout the world. To achieve this goal, the WHO publishes international health statistics, recommendations, and documents; has committees to work on the standardization of therapeutic substances, atomic energy, and health laboratory methods; and documents worldwide outbreaks of disease. It sets international quarantine measures and collects and disseminates epidemiological data. WHO is a world clearinghouse for health care information and sets worldwide health standards and practices. WHO is actively involved in coordinating international AIDS research and information. The world headquarters of WHO are located in Geneva, Switzerland.

United Nations' Children's Fund (UNICEF)

UNICEF attempts to meet the emergency and ongoing needs of children, particularly children in developing countries. It has improved maternal and child health and welfare conditions by combating malnutrition (food programs), preventing and controlling communicable diseases (immunization and treatment programs), compiling statistics, supporting research, and providing shelter and other basic welfare needs. WHO and UNICEF work closely together to promote services for at-risk mothers and children throughout the world.

Peace Corps

The Peace Corps was established in 1961 and was made an independent agency by the International Security and Development Act of 1981. The corps is charged with promoting world peace and friendship by helping to meet the needs of other countries for trained labor and by promoting a better understanding of the American people. Corps members serve in a volunteer capacity. Main headquarters are in Washington, D.C., with three regional recruitment centers, 16 area offices, and services in over 60 countries.

Men and women of all ages and from all walks of life serve as volunteers in the Peace Corps. Thousands of Corps volunteers serve in Latin America, Africa, the Near East, Asia, and the Pacific. Volunteers often work in the areas of rural development and agriculture, small business assistance, health, natural resources conservation, and education. The Peace Corps serves as the sponsor for U.S. citizens who serve in the United Nations Volunteer Program. Its Partnership Program provides opportunities for elementary, junior and senior high schools, civic groups, neighborhood, and youth organizations in the United States to sponsor assistance to an overseas community.

STATE AND LOCAL GOVERNMENT: PUBLIC HEALTH SERVICES RELATIONSHIP

Each state is responsible for providing for the health of its residents. Each state has a public health code that authorizes public health activities, and an agency, a state authority, to deal with health. In this text, the terms *state health authority (SHA)* and *local health department (LHD)* refer to official government health departments. These agencies are supported by general tax revenues and provide services at little or no cost to the general public. The services they offer are discussed later in this chapter; they vary greatly from state to state and community to community.

Each state health authority has local affiliates. State public health codes establish what type of relationship will evolve between SHAs and LHDs. Miller, Brooks, DeFriese, Gilbert, Jain, and Kavaler (1977, p. 47) found that these relationships had definite patterns of organization.

Patterns of Organizational Structure between State Health Authorities and Local Health Departments

Three organizational patterns characterize the administrative relationships between state and local health departments (Miller, Brooks, DeFriese, Gilbert, Jain, and Kavaler, 1977, p. 932):

1. Centralized organization: a state health authority of public health or a state board of health operates local health units that function directly under the state's authority, sometimes through regional administration.
2. Decentralized organization: local government (geopolitical unit of: city, township, county, or some combination) operates a health department. The state health authority offers consultation and advice to the local agency.
3. Shared organizational control: state health authorities and local health departments share public health responsibilities, and the state may retain appointive and line authority over local health officers (who are also responsible to local boards or commissions). Sometimes the local departments must submit programs, plans, and budgets to the state health department in order to qualify for federal or state funds.

The relationships between state and local health departments are seldom explicit. Authority for the promulgation of health rules and regulations is shared by state and local health departments in 68 percent of the states and held exclusively by state health departments in 30 percent (Miller, Brooks, DeFriese, Gilbert, Jain, and Kavaler, 1977, p. 935). State health departments usually share in the cost of local health department services, but the cost-sharing ratio varies greatly. Services provided by state and local health departments vary. Some common service areas are discussed here.

State Health Authorities and Local Health Departments: Service Functions

An overall goal of state health authorities and local health departments is to enhance personal and community health. This is done through provision of public health services such as:

1. Administrative
2. Communicable disease control
3. Personal health (maternal-child health and adult health)
4. Environmental health and safety
5. Occupational health
6. Vital statistics
7. Laboratory
8. Health education and training
9. Research
10. Emergency and special medical

Public health services are established in the state's public health code. States are often slow to revise these codes and many still deal primarily with communicable disease control.

STATE HEALTH AUTHORITY (SHA)

The U.S. Constitution empowers state governments to protect the health and welfare of their citizens. States are the central authorities in the nation's public health system and they have the primary public sector responsibility for public health (Institute of Medicine, 1988, p. 8).

The Institute of Medicine's Committee for the Study of the Future of Public Health recommended that the public health duties of states should include, in addition to the core activities, the following (Institute of Medicine, 1988, p. 12):

- Assessment of health needs in the state based on statewide data collection
- Assurance of an adequate statutory base for health activities in the state
- Establishment of statewide health objectives, delegating power to local health departments (LHDs) as necessary and holding them accountable
- Assuring statewide efforts to develop and maintain essential personal, educational, and environmental health services, provision of access to necessary services, and problem solving for public health
- Guaranteeing a minimum set of essential health services

• Supporting of local service capacity, especially when disparities in local ability to raise revenue and/or administer programs exists

The Public Health Foundation (PHF), founded by the Association of State and Territorial Health Officials (ASTHO), is one excellent source of information on state health (agencies). The ASTHO reporting system on state health departments started in 1970 as an amendment to the Public Health Service Act. This reporting system was designated as the uniform, national health program reporting system on state health departments and was intended to provide comprehensive data, on a national basis, about public health programs and expenditures of state and territorial health agencies (ASTHO, 1983, Public health agencies, iii). ASTHO publishes on a yearly basis (1) *Public Health Agencies: An Inventory of Programs and Block Grant Expenditures* and (2) *Public Health Chartbook.* ASTHO has done an admirable job; these publications are thorough and informative. The state-by-state information given is extremely beneficial in evaluating national health programs and activities.

There are 55 state and territorial health agencies (PHF, 1989, 1989 Public health agencies, p. 2). Most states have a separate department of public health, but some states have gone to a superagency approach, similar to the federal government's DHHS.

A major drawback to superagencies is the blending of health, welfare, and sometimes environmental and mental health services under one agency, with one detracting from another, and with little emphasis placed on health issues. The Institute of Medicine's Committee for Study of the Future of Public Health (1988, p. 152) recommended that public health and income maintenance be organizationally separate agencies while maintaining close and cooperative ties. Fifteen SHDs are also designated as the state mental health agency, 10 as the state Medicaid agency, 12 as the state environmental health agency, and 42 as the designated state crippled children's agency (PHF, 1989, Public health agencies, p. 7).

The chief executive of the department is often called the health officer or the director. The impact of politics is clearly evident with these positions: state health officers are frequently political appointees with an average term of 2 years (Institute of Medicine, 1988, p. 148). There is definitely a need for greater continuity of professional leadership in such positions. Most SHA health officers are physicians, but less than half have had public health training or experience (Institute of Medicine, 1988, p. 174). Some states are now requiring that the executive health officer have public health education on the graduate level. Health professionals from various disciplines with training or experience in public health administration are being considered for state health officer positions in some states. In these states physicians have positions as medical directors.

Each state authorizes specific public health services through its public health code: all state public health codes include communicable disease control and collection of vital statistics; 92 percent of them include venereal disease (VD) control and quarantine; 82 percent include refuse disposal; and only 26 percent include family planning services (Miller, Gilbert, Warren, Brooks, DeFriese, Jain, and Kavaler, 1977, p. 943). The state health department can delegate authority and responsibility for certain health activities to local health departments, but ultimate responsibility rests with the state.

The structure of state health departments differs from state to state. Figure 5-3 is an organizational chart depicting how a state health department may be organized.

SHAs spends billions of dollars each year, though budgets vary from state to state. In 1987 SHAs spent $8.1 billion, approximately $33.48 per state resident (PHF, 1989, SHA spending, p. 1). Of SHA expenditures, approximately 74 percent were for personal health expenditures, 6 percent for health, 3 percent for laboratory services, 6 percent for administration, and 9 percent for miscellaneous expenses (PHF, 1988, Public health chartbook, Figure 6). SHA spending was financed primarily from state and federal funds with 45 percent coming from state funds, 30 percent from federal funds, 13 percent from local

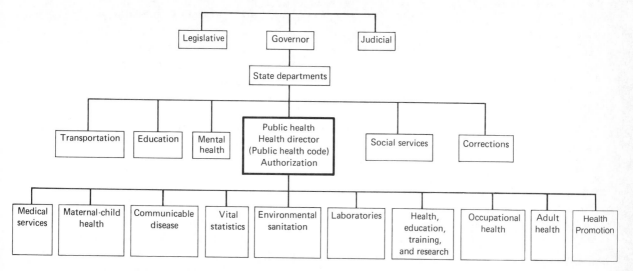

Figure 5-3   Organizational chart of a state health authority.

funds, and 8 percent from fees and reimbursement (PHF, 1989, SHA spending, p. 1). The amount of financing from fees for service has increased since 1986 (PHF, 1989, Fee income, p. 1). The Supplemental Food Program for Women, Infants, and Children (WIC) amounted to 20 percent of all public health expenditures for SHA in 1987 (PHF, 1989, SHA spending, p. 1). The combined spending of the SHAs of California, Maryland, and New York made up one fourth of all SHA public health expenditures in 1987 (PHF, 1989, SHA spending, p. 1).

Service Functions

The state health authority is charged with furnishing the leadership and funding to meet state public health needs. It carries out this charge through the service functions described below.

Administrative

Promulgation and enforcement of health standards, regulations, and policies are primary functions of SHAs. Sixteen states have policy analysis and development units (Institute of Medicine, 1988, p. 176). States ensure a statutory base for public health activities. They set legally enforceable health standards, regulations, and policies.

These frequently include establishing and enforcing public health codes; determining state public health policy; providing a state public health program with clear goals and objectives; establishing communicable disease regulations; licensing of health facilities; and monitoring state health insurance laws. Thirty-seven SHAs set standards for LHDs (Institute of Medicine, 1988, p. 177). States may delegate enforcement of public health law and regulations to local health agencies, but this function is overwhelmingly assigned to states in the public health codes. The state health department may take action against a local health department that is not adhering to state health policies. State health departments also develop standardized forms for statewide use in obtaining statistical information on births, marriages, and morbidity and mortality events. The licensing of health facilities is another important state function.

Working with local health departments to promote comprehensive, coordinated services in accordance with state health policy is extremely important. The state health department advises local health departments on health planning, programming and enforcement, budget review, and personnel policies. It can assist them in obtaining staff members and may approve their plan of organization and function. In some states, the state health department establishes the qualifications for local health officers. It may share the cost of service provision with local health departments, often on a per capita or straight percentage basis (e.g., 20 percent of cost).

Consultation services are provided to local health departments and other health agencies. Consultants are available in such fields as maternal-child health, nutrition, epidemiology, community health nursing, mental health, occupational health, and environmental health. These consultant activities are usually well utilized and are a major state health department service.

Administration of federally aided programs is an important function of state health authorities. The federal government provides funding for health programs, many through a block grant method of financing. These block grant areas include *preventive health services* (health education and risk reduction, health incentive grants, emergency medical services, fluoridation, hypertension, rape prevention and counseling); *maternal and child health* (specific maternal and child health programs, crippled children, SSI-Disabled Children's Program, lead-based paint poisoning, and sudden infant death syndrome); *alcohol and drug abuse;* and *primary health care* funding for community health centers. Some programs, such as immunization and family planning services, have not been incorporated into block grants; the states would be responsible for administering and accounting for these monies separately.

Health planning activities are also carried out by the SHA. These include assessment of state health needs, program development, and ongoing program evaluation, and quality assurance. States participate in comprehensive health planning activities and work with private and governmental agencies to utilize health care resources to their fullest potential.

Coordination of federal, state, and local health programs and services is another function assumed by the SHA. Data are compiled on available health resources and services offered throughout the state.

Legislation for health is promulgated and en-forced at the state and federal levels. Health legislation that represents and meets the needs of the people is promoted and developed. Representatives of the SHA may meet regularly with state legislators and congressmen.

Personnel policies, including hiring and promotional guides, grievance procedures, position descriptions, and manuals are developed by the state health department. A roster of available health personnel may be kept to help local health departments and other agencies recruit new staff.

Control of Communicable Disease

Communicable disease control is a major service function of SHAs. The state establishes immunization schedules, quarantine measures, and reportable communicable diseases, provides policies for epidemics and laboratory diagnostic services, and may supply local health departments with biologics. Local health departments must adhere to state communicable disease policies and report cases of communicable disease as determined by the state. Control of communicable disease is an extremely important function, even though the extent of communicable diseases has significantly decreased in the last century.

Personal Health Services

Personal health services *are all services delivered to individuals, except those related to environmental health.* These include maternal-child health services, such as family planning, the Medicaid program of Early, Periodic Screening, Diagnosis, and Treatment (EPSDT), and services to crippled children and children with mental retardation and other developmental disabilities. The state provides consultation for many maternal-child health programs that are offered at the local level.

Adult health activities include administering federal programs for heart disease, cancer, stroke, kidney disease, arthritis, and mental health. Again, these programs are brought to a direct service level through the local health department.

Environmental Health

Some SHAs administer federal environmental legislation: the Clean Air Act is administered by 12 SHAs, the Clean Water Act by 11, the Safe

Drinking Water Act by 32, the Conservation and Recovery Act by 14, the Superfund Legislation by 14, the Toxic Substance and Control Act by 11, and the Federal Hazardous Substance Act by 13 (PHF, 1988, Public health chartbook, Figures 2, 2A, and 2B). However, many environmental concerns and the authority to deal with them have been removed from public health agencies. This had led to diffuse patterns of responsibility, lack of coordination, and inadequate handling of environmental problems. State public health authorities must strengthen their capacities for identification, understanding, and control of environmental problems as health hazards (Institute of Medicine, 1988, pp. 150-151).

SHAs are also involved in setting and enforcing state environmental health standards. Increasingly, it is being recognized that there are major environmental health concerns in the United States that must be addressed.

Occupational Health

State health officials are assuming a more prominent role in occupational health and safety, an area often reserved for labor officials (PHF, 1988, SHAs expand, p. 2). However, SHAs are the lead agency for occupational health in only five states: New Jersey, New Mexico, North Dakota, Rhode Island, and Texas (PHF, 1988, Public health chartbook, Figure 2B). State occupational health and safety standards must be *equal to or exceed* federal standards. Thirty-one SHAs code occupation information on death certificates, 14 collect data on the parents' occupation on birth certificates to help pinpoint causes of congenital malformations and disorders, 11 collect occupational histories for all cancer patients, and 7 mandate registries for occupational diseases other than cancer (PHF, 1988, SHAs expand, p. 2).

Vital Statistics

Vital statistics are collected and disseminated by the SHA. Thirty-one SHAs have centers for health statistics (Institute of Medicine, 1988, p. 176). The state develops standardized forms, including certificates of birth, death, fetal death, marriage, and divorce; licenses for marriage; and epidemiologic reporting forms. The state also disseminates statistical information to individuals and agencies, including the National Center for Health Statistics. The state health department has an abundance of statistical information about the health status of its population and the health work force and resources within the state. This is valuable information and available to the general public on request.

Laboratory Services

Laboratory services are operated by most SHAs. Specimens are sent there for analysis; the diagnostic services rendered are primarily in relation to communicable disease control and environmental sanitation. Local health departments and private physicians often utilize these services on behalf of clients. There is usually no fee, or a minimal fee, to the public for laboratory analysis of reportable communicable diseases. The laboratory also certifies vaccines and other biologics.

Health Education and Training

Education, training, and research are carried out by the SHA. The state promotes the development of new health knowledge through the support of state colleges and universities and research agencies; the dissemination of health information to the general public (printed materials, classes, and media programs); the development of training and inservice programs for state and local health department personnel; and involvement in research activities. Local health departments find SHAs to be valuable resources when health information and audiovisual media are needed.

Research

State health departments promote the development of new health care research. They carry out research studies and subsidize research activities. Health policies of the future are influenced by this research. Research funds need to be advocated for and carefully guarded; however, these funds are often the first monies included in budget cuts.

Emergency and Special Medical Services

Special medical services include the provision of hospital and institutional services for chronic or long-term conditions, such as mental retardation, mental illness, and tuberculosis. In the event of emergencies such as epidemics and natural disasters, emergency services ensure that the necessary public health care is made available to the community in need. Seventeen states operate public hospitals or long-term care facilities (PHF, 1989, Public health agencies, p. 7).

Staff

The state health department is headed by a chief executive (health officer or other title) who is usually appointed by the governor; this person is traditionally a physician. Other staff members include administrators, clerical workers, and consultants in fields such as community health nursing, occupational health, mental health, epidemiology, statistics, maternal-child health, health education, and nutrition. State health departments have legal counsel available to them, often through the state attorney general's office. States may have regional directors who serve as intermediaries between their regions and the state department. Most state health department personnel, except for the chief executive, are civil service employees.

Community health nurses are a valuable part of state health department staffs. They are hired on a consultant basis and help to establish state health policies, particularly in relation to maternal-child health and adult health services. They work closely with local health departments to improve the quality of care delivered to individuals, families, and populations at risk. Generally, community health nurses who work for state health departments are prepared at the master's or doctoral level and have past community health nursing experience.

LOCAL HEALTH DEPARTMENT (LHD)

There are over 3000 local health departments in the United States (PHF, 1989, Public health agencies, p. 1). No local health departments exist in 5 states (Arkansas, Delaware, the District of Columbia, Rhode Island, Vermont), and in the territories of American Samoa and Guam (PHF, 1989, Public health agencies, p. 144). Where local health departments do not exist, services are offered through the state or territorial health authorities.

The Institute of Medicine's Committee for the Study of the Future of Public Health recommends that in addition to the core public health functions (refer to the section on federal government functions in this chapter) LHDs are also responsible for the following (Institute of Medicine, 1988, pp. 9-10):

- Assessment, monitoring, and surveillance of local health problems and needs and resources for dealing with them
- Policy development and leadership that foster local involvement and a sense of ownership, that emphasize local needs and that advocate equitable distribution of public resources, and complementary private activities commensurate with community needs
- Assurance that high-quality services, including personal health services, needed for the protection of public health in the community are available and accessible to all persons; that the community receives proper consideration in the allocation of federal and state as well as local resources for public health, and that the community is informed about how to obtain public health, including personal health, services, or how to comply with public health regulations

The *local health department is the basic unit for the delivery of public health services.* It has responsibility for a specific jurisdiction; often a geopolitical jurisdiction such as a city, town, or county. In the United States, approximately 47 percent of local health departments represent one county (an additional 8 percent represent two or more counties), 14 percent represent a city, and 9 percent represent a town (Miller, Brooks, DeFriese, Gilbert, Jain, and Kavaler, 1977, p. 933). Most Americans benefit directly or indirectly from health department services.

Local health departments receive their funding from a number of sources, primarily from federal, state, and local tax dollars. Approximately 34 percent of their funding is local, 29 percent is state,

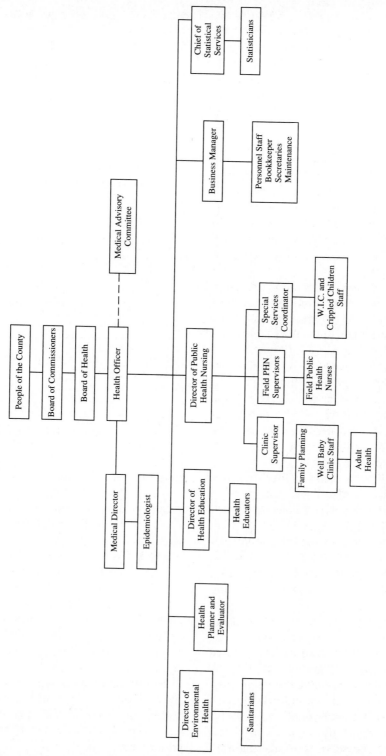

Figure 5-4   Organizational chart of a local health department.

and 19 percent is federal (PHF, 1988, Public health chartbook, Figure 23). Approximately 11 percent comes from fees, contracts, and other sources, and the remainder is from miscellaneous funding. In 1986, local health departments spent over $3.6 billion nationwide (PHF, 1988, Public health chartbook, Figure 23). Local health departments can provide a number of services at low or no cost to the general public. Many people in the community are not aware of this or of the services available at their LHD. A major function of the community health nurse is to assist the public in both learning about and utilizing the services of local health agencies. Some clients would be more likely to utilize LHD services if they knew that they have already supported them through their tax dollars.

Rural areas may have a difficult time obtaining enough tax funds, population, and health professionals to support a health department. There is a growing trend, in rural areas as well as large cities and counties, toward merger of city and county health departments or several county health departments merging. It is believed that the formation of district health departments will bring about greater efficiency and improved public services (Hanlon and Pickett, 1984, p. 146). Increasingly it is being found that the health needs of rural citizens are not being met.

LHDs usually have a board of health and a chief executive or health officer. An example of an organizational structure for a local health department is given in Figure 5-4. Each local health department establishes its own organizational pattern.

Just as each LHD establishes its own organization, each also determines its own services and methods of service provision. Thus, there is great variation between the services offered by local health departments. Table 5-4 presents an overview of the types of services consistently offered by local health departments and includes the percentage of departments providing these services.

A Public Health Foundation survey revealed that the quantity and quality of the nation's LHDs vary widely, that little is known at the national level about the services of the nation's

TABLE 5-4 Percent of U.S. health departments providing selected services

Services	Percent providing each service	Percent serving as sole provider of each service
Immunization programs	96.3	62.3
Environmental surveillance	96.0	70.4
Tuberculosis control	93.9	63.3
Maternal and child health	89.4	48.5
School health programs	89.2	38.5
Venereal disease control	88.0	57.7
Chronic disease programs	84.3	25.7
Home care	76.7	44.8
Family planning	63.3	38.0
Ambulatory care	50.3	7.6
Mental health	47.4	5.4
Chronic institutional care	11.8	1.5
Acute institutional care	8.4	1.4

From Miller CA, Brooks EF, DeFriese GH, Gilbert B, Jain SC, and Kavaler F: A survey of local health departments and their directors, Am J Public Health 67:934, 1977.

LHDs, and that many SHAs reported they have no system for collecting information on LHD activities (PHF, 1989, Survey shows, p. 2). Some SHAs are improving LHD reporting in their states. Alabama, Kentucky, Mississippi, and Tennessee are implementing automated information systems that gather data through patient encounter forms, allow for timeliness of reporting and patient tracking, and provide essential information to SHAs (PHF, 1989, Survey shows, p. 2).

Two concepts relatively new to the operation of LHDs are (1) model standards and (2) provision of primary care. It has been proposed that states should establish model health standards, but this is a long way from occurring nationwide. However, there could be a trend in this direction in the near future.

Traditionally, most LHDs have not actively engaged in the provision of ongoing, primary health care services. Many people in this country are medically underserved and could benefit from primary care services being provided at low or no cost through local health departments. The provision of direct patient care services is more popular in the southeastern part of the country. Many LHDs in this area are establishing clinic services to address the growing need for ongoing primary care services for disadvantaged populations. (PHF, 1989, Survey shows).

It will be interesting to note the future role played by LHDs in the provision of primary health care services. The Institute of Medicine's Committee for the Study of the Future of Public Health (CSFPH) cautions us that provision of such service may drain vital resources away from population-wide services, that the U.S. public health system is inadequately equipped to address these needs, and that this provision of care may pose a threat to the maintenance of crucial disease prevention and health promotion efforts (Institute of Medicine, 1988, pp. 13, 152-153). The committee endorsed the idea that the ultimate responsibility for ensuring equitable access to health care for all rests with the federal government. However, until this federal government responsibility is fulfilled, LHD efforts will help to fill a gap in our health care system. Currently, LHDs are meeting this challenge by providing direct patient care services themselves (refer to Chapter 20) or through contracting for the delivery of primary care with private providers.

Service Functions

Local health departments have functions similar to those carried out by the state health department, but the services they provide are more *direct*. Direct services offered by local health departments are extensive.

Administrative

The administrative functions of the local health department are identical in coverage to those implemented by the state health department, but the specific services vary.

Promulgation and enforcement of health standards, regulations, and policies are responsibilities carried out by the LHD for the jurisdiction it serves. The standards established by a local health department usually relate to public food handling,

storage, preparation, and disposal; and to public water supplies, including wells, septic systems, and pools or lakes at recreational facilities. LHDs also supervise and license local health facilities such as hospitals and nursing homes. Extensive health data, in relation to these functions, are frequently collected and available for health planning purposes (refer to Chapter 12).

Working cooperatively with local health agencies is a function of the health department. Coordinating private and official health care resources and providing advice on health matters are functions that the LHD does not always maximize to fullest potential. However, interagency planning is increasingly being done.

Consultation services are offered by the local health department to agencies and individuals. These activities usually involve consulting services from community health nurses, environmental engineers, nutritionists, and epidemiologists. Consultation in relation to health policy, environmental safety, and personal health services is often offered to schools, industry, hospitals, and nursing homes within the health department's jurisdiction.

Health planning activities within the LHD include analyzing and determining the public health needs of the people within its jurisdiction and planning health action strategies to meet these needs. The health department also carries out an ongoing evaluation of its programs and participates in statewide health planning activities and interagency planning (refer to Chapter 12).

Coordination of health services with other community agencies is an important function of the local health department. Often the health department provides leadership for resource coordination and development within the local community. Community involvement should be encouraged, and consumers should be involved in health affairs.

Legislation is guided and influenced by this department, primarily on a state level. The local health department makes its legislative needs known to the state legislators and members of congress. It is imperative that local health departments assume leadership in the formulation of health policy, because they are the direct service providers and have first-hand knowledge of client needs. If local health departments do not become involved in policy making, important preventive health care services may be lacking in a community.

Personnel policies, promotion guides, position descriptions, grievance policies, and manuals are developed by local health departments to facilitate effective and efficient management of the organization. Staff turnover and job satisfaction are often directly related to how well an organization is managed (refer to Chapter 21). Some position descriptions and qualifications, such as health officer, may be determined by the SHA and followed by the LHD. Some health departments use state services to recruit qualified personnel. Many LHDs are involved in working with staff unions and other collective bargaining groups. Local health department employees are frequently civil service employees.

Control of Communicable Disease

Communicable disease control is a major emphasis of the LHD. Each local health authority, in conformity with regulations of higher authority (state, national, and international), will determine what diseases are to be routinely and regularly reported, who is responsible for reporting, the nature of the reports, and the manner in which the reports are to be forwarded (Benenson, 1990, p. xxiv). Reportable communicable diseases that are required by international health regulations are cholera, plague, smallpox, and yellow fever, and those diseases under surveillance by WHO: louse-borne typhus fever and relapsing fever, paralytic poliomyelitis, viral influenza, and malaria (Benenson, 1990, p. xxv).

Communicable diseases reportable to the local health authority will vary, and their selection is often dependent on the severity and frequency of the disease. Some communicable diseases will be reported on the basis of individual cases and some only if epidemics occur. Some commonly reportable individual cases of communicable diseases are viral hepatitis, infectious hepatitis, rubella, salmonellosis, venereal syphilis, diphtheria, gon-

orrhea, leprosy, rubeola, meningococcal meningitis, Q fever, rabies, shigellosis, tetanus, tuberculosis, typhoid, and whooping cough. Some commonly reportable disease epidemics are ringworm, conjunctivitis, staphylococcal food poisoning, viral gastroenteritis, giardiasis, bacterial pneumonia, staphylococcal disease, streptococcal disease, and botulism.

The communicable disease services of LHDs include prevention, case finding, early diagnosis, and treatment. Many operate sexually transmitted disease, tuberculosis, and immunization clinics. These services are provided at no or little cost to the general public. Biologics for immunizations are distributed to private physicians by the health department. The department also makes epidemiological studies of suspected or reported cases of communicable disease, and the community health nurse is actively involved in this follow-up (refer to Chapter 10).

The health department provides other communicable disease measures, such as enforcing quarantines; conducting public food, water, and refuse disposal inspections; controlling rabies; and maintaining communicable disease statistics. The environmental health division is extensively involved in these measures. Continuing surveillance and prevention of communicable diseases should be stressed (Benenson, 1990, p. xxii). It is too easy to become lax about this surveillance when there has been no recent outbreak of disease.

Personal Health Services

Personal health services are a major component of LHD services. They include both maternal-child health and adult health activities. To carry out these activities, the health department offers an extensive array of clinics, classes, and home visit services.

School health is a major component of maternal-child health services on the local level. Community health nurses employed by the health department often function in schools to provide health education, counseling, and direct care services to pupils. They may conduct screening programs, such as hearing, vision, and scoliosis, to identify children who have health needs. School health services and the role of the school nurse are discussed in Chapter 14.

Many other maternal-child health services are provided by the LHD. Clinic services for these two segments of the population include family planning, immunization, sexually transmitted disease control, well-child, and Early, Periodic Screening, Diagnosis, and Treatment (EPSDT). A variety of other services are offered including classes for expectant and new parents and home visits to follow up on antepartal and postpartum clients, crippled children, and high-risk infants and mothers. Counseling and health teaching in relation to immunizations, growth and development, and community resources are a few examples of the types of services provided by community health nurses when they make home visits. In addition, programs such as the nutrition program for Women, Infants, and Children (WIC), dental health, and hearing-vision conservation are often established by the LHD in order to reduce maternal and child health morbidity and mortality. State consultants are often available to facilitate implementation of these services.

Adult health services also involve clinics, classes, and home visit services by the community health nurse. Community health nurses frequently visit adults to provide information about health conditions, including chronic conditions such as heart disease, diabetes, cancer, accidents, arthritis, stroke, alcoholism, and drug abuse. In work with clients who have chronic conditions, interventions should focus on prevention, detection, treatment, and rehabilitation in an attempt to fend off the need for long-term, institutional care and to encourage development of community support services. The community health nurse's major goal when working with adult clients is to enhance their self-care capabilities.

Classes in relation to such conditions as diabetes and hypertension are also conducted by the community health nurse or other health department personnel. In addition, clinics for sexually transmitted disease, family planning, immunization, blood pressure screening, breast cancer screening, and geriatric multiphasic screening are offered to promote wellness in adults. Programs in

dental health, substance abuse, accident prevention, and nutrition are essential to an effective program of personal health services (Pickett and Hanlon, 1990). The community health nurse works closely with community resources to assist the adult in meeting health care needs.

Environmental Health

Many of the public health successes we have had in the past in relation to communicable disease control have come about as a result of effective environmental health practices (e.g., safe water management, safe sewage disposal). Traditionally, health departments have been involved in environmental health as it relates to air and water quality, land use, environmental safety, building codes and safety, noise pollution, waste management, sanitation, food quality and protection, and vector and animal control. Environmental concerns dealing with radiation control and toxic and hazardous substances have recently emerged. There are thousands of hazardous chemicals manufactured and used in the United States today. The EPA has been ordered to set standards, monitor, and inventory 328 of these. These hazardous chemicals are a major cause of pollution in the United States because they contaminate land, air, and water supplies. Health departments are developing programs to safeguard their residents from such hazards.

Local health departments include environmental health services that deal with these traditional and evolving issues. Increasingly, both health care professionals and consumers are recognizing the importance of safeguarding our environment. We are all aware of situations where people have been forced to leave their homes due to improperly disposed of chemicals, advised not to eat polluted fish and game, warned about polluted streams and rivers and the dangers of pesticide and lead poisoning, and shocked by the damage from oil spills. More than three fourths of all Americans worry about chemical additives and residues in their food (Associated Press, 1984, p. A10).

The areas that environmental health deals with show some staggering statistics (Smolensky 1982; Kalette, 1989; Taking inventory, 1989):

- Since 1980 there have been 11,048 documented toxic chemical accidents in the United States, resulting in 309 deaths, 11,000 injuries and evacuation of more than half a million people; and concern is that a situation like the tragedy that occurred in Bhopal, India, may occur in the United States in the near future.
- In 1987 factories in the United States discharged more than 7 billion pounds of toxic substances into the air, water, and land (232 million pounds of toxins were poured into the Mississippi River alone in 1987).
- In a major U.S. earthquake there are likely to be more deaths from inhaling the toxic gases that are released than from all other causes.
- Air pollution is implicated in about one percent of all U.S. deaths each year with automobile emissions contributing up to one fourth of this pollution (4000 deaths).
- The average per capita production of refuse in the United States is 4 lb per day; this means that a small city of 10,000 would have to dispose of 20 tons of refuse a day.
- New York City is expected to run out of all its feasible landfill sites before the turn of the century.

Preserving our natural resources (refer to Figure 5-5) is a major challenge that must be addressed by public health professionals across the country.

The American Public Health Association's most current statement (1975) on LHA responsibilities has outlined a number of environmental health programs that should be undertaken by LHAs; Table 5-5 presents these environmental health programs.

Appendix 4-4 presents an overview of environmental health legislation in the United States. When reviewing this legislation, one can quickly see that there is not one all-encompassing piece of environmental legislation. The legislation is diverse and sometimes confusing, but does show a pattern in the establishment of environmental programs in the United States. Many of these acts have been amended. Often, when environmental legislation is enacted and amended, insufficient funds are allocated for enforcement purposes.

Occupational Health

Occupational health services are usually not carried out extensively on a local level. The Occupational Safety and Health Act of 1970 allows states to establish their own occupational safety and health administrations, but occupational health activities are largely conducted on a state level. Some industries are contracting with local health departments to route workers through health department diagnostic and screening programs. Some occupational health nurses, especially those in small industries, are seeking consultation from the nursing staff in the local health department for the development of health policies and procedures and the management of clinic facilities. Although this would seem to be a natural area for LHDs, there is little involvement by them.

Vital Statistics

Vital statistics in relation to the population that the health department serves are collected and disseminated to individuals, interested groups, and the SHA. The LHD keeps statistics on births, deaths, and reportable communicable diseases, maintains registers of individuals known to have specific communicable diseases where carrier states exist (typhoid), conducts morbidity and mortality surveys as necessary, and maintains records on jurisdictional health facilities.

Laboratory Services

Laboratory services are provided by the LHD. However, many do not have their own laboratories and use state facilities. Laboratory services may be extended to hospitals, clinics, and private practitioners on a contractual, fee-for-service basis. Laboratory services include water analysis, serology, urology, parasitology, identification of microorganisms, x-ray services for tuberculosis control, sanitation laboratory services, and metabolic and genetic screening for conditions such as phenylketonuria (PKU) and sickle cell anemia. These services are essential for communicable disease control and environmental sanitation and safety, as well as for the treatment of genetic and metabolic disorders and genetic counseling related to these conditions.

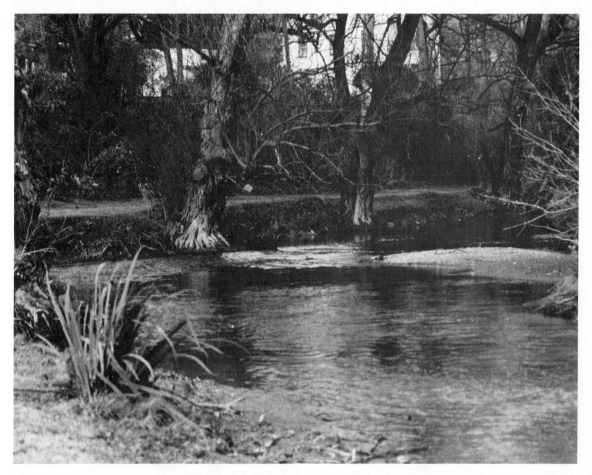

Figure 5-5   Safeguarding our natural resources is a major public health need. Despite all our modern technology, our nation has not been effective in controlling disease outbreaks related to environmental pollutants. In recent years, there has been a dramatic rise in the number of disease outbreaks from contaminated water. (Courtesy of photographer, Henry Parks.)

Health Education and Training

Education and training are a part of LHD services. The LHD provides health education services directly to individual clients, develops and carries out community health education programs, distributes health education materials, provides classes, and serves as a health information center. Master's-prepared health educators are often hired by LHDs to coordinate health education activities.

Training activities largely involve staff in-service and continuing education programs. Some health departments offer tuition reimbursement for university course work in public health or related fields as a staff benefit.

Research

Research is engaged in by LHDs to promote the health of population groups and the community and to strengthen the health care delivery system. Research is carried out by a variety of staff members and can be done in conjunction with program evaluation studies.

Research activities often include morbidity, mortality, and program evaluation studies. State health departments are usually more actively in-

TABLE 5-5 Categories of environmental concern in the United States and suggested environmental health programs for local health agencies

Categories of environmental concern	Programs	Program purpose
Air	Air quality management	To assure a community air resource conducive to good health, which will not injure plant or animal life or property, and which will be esthetically desirable
Water	Water supply sanitation	To assure the provision of safe public and private water supplies, adequate in quantity and quality for every person
	Water pollution control	To assure the cooperation with state water pollution control agencies, that surface and subsurface water supplies meet all state and local standards and regulations for water quality
Waste	Solid waste management	To assure that all solid wastes are stored, collected, transported, and disposed of in a manner which does not create health, safety, or esthetic problems
	Liquid waste control	To assure the treatment of liquid wastes in such a manner as to prevent problems of sanitation, public health nuisances, or pollution
Food	Food protection	To assure that all people are adequately protected from unhealthful or unsafe food or food products. This necessitates a comprehensive food protection program covering every facility where food or food products are stored, transported, processed, packaged, served, or vended, and regulating sanitation, wholesomeness, adulteration, advertising, labeling weights and measures, and fill-of-containers
Recreation	Swimming pool sanitation and safety	To assure the safety and sanitation of public, semipublic, and private swimming pools
	Recreational sanitation	To assure that all public recreational areas are operated so as to prevent health and safety problems
Hazardous substances/ products	Hazardous substances and product safety	To assure that all people are adequately protected from unhealthful or unsafe substances or products in the home, business, and industry
	Radiation control	To prevent unnecessary or hazardous radiation exposure from the transportation, use, or disposal of all types of radiation-producing devices and products
Occupational	Occupational health and safety	To assure, in cooperation with state officials, the health and safety of workers in places of employment, through controlling relevant environmental factors
Vectors	Vector control	To control all insects, rodents, and other animals which adversely affect our health, safety, or comfort
Noise	Noise pollution control	To prevent hazardous or annoying noise levels in residential, business, industrial, and recreational structures and areas
Accidents	Environmental injury prevention	To influence or regulate planning, design, and construction in such a manner as to reduce the possibility of accidents through proper management of the environment
Housing/facilities	Housing conservation and rehabilitation	To assure programs which will provide decent, safe, and healthful housing for all people
	Institutional sanitation	To assure that institutions such as hospitals, schools, nurseries, jails, and prisons are operated so as to prevent sanitation and safety problems

Adapted from American Public Health Association: Position paper: the role of official local health agencies, Am J Public Health February 65:189-193, 1975.

volved in research, but increasingly, LHDs are recognizing the need for such activity. Research studies related to service effectiveness and cost containment are especially emphasized at the local level. Staff should be encouraged to engage in research, and research activities should be an ongoing function of the agency.

Emergency and Special Medical Services

Special and emergency medical services offered by the LHD usually involve catastrophic medical care during a natural disaster or an epidemic, compulsory hospitalization through judicial admissions for acute communicable diseases such as tuberculosis, and environmental accidents (e.g., hazardous chemical spills or contamination). Health department personnel are also involved in health planning activities designed to meet the emergency needs of community citizens. In order to carry out these diverse functions and meet emergency and special needs, LHDs employ staff members from a variety of disciplines.

Staff

Staff will vary from one LHD to another. The minimum staff includes (1) a health officer, (2) a community health nurse, (3) an environmental engineer (sanitarian), and (4) a clerk. Additional personnel include statistician, epidemiologist, health educator, physical therapist, occupational health specialist, nutritionist, dentist, dental hygienist, veterinarian, and social worker. To provide comprehensive community health services, a basic, multidisciplinary staff is necessary. Historically, the following staff-to-community population ratio was recommended (Hanlon and Mc-Hose, 1971, p. 56):

Staff	Population
Health officer/medical personnel	1:50,000
Sanitarians (environmental engineers)	1:15,000
Community health nurses	1:5,000
Office personnel (clerk)	1:15,000

The above ratios were not and often are not achieved in many local communities. It is being found, however, that estimating the number of community health personnel needed in a local area is not as simple as previously thought. Multiple factors, such as current health problems in the community and the type and supply of health professionals in an area, influence work force planning. Staffing needs are based on service delivery needs as well as available community resources. If staffing patterns are less than ideal, LHDs must establish priorities based on available resources and needs.

Health Officer

Traditionally a health officer was a physician with public health training who was licensed to practice in the state. Today, the majority of health officers are still physicians, but the field is opening up to other health professionals such as nurses and public health administrators. If the health officer is not a physician, a medical director is hired to provide medical direction and consultation for maternal-child health and adult health service programs. The health officer administers the agency; prepares and submits budgets; appoints and hires personnel; takes part in program planning, implementation, and evaluation; and serves as a consultant to health department staff and community agencies. The health officer is responsible for seeing that all divisions in the local health department are run effectively and efficiently.

Community Health Nurse

Community health nurses carry out a variety of health activities, which are discussed throughout this text. Community health nurses utilize a synthesis of nursing and public health theory to facilitate client use of services in industry, schools, home, classes, clinics, and the community as a whole. They are the *backbone* of the personal health services of the health department and are extensively involved in most health department programs. The types of services offered by the nursing division in a LHD vary, depending on the work force available and other community resources that have been developed to meet the health care needs of community citizens.

If the LHD has a home care program, the community health nurse will provide skilled nursing care in the home. Community health nurses are extensively involved in health education activities and conduct a variety of classes (e.g., expectant parent classes, diabetic classes, and family planning information sessions). Professionals in the field recommend baccalaureate preparation for entry level positions in community health (Anderson and Meyer, 1985; Jones, Davis, and Davis, 1987), because baccalaureate-prepared nurses have more extensive community health nursing content during their educational preparation than other beginning levels of nursing education.

Environmental Engineer

The environmental engineer (sanitarian) is responsible for the elimination or reduction of hazards in the environment. Environmental engineers apply principles of public health, toxicology, education, and law enforcement and use practical and technical measures to eliminate or control environmental health problems (Smolensky, 1982, p. 159). The environmental health areas covered in this chapter illustrate the diversity of practice of the environmental engineer.

Clerk

The clerk is responsible for the clerical and secretarial aspects of maintaining the health department. These services are invaluable. It is extremely important to keep in mind that the clerical staff may need to be increased as new programs are developed in the health department. Without an adequate clerical staff, it is extremely difficult to effectively and efficiently manage health department services.

STATE AND LOCAL GOVERNMENT WELFARE ORGANIZATION

The provision of welfare assistance and insurance programs in every state and locality is legally mandated as a result of the Social Security Act of 1935 and other legislation. The specific services provided under the Social Security Act are discussed in Chapter 4.

The primary purpose of official welfare agen-cies is to assist indigent individuals in meeting their basic needs of food, shelter, and clothing. Benefits provided by these agencies are either cash or service (food and shelter). Official welfare services are organized in much the same manner as official health services. There is usually a department, such as the state department of social or human services, to establish rules and regulations, to set guidelines for service provision, and to administer services, as well as a local department of social services to provide direct services to clients. Local departments of social services administer state-subsidized programs such as Aid to Families of Dependent Children, food stamps, General Assistance, and Medicaid. Old Age, Survivors & Disability Insurance (OASDI) and Supplemental Security Income (SSI) are administered by the federal government through Social Security Administration offices (refer to Chapter 4). Protective services for children and adults are often administered through departments of social service.

The money spent on welfare assistance programs is enormous. State and local governments spent over $41 billion on public welfare in 1987 (Bixby, 1990, p. 14).

PRIVATE HEALTH, WELFARE, AND ENVIRONMENTAL ORGANIZATION

The United States abounds in private health and welfare resources. These resources can be classified as either profit or nonprofit. Historically, there has been limited coordination between these and government resources. In addition, there is no central coordination of all private health and welfare resources. Both profit and nonprofit resources exist in the private health and welfare sectors.

Private profit health and welfare services include an increasing number of hospitals, a large percentage of nursing homes, health and welfare professionals in private practice, pharmacies, health business companies (medical equipment companies, hospital supplies), and proprietary social service agencies. These services are available on a fee-for-service basis and are organized primarily as companies and independent businesses.

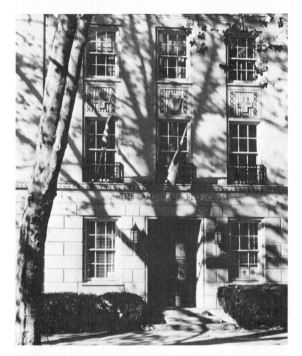

Figure 5-6 For over 100 years, the American Red Cross, a voluntary, nonprofit organization has initiated the development of and has provided health and welfare services. Established originally to assist and support military men and their families during times of war and to aid victims of disasters, this agency continues to make significant public health contributions. Some of its current efforts include the promotion of health education through formal classes and publications, the collection and distribution of whole blood products, and the provision of selected health and welfare services, based on community need. Friendly visiting to senior citizens, the provision of transportation for medical appointments, and the donation of clothing for needy families are examples of such services. In addition, the American Red Cross continues to provide relief for disaster victims and to serve military families. Local chapters of this organization can be found in most major cities across the United States. (Courtesy of photographer, Henry Parks.)

Private nonprofit resources are usually voluntary resources. They are not mandated by any law and provide services on a nonprofit basis. They are represented by individuals, professional societies, service organizations, agencies, and facilities. Their services augment official (government) services. Voluntary resources are uniquely American. Individual voluntary efforts (volunteerism) have likely been with us since this country was founded. One of the earliest voluntary associations, the American Red Cross, was established in 1882 and continues to provide significant health and welfare services for communities throughout the United States (refer to Chapter 1 and Figure 5-6). The International Red Cross provides health and welfare services throughout the world.

Since 1882, many other voluntary associations have emerged. Voluntary efforts have aided the development of American health and welfare resources, provided services that otherwise may not have been possible, and advocated health and welfare reform. The box below briefly summarizes the characteristics of voluntary resources that exist in the United States.

The functions of voluntary, nonprofit health agencies were studied in the classic Gunn-Platt Report (1945). The functions of these agencies were described as pioneering and include explor-

---

Voluntary Resources: Characteristics, Classifications and Examples

CHARACTERISTICS

Voluntarily organized

Governed by a board of directors which includes lay and/or professional members

Have no legal powers

Support received primarily from voluntary contributions, fees for service, third party payers, and grants

Usually provide services to a defined geographic location

CLASSIFICATIONS

Professional Societies: American Nurses Association (ANA), American Public Health Association (APHA)

Service Agencies: Visiting Nurse Association (VNA), American Cancer Society, American Red Cross, Alcoholics Anonymous, Rockefeller Foundation, United Community Services

Facilities: Universities, public museums, and libraries

Individuals

Adapted from Black L: Community health and administration, Ann Arbor, 1977, University of Michigan School of Nursing.

ing and surveying for unmet needs, demonstration, education, supplementation of official activities, guarding of citizens' interest in health, promotion of health legislation, planning and coordination, and development of well-balanced community health programs (Gunn and Platt, 1945). These functions have not altered over time and are becoming increasingly more significant in this era of federal cost containment.

Millions of Americans volunteer their services to assist health and welfare programs each year. Operating funds for voluntary resources come largely from individual contributions, fees-for-service, membership dues, investment earnings, sales of goods and publications, bequests, grants, contracts for service, and tax funds. Fund raising is of vital importance to these organizations, and monies are often raised through donation campaigns. One voluntary service agency, the *United Way,* represents a large number of local, voluntary resources with a central fund-raising campaign. Giving to the United Way campaign means giving to many voluntary resources with one donation. The federal government has encouraged private philanthropic giving to voluntary organizations by permitting contributions to be deducted from personal and corporate income tax.

There are usually many voluntary resources in local communities. Private profit-oriented health care agencies are emerging with increasing frequency. The Visiting Nurse Association and other home health care programs are discussed below, because home health care is becoming one of the major responsibilities of nurses in the community setting (refer to Chapter 19). Limiting discussion to these types of private health and welfare organizations is not meant to imply that other private agencies do not provide a valuable service to the community.

Visiting Nurse Associations (VNAs)

Visiting Nurse Associations are especially significant voluntary organizations in community health. VNAs began with the Women's Branch of the New York City Mission, organized in 1877 to teach hygiene in the homes of the underprivileged. The first visiting nursing associations were

established in Buffalo in 1885 and in Boston and Philadelphia in 1886 (Pickett and Hanlon, 1990, p. 510). In the early 1900s, because of the strong leadership of Lillian Wald and other nursing leaders, visiting nurse associations expanded rapidly across the country. Lillian Wald encouraged the development of visiting nurse services in rural as well as urban communities (Kaufman, Hawkins, Higgins, and Friedman, 1988). Chapter 1 discusses the historical development of these voluntary organizations. Today's VNA organizations still model the strong professional community health nursing service promoted by Wald in the early 1900s.

Visiting Nurse Associations augment the services of the official health department, primarily by providing skilled nursing services (home care nursing). Historically, there has been coordination between these agencies and official health departments. In some instances, combined agencies were formed. *Combination agencies* are a consolidation under one centrally administered agency of official and voluntary health agency structure, function, funding, and staffing.

The organization and staffing of VNAs vary based on their size and the type of services provided. Nurses are the largest direct service group in these agencies. Visiting Nurse Associations often employ nurses who have received a master's degree in consultant and administrative positions. The VNA is administered by an executive director or chief executive officer (CEO) who operates under the authority of a board of directors. The board establishes policy and program emphasis and is responsible for various fund-raising activities. In contrast to the health department, the program emphasis is usually on secondary and tertiary preventive activities, rather than on primary prevention. However, staff nurses do engage in primary prevention counseling as they provide skilled nursing care. For example, they discuss accident prevention when they assist clients with mobility.

A variety of interdisciplinary personnel provide leadership in VNAs. A VNA may have an executive director, a director of nursing or clinical services, a medical director, a quality assurance

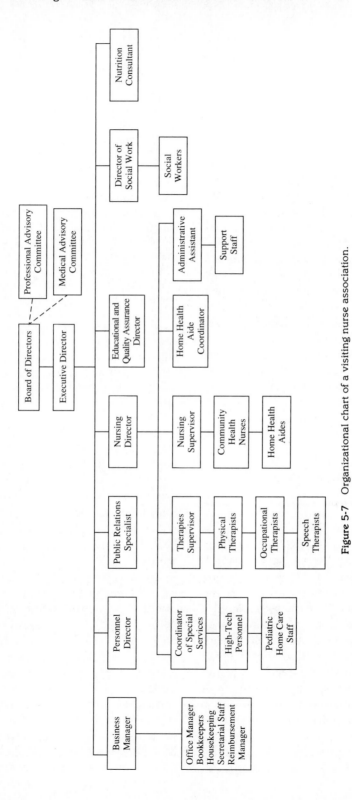

Figure 5-7   Organizational chart of a visiting nurse association.

and educational coordinator, a public relations specialist, nursing, physical therapy and speech therapy supervisors, a business manager, and a personnel director. A medical advisory committee assists the board of directors and administrative staff in formulating sound professional policies and provides consultation in relation to professional practice. A professional advisory committee helps agency staff with overall agency evaluation and provides advice about agency programming and functioning. Figure 5-7 presents a sample organizational chart for a VNA.

Home Health Care Programs

Home health care programs are organized in both the private for-profit and nonprofit sectors. Their services are delivered to individuals in their homes and help to maintain the individual in an independent living situation. Decreasing hospital stays and reducing readmission and admission to hospitals are also goals of these programs; clients who use the services of home health care agencies are often elderly and disabled. These programs are rapidly growing in numbers and are providing much competition to the long-standing VNA. They are discussed in depth in Chapter 19.

COORDINATION OF HEALTH, WELFARE, AND ENVIRONMENTAL RESOURCES

The diversity of health, welfare, and environmental resources and services should now be clear. The lack of coordination between these services can present a multitude of problems for both providers and recipients of service. Providers of service may become frustrated because they find it difficult to know about the many resources available and to effect change in the system. Recipients of service are frustrated because they are not aware of resources, do not understand how to utilize them, and often receive fragmented care. A major role of the community health nurse is to explain and coordinate community services. Lack of resource coordination can adversely affect the quality of care delivered to clients. This is demonstrated in the following case situation:

John Falta, age 19, was in a motorcycle accident that necessitated an amputation below the right knee. He was hospitalized for 6 weeks and upon discharge was referred to a local VNA for skilled nursing services, the Office of Vocational Rehabilitation for rehabilitation training, and the Department of Social Services for assistance with his medical expenses. In addition, a physical therapist from the hospital saw John on a weekly basis at home, and a volunteer from a local amputee self-help group visited him regularly to help him adapt to the changes that had occurred in his life. Each of these health and welfare resources provided a valuable service, but because they were not initially coordinated, John found it difficult to understand why so many people were involved in his care. He told the visiting nurse that he was confused and depressed about the onslaught of so many "helping agencies" and the different goals that had been set for him. The nurse suggested that a conference be arranged between John, his family, and the involved resources; John agreed that this was necessary. The conference helped to coordinate John's care as well as to stimulate John's involvement in the rehabilitation process. Because he had a clearer picture about what was happening, his depression decreased and he actively participated in establishing goals for his future.

It is not uncommon to encounter clients like John Falta in community health nursing practice. Health and welfare personnel meet too infrequently to plan for coordinated service delivery. When such meetings do occur, they are often arranged to deal with individual client problems rather than to *plan* for coordinated preventive health, welfare, and environmental resources and services.

Lack of coordination occurs between the health, welfare, and environmental resources. A classic example of lack of coordination in this country between health and welfare systems is the administration of the government health insurance program of Medicare and the health assistance program of Medicaid. These programs are administered by official agencies that are traditionally considered to be welfare agencies: the Social Security Administration and state departments of social service. Official and private health agencies have little input into, control over, or administration of these two major government health programs. The case situation of John Falta also evidenced such lack of coordination; health care and welfare professionals were not communicating with one another or with professionals from other systems.

Lack of coordination of services has been evident in all sectors of our health and welfare systems for decades. The National Commission on Community Health Services (1966, p. 132) identified that there was minimal coordination between official (government) and private health care agencies. The National Health Planning and Resource Development Act of 1974 (Public Law 93-641) was passed to improve the delivery and coordination of government health care services to all segments of the population. However, in 1981, the Omnibus Budget Reconciliation Act was passed, which ended the federal mandate for Public Law 93-641 planning. It is now hoped that federal block grant program funding will improve the coordination of services (refer to Chapter 12).

Community health nurses are in a unique position to influence coordination of care on both an individual level with clients and a community level with health planners. On an individual level, community health nurses are frequently the primary providers in the home setting. At this level, one of their major functions is coordination of community resources for the families they visit. The John Falta case illustrates this. On a community level, community health nurses are currently writing grants to obtain block grant funding for community health services. The holistic philosophy of community health nurses provides them with the skills needed to integrate service delivery issues.

SUMMARY

The Institute of Medicine's Committee for the Study of the Future of Public Health found that public health is a vital function that is in trouble in the United States. Public health agencies have many challenges to face such as AIDS, chronic disease, an aging population, leadership, financing, policy development, and funding.

The federal government has taken a leadership role in establishing national health objectives and supporting model public health standards. States need resources and better reporting mechanisms to implement and evaluate these standards. The nation as a whole needs to make a concerted effort to ensure the stability of the public health system. Public health can no longer be taken for granted. Americans must not be lax in their public health practices, or attempt to divest themselves of public health issues.

The community health nurse needs to be aware of national health objectives and model standards as discussed in this chapter. The nurse must understand how health, welfare, and environmental services are organized on both governmental and private levels to enhance service delivery and coordination effectively, and to familiarize clients with the service delivery system. Community health nurses must know what services are offered by state and local health agencies. They must be able to wrok with communities to promote public health, and to help instill in communities the belief that public health is too important a function to be taken for granted or neglected.

REFERENCES

American Public Health Association: Position paper: the role of official local health agencies, Am J Public Health 65:189-193, 1975.

American Public Health Association: Model standards: a guide for community preventive health services, ed 2, Washington, DC, 1985, The Association.

Anderson E and Meyer AT: Consensus conference on the essentials of public health nursing practice and education, Rockville, Md, 1985, USDHHS Public Health Service.

Associated Press: Chemicals in food real worry, poll says, Knoxville Journal, March 27, 1984, p A-10.

Association of State and Territorial Health Officials (ASTHO): Public health agencies 1981. A report on their expenditures and activities, Kensington, Md, 1983, The Association.

Benenson AS, ed: Control of communicable diseases in man, ed 15, Washington, DC, 1990, American Public Health Association.

Bixby AK: Public social welfare expenditures, fiscal years 1965-1987, Social Sec Bull 53(2):10-26, 1990.

Black L: Community health administration, Ann

Arbor, 1977, University of Michigan College of Nursing—Community Health Nursing.

Bureau of Census: County spending, USA Today March 19, 1984.

Gunn SM and Platt PS: Voluntary health agencies: an interpretative study, New York, 1945, Ronald Press.

Hanlon JJ, and McHose E: Design for health, ed 2, Philadelphia, 1971, Lea & Febiger.

Hanlon JJ and Pickett GE: Public health administration and practice, ed 8, St Louis, 1984, Times Mirror/Mosby.

Harmon RG: Macroviewpoint: the future of public health, Public Health Macroview 1(5):4, 1988.

Institute of Medicine—Committee for the Study of the Future of Public Health: The future of public health, Washington, DC, 1988, National Academy Press.

Jones DC, Davis JA, and Davis MC: Public health nursing education and practice (accession number HRP-0909092), Springfield, Va, 1987, National Technical Information.

Kalette D: Toxic disaster is possible here, USA Today August 1, 1989, p A-6.

Kaufman M, Hawkins JW, Higgins LP, and Friedman AH, eds: Dictionary of American nursing biography, New York, 1988, Greenwood Press.

Miller CA, Gilbert B, Warren DG, Brooks EF, DeFriese GH, Jain SC, and Kavaler F: A survey of local public health departments and their directors, Am J Public Health 67:931-939, 1977.

Miller CA, Brooks EF, DeFriese GH, Gilbert B, Jain SC, and Kavaler F: Statutory authorizations for the work of local health departments, Am J Public Health 67:940-945, 1977.

National Commission on Community Health Services: Health is a community affair, Cambridge, Ma, 1966, Harvard University Press.

Office of the Federal Registry: United States government manual, 1988/89, Washington, DC, 1988, US Government Printing Office.

Pickett G and Hanlon JJ: Public health administration and practice, ed 9, St Louis, 1990, Times Mirror/Mosby College Publishing.

Public Health Foundation (PHF): USDA provides 57% of SHAs' federal funding, Public Health Macroview 1(4):1, 1988.

Public Health Foundation: SHAs expand occupational role, Public Health Macroview 1(4):2, 1988.

Public Health Foundation: Status report: state progress on 1990 health objectives for the nation, Washington, DC, 1988, The Foundation.

Public Health Foundation: Public health chartbook, Washington, DC, 1988, The Foundation.

Public Health Foundation: Public health agencies 1989: an inventory of programs and block grant expenditures, Washington, DC, 1989, The Foundation.

Public Health Foundation: Fee income: a small but growing source of support for SHAs, Public Health Macroview 2(3):1, 1989.

Public Health Foundation: Survey shows wide variation in LHD reporting, Public Health Macroview 2(3):2, 1989.

Public Health Foundation: SHA spending in brief, Public Health Macroview 2(2):1, 1989.

Public Health Foundation: Year 2000 health objectives to be published for comment, Public Health Macroview 2(2):2-3, 1989.

Smolensky J: Principles of community health, ed 5, Philadelphia, 1982, Saunders.

Taking inventory of 7 billion toxic pounds: USA Today, August 2, 1989, p A-7.

Turner JB, ed: Encyclopedia of social work, Washington, DC, 1977, National Association of Social Workers.

US Department of Health, Education, and Welfare: Healthy people. The Surgeon General's report on health promotion and disease prevention, Washington, DC, 1979, US Government Printing Office.

US Department of Health and Human Services: Promoting health/preventing disease. Objectives for the nation, Washington, DC, 1980, US Government Printing Office.

US Public Health Service: The 1990 health objectives for the nation: a midcourse review, Washington, DC, 1986, US Government Printing Office.

US Statutes-at-Large (selected years): Washington, DC, US Government Printing Office.

Wilner DM, Walkley RP, and O'Neill E: Introduction to public health, New York, 1978, Macmillan.

World Health Organization (WHO): Four decades of achievement: highlights of the work of WHO, Geneva, Switzerland, 1988, The Organization.

SELECTED BIBLIOGRAPHY

Battista RN and Lawrence RS, eds: Implementing preventive services, New York, 1987, Oxford University Press. Papers prepared for the International Symposium on Preventive Services in Primary Care: Issues and Strategies, October 4-6, 1987, L'Esterel, Quebec.

Cohen WJ: Current problems in health care, N Engl J Med 281:193-197, 1969.

Houle CO: Governing boards, San Francisco, 1989, Jossey-Bass Publishers.

Kennedy EM: In critical condition: the crisis in American health care, New York, 1973, Pocket Books.

Lorsch RL: State and local politics. The entanglement, Englewood Cliffs, NJ, 1983, Prentice-Hall.

Public Health Foundation: SHA staffing declines 8% from 1979-1985, Public Health Macroview 1(4):5, 1988.

Public Health Foundation: New block grant legislation mandates reporting/modifies spending restrictions, Public Health Macroview 2(2):7, 1989.

Public Health Foundation: Progress on the 1990 national health objectives: high blood pressure, Public Health Macroview 2(3):4-5, 1989.

United Hospital Fund of New York: A guide to citizen action for health, New York, 1980, United Hospital Fund.

US Public Health Service: Setting nationwide objectives in disease prevention and health promotion: the United States experience, [monograph series], Washington, DC, 1987, US Government Printing Office [Reprint from McGinnis JM: Oxford textbook of public health, vol 3, Investigative methods in public health, Oxford, 1985, Oxford University Press, pp 385-401.]

Wilson FA and Neuhauser D: Health services in the United States, ed 2 revised, Cambridge, Ma, 1985, Ballinger.

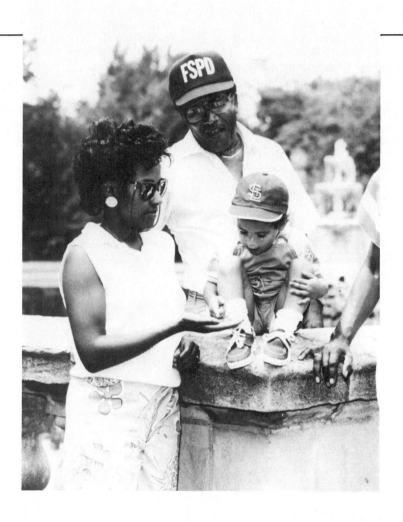

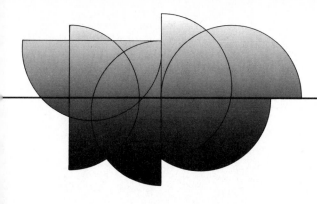

PART TWO

Working with Families in the Community Setting

Family-centered care was historically and is still a key principle in community health nursing practice. Community health nurses believe that the health needs of individuals cannot be isolated from the interactions of the family and that stresses experienced by individual family members affect the entire family unit. They recognize that the family greatly influences the beliefs, values, attitudes, and health behaviors of its members and determines when family members will seek assistance from health care professionals.

Community health nurses use the nursing process to help families and individuals analyze the multiple forces that inhibit or facilitate their growth and to plan intervention strategies that will strengthen their self-care capabilities. Part 2 presents the theoretical concepts essential for understanding family functioning and for effectively utilizing the nursing and referral processes to provide comprehensive, continuous nursing services in the community setting. It is important to recognize that nurses use multiple strategies when working with families in the community.

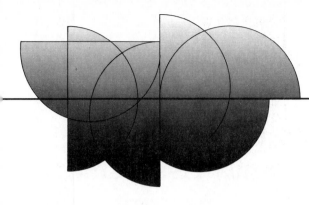

UNIT THREE

Family-Centered Approach to Community Health Nursing Practice

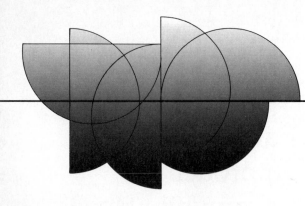

6

Foundations for Family Assessment: Basic Concepts and Tools

The ancient trinity of father, mother, and child has survived more vicissitudes than any other relationship. It is the bedrock underlying all other family structures. Although more elaborate family patterns can be broken from without or may even collapse of their own weight, the rock remains. In the Götterdammerung which otherwise science and overfoolish statesmanship are preparing for us, the last man will spend his last hours searching for his wife and child.

LINTON *(1959, p. 52)*

OBJECTIVES

Upon completion of this chapter, the reader will be able to:

1. Construct a personal definition for the term family.

2. Identify variations in family structure in the United States.

3. Discuss the meaning of the phrase, "the family is the unit of service."

4. Explain how theoretical frameworks for family study enhance family-focused community health nursing practice.

5. Discuss the structural and process parameters for family assessment and their relevance to community health nursing practice.

6. Discuss how cultural factors influence health and health behaviors.

7. Formulate guidelines for completing a cultural assessment.

8. Describe tools used to facilitate the family assessment process.

Major societal changes in the past 30 years have resulted in various family forms and lifestyles; however, the family is still the basic social unit in our society. Even though family structures and functions have changed, "the family continues to play a vital role in today's world. Most Americans still regard the family as central to their well-being and happiness" (Thornton and Freedman, 1983, pp. 36-37). "The family continues to be of central importance in American society because of its contribution to both family members' and society's goals and purposes" (Nickols and Nickols, 1983, p. 14). The bureaucratic organizations of our society cannot fulfill the emotional support and nurturing needs required by all human beings.

Families must survive if individuals are to achieve emotional health and well-being. "Families are America's most precious resource and most important institution. Families have the most fundamental, powerful, and lasting influence on our lives. The strength of our families is the key determinate of the health and well-being of our nation, of our communities, and of our lives as individuals" (White House Conference on Families, 1978, p. 286).

THE AMERICAN FAMILY

Diversity is the term which best describes the American family. Cultural backgrounds, socioeconomic levels, and family structures differ throughout the country. The nuclear family unit—mother, father, and children—established through the legal sanction of marriage, is no longer the only acceptable form for family life. Alternative life-styles are becoming increasingly prevalent. Changes in societal values and attitudes are affecting both family structures and modes of living.

Scientific, technological, and sociological advances have greatly influenced societal attitudes and values about American family life. The discovery of effective contraceptive methods, increased social mobility due to improved transportation, the women's movement, which promotes equal opportunities for women in the job market, the redefinition of sex roles, and increased health and welfare legislation have all made an impact on the American family. As a result of these events, transitions in family structure and function have occurred. Family size has decreased, with some couples choosing not to have children. More women are becoming involved in careers outside the home. The role of the father in parenthood is examined more carefully (refer to Figure 6-1). Families are changing their place of residence with increasing frequency. Legislation is broadening the opportunities for education, health services, and changes in marital status.

All of the above changes have provided more options for families. They have also brought new problems and stresses which require different coping mechanisms. A cultural lag between social policy and norms for families and changing societal values has influenced the development of these concerns.

New problems have emerged for families as well as our society. Families need to deal with child care arrangements that are often very complicated, have to coordinate family and work roles and intergenerational relationships, and must address problems such as drug abuse and premarital sexuality issues not commonly experienced by other generations. On the other hand, society needs to deal with issues such as the increasing number of people living in poverty, the dramatic rise in premarital childbearing, and maintaining the viability of nonprofit organizations as volunteer workers become less available (Spanier, 1989; Bengtson and Dannefer, 1987; Yogman and Brazelton, 1986; Thornton & Freedman, 1983).

An example of this is the nuclear family's difficulty in assuming all of the responsibilities once shared by the extended family. Changes in health, welfare and educational legislation and programs are needed to prepare families to handle their responsibilities and to make resources available during critical transition periods. Social policy must take into consideration the needs of varying family forms and life-styles because the American family is changing.

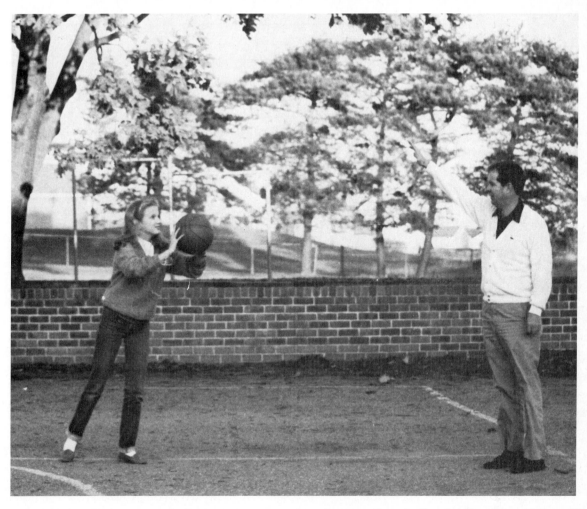

Figure 6-1 Increasingly, fathers are becoming more involved in parenting and are significantly influencing a child's socialization. (Courtesy of photographer, Henry Parks.)

Variations in Family Structures

Currently, several family structural forms exist in the United States. These are presented in Table 6-1. Even though all these family forms are not widely accepted, they are becoming more evident in our society. The number of unmarried couples living together has, for example, increased 63 percent between 1980 and 1988 (U.S. Bureau of the Census, 1989, p. 3).

It is obvious from reviewing Table 6-1 that what actually constitutes a family is no longer easy to define. Various family organizational structures have made the concept of the family an elusive one, open to numerous definitions depending on one's value system. The traditional definition of this term—a group of two or more persons related by blood, marriage, or adoption and residing together—is no longer adequate for understanding and studying the needs of the American family. It is extremely important that practitioners in the helping professions remain flexible in their interpretation of the word *family*

TABLE 6-1 Variations in family life-styles in the United States

Traditional family structures	Emerging experimental family structures

1. *Nuclear family*—husband, wife, and offspring living in a common household, established through the legal sanction of marriage
 	
  a. Single career
 	
    (1) Husband breadwinner, wife at home
 	
    (2) Wife breadwinner, husband at home (usually this pattern is accepted by society only if the husband is ill, is obtaining advanced education, or is unemployed and looking for employment)
 	
  b. Dual career
 	
    (1) Both parents gainfully employed from the outset of the marriage
 	
    (2) Wife's career interrupted due to child-rearing responsibilities
 	
    (3) Wife starts career after children enter school
 	
2. *Reconstituted nuclear family*—remarried men and women, living in a common household with children from both previous marriages, children from one previous marriage, or children from previous marriages and children from current marriage
 	
  a. Single career
 	
  b. Dual career
 	
3. *Dyadic nuclear family*—childless husband and wife; one or both parents gainfully employed
 	
4. *Single-parent family*—one parent, as a consequence of divorce, abandonment, or separation (with financial aid rarely coming from the second parent), and usually including preschool, school-age children; or both
 	
  a. Parent working
 	
  b. Parent not working, supported by government funds (welfare or social security), family or life insurance, and savings
 	
5. *Single adult*—living alone, usually with a career, who may or may not desire to marry
 	
6. *Three-generation family*—three generations or more living in a household
 	
7. *Middle-aged or aging couple*—husband as provider, wife at home (children have been "launched" into college, career, or marriage)
 	
8. *Kin network*—nuclear households or unmarried members living in close geographical proximity and operating within a reciprocal system of exchange of goods and services
 	
9. *"Second-career" family*—the wife entering the work force when the children are in school or have left the parental home
 	
10. *Institutional family*—children in orphanages, residential schools, or correctional institutions
	1. *Binuclear family*—divorced parents assuming joint custody and coparenting responsibilities for a minor child; the child is part of a family system consisting of two nuclear households.
	
	2. *Commune family*
	
	  a. Monogamous—household of more than one monogamous couple with children, sharing common facilities, resources, and appliances; socialization of the child is a group activity
	
	  b. Group marriage—household of adults and offspring known as one family, where all individuals are *married* to each other and all are *parents* to the children; usually develops a status system with leaders believed to have charisma
	
	3. *Unmarried-parent-and-child family*—usually mother and child, where marriage is not desired or possible
	
	4. *Unmarried-couple-and-child family*—usually a commonlaw marriage with the child their biological issue or informally adopted
	
	5. *Dyadic nuclear family*—husband and wife who have voluntarily chosen not to have children (national support groups are forming to help these couples maintain their position); one or both partners gainfully employed
	
	6. *Homosexual families*—a homosexual couple, male or female, living together with or without children; children may be informally or legally adopted
	
	7. *Cohabiting retired couple*—an unmarried retired couple living together, usually because financial hardship would result if they married (retirement benefits would decrease)

Adapted from Sussman MB (Chairperson): Changing families in a changing society, 1970 White House Conference on Children, Forum 14 report, Washington, DC, 1971, US Government Printing Office, pp 228-229; Ahrons CR: The binuclear family: two households, one family, Alternative Lifestyles 2:449-515, 1979.

so that social policies which enhance the growth of all types of families are developed. Families who are not legally bound together by marriage have the same needs as families who are. They need financial resources, social and educational opportunities, and health services to meet their basic needs. Denying them options to strengthen their family life does not strengthen our nation, and is not sensitive to their needs.

In addition to reexamining the definition of the word *family,* community health nurses must also carefully identify their attitudes and values about family life. Although community health nurses may not choose a particular mode of living for themselves, their personal preferences should not influence their clinical judgments about the adequacy of family functioning when they work with families whose life-styles differ from theirs. Data collected from the family should be the key factor by which the community health nurse determines family strengths and needs. A single-parent mother, for instance, may be meeting the needs of her child much more appropriately than married couples who are having conflicts in their marriage. Assumptions about how well a family is providing for its members should not be made solely on the basis of the family's organizational structure.

THE FAMILY AS A UNIT OF SERVICE

Despite the changing nature of the American family, community health nurses still subscribe to the philosophy that the family is the basic unit of service in community health nursing practice. They recognize that the family, as the major socializing unit of society, determines how its individual members relate and act in our culture. They believe that the family greatly influences the beliefs, values, attitudes, and health behaviors of its members and realize that the health of individual family members affects the health of the entire family unit. They see that the family provides support and encouragement at times of stress and joy. They value the role the family has in facilitating the physical and psychosocial growth of its members.

Ronald Peterson (1978) put into very simple, but impressive terms, the significance of the family in promoting the growth of its individual members when he presented the following concept of the family at a national conference on the chronic mentally ill client:

A family is a place where I think a lot of things go on. You really don't feel you're being "raised," that people are doing things to you, to raise you. Your life seems "real" and most of the time, almost everything that happens to you, you talk about it. Sometimes you have good news, sometimes you have bad news. But most of the time, it's just talking about what is going on.

It's a place you go from, to the doctor or to the hospital or the dentist, or school, or to the movies or to a job. But it's a place where you belong, where you somehow learn a lot. You change I'm sure, but usually without knowing it. And you certainly are not looked at as a patient or one who is being rehabilitated. You don't get discharged or terminated, and even when you grow up and get a job of your own and move away, it's a place you keep in touch with and visit. There's always an interest, and that's what makes the difference.*

Community health nurses have found, like Peterson, that families do make a difference; families provide supportive and nurturing services in a way that no other social institution provides. Families influence health beliefs and attitudes, even when they are not physically present. They often extend themselves much further in providing assistance than would friends or health care professionals. It is for these reasons that community health nurses believe in the family-centered approach to nursing care.

Historically, the family-centered approach to community health nursing practice grew out of the recognition that the physical care of an individual client could not be divorced from all other aspects of a client's functioning. Innovative community health nursing leaders of the early 1900s recognized that a preventive, holistic approach to the delivery of nursing services was essential if the

---

*Peterson R: What are the needs of the chronic mental patients? Presented at the APA Conference on the Chronic Mental Patient, Washington, DC, January 11-14, 1978.

health of an individual, the family, and the community was to be maintained and enhanced. They saw the need to work with the family and the community in order to achieve their goals with individual clients.

The concept of family-centered care has evolved over time. Initially, focus was placed on analyzing how the family could assist its members to achieve health and well-being. Gradually, the enhancement of the health and well-being of the entire *family unit* became the primary objective for community health nursing visits, with emphasis placed on analyzing family dynamics, as well as on identifying the health status of all family members.

Clinical practice and research has sufficiently demonstrated the value of the family-centered approach to community health nursing practice. "The family constitutes perhaps the most important social context within which illness occurs and is resolved. It consequently serves as a primary unit in health and medical care" (Litman, 1974, p. 495). The family influences the development of health behavior, the utilization of health services, and health outcomes for individuals (Barnard, 1988; Schor, Starfield, Stidley, and Hankin, 1987; Pratt, 1976; Litman, 1974).

Although the family-centered approach to nursing care is valued, it is not fully realized in the clinical setting. Lack of knowledge regarding family processes, federal legislation which financially supports individual services, insufficient criteria for judging family health, and heavy caseload demands, impede nurses' efforts to implement family care. Research, advocacy activities, and continuing education programs could alter this trend. Research is needed to document the value of preventive health care to families and to establish criteria for evaluating family health. Advocacy efforts which support the need for reimbursing family health care services are essential since traditionally health legislation has encouraged the delivery of curative, individual health care services. Continuing education activities aimed at increasing nurses' theoretical base concerning family processes are necessary because many nurses have not had the opportunity to examine family theory in the educational setting.

Community health nursing leaders of the past were truly creative and innovative. They were far ahead of their time when they subscribed to the belief that family care was a key principle in community health nursing practice. It was not until the 1950s that most professional disciplines actually began to focus attention on working with families rather than with individual clients. It was only at this time that social scientists initiated systematic theory building in relation to family processes. Thus, it is no wonder that the family-centered approach to nursing care is not completely operationalized in the practice setting. Theoretical knowledge to guide one's clinical judgments and the support for its use are needed before a particular nursing care approach can be fully implemented.

New knowledge gained about family functioning since the 1950s has made it easier for nurses to analyze family strengths and needs and to intervene appropriately with families. Selected theoretical frameworks currently being used to study the family are briefly summarized below. These frameworks help nurses to organize the family assessment process systematically and to identify the range of variables essential for understanding family relationships. They do not ensure, however, that family-centered care will be implemented. The community health nurse must internalize the belief that working with the family as a unit is important; otherwise, the goal of family-centered practice will be compromised.

THEORETICAL FRAMEWORKS FOR FAMILY STUDY

The family can be analyzed from multiple perspectives. Duvall and Miller (1985), who partially listed the kinds of family studies currently being conducted, identified 16 disciplines (e.g., anthropology, demography, history, law, and public health) involved in family study. Burr and Leigh (1983) found at least 19 disciplines, including nursing, that shared an interest in developing a knowledge base related to the family. The field of family study has had an interdisciplinary focus since its origin. According to Duvall and Miller (1985), an interdisciplinary focus adds depth to family study because concepts about several facets of family life are synthesized. Generally, scholars from the different behavioral sciences focus attention on only limited aspects of family life. Interdisciplinary research helps to bring together the various theoretical frames of reference used by different disciplines. This, in turn, gives a more comprehensive view of family functioning.

Theory building, in relation to the family, is a relatively new phenomenon. It was only four decades ago that family scholars developed an interest in theory construction. At that time there began a much greater emphasis on *scientific* study to discover relationships between family concepts which could be generalized across cultures. In addition, for the first time, focus was placed on examining how cultural variables affected family dynamics (Christensen, 1964, p. 10).

The quantity and quality of family research has increased since the original thrust in the 1950s. In the 1960s, substantive theory building in relation to the family expanded (Broderick, 1971). During the 1970s, the field of family research and theory building experienced phenomenal growth (Berardo, 1980; Holman and Burr, 1980), as new areas of family research such as domestic violence, teenage parenthood, sex roles, and family stress and coping emerged (Berardo, 1980). An increasing interest in family-focused research among nurses also occurred during this time (Murphy, 1986; Barnard, 1984; Feetham, 1984; Gilliss, 1983). The Family Nursing Continuing Education Project, a 3-year project begun in 1987, was designed to foster a nationwide network of family nurses who hope to achieve a common knowledge and research base for their practice (Krentz, 1989, p. 4). Currently, nursing borrows family concepts/models/theories from other fields of family study (Hanson, 1987).

It is important for practitioners to have an awareness of trends and developments in family research and theory building, because as research becomes more refined, conceptual frameworks for clinical practice emerge. Research on family stress and coping has, for example, provided a conceptual framework which assists practitioners in identifying families who are having difficulty coping and the factors involved in successful crisis resolution (refer to Chapter 7).

Historically, five conceptual frameworks were utilized to study the family: interactional, structural-functional, situational, institutional, and developmental. These were first delineated by Hill and Hansen in their landmark 1960 article, "The Identification of Conceptual Frameworks Utilized in Family Study." In 1964, Christensen devoted several chapters in his book *Handbook of Marriage and the Family* to the analysis of these frameworks. Both of these writings are now considered classics in the field of family study, because they had a tremendous influence on the development of family theory in the 1960s.

Carlfred B. Broderick, after an extensive review of marriage and family living literature, concluded that three of the five original frameworks survived in the 1960s. These were interactional, structural-functional, and developmental (Broderick, 1971, p. 141). In addition, he saw several new conceptual frameworks for family analysis emerging: balance theory, game theory, exchange theory, and general systems theory.

Holman and Burr (1980), upon reviewing the growth of family theories in the 1970s, found that symbolic interaction theory, exchange theory, and systems theory emerged as the major schools of thought. The interactionist approach was the most influential framework in the 1970s and maintains stability in its use over time. While some work was done on the developmental framework during this time period, major study to expand and refine it did not occur (Holman and Burr, 1980, pp. 731-732).

Presented below is a brief overview of some of the theoretical frameworks which have guided clinical practice in recent years. Practitioners generally find that an eclectic approach, or one that integrates concepts from several frameworks, best meets their needs when completing a family assessment.

Structural-Functional Approach

The structural-functional framework was developed by social scientists from sociology and social anthropology. It views the family as a social system which interacts with other social systems within society. It focuses on the analysis of family interplay between collateral systems, such as school, work, or health care worlds, and the transactions between the family and its subsystems (husband-wife dyad, the sibling cliques, and personality systems of individual family members). With this approach, emphasis is placed on examining the functions society performs for the family, as well as the functions the family performs for society and its individual family members. In addition, this framework looks at how the structure (organization) of systems affects their functioning (Hill and Hansen, 1960, pp. 303-304).

The family in the structural-functional approach is seen as *open* to outside influences and transactions, but both the family and its individual family members are considered to be reactive, passive elements of systems rather than active agents of change. This framework deals poorly with social change processes and dynamics. It handles well the relationships between the family and other social systems (Hill and Hansen, 1960, pp. 303-304).

Although the structural-functional approach is no longer considered a major research framework in the field of family studies, it continues to be a meaningful framework for guiding family assessment in the clinical setting. The broad scope of this framework allows for the analysis of the multiple environmental forces which influence family functioning as well as family interactions and transactions (Aldous, 1978, p. 14). The changing nature of the American family makes it increasingly critical for the practitioner to examine the interplay between the family and its external environment. Many functions once assumed primarily by the family system, such as child-rearing responsibilities, are now being shared by collateral systems in the community.

Interactional Approach

Frequently labeled as the *symbolic* interactional frame of reference, this approach comes from sociology and social psychology. The interactionalist views the family as a unity of interacting personalities within which individual family members occupy a position or positions, such as husband-father, wife-mother, and daughter-sister.

A cluster of roles—such as provider, homemaker, companion, and sex partner—are assigned to each of these positions, and a set of social norms or behavioral role expectations is perceived for each of these roles by the individual fulfilling them. Perceptions about role expectations emerge from an individual's self-concept and from an individual's reference group. As each individual carries out the various roles, role expectations are retained, modified, or discarded based upon the reactions of others within the family environment (Aldous, 1978, pp. 10, 14).

Interactionalists view the family as being relatively *closed* to outside systems. Family members are seen as actors and reactors, who interact with their environment through symbolic communication. As a reactor, an individual does not simply respond to stimuli from the external environment. Symbolic communication evolving from the self and the environment helps individuals to interpret and select the environment to which they respond. Based on this assumption, interactionalists stress that investigators or clinicians must see the world from the point of view of the individual (Stryker, 1964, pp. 134-135).

The interactional framework emphasizes analysis of the internal aspects of family functioning, but neglects the family's relationships with other social systems. This framework identifies how relationships with others affect an individual's functioning. In addition to role analysis, interactionalists examine communication, decision-making and problem-solving processes, conflict, reactions to stress, and other family situations—such as divorce and domestic violence—which are influenced by family interactions and interactive processes (Aldous, 1978, p. 14; Hill and Hansen, 1960, pp. 302-303).

Developmental Approach

Concepts from various disciplines and approaches (rural sociology, child psychology, human development, sociology, and structural-functional and interactional approaches) were synthesized to create the developmental approach to family study. This approach looks at family development throughout its generational life cycle. It examines developmental tasks and role expectations for children, parents, and the family as a unit and how they change throughout family life (Hill and Hansen, 1960, pp. 307-308).

Duvall and Miller (1985) summarize the key features of the developmental approach to family study as follows. The developmental approach:

1. Keeps the family in focus throughout its history
2. Sees each family member in interaction with all other members
3. Watches the ways in which individuals and the family unit influence one another
4. Recognizes what a given family is going through at any particular time
5. Highlights critical periods of personal and family growth and development
6. Views both the universals and the variations among families
7. Beams in on the ways in which the culture and families influence each other
8. Provides a basis for forecasting what a given family will be going through at any period in its life-span

Exchange Theory

Developed by sociologists and behavioral psychologists, exchange theory achieved a place of prominence in the field of family study in the 1960s (Broderick, 1971, p. 144). This theory examines human behavior from an exchange relationship perspective. The basic assumption in this framework is that human beings maintain involvement in relationships on the basis of rewards and costs. Rewarding situations are developed and maintained; nonrewarding situations are avoided or ended. For a relationship to last, each person must believe that he or she is receiving rewards equivalent to or greater than the costs. Implicit in this exchange is the principle of reciprocity—to receive, one must give (Eshleman and Clarke, 1978, pp. 12-13).

Rewards, according to exchange theorists, are not necessarily tangible objects like money or presents. A woman giving affection to her husband and children, a man sharing his time for a family outing, or an employer providing praise for a job well done are some examples of rewards in social interactions which are just as significant as tangible objects. Rewards, whether tangible or intangible, must be valued by the other person in order for them to be perceived as rewards.

Exchange theory is used to analyze interactions between people. It helps to determine why certain patterns of behavior have developed between individual family members. It also assists in explaining why some relationships are positive and others negative within the family unit. In addition, it offers a rationale for why interactions change over time; individuals who perceive that they are not being rewarded often end a relationship through divorce, separation, abandonment, or termination.

General Systems Theory

First introduced by biologist Ludwig von Bertalanffy (1968, p. 11), systems theory is currently being used in many disciplines. General systems theory is a "science of wholeness." "Its subject matter is the formulation of principles that are valid for 'systems' in general, whatever the nature of their component elements and the relations or 'forces' between them" (von Bertalanffy, 1968, p. 37). The goals of general systems study are to develop a theory which unites scientific thinking across disciplines and which provides a framework for analyzing the "whole" of any given system.

Von Bertalanffy (1968, p. 83) defines a system "as a complex of elements in interaction." Although the definition of systems varies slightly from author to author, several commonalities emerge. It is generally agreed that a system consists of two or more connected elements which form an organized whole and which interact with each other.

Churchman (1968, p. 29) proposes five basic considerations that must be kept in mind when one is thinking about the meaning of a system:

1. The total system objectives and, more specifically, the performance measures of the whole system

2. The system's environment: the fixed constraints
3. The resources of the system
4. The components (elements or subsystems) of the system, their activities, goals, and measures of performance
5. The management of the system

Churchman, like many system scientists, uses an input-process-output-feedback model to depict the structural relationships of a system. An example of this type of model is shown in Figure 6-2. In simplistic terms, this model illustrates that all systems have *inputs* or resources which, when *processed,* help the system to achieve its goals or *outputs.* It further shows that a system is cyclical in nature and continues to be so as long as the four parts keep interacting. If, however, there are changes in any one of the four parts, there will be changes in all of the parts. *Feedback* from within the system or the *environment* provides information which helps a system to determine whether it is meeting its goals.

When analyzing any system, it is extremely important to recognize that all systems have fixed constraints from the environment, as well as choices that can be made about how the system will use its resources (inputs). Families, for example, must send their children to school after

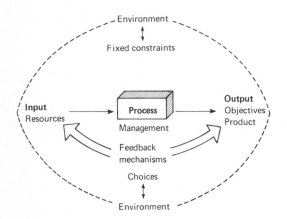

Figure 6-2   Structural arrangements of a system. (Adapted from Clemen SJ: Introduction to health care facility: food service administration, University Park, 1974, Pennsylvania State University Press, p 24.)

they reach a certain age. This is a *legal constraint,* not easily altered by a family system. To change this constraint would require consensus action by multiple systems. A family system does have some choice, however, about where the children will attend school. If a family does not like a particular public school district, this family may decide to move to another school district or to enroll the children in a private school.

No system can function in a vacuum. The environment of any system greatly affects how the system is able to function. Families' choices about educational opportunities for their children vividly illustrate this point. Some families may want to send the children to private school but are unable to do so because of *educational constraints* placed on them from the environment; in some settings private schools are unavailable. Other families may not be able to choose private school education because of *economic constraints* placed on them from the environment; their incomes may be insufficient to meet the financial requirements of a private educational system.

The processing of inputs (resources) received from the environment requires a series of dynamic, interrelated transactions. These transactions link together the environment, the system inputs, and the system outputs.

Processes are simply "the actions needed to get the job done" (Clemen, 1974, p. 26). Different types of processes are needed to accomplish particular tasks. Those processes of special interest to community health nurses are discussed throughout this text. Processes used by families to maintain healthy family functioning are discussed in a later section of this chapter. Presented in Chapter 8 (nursing process) and Chapter 9 (referral process and discharge planning) are the dynamic actions used by community health nurses to enhance client growth. Examined in Chapter 10 (epidemiological process), Chapter 11 (community diagnosis process), and Chapter 12 (planning process) are the dynamic actions integrated by community health nurses to plan and implement services for populations at risk. Covered in Chapter 21 (management process) and Chapter 22 (quality assurance process) are the dynamic actions carried out by community health nurses to ensure effective and efficient utilization of nursing time and the delivery of quality care.

The feedback mechanism is the most significant aspect of a system. It assists the system in identifying its strengths and needs and in evaluating how well it is accomplishing its goals. Feedback provides data essential for effective adaptation to internal and external system changes. It provides information which helps the system to select corrective actions when problems exist.

A system needs a mechanism that facilitates the sharing of both positive and negative feedback. A family system which discourages negative input often remains static or develops dysfunctional patterns. This can lead to disorganization, confusion, or chaos. Lack of positive feedback, however, can also lead to dysfunctional behavior. Positive feedback helps families to maintain healthy patterns of functioning and to stimulate creative ideas. If members of a family system receive only negative feedback, they become discouraged and find it difficult to utilize their creative talents.

In addition to the input-process-output-feedback element, there are several other characteristics of all systems. The following list briefly summarizes some of the more significant ones:

1. *Boundaries.* Every system has filtering mechanisms, or boundaries, which regulate the flow of energy to and from other systems. Boundaries in a system are not physical barriers. Rather, they are *abstract* entities such as norms, values, attitudes, and rules which inhibit or facilitate human transactional processes between systems.

2. *Exchange of energy.* Energy transport is crucial to the survival of any system. Without it, dysfunction results. An effectively functioning system uses energy to obtain resources (inputs) from the outside, to process resources to achieve its goals, and to release outputs into the environment. Energy that promotes order in a system is labeled *negentropy.* Energy that results in chaos or disorganization, is termed *entropy* (von Berta-

lanffy, 1968; Wiener, 1968). All living systems contain entropy and negentropy. A system becomes distressed if extreme entropy exists for a considerable length of time. Family systems which are ineffectively dealing with crisis situations may reflect the concept of entropy. These families frequently lack energy to carry out their normal patterns of functioning and thus chaos or disorganization results.

3. *Hierarchic order.* In all systems, there is order and patterning. Von Bertalanffy (1968, p. 27) noted that fundamental to general systems theory is the concept of hierarchic order in structure (order of parts) and function (order of processes). This implies that all systems are interconnected through a complex array of processes with other systems (families), their subsystems (the family members), and suprasystems (community) and that there is a logical relationship among the parts of all systems.

4. *Open or closed systems.* *Open* and *closed* are terms used in general systems theory to describe how a system interfaces with its environment. A system which isolates itself from others is viewed as a closed system. A system which exchanges energy and resources with other systems is an open system. All living systems are open systems. The degree of their openness varies, however, depending on how well they transport energy to maintain themselves.

5. *Self-regulation.* An open system, through its feedback mechanism or its information processing element, obtains data needed to adjust to its environment. The circular nature of its input-process-output-feedback unit helps a system to adapt the flow of inputs and outputs so that it can achieve a balance between what is taken from the environment and what is released into the environment. It helps the system to maintain homeostasis and to promote growth (von Bertalanffy, 1968, pp. 160-163).

Increasingly, health care professionals and

family scholars are applying the concepts, principles, and models of system theory to the study of the family. General systems theory provides a conceptual framework which is consistent with the holistic nature of humankind and professional practice. It offers a logical way to integrate all the factors that make an impact on family functioning and link the family together into a meaningful whole. It provides the basis for a humanistic philosophy of professional practice. The reason it does so is that family analysis from a systems perspective examines the family as a whole, rather than from isolated cause-and-effect relationships. Functional and dysfunctional patterns of behavior are considered to be products of system functioning. Family structure, functions, and processes are analyzed to determine why adaptive or maladaptive behavior is occurring within the family. This, in turn, negates individual blame and focuses attention on how the system must change in order to achieve productive functioning.

Use of Theoretical Frameworks in the Practice Setting

Theoretical frameworks help the practitioner to assess family structure and processes in an organized and logical fashion. They provide parameters to consider when collecting data about client situations. They facilitate the synthesis of data so that family strengths and needs can be identified. They help to explain family dynamics, which, in turn, assist the practitioner in developing appropriate intervention strategies. When a conceptual framework is lacking, it is extremely difficult to group data and to identify the relationships between the multiple variables that make an impact on the client.

Community health nurses generally utilize a combination of several theoretical frameworks to guide the family assessment process. This is appropriate since the needs of clients are varied and because there is no one framework which explains all family phenomena. Research frameworks, such as those previously discussed, tend to focus attention on some aspects of family life more than on others. In the clinical setting, it is essential for the nurse to examine the multiple aspects of internal family functioning as well as the family's relationships with other social systems. An effective management plan can be developed only after both of these areas have been assessed.

PARAMETERS TO CONSIDER DURING THE FAMILY ASSESSMENT PROCESS

In terms of the family, parameters related to both family structure and process should be considered during the family assessment process. This is true no matter what conceptual framework or combination of frameworks is selected to guide community health nursing practice. These parameters assist the nurse in obtaining a holistic view of the family. They help the nurse to identify who the family is and how family members interact to carry out their family functions.

Structural Parameters for Family Assessment

Structural components of a family are those variables which provide organization for the family system. They assist the family in coordinating their activities so that family and individual needs are met. Briar (1964, pp. 251-254) identified eight major structural characteristics of families: (1) division of labor, (2) distribution of power and authority, (3) communication, (4) boundaries of family world, (5) relations with other groups and systems, (6) ways of obtaining and giving emotional support, (7) rituals and symbols, and (8) a set of personal roles. These, as well as cultural values and attitudes and religious beliefs, are described below. Briar's delineation of the structural components of a family continues to be consistent with recent notions about the structural parameters of family life.

Division of Labor

Families allocate leadership responsibilities for maintaining their household in a variety of ways. Some follow traditional norms, with the man assuming major responsibility for the provider role and the woman for the homemaker role, regardless of the other role responsibilities each person has in the partnership. Some divide tasks according to their likes and dislikes or the level of competence each person has in relation to a particular task. Others share responsibilities equally, based on the demands each person has from other role positions. Nye (1976), in his text *Role Structure and Analysis of the Family,* discusses extensively the allocation of roles and the division of labor in family systems. This is a valuable reference for one who wants to review or expand knowledge in relation to role theory.

Families who rigidly define either the provider or homemaker role tend to experience more stress when family members are unable to perform their expected tasks than do families who have a flexible division of labor (Otto, 1963; Lewis, Beavers, Gossett, and Phillips, 1976; Pratt, 1976; Beavers, 1977). It is also extremely difficult for families who have rigid patterns of functioning to mobilize new coping mechanisms when experiencing a crisis. Health care professionals, for instance, often observe confusion and disorganization when a spouse dies. This confusion is heightened if the man or woman has not been prepared to deal with the demands of daily living. Assuming responsibilities for tasks one is not accustomed to performing is difficult at any time, but especially when one is experiencing a crisis.

Identifying how the division of labor is handled by a family helps the community health nurse to understand the stresses family members are experiencing when changes have occurred. Role strain results when families do not take into consideration that role responsibilities change over time. Mothers, for example, are often confronted with excessive role demands after the birth of a child. This is especially true if husbands do not share the responsibility for housekeeping and child-care tasks. Role strain also occurs when family members are unable to perform the activities related to a given role. This is particularly noticeable when role modifications are needed because of the prolonged absence of one family member. Absences that are a result of illness, divorce, separation, or vocational responsibilities frequently require drastic modifications in a family's division of labor and result in role strain.

All family members can experience role strain.

Children may be required to assume adult responsibilities which are excessive for their age and level of growth and development. This most often occurs during times of crisis or when parents have not assumed adult leadership responsibilities required to maintain their household. It has been found, that role-reversal behavior between parents and children is often present when child abuse occurs (Flanzraich and Dunsavage, 1977, p. 13). It is important for community health nurses to recognize that children do experience role strain when they assume parental functions, and to avoid reinforcing role-reversal patterns. It is easy to praise a child who is functioning beyond his or her chronological age. This praise, however, may support the continuance of family patterns which are unhealthy and which adversely affect a child's emotional growth and development.

Distribution of Power and Authority

Power was conceptualized by Bredemeir and Stephenson (1965, p. 50) "as the capacity to carry out, by whatever means, a desired course of action despite the resistance of others and without having to take into consideration their needs. When power is institutionalized through respect, fear, esteem, or position, it is referred to as authority."

Several variables affect who will have power in the family system. The position of power can be *culturally* prescribed, usually with the father being in a position of authority by virtue of his role as a male. This is frequently seen in Spanish-American and Asian cultures, where male dominance is the norm. Power can also be *situationally* prescribed when family members do not necessarily follow cultural norms but develop a power structure based on their circumstances and personal interactions. The continuum of family power based on cultural and situational variables ranges from complete dominance to complete absence of power, both of which can produce dysfunctional family patterns. Complete dominance by one family member poses a threat to the self-esteem of other family members and makes it difficult for individuals to resolve the independence-dependence conflicts which arise during adolescence and young adulthood. Complete absence of power in a family system tends to produce confusion, disorganization, and chaos. Dysfunctional families frequently exhibit power structures on either end of the continuum. Healthy families usually fall in the middle of the continuum, where power is shared by adult members, and children are involved in the decision-making process.

Exchange theory helps to explain why an equal or unequal distribution of power evolves in a family system. Sharing of power is more likely to occur when all family members perceive that they have resources to contribute which enhance the family's ability to achieve its goals and to meet the needs of individual family members. Family members who do not value their contributions or whose contributions are not valued by other family members will probably not have power within the family system.

Understanding the relationship between issues of power and decision making is essential to effect permanent changes within a family system. If the power and authority structure of a family is ignored, nursing interventions are often inappropriate and place additional stress on family members who lack the power to make decisions about needed health actions. Family members who have power must be consulted if changes in health behavior are to occur. One community health nurse, for instance, realized after several home visits to a Spanish-American family that the only way she would influence the family to obtain needed surgery for their 4-year-old preschooler was to talk with the child's father. Although the mother stated frequently that she felt it was important for her son to have surgery, no action was taken. When the mother was finally asked how her husband felt about this matter, the nurse discovered that he felt surgery was unnecessary and that he was the one who made the final decision about needed health care.

In situations where the dominant family member is temporarily immobilized, it is extremely important for the community health nurse to recognize that the family may reassign the dominant position to the nurse. Because of the nurse's professional status, families who are under stress may initially allow a nurse to assume a position of au-

thority within the family structure. They may follow the nurse's suggestions to relieve the anxiety they are experiencing at the time. These suggestions may not necessarily be appropriate for the family, but the family may follow through on them because its anxiety level is so high. A family under stress will frequently try anything to reduce its level of discomfort. It is significant for a nurse to recognize that this does happen, because when families are experiencing pain it is easier at times to do things for them than to foster family decision making. Taking over decision making for a family is not therapeutic.

Communication Patterns

Verbal and nonverbal interactions within a family usually display significant regularities or patterns. Norms involving what is shared and not shared, as well as who shares with whom, are implicitly, if not explicitly, known by all family members. Messages are provided in a variety of ways to let family members know how to communicate within and outside the family system.

The ability to communicate accurately and effectively is essential to all aspects of family functioning because communication is an integral part of daily living. It helps the family to carry out its functions, to meet the needs of individual family members, and to move toward achieving its goals.

Communication is an extremely complex process, involving not only what is said but also *how* it is said, and the *behavioral interactions* which occur during the course of a conversation. An individual can communicate even when verbal information is not shared. Watzlawick, Beavin, and Jackson (1967, pp. 48-49) noted that because all behavior in an interactional situation has message value, it is impossible for one not to communicate. They believe that "activity or inactivity, words or silence, all have message value which influence others; others, in turn, cannot avoid responding to these communications and are thus, themselves communicating." Even silence conveys a message to an individual who is sharing thoughts, ideas, or feelings.

Communication-oriented theorists believe that

family communication patterns need to be analyzed along several dimensions (Haley, 1971; Jackson, 1968; Satir, 1972; Watzlawick, Beavin and Jackson, 1967). Verbal, nonverbal, and behavioral processes should be observed to identify the following aspects of a family's communication patterns.

1. *Content.* What actually is conveyed is known as the content of communication. Observations should be made to determine what is being shared as well as what is not being shared. It is not unusual for individuals to feel uncomfortable about sharing information concerning personal topics such as sexuality, finances, and troubled relationships with significant others. A health care professional needs to "listen between the lines" in order to help clients verbalize areas of concern beyond those which are explicitly expressed.

2. *How content is shared.* The sharing of content does not necessarily convey to the receiver accurate knowledge, facts, or ideas, or help the receiver to understand the message one is attempting to share. Content becomes functional when there is clarity of thought, organization of ideas, and accuracy and completeness of facts. It is difficult for the receiver to understand what is being said when information is being withheld, when an overabundance of data is being shared, or when conflicting messages are being conveyed. These problems tend to distort reality and confuse the listener. They can lead to a lack of responsiveness or hostile interchange.

3. *Behavioral interactions.* How an individual responds, either verbally or nonverbally, during a conversation provides clues to others about how this individual views what is being said or how he or she regards the sender. Body mannerisms, eye contact, silence or responsiveness to content, vocal characteristics, and ways of eliciting information all provide behavioral messages which guide the course of a conversation.

Behavioral messages are often *far more meaningful* in a positive or negative sense than verbal content. They may provide "double-level messages, with the voice saying one thing and the rest of the person saying something else" (Satir, 1972, p. 60). Healthy families tend to share fewer "double-level" messages than nonhealthy families.

4. *Interpretation of content and behavioral interactions.* How information and interactions are interpreted varies from one individual to another. Perceptions about messages being conveyed are influenced by several factors, including such things as previous experiences when communicating with others, the motivations of persons involved in a conversation, feelings about oneself, and current stresses being experienced. Persons, for example, who have low self-esteem frequently find it difficult to interpret messages positively; praise is often not heard or is negated. The interpretation of messages is a key factor which determines the difference between healthy and pathological communication. When assessing family communication patterns, it is extremely important to note whether real-life events and the feelings and thoughts of others are accurately perceived. When healthy communication patterns exist, clarification is sought if individuals do not understand what is being said. Feelings such as sadness, joy, or anger are not attributed to others without validation.

5. *Ways utilized to communicate.* Satir (1975, pp. 141-149) noted that individuals use five major transactional modes to communicate when they are under stress. These are placating, blaming, superreasonable, irrelevant, and congruent modes.

   a. *Placating* refers to a mode of communication which entails agreeing with what is being said, even when one does not inwardly desire to do so. The placater is trying to please others and does not share personal feelings and reactions. Placating may occur if an individual does not wish to engage in a conversation.

b. *Blaming* patterns of behavior result when an individual has a need to prove that he or she is strong. Techniques such as fault-finding, dictatorship, or cutting remarks are used to demonstrate that one has power. Individuals who use blaming techniques are usually very insecure. Often, they exert control over others, in order to achieve a sense of security through power.

c. *Superreasonable* communication occurs when a person intellectualizes and avoids the sharing of feelings and emotions. Individuals who are afraid to deal with feelings and emotions frequently do not recognize the need to make constructive changes in their lives; they suppress feelings of anxiety which are needed to motivate them to examine dysfunctional patterns of behavior.

d. *Irrelevant* transactions are illogical from the perspective of what is happening in an individual's environment. Irrelevant communication patterns affect the flow of a conversation as well as problem-solving and decision-making processes.

e. *Congruent* interactions result when feelings and content are integrated and information sharing is logical in relation to what is happening in the environment. When using congruent communication, an individual is "real." That is, there is a consistency between what the individual outwardly shares and what is inwardly felt; this is the most functional way to interact with others. Satir (1975, p. 48) has found that when the other transactional modes of communication become patterned, psychosomatic and other illnesses often result.

6. *Linguistic characteristics.* Families have varying dialects or language differences, depending on their cultural background, their socialization process, and their geographic location. It is important for a community health nurse to note these differences, be-

cause they can interfere with communication, especially when a family's or a nurse's dialect is incongruent with the dialect of others in their environment. Generally, clients are more than willing to help health care professionals understand language differences, if the health care professional shows an interest in learning about them.

The primary goal of observing family communication patterns is to determine if the patterns established by a particular family are functional. That is, do they help the family to carry out its functions, to relate effectively to the environment, to meet the needs of individual family members, and to achieve its goals? It is important to remember that ways of achieving functional communication between family members can vary from one family to another. In recent professional and lay literature, there has been a tendency to idealize frank, honest self-disclosure (Briar, 1964, p. 252). Frankness may not always be functional, however; stating what one thinks without taking into consideration another person's feelings can be irresponsible. Honest interchanges in communication can occur without frank disclosure. Being honest is saying only what you mean, not everything (Hacker, 1985).

Hacker (1985), a health educator who specializes in sexuality counseling, has found that both clients and health care professionals are often afraid of handling sensitive topics because they are confused about the difference between honesty and self-disclosure. To her, an honest individual is one who says what he or she means and is comfortable with what is not shared. Self-disclosure is the frank sharing of one's private feelings, thoughts, and actions, often without evaluating the appropriateness of doing so in one's current situation. Hacker has found that self-disclosure is not necessarily the key to the successful handling of sexuality issues. Rather, she believes that one needs to be honest with oneself about personal sexuality concerns. Only then will one be able to deal with value issues and feelings. Shakespeare was wise when he said in *Hamlet,* "This above all: to thine own self be true,/ And it must follow, as the night the day,/ Thou canst not then be false to any man" (*Hamlet,* act 1, sc. 3).

Boundaries of Family World

Boundary development and maintenance is essential for family survival and growth. Families must have effective filtering mechanisms so that the exchange of energies corresponds to the needs of the family. Energy exchanges which occur too rapidly or too slowly can be disruptive to the family system. Families need to bring inputs into their system and release outputs into the environment so that they can carry out their functions. However, they also need to limit the amount of input from the environment to prevent system overload and to limit the release of outputs to prevent energy depletion.

The rate of energy flow between the family and the environment must vary in order for the family to maintain the integrity of its system. Families who do not adjust their energy flow to correspond to their current circumstances have difficulty handling stress and change. In times of family stress and change, limiting the exchange of inputs and outputs conserves energy needed to carry out activities of daily living. A new mother or father, for instance, may need to reduce working hours (output) in order to conserve energy for child-care activities and to provide emotional support for others in the family system.

It is not uncommon for community health nurses to work with families who are having difficulty adjusting energy flow to and from their family system. Some of the most frequent difficulties in relation to boundary maintenance issues which will be encountered in clinical practice are summarized below:

1. *Boundaries too loose.* Disorganized, multi-problem, and crisis-prone families tend to take little control over what enters or exits their environment. They have numerous outsiders, such as health care professionals or legal authorities (inputs), working with them, and often they do not set rules about how and when family members should interact outside the family system. These fam-

ilies usually come to the attention of health care professionals because their outputs are not acceptable to the suprasystem (community). It is not unusual for such families to be referred to the community health nurse when their children enter school, because they lacked the energy to fulfill the health requirements (immunizations and physical examinations) mandated by the educational system for school entry. In these situations, families' energies are often used to deal with outsiders or crises rather than to take care of the needs of individual family members.

2. *Boundaries too rigid.* Some families allow few inputs to cross their boundaries. They isolate themselves from the larger community and may not obtain the resources needed for family growth. Families from differing cultural backgrounds or families who have members with a mental or physical handicap may limit inputs from the environment because they are afraid that the larger society will not accept their differences. Conflicts between these families and their environment arise when they do not release outputs (do not send their children to school) or when their outputs are inadequate (children not prepared to handle environmental demands and pressures).

3. *Boundaries not agreed upon.* At times, community health nurses find that there is a discrepancy between the views of one family member and another regarding boundary maintenance. Families may have some boundaries which are well defined and others which are unclearly defined. They may, for example, use community resources appropriately but may not agree on how often and when they should interface with friends and the extended family. Lack of agreement on boundary maintenance issues can lead to conflict, disequilibrium, and system disintegration.

Relations with Other Groups and Systems

The development of relationships with other groups, such as extended kin or neighbors, and other systems, such as church, school, or health care agencies, is directly related to the way the family handles its boundary maintenance functions. Family boundaries can facilitate or inhibit the establishment and maintenance of interpersonal relationships with others outside the family system. Families with rigid boundaries have few contacts wth persons outside their family system. Families with flexible boundaries tend to encourage close interactions with others.

When assessing family relationships outside the family system, it is important to look at the *type* of relationships they have as well as the contact allowed. Interaction with numerous people does not necessarily mean that the family is meeting their support, companionship, and growth needs. Some families develop relationships which involve more giving than receiving. In these situations, family energies are devoted to helping others, but the family receives very little support in return. In other families, individual family members are allowed to interact with anyone, even though their interactions may not be positive. Children, for example, may encounter legal difficulties because there are no controls placed on their relationships with people who are engaging in illegal activities.

Ways of Obtaining and Giving Emotional Support

Families need to achieve a balance between their relationship with others and their relationship with family members. If the family excludes itself from its external environment, there may be a lack of support from others during times of stress and crisis. If, on the other hand, the family devotes all its energy to helping others, it is highly unlikely that the family will be able to meet the emotional needs of individual family members.

Families meet their emotional needs in a variety of ways. They develop norms which regulate sources of support, provide guidelines for giving support, and define when support will be given. When assessing the ways a family obtains and gives emotional support, the following factors should be considered:

1. *Distribution of support.* All family members need support, encouragement, and praise. If support is not evenly distributed, family members who are not receiving what they need may seek support from their environment and isolate themselves from the family system. Or they may withdraw and limit contact with others outside the family as well as within the family system.

2. *When support is given.* Some families provide support only during times of stress and crisis. Others are supportive during times of stress but also during normal functioning periods. The sharing of love, attention, and affection only when family members are distressed can be dysfunctional in that it may reinforce such behaviors as illness, truancy, and other destructive activities. All human beings need emotional care and nurturing. If they are unable to obtain emotional support without manifesting symptoms of distress, they may develop physical or psychosocial difficulties in order to receive the attention needed for emotional survival. Often, such individuals are unaware that they are doing this.

3. *Acceptance of family members.* How an individual family member is viewed by other family members greatly affects the amount of emotional support the individual will receive. Family goals which define desired achievements, norms which regulate acceptable and unacceptable behavior, and the emotional maturity of the family all influence how well individual family members will be accepted by other family members. Individuals within the family who do not conform to family norms and goals usually receive less support than those who do. Illustrating this is the teenager from a family with high educational aspirations who does not share these aspirations and decides not to go to college. This teenager very quickly receives a message from other family members that this is an inappropriate decision. If she or he does not alter these views, family members may withdraw support and encouragement, even if the family member

succeeds outside the educational environment.

4. *How support is given.* Families use both verbal and nonverbal communication to provide support for their members. Some share support spontaneously, whereas others are more reserved and do not give support until it is elicited from them. Individuals from families who spontaneously share with each other may sense a lack of support if they marry individuals from families who were reserved in their interactions with others. This can also occur when individual family members observe how their friends' families provide support for their members. Children, for instance, may perceive that they are not loved by their parents if they observe spontaneous sharing in the homes of their friends.

Set of Personal Roles

Every family has the task of organizing its roles in a way that helps the family to achieve its goals and to carry out its functions. There is no one role-allocation pattern that works for all families. Families must allocate and differentiate roles in a manner which facilitates their functioning.

Personal roles as well as family roles evolve when families organize their role structure. Some common examples of personal roles are "the 'baby' in the family; the 'good' child; the 'bad' child; the scapegoat; the strict parent; and the 'sickest' member of the family. Such roles, even when they emerge fortuitously, can become patterned very quickly. As a result, the person may be 'locked' in the role, with important consequences for how others will treat him and what they will expect of him" (Briar, 1964, p. 254). When one is assessing family dynamics, it is extremely important to identify how personal role allocation has influenced the behavior of all family members. The "sick" member of the family, for example, is often not allowed to do things that he or she is capable of doing. Frequently, family members "take care" of this person so well that he or she never learns how to function independently.

Rituals and Symbols

Family rituals and symbols come from two major sources. First, some are adopted from the culture as a whole or a subculture within the wider culture. Second, they develop from human transactional processes which have occurred within the family system (Briar, 1964, pp. 253-254).

Family rituals and symbols develop around multiple aspects of family life. They help family members and outsiders to identify what the family views as important. They provide structure for activities of daily living and for special occasions.

Examples of the types of rituals and symbols which develop in family systems are shared below. Although some of the rituals within a family appear very similar to societal ones, family rituals usually have some very specific, unique characteristics.

1. Mealtimes: designating times for meals, seating arrangements during meals, and conversation sharing
2. Family names: giving nicknames to all family members or naming children for specific family members
3. Holidays: serving specific types of food or carrying out certain kinds of activities (refer to Figures 6-3 and 6-4)
4. Religious observances: saying prayers at mealtime or bedtime or engaging in specific activities when a family member has died

Family rituals and symbols are extremely significant and are usually valued highly by families. They are often continued even when individual family members do not view them as important. Frequently, pressure is placed on family members to conform to family rituals and symbols until the entire family unit alters its views about them.

Cultural Values and Attitudes

There are numerous factors which influence the biological, psychosocial, and spiritual development of all human beings. Human growth and development begins with genetic characteristics inherited from parents but then branches off in different directions as one interacts with one's environment. Within this environment, the caring

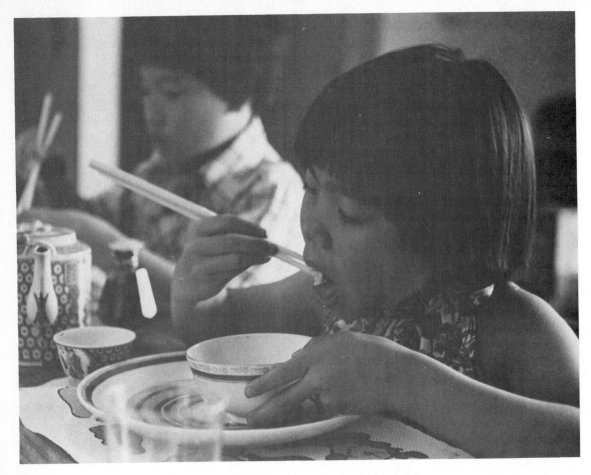

Figure 6-3   Cultural values and attitudes provide a foundation for activities of daily living.

and nurturing by significant others greatly affects how growth progresses and what decisions are made about how to handle activities of daily living. Through environmental conditioning, people learn patterns of behavior which influence how they relate to others, how they act in social situations, and how they make decisions about significant issues. Because these patterns of behavior provide stability and security, they are not easily altered; they continuously influence the direction of one's life. They shape beliefs and values which provide a foundation for future decision making.

Culture is the term used to describe the values, attitudes, and patterns of behavior which are transmitted to all individuals in a particular social environment. Social scientists have defined culture in many ways, but most of these definitions have three central themes: (1) beliefs, values, and patterns of behavior are learned and passed on from one generation to the next; (2) culture provides a prescription for daily living and decision making; and (3) the components of a culture are valued by members of the culture and are considered to be right and not open to questioning.

Every culture has a schema, composed of specific components, which shapes such things as family structure, dietary habits, religious practices, the development of art, music, and drama, ways of communicating, dress, and health behavior (refer to Figure 6-3). A culture schema, for in-

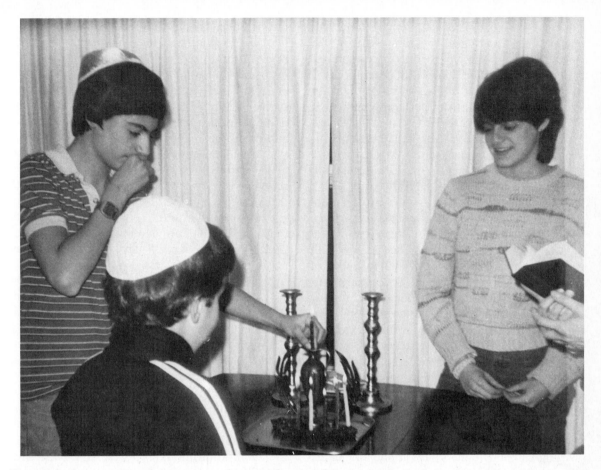

Figure 6-4   For centuries, religious systems have significantly influenced the development of customs and rituals within family systems and have preserved and transmitted these traditions from one generation to another. Hanukkah, a festive Jewish holiday lasting 8 days in early December, has been celebrated for centuries in memory of the rededication of the temple of Jerusalem under the Maccabees in 164 B.C. Hanukkah is a celebration of freedom—freedom to practice one's own religion. It is a joyous time which includes a symbolic lighting of candles, the sharing of gifts, and the serving of special foods.

stance, affects how one perceives health and illness and when and from whom one seeks health care. Because the Jewish culture values the sacredness of human life and health, members of this particular cultural group have traditionally respected health care providers and have engaged in activities, regardless of the expense, to restore health. The value the Jewish culture places on health is reflected in a favorite Yiddish parting phrase, *Sei gesund,* "be well" (Kensky, 1977, p. 197). In contrast to the health values held by the Jewish culture are the beliefs and values transmit-

ted by the Mexican-American culture. Many individuals from this culture are influenced by a folk system which encourages the use of folk medicine and supports the belief that one has very little control over one's life; it is felt that supernatural forces cause disease and that one can do very little to prevent illness. Mexican healers, *curanderos(as),* rather than health care professionals are used by some Mexican-American families when health care services are needed (Baca, 1973; Prattes, 1973; Samora, 1978).

A rich diversity of cultural values and attitudes

exists in our nation. In community health nursing practice, encountering clients who have beliefs which differ from those of the health care professional is a common occurrence. In order for community health nurses to work effectively with such clients, they must develop an appreciation for the inherent worth of different cultural patterns. This involves a process which not only increases one's knowledge about various cultural schemata but also increases one's acceptance of all human beings and their cultures.

Developing cultural sensitivity in clinical practice is not an easy task. Health care professionals, like clients, are influenced by their own social conditioning, which has a long-lasting effect on everything they do. It is often difficult to recognize the effects of earlier influences, because patterns of functioning derived from social conditioning become a way of life. These patterns subtly influence behavior even when they are no longer recognized on a conscious level. Hence, health care professionals need to examine carefully how their values and attitudes are affecting their clinical judgments. This process can be painful, especially when it is identified that one's interventions are not therapeutic because the client's health beliefs have been discounted. Remember, if this happens, that all practitioners have at one time or another experienced professional situations in which they have not been effective because of value conflicts. Being able to identify that one's behavior is adversely affecting professional interactions and to take action to alter nontherapeutic intervention is one of the characteristics of a sensitive professional.

When learning about specific cultural beliefs, it is best to seek information about these beliefs from members of the particular culture being studied. Many cultural patterns are not written or recorded. Most, in fact, are transmitted from one generation to another through oral communication and behavioral transactions. When one is receiving input from individuals who represent a given cultural group, it is extremely important to remember that diversity exists within cultures as well as between cultures. Knowledge about cultural values and attitudes helps one to identify

factors to consider when collecting data about family functioning. This knowledge, however, *never replaces the need to obtain specific data from individual families during the assessment process.* When working with families in the community setting, a cultural assessment should be done to determine their unique characteristics and needs.

Cultural assessments assist nurses in individualizing family care. When conducting a cultural assessment, community health nurses need to focus on collecting basic cultural data which identify major family values, beliefs, customs, and behaviors that influence and relate to health needs, health care practices, and family attitudes about health and illness, health care providers, and health care systems (Orgue, Bloch, and Monrroy, 1983, p. 55; Tripp-Reimer, Brink, and Saunders, 1984, p. 79). According to Tripp-Reimer, Brink, and Saunders (1984, p. 79), "basic cultural data include: ethnic affiliation, religious preference, family patterns, food patterns, and ethnic health care practices."

Displayed in Appendix 6-1 is a cultural assessment tool developed by Bloch (1983) to facilitate cultural assessments in the clinical setting. This tool identifies content areas such as race, language and communication processes, and nutritional variables to be considered when making a cultural assessment. In their text, *Ethnic Nursing Care,* Orgue, Bloch, and Monrroy examine specific factors to consider when providing nursing care for Black, Raza/Latina, Filipino American, Chinese American, Japanese American, South Vietnamese, and American Indian clients. Referring to this text will help the reader to plan appropriate nursing interventions when working with families from the above ethnic minority groups.

When using Bloch's cultural assessment guide, one must remember that a barrage of questions related to the cultural content areas on this tool is inappropriate. This type of interviewing inhibits communication and adversely affects the nurse-client relationship. When collecting any type of information during the assessment phase of the nursing process, the community health nurse must focus on building a therapeutic relationship as well as obtaining data (refer to Chapter 8). Brownlee (1978), in *Community, Culture and Care,* provides some valuable guidelines to consider when collecting cultural data.

Religious Beliefs

Cultural values and attitudes are often shaped and maintained by religious systems. From earliest times, religious systems have preserved and transmitted traditions from one generation to another, and have greatly influenced the development of norms for social behavior. Spiritual beliefs valued by these systems have provided a foundation for moral behavior in societies; they have also helped to maintain order and cohesiveness in social groups.

Despite major changes in our religious systems in the past two decades, spiritual beliefs still affect the lives of most individuals. They influence such things as contraceptive practices, dietary habits, developmental transitions through rites of passage, selection of marriage partners, reactions to health and illness, and the development of customs and rituals (refer to Figure 6-4).

Spiritual beliefs of clients are often not addressed in the clinical setting. This is unfortunate, because these beliefs frequently bring comfort to distressed individuals and help them to cope with illness and crisis. Involving spiritual leaders in a client's care and allowing clients to verbalize their feelings about their religious values can strengthen the relationships between health care professionals and clients and can promote effective decision making about needed health care services.

Process Parameters for Family Assessment

Basic to the understanding of family functioning is the analysis of family processes. Family processes are methods used by families to determine how their structure evolves, how decisions are made, and how the family carries out its functions to maintain stability and to promote growth within the family unit.

There are several parameters to consider when assessing family processes:

1. How the family integrates its role relationships
2. How the family utilizes information from the environment
3. How the family adapts to changes within the family system and its environment
4. How the family makes and implements decisions
5. How the family deals with conflict or disagreement
6. How the family maintains the integrity of the family unit, as well as the personal autonomy of family members

Family health is a function of process rather than outcome. It is family process which helps the family to manage stress, to survive crises, to deal with conflict, and to organize itself so that it can achieve its goals. Usually, however, a family comes to the attention of the health care professional because its outputs are inadequate or because the family perceives it is having difficulty meeting its goals. When one is assessing family functioning, it is extremely important to examine process variables as well as outcomes desired by a family; family processes frequently need to be altered before desired outcomes can be reached.

Direct observation of the family system is the best way to gain an understanding of family processes. This is especially true during times of crisis, because it is during these periods that functional or dysfunctional behaviors become more evident. Decision-making as well as communication patterns should be analyzed carefully in an assessment of family processes. Chapter 7 presents the concepts of stress and crisis and examines some of the factors which affect decision making when people are distressed. Parameters to observe when one is looking at family communication patterns have been discussed previously in this chapter. Publications by Ackerman (1959, 1970), Bowen (1973), Haley (1971), Jackson (1968), Minuchin (1974), Satir (1972), and Watzlawick, Beavin, and Jackson (1967) provide an in-depth analysis of family processes and are very useful references for practitioners who view the family as their unit of service.

TABLE 6-2   The North American Nursing Diagnosis Association: Altered family processes

Diagnostic label	Definition	Etiology/Related factors	Defining characteristics
Altered family processes	Inability of family system (household members) to meet needs of members, carry out family functions, or maintain communications for mutual growth and maturation	Situational crisis or transition Developmental crisis or transition	Inability of family members to relate to each other for mutual growth and maturation
			Failure to send and receive clear messages
			Poorly communicated family rules, rituals, symbols; unexamined myths
			Unhealthy family decision-making processes
			Inability of family members to express and accept wide range of feelings
			Inability to accept and receive help
			Does not demonstrate respect for individuality and autonomy of members
			Rigidity in functions and roles
			Fails to accomplish current (or past) family developmental tasks
			Inappropriate (nonproductive) boundary maintenance
			Inability to adapt to change
			Inability to deal with traumatic or crisis experience constructively
			Parents do not demonstrate respect for each other's views on child-rearing practices
			Inappropriate (nonproductive) level and direction of energy
			Inability to meet needs of members (physical, security, emotional, spiritual)
			Family uninvolved in community activities

From Gordon M: Manual of nursing diagnosis 1988-1989, St Louis, 1989, CV Mosby Co, pp 234, 236.

Table 6-2 presents characteristics which reflect dysfunctional processes in a family unit. These behaviors were identified by the North American Nursing Diagnosis Association, a national organization established to develop standard nursing diagnoses for the profession. Having an understanding of these behaviors assists the community health nurse in identifying families who need nursing intervention.

TOOLS THAT FACILITATE THE FAMILY ASSESSMENT PROCESS

There are a variety of tools a community health nurse can use to facilitate family assessment. Some of these tools are discussed below. They are designed to help the practitioner elicit data about certain aspects of family structure, function, and process and aid the health professional in determining major family concerns, needs, and strengths. Assessment tools, however, are only guides, and before using them, one needs to have an understanding of family theory and of communication processes that enhance effective nurse-client relationships.

Family Assessment Guides

Many community health agencies have developed family assessment guides so that staff members can focus attention on family functioning as well as on the health status of individual family members. Appendix 6-2 is an example of such a tool.

When completed, it provides a quick visual summary of family strengths, family behaviors which need to be altered, and anticipated guidance needs.

Generally, family assessment guides examine both the family's relationships with its environment and its internal functioning. It is extremely important when designing guides to facilitate the data collection process to take into consideration the need to identify both functional and dysfunctional behaviors within a family system. It is very easy to focus only on family problems. When this is done, areas of family dysfunctioning may be overemphasized. This can have a devastating affect on the family and the nurse and lead to frustration, discouragement, and a feeling of hopelessness for all. Nurses who are unable to see family strengths "burn out" quickly; families who never receive positive feedback for what they are handling well question their ability to adequately maintain themselves and often become dependent on others for decision making.

Before constructing a family assessment guide, an agency needs to make a careful analysis of its philosophy of nursing practice, so that it is reflected in the assessment tool being developed. For instance, a belief in preventive health behavior would be operationalized if staff members were encouraged to discern anticipatory guidance needs and then to plan nursing intervention strategies which might prevent future health problems. Perhaps hazards in the environment have not yet caused an accident; however, if hazards such as medications left where small children can reach them are not eliminated, a serious health problem may result. Health counseling assists parents in realizing how much of a threat medication might be to small children, and it may be the impetus which influences preventive health changes in a family's environment.

The community health nurse should be allowed to use a variety of assessment methodologies when implementing an agency's philosophy of practice. If a tool interferes with a practitioner's clinical style, it is highly unlikely that it will be used. Or, if the practitioner does attempt to use it, even though it does not relate to the practitioner's frame of reference, the nurse-client relationship may be distorted. Family assessment tools should be used to provide guidelines for data collection only. They should not tie a nurse into a particular interactive style or theoretical framework for family assessment.

A family assessment tool must be easily utilized by the practitioner. Tools which take a minimal amount of time to complete and which provide a composite picture of family strengths and needs are most beneficial. Many community health nurses have heavy caseload demands and become frustrated if they are asked to fill out a lengthy assessment form.

Family assessment tools are useful only when the practitioner has the theoretical background to handle them. Having knowledge about such things as role theory, cultural values and attitudes, family decision making, and concepts of stress and crisis is essential before an assessment guide can be used effectively. Assessment tools can never replace a genuine understanding of theories which analyze family functioning or which describe how nurse-client interactions affect the therapeutic process.

Genograms

A genogram is a tool which aids the community health nurse in collecting generational information about family structure and processes. It visually portrays to the nurse and the family how the family has evolved. It very quickly helps the community health nurse to identify the relationships between significant family members, the health status of individual family members, and the family's reactions to sociocultural and spiritual variables which have affected their lives.

Illustrated in Figure 6-5 is a partial genogram constructed by a community health nurse during her sixth home visit to the Z. family. Prior to doing the genogram, the nurse had been helping the family members deal with their feelings about the son's recent diagnosis of allergies. She identified that there was a discrepancy in how each parent viewed the son's health status. Wondering whether this was related to previous life experiences, the nurse completed a genogram with the

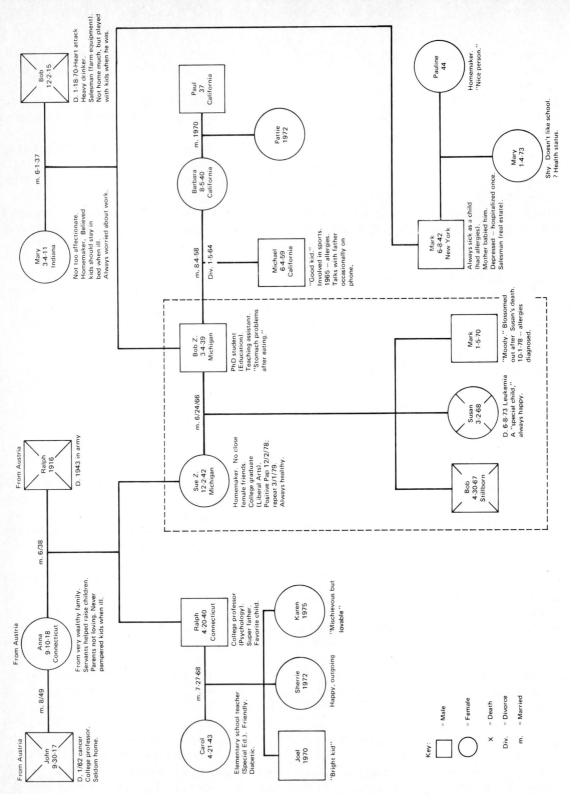

Figure 6-5 Sample genogram of the Z. family.

From Austria
John
9-30-17
D. 1/62 cancer
College professor.
Seldom home.

From Austria
Anna
9-10-18
Connecticut
From very wealthy family.
Servants helped raise children.
Parents not loving. Never
pampered kids when ill.

m. 8/49

From Austria
Ralph
1916
D. 1943 in army

m. 6/38

Bob
12-2-15
D. 1-18-70-Heart attack
Heavy drinker.
Salesman (farm equipment).
Not home much, but played
with kids when he was.

m. 6-1-37

Mary
3-4-11
Indiana
Not too affectionate.
Homemaker. Believed
kids should stay in
bed when ill.
Always worried about work.

Barbara
8-5-40
California

m. 1970

Paul
37
California

Pattie
1972

Michael
6-4-59
California
"Good kid."
Involved in sports.
1965 — allergies.
Talks with father
occasionally on
phone.

m. 8-4-58   Div. 1-5-64

Pauline
44
Homemaker.
"Nice person."

Mark
6-8-42
New York
Always sick as a child
(had allergies).
Mother babied him.
Depressed — hospitalized once.
Salesman (real estate).

Mary
1-4-73
Shy. Doesn't like school.
? Health status.

Bob Z.
3-4-39
Michigan
PhD student
(Education).
Teaching assistant.
"Stomach problems
after eating."

Sue Z.
12-2-42
Michigan
Homemaker. No close
female friends.
College graduate
(Liberal Arts).
Positive Pap 12/2/78:
repeat 3/1/79.
Always healthy.

m. 6/24/66

Bob
4-30-67
Stillborn

Susan
3-2-68
D. 6-8-73 Leukemia
A "special child."
always happy.

Mark
1-5-70
"Moody." "Blossomed
out after Susan's death.
10-1-78 — allergies
diagnosed.

Ralph
4-20-40
Connecticut
College professor
(Psychology).
Super father.
Favorite child.

Carol
4-21-43
Elementary school teacher
(Special Ed.). Friendly.
Diabetic.

m. 7-27-68

Joel
1970
"Bright kid"

Sherrie
1972
Happy, outgoing

Karen
1975
"Mischievous but
lovable"

Key:
□ = Male
○ = Female
X = Death
Div. = Divorce
m. = Married

family. By doing this, the nurse was able to trace each parent's attitudes about health and illness. She was also able to identify that the family lacked a significant support system, that both parents had had an unhappy childhood, and that they were afraid that they were "going to raise their son wrong." In addition, it was discovered that the family was having difficulty adjusting to recent role changes and that all family members had unresolved feelings about the death of two children in the family. The community health nurse who constructed the genogram shown in Figure 6-5 found that this tool helped both her and the family to focus more clearly on current significant events as well as to gain an appreciation for how past happenings were influencing present health behavior. The development of the genogram provided structure for the interviewing process and helped the community health nurse to obtain an extensive family history very rapidly.

Genograms schematically depict a family tree. Geneticists, physicians, and nurse clinicians have used them to trace genetic disorders in families. They are now being used by health care professionals to integrate health and sociocultural data. A family tree drawn by a professional differs from the one drawn by a family in that the professional uses theory as a basis to elicit data about family structure, function, and process. Normally a family tree done by a lay person illustrates only structural information.

The interview process is the most critical component to consider when one is completing a genogram. If information concerning child-rearing practices, health beliefs and attitudes, significant social data, and traditions passed on from one generation to another is not obtained, the genogram has very little meaning. Completing the actual drawing of a genogram takes minimal skill; focusing the conversation on relevant aspects of family functioning requires not only interviewing skill but also knowledge of family dynamics.

Eco-Map

An eco-map is another tool used by health care professionals which schematically portrays factual data about family relationships. It helps the family and the nurse to visually analyze a family's interactions with its external environment. Presented in Figure 6-6 is an eco-map developed by Dr. Ann Hartman for workers in a child welfare practice (Hartman, 1978, p. 466). Based on a systems theoretical framework, Hartman's tool examines boundary-maintenance aspects of family functioning. It dramatically illustrates the amount of energy used by a family to maintain its system as well as the presence or absence of situational supports and other family resources. By utilizing this tool, for example, families can be helped to identify that their energies are being used to handle stressful encounters with external systems rather than to enhance positive, supportive relationships with others. For instance, if a family's flow of energy as depicted on the eco-map reflects only an outward directional process ($\rightarrow\rightarrow\rightarrow$), the family may recognize why its goals are not being achieved.

Community health nurses have found the use of the eco-map beneficial because they are frequently involved with clients who have encounters with numerous health and welfare agencies, who have few support systems, or who "lack energy" to maintain their family system. An eco-map assists a family in visualizing how their relationships with external systems are affecting their state of well-being. One community health nurse decided to use this tool with a family because its multiple relationships with agencies were unclear and because the family members were having difficulty verbalizing their feelings about their "hopeless" family situation. "We have tried everything, and still our situation gets worse." The use of the eco-map increased the family's involvement in the therapeutic process and gave them something concrete to do, which relieved at least some of their anxiety about their "hopeless" state of affairs. When the eco-map was completed, it was obvious to both the nurse and the family that there were numerous stressors that were affecting the family's feelings about itself. The family was allowing health and social agencies to take over its affairs, extended-family members gave only negative feedback, friends seldom visited, and the family had few leisure activities. The eco-

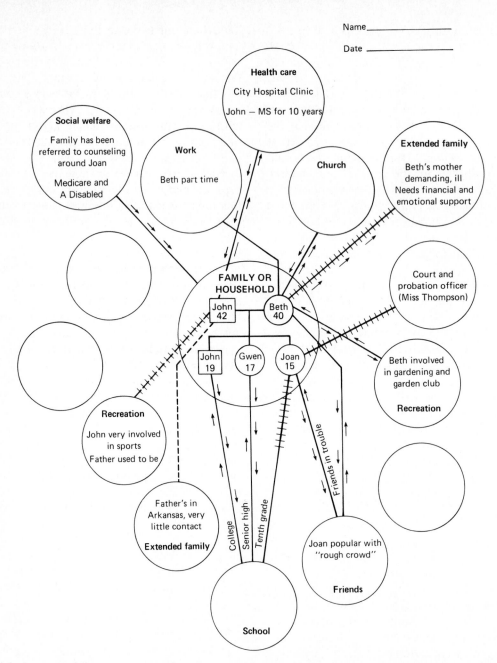

Figure 6-6 Eco-map. Fill in connections where they exist. Indicate nature of connections with a descriptive word or by drawing different kinds of lines. ———— for strong; ---------- for tenuous; ╫╫╫╫ for stressful. Draw arrows along lines to signify flow of energy, resources, and so on (→→→). Identify significant people and fill in empty circles as needed. (Hartman SA: Diagrammatic assessment of family relationships, Soc Casework, 59:470, 1978.)

map pointed out to the family the multiple problems they were encountering and assisted the nurse in planning her intervention strategies as well.

It is impossible to function effectively in the community health setting without looking at how the family interfaces with its external environment. The eco-map enhances the community health nurses's ability to gain this type of information. It is an especially useful tool because it summarizes, on one page, family strengths, conflicts, and stresses in relation to its interactions with individuals and agencies outside the family system.

Family-Life Chronology

Community health nurses may encounter families who are experiencing relationship problems, a situation which makes it difficult for them to concentrate on health concerns or to take needed health actions. These families can find it hard to examine objectively what is happening in their relationships or to make a decision about seeking counseling. Satir's (1967, p. 135) family-life chronology model (Figure 6-7) helps the community health nurse and the family to identify interactive processes that have evolved. Stresses are often related only to current family changes, such as a chronic health problem, an additional family member, or financial difficulties. Helping a family's members to look at how successful they have been in handling interpersonal interactions up to this point may provide the positive reinforcement they need to examine how they can alter their current behavior to reduce existing stresses. Sometimes, however, it will be found that a family has had long-standing relationship problems. Helping family members to identify the chronic nature of their current difficulties may assist them in seeing the need for psychosocial counseling.

The process for collecting a family-life chronology is discussed in Satir's book, *Conjoint Family Therapy* (1967). Community health nurse practitioners have found this book to be a valu-

To mates

Asks about how they met, when they decided to marry, etc.

To wife	**To husband**
Asks how she saw her parents, her sibs, her family life	Asks how he saw his parents, his sibs, his family life
Brings chronology back to when she met her husband	Brings chronology back to when he met his wife
Asks about her expectations of marriage	Asks about his expectations of marriage

To mates
Asks about early married life; comments on influence of past

To mates as parents
Asks about their expectations of parenting; comments on the influence of the past

To child
Asks about the child's views of the parents, how he or she sees them having fun, disagreeing, etc.

To family as a whole
Reassures family that it is safe to comment; stresses need for clear communication; gives closure, points to next meeting, gives hope

Figure 6-7   Main flow of family-life chronology. (From Satir V: Conjoint family therapy, a guide to theory and technique, Palo Alto, Ca, 1967, Science and Behavior Books, p 135.)

able reference that helps them work more effectively with families who are experiencing distress in their relationships.

A community health nurse cannot ignore relationship problems when working with families in their homes. Such difficulties can disrupt all parameters of family functioning and are often the key factor in preventing a family from taking needed health action. If these difficulties are not addressed, nursing intervention strategies can be ineffective. Dealing with the symptoms of distress, such as physical health problems, complaints about lack of time for leisure activities, or feelings of depression, rather than with the relationship difficulties themselves, will not alter a family's functioning in any lasting way. One mother, for example, complained to the community health nurse that she had no time for herself and that she found caring for three children, 4, 6, and 8 years old, very restrictive. Suggestions by the community health nurse on how she might care for her children and still have time for leisure activities were ignored. The mother finally shared with the nurse that her husband felt that "a woman's place was in the home. Even if I enrolled my 4-year-old son in a nursery school, I still could not get out of the house. My husband gets very upset if I am gone from home without him." This woman was depressed and discouraged. She loved her children but also wanted to explore adult interests; the only way she was able to accomplish this was to deal with the conflicts between herself and her husband.

The above situation illustrates that in working with individual family members, a nurse must determine how other members of the family view the issues being raised. Otherwise, significant data will be missed and interventions will be planned that are inappropriate to the needs of the family. It is best to obtain the ideas and opinions of all family members by seeing them together. If this cannot be arranged, asking questions such as "How does your husband react when you talk about getting a job?" provides clues about family interactions and differing value systems. It must be emphasized that family meetings can be arranged more frequently then they are; often

nurses do not suggest this strategy because they do not feel comfortable in dealing with family dynamics.

Recent Experience Life Change Questionnaires

Research since the early sixties has documented that significant life changes can adversely affect the health status of individuals (Rahe, 1972, p. 62). The Life Change Questionnaire (see Table 6-3) developed by Holmes, Rahe, Masuda, and others, has been used throughout the United States and in foreign countries to demonstrate the relationships between a cluster of events requiring life changes and illness. It has been shown that individuals whose life change units (LCU) are greater than the value of 150 in a year's time are more susceptible to illness than individuals whose life change units are below this value. Studies conducted by Rahe while at the University of Washington in Seattle, for instance, demonstrated that 50 percent of the individuals whose life change units ranged from 150 to 300 LCU had an illness within the following year. In addition, 70 percent of those individuals whose LCU values exceeded 300 had an illness the following year (Rahe, 1972).

Practitioners as well as researchers have used the Life Change Questionnaire to identify persons at risk for illness. When they discover individuals who have high LCU values, they discuss the impact of several life changes on one's health status and the importance of not making other major life changes at this time.

Increasingly, based on the recognition that the types of life-change events which produce stress vary across the life-span, research is being conducted to increase the relevance of the life-event questionnaire for a particular developmental age group or for specific population groups. Norbeck (1984) has modified the life-event questionnaire to address the needs of adult females of childbearing age. Norbeck's modified tool includes items which deal with significant concerns of women such as having difficulties with contraception, changing child care arrangements, being the victim of violent acts (rape, assault, and so on), and parenting conflicts (Norbeck, 1984, p. 64).

TABLE 6-3   Life change events

Events	LCU values	Events	LCU values
Family		Major revision of personal habits	24
Death of spouse	100	Changing to a new school	20
Divorce	73	Change in residence	20
Marital separation	65	Major change in recreation	19
Death of a close family member	63	Major change in church activities	19
Marriage	50	Major change in sleeping habits	16
Marital reconciliation	45	Major change in eating habits	15
Major change in health of family	44	Vacation	13
Pregnancy	40	Christmas	12
Addition of new family member	39	Minor violations of the law	11
Major change in arguments with wife	35		
Son or daughter leaving home	29	*Work*	
In-law troubles	29	Being fired from work	47
Wife starting or ending work	26	Retirement from work	45
Major change in family get-togethers	15	Major business adjustment	39
		Changing to different line of work	36
Personal		Major change in work responsibilities	29
Detention in jail	63	Trouble with boss	23
Major personal injury or illness	53	Major change in working conditions	20
Sexual difficulties	39		
Death of a close friend	37	*Financial*	
Outstanding personal achievement	28	Major change in financial state	38
Start or end of formal schooling	26	Mortgage or loan over $10,000	31
Major change in living conditions	25	Mortgage foreclosure	30
		Mortgage or loan less than $10,000	17

From Rahe RH: Subjects' recent life changes and their near-future illness reports, Ann Clin Res 4:250-265, 1972. This study report was supported by the Bureau of Medicine and Surgery, Department of the Navy, under Research Work Unit MF51.524.002-5011-DD5G (Report No. 72-31). Opinions expressed are those of the author and are not to be construed as necessarily reflecting the official view or endorsement of the Department of the Navy.

Barnard's (1988) Difficult Life Circumstance (DLC) scale was designed to ascertain the existence of chronic family problems among high-risk families dealing with pregnancy. The items on the DLC scale address such things as domestic violence, child abuse, long-term illness, and problems with alcohol and drug use. Barnard found that families with a high DLC score (a score reflecting the existence of several difficult life circumstances) had less favorable maternal and family outcomes than families with a low DLC score.

Beall and Schmidt (1984) have developed a tool for use with adolescents (refer to Figure 6-8). The Youth Adaptation Rating Scale is not designed to be used as a predictor of illness. Rather, it was developed "to measure the causes of adolescent adaptation and to provide parents, teachers, and adolescents with a clearer perception of

☐ Graduation (.57)

☐ Pet dies (.55)

☐ Fights with parents (.67)

☐ Getting pressure about having sex (.63)

☐ Caught cheating or lying repeatedly (.73)

☐ Getting a major illness/injury/car accident (.81)

☐ Becoming religious or giving up religion (.63)

☐ Referral to the principal's office (.47)

☐ Getting acne/warts (.45)

☐ Trouble getting a date when it was not a problem before (.61)

☐ Problems developed with teachers/employers (.59)

☐ Making career decisions (college, majors training, etc.) (.64)

☐ Starting to go to weekend parties/rock concerts (.35)

☐ First day of school (.37)

☐ Going on first date/starting to date (.53)

☐ Death of a parent/guardian (.95)

☐ Not getting promoted to next grade (.76)

☐ Getting caught using drugs (.86)

☐ Getting attacked/raped/beat up (.84)

☐ Getting a ticket or other minor problems with law (.58)

☐ Parents getting a divorce/separation (.83)

☐ Getting expelled/suspended (.71)

☐ Fad pressure (.43)

☐ Breaking up with boy/girlfriend (.57)

☐ Getting minor illness (cold, flu, etc.) (.30)

☐ Arguments with peers/brothers/sisters (.46)

☐ Starting to perform (speeches, presentations, musical or drama performances) (.60)

☐ Getting a bad report card (.59)

☐ Getting fired from a job (.63)

☐ Going into debt (.72)

☐ Being stereotyped/discriminated/having bad rumors spread about you (.70)

☐ Death of a close family member (.94)

☐ Death of a boy/girlfriend/close friend (.94)

☐ Getting V.D. (.86)

☐ Getting someone pregnant/getting pregnant (.92)

☐ Taking finals/SAT test (.61)

☐ Moving to a different town/school/making new friends (.67)

☐ Getting a car (.35)

☐ Trying to get a job/job interview (.49)

☐ Getting an award, office, etc. (.36)

☐ Making a team (drill, athletic, debate) (.44)

☐ Getting married (.73)

☐ Getting beat up by parents (.86)

☐ Taking the driver license test (.55)

☐ Getting a new addition to the family (.45)

☐ Going to the dentist or doctor (.37)

☐ Going to jail/reform school (.88)

☐ Starting to use drugs (.82)

☐ Getting braces (.45)

☐ Going on a diet (.41)

☐ Losing or gaining weight (.49)

☐ Changing exercise habits (.21)

☐ Pressure to take drugs (.71)

☐ Moving out of the house (.56)

☐ Falling in love (.66)

☐ Getting a bad haircut (.57)

☐ Getting glasses (.49)

☐ Family member moving out (.47)

Figure 6-8 Youth adaptation rating scale. The number after each item is the ratio value or degree of severity. This ratio value was determined by dividing the total value for each item by the highest possible score. Events with a high ratio value produce greater stress and require a greater degree of adaptation than do events with a lower ratio value. (From Beall S and Schmidt G: Development of a youth adaptation rating scale, J School Health 54(5):197-200, 1984, © 1984, American School Health Association, Kent, Ohio, 44240.)

events that may cause stress during the adolescent years" (Beall and Schmidt, 1984, p. 197). This tool was tested in a variety of settings and by six ethnic groups. Adolescents were asked to rank each item on the tool using a five-point descriptive scale with a zero indicating that the event was not stressful at all and the number five reflecting a very stressful event that would require a major change in one's life. No significant differences existed between the ethnic groups or the adolescents from communities of different sizes. It was found, however, that the need for adaptation or the recognition of that need becomes more evident as the adolescent grows older and matures (Beall and Schmidt, pp. 199-200).

The Life Change Questionnaire and the developmental and aggregate specific tools such as those developed by Barnard, Norbeck, and Beall and Schmidt can be used to facilitate nursing assessment as well as teaching or learning processes. Use of these tools can help community health nurses to quickly discern individuals who are experiencing multiple stressors. These tools can also assist community health nurses in teaching about normative life events, which contribute to stress during a specific developmental stage, and coping strategies for dealing with stress.

Clinically, it has been found that clients who have encountered several major life changes frequently do not recognize that this has happened. Life change questionnaires can help clients to visualize the relationship between their feelings of distress and the events that have been occurring in their lives. This recognition often promotes the development of effective stress management techniques.

Videotaping

Videotaping is another tool which has helped the community health nurse to identify family dynamics. It has been used in some community health nursing settings to assess family interactions when a handicapped child is performing activities of daily living. Community health nurses have used videotaping in these situations to observe simultaneously the interactions of a child and family, as well as the functional capabilities

of the client being assessed. It is important to observe both the client and significant others during a functional assessment, because behavior of significant others either inhibits or enhances functional capabilities.

Videotaping provides specific data about family dynamics and a child's functional abilities which are often missed during a home visit. It is easy to overlook small accomplishments of a child when other things are occurring in the environment. It is equally easy to miss nurse or family behaviors which negatively affect a child's performance. For instance, use of videotaping enabled one nurse to identify that she had not given the 4-year-old child she was assessing sufficient time to complete the tasks she asked him to perform. A repeat assessment on her next home visit provided her with more accurate data in relation to the child's level of functioning. Without videotaping, this child's level of performance would have been assessed inappropriately.

Families are usually receptive to videotaping, especially when the community health nurse explains that a more accurate evaluation of a child's abilities may be obtained through the use of this tool. Assuring them that confidentiality will be maintained also relieves their anxiety.

A videotaped child assessment can be very motivating to families because it dramatically illustrates a child's strengths and needs. Videotaping helps a family to identify positive and negative behaviors which are promoting or inhibiting a child's growth. The impact of seeing actual behaviors is not quickly forgotten.

SUMMARY

Despite its changing nature, the family is still considered the basic unit of service in community health nursing settings. Historical evidence from clinical practice and research have sufficiently demonstrated that family-centered nursing services more effectively meet the needs of individuals, families, and communities than do services delivered only to individual clients. Viewing the family from the traditional perspective, however, is no longer appropriate because alternative family life-styles are becoming more evident in our culture. The nuclear family unit is no longer the only acceptable form of family life.

It is essential for community health nurses to have an understanding of family theory in order to implement a family-centered preventive health approach to nursing care. Theory helps the practitioner to assess family structure, function, and process in an organized and logical fashion. It provides parameters to consider when one is collecting data about client situations. It assists in ex-

plaining the phenomena that are occurring within a family, which in turn helps one to plan effective intervention strategies.

Tools such as the genogram, the eco-map, and the Life Change Questionnaire are available for facilitating the family assessment process. These tools do not, however, take the place of a genuine understanding of family dynamics. They only provide guidelines for the organization and collection of data.

APPENDIX 6-1

Bloch's Ethnic/Cultural Assessment Guide

Categories	Guideline questions/instructions	Data collected
Cultural		
Ethnic origin	Does the patient identify with a particular ethnic group (e.g., Puerto Rican, African)?	
Race	What is the patient's racial background (e.g., Black, Filipino, American Indian)?	
Place of birth	Where was the patient born?	
Relocations	Where has he lived (country, city)? During what years did patient live there and for how long? Has he moved recently?	
Habits, customs, values, and beliefs	Describe habits, customs, values, and beliefs patient holds or practices that affect his attitude toward birth, life, death, health and illness, time orientation, and health care system and health care providers. What is degree of belief and adherence by patient to his overall cultural system?	
Behaviors valued by culture	How does patient value privacy, courtesy, respect for elders, behaviors related to family roles and sex roles, and work ethics?	
Cultural sanctions and restrictions	*Sanctions*—What is accepted behavior by patient's cultural group regarding expression of emotions and feelings, religious expressions, and response to illness and death?	
	Restrictions—Does patient have any restrictions related to sexual matters, exposure of body parts, certain types of surgery (e.g., hysterectomy), discussion of dead relatives, and discussion of fears related to the unknown?	
Language and communication processes:	What are some overall cultural characteristics of patient's language and communication process?	
Language(s) and/or dialect(s) spoken	Which language(s) and/or dialect(s) does patient speak most frequently? Where? At home or at work?	
Language barriers	Which language does patient predominantly use in thinking? Does patient need bilingual interpreter in nurse-patient interactions? Is patient non-English-speaking or limited English-speaking? Is patient able to read and/or write in English?	
Communication process	What are rules (linguistics) and modes (style) of communication process (e.g., "honorific" concept of showing "respect or deference" to others using words only common to specific ethnic/cultural group)?	
	Is there need for variation in technique of communicating and interviewing to accommodate patient's cultural background (e.g., tempo of conversation, eye/body contact, topic restrictions, norms of confidentiality, and style of explanation)?	
	Are there any conflicts in verbal and nonverbal interactions between patient and nurse?	
	How does patient's nonverbal communication process compare with other ethnic/cultural groups, and how does it affect patient's response to nursing and medical care?	
	Are there any variations between patient's interethnic and interracial communication process or intracultural and intraracial communication process [e.g., ethnic minority patient and White middle-class nurse, ethnic minority patient and ethnic minority nurse; beliefs, attitudes, values, role variations, stereotyping (perceptions and prejudice)]?	

Continued.

APPENDIX 6-1

Bloch's Ethnic/Cultural Assessment Guide—cont'd

Categories	Guideline questions/instructions	Data collected
Healing beliefs and practices Cultural healing system	What cultural healing system does the patient predominantly adhere to (e.g., Asian healing system, Raza/Latina Curanderismo)? What religious healing system does the patient predominantly adhere to (e.g., Seventh Day Adventist, West African voodoo, Fundamentalist sect, Pentacostal)?	
Cultural health beliefs	Is illness explained by the germ theory or cause-effect relationship, presence of evil spirits, imbalance between "hot" and "cold" (yin and yang in Chinese culture), or disequilibrium between nature and man?	
	Is good health related to success, ability to work or fulfill roles, reward from God, or balance with nature?	
Cultural health practices	What types of cultural healing practices does person from ethnic/cultural group adhere to? Does he use healing remedies to cure *natural* illnesses caused by the external environment [e.g., massage to cure *empacho* (a ball of food clinging to stomach wall), wearing of talismans or charms for protection against illness]?	
Cultural healers	Does patient rely on cultural healers [e.g., medicine men for American Indian, Curandero for Raza/Latina, Chinese herbalist, hougan (voodoo priest), spiritualist, or minister for Black American]?	
Nutritional variables or factors	What nutritional variables or factors are influenced by the patient's ethnic/cultural background?	
Characteristics of food preparation and consumption	What types of food preferences and restrictions, meaning of foods, style of food preparation and consumption, frequency of eating, time of eating, and eating utensils are culturally determined for patient? Are there any religious influences on food preparation and consumption?	
Influences from external environment	What modifications if any did the ethnic group patient identifies with have to make in its food practices in White dominant American society? Are there any adaptations of food customs and beliefs from rural setting to urban setting?	
Patient education needs	What are some implications of diet planning and teaching to patient who adheres to cultural practices concerning foods?	
Sociological		
Economic status	Who is principal wage earner in patient's family? What is total annual income (approximately) of family? What impact does economic status have on life-style, place of residence, living conditions, and ability to obtain health services?	
Educational status	What is highest educational level obtained? Does patient's educational background influence his ability to understand how to seek health services, literature on health care, patient teaching experiences, and any written material patient is exposed to in health care setting (e.g., admission forms, patient care forms, teaching literature, and lab test forms)?	
	Does patient's educational background cause him to feel inferior or superior to health care personnel in health care setting?	
Social network	What is patient's social network (kinship, peer, and cultural healing networks)? How do they influence health or illness status of patient?	

APPENDIX 6-1

Bloch's Ethnic/Cultural Assessment Guide—cont'd

Categories	Guideline questions/instructions	Data collected
Family as supportive group	Does patient's family feel need for continuous presence in patient's clinical setting (is this an ethnic/cultural characteristic)? How is family valued during illness or death?	
	How does family participate in patient's nursing care process (e.g., giving baths, feeding, using touch as support [cultural meaning], supportive presence)?	
	How does ethnic/cultural family structure influence patient response to health or illness (e.g., roles, beliefs, strengths, weaknesses, and social class)?	
	Are there any key family roles characteristic of a specific ethnic/cultural group (e.g., grandmother in Black and some American Indian families), and can these key persons be a resource for health personnel?	
	What role does family play in health promotion or cause of illness (e.g., would family be intermediary group in patient interactions with health personnel and making decisions regarding his care)?	
Supportive institutions in ethnic/cultural community	What influence do ethnic/cultural institutions have on patient receiving health services (i.e., institutions such as Organization of Migrant Workers, NAACP, Black Political Caucus, churches, schools, Urban League, community clinics)?	
Institutional racism	How does institutional racism in health facilities influence patient's response to receiving health care?	
Psychological		
Self-concept (identity)	Does patient show strong racial/cultural identity? How does this compare to that of other racial/cultural groups or to members of dominant society?	
	What factors in patient's development helped to shape his self-concept (e.g., family, peers, society labels, external environment, institutions, racism)?	
	How does patient deal with stereotypical behavior from health professionals?	
	What is impact of racism on patient from distinct ethnic/cultural group (e.g., social anxiety, noncompliance to health care process in clinical settings, avoidance of utilizing or participating in health care institutions)?	
	Does ethnic/cultural background have impact on how patient relates to body image change resulting from illness or surgery (e.g., importance to appearance and roles in cultural group)?	
	Any adherence or identification with ethnic/cultural "group" identity? (e.g., solidarity, "we" concept)?	
Mental and behavioral processes and characteristics of ethnic/cultural group	How does patient relate to his external environment in clinical setting (e.g., fears, stress, and adaptive mechanisms characteristic of a specific ethnic/cultural group)? Any variations based on the life span? What is patient's ability to relate to persons outside of his ethnic/cultural group (health personnel)? Is he withdrawn, verbally or nonverbally expressive, negative or positive, feeling mentally or physically inferior or superior?	
	How does patient deal with feelings of loss of dignity and respect in clinical setting?	

Continued.

APPENDIX 6-1

Bloch's Ethnic/Cultural Assessment Guide—cont'd

Categories	Guideline questions/instructions	Data collected
Religious influences on psychological effects of health/illness	Does patient's religion have a strong impact on how he relates to health/illness influences or outcomes (e.g., death/chronic illness, cause and effect of illness, or adherence to nursing/medical practices)?	
	Do religious beliefs, sacred practices, and talismans play a role in treatment of disease?	
	What is role of significant religious persons during health/illness (e.g., Black ministers, Catholic priests, Buddhist monks, Islamic imams)?	
Psychological/cultural reponse to stress and discomfort of illness	Based on ethnic/cultural background, does patient exhibit any variations in psychological response to pain or physical disability of disease processes?	
Biological/Physiological		
(Consideration of *norms* for different ethnic/cultural groups)		
Racial-anatomical characteristics	Does patient have any distinct racial characteristics (e.g., skin color, hair texture and color, color of mucous membranes)?	
	Does patient have any variations in anatomical characteristics (e.g., body structure [height and weight] more prevalent for ethnic/cultural group, skeletal formation [pelvic shape, especially for obstetrical evaluation], facial shape and structure [nose, eye shape, facial contour], upper and lower extremities)?	
	How do patient's racial and anatomical characteristics affect his self-concept and the way others relate to him?	
	Does variation in racial-anatomical characteristics affect physical evaluations and physical care, skin assessment based on color, and variations in hair care and hygienic practices?	
Growth and development patterns	Are there any distinct growth and development characteristics that vary with patient's ethnic/cultural background (e.g., bone, density, fatfolds, motor ability)?	
	What factors are important for nutritional assessment, neurological and motor assessment, assessment of bone deterioration in disease process or injury, evaluation of newborns, evaluation of intellectual status, or capacity in relationship to motor/sensory development in children?	
	How do these differ in ethnic/cultural groups?	
Variations in body systems	Are there any variations in body systems for patient from distinct ethnic/cultural group (e.g., gastrointestinal disturbance with lactose intolerance in Blacks, nutritional intake of cultural foods causing adverse effects on gastrointestinal tract and fluid and electrolyte system, and variations in chemical and hematological systems [certain blood types prevalent in particular ethnic/cultural groups])?	
Skin and hair physiology, mucous membranes	How does skin color variation influence assessment of skin color changes (e.g., jaundice, cyanosis, ecchymosis, erythema, and its relationship to disease processes)?	
	What are methods of assessing skin color changes (comparing variations and similarities between different ethnic groups)?	

APPENDIX 6-1

Bloch's Ethnic/Cultural Assessment Guide—cont'd

Categories	Guideline questions/instructions	Data collected
	Are there conditions of hypopigmentation and hyperpigmentation (e.g., vitiligo, mongolian spots, albinism, discoloration caused by trauma)? Why would these be more striking in some ethnic groups?	
	Are there any skin conditions more prevalent in a distinct ethnic group (e.g., keloids in Blacks)?	
	Is there any correlation between oral and skin pigmentation and their variations among distinct racial groups when doing assessment of oral cavity (e.g., leukoedema is normal occurrence in Blacks)?	
	What are variations in hair texture and color among racially different groups? Ask patient about preferred hair care methods or any racial/cultural restrictions (e.g., not washing "hot-combed" hair while in clinical setting, not cutting very long hair of Raza/Latina patients).	
	Are there any variations in skin care methods (e.g., using Vaseline on Black skin)?	
Diseases more prevalent among ethnic/cultural group	Are there any specific diseases or conditions that are more prevalent for a specific ethnic/cultural group (e.g., hypertension, sickle cell anemia, G6-PD, lactose intolerance)?	
	Does patient have any socioenvironmental diseases common among ethnic/cultural groups [e.g., lead paint poisoning, poor nutrition, overcrowding (prone to tuberculosis), alcoholism resulting from psychological despair and alienation from dominant society, rat bites, poor sanitation]?	
Diseases ethnic/cultural group has increased resistance to	Are there any diseases that patient has increased resistance to because of racial/cultural background (e.g., skin cancer in Blacks)?	

From Bloch B: Bloch's assessment guide for ethnic/cultural variations. In Orgue MS, Bloch B, and Monrroy LSA, editors: Ethnic nursing care: a multicultural approach, St Louis, 1983, CV Mosby Co, pp 63-69.

APPENDIX 6-2
Family Assessment Guide

Family name _____ Family ID no. _____

Source of referral _____

Reason for referral _____

Occupational status _____

Health insurance _____

Medical emergency plan _____

Preventive health care _____

Family composition: Map family constellation; include health problems of individual members.

Date		Assessment parameters	Rating		Significant data
1st	*2d*		*1st*	*2d*	
		1. *Structural characteristics*			
		a. Financial resources			
		b. Educational experiences			
		c. Allocation of family and personal roles			
		d. Division of labor			
		e. Distribution of power and authority			
		f. Cultural influences			
		(1) Health beliefs and attitudes			
		(2) Family goals			
		(3) Norms for social behavior			
		(4) Spiritual beliefs			
		(5) Beliefs about folk diseases and medicine			
		g. Activities of daily living			
		(1) Dietary habits			
		(2) Child-rearing practices			
		(3) Housekeeping			
		(4) Sleeping arrangements			
		(5) Laundry facilities			
		(6) Transportation			
		(7) Care of ill family members			
		(8) Knowledge of health problems			
		(9) Understanding of health promotion practices			

Date		Assessment parameters	Rating		Significant data
1st	2d		1st	2d	
		2. *Process characteristics*			
		a. Atmosphere of home			
		b. Communication patterns			
		c. Decision-making processes			
		(1) How decisions made			
		(2) How decisions implemented			
		d. Conflict negotiation			
		e. Achievement of developmental tasks			
		f. Adaptation to change			
		g. Autonomy of individual family members			
		3. *Relationships with external systems*			
		a. How family boundaries established			
		b. Utilization of information from environment			
		c. Contact with extended families			
		d. Interactions with friends and neighbors			
		e. Attitudes about community systems			
		(1) Health			
		(2) Welfare			
		(3) Educational			
		(4) Others (describe)			
		f. Use of the referral process			
		(1) Ability to seek assistance			
		(2) Level of independence			
		4. *Environmental characteristics*			
		a. Neighborhood			
		(1) Accessibility of facilities to meet basic needs			
		(2) Availability of recreational, educational, religious, and other resources			
		(3) Safety (physical and psychosocial)			
		b. Housing			
		(1) Suitability in relation to family needs			
		(2) Condition of structural components			
		(3) Suitability of home furnishings			
		(4) Sanitation (water source and sewage and garbage disposal and housekeeping practices)			

Continued.

APPENDIX 6-2

Family Assessment Guide—cont'd

Date		Assessment parameters	Rating		Significant data
1st	*2d*		*1st*	*2d*	
		(5) Accident hazards			
		(6) Barriers to family mobility			

Professionals and volunteers working with family (identify person and agency)

Summary of family strengths (based on categories rated No. 1)

Description of family priorities and assistance desired

Specific factors to consider when developing and implementing a management plan

Assessor _____ Date_____
Assessor _____ Date_____
Assessor _____ Date_____

NOTE: Code for recording assessment data—use a different-color ink for the first and second assessment or rating (generally it takes several home visits to complete a family assessment). Rating scale: 1 = strength; 2 = problem; 3 = anticipatory guidance warranted; 4 = problem—family does not wish to change this area of functioning at this time; 5 = not applicable. Family functioning should be rated every 4 months to assist in evaluating family progress and nursing intervention strategies.

REFERENCES

Ackerman NW, ed: The psychodynamics of family life: diagnosis and treatment of family relationships, New York, 1959, Basic Books.

Ackerman, NW, ed: Family process, New York, 1970, Basic Books.

Ahrons CR: The binuclear family: two households, one family, Alternative Lifestyles 2:449-515, 1979.

Aldous J: Family careers: developmental change in families, New York, 1978, Wiley.

Baca JE: Some health beliefs of the Spanish speaking. In Reinhardt A and Quinn M, eds: Family-centered community nursing: a sociocultural framework, St Louis, 1973, CV Mosby Co.

Bane MJ: Here to stay—American families in the twentieth century, New York, 1976, Basic Books.

Barnard KE: MCN keys to research: the family as a unit of measurement, MCN 9:21, 1984.

Barnard KE: Difficult life circumstances (DLC). In Krentz LG, ed: Nursing and the promotion/protection of family health: workshop proceedings, Portland, Or, September 1988, Oregon Health Sciences University.

Beall S, and Schmidt G: Development of a youth adaptation rating scale, School Health 54:197-200, American School Health Association, Kent, Oh, © 1984.

Beavers WR: Psychotherapy and growth: a family systems perspective, New York, 1977, Brunner/Mazel.

Bengtson UL and Dannefer D: Families, work, and aging: implications of disordered cohort flow for the twenty-first century. In Ward RA and Tobin SS, eds: Health in aging: sociological issues and policy directions, New York, 1987, Springer.

Berardo FM: Decade preview: some trends and directions for family research and theory in the 1980s, J Marriage Family 42:723-728, 1980.

Bernard J: The adjustments of married mates. In Christensen HT, ed: Handbook of marriage and the family, Chicago, 1964, Rand McNally, pp 675-739.

Bloch B: Bloch's assessment guide for ethnic/cultural variations. In Orgue MS, Bloch B, and Monrroy LSA, eds: Ethnic nursing care: a multicultural approach, St Louis, 1983, CV Mosby Co, pp 49-75.

Bowen M: Toward the differentiation of a self in one's own family. In Framo JL, ed: Family interaction: a dialogue between family researchers and family therapists, New York, 1973, Springer.

Bredemeir HC and Stephenson RN: The analysis of social systems, New York, 1965, Holt.

Briar S: The family as an organization: an approach to family diagnosis and treatment, Soc Service Rev 38:247-255, 1964.

Broderick CB: Beyond the five conceptual frameworks: a decade of development in family theory, J Marriage Family 33:139-159, 1971.

Brownlee AT: Community, culture and care: a cross-cultural guide for health workers, St Louis, 1978, CV Mosby Co.

Burr WR and Leigh GK: Famology: a new discipline, J Marriage Family 45:467-480, 1983.

Castles MR: Game theory as a conceptual framework for nursing practice. In Hymovich DP and Barnard MU, eds: Family health care, New York, 1973, McGraw-Hill.

Christensen HT, ed: Handbook of marriage and the family, Chicago, 1964, Rand McNally.

Churchman CW: The systems approach, New York, 1968, Dell.

Clemen SJ: Introduction to health care facility: food service administration, University Park, Pa, 1974, Pennsylvania State University Press.

Duvall EM and Miller BC: Marriage and family development, ed 6, New York, 1985, Harper & Row.

Eshleman JR and Clarke JN: Intimacy, commitments, and marriage: development of relationships, Boston, 1978, Allyn and Bacon.

Feetham SL: Family research: issues and directions for nursing. In Werley HH and Fitzpatrick JJ, eds: Annual review of nursing research, vol 1, New York, 1984, Springer, pp 3-25.

Flanzraich M and Dunsavage I: Role reversal in abused/neglected families, Children Today 6:13-15, 1977.

Gilliss CL: The family as a unit of analysis: strategies for the nurse researcher, Adv Nurs Sci 5(3):50-59, 1983.

Gordon M: Manual of nursing diagnosis 1988-1989, St Louis, 1989, CV Mosby Co.

Hacker S: The primary task of the health professional in dealing with adolescent sexuality, Int J Adolescent Med Health 1(1,2):73-80, 1985.

Haley J, ed: Changing families, New York, 1971, Grune & Stratton.

Hanson SM: Family nursing: past, present and future. In Krentz LG, ed: Nursing of families in transition, Portland, Or, 1987, Oregon Health Sciences University.

Hartman A: Diagrammatic assessment of family relationships, Soc Casework 59:465-476, 1978.

Hill R and Hansen DA: The identification of conceptual frameworks utilized in family study, Marriage Family Living 22:299-311, 1960.

Holman TB and Burr WR: Beyond the beyond; the growth of family theories in the 1970s, J Marriage Family 42:729-741, 1980.

Jackson DD, ed: Communication, family and marriage, vol 1, Palo Alto, Ca, 1968, Science and Behavior Books.

Kensky AD: Cultural influences on the Jewish patient. In Clemen SA and Will M, eds: Family and community health nursing: a workbook, Ann Arbor, 1977, University of Michigan Press.

Krentz LG: Nursing of families and the health care delivery system: workshop proceedings, Portland, Or, 1989, Oregon Health Sciences University.

Lewis J, Beavers R, Gossett JT, and Phillips VA: No single thread: psychological health in family systems, New York, 1976, Brunner/Mazel.

Linton R: The natural history of the family. In Anshen RN, ed: The family: its function and destiny, revised ed, New York, 1959, Harper & Row.

Litman TJ: The family as a basic unit in health and medical care: a social-behavioral overview, Soc Sci Med 8:495-519, 1974.

Minuchin S: Families and family therapy, Cambridge, Ma, 1974, Harvard University Press.

Murphy S: Family study and nursing research, Image: J Nurs Scholar 18(4):170-174, 1986.

Nickols SY and Nickols SA: Family: its worth, diversity, persistence. In College of Home Economics, ed: Families of the future: continuity and change, Ames, Ia, 1983, Iowa State University Press.

Norbeck J: Modification of life event questionnaires for use with female respondents, Res Nurs Health 7:61-71, 1984.

Nye FI: Role structure and analysis of the family, Beverly Hills, 1976, Sage.

Orgue MS, Bloch B, and Monrroy LSA: Ethnic nursing care: a multicultural approach, St Louis, 1983, CV Mosby Co.

Otto H: Criteria for assessing family strengths, Family Process 2:329-338, 1963.

Peterson R: What are the needs of the chronic mental patients? Presented at the APA Conference on the Chronic Mental Patient, Washington, DC, January 1978.

Pratt L: Family structure and effective health behavior: the energized family, Boston, 1976, Houghton Mifflin.

Prattes O: Beliefs of the Mexican-American family. In

Hymovich D and Barnard M, eds: Family health care, New York, 1973, McGraw-Hill.

Rahe RH: Subjects' recent life changes and their near-future illness reports, Ann Clin Res 4:250-265, 1972.

Samora J: Conceptions of health and disease among Spanish-Americans. In Martinez RH, ed: Hispanic culture and health care: fact, fiction, folklore, St Louis, 1978, CV Mosby Co.

Satir V: Conjoint family therapy: a guide to theory and technique, Palo Alto, Ca, 1967, Science and Behavior Books.

Satir V: Peoplemaking, Palo Alto, Ca, 1972, Science and Behavior Books.

Satir V: You as a change agent in helping families to change. In Satir V, Stachowiak J, and Taskman H, eds: Helping families to change, New York, 1975, Jason Aronson.

Schor E, Starfield B, Stidley C, and Hankin J: Family health: utilization and effects of family membership, Med Care 25(7):616-625, 1987.

Spanier GB: Bequeathing family continuity, J Marriage Family 51(2):3-13, 1989.

Stryker SL: The interactional and situational approaches. In Christensen HT, ed: Handbook of marriage and the family, Chicago, 1964, Rand McNally, pp 125-170.

Sussman MB, chairperson: Changing families in a changing society, 1970 White House Conference on Children, Forum 14 report, Washington DC, 1971, US Government Printing Office.

Thornton A and Freedman D: The changing American family, Population Bull 38(4), Washington DC, 1983, Population Reference Bureau.

Tripp-Reimer T, Brink PJ, and Saunders JM: Cultural assessment: content and process, Nurs Outlook 32:78-82, 1984.

US Bureau of the Census: Population profile of the United States: 1989, Current population reports, Series P-23, No. 159, Washington, DC, 1989, US Government Printing Office.

von Bertalanffy L: General systems theory, New York, 1968, George Braziller.

Watzlawick P, Beavin JH, and Jackson DD: Pragmatics of human communication: a study of interactional patterns, pathologies, and paradoxes, New York, 1967, Norton.

White House Conference on Families, 1978, Joint hearings before the Subcommittee on Child and Human Development of the Committee on Human Resources, US Senate and the Subcommittee on Select Education of the Committee on Education and

Labor, House of Representatives, Ninety-fifth Congress, Washington, DC, 1978, US Government Printing Office.

Wiener N: Cybernetics in history. In Buckley W, ed: Modern systems research for the behavioral scientist, Chicago, 1968, Aldine.

Yogman M and Brazelton TB: In support of families, Cambridge, Ma, 1986, Harvard University Press.

SELECTED BIBLIOGRAPHY

Burr WR, Hill R, Nye FI, and Reiss IL, eds: Contemporary theories about the family, vol 2, General theories/theoretical orientations, New York, 1979, Free Press.

Burr WR, Hill R, Nye FI, and Reiss IL, eds: Contemporary theories about the family, vol 1, Research-based theories, New York, 1979, Free Press.

Clements IW and Roberts FB: Family health: a theoretical approach to nursing care, New York, 1983, Wiley.

Frederick RF and Herrick J: Family rules: family life styles, Am J Orthopsychiatry 44:61-69, 1974.

Friedman MM: Family nursing: theory and assessment, New York, 1981, Appleton-Century-Crofts.

Galvin KM and Brommel BJ: Family communication: cohesion and change, Glenview, Il, 1982, Scott, Foresman.

Gilliss CL, Highley BL, Roberts BM, and Martinson IM: Toward a science of family nursing, Menlo Park, Ca, 1989, Addison-Wesley.

Glick PC: How American families are changing, Am Demographics 6:20-27, 1984.

Handel G, ed: The psycho-social interior of the family, Chicago, 1967, Aldine-Atherton.

Hareven TR, ed: Transitions: the family and the life course in historical perspective, New York, 1978, Academic Press.

Hill RA: The strengths of black families, New York, 1972, Emerson Hall.

Macklin ED: Nontraditional family forms: a decade of research, J Marriage Family 42:905-922, 1980.

Martin M and Henry M: Cultural relativity and poverty, Public Health Nurs 6(1):28-34, 1989.

Nye FI: Fifty years of family research, 1937-1987, J Marriage Family 50:305-316, 1988.

Petze CF: Health promotion for the well family, Nurs Clin North Am 19(2):229-237, 1984.

Speer JJ and Sachs B: Selecting the appropriate family assessment tool, Pediatr Nurs 11:349-355, 1985.

Whall AL: The family as the unit of care in nursing: a historical review, Public Health Nurs 3:240-249, 1986.

Whall AL: Family therapy theory for nursing: four approaches, Norwalk, Ct, 1987, Appleton-Century-Crofts.

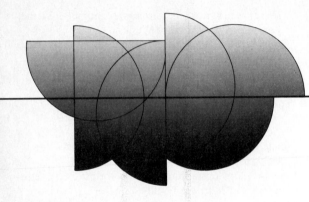

7

Foundations for Family Intervention: Families under Stress

Accept me as I am so I may learn what I can become.

―――――――――――――――― OBJECTIVES ――――――――――――――――

Upon completion of this chapter, the reader will be able to:

1. *Discuss the concepts of stress and crisis as they relate to family functioning.*
2. *Describe factors that affect the outcome of a family crisis.*
3. *Identify characteristics that signal ineffective individual or family coping during periods of stress and crisis.*
4. *Differentiate between developmental and situational crises and give examples of each type of crisis.*

5. *Describe general principles that the community health nurse should apply when giving constructive assistance to families in crisis.*
6. *Explain nursing intervention strategies used by community health nurses to promote effective family functioning during periods of stress and crisis.*

A major preventive responsibility of the community health nurse is to help individuals and families handle stressful life events so that their energies can be used to achieve self-fulfillment and to develop a capacity to extend themselves to others. Some stress is normal and essential for life and growth. Stress provides the stimulus needed to adapt to the everchanging conditions of life. Too much stress, however, prevents people from seeing what "they can become."

Selye (1975, p. xv), has found that any emotion or activity, whether it produces joy or sadness, causes stress. He believes that stressful life events (refer to Table 6-3) will more likely result in disease and unhappiness when individuals and families are not prepared to deal with them. Persons who are not prepared to handle the pressures and experiences encountered throughout life often do not recognize signals of distress that reflect a need to mobilize different coping mechanisms.

Community health nurses are in a key position to help individuals and families adapt to new or threatening life changes. In their work in the home and other settings, they encounter clients who are experiencing various degrees of stress. Many times these clients have not had life experiences or exposure to knowledge that would assist them in altering patterns of functioning that intensify stress. Most parents, for instance, have not been prepared to handle children whose growth and development significantly deviate from normal patterns of functioning. Hence, they experience heightened distress and are frequently open to professional intervention. Illustrative of this is the situation encountered by a community health nurse when she visited the Slavovi family for the first time:

The Slavovi family was referred to the community health nurse for health supervision follow-up after the birth of their fourth child, Stephanie, who had multiple handicaps. Even though this was the family's first exposure to community health nursing service, Mr. and Mrs. Slavovi talked freely when the nurse visited. Both manifested high levels of anxiety and confusion about how to care for their newborn infant. Angel and Maria Slavovi had always taken great pride in being good parents. Stephanie's physical and mental handicaps were

particularly distressing to them: "We don't know how to help her. She continues to cry even when we hold her and seems to hurt all the time. Children need loving. Why doesn't Stephanie want us to hold her? We must be doing something wrong."

Having an understanding of the concept of stress helps the community health nurse to intervene more effectively with clients like the Slavovis. Stress theory provides the foundation for identifying signs and symptoms of distress and for recognizing potential stressors. It also provides clues about how to bring about change when a client's usual methods of coping are no longer effective.

For at least 50 years, the concept of stress has been discussed in the literature (Knapp, 1988). Several authors have written extensively about this concept, including Cannon (1929, 1935); Cassel (1974, Psychiatric; 1974, Psychosocial); Figley and McCubbin (1983); Hill (1949); Lazarus (1966, 1981); Lazarus and Folkman (1984); McCubbin, Cauble, and Patterson (1982); McCubbin and Figley (1983); and Selye (1975, 1976). Since only a very brief overview of the concept of stress will be presented in this text, the reader may wish to refer to the writings of the above authors for further study.

THE STRESS PHENOMENON

Selye (1975, p. 1) has defined stress "as the non-specific response of the body to any demand." It is a dynamic state triggered by stressors which help to maintain an internal balance within human systems. Stressors are "anything which produce stress" (Selye, 1975, p. 78).

Stress theory is based on the concepts of homeostasis (state of physiologic balance) and adaptation. Because stress is an inherent and integral part of life, individuals and families must constantly readjust to maintain themselves. One's state of balance is maintained when one learns to recognize the signals of distress and then adapts or changes functioning to meet the demands of the stress encountered. *Distress,* as defined by Selye, "is unpleasant or disease-producing stress" (Selye, p. 465). In contrast, "eustress is seen as good,

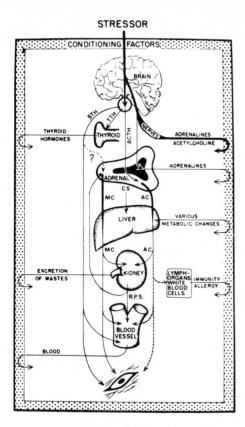

Figure 7-1 Physiological responses to stress. (Selye H: The stress of life, New York, 1976, McGraw-Hill, p 15.)

pleasant, or curative stress" (Selye, 1975, p. 466).

Physiological responses (Figure 7-1) in the nervous and endocrine systems alert individuals to the occurrence of distress or eustress. These responses produce feelings such as joy, fatigue, or uneasiness. They help individuals to identify that their steady state is being threatened.

The physiological changes that occur in response to stress are nonspecific. They produce changes that affect a person's entire body and that happen any time an individual is experiencing stress, no matter what the cause. According to Selye (1975, p. 163), the nonspecific responses to stress evolve in three stages, which he has labeled the *general adaptation syndrome* (GAS):

1. The *alarm reaction,* during which defense mechanisms are mobilized
2. The *stage of resistance,* when adaptation is

acquired because optimum channels of defense were developed
3. The *stage of exhaustion,* which reflects a depletion of adaptation energy necessary to cope with prolonged and intensified stress

Although stress is essential for life and growth, every individual has limits beyond which stress is no longer healthy. When these limits are reached, exhaustion occurs and energies needed to deal with activities of daily living become depleted. All individuals have the capacity to deal with distress; however, they need to learn the limits of stress they can tolerate and adaptive mechanisms that will help them to maintain homeostasis and to promote growth.

Our bodies provide numerous physiological and psychological signals that reflect disruption of homeostasis. Examples of these signals are presented in the box on p. 232.

In terms of the family, stress is manifested by dysfunctional family patterns, as well as by the occurrence of the above signs and symptoms in its individual family members. Child abuse and neglect, domestic violence, strained communication patterns and decision-making conflicts are a few such dysfunctional patterns that may result when a family is under stress. Others are shared in Table 6-2.

Individuals and families who learn that the above signs and symptoms result when they are experiencing stress beyond tolerable limits may be able to mobilize or adjust their coping mechanisms in a way that increases their resistance to stress. Persons who ignore signals of distress or who do not initiate appropriate defense mechanisms experience crisis.

THE CRISIS PHENOMENON

Crisis, like stress, is an elusive concept which can be identified only by recognizing the manifestations or characteristic signs and symptoms of the crisis state. That is why it is so important for nurses to have a firm understanding of the crisis sequence. Concepts of crisis help the practitioner to quickly recognize clients who need to adjust their coping mechanisms. It is especially critical

---

Examples of Physiological and Psychological Signals of Stress

PHYSIOLOGICAL SIGNALS

Pounding of the heart

Dryness of the throat and mouth

Sweating

Frequent need to urinate

Diarrhea, indigestion, vomiting

Migraine headaches

Missed menstrual period

Loss of or excessive appetite

Increased smoking and alcohol and drug use

Increased use of legally prescribed drugs (e.g., tranquilizers or amphetamines)

Pain in neck or lower back

PSYCHOLOGICAL SIGNALS

General irritability, hyperexcitation or depression

Impulsive behavior, emotional instability

Overpowering urge to cry or run and hide

Inability to concentrate, flight of thoughts, and general disorientation

Floating anxiety

Trembling, nervous tics

Nightmares

Neurotic or psychotic behavior

Accident proneness

From Selye H: Stress in health and disease, Boston, 1976, Butterworths, pp 174-177.

---

for community health nurses to be well grounded in crisis theory, because they frequently encounter clients, such as the Slavovi family, in the home environment who are dealing with new, different, or threatening stressful events. Early identification of those clients who are having difficulty coping with these events could prevent an intensified crisis state.

A preventive health philosophy stimulated the development of crisis theory and intervention.

Erich Lindemann (1944), through his classic study of grief reactions, identified the need for *preventive counseling* with clients experiencing loss through death or separation. After investigating the responses of clients who had lost a relative in the famous Coconut Grove fire in Boston, he concluded that appropriate psychiatric intervention with clients who were experiencing grief could prevent prolonged and serious social maladjustment (Lindemann, 1944, p. 147). He further concluded, after observing clients who experienced an "anticipatory grief reaction," that prophylactic counseling could prevent family crisis (Lindemann, 1944, p. 148). Anticipatory grief reactions occur when there is a threat of death, such as when soldiers engage in war activities. Clients in these situations go through all the stages of grief. It has been found in some cases that wives of soldiers in the war handled the grief process so effectively that they emancipated themselves from their spouse. This precipitated a crisis if husbands returned from the war, because their wives needed to reestablish marital relationships before they could express feelings of love and caring. Husbands in these situations felt that their wives no longer loved them and frequently asked for a divorce (Lindemann, 1944, pp. 147-148).

Crisis reactions, such as those described by Lindemann, can be predicted and often prevented. Lindemann, Caplan, and other crisis theorists have delineated a sequence of events that occur when a client is experiencing a crisis, as well as factors that intensify the crisis state. In addition, these theorists have identified situations that frequently precipitate a crisis during the developmental life cycle of a family. They also discovered therapeutic processes that have a positive influence on client functioning when the family is experiencing a crisis.

The Crisis Sequence

Gerald Caplan (1961, p. 18), the father of preventive psychiatry, describes *crisis* as a state "provoked when a person faces an obstacle to important life goals that is, for a time, insurmountable through the utilization of customary methods of problem solving. A period of disorganization ensues, a period of upset, during which many different abortive attempts at solution are made. Eventually some kind of adaptation is achieved, which may or may not be in the best interests of that person and his fellows."

When describing the normal sequence of events that occur during a crisis, Caplan (1964, pp. 40-41) identifies four characteristic phases:

1. An initial phase when an individual's tension rises as he or she uses habitual problem-solving responses to achieve emotional homeostasis.
2. A second stage in which tension increases and the individual becomes ineffective and upset because normal coping mechanisms were not effective in resolving the state of crisis.
3. A third threshold when tension mounts and stimulates the mobilization of new and emergency problem-solving mechanisms. The problem may be resolved if an individual can redefine the situation in order to cope with it and can adjust to role changes that have occurred.
4. A final phase when tension mounts beyond the limits an individual can tolerate; major disorganization results.

Inherent in Caplan's description of a crisis are several key ideas: (1) change which threatens an individual's ability to meet life goals disrupts the individual's homeostasis; (2) crisis results when an individual's customary methods of adaptation are ineffective in handling change; (3) disorganization occurs during the crisis state; (4) crisis is self-limiting, with a subsequent reduction of emotional tension (adaptation); (5) biopsychosocial homeostasis following a crisis may be at a level the same as, better than, or worse than the precrisis level. The goal of crisis intervention is to help the client to maintain a level of functioning equal to or better than the precrisis level.

It is not uncommon for community health nurses to work with families who have been unable to return successfully to their precrisis level of functioning after experiencing a crisis. When first encountered by the community health nurse, these families often present multiple difficulties, ineffective problem-solving methods, and feelings of helplessness and hopelessness.

Community health nurses also encounter families who not only return to precrisis levels of functioning but, in addition, *experience growth during crisis situations.* Many families develop new methods of coping which provide alternative ways for handling future stresses. Many also develop a cohesive family unity which increases the supportive and nurturing aspects of their family life-style and which encourages risk taking. Risk taking may expose individuals and families to other growth-producing opportunities.

There are several factors that affect how well a family handles stress and deals with crises (Choi, Josten, and Christensen, 1983). Community health nurses who understand these variables are better able to help families achieve successful resolution and growth during a crisis state.

Factors Affecting the Outcome of a Crisis

Aquilera (1989, p. 65) contends that there are three balancing factors that relate to the precipitation and successful resolution of a crisis. These are *perception of the event, available support systems,* and *adequate coping mechanisms.* Figure 7-2 presents the paradigm developed by Aquilera (1989, p. 66) to study the influence of these balancing factors during times of stress. It illustrates that clients must achieve a realistic perception of the event, develop adequate situational supports, and mobilize coping mechanisms to achieve successful adaptation during periods of disequilibrium.

Aquilera's paradigm provides a logical and useful model for analyzing a client's ability to adjust when experiencing stress. The paradigm provides a framework for identifying significant parameters to assess when working with individuals and families who have encountered threatening life events. A data base relative to each of Aquilera's balancing factors should be obtained when working with such persons. In her text, *Crisis Intervention: Theory and Methodology,* Aquilera has shared several case situations which illustrate the

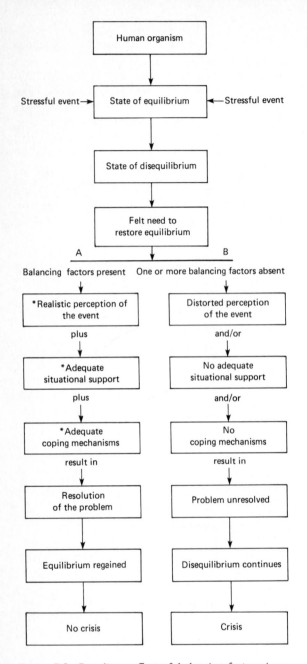

Figure 7-2 Paradigm: effect of balancing factors in a stressful event; * = balancing factors. (Aquilera DC: Crisis intervention; theory and methodology, ed 6, St Louis, 1989, CV Mosby Co, p 66.)

significant influence these balancing factors have during times of stress.

Perception of the Event

Crisis is the emotional reaction that occurs in relation to a new, different, or threatening event, not the event itself. Basically, the extent of this emotional reaction is determined by how the client (individual, family, population group) defines his or her particular circumstances (Aquilera, 1989; Burr, 1973; Caplan, 1964; Hansen and Hill, 1964; Rahe, 1974).

A number of factors influence how a client perceives a hazardous situation. Specifically, the practitioner should analyze the following variables when working with clients who have intensified stress:

1. Number of stressors client is experiencing
2. Client's past experiences in handling current stressor(s)
3. Biopsychosocial status of the client prior to encountering hazardous event(s)
4. Duration of exposure to current stressor(s)
5. Magnitude or seriousness of current event(s)
6. Suddenness of the event(s)
7. Client's understanding of the stressor event(s)

Even though the responses of individuals and families to hazardous events are highly variable, there is evidence which supports the theory that distress increases when one encounters multiple stressors (Rahe, 1974), experiences the stressor or stressors for a prolonged length of time (Selye, 1975), is exposed to a stressor with little or no time for anticipating problem solving (Hansen and Hill, 1964), faces an event that is highly ambiguous (McHugh, 1968), or encounters a situation that presents hardship or has serious consequences, such as death (Hill, 1949). When distress heightens, clients are more likely to have a distorted view of the current stressor. They may experience such feelings as helplessness, hopelessness, anxiety, fatigue, or depression. It must be emphasized, however, that even when one or more of the above factors exist in stressful occurrences, the perceived meaning of occurrences varies from one individual to another. The above factors only place individuals more at risk for developing crisis.

Caplan (1964, pp. 42-43) has found that for a stressor to become problematic, "it must be perceived as a threat or loss to need satisfaction or as a challenge." He believes that two major variables, personality and sociocultural factors, significantly affect how one perceives life events. These variables determine the type of life experiences one has, prescribe the limits of acceptable behavior when dealing with stress, and influence how one feels about one's abilities to handle changes in life. Case situations can best illustrate how the variables of personality and sociocultural influences affect one's perception of an event.

Mrs. Farias was 34 years old and left with two sons, 8 and 10 years old, and one daughter, age 14, when her husband was killed in a car accident. The community health nurse had encountered the Farias family prior to Mr. Farias's death, because Carmelina, their 14-year-old daughter, needed orthopedic follow-up for a scoliosis problem discovered through health screening at her high school. During a home visit 8 months after Mr. Farias's death, the community health nurse became concerned about Mrs. Farias's physical and psychological health. She looked uncared for, her home was untidy, and she had no interest in talking about Carmelina's health problems. Weeping, Mrs. Farias shared with the nurse that "nothing was going right lately; the children don't obey, I can't get my husband's life insurance, and my friends haven't visited lately." She became particularly distressed when she talked about how she was going to feed her family in the future. "Our savings are almost gone. I can't get a job. What will I do? I have never worked, because Julio thought that a wife should stay at home. My folks thought that girls should marry and raise a family. I never was good at much except maybe cooking, housekeeping, and loving the kids. My family thinks it is wrong to take money from the welfare department. They say they will help me until I remarry, but I know they don't have anything extra. Besides, I am too old to remarry. Most men I know want their own children, not someone else's. You can't meet men when you are my age."

Another case situation illustrates different family reactions to the death of its male provider.

Mrs. Ulisses was a 33-year-old widow with two daughters, 2 and 6 years of age, and two sons, ages 8 and 11. Her husband was killed while hunting. The community health nurse started visiting Mrs. Ulisses after she brought her 2-year-old to the well-baby clinic, 6 weeks after her husband's death. At that time, she expressed a desire to obtain information about day-care centers. The nurse visited regularly for a year to help Mrs. Ulisses sort out what she would like to do in the future. She and her husband were never able to save much, so Mrs. Ulisses applied for financial assistance from the Department of Social Service. She did not like receiving Aid to Families of Dependent Children funds, but felt that she needed time to make child-care arrangements before she went back to work. Seven and a half months after her husband's death, Mrs. Ulisses enrolled in college. "I know I can find a job, because I have worked off and on since age 15. If I had some training, however, I would be more secure in the future. I am still not sure if I want to get married again, so I better prepare myself to care for my family."

Both Mrs. Farias and Mrs. Ulisses were facing similar situations. They experienced the loss of a significant other who had assumed the provider role in their family system when he was living. Mrs. Farias, however, was more threatened by her circumstances because past and current cultural influences affected her ability to be flexible when role changes were needed. In addition, Mrs. Farias lacked confidence (personality factor) in her abilities to succeed in work and social settings. Her life experiences were focused on preparing her for traditional female roles only.

Mrs. Ulisses, on the other hand, was discouraged at times, but was actively involved in planning for a future career. She was better prepared to assume the provider role, having worked off and on since her teenage years, and felt more confident about her abilities to succeed outside the home setting. Her life experiences provided her with a different perception of her female role.

Situational Supports

It has long been recognized that meaningful human relationships assist individuals to cope with the stresses of life (Cobb, 1976; Kaplan, Cassel, and Gore, 1977). It has been demonstrated that presence of social support can play a significant role in "modifying the deleterious health effects of stress, in influencing the use of health services, and in affecting other aspects of health behavior such as compliance with medical regimens" (Hamburg and Killilea, 1979, p. 256). A review of studies related to social support, stress, and health and illness outcomes by Hamburg and Killilea (1979, pp. 256-257), shows that social supports can:

1. Reduce the number of complications of pregnancy for women under high life stress (Nuckolls, Cassel, and Kaplan, 1972)
2. Help prevent posthospital psychological reactions in children after a tonsillectomy (Jessner, Blom, and Waldfogel, 1952)
3. Aid recovery from surgery (Egbert, Battib, Welch, and Bartlett, 1964)
4. Aid recovery from illness (Chambers and Reiser, 1953; Chen and Cobb, 1960; Mather, 1974)
5. Reduce the need for steroids in adult asthmatics in periods of stress (deAraujo, Van Arsdel, Holmes, and Dudley, 1973)
6. Protect against clinical depression in the face of adverse events (Brown, Bhrolchain, and Harris, 1975)
7. Reduce psychological distress and physiologic symptoms following job loss and bereavement (Burch, 1972; Cobb, 1974; Gore, 1973; Maddison and Walther, 1967; Parkes, Benjamin, and Fitzgerald, 1969)
8. Protect against the development of emotional problems which can be associated with aging (Blau, 1973; Lowenthal and Haven, 1968)
9. Reduce the physiologic symptomatology in those working in highly stressful job environments (Cobb, 1974; Cobb, Kasl, and French, 1969)
10. Help patients to continue needed medical treatment and promote adherence to needed medical regimens (Bakeland and Lundwall, 1975; Caplan, Robinson, French Jr., Caldwell, and Shinn, 1976; Haynes and Sackett, 1974).

Social supports can have a direct effect on health.

They provide a *buffer* against the effects of high stress and have a *mediating effect* which stimulates the development of coping strategies and promotes mastery. Lack of social supports can exacerbate the impact of stressful life events (Hamburg and Killilea, 1979, p. 257).

Since significant others (family, friends, relatives, professionals, and other supports) can increase or decrease an individual's vulnerability to crisis during times of stress, it is important to ascertain information about the *quality of the interactions* that clients have with others. It is also crucial to assess the *amount of contact* clients have with social supports. During periods of disequilibrium, persons need supportive relationships that allow them to verbalize feelings and encourage them to sort out the realities of their situation. Clients also need assistance with problem solving. In addition, concrete help is frequently needed to facilitate their ability to obtain resources, such as financial assistance, from their environment (refer to Chapter 9). Behaviors that support a client's distorted perception of the event are not helpful. A friend, for example, who reinforces a client's blaming behaviors inhibits client growth and successful resolution of a crisis; this type of behavior supports the client's current ineffective coping style, which in turn prevents the client from mobilizing more effective coping mechanisms.

When working with clients who are experiencing a crisis, it is extremely important to remember that their significant others may also be in crisis. Often the practitioner finds that others in a client's social network are experiencing as much or more distress than the client. Thus, they are unable to provide the assistance needed by the client to achieve healthy adaptation and may, in fact, be reinforcing maladaptive behaviors. Because of this, significant others are often included in the therapeutic process so that they do not inhibit a client's growth and so that they receive the help they themselves need to cope with the stressful changes being experienced.

Adequate Coping Mechanisms

The stress-crisis sequence evolves when an individual's usual coping mechanisms or ways of reducing stress are inadequate to deal with the threatening event(s) being encountered. If the client becomes immobilized, he or she will probably emerge from the crisis functioning at a level lower than the precrisis state. On the other hand, if the client is able to mobilize untapped, inner strengths or resources, positive outcomes may result; the client could resolve problem(s) and learn new ways of coping with stress in the future. The client could also experience growth.

During the crisis sequence, clients generally experience heightened anxiety, which often results in two types of behavior. First, the client will attempt, sometimes frantically, to use previously learned patterns of coping to alleviate discomfort. Clients usually cling to the familiar during a state of anxiety because it provides a sense of stability, even if real stability does not exist. Second, because a high level of anxiety is accompanied by feelings of helplessness and hopelessness, clients are frequently more amenable to outside influence and assistance. This is especially true during the period of disequilibrium. When reorganization and equilibrium begin to occur and new adaptive or maladaptive defense patterns evolve, this is less true. That is why crisis theorists stress the importance of high-quality therapeutic intervention during the time the person in crisis is establishing new coping mechanisms. Caplan (1964, p. 53) has found that intervention at this time can be the critical balancing factor in helping clients to achieve positive outcomes during crisis states.

The major task for an individual family that is experiencing a crisis is to recognize that customary coping mechanisms are ineffective and that new patterns for coping must be established. Some clients, particularly those who have adequate situational supports and who have been flexible in the past, are able to accomplish this task with little or no assistance. Other clients, especially those who have few or no situational supports, who rigidly define role patterns, and who lack maturity because of past experiences, will need help from others in developing new ways for handling stress. These persons are frequently unable to identify the nature of the stress they are

experiencing or why their patterns of functioning are ineffective.

It should be obvious at this point that the balancing forces in Aquilera's paradigm (Figure 7-2) are interrelated and must be viewed as a composite of forces rather than isolated elements. If this view is not taken, nursing interventions may be inappropriate to meet the needs of the client. Ms. Himes's case situation is a good example. She called the county health department and requested nursing service for her mother. Without emotion she stated that "someone needs to show me how to care for her. I don't know what to do any longer."

Sally Himes was a 50-year-old single woman. She lived with her 85-year-old mother, who had had a CVA 15 years ago which left her paralyzed and unable to speak. Before her father's death, Ms. Himes had promised him that she would always take care of her mother. When the community health nurse arrived at the Himes home, Sally immediately took her into the bedroom to see her mother, who appeared very comfortable in her current surroundings. Sally insisted, however, that the nurse check her over. "I am doing something that is not right. The doctor needs to visit more frequently to give mother shots for water in her lungs." The nurse examined Sally's mother carefully and, finding nothing seriously wrong, decided to spend the rest of the visit talking with Sally.

After the nurse provided positive reinforcement for how well Sally was caring for her mother, Sally replied, "The mailman came today." It took several probing questions like, "Was there something special about the mailman's visit?" before Sally identified that she had received an invitation to her niece's wedding. She was distressed because her mother had not also been invited. "They don't care about her anymore." Further interviewing revealed that for the past 2 years Sally had isolated herself from family and friends because she felt her mother's condition was deteriorating and that significant others were too busy. "I can't leave her. No one else knows what to do. Besides, my family has lots of other responsibilities. I always thought they cared about mother, but now I wonder. If they really cared, they would have invited her to Sue's wedding. Sometimes I really get discouraged. I wonder if my family and friends care about me."

The invitation Sally had received from her

family challenged her thought processes. It brought to a conscious level feelings of noncaring, which was fortunate because Sally had been coping with these feelings by withdrawing. She was no longer able to ask for assistance from her family and friends and increasingly limited most of her social contacts. With the help of the community health nurse, she was able to identify why she had become so upset when the invitation was delivered. She was also able to recognize that she needed to make changes in her situation so that her own needs could be met. One nursing intervention strategy, arranging a conference with the entire family, resulted in a plan in which all family members would share the responsibility for the care of Sally's mother. This would not have happened if the community health nurse had focused only on helping Sally to see that her perceptions about how well she was caring for her mother were distorted. Changes in Sally's situation would also not have occurred if emphasis had been placed on examining only Sally's feelings about who was invited to Sue's wedding. Helping Sally to recognize that she needed situational supports was critical to the successful resolution of her crisis.

When nurses work with clients who are experiencing heightened stress, they find that a *triggering event* (e.g., the invitation to Sue's wedding) stimulates the development of a crisis. This event produces additional stress to the point where the client is no longer able to adapt. The triggering event must be recognized as a signal of distress, otherwise clients will not be helped to develop new ways of coping. At times it is easy to miss symptoms of distress because the triggering event is a very minor occurrence. For example, a child who comes sobbing into the health clinic at school because of a shove by peers on the playground could need just a little extra attention. On the other hand, if this child perceives the push to mean that he or she is not liked, the child may be having difficulty developing social relationships. The sobbing could be a cry for help. Taking time to collect sufficient data helps a nurse to discriminate between simple and serious difficulties such as those described above. It is usually wise for a

community health nurse to obtain information about the client's daily functioning, support systems, and recent life changes, when she or he believes that an emotional reaction to an event is disproportionate to what one would expect. Family assessment tools and life change questionnaires, like those presented in Chapter 6, can facilitate collection of such information.

It will also be found when working with clients, particularly those who tend to perceive all difficulties as crises, that problems from the past are reactivated during the crisis state. This happens because these clients have been unsuccessful in dealing with these problems and thus have developed ineffective coping mechanisms (Caplan, 1964, p. 41). This can compound the effects of the current threatening event but can also provide an opportunity for growth. Clients, during times of crisis, can be helped to resolve old as well as new problems and can learn coping strategies which promote growth.

Having an awareness of behaviors which are commonly observed when individuals and families have developed ineffective coping mechanisms, enhances the community health nurse's ability to quickly identify clients who are experiencing distress, crisis, or dysfunctional family dynamics. In 1984 and 1988, the North American Nursing Diagnosis Association identified characteristics of individuals and families who have ineffective coping patterns, when it accepted "individual and family coping" as appropriate nursing diagnostic categories. These characteristics are displayed in Tables 7-1 and 7-2, and can assist community health nurses in determining when individuals and families are having difficulty handling stress. The ineffective behaviors presented in Table 7-2 are primarily identified in terms of how a family relates to a client with an identified problem. During times of distress and crisis, families may also develop dysfunctional patterns of functioning which affect the entire family unit. Deceptive, confused, or secretive communication, inability to meet basic needs of family life (e.g., impaired home management), inappropriate or lack of decision making and problem solving, and family interactions characterized by constant con-

TABLE 7-1 The North American Nursing Diagnosis Association: Ineffective individual coping diagnostic category

Diagnostic label	Definition	Etiology	Defining characteristics
Ineffective coping: Individual	Impairment of adaptive behaviors and problem-solving abilities for meeting life's demands and roles. Methods of handling stressful life situations are insufficient to control anxiety, fear, or anger.	Situational crisis (specify type) Maturational crises (specify type) Personal vulnerability Knowledge deficit (specify) Problem-solving skills deficit	*Verbalization of inability to cope *Inability to ask for help Inability to solve problem effectively Anxiety, fear, anger, irritability, tension Presence of life stress Inability to meet role expectations Inability to meet basic needs Alteration in societal participation Destructive behavior toward self and others Inappropriate or ineffective use of defense mechanisms Change in usual communication patterns High rate of accidents Verbal manipulation Excess food intake, alcohol consumption; smoking Digestive, bowel, appetite disturbance; chronic fatigue or sleep pattern disturbance

*Denotes critical or major defining characteristics.
From Gordon M: Manual of nursing diagnosis, 1988-1989, St Louis, 1989, CV Mosby Co, p 272.

flict, are a few examples of such patterns. Others are shared in Table 6-2.

Types of Crises

Although crisis is basically an individual perceptual matter, certain life events have frequently been found to produce or increase the potential for crisis. These events are viewed as developmental, situational, or a combination of the two. They encompass change, either internally or externally produced, which necessitates altering one's thinking, feelings, and coping style.

Developmental or maturational crises occur across the life spectrum. They relate to critical transition points in the course of normal human development which involve many physical, psychological, and social changes. These transition stages, such as entry into school, puberty, starting a career, leaving home, marriage, parenthood, middlescence, retirement, and facing one's own

death and that of others due to aging, require many role changes and produce heightened stress. The role changes that occur during these anticipated crises are discussed in Chapters 13 through 18.

Situational crises also occur across the lifespan, but they are usually not anticipated and do not relate to normal maturational processes. They are precipitated by such things as divorce, illness, accidents, changes in social status, cultural relocation, and early death of a significant other. Since situational crises are frequently sudden and unexpected, an individual or family faces this type of crisis situation without benefit of anticipatory problem solving. This puts the individual or family more at risk for developing distress, because they are unprepared to deal with the changes that accompanied these life events.

Sometimes situational and developmental crises occur simultaneously. When this happens, an

TABLE 7-2 The North American Nursing Diagnosis Association: Ineffective family coping diagnostic categories

Diagnostic label	Definition	Etiology	Defining characteristics
Ineffective family coping: Compromised	Usually supportive primary person (family member or close friend) providing insufficient, ineffective, or compromised support, comfort, assistance, or encouragement which may be needed by client to manage or master adaptive tasks related to health challenge	Knowledge deficit Emotional conflicts Exhaustion of supportive capacity Role changes (family) Temporary family disorganization Developmental or situational crises	Client expresses concern or complaint about significant other's response to his/her health problem Significant person describes preoccupation with personal reactions (e.g., fear, guilt, anticipatory grief, anxiety) to client's illness, disability, or other situational or developmental crises Significant person describes or confirms inadequate understanding of knowledge base which interferes with effective assistive or supportive behaviors Significant person attempts assistive or supportive behaviors with less than satisfactory results Significant person withdraws or enters into limited or temporary personal communication with client at time of need Significant person displays protective behavior disproportionate (too little or too much) to client's abilities or need for autonomy
Ineffective family coping: Disabling	Behavior of significant person (family member or primary person) disables own capacities and client's capacities to effectively address tasks essential to either person's adaptation to the health challenge	Chronically unexpressed guilt/anxiety/hostility/ etc. (significant other) Dissonant discrepancy of coping styles (for dealing with adaptive tasks by the significant person and client or among significant people) Highly ambivalent family relationships Arbitrary handling of family's resistance to treatment (which tends to solidify defensiveness as it fails to deal adequately with underlying anxiety)	Neglectful care of client in regard to basic human needs and/or illness treatment Distortion of reality regarding client's health problem including extreme denial about existence or severity Intolerance Rejection Abandonment Desertion Carrying on usual routines disregarding client's needs Psychosomaticism Taking on illness signs of the client Decisions and actions by family which are detrimental to economic or social well-being Agitation, depression, aggression, hostility, anxiety, despair, guilt Impaired restructuring of a meaningful life for self, impaired individuation, prolonged overconcern for client Neglectful relationships with other family members Client's development of helpless, inactive dependence

From Gordon M: Manual of nursing diagnosis, 1988-1989, St Louis, 1989, CV Mosby Co, pp 288, 290, 292, 294.

individual's or a family's adaptive energies are seriously overtaxed. Multiple stressors make it more difficult for these persons to evaluate realistically the changes that are occurring and to adjust their coping style to accommodate them. For example, a 5-year-old child who has recently changed cultural settings must deal with stresses related to school entry as well as those related to living in a new environment. School entry is in itself often very traumatic. This, coupled with the pressures that result from relocation, such as learning a different language, developing all new friendships, and adjusting to an unfamiliar lifestyle, can be overwhelming.

Several developmental and situational crises such as teenage parenthood, changing careers, and a newly diagnosed chronic illness are discussed in Chapters 13 through 18. When community health nurses work with families who are experiencing such crises, each family member's level of stress should be assessed. A system's framework (refer to Chapter 6) can be especially helpful in identifying the impact of a crisis on the entire family unit. Both structural and process parameters of family functioning as well as the biopsychosocial components of individual functioning should be examined during times of stress. During the assessment process, it is important to focus on what is occurring and how the family is handling its feelings and the activities of daily living. At times, individuals and families attempt to establish blame elsewhere to relieve anxiety. Blaming behavior does not lead to healthy coping.

Because community health nurses are frequently present when crisis-producing events are occurring, they are in a favorable position to initiate supportive interventions that will enhance a client's ability to adapt. In order to do so, they must know about life events which can precipitate crisis, must recognize signs and symptoms which signal distress, and must develop skill in utilizing several types of intervention strategies with clients who are experiencing stress or crisis.

NURSING INTERVENTION STRATEGIES

Community health nurses use a variety of intervention approaches to facilitate adaptation during times of stress and to enhance successful resolution of crisis. Some of these approaches will be briefly summarized under three major categories: supportive, educative and problem-solving. Separating strategies into categories is an artificial technique which is used here only to focus discussion about ways to effect client change. In reality, community health nurses find that often they must integrate several intervention approaches in order to intervene effectively with clients.

Establishing rapport and collecting adequate data to identify the task to be accomplished are the essential first steps in any intervention process. These steps are discussed in Chapters 6 and 8 and are not repeated here. They should, however, be kept in mind when one is selecting a particular intervention modality.

Supportive Approach

The multiple symptoms that clients experience during distress and/or crisis were previously discussed in this chapter. These symptoms can be very unpleasant and can create great discomfort. Often, they are difficult for clients to understand. Some clients, when experiencing these symptoms, fear that something is seriously wrong with them. This tends to increase their anxieties and fears.

Clients who are experiencing symptoms of distress need to reduce these symptoms before they can actively engage in activities which will lead to problem resolution. Supportive intervention by significant others (family, friends, and professionals) can assist clients in dealing with symptoms of distress. Two types of support are especially helpful: (1) providing an opportunity for the client to share feelings with persons who are accepting and nonjudgmental and (2) assisting the client with concrete daily tasks, such as home management and keeping health appointments. Community health nurses frequently help clients who are experiencing crisis with concrete tasks by making referrals for homemakers or home health aides, or by helping the client to mobilize family resources. At times, they also provide this assistance themselves during home visits. They may, for example, feed an infant while talking to a distressed mother.

It is important to remember that clients who

are experiencing distress often need time to deal with their feelings and to sort out realities before they can engage in problem solving and the learning of new knowledge. Ignoring the feeling levels of clients during these times can disrupt the therapeutic relationship and may result in the client withdrawing or becoming increasingly distressed. Following the principles of crisis intervention delineated by Caplan (discussed later in this chapter) helps to develop a caring, trusting, professional relationship with clients in crisis.

Educative Approach

Health education has traditionally been a function of the community health nurse. Lillian Wald cared for the sick in the home and also provided instruction so that families were better equipped to assist their ill members. Lina Rodgers taught personal hygiene to school-age children and their families and as a result the spread of disease was reduced and wellness was promoted. Funds were made available through Federal Maternal and Child Health Grants in the '20s and '30s so that community health nurses could be hired to provide health teaching in relation to child care, nutrition, and family-life education. Monies were also allocated at this time for preventive health teaching services aimed at combating communicable diseases such as tuberculosis and childhood illnesses.

The health education function of nurses in the community setting has remained viable over the years. It is still a major focus of all community health nurses, regardless of the setting in which they practice, because practitioners in the field have clearly demonstrated the value of this activity.

Health beliefs and behavior are the targets of teaching or the educative approach in nursing practice (Redman, 1988). Health education activities are designed to promote wellness and to prevent illness. They are used to prepare clients to deal with maturational and situational events that produce stress. They are also used to promote personal habits that foster optimal health, including obtaining immunizations to prevent communicable disease, eating balanced meals, and seeking medical care when ill. Psychosocial as well as physical aspects of health and disease are taken into consideration when the community health nurse utilizes this intervention strategy.

The educative strategy has two major components: (1) increasing the learner's understanding of new events and his or her healthy functioning through the acquisition of knowledge and (2) helping the learner to apply the new information. Readiness of the learner must be assessed and established before either of these components can be implemented successfully. Sharing information the client does not wish to assimilate does not increase client understanding. In fact, when this happens clients frequently do not hear what is being shared.

The concept of learner readiness or motivation is a complex, multidimensional phenomenon. It involves the interaction between multiple, interrelated variables such as clients' perceptions of health and illness, family patterns of health care, and availability and accessibility of resources. Various models have been proposed by social scientists and nurses to explain why clients are or are not motivated to engage in health behaviors (Cox, 1982; Fishbein and Ajzen, 1975; Kulbok, 1985; Pender, 1987, Health promotion in practice; Rosenstock, 1966, 1974; Rotter, 1966). The most widely used model, the *Health Belief Model,* examines why individuals engage in diagnostic and other disease-prevention activities (Rosenstock, 1974). In the mid-1960s, Rosenstock stimulated significant interest among health professionals in the use of this model when he examined in the literature why people use health services (Rosenstock, 1966). The Health Belief Model, developed by a group of social scientists, advances the idea that readiness to take health action is dependent on several variables including (a) perceived susceptibility to a specific condition, (b) perceived seriousness of a given health problem, (c) perceived benefits and barriers to taking action, and (d) cues to action such as knowledge that someone else has become affected by the condition. The Health Belief Model emphasizes that the beliefs that define readiness have both cognitive and emotional components and the motivational variables that promote disease-oriented, preventive health action are individually defined (Rosenstock, 1966).

The Health Belief Model is useful in explaining health-promoting behaviors that are triggered by an interest in preventing disease occurrence. Other conceptual models have been developed to examine health-promoting behaviors that are wellness oriented rather than disease focused. An example of such a model is the Health Promotion Model developed by Pender (1987, Health and health promotion). In this model, "cognitive-perceptual factors are considered to be the primary determinants of behavior and are identified as (1) importance of health; (2) perceived control of health; (3) perceived self-efficacy; (4) definition of health; (5) perceived health status; (6) perceived benefits of health-promoting behaviors; and (7) perceived barriers to health-promoting behaviors. Demographic characteristics, biologic characteristics, interpersonal influences, situational factors and behavioral factors are hypothesized as influencing health behaviors through cognitive-perceptual processes. As in the Health Belief Model, cues to action are considered important in the initiation of health actions" (Pender, 1987, Health and health promotion, pp. 13-14). An in-depth discussion of this model can be found in Pender's (1987) book, *Health Promotion in Nursing Practice.*

Health behavior models such as those just discussed emphasize the importance of assessing more than just cognitive understanding or knowledge when determining learner readiness. Often, underlying psychosocial factors are the key variables which influence why people do or do not engage in positive health action. If that is the case, these factors must be dealt with before the health professional initiates cognitive teaching strategies.

Use of the nursing process (refer to Chapter 8) combined with an understanding of the principles of teaching and learning aids the community health nurse in assessing learner readiness. These factors also help to individualize educational plans based on client needs and circumstances. Writings by Brill (1978), Pohl (1978), and Redman (1988) are valuable resources if one wants to review or expand knowledge in relation to the principles of teaching and learning.

After community health nurses establish learner readiness, they and their clients develop teaching and learning goals. Together they also select from a variety of alternative intervention options a teaching strategy which best fits the client's needs and circumstances. Frequently a combination of two or more teaching methods is used. For example, a community health nurse might combine discussion, demonstration, and use of pamphlets to teach new parents how to bathe a baby. Or the nurse might use group process, audiovisual aids, self-instructional materials, and a baby bath demonstration to teach this same procedure. Whatever techniques are selected, the learner should have the opportunity to obtain new knowledge as well as to apply the knowledge gained. For instance, understanding how to bathe a baby does not always increase a new parent's level of comfort when doing so. Being allowed to demonstrate what has been learned when assistance is available is more likely to promote ease with such a procedure.

Developing specific, measurable, client-centered goals for the teaching and learning process is essential for several reasons. Specific goals help to determine what content or information is needed by the client. They also aid in developing and implementing teaching techniques that are relevant to the client's needs. In addition, they facilitate evaluation of the learning process because they define what the client desires to learn. A global goal such as "learning about growth and development" does none of these things. It does not define what information parents need in order to handle the developmental needs of their child more effectively. A goal which states that "Jean will verbally identify the developmental tasks of a 1-year-old" is much clearer.

Individualizing teaching and learning plans is crucial, because client needs vary even when different people encounter similar situations. Some parents understand normal growth-and-development processes very well but have difficulty handling the physical aspects of child care. Others are at ease with feeding, bathing, and clothing their infant but become frustrated when the child does not achieve developmental tasks, even if it is too soon for him or her to accomplish them. Differences like these are not uncommon among clients who are experiencing similar situations.

Opportunities to use the educative strategy in the community health setting are endless. Teaching a child at school how to prevent infection when hurt, discussing sexuality issues with a mother who has preadolescent children, and sharing information about the hereditary aspects of diabetes when a family history reflects a need are a few examples of when a community health nurse uses the educative strategy. Education is not always needed, however, and can be misused. This happens particularly when the nurse makes an assumption about what the client needs to learn without first collecting data, or when the nurse imposes information on the client because of value conflicts. Some parents who have several children, for example, desire to have more. Continuing to teach about family planning after it has been validated that the parents know how to prevent pregnancy and understand the pros and cons of increasing their family size is meeting the nurse's needs, not the family's needs.

Problem-Solving Approach

In the community health setting, nurses encounter clients who are having difficulty making decisions about a variety of personal life events. Specifically, community health nurses help clients to make decisions about such things as career choices, maintaining or establishing intimate relationships with others, when and where to obtain preventive and curative health care services, how to deal with family conflicts, how to handle financial crises, or how to provide needed care for aging family members. At times, clients dealing with situations such as these have difficulty identifying why they cannot make a decision about what to do. They know that something is wrong because symptoms of anxiety are present, but they are unable to take action to reduce their stress.

There are various reasons why clients are unable to alter their behavior in a way to help them resolve their stress appropriately. Examples are illustrated in the case situations below.

Client Has Not Specifically Identified the Nature of the Problem

Barb Lehi, a 28-year-old wife and the mother of two children, returned to work when her youngest child entered school. Her family adjusted well to her role change because joint decision making occurred prior to Barb's employment. Barb was enjoying what she was doing but began to have tension headaches 2 months after she started her new job. She felt her headaches were related to the adjustments she had to make in her daily routine, and assumed that they would go away shortly. They did not, however, until she was able to identify that she was having guilt feelings about being a working mother.

Client Has a Vested Interest in Not Identifying the Problem

Mrs. Jackson, a 68-year-old widow living by herself, kept finding reasons why she should not see a physician after she started having "fainting spells." Her family became frustrated and worried and asked the community health nurse to visit. Referral for medical evaluation was successfully implemented only when Mrs. Jackson was able to verbalize that being ill was the only way she could get attention from her family. Her family visited very sporadically when she was well but daily when she was ill.

Client Is Unable to Acknowledge Feelings

Gail Hayes, a 31-year-old mother and wife, provided no stimulation for her 2-year-old daughter who was retarded due to rubella exposure in utero. The community health nurse became involved after hearing from a neighbor that Gail left her daughter alone in the house when she visited friends and neighbors. After several home visits, the nurse discovered that Gail did so because "I can't stand to be with her. She is such a fussy child and wants attention all of the time. I hate seeing her so deformed and feel guilty because if I hadn't gotten measles while pregnant, she would be all right." Gail had never before acknowledged these feelings. When she did, she was able to use the help offered by others and to relate more effectively to her daughter.

Client Does Not Assume Accountability for Feelings

Bob Woodrow, a 40-year-old construction worker, was referred to the health department for rehabilitative services after a myocardial infarction. Because of the strenuous nature of construction work, it was recommended that he seek other employment. He verbalized an interest in obtaining job training through the Division of Vocational Rehabilitation but took no action. When the community health nurse questioned why, he responded by placing the blame on others. "My wife thinks it is too soon and nags me about not going back to work. I am not sure if my physician thinks I should, because he is always so vague about what is happening with my heart. My car needs fixing before I can use it regularly, and we don't have the money to get it fixed." It took several months for Bob to see that he was not taking action because of his own fears about having another heart attack and about not being able to succeed in a new line of work.

Client Cannot Distinguish between Feelings and Facts

Carol Strang, a 17-year-old junior, repeatedly visited the school nurse for minor physical concerns. Assessments made by the nurse revealed that this occurred when Carol felt that she was not performing well academically. In reality, Carol was very successful in her schoolwork, ranking in the top 5 percent of her class. In addition, she had several close friends who provided praise for her academic achievements. Carol, however, perceived that she was achieving satisfactorily only when she received straight As. When she received anything less than an A, she expressed feelings associated with failure.

Client Lacks Experience with Problem Solving

Mrs. Raabe, a 71-year-old widow, became confused and severely upset after her husband's death. All her life she had been cared for by others. Her parents and her brothers anticipated her needs because she was the "baby" of the family and "helpless." Because her husband assumed the same role as her family, Mrs. Raabe felt lost when he died. She found managing her finances particularly stressful since she had never taken care of the family budget. She needed help with such basics as writing a check, depositing money in the bank, and balancing her income and expenses.

Client Has Undetected Physical or Perceptual Problems

Mrs. La Rosa, a 37-year-old divorced mother of six children, was referred to the health department by her caseworker from the Department of Social Service. Her caseworker believed that Mrs. La Rosa was neglecting her children and felt that environmental conditions were dangerous to the family's health. Mrs. La Rosa told the community health nurse that "I know I should keep my home more tidy, but I am just too tired to keep up with things that need to be done around the house. Sometimes all I want to do is sleep." The community health nurse assisted her in obtaining a medical evaluation. It was found during this evaluation that Mrs. La Rosa had hypertension and diabetes. When both of these conditions were under control, home management and child care skills improved.

Client Missed Essential Steps in Skill Development

Mr. and Mrs. Lueck were extremely upset when their 10-year-old retarded son was sent home from camp because he could not handle activities of daily living such as bathing and toileting. "Tommie always does these things at home. They just don't know how to work with retarded kids." Upon talking with the Luecks, the community health nurse discovered Tommie did wash himself when bathing at home, but that family members helped him with most of the activities necessary for completing a bath. For example, the family ran his bath water for him; assembled the materials he needed to take a bath, including soap, washcloth, and towel; and selected the clothing he would wear afterward. It was obvious to the nurse but not the parents that Tommie never really learned how to handle his personal hygiene needs. He had skill in washing body parts, but lacked decision-making skill about how and when to carry out these activities.

Client Is Unable to Generate Alternative Options during Problem Solving or Fears the Consequences of a Newly Generated Alternative

Amy Schmidt, wife and mother of two preschoolers, was physically abused by her husband regularly and expressed a desire to leave him. She found it difficult to take this action because she thought that it was impossible for her to do so. She felt trapped because she had no job skills and her family and friends were unable to assist her financially. In addition, she felt that the abuse would not stop, even if she left home, because her husband could always find her. The community health nurse assisted Mrs. Schmidt in identifying ways to obtain financial aid as well as legal assistance to control her husband's behavior. Mrs. Schmidt was also helped to see that living alone could be less frightening for her and her children than being physically abused.

The situations presented above are far more complex than indicated by the discussion. They are briefly summarized to illustrate that there are many reasons why established problem-solving patterns are ineffective during times of stress and crisis. Identifying the specific reason(s) for each client's stress is the essential first step when the community health nurse utilizes the problem-solving approach to enhance client growth.

A community health nurse has two major goals when using the problem-solving approach: (1) to assist the client in solving immediate problem(s) and (2) to help the client increase independent problem-solving abilities. Implicit in these goals is the belief that clients *can learn* skills which will help them to make decisions wisely and to alter behavior accordingly. A community health nurse who has difficulty *internalizing* this belief will find it hard to move a client toward independence. This nurse is more likely *to do for* the client than *to work with* the client.

A variety of techniques can be used to help a client enhance his or her problem-solving abilities, including such things as individual counseling, group work, role modeling, and behavioral programming. When using any one of these techniques, the community health nurse should focus on helping the client to identify the nature of the problem(s), to discover alternative options for problem solving, to make decisions about which option is most appropriate, and to take action to resolve the problem(s). The community health nurse should not assume that the client will take action after making a decision about the most ap-

propriate option and prematurely close the family to service. Taking action is often the most difficult step in the problem-solving process because it is at this point that the client is giving up the "secure" familiar for the "threatening" unknown.

Clients must be allowed to make decisions and to take action for themselves before they are able to achieve independent problem-solving abilities. It is natural to want to "rescue" clients when they are experiencing pain. *Rescue behavior, such as giving advice and doing for the client, reduces anxiety only temporarily, because the client is not prepared to handle stress in the future.* It can be helpful for the community health nurse to share alternative ways for handling stresses, but the client should be encouraged to evaluate suggestions in terms of his or her own circumstances. The client should be given the message that no one way is being advocated but that these options have worked with others in the past.

When clients are experiencing crisis, they often desperately want others to make decisions for them. Cadden (1964, pp. 293-296) has delineated several principles of crisis intervention that help a community health nurse avoid rescue activities and provide constructive aid to the family. These are:

1. *Help the client confront the crisis* by supporting expression of feelings and emotions such as fear, guilt, and crying.
2. *Help the client confront the crisis in manageable doses* without dampening the impact of the crisis to a point where the client no longer recognizes the need to alter coping mechanisms. Drugs and diversional activities are helpful when they are used to decrease unmanageable stress. They are harmful when they prevent the client from looking at the realities of his or her situation.
3. *Help the client to find the facts,* because truth is less frightening than the unknown. Clients may need frequent visits during periods of crisis because they may not have the energy to analyze all the stresses they are experiencing during one home visit.
4. *Do not give the client false reassurance* be-

cause this leads to mistrust and maladaptive coping behaviors. To succeed in resolving a crisis, a client needs reassurance which supports his or her ability to handle the crisis situation.

5. *Do not encourage the client to blame others,* because blaming only reduces tension momentarily and can help the client to suppress feelings. This can result in maladaptive behaviors that decrease the client's level of functioning after crisis resolution.

6. *Help the client to accept help* because some clients avoid confronting a crisis by denying that they need help and that a problem exists. If the client does not face the crisis, he or she will not mobilize coping mechanisms that will enhance growth.

7. *Help the client with everyday tasks* in a manner that reflects kindness and thoughtfulness rather than one that gives a message that the client is weak or incompetent. Clients need help with everyday tasks because it takes considerable energy to resolve a crisis; thus, clients often lack sufficient energy to handle daily activities as well.

Problem solving takes time. Both the client and the community health nurse must guard against expecting change too rapidly. When progress is slow, a client may question if the nurse can really help, and the nurse often begins to wonder whether or not the client really wants to change. At times, both of these feelings are justified. More frequently, however, the need is for the client and nurse to recognize that well-established patterns of behavior cannot be changed immediately.

Community health nurses cannot help all clients to learn to make decisions wisely. Some situations are beyond their competence and must be referred to others who are better qualified. Because competence varies from one community health nurse to another as a result of differences in academic preparation and work experiences, nurses must learn how to discriminate between situations that they can and cannot handle. Peer and supervisory conferences will assist a new nurse to objectively evaluate her or his skills.

Underestimating one's ability to help a client, rather than overestimating competency, is often more of a problem when nurses begin practice in the community health setting. Most clients experiencing stress and crisis do not need psychotherapy. Instead, they need someone who cares and who will provide supportive guidance and positive reinforcement for the strength they have.

SUMMARY

The community health nurse is often the primary source of assistance when an individual or a family is experiencing stress. Stress is a normal, human phenomenon necessary for survival and growth. It triggers the general adaptation syndrome which helps people to adapt to the demands and pressures of life. Although stress is essential for survival and growth, every individual has limits beyond which stress is no longer tolerated. Prolonged and intensified stress results in crisis, especially when an individual's coping mechanisms are inadequate to reduce disequilibrium.

A person in crisis experiences disorganization and heightened stress. Crisis is self-limiting but biopsychosocial homeostasis following a crisis may be at a level equal to, better than, or lower than the precrisis level. Timely supportive intervention may be the critical factor that determines if an individual or family has a positive or negative outcome during periods of crisis.

REFERENCES

Aquilera, DC: Crisis intervention: theory and methodology, ed 6, St Louis, 1989, CV Mosby Co.

Bakeland F and Lundwall L: Dropping out of treatment: a critical review, Psychol Bull 82:738-783, 1975.

Blau ZS: Old age in a changing society, New York, 1973, New Viewpoints.

Brill NI: Working with people: the helping process, Philadelphia, 1978, Lippincott.

Brown GW, Bhrolchain MN, and Harris TO: Social class and psychiatric disturbance among women in an urban population, Sociology 9:225-231, 1975.

Burch J: Recent bereavement in relation to suicide, J Psychosom Med 16:361-366, 1972.

Burr WR: Theory construction and the sociology of the family, New York, 1973, Wiley.

Cadden V: Crisis in the family. In Caplan G, ed: Principles of preventive psychiatry, New York, 1964, Basic Books, pp 228-296.

Cannon WB: Bodily changes in pain, hunger, fear, and rage, New York, 1929, Appleton.

Cannon WB: Stresses and strains of homeostasis, Am J Med Sci 189:1-14, 1935.

Caplan G: An approach to community mental health, New York, 1961, Grune & Stratton.

Caplan G: Principles of preventive psychiatry, New York, 1964, Basic Books.

Caplan RD, Robinson EAR, French JRP Jr, Caldwell JR, and Shinn MB: Adhering to medical regimens: pilot experiments in patient education and social support, Ann Arbor, 1976, University of Michigan, Institute for Social Research.

Cassel JC: Psychiatric epidemiology. In Caplan G, ed: American handbook of psychiatry, vol 2, New York, 1974, Basic Books.

Cassel JC: Psychosocial processes and stress: theoretical formulation, Int J Health Serv 4:471-482, 1974.

Chambers WN and Reiser MF: Emotional stress in the precipitation of congestive heart failure, Psychosom Med 15:38-60, 1953.

Chen E and Cobb S: Family structure in relation to health and disease, J Chron Dis 12:544-567, 1960.

Choi T, Josten L, and Christensen ML: Health-specific family coping index for noninstitutional care, Am J Public Health 73:1275-1277, 1983.

Cobb S: Physiological changes in men whose jobs were abolished, J Psychosom Res 18:245-258, 1974.

Cobb S: Social support as a moderator of life stress, Psychom Med 38:300-314, 1976.

Cobb S, Kasl SV, French JRP, and Norstebo G: The intrafamilial transmission of rheumatoid arthritis VII, Why wives with rheumatoid arthritis have husbands with peptic ulcer? J Chron Dis 22:279-293, 1969.

Cox C: An interaction model of client health behavior: theoretical prescription for nursing, Adv Nurs Sci 5:41-56, 1982.

de Araujo G, Van Arsdel PP, Holmes TH, and Dudley DL: Life change, coping ability and chronic intrinsic asthma, J Psychosom Res 17:359-363, 1973.

Egbert LD, Battib GE, Welch CE, and Bartlett MK: Reduction of post-operative pain by encouragement and instruction of patients, N Engl J Med 270:825-827, 1964.

Figley, CR and McCubbin HI: Stress and the family, vol II, Coping with catastrophe, New York, 1983, Brunner/Mazel.

Fishbein M and Ajzen I: Belief, attitude, intention and behavior: an introduction to theory research, Reading, Ma, 1975, Addison-Wesley.

Gordon M: Manual of nursing diagnosis, 1988-1989, St Louis, 1989, CV Mosby Co.

Gore S: The influence of social support and related variables in ameliorating the consequence of job loss, Doctoral dissertation, Philadelphia, 1973, University of Pennsylvania.

Hamburg B and Killilea M: Relation of social support, stress, illness, and use of health services. In Hamburg D, ed: Healthy people: the Surgeon General's report on health promotion and disease prevention, DHEW PHS Pub. No. 79-55071A, Washington, DC, 1979, US Department of Health, Education, and Welfare.

Hansen DA and Hill R: Families under stress. In Christensen HT, ed: Handbook of marriage and the family, Chicago, 1964, Rand McNally, pp 783-819.

Haynes RB and Sackett DL: A working symposium: compliance with therapeutic regimens, annotated bibliography, Hamilton, Ont, 1974, McMaster University Medical Center, Department of Epidemiology and Biostatistics.

Hill R: Families under stress, New York, 1949, Harper & Row.

Jessner L, Blom GE, and Waldfogel S: Emotional implications of tonsillectomy and adenoidectomy on children, Psychoanal Study Child 7:126-169, 1952.

Kaplan BH, Cassel JC, and Gore S: Social support and health, Med Care 15(5, suppl):47-58, 1977.

Knapp TR: Stress versus strain: methodological critique, Nurs Res 37:181-184, 1988.

Kulbok PP: Social resources, health resources, and preventive health behavior: patterns and predictions, Public Health Nurs 2:67-81, 1985.

Lazarus RS: Psychological stress and the coping process, New York, 1966, McGraw-Hill.

Lazarus RS: The stress and coping paradigm, In Eisdorfer C, Cohen D, Kleinman A, and Masim P, eds: Models for clinical psychopathology, New York, 1981, Spectrum, pp 177-214.

Lazarus RS and Folkman S: Stress, appraisal and coping, New York, 1984, Springer.

Lindemann E: Symptomatology and management of acute grief, Am J Psychiatry 101:141-148, 1944.

Lowenthal MF and Haven C: Interaction and adoption intimacy: a critical variable, Am Sociol Rev 33:20, 1968.

Maddison DC and Walther WL: Factors affecting the outcome of conjugal bereavement, Br J Psychiatry 113:1057-1067, 1967.

Mather HG: Intensive care, Br Med J 2:322, 1974.

Mather HG, Pearson NG, Read KLQ, Shaw DB, Steed GR, Thorne MG, Jones S, Guerrier CJ, Eraut CD, McHugh PM, Chowdhury NF, Jafary MH, Wallace TJ: Acute myocardial infarction: home and hospital treatment, Br Med J 3:334-338, 1971.

McCubbin H, Cauble E, and Patterson J, eds: Family stress in coping, and social support, Springfield, Il, 1982, Charles C Thomas.

McCubbin H and Figley CR: Stress and the family, vol I, Coping with normative transitions, New York, 1983, Brunner/Mazel.

McHugh P: Defining the situation: the organization of meaning in social interactions, Indianapolis, 1968, Bobbs-Merrill.

Nuckolls KB, Cassel JC, and Kaplan BH: Psycho-social assets, life crisis and prognosis of pregnancy, Am J Epidemiol 95:431-441, 1972.

Parkes CM, Benjamin B, and Fitzgerald RE: Broken heart: a study of increased mortality among widowers, Br Med J 1:740, 1969.

Parkes CM: Bereavement: studies of grief in adult life, New York, 1972, International Universities Press.

Pender NJ: Health and health promotion: conceptual dilemmas. In Duffy ME and Pender NJ, eds: Conceptual issues in health promotion: report of proceedings of a wingspread conference, Indianapolis, 1987, Sigma Theta Tau, pp. 7-23.

Pender NJ: Health promotion in nursing practice, Norwalk, Ct, 1987, Appleton-Century-Crofts.

Pohl ML: The teaching function of the nursing practitioner, Dubuque, 1978, Wm C Brown.

Rahe RH: The pathway between subjects' recent life changes and their near-future illness reports: representative results and methodological issues. In Dohrenwend BS and Dohrenwend BP, eds: Stressful life events, New York, 1974, Wiley.

Redman BK: The process of patient education, ed 6, St Louis, 1988, CV Mosby Co.

Rosenstock IM: Why people use health services, Milbank Q 44:94-127, 1966.

Rosenstock IM: Historical origins of the health belief model, Health Education Monograph 2(4):328-335, 1974.

Rotter JB: Internal versus external control of reinforcement, Psychological Monograph 80(1), 1966.

Selye H: The stress of life, New York, 1975, McGraw-Hill.

Selye H: Stress in health and disease, Boston, 1976, Butterworths.

SELECTED BIBLIOGRAPHY

Allan JD: Identification of health risks in a young adult population, J Commun Health Nurs 4:223-233, 1987.

Antonousky A: Health, stress, and coping, San Francisco, 1979, Jossey-Bass.

Family Nursing Continuing Education Project: Nursing of families in transition: workshop proceedings, Portland, Or, 1987, Oregon Health Sciences University.

Family Nursing Continuing Education Project: Nursing of families with acute or chronic illness: workshop proceedings, Portland, Or, 1988, Oregon Health Sciences University.

Hyman RB and Woog P: Stressful life events and illness onset: a review of crucial variables, Res Nurs Health 5:155-163, 1982.

Johnson JE and Lauver DR: Alternative explanations of coping with stressful experiences associated with physical illness, Adv Nurs Sci 11(2):39-52, 1989.

Krentz LG, ed: Nursing and the promotion/protection of family health: workshop proceedings, Portland, Or, 1988, Oregon Health Sciences University.

Laffrey SC, Loveland-Cherry CJ and Winkler SJ: Health behavior: evolution of two paradigms, Public Health Nurs 3:92-100, 1986.

Manfredi C and Pickett M: Perceived stressful situations and coping strategies utilized by the elderly, J Commun Health Nurs 4:99-110, 1987.

McCubbin HI, Joy CB, Cauble AE, Comeau JK, Patterson JM, and Needle RH: Family stress and coping: a decade of review, J Marriage Family 42:855-871, 1980.

McHatton M: A theory of timely teaching, Am J Nurs 7:798, 1985.

Parad HJ ed: Crisis intervention: selected readings, New York, 1965, Family Service Association of America.

Rolland JS: Chronic illness and the life cycle: a conceptual framework, Family Process 26:203-221, 1987.

Silverman MM, Lalley TL, Rosenberg ML, Smith JC, Parron D, and Jacobs J: Control of stress and violent behavior: mid-course review of the 1990 health objectives, Public Health Rep 103: 38-48, 1988.

Stone GC, Cohen F, and Adler NE: Health psychology, San Francisco, 1979, Jossey-Bass.

Wismont JM and Reame NE: The lesbian childbearing experience: assessing developmental tasks, Image: J Nurs Scholarship 21:137-141, 1989.

Wright LM and Leahey M: Families and chronic illness, Springhouse, Pa, 1987, Springhouse Corporation.

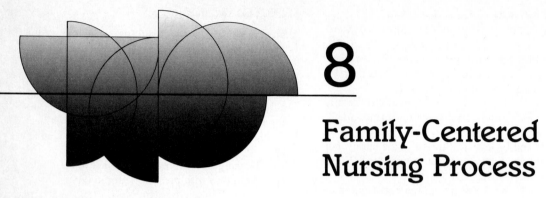

8

Family-Centered Nursing Process

For a green plant to survive, it must reach sunlight. So nature provides that if the plant's growth is blocked in one direction, it can grow in another.

CONOCO OIL COMPANY

_____ OBJECTIVES _____

Upon completion of this chapter, the reader will be able to:

1. *Discuss four key elements inherent in the definition of the family-centered nursing process.*
2. *Distinguish between the phases of the family-centered nursing process.*
3. *Describe the relationship between the phases of the family-centered nursing process.*
4. *Compare and contrast the family-centered nursing process and the individual-focused nursing process.*
5. *Identify the importance of applying theoretical concepts as a basis for decision making in practice and theory bases applicable to community health nursing.*
6. *Summarize the nursing responsibilities related to a home visit and the importance of each to the*

development of a therapeutic *nurse-family relationship.*
7. *Describe client rights and related agency obligations throughout the provider/client relationship.*
8. *Formulate criteria for assessing healthy and dysfunctional family behaviors.*
9. *Construct examples of family-centered nursing diagnoses, interventions, and evaluation statements.*
10. *Discuss the philosophy underlying the use of contracting as a community health nursing intervention strategy and provide examples of contracting with families.*

People, like green plants, can grow in multiple directions. Stumbling blocks along the way do not necessarily stop growth (refer to Figure 8-1). Caring, support, and assistance from significant others can help humanity to change the course of its development when barriers are inhibiting the growth process.

Although human growth follows a predictable pattern, all individuals are still unique. As they develop, they make choices about pathways to take to reach sunlight and to achieve happiness. Although physiological, psychosocial, cultural, and spiritual forces influence individual decision making about what brings a rich and satisfying life, every human being also needs the opportunity to define which pathways lead to personal growth and self-fulfillment. Individuals who encourage others to make independent decisions about life choices are more likely to facilitate growth than individuals who impose on others their beliefs about appropriate life pathways.

Community health nurses can facilitate the human growth process. They work to develop trusting, supportive relationships so that clients can reach out and use their help when needed. Some clients will not seek assistance from com-

Figure 8-1 Nature doesn't explore just one path to reach a goal. Neither should man. (Conoco Oil Company.)

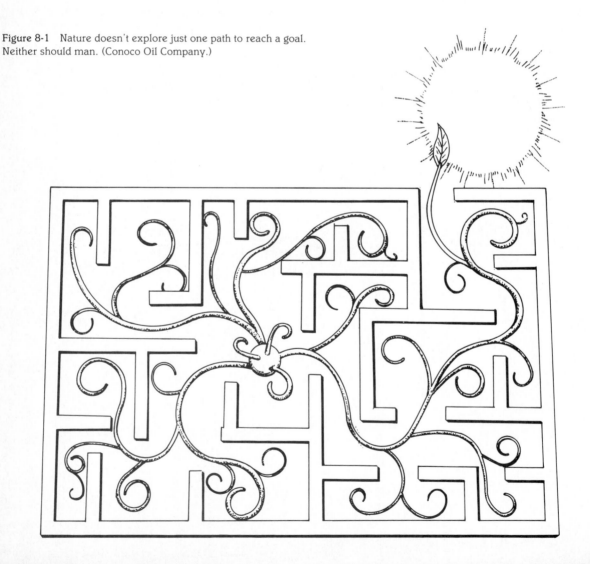

munity health nurses because they have found other support systems more relevant to them. However, when a client does accept the help offered by a community health nurse, it is extremely important for the nurse to recognize that her or his role is to help the client determine which pathways to brightness are appropriate for that individual. The nurse cannot know what is best for other human beings. Taking away an individual's independence leads to darkness, not light.

Increasingly, nurses and other health care professionals have accepted the client's right of self-determination in relation to decision making and change. They have identified that doing *for* the client instead of working *with* him or her can result in client dependence and other modes of limited behavioral action. Clients must internalize the need for change before they will alter their behavior. Take, for example, a 40-year-old man with a cardiac problem who has been advised to modify his diet. In the hospital he was served low-sodium food. If this client does not understand his diet or why it is necessary, he is likely to resume his previous eating patterns once he returns home. In his own environment, the client makes decisions about what he will eat. Nurses can influence client change but only the client can alter his behavior.

At times, the concept of individual self-determination is difficult to operationalize, because a professional's personal feelings can influence the interactions between that person and the client. It is easy for a nurse to feel like a failure when a client does not alter health actions, especially when this behavior is adversely affecting the client's health status. Viewing oneself as a client often helps. Stop and think for a while how you make changes in your life-style. For most people, being ordered to change produces feelings of resentment and increases resistance. People want to believe that they are capable of making decisions about their lives, and they want the freedom to make choices even if the choices have negative consequences. Depending on the situation, clients may want or need varying degrees of guidance and support, but at all times they should be given a message that they are capable of independent decision making.

To function effectively in the community setting, a nurse must accept the fact that clients are responsible for their health behavior, even when they choose a plan of action that the nurse would not choose. Nurse-defined goals for clients are seldom achieved. Goals defined by the client are more frequently accomplished. The nurse who takes over for clients quickly becomes frustrated with the lack of client response and may "burn out."

The nursing process helps the community health nurse to facilitate client goal setting. This therapeutic process is used by nurses in all settings. However, it is labeled the *family-centered nursing process* in the community health setting because community health nurses use it to analyze family functioning and to extend services to all family members. This focus is based on the belief that the family is the basic unit for nursing service: family functioning affects the health of all

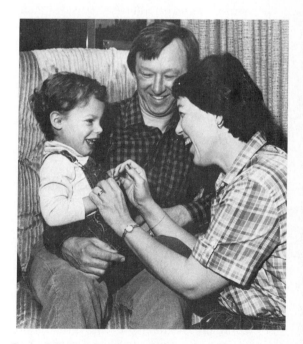

Figure 8-2 The family-centered approach to nursing care focuses on the family as the unit of service. When utilizing the nursing process in the community setting, nurses assess family dynamics as well as individual functioning and establish client-centered goals relevant to the needs of the entire family unit.

family members by inhibiting or facilitating the growth process and by influencing when family members will accept help from community systems (refer to Figure 8-2).

FAMILY-CENTERED NURSING PROCESS DEFINED

The family-centered nursing process is a systematic approach to scientific problem solving, involving a series of circular dynamic actions—assessing, analyzing, planning, implementing, evaluating, and terminating—for the purpose of facilitating optimum client functioning. There are four key elements in this definition:

- *Systematic approach:* This process enables the community health nurse to function in an orderly, logical manner. The nurse *plans* her or his actions to achieve specific goals and recognizes that time and efforts are often wasted if a "hit-or-miss" approach is used.
- *Scientific problem solving:* Decisions made about client needs and appropriate nursing interventions are based on scientific principles. The problem-solving approach is used in everyday life. The nursing process differs from simple problem solving: scientific knowledge gained from advanced study assists the nurse in refining the data analysis process in relation to health, illness, and prevention, and in expanding intervention options which aid clients in maximizing their self-care capabilities. McCain (1965, p. 82), in her classic article on the nursing process, stressed that this process helps nurses to function in a deliberative rather than an intuitive way.
- *Series of circular, dynamic actions:* No one action alone helps the community health nurse to enhance client growth. All phases of the nursing process must be carried out in order for sound decision making and effective nursing intervention to occur. *Dynamic* implies that care plans are revised when assessment and evaluation data reflect needed change. The nursing process is circular in nature because each phase provides data which either validate or alter original nursing diagnoses, goals, and plans.

- *Purpose of facilitating optimum client functioning:* Nursing interventions should help the client to resolve his or her health care needs and to achieve specific, client-defined goals and objectives. A helping interactive process whereby the *client* and the nurse share data for the purpose of identifying ways to make things less difficult for the client facilitates this process. To effectively facilitate client functioning, the nurse must individualize nursing actions, since clients define optimum functioning differently.

A community health nurse using the nursing process is much like a master chef using a recipe to bake a cake. The master chef does not just throw things together, as can be seen in Figure 8-3. The chef, unlike his juggler friend, knows that the right ingredients in correct proportion must be thoroughly mixed and baked at the proper time and temperature. Through knowledge and experience, he has learned how to adjust his ingredients to add a special flavor to his cake.

An effective nurse, like a master chef, learns that by using a systematic process, more satisfying results can be obtained. The nurse knows that it is necessary to have guidelines to follow (scientific knowledge), the right ingredients in correct proportion (adequate data), thorough mixing (analysis of data), a specific cake form (specific client goals and nursing interventions), and testing of the finished product (evaluation). Illustrative of this are the factors the nurse takes into consideration when working with a child who has juvenile diabetes. Based on scientific information, it is known that this child needs such things as:

- Adequate nutrition
- Proper hygiene
- Insulin injections
- Regular urine testing
- Adequate exercise
- Socializing experiences like interactions with peers

Teaching about these needs could lead to a jumbled mess, just like the juggler's cake, unless the nurse considers the:

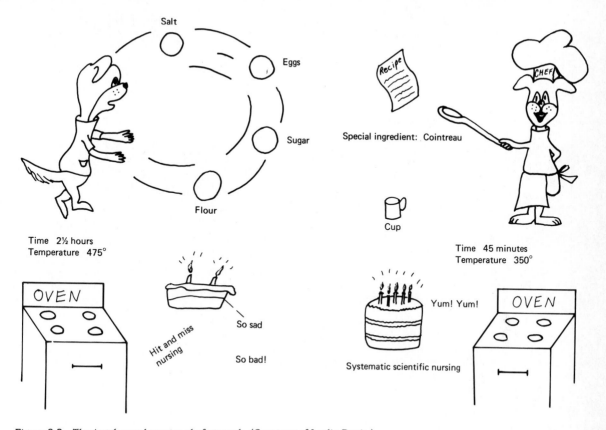

Figure 8-3   The juggler and master chef at work. (Courtesy of Leslie Davis.)

- Family's financial situation
- Family's daily living patterns and how these patterns may need to be altered to provide adequate nutrition, proper hygiene, and appropriate medication for the child
- Family's perceptions of the child's health and knowledge about his or her health status
- Child's emotional reaction to the diabetic condition and knowledge about his or her health status

In order to achieve desired goals relative to the child's needs, the nurse must take all the knowledge available about diabetes and mix it well within the framework of the child's family situation. All good cooks know how to adjust their actions to fit individual situations, and so must a community health nurse. The family's perceptions of their child's health, along with the child's emotional reaction to his or her condition, are two critical factors that nurses consider when individualizing management plans. Intervention strategies are often ineffective until these variables are analyzed. One community health nurse, for instance, visited intensively the family of a 6-year-old child who had brittle diabetes. The child did not follow her prescribed diabetic regimen and one consequence was frequent hospitalizations for treatment of diabetic coma. When the nurse finally questioned the parents about their perceptions of their child's health condition, she discovered that they were not ready to accept the diagnosis as permanent. Denying the diagnosis was their way of coping with it. The nurse had to help the parents handle their feelings of guilt and anger before she could discuss treatment plans with them.

The family-centered nursing process facilitates the analysis of psychosocial influences as well as physiological ones. Looking more closely at the

TABLE 8-1 Relationships among the phases of the family-centered nursing process

Assessing	Analyzing	Planning	Implementing	Evaluating	Terminating
Process for obtaining a data base	A cognitive data-ordering process for the purpose of identifying nursing diagnoses	Formulation of desired family outcomes (goals) and identification of actions (intervention strategies) to achieve goals	A systematic approach to action used by the family and nurse to achieve desired family outcomes	A continuous, concurrent process used to critique each component of the nursing process	A therapeutic process that helps the client and the nurse to end their relationship

Triangle of family health

Assessing

1. Develop a trusting relationship
   a. Explain purpose of community health nursing visit
   b. Describe what community health nurse has to offer
   c. Facilitate the sharing of thoughts, feelings, and data
   d. Set time parameters for evaluation and frequency and length of visits

Analyzing

1. Make differential conclusions about family needs by:
   a. Using theoretical knowledge to identify significant signs and symptoms
   b. Grouping data to show relationships between assessment categories and to identify *patterns* of behavior
   c. Relating family

Planning

1. Consider three key principles:
   a. Individualization of client care plans
   b. Active client participation
   c. Client's right of self-determination
2. Formulate client-centered goals and objectives
   a. Establish realistic goals consistent with the data base and nursing diagnoses

Implementing

1. Base nursing actions on data obtained during the assessment phase; family needs, knowledge receptivity, and level of understanding
   a. Demonstrate awareness of proper timing when carrying out intervention activities
   b. Adapt or modify intervention

Evaluating

1. Elicit ongoing feedback from client to determine if goals, plans, and interventions are appropriate
2. Identify the results of intervention activities taken by:
   a. Client
   b. Community health nurse
   c. Other health care professionals
3. Determine why intervention activities have been

Terminating

1. Deal with feelings associated with termination
2. Review client achievements
3. Discuss what the therapeutic process has meant
4. Plan carefully the termination of visits
5. Share with client how to

2. Collect data in variety of ways
   a. Observation
   b. Interview
   c. Inspection
   d. Contact with secondary sources
   e. Review of records
3. Assess all parameters of family functioning
   a. Family dynamics
   b. Health status— individual family members
   c. Physiological data
   d. Psychosocial data
   e. Sociocultural data
   f. Environmental data
   g. Preventive health practices
4. Obtain data from multiple sources
   a. Client, family
   b. Health team members
   c. Community agencies
   d. Significant others
   e. Relevant records
5. Use standards of care to focus the interviewing process (refer to Chapter 22)

data to relevant clinical and research findings
   d. Comparing nursing diagnoses with diagnoses of other health professionals
2. Formulate specific nursing diagnoses
   a. Base diagnoses on a strong data base
   b. Identify the functional aspects of a client's current health status
   c. Determine various levels of family functioning
      (1) Strengths
      (2) Needs
      (3) Anticipatory guidance warranted
   d. Identify when data are insufficient to make a nursing diagnosis

   b. State goals and objectives in specific, achievable, and measurable terms
   c. Develop goals and objectives in collaboration with the family (contracting)
   d. Identify family as well as individual goals and objectives
   e. Formulate cognitive, affective, and psychomotor objectives when appropriate
   f. Distinguish between nurse-focused goals and client-focused goals
3. Identify alternative intervention strategies
   a. Identify various intervention activities based on assessment data, nursing diagnoses, and client goals and objectives
   b. Determine activities which the client, the nurse, and other health professionals might carry out to help the client to achieve desired goals and objectives

strategies when client situation changes
   c. Modify activities to accommodate factors in the home
2. Recognize social, cultural, economic, and environmental barriers, and work within these limitations (refer to Chapter 9)
3. Carry through with planned interventions
   a. Performing nursing care activities
   b. Engaging the family in the referral process
   c. Implementing teaching, learning plans
   d. Helping family to problem solve
   e. Providing supportive intervention
   f. Keeping appointments with the family
4. Base intervention activities on scientific principles and knowledge
   a. Review literature to obtain knowledge in relation to content being taught or situation being encountered

ineffective, if warranted
4. Modify the management plan when appropriate
5. Use a variety of methods to evaluate
   a. Obtain feedback from client
   b. Consult with peers, supervisors, and other health care professionals
   c. Summarize records
   d. Conduct nursing audits (refer to Chapter 22)

restablish contact if needed
6. Discuss with client self-care requirements upon discharge

Continued.

TABLE 8-1 Relationships among the phases of the family-centered nursing process—cont'd

Assessing	Analyzing	Planning	Implementing	Evaluating	Terminating
		c. Identify pros and cons of each intervention strategy d. Assist the client in identifying alternative courses of action and in making decisions about actions to be implemented 4. Establish priorities in relation to client goals and intervention strategies a. Differentiate between problems that need immediate action and those that can wait b. Consider the health and safety of the client c. Use theory and the family data base to identify potential crisis situations 5. Identify criteria for evaluating goal attainment	b. Consult with peers, supervisor, and other health care professionals to expand knowledge and to evaluate appropriateness of nursing interventions		

nursing process, the reader can find that it consists of the following six phases:

- Assessing
- Analyzing
- Planning
- Implementing
- Evaluating
- Terminating

Although each phase is discussed separately, it should be remembered that they interrelate and overlap. The interrelated nature of these phases, along with nursing activities during each phase, is presented in Table 8-1. When examining this diagram, it is important to note the relationships between the data-collection phase and the triangle of family health. Collected data should always be validated with the family before nursing diagnoses, goals, and intervention strategies are formulated. The family-centered nursing process is a client-oriented not a nurse-oriented process.

THEORY GUIDES PRACTICE

The ANA (1986) standards of community health nursing practice specify that "the nurse applies theoretical concepts as a basis for decisions in practice" (p. 5). In order to function effectively in community health, the nurse must integrate skills and knowledge relevant to both nursing and public health (ANA, 1986, p. 1). Public health knowledge includes concepts from epidemiology, biostatistics, environmental health, social sciences, and public health administration. Core concepts from the epidemiological model (host, agent, and environment) and levels of prevention (primary, secondary, and tertiary) guide public health practice.

Historically, the major focus of epidemiology was on the investigation of epidemics or disease outbreaks. Today, public health professionals examine variables that keep people healthy, as well as factors that cause the occurrence of disease and unhealthy conditions. Concepts from epidemiology help the nurse to identify at-risk clients (individuals, families, and communities) for the purposes of identifying or preventing disease and

rehabilitating clients with active disease or disability. During the assessment phase of the nursing process, nurses complete a health risk appraisal. As previously discussed, a *health risk appraisal* is a process whereby data are collected and analyzed to identify characteristics which may make clients vulnerable to illness, premature death, or unhealthy conditions (e.g., hereditary links to disease such as diabetes; behaviors which increase the potential for disease occurrence or premature death; and risk factors related to unhealthy conditions such as child maltreatment). Once a risk profile is established, nurses initiate educational strategies to help clients acquire knowledge about ways to reduce health risks. The at-risk concept and other epidemiological concepts are discussed extensively in Chapter 10.

Nursing conceptualizations focus on four essential concepts—person, environment, health, and nursing (Fawcett, 1984; Flaskerudt and Halloran, 1980). Nursing models specify the nursing perspective related to these concepts and their interrelatedness. A nursing "conceptual model comprises abstract, general concepts, and statements that describe and link the concepts. Each conceptual model of nursing represents a particular frame of reference within which patients (persons/clients), their environments and health states, and nursing activities are viewed, and thus it presents a comprehensive holistic view of nursing care" (Fawcett and Carino, 1989, p. 2).

Several nursing models have been developed in an attempt to capture a comprehensive, holistic view of nursing care. They have met with varying degrees of success. Examples of such models include Johnson's Behavioral System Model, King's Conceptual Framework of Nursing, Neuman's Health Care Systems, Orem's Self-Care Framework, Rogers' Science of Unitary Human Beings, Roy's Adaptation Model, White's Model for Public Health Nursing Practice (refer to Chapter 2) and Anderson's Community as Client Model (refer to Chapter 3). Although most of the nursing models focus on the individual as the unit of analysis, rather than the family and the community, some concepts being advanced by nurse theorists can be applied in the community health nursing

TABLE 8-2   Examples of nursing theory bases applicable to community health nursing

Applicable content	Name of nursing theory base	Primary author	Nursing examples
Client's self-care ability changing with state of health	Self-Care Framework	Orem, 1971, 1980, 1985; Orem and Taylor, 1986	Blazek and McCaellen, 1983; Bliss-Holtz, 1988; Campbell, 1986; Chang, Uman, Linn, Ware and Kane, 1985; Galli, 1984; Hanchett, 1988; Harper, 1984; Kearney and Fleisher, 1979; Kruger, Shawver, and Jones, 1980; Maunz and Woods, 1988; Michael and Sewall, 1980; Nunn and Marriner-Tomey, 1989; Pridham, 1971; Walborn, 1980
Maintaining stressors within client's adaptation Interdependence and role function modes of person re family	Adaptation Model	Roy, 1970, 1976, 1983, 1984, 1987, 1988; Roy and Roberts, 1981	Fawcett, 1981; Hanchett, 1988; Kehoe, 1981; Limandri, 1986; Schmitz, 1980, Wagner, 1976
Primary, secondary, tertiary prevention Lines of defense	Health Care Systems Model	Neuman, 1972, 1980, 1982, 1989	Beitler, Tkachuck, and Aamodt, 1980; Benedict and Sproles, 1982; Bigbee, 1984; Buchanan, 1987; Hoch, 1987; Pinkerton, 1974; Story and Ross, 1986; West, 1984
Holistic health Time perception	Science of Unitary Human Beings	Rogers, 1970, 1980, 1983, 1986, 1987	Boyd, 1985; Fawcett, 1977; Hanchett, 1979, 1988; Laffrey, 1985; Levine, 1976; Rawnsley, 1977; Whall, 1981; Wood and Kekahbah, 1985

Developed by J. Atwood, Professor and Director, NRSA Pre- and Post-Doctoral Institutional Instrumentation Fellowship Program, College of Nursing and Cancer Prevention and Control, Behavioral Sciences Coordinator, Arizona Cancer Center, University of Arizona, Tucson, Az, 1990.

arena (refer to Table 8-2). Recent work has begun to provide an understanding of conceptual nursing models as they relate to the community as client (Hanchett, 1988) and the family as client (Clements and Roberts, 1983; Hanson, 1984; Riehl-Sisca, 1985; Whall, 1981, 1987).

Community health nursing focuses on the three levels of prevention (primary, secondary, and tertiary), values the holistic nature of humankind, and recognizes the importance of increasing a client's self-care capabilities to promote independence. Community health nurses use a variety of assessment strategies to obtain a holisitc perspective about an individual's health status and family dynamics, including a family's role functions and interdependence behaviors (refer to Chapter 6). Based on assessment data, commu-

nity health nurses implement intervention strategies that assist clients in maintaining stress at a functional level (within a client's adaptation zone or lines of defense). For example, they coordinate resources for clients who are experiencing stress to decrease the input clients must handle.

Since a comprehensive discussion about nursing theory is beyond the scope of this text, the reader is encouraged to examine writings by the primary author to obtain an accurate understanding of the theoretical and conceptual bases in each nursing model. Examining how others have discussed the application of these models in practice, research and education can also be beneficial. Table 8-2 provides nursing examples related to community health nursing practice which have applied nursing theory.

PHASES OF THE FAMILY-CENTERED NURSING PROCESS

It may be found that phases and terms within the nursing process are labeled differently from what the reader has seen before. There are hundreds of books and articles written on the nursing process, and terminology varies from one author to another. The dispute over terminology serves to confuse practitioners and makes it difficult to recognize that it is the *process,* not the terminology, that is significant. Focusing on the process aspects of the phases as they are discussed will allow the reader to effectively implement the family-centered nursing process regardless of the terminology used in different practice settings.

Assessing

The assessment phase involves a systematic data collection process which provides the foundation for making nursing diagnoses. During this phase, the community health nurse places emphasis on collecting specific data about client (family) functioning so that objective conclusions regarding the client's health status can be made. Inferences about a client's level of functioning should only be made after a sufficient data base has been obtained.

The primary responsibilities of the community health nurse during the assessment phase are threefold: (1) developing a trusting, therapeutic relationship; (2) using a variety of data collection methods to obtain client information from all available resources; and (3) assessing all parameters of family health, including family dynamics, family resources, health status of individual family members, and environmental factors which influence family health. Careful attention given to all three of these activities helps the community health nurse to clearly delineate client needs and goals and intervention strategies which may enhance client growth.

First Home Visits

"Home visiting is a long-established method of helping families cope with changes in their lives" (National Commission to Prevent Infant Mortal-ity, 1989, p. 1). Despite a recent trend emphasizing population-based interventions such as groupwork and clinic or school services, home visiting continues to be a significant component of community health nursing practice. In the home health care setting, it is the principal means by which community health nurses provide services for clients and their families.

Making first home visits to families can be stressful, especially for a nurse entering an unknown environment which is controlled by the client rather than the health care professional. First home visits can also be challenging, particularly if the nurse recognizes that he or she is providing a valuable service. In general, families are receptive and interested in the services community health nurses have to offer. There may be times, however, when a family prefers to handle its health care needs within the family unit without assistance from "outsiders." If this is the preferred family pattern of functioning, the community health nurse accepts the family's decision and does not view this as a personal failure. Sometimes families do not appear interested in home visits because they are unaware of how a community health nurse may assist them. A nurse who is clear about his or her role, and who relates role responsibilities to the family situation can often help families recognize the value of home visits. For example, when community health nurses receive a referral for antepartum follow-up on a low-income family, they frequently share with these families that they can assist them in using community resources which would be helpful to them.

First home visits can influence families' receptivity to future home visits. Carefully planned first visits can facilitate relationship building and assist nurses to demonstrate the contributions they can make in helping families to deal with their current health needs. Table 8-3 outlines how to prepare for a first home visit, tasks to initiate during the visit, and postvisit activities. The goals for the first visit should be to establish a positive client/nurse working relationship, obtain baseline data on the family, and address the immediate concerns of the family. The extent to which one carries out

TABLE 8-3 First home visits: responsibilities and tasks

Responsibility	*Tasks*
I. Previsit preparation	Review available family data including referral information and previous family records.
	Clarify data with others if unclear (e.g., contact family physician and/or other referral sources or talk with intake nurse).
	Establish a plan for the visit.
	Consider appropriate community resources.
	Review theory related to identified family problems.
II. Establish contact with family	Contact family via the phone, if available.
	Identify self, including name and agency you are representing.
	Explain who referred family to agency and purpose of referral.
	Discuss briefly services CHN can provide such as sharing data about available community resources.
	Identify family's need for CHN services and willingness to have nurse visits.
	Schedule home visit at a time convenient for family.
III. Home visit intervention A. Relationship-building period	Introduce self and role.
	Introduce agency, agency obligations, and programs and services.
	Explain purpose of home visit.
	Build a nurse/client relationship.
	Discuss client rights and responsibilities.
	Assess safety of care plan: Is a primary caregiver present and available if needed?
B. Intervention period	Carry out a client assessment.
	Carry out a family assessment.
	Carry out an environmental assessment, especially in relation to client safety and health needs.
	Elicit family's perceptions of how a CHN can assist.
	Assess doctor's orders and need for changes if appropriate.
	Assess appropriateness of stated third-party reimbursement.
	Assess need for other services such as physical therapy or referral to a community agency for parenting classes.
	Assess need for equipment and supplies.
	Confirm medication orders, dosages, and client knowledge of medications.
	Identify client's knowledge base related to identified problems (e.g., disease process or care of infant).
	Discuss estimated length of service.
C. Closing period	Summarize visit activities with family.
	Together decide what the client/family will be doing between now and the next visit.
	Inform client/family how to reach nurse between visits.
	Set time for next visit.

TABLE 8-3 First home visits: responsibilities and tasks—cont'd

Responsibility	*Tasks*
IV. Postvisit activities	Begin the nursing care plan.
	Document visit.
	Make contacts on behalf of client/family if needed (e.g., initiate other services, contact physician regarding needed change in order, or inform vendors about needed equipment and supplies).
	Complete agency reporting forms and paperwork for third-party reimbursement.
	Evaluate visit progress.

the tasks identified in Table 8-3 during the initial visit will vary depending on the family's circumstances. Some tasks will not be done at all, because they are not appropriate for the client's situation. For example, doctor's orders are not required for families receiving only health promotion services. On the other hand, nurses do not provide home health or care of the sick services without a doctor's order. It is critical to remember that the assessment phase of the nursing process is ongoing and should extend throughout the length of the nurse/client relationship. *It is not feasible or appropriate to obtain all needed data during the initial contact.*

Community health nurses encounter a variety of situations on first home visits, such as families who want parenting education or elderly couples who have requested assistance with care of an ill family member. While the major focus on these visits may vary from care of the sick to health teaching, the provision of health promotion services is a primary component of all community health nursing visits. Health promotion activities should not be neglected during care of the sick visits. Examples of health promotion interventions implemented during these type of visits are teaching to increase the client's self-care capabilities, environmental assessment to prevent home accidents and referral for respite services to prevent caregiver burnout.

Relationship Building

The type of relationship established during the assessment phase can be the critical factor in helping the client determine whether or not to accept

the assistance offered by the community health nurse. It is natural for clients to evaluate their interactions with community health nurses during the assessment phase. Most people take time to assess how others respond to them before they develop a trusting relationship which allows disclosure of personal thoughts, feelings, and problems.

Explaining the purpose of community health nursing visits, describing services the community health nurse can provide, and fostering a nonthreatening atmosphere which allows the client to share data at his or her own pace often promote trust between the nurse and the client. Clarifying why the community health nurse is visiting is essential. When clients do not understand the purpose of nursing visits, it is hard for them to become involved in the therapeutic process. Lack of clarity in the therapeutic relationship can result in frustration and mistrust and inhibit the expression of thoughts, feelings, and data. Clients usually do not share information freely until they understand why the information is needed.

Sharing with clients their rights and responsibilities and agency obligations can help to clarify the purpose of home visits. All clients have the right to be active participants in the care process, including continuity of care decisions, and to have their privacy and property respected. They also have the right to voice complaints without fear of reprisal. Table 8-4 delineates specific client rights and responsibilities and related agency obligations as defined by the Health Care Financing Administration (HCFA) and the National Association for Home Care (NAHC).

Clients are more likely to develop a trusting re-

TABLE 8-4 Client rights and responsibilities and related agency obligations

Rights/obligations	Client rights	Agency obligations
Notice of rights	To be fully informed of all his or her rights and responsibilities	Provide client with a written notice of rights in advance of initiating care.
		Obtain signed verification from client or client's caregiver that they have received written notice of rights.
Exercise of rights and respect for property and person	Have property treated with respect	Investigate complaints made by client or client's family or guardian.
	Voice grievances and suggest change in service without fear of reprisal or discrimination	Document existence of complaint and resolution of complaint.
	Have family or guardian voice grievances when judged incompetent	
	Right to privacy	
To be informed and to participate in planning care and treatment	Receive appropriate and professional care related to physician orders.	Admit client for service only if the agency has the ability to provide safe professional care at the level of intensity needed.
	Choice of care provided	Share with client physician orders.
	Receive information necessary to give informed consent prior to the starting of any care	Advise client in advance of care, the disciplines that will furnish care and the frequency of visits.
	Know how to reach agency staff 24 hours a day, 7 days a week, and what to do in an emergency	Advise client in advance of any changes in care.
	Refuse treatment within the confines of the law and to be informed of the consequences of this action	Involve client in the planning of care.
	Reasonable continuity of care	Inform client of agency policies and procedures.
	To be informed in reasonable time of anticipated termination of service and plans for transfer to another agency	
Confidentiality of medical record	Agency maintains confidentiality of the clinical records	Advise client of agency's policies and procedures regarding disclosure of information in clinical records.
Liability for payment	Receive information regarding charges for services, the client's potential liability for these charges, and client's eligibility for third party reimbursements	Inform client orally and in writing and in advance of care the extent to which third party reimbursement may pay for care and charges client may have to pay.
	Right of referral if service denied solely on the inability to pay for service	Notify client orally and in writing changes in eligibility for services from third party reimbursement.
Home health hotline	Know about the availability of a toll-free HHA hotline in the state to voice complaints about agency services or to have questions answered about home care	Inform client in writing how to reach the home health hotline.

From Health Care Financing Administration (HCFA): Conditions of participation: home health agencies, 42CFR Part 484, Sections 484.1 through 484.52, Washington, DC, October 1989, Department of Health and Human Services, Section 484.10; and National Association for Home Care (NAHC): Code of ethics, Washington, DC, 1982, The Association, pp 1-2.

lationship with professionals who are open and honest and who show a genuine concern for their welfare than with professionals who do not demonstrate these characteristics. An interview style which reflects sensitivity, a nonjudgmental, accepting attitude, and a respect for the client's rights facilitates the development of a trusting relationship. A skillful interviewer avoids barriers to communication such as false reassurance, advice giving, excessive talking, and the showing of approval or disapproval. At times, this is not easy. For example, when families are under stress they may press for advice. Frequently a family member will say, "What would you do if you were me?" An empathic interviewer responds to the family's feelings of distress but supports its ability to make its own decisions. Advice giving can lead to an unhealthy dependency.

The community health nurse needs to be careful not to foster inappropriate dependency. However, it is important to realize that interdependency is not negative and that clients may request assistance with problem solving. A mature adult *recognizes* and *acts* on the need for support, caring, and assistance from others while maintaining independent decision making. Sometimes a professional's fear of dependency can be detrimental to the client-professional relationship. It can prevent the professional from demonstrating to clients a genuine interest in helping.

Numerous books discuss interviewing techniques that promote a therapeutic relationship. Readers are encouraged to examine various theoretical viewpoints of counseling in order to determine which style fits their needs. Whatever interviewing or counseling style is used, however, it must be individualized for each unique client. For example, some individuals do not verbalize spontaneously: they share what they feel is important to share and then are silent until further information is requested. A nurse who firmly believes in a nondirective approach would have difficulty relating to such clients, if he or she did not adjust the interviewing style.

Family Interviews

Working with families presents special interviewing challenges for the community health nurse be-

cause families are composed of several "unique" individuals who have varying needs, concerns, and communication styles. Since the goal of community health nursing service is to help the family as a unit, rather than to help each individual family member separately, the nurse must become a "third ear of the family, listening for the effect of a person's statements on other people" (Haley, 1971, p. 281). The nurse needs to facilitate effective interaction between all family members in order to promote the family's nurturing and decision-making processes. At times this can be difficult, especially when there are conflicting interests that need to be negotiated between individual family members.

When a nurse is allowed to cross the family boundaries and is accepted by the family system, the influences the nurse has on that system must be examined carefully. The nurse needs to watch closely her or his own interactions with the family, as well as interactions between individual family members. Haley suggests that counselors (nurses) should view themselves as part of the "diagnostic unit because the way the family is behaving is influenced by the ways the counselor (nurse) deals with them" (Haley, 1971, p. 282). Nurse bias in family counseling can disrupt the family system. Sills (1975, p. 16) believes "bias occurs when there is unwitting or unintentional and unwanted social influence introduced into the family therapy session by the therapist." From clinical practice she has developed three categories of bias which negatively influence family functioning. These are "coalition biases, dynamic biases, and social biases" (Sills, 1975, p. 17).

Coalition biases occur when a nurse unknowingly forms an alliance with one family member and closes out other family members. Age and sex of the nurse and identification with the labeled client can influence the development of such coalitions within the family system (Sills, 1975, p. 18). For instance, a nurse who firmly believes that all women need a career outside the home may strongly support a female client's desires to work without allowing her husband to verbalize his concerns. This may disrupt joint decision making for the couple.

It is particularly easy for community health

nurses to form coalition biases because they are not always able to see the entire family unit together. When interviewing only one family member, it can be difficult not to take sides. Taking sides is not therapeutic, however, because it may reinforce dysfunctional family patterns. If the family is having difficulty negotiating conflicting issues, it does not help the family to deal with these issues when the nurse supports one member's viewpoint. This type of behavior by the nurse only serves to give one family member ammunition to use against other family members, which in turn discourages analysis of all viewpoints and family decision making. If communication, decision-making, or relationship difficulties are presented as the major family concern, every effort should be made by the community health nurse to see all family members together.

Dynamic biases may result when a nurse attempts to change his or her theoretical orientation about family counseling. For example, in moving from a concept of a "problem" family member to a concept that views the family system as the "problem," a nurse may unintentionally focus on a "problem" family member before becoming comfortable with the systems approach. In addition, a nurse who acts on intuitive diagnoses without confirming them by collected data from the family is engaging in a dynamic bias (Sills, 1975, p. 20). Inappropriate methods of professional intervention result from this type of action. One community health nurse, for instance, felt a mother needed nutritional counseling after she observed one family meal and discovered that a child in this family had severe nutritional anemia. She later found out that this child refused to eat solid foods. The mother had a good understanding of the "basic four," but needed assistance with feeding techniques and child discipline.

Social biases stem from the "social positions and social roles that the therapist occupies in addition to his professional role" (Sills, 1975, p. 21). Nurses who are wives and mothers or husbands and fathers develop their own perceptions of how these roles should be implemented. Unconsciously, they may label behavior as dysfunctional if it does not correspond with their role perceptions.

Values, attitudes, and beliefs can and frequently do influence the dynamic interactive processes that occur between people. Use of peer collaboration, professional supervision, and self-scrutiny helps the professional nurse to identify when personal values, attitudes, and beliefs are adversely affecting the therapeutic process. It is not uncommon for families to be viewed as "hopeless" because they do not change in the way professionals would like them to change. When this happens, both nurses and clients become frustrated. An objective third party (colleague, supervisor, or consultant) can often help professionals to identify why frustration occurs in the therapeutic process and how to alter their perceptions of the situation.

Sources and Methods for Collecting Data

During the assessment phase, both primary and secondary data are collected from all available sources to determine how well the client is coping with the encountered stressors. Primary data are those data which the community health nurse actually obtains from the client or sees, hears, feels, or smells in the client's environment. An astute community health nurse carefully notes observations as well as verbal information received from the client. It is often found that significant clues about a client's level of functioning are obtained by observing how the client interacts with the environment. It is not unusual for the community health nurse to discern a child discipline problem by repeatedly watching parents interact with their children during home visits. When a nurse observes client functioning, it is important to remember that inferences about client problems should be based on *patterns* of behavior rather than isolated incidents of behavior. Labeling behavior dysfunctional after one observation is a dangerous practice and can adversely affect the nurse-client relationship.

In the community health setting, secondary data are obtained from a variety of sources such as significant others, personnel from health and social agencies, the family's physician, spiritual leaders, and health records. When these data are recorded, the source of the information should also be recorded. Generally, the community health nurse receives either verbal or written permission from the client before making contact with secondary sources of data outside the family system. This practice not only protects the client's right of privacy, but also promotes honesty and trust in the therapeutic relationship. In addition, seeking a client's permission to obtain information from others demonstrates to the client that the nurse does respect the client's right of self-determination.

When using secondary data, the nurse must recognize that this type of data may not accurately reflect *clients' perceptions* of themselves or their needs. Instead, secondary data may reflect what others perceive about clients and their needs. This point is particularly significant for a community health nurse to keep in mind, because frequently secondary data about the problems of family members are obtained when these individuals are not present. When this occurs, the community health nurse often finds it necessary to make arrangements to obtain primary data. She or he may visit a child in school or schedule a home visit after school hours in order to identify how this child is reacting to a newly diagnosed health problem.

Various assessment methodologies should be used to collect primary and secondary data. Interview, observation, direct examination (auscultation, percussion, palpation, inspection, and measurement), contact with secondary sources of data, and review of relevant records are methods used by the community health nurse to obtain an accurate and a complete profile of a client's situation. These methods are used to identify client *strengths* as well as client needs.

The significance of utilizing a variety of methods to collect data about family functioning cannot be overstated. No one data collection method provides the community health nurse with all the information needed to formulate accurate nursing diagnoses. The Daniels family case situation which follows illustrates this fact by showing the difference between the type of data one nurse obtained from interview and from direct observation.

Following hospitalization of Mr. Daniels for an acute exacerbation episode of multiple sclerosis, the Daniels family was referred to the health department for health supervision follow-up. Ms. Garitt, hospital social worker, requested that a community health nurse assess this family's needs in relation to its understanding of multiple sclerosis, its ability to handle activities of daily living, and its knowledge of community resources. While Jane Mathews, CHN, was interviewing the family and collecting data on the entire family situation, she asked Mr. and Mrs. Daniels how they were managing Mr. Daniels' exercises. Both related that they were doing them regularly. Mrs. Daniels accurately described how the exercises should be done and verbalized that she felt comfortable handling them, since she was instructed how to do so by hospital staff. While Mrs. Daniels was demonstrating what she had learned, it was found that she did have an understanding about the proper exercises for her husband. However, her body mechanics were inappropriate and this caused severe backache which she failed to mention during the interviewing process. In addition to Mrs. Daniels' poor body mechanics, the nurse also discovered that Mr. Daniels was very demanding of his wife, expecting her to do exercises for him that he could do independently. Further exploration revealed that Mr. Daniels was doing very little for himself. Before his illness he had been the "man of the house. Now I can't do anything." Through demonstration and return demonstration, the nurse showed Mr. Daniels that he was not helpless and assisted Mrs. Daniels in learning how to position herself appropriately when helping her husband.

If the community health nurse, in the above situation, had not observed Mr. and Mrs. Daniels's functioning, it could have taken her a considerable length of time to collect the data needed to accurately identify the real concerns in this family situation. Observing family interactions provided this nurse with data about family functioning that were not obtained through interview.

Assessing All Parameters of Family Health

The family-centered approach to nursing care focuses on the family as a "unit of people," rather than a collection of individual family members. This implies that the family is viewed as a system, in which the actions and health status of one family member always affect the behavior and health status of all other family members. Thus, when

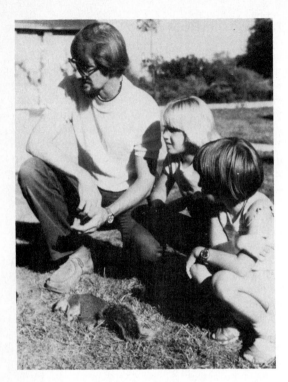

Figure 8-4 Family dynamics influence how well individual family members handle critical life events. The ability to provide support and security during times of stress (the loss of a loved one) is a family strength which should be reinforced.

community health nurses assess family health, they not only examine the health status of individual family members but look at *family dynamics* as well (refer to Figure 8-4). Chapter 6 presents guidelines for examining family dynamics and includes a family assessment tool (refer to Appendix 6-2) which facilitates the collection of family functioning data.

Family dynamics. To discern functional and dysfunctional characteristics of family dynamics, a community health nurse must establish criteria for evaluating family health to use for comparison purposes. In addition, a community health nurse must identify what type of data are needed for analyzing family functioning in order to focus assessment procedures. As previously mentioned, a conceptual framework should be used to organize the collection of family functioning data. It is also

important to remember that if major emphasis is placed on the biological aspects of a family's health status during the beginning phase of a relationship, it may be difficult to refocus the family when the nurse wants to assess other parameters of family functioning. Explaining early in the therapeutic process why data about family dynamics are needed facilitates the collection of this type of information.

Identifying criteria for evaluating "family health" involves a process where one examines one's conceptual beliefs about health and about people and then delineates specific behaviors which reflect healthy functioning in relation to the family. Throughout this text, emphasis has been placed on viewing health "not merely as the absence of disease, but as a state of complete physical, mental, and social well-being" (WHO, 1947). Dunn (1961), in his classic writings, focused on wellness when discussing the concept of complete well-being. He believed that implicit in this concept is the idea of high-level wellness, which he defines as "an integrated method of functioning which is oriented toward maximizing the potential of which the individual is capable, within the environment where he is functioning." He saw wellness as being influenced by variables which are both internal and external to individual systems. "Well being both in body and mind and within the family and within community life should be interrelated in order for the individual to achieve a zest for life." Wellness, according to Dunn, is a dynamic state, "ever-changing in its characteristics." "What is complete today, may be incomplete tomorrow" (Dunn, 1961, pp. 2-4). This implies that one always has the potential for growth, a philosophy which promotes a humanistic or caring approach to all humankind. It is believed by the authors that all clients should be approached in this way.

Inherent in Dunn's concept of "high-level wellness" for an individual is a conceptualization of family health. He saw the individual being influenced by his "inner and outer [family] worlds" (Dunn, 1961, p. 25). Because families are responsible for meeting the needs of their individual family members, as well as for maintaining a

TABLE 8-5 Criteria to consider when assessing "healthy" family functioning: three authors' viewpoints

Assessment parameters	Authors		
	Otto (1963): Family strengths	Pratt (1976): Family structure and health behavior characterizing the energized family	Curran (1983): Traits of a healthy family
Adaptive abilities	The ability to provide for the physical, emotional, and spiritual needs of a family The ability to use a crisis or seemingly injurious experience as a means of growth Ability for self-help, and ability to accept help when appropriate An ability to perform family roles flexibly The ability to communicate effectively	Combined health behaviors of all family members are energized; all family members tend to care for their health Actively and energetically attempt to cope with life's problems and issues Flexible division of tasks and activities	The healthy family admits to and seeks help with problems The healthy family communicates and listens
Atmosphere and affect	The ability to be sensitive to the needs of family members The ability to provide support, security, and encouragement	Responsive to the particular interests and needs of individual family members Regular and varied interaction among family members	The healthy family teaches respect for others The healthy family has a sense of play and humor The healthy family shares leisure time The healthy family fosters table time and conversation
Individual autonomy and integrity of family system	Mutual respect for the individuality of family members A concern for family unity, loyalty, and interfamily cooperation	Egalitarian distribution of power Provide autonomy for individual family members	The healthy family respects the privacy of individual members The healthy family affirms and supports individual members The healthy family maintains a balance of interaction among members The healthy family has a strong sense of family in which rituals and traditions abound The healthy family exhibits a sense of shared responsibility The healthy family develops a sense of trust The healthy family has a shared religious core
Relationships with others	The ability to initiate and maintain growth-producing relationships and experiences within and without the family The capacity to maintain and create constructive and responsible relationships in the neighborhood, school, town, and local and state government	Provide regular links with the broader community through active participation in community activities	The healthy family values service to others The healthy family teaches a sense of right and wrong

Adapted from Otto H: Criteria for assessing family strength, Family Process, 2:333-336, 1963; Pratt L: Family structure and effective health behavior: the energized family, Boston, 1976, Houghton Mifflin, pp 84-92; Curran D: Traits of a healthy family, copyright by Doris Curran, Minneapolis Mn, 1983, Winston Press, pp 23-24. All rights reserved. Used with permission.

functional family unit, family health can be defined as:

"An integrated method of functioning which is oriented toward maximizing the potential" (Dunn, 1961, p. 4) of individual family members throughout the life-span while maintaining the integrity of the family as a system.

To be useful for comparison purposes, this global definition of family health must be translated into criteria which identify growth-producing family behaviors. Potential for growth is unique for each individual and each family unit. Client behavior must be analyzed from the client's perspective, because dysfunctional or maladaptive behavior in one family can be functional or adaptive in another. The family's perceptions about how well it is functioning must be the key factor which helps a nurse to determine whether or not a family is reaching its potential. If the family's perceptions are not understood, the community health nurse cannot influence a family to alter these perceptions.

Reviewing writings by Beavers (1977), Curran (1983), Lewis, Beavers, Gossett, and Phillips (1976), Otto (1963), and Pratt (1976), and examining the Family Coping Index, a tool developed by the Richmond-Hopkins Cooperative Nursing Study (Freeman and Lowe, 1964), will help the reader to delineate criteria for evaluating family health. The similarities between these authors' findings are striking. Flexible role patterns, responsiveness to the needs of individual members, active problem-solving mechanisms, ability to accept help, open communication patterns, and the provision of a warm, caring atmosphere were some of the main commonalities found in healthy families in these authors' studies. Table 8-5 presents an outline of the specific variables identified by Otto, Pratt, and Curran. Although these variables are not intended to be normative, they do provide guidelines for data comparison purposes.

Since culture affects how one perceives health and illness and the manner in which clients seek health care, it is important to examine the family's cultural beliefs, values, and practices when assessing family functioning. "Cultural assessments are performed to identify patterns that may assist or interfere with a nursing intervention or treatment regimen" (Tripp-Reimer, Brink and Saunders, 1984, p. 81). Cultural assessments help the community health nurse to individualize the nursing care plan for each family. Chapter 6 provides guidelines for completing a cultural assessment.

Individual functioning. The purpose of a family health assessment is to obtain pertinent data about the functioning of individual family members as well as the family system. In keeping with the view of health presented above, family members are viewed from an integrated, holistic, individual perspective. Biological, psychological, sociocultural, spiritual, developmental, and environmental parameters of functioning are assessed in order to determine the client's perception of his or her health status.

In general, clients do not think systematically about all the variables that affect their health. A major role of the community health nurse when completing an individual health assessment is to increase the client's awareness of all the factors that influence healthy functioning. A health assessment should be purposeful, meaningful, and goal directed and should provide the client with an opportunity to identify both personal strengths and needs in relation to the individual's current level of functioning. Data about preventive health practices and healthy aspects of coping along with information about ways in which the client handles illness should be elicited.

The vehicles used for organizing an individual functional assessment are the health history and the physical examination. Exploring the techniques of physical appraisal is beyond the scope of this text. Writings by Bowers and Thompson (1988); Fox (1981); Guzzetta, Bunton, Prinkey, Sherer, and Seifert (1989); and Malasanos, Barkauskas, and Stoltenberg-Allen (1989) discuss extensively the physical examination process. It is essential for community health nurses to have skill in completing a gross physical appraisal, since clients may not have a regular source of medical care even though they may have health problems. Community health nurses must have the ability to distinguish between *abnormal* and *normal* health findings. Price and Wilson (1986) provide a theoretical basis for analyzing health assessment findings. In addition community health nurses need skill in the use of the referral process (refer to Chapter 9) in order to help clients obtain needed health care services when abnormal findings are identified.

"A nursing health history differs from a medical health history in that it focuses on the meaning of illness and hospitalization [health care] to the patient [client] and his family as a basis for planning nursing care. The medical history is taken to determine whether pathology is present as a basis for planning medical care" (McPhetridge, 1968, p. 68). When completing a health history, the community health nurse explores carefully the client's perceptions of his or her health status and how current stressors are affecting functioning; emphasis is placed on identifying the client as a *unique individual* rather than as a person who has a specific disease process.

Components included in a health history vary slightly from one author to another. Basically, the goal of a health history is to determine how well the client is meeting health needs and how activities of daily living have been altered to meet these needs. A comprehensive review of the client's past and current health status is elicited to identify an accurate and complete composite of the client's health functioning. With this information, the client and the nurse can explore ways for increasing the client's self-care capabilities.

Mahoney, Verdisco, and Shortridge (1982, pp. 6-7) identify the following seven components of an individual health history:

1. *Reason for contact:* Why the client is seeking help at this time
2. *Biographical data:* Structural variables common to all clients such as name, age, sex, marital status, religious preference, ethnic background, educational level, occupational status, health insurance, and social security information
3. *Current health status:* The client's perceptions of his or her health, with a specific delineation of current complaints and activities of daily living

4. *Past health history:* Data relative to the previous health or illness state of the client and contact with health care professionals, including a description of developmental accomplishments, health practices, known illnesses, allergies, restorative treatment, and social activities such as foreign travel which might be related to the client's current health status
5. *Family history:* A description of the current health status of each family member, relationships among family members, and a genetic history in relation to health and illness
6. *Social history:* An accounting of intrapersonal and interpersonal factors which influence the client's social adjustment, including environmental stressors which may be increasing or decreasing the client's vulnerability to crisis during times of stress
7. *Review of systems:* A systematic assessment of biological functioning from head to toe

When one is completing a health history, it is extremely important to elicit the client's expectations of the health care provider. If the client's and the professional's expectations are inconsistent, frustration results for all parties involved. For instance, a client who has diabetes and is expecting a cure will likely have difficulty working with a health care professional whose goal is to help the client live a normal life within the limitations of his or her condition. If the discrepancy between these two goals is not resolved, neither of these goals will be reached.

Every nurse must decide on a format which will facilitate data collection. Although formats may vary, it is crucial to collect data in an *orderly* fashion on all parameters of client functioning before a nursing care plan is developed. There are times when a crisis situation warrants dealing with the immediate concerns of the client before all data are collected. In order to intervene effectively during times of crisis, the health care professional needs an *adequate* data base. Without this data base, it is impossible to help the client to make appropriate choices about solutions for resolving current health stress.

Assessment guides can help the community health nurse collect health data in an orderly fashion. Assessment tools designed to collect information about the health status of individual family members should help the nurse to examine multiple aspects of a client's functioning. Appendixes 8-1, 8-2, and 8-3 are three assessment forms (antepartum, postpartum, and newborn) developed by community health nurses at the Seattle King County Department of Public Health. These tools aid the nurse in identifying psychosocial as well as physical components of a client's health status. In addition, they help a nurse to integrate individual and family functioning by raising issues pertinent to the needs of all family members.

Assessment tools have limitations and must be used only as guides to focus a nurse's attention on significant parameters to assess during the health interview and the physical examination process. Spontaneous interchange between the nurse and the client must always be allowed so that the client can fully express needs and can determine priorities which relate to her or his life-style. A barrage of questions from an assessment form stifles communication.

Analyzing

Once individual and family data are collected, the analysis phase of the nursing process begins. This phase encompasses a cognitive data ordering process, which results in the formation of nursing diagnoses. Nursing diagnoses are inferences made about "the individual's, the family's, or the community's health problem/condition and the primary etiological or related factor(s) contributing to the problem/condition that is the focus of nursing treatment" (Gordon, 1989, p. xiii).

Nursing diagnoses are based on *patterns* reflected in assessment data and identify actual or potential client problems amenable to nursing interventions (Gordon, 1989). They also delineate client strengths which should be reinforced when the nurse is helping the client to enhance his or her self-care capabilities. In the community health setting, nursing diagnoses examine the needs and strengths of family units as well as the needs and strengths of individual clients. If the identified needs of a family or individual clients are not amenable to nursing intervention, the community health nurse makes a referral to an appropri-

ate care provider (refer to Chapter 9).

In order to formulate nursing diagnoses, the community health nurse must group data so that relationships between assessment categories can be analyzed and patterns of behavior can be identified. Establishing relationships between assessment categories involves looking at all parameters of individual as well as family functioning. It requires a synthesis of data to determine the unique combination of biologic, psychosocial, developmental, spiritual, and environmental factors that are making an impact on a specific family unit. It is important to synthesize data collected from a family, as client needs vary even when clients are experiencing similar situations. For example, one community health nurse was visiting two families who were both expressing concern about a child who cried when preparing to leave for school. In one family situation, the nurse's diagnosis of this behavior was anticipatory anxiety (Susie was distressed as a result of family illness). Assessment data revealed that (1) Susie had enjoyed school until her father had a heart attack; (2) Susie's father had his heart attack while she was at school; and (3) Susie had been asking lately if her father was going to die. In the other family situation, the nursing diagnosis in relation to the child's crying was quite different. It read, altered growth and development, social skills (Bonnie's dependency on her mother was inhibiting her psychosocial development). The community health nurse came to this conclusion after the parents shared that (1) Bonnie started school a year late because she was "immature" for her developmental age; (2) Bonnie had never enjoyed school; (3) Bonnie spent most of her free time with her mother, even when children her own age were around; and (4) Bonnie would cling to her mother when babysitters came to the house.

Nursing diagnoses must be based on a strong data base validated by the client and data must be synthesized before nursing diagnoses are established. Formulating diagnoses without adequate information, or in relation to fragmented pieces of data, leads to invalid diagnoses and inappropriate client goals and nursing interventions. A nursing diagnosis, which is based only on environmental observations (fragmented data) and which focuses on "unsafe housekeeping practices," provides very little direction for client and nursing intervention. Unsafe housekeeping practices can result from several factors, including lack of home management skill, energy depletion due to maturational and situational crises, and differing values about environmental safety. How a community health nurse would intervene when unsafe housekeeping practices are encountered is greatly influenced by the data base obtained and the nursing diagnosis developed. For example, an educative strategy is used when a client lacks home management skill, whereas a crisis intervention approach is initiated when a client's energies are depleted because of crisis.

Use of scientific knowledge such as Maslow's hierarchy of needs, theories of growth and development, and concepts of stress and crisis enhances a community health nurse's ability to synthesize data and to formulate an appropriate nursing diagnosis. Scientific knowledge helps a nurse to identify significant signs and symptoms of distress and to organize collected data into a meaningful whole. Grouping the symptoms presented by a client and then comparing them to clinical and research findings such as those presented in Chapter 7 aids the nurse in determining when a client may be in a state of crisis or vulnerable to crisis.

When comparing collected data with relevant clinical and research findings, it is important to identify nursing diagnoses in relation to client strengths as well as client needs. Discerning client strengths helps the community health nurse to reinforce self-sufficiency skills, which in turn aids the nurse in avoiding dependency-building nursing activities. In the community health nurse setting, special emphasis is placed on identifying nursing diagnoses that relate to situations or potential problems which warrant anticipatory guidance counseling. This emphasis is based on the belief that primary prevention should be a major focus in community health nursing practice. Situations throughout one's life-span that warrant anticipatory guidance are covered in Chapters 13 through 19.

Synthesizing data and formulating nursing diagnoses can be difficult when the nurse works with clients in the community health setting because data about several individuals as well as family dynamics must be integrated. Peer consultation, supervised clinical practice, and comparison of nursing diagnoses with diagnoses of other health professionals can help practitioners to increase their diagnostic abilities. Knowing when to seek assistance from others is one earmark of a professional nurse.

Nursing Classification Systems

Use of nursing classification systems can also help practitioners to refine their diagnostic skills and to document the effectiveness of nursing interventions. In addition, these systems can facilitate the collection of assessment data and can assist in organizing these data. Two such systems, one developed by The North American Nursing Diagnosis Association and the other by the Visiting Nurse Association of Omaha, Nebraska, are being used by nurses across the country. Other nursing classification systems are shared in Chapter 22.

The North American Nursing Diagnosis Association was established in St. Louis, Missouri in 1973, for the purpose of developing a standard nomenclature for describing health problems amenable to treatment by nurses (Kim and Moritz, 1982, p. xvii). Since its inception, this association has sponsored several National Nursing Diagnosis Conferences, which have resulted in the identification of appropriate *nursing* diagnostic categories for practitioners. Currently, there are 99 nursing diagnoses which have been accepted for clinical testing by the North American Nursing Diagnosis Assoication (refer to Table 8-6). These diagnoses are grouped under 11 diagnostic categories which were derived from significant functional health patterns. These functional health patterns provide a format for an admission assessment and a data base for nursing diagnosis (Gordon, 1989). Gordon (1989), in *Manual of Nursing Diagnosis, 1988-1989,* explicates in more detail how to use the classification system and the functional health patterns to facilitate nursing assessments and the identification of nursing diag-

TABLE 8-6 The North American Nursing Diagnosis Association: Nursing diagnostic categories and diagnoses accepted for clinical testing, 1988*

Diagnostic categories	*Nursing diagnoses*
Health-perception-health-management pattern	**Altered Health Maintenance**
	Total Health Management Deficit
	Health Management Deficit (Specify)
	Health-Seeking Behaviors (Specify)
	Noncompliance (Specify)
	Potential Noncompliance (Specify)
	Potential for Infection
	Potential for Injury
	Potential for Poisoning
	Potential for Suffocation
Nutritional-metabolic pattern	**Altered Nutrition: Potential for More than Body Requirements** or Potential Obesity
	Altered Nutrition: More than Body Requirements or Exogenous Obesity
	Altered Nutrition: Less than Body Requirements or Nutritional Deficit (Specify)
	Ineffective Breastfeeding
	Impaired Swallowing
	Potential for Aspiration
	Altered Oral Mucous Membranes
	Potential Fluid Volume Deficit
	Fluid Volume Deficit (Actual) (1)
	Fluid Volume Deficit (Actual) (2)
	Fluid Volume Excess
	Potential for Impaired Skin Integrity or Potential Skin Breakdown
	Impaired Skin Integrity
	Decubitus Ulcer (Specify Stage)
	Impaired Tissue Integrity
	Potential for Altered Body Temperature
	Ineffective Thermoregulation
	Hyperthemia
	Hypothermia
Elimination pattern	**Constipation** or Intermittent Constipation Pattern
	Colonic Constipation
	Perceived Constipation
	Diarrhea
	Bowel Incontinence

*Diagnoses accepted by the North American Nursing Diagnosis Association appear in boldface type. Diagnoses found to be useful in clinical practice but not yet accepted are in roman type.

From Gordon M: Manual of nursing diagnosis, 1988-1989, St Louis, 1989, CV Mosby Co., pp iii-viii.

TABLE 8-6   The North American Nursing Diagnosis Association: Nursing diagnostic categories and diagnoses accepted for clinical testing, 1988—cont'd

Diagnostic categories	*Nursing diagnoses*
	Altered Urinary Elimination Pattern
	Functional Incontinence
	Reflex Incontinence
	Stress Incontinence
	Urge Incontinence
	Total Incontinence
	Urinary Retention
Activity-exercise pattern	**Potential Activity Intolerance**
	Activity Intolerance (Specify Level)
	Fatigue
	Impaired Physical Mobility (Specify Level)
	Potential for Disuse Syndrome
	Total Self-Care Deficit (Specify Level)
	Self-Bathing—Hygiene Deficit (Specify Level)
	Self-Dressing—Grooming Deficit (Specify Level)
	Self-Feeding Deficit (Specify Level)
	Self-Toileting Deficit (Specify Level)
	Altered Growth and Development: Self-Care Skills (Specify Level)
	Diversional Activity Deficit
	Impaired Home Maintenance Management (Mild, Moderate, Severe, Potential, Chronic)
	Potential Joint Contractures
	Ineffective Airway Clearance
	Ineffective Breathing Pattern
	Impaired Gas Exchange
	Decreased Cardiac Output
	Altered Tissue Perfusion (Specify)
	Dysreflexia
	Altered Growth and Development
Sleep-rest pattern	**Sleep-Pattern Disturbance**
Cognitive-perceptual pattern	**Pain**
	Chronic Pain
	Pain Self-Management Deficit (Acute, Chronic)
	Uncompensated Sensory Deficit (Specify)
	Sensory-Perceptual Alternation: Input Deficit or Sensory Deprivation
	Sensory-Perceptual Alternation: Input Excess or Sensory Overload
	Unilateral Neglect

Continued.

TABLE 8-6 The North American Nursing Diagnosis Association: Nursing diagnostic categories and diagnoses accepted for clinical testing, 1988—cont'd

Diagnostic categories	Nursing diagnoses
	Knowledge Deficit (Specify)
	Uncompensated Short-Term Memory Deficit
	Potential Cognitive Impairment
	Impaired Thought Processes
	Decisional Conflict (Specify)
Self-perception–self-concept pattern	**Fear (Specify Focus)**
	Anticipatory Anxiety (Mild, Moderate, Severe)
	Anxiety
	Mild Anxiety
	Moderate Anxiety
	Severe Anxiety (Panic)
	Reactive Depression (Situational)
	Hopelessness
	Powerlessness (Severe, Moderate, Low)
	Self-Esteem Disturbance
	Chronic Low Self-Esteem
	Situational Low Self-Esteem
	Body Image Disturbance
	Personal Identity Disturbance
Role-relationship pattern	**Anticipatory Grieving**
	Dysfunctional Grieving
	Disturbance in Role Performance
	Unresolved Independence-Dependence Conflict
	Social Isolation
	Social Isolation or Social Rejection
	Impaired Social Interaction
	Altered Growth and Development: Social Skills (Specify)
	Translocation Syndrome
	Altered Family Processes
	Potential for Altered Parenting
	Altered Parenting
	Parental Role Conflict
	Weak Mother-Infant Attachment or Parent-Infant Attachment
	Impaired Verbal Communication
	Altered Growth and Development: Communication Skills (Specify)
	Potential for Violence

TABLE 8-6 The North American Nursing Diagnosis Association: Nursing diagnostic categories and diagnoses accepted for clinical testing, 1988—cont'd

Diagnostic categories	Nursing diagnoses
Sexuality-reproductive pattern	**Sexual Dysfunction**
	Altered Sexuality Patterns
	Rape Trauma Syndrome
	Rape Trauma Syndrome: Compound Reaction
	Rape Trauma Syndrome: Silent Reaction
Coping-stress-tolerance pattern	**Ineffective Coping (Individual)**
	Avoidance Coping
	Defensive Coping
	Ineffective Denial or Denial
	Impaired Adjustment
	Post-Trauma Response
	Family Coping: Potential for Growth
	Ineffective Family Coping: Disabling
	Ineffective Family Coping: Compromised
Value-belief pattern	Spiritual Distress (Distress of Human Spirit)

noses. She also provides a functional health patterns assessment tool which can be used to guide the nursing assessment process. Gordon stresses that the nursing diagnoses accepted for clinical testing by the North American Nursing Diagnosis Association are in process of development and need to be refined. All professional nurses are encouraged to submit refinements of accepted diagnoses to the North American Nursing Diagnosis Association, c/o Clearinghouse for Nursing Diagnoses, St. Louis University School of Nursing, 3525 Caroline Avenue, St. Louis, Missouri 63104 (Gordon, 1989).

The classification system developed by the Visiting Nurse Association of Omaha was designed to provide an organizing framework for client problems diagnosed by nurses in the community health setting. This classification scheme, based upon the ANA definition of community health nursing, is an orderly arrangement of a nonexhaustive list of client problems which are grouped into four major domains: environmental, psychosocial, physiologic, and health behaviors. Definitions for each of these domains are as follows (Simmons, 1980, pp. 6, 8):

1. *Environmental*—Refers to the material resources and physical surroundings of the home, neighborhood, and broader community in which the client lives. This domain focuses on factors external to the client which affect the health or illness of that client.

2. *Psychosocial*—Refers to patterns of behavior, communication, relationship, and development. This domain includes problems which address the relationships of the client as an individual or the family with other persons. These persons may be immediate or extended family members, significant others, neighbors, acquaintances, or community workers. Thus, this group of problems often reflects inability of the individual or family to interact positively with persons inside or outside the family unit.

3. *Physiological*—Refers to the functional status of

TABLE 8-7   The Visiting Nurse Service of Omaha, Nebraska: organization of classification scheme for client problems in community health nursing, selected examples

Domain	Problem label	Modifier	Sign or symptom
Environmental	Income	Deficit	Low/no income
			Uninsured medical expenses
			Inadequate money management
			Able to buy only necessities
			Difficulty buying necessities
			Other (specify)
Psychosocial	Communication with community resources	Impairment	Unfamiliar with options/procedures for obtaining services
			Difficulty understanding roles/regulations of service provider
			Dissatisfaction with services
			Language barrier
			Inadequate/unavailable resources
			Other (specify)
Physiological	Hearing	Impairment	Difficulty hearing normal speech tones
			Absent/abnormal response to sound
			Abnormal results of hearing screening test
			Other (specify)
Health-related behaviors	Nutrition	Impairment	Weighs 10 percent more than average
			Weighs 10 percent less than average
			Lacks established standards for daily caloric/fluid intake
			Unbalanced diet
			Improper feeding schedule for age
			Nonadherence to prescribed diet
			Other (specify)

From Simmons DA, Martin KS, Crews CC, and Scheet NJ: Client management information system for community health nursing agencies, NTIS Accession No HRP-0907023, Springfield, Va, 1986, National Technical Information Service, pp 60, 61, 64, 68.

processes that maintain life. Because of the focus of the problems in this domain, the labels tend to be referenced to the client as an individual rather than to the client as a family unit.

4. *Health behaviors*—Refers to activities which maintain or promote wellness, promote recovery, or maximize rehabilitation. The problems address health-seeking behaviors which have the potential of improving the quality of the client's life. Personal motivation on the part of the client is especially critical in resolving this group of problems, since he or she must change health behavior appropriately, often without rapid or visible benefits.

Within each of these domains are the names of identified problems which may be actual or potential, modifiers of these problems and signs or symptoms of the problems. The signs and symptoms are general statements which condense more specific information about a client. Additionally, problems may be referenced to either an individual or to a family. Presented in Table 8-7 are examples of how the classification scheme, developed by the Visiting Nurse Service of Omaha, is organized according to domain, problem label, modifier, and sign or symptom.

Directly related to the problem classification

scheme and the nursing process is a problem-rating scale which helps nurses to evaluate client outcomes at regular time intervals and a nursing intervention scheme consisting of nursing activities aimed at addressing specific nursing problems (Simmons, Martin, Crews, and Scheet, 1986).

The structure of the Omaha classification scheme easily adapts to a computerized system of record keeping (Simmons, Martin, Crews, and Scheet, 1986). Data can be efficiently stored and retrieved, and each client problem can be identified by a numerical code. Computerized management information systems are becoming the norm across the country (refer to Chapters 21 and 22).

Planning

After nursing diagnoses are established and *validated with the client,* the community health nurse and the client move into the planning phase of the nursing process. Two major activities occur during this phase: (1) client-centered goals and objectives (criteria) for evaluating goal attainment are formulated and (2) alternative interventions are identified and evaluated. A goal is a broad desired *outcome* toward which behavior is directed, such as "the family will value preventive health care services." An objective delineates *client behaviors* which reflect that a goal has been reached. "The family will obtain a regular source of medical care by September" might be one objective established to determine if the above goal has been accomplished. Alternative interventions are *activities* which may be implemented by the client, the nurse, and other health care professionals to help the client achieve the desired goals. For example, in relation to the above objective, the nurse might discuss with the client the services of all the available medical resources in the community and assist the client in obtaining transportation if necessary.

All goals and objectives should be stated in specific and realistic terms and relate to the nursing diagnoses that have been established. They should not include expectations that are beyond the professional's or client's resources or capabilities. A goal of a severely retarded child achieving normal growth and development is extremely unrealistic. It is very appropriate to work toward maximizing this child's potential but inappropriate to expect that this child will reach normal growth and development parameters.

Goal statements and objectives that are written in positive terms provide direction for nursing interventions more effectively than those that have a negative orientation. Negative goal statements such as "parents will not use harsh disciplinary measures with their children" tend to focus on family weaknesses rather than on family strengths, which can be mobilized to reduce current stresses. Positive goal statements, such as "parents will talk with their children when the children act out," lead to the development of more positive interventions for achieving goals.

The nurse may find after client-centered goals are developed that the client finds it impossible to work on all of them immediately. When this happens, the nurse and the client should work together to differentiate between problems that require immediate action and those that are of less concern to the client. When establishing priorities in relation to client goals, the nurse must keep in mind that the client has the right to make the final decision about goals to focus on. The nurse does have a responsibility to share concerns when she or he believes that client actions are unsafe or are precipitating a crisis situation.

After client-centered, positively stated goals have been established and priorities determined, behavioral objectives that can be measured should be written. The importance of formulating specific objectives for evaluating goal attainment must be stressed. Broad, general goals do not provide sufficient direction for planning intervention strategies. "Maximizing the potential" of a child who has a developmental lag, for example, does not specifically identify needed areas of improvement. Objectives such as those listed below more appropriately facilitate the development of intervention strategies because they focus on specific developmental needs of the client:

- Joel will achieve daytime bladder and bowel control by December.

- Joel will eat solid foods by October.
- Joel's family will share their feelings about Joel's condition.
- Joel's family will verbally identify how their feelings about Joel's condition positively or adversely affect his growth and development.

Interventions, like objectives, should be specific and based on sound scientific knowledge. "Teaching about growth and development" is not a specifically stated intervention. It is extremely global and does not take into account the individual needs of a particular family. A community health nurse could better prepare for family visits if the above intervention was stated as follows: "discuss various ways to achieve daytime bladder and bowel control."

When delineating a plan for intervention, both family and nurse activities should be identified. If only nursing actions are established, the client cannot be an active participant in the therapeutic process. Unfortunately, family resources are frequently overlooked when intervention strategies are developed. For instance, plans are too often made to involve community resources in the client's care even though friends or family members are available and would be more than willing to assist the client in achieving goals.

When intervention strategies are discussed, it may be found that referral to other health care professionals can best help the client to meet his or her needs. In these instances, the community health nurse should discuss with the family how essential data about their situation can be shared. The family's permission should be obtained before releasing any information to other health care agencies. The client has the right to determine what data, shared in confidence with the nurse, should or should not be shared with others. Indiscriminate exchange of client information among professionals violates the client's right to confidentiality and usually promotes mistrust and resistance to professional intervention. The principle of confidentiality is most often violated when goals are not mutually established and the nurse shares or seeks data to validate nurse-focused goals.

Interdisciplinary collaboration is appropriate and often essential. The family must, however, support the need for such an approach before it can be fully successful. Application of the principles of the referral process which are discussed in Chapter 9 usually help a nurse to reduce resistance to interdisciplinary collaboration.

Three key principles must be taken into consideration during all phases of the planning process. These are (1) individualization of client care plans; (2) active client participation; and (3) the client's right of self-determination. The family-centered nursing process is a scientific process designed to meet the needs of *clients.* Inherent in this concept is the belief that clients have unique needs and, thus, care cannot be standardized. Unique needs of clients can be discovered only by actively involving the client in the therapeutic process. Active client participation also promotes client commitment to goal attainment and decreases resistance to change. Taking over for a client may reinforce a client's feelings of inadequacy or increase the client's resentment of authority figures. These types of feelings can foster dependency or rejection of aid offered by the community health nurse.

For clients to fully participate in the therapeutic process, they must have the right to refuse any course of action they deem inappropriate for them. The community health nurse can help a client to examine the pros and cons of certain health actions or the consequences of continuing a particular pattern of functioning. The nurse should not make decisions for the client or expect the client to make decisions in the way the nurse would make them. This is not meant to imply that the nurse should reinforce behavior which could be harmful to the client. Rather, it emphasizes that clients are responsible for the decisions they make and that they should not be rejected (e.g., viewed as "hopeless" or "resistant to change") if they do not make decisions in the way the health care professional would make them. Occasionally the community health nurse does intervene without a client's consent because the client is a threat to others (e.g., child abuse, spread of communicable disease) or to herself or himself (suicidal). Even in these situations the community health nurse works with the client, if possible, to help reduce the distress being experienced and to develop new patterns of coping.

To effectively apply the principles of individualization, active participation, and self-determination, the community health nurse must *internalize* the belief that all clients are unique and capable of making decisions about health care issues. Nurses must also consistently examine how personal attitudes, beliefs, motivations, and conditioning are influencing their professional relationships. Personal biases can and do subtly influence how professionals interact with clients. One community health nurse, for instance, found it difficult to maintain a therapeutic relationship with families when the male provider in the family had a "drinking problem." She would support the female's viewpoints without helping her to analyze how she might be reinforcing her husband's dysfunctional behavior. The nurse recognized that this was happening and was able to verbalize that she felt her sister died prematurely as a result of stress associated with her husband's drinking problem. When the nurse was conscious of her feelings, she was able to deal with them and better assist clients in these situations.

Professional Contracting

Contracting with clients is one way of consistently monitoring professional biases and applying the principles of individualization, active participation, and self-determination. A contract, a mutual agreement between two or more persons for a specific purpose, provides a framework for evaluating the interactions which are occurring between people. It does so because a contract clearly identifies what each person in the relationship can expect from the other person in the relationship.

Contracts are used for a variety of reasons. They may be formal, legally binding, long-term agreements, such as when a couple buys a home, or they may be casual, short-term commitments, such as when a friend consents to dog-sit while the dog's owner is gone on vacation. Contracts are also being used effectively by health care professionals to encourage their clients to participate more actively in dealing with their own health care needs. In these situations, the contract assumes a different purpose. It becomes a method of professional intervention that facilitates the helping relationship with clients. Contracting has been used by health care professionals more frequently in recent years, because there is a growing interest in promoting a philosophy of professional practice which supports the client's self-care capabilities. Increased use of contracting has also occurred because it has been found that clients who are actively involved in identifying their own health needs and in formulating health care goals are more likely to change their health behaviors than clients who have no voice in these decisions.

A professional contract may be defined very simply as a mutually agreed upon working understanding that relates to the terms of treatment and is continuously negotiable between the nurse and the family (Maluccio and Marlow, 1974; Seabury, 1976). The contract may be either written or oral, but it must be clear and explicit to all parties involved. When methods for *reinforcing* clients' actions are explicitly spelled out, the contract is labeled a *contingency contract*. The contingency contracting process is based on theories of behavior modification, which postulate that reinforcers or rewards increase the probability that a desired response will occur. Before implementing contingency contracting, the professional should have a firm understanding of the principles of behavior modification.

The professional using the contracting method of intervention must feel comfortable with the philosophy that all individuals have the potential for growth and that they are capable of effective decision making. The professional must also believe that the client has the right to determine which course of action will best meet his or her health care needs. In essence, contracting is a *philosophy of practice* that governs how the community health nurse implements the family-centered nursing process. The nurse who believes in contracting involves the client in all aspects of care. She or he makes an agreement with the client which spells out explicitly the responsibilities of both nurse and client in achieving mutually defined, client-centered goals. The quality of explicitness implies that terms of intervention are known to both the client and the nurse. When contracting occurs, all involved parties have a mutual understanding about:

1. Purpose of client-nurse interactions
2. Nursing diagnoses
3. Desired outcomes (goals) toward which behavior is directed
4. Priority needs in relation to client goals
5. Methods of intervention
6. Specific activities each party will carry out to achieve stated goals
7. Established time parameters for evaluation and the frequency and length of visits

Contracting increases the clarity in nurse-client interactions. Specific commitments are made orally so that each party is aware of its role in the therapeutic process. Increased clarity often enhances the therapeutic relationship. This is especially true when clients have multiple problems or are unable to identify the nature of their problems. A case situation can best illustrate this point.

The Beech family, two parents with five children, had been visited by community health nurses for years. The family folder reflected many problems; marital stress, financial difficulties, poor nutrition, lack of preventive health care for family members, irregular school attendance, and frequent childhood infections were the primary problems with which the family was dealing. Infrequent visits were made by the community health nurse because the family continually failed to deal actively with health care needs. Because they moved frequently, the Beech family never had consistent contact with one nurse for any length of time. Finally the community health nurse decided to talk with Mrs. Beech about terminating nursing service because she believed that the family did not desire assistance. To her surprise, Mrs. Beech verbalized that her family did need help and that she really wanted the nurse to continue visiting. She further shared that she had difficulty concentrating on anything because the family had so many problems to handle. The nurse agreed with Mrs. Beech that it was an impossible task to solve all the family problems at once. She proposed that it might be helpful if the family and the nurse could work together to resolve the one health problem Mrs. Beech felt was most

distressing at that time. Mrs. Beech had trouble focusing on one particular concern, because she had never before attempted to do so. Because she spent a considerable amount of time talking about Mary, her 10-year-old who had recently failed a hearing test at school, the nurse questioned if Mrs. Beech might want to explore ways to resolve this health care problem. The nurse also suggested that it might be helpful to order the family's health problems from most significant to least significant. Since these suggestions were acceptable to Mrs. Beech, the following contract was established:

- *Purpose of client-nurse interactions:* The community health nurse will help the family to establish priorities in relation to their health problems and to handle their problems in manageable doses.
- *Priority need:* Mary's failure of hearing test at school.
- *Mutual goal:* Mary's hearing problem will be evaluated by a physician.
- *Method of intervention:* Family will take Mary to the hearing specialist she had seen before. (This decision was made after the nurse discussed all the possible resources where Mary could obtain care and Mrs. Beech shared that Mary had had hearing problems in the past.)
- *Responsibilities of family:* (1) Make appointment with the doctor; (2) arrange for child care for their two preschoolers for the afternoon of the appointment; (3) arrange for transportation; (4) together with the nurse, make list of questions to ask the doctor during the visit.
- *Responsibilities of nurse:* Contact the physician to share the results of Mary's hearing test and Mrs. Beech's fears about health care professionals. (Mrs. Beech had been frequently criticized by health care professionals in the past for waiting too long before she sought medical help.) Visit weekly to evaluate how plans for Mary's care are progressing and to help the family establish priorities for health care action.
- *Time limits:* Mary to see the physician by the end of the month.

Mary saw the physician within the appropriate time frame; it was determined that she would need ear surgery. Since the contracting method of intervention helped Mrs. Beech to achieve her first goal, Mrs. Beech and the nurse agreed to renegotiate for follow-up based on the doctor's recommendation. Many other contracts were made before this family case record was closed. Accomplishing resolution of one problem helped family members to see that their situation was not hopeless. Setting priorities in relation to goal attainment decreased the family's anxiety about all the problems they had to handle.

Contracting is a dynamic, complex process which gradually evolves as the therapeutic relationship is strengthened. It should not be viewed as a simple procedure, involving only a discussion about goals, intervention strategies, and time limits. To successfully engage a family in the contracting process, the community health nurse must help the family to gain a clear understanding of its needs. The nurse must also explain the nature of a therapeutic relationship and explore with the client the range of alternative interventions that are available.

It is important to remember when thinking about contracting with clients that clients may not know about all the resources available to them. They also may not know why they are experiencing distress at this time. A new mother, for example, may recognize that she is concerned about the physical aspects of child care, but she may not realize that some of her stress is related to role changes associated with parenthood.

Initially a contract may be very general and include only an agreement to explore the nature of the client's problems and the meaning of a therapeutic relationship. The terms of a contract become more inclusive as specific data are obtained. Establishing time parameters is important even when a general contract is developed, because they emphasize the need for reviewing progress made in relation to goal attainment.

Contracting is an effective way to involve families in their own health care. Contracting can reinforce dysfunctional family patterns, however, if the nurse does not analyze carefully family dynamics. When a contract supports unhealthy family functioning, it is labeled a *corrupt contract* (Beall, 1972, p. 77). A corrupt contract might evolve, for instance, when a community health nurse is working with a family who would like their aging parents to move to a nursing home. Sometimes families push for nursing home placement to meet their own needs rather than the needs of their aging parents. If the community health nurse supports the family's decision and encourages the parents to move without talking to them about their needs and desires, he or she is violating the rights of the aging parents and the principles of contracting.

During the contracting process, a community health nurse may identify problems such as lack of protection against communicable diseases or inadequate dental care that do not seem to be of concern to the family. In these situations, a nurse-centered goal rather than a client-centered goal is formulated. A nurse-centered goal should be stated as such and should not emphasize family action like the "family will make an appointment at the immunization clinic." Instead, it should focus on increasing the family's awareness of the problem and be stated in such terms as "the family will verbalize the need for immunizations." Distinguishing carefully between nurse goals and family goals helps the community health nurse to prevent imposing personal values on clients and helps the nurse to focus on the problems and goals important to the family. Generally, families do not explore problems identified by the nurse that they do not see as problems until they have achieved their own client-centered goals.

Throughout the contracting process, the community health nurse must clearly document on the family record assessment data, goals, objectives, intervention strategies, and evaluation findings. Written data are retrievable, whereas oral information can be easily lost or misinterpreted. The family service record should provide concrete data, organized in such a manner that they can be easily analyzed. Lack of documentation discourages effective evaluation of nursing care and client goal attainment. It is often indicative of inadequate data analysis and insufficient planning. In Chapter 22, the significance of accurate recording in relation to the development of a sound quality assurance program is discussed. The record system used in the community health setting is extremely important, and a variety of formats can be effectively used to document all aspects of the nursing process.

It is crucial that the record format represents and shows the flow between all aspects of the nursing process presented in Table 8-1. This is not an easy task, but it must be addressed. The quality of the record system will affect the quality of care given to a client, especially in relation to continuity of care. It is often helpful to place diagnoses, goals, plans, interventions, and evaluation findings on one sheet in the record so that the relationship between each phase and the next one can be easily identified. If the phases of the nursing process are on different pages of the record, it is difficult to coordinate diagnoses, goals, plans, interventions, and evaluation findings.

Implementing

The implementation phase of the nursing process deals specifically with how activities are carried out to achieve client goals. Together, the client and the nurse select and test intervention strategies to determine their appropriateness in helping the client move toward problem resolution. Priorities concerning when actions will be taken are established so that the client can deal with his or her problems in manageable doses. If needed, other resources are mobilized to help the client handle the change process.

Because change is often threatening, a warm, caring, supportive atmosphere which reinforces client accomplishments should be fostered. Focusing on what remains to be accomplished rather than emphasizing positive results that have already occurred serves only to discourage the client. Honest, positive feedback can be the motivating factor that promotes client involvement in the therapeutic process. Positive feedback can also help to increase clients' self-esteem and confidence in their ability to assume responsibility for maintaining and promoting their health status.

The community health nurse utilizes a variety of intervention strategies to help clients alter those aspects of life they desire to change. Some of these are discussed in Chapter 7, where the supportive, educative, and problem-solving strategies were explored. Nursing actions should be based on sound scientific principles and knowledge. If a planned intervention, for instance, is to increase the

client's understanding of how to prepare nutritious meals, the teaching methodology chosen should take into consideration specific client characteristics, such as financial resources, demands on the homemaker's time, nutritional needs of all family members, and cultural preferences in relation to food likes and dislikes. It should also reflect current knowledge about nutritional requirements and appropriate application of the principles of teaching and learning.

All other phases of the nursing process are usually carried out during the implementation phase. While clients are actively participating in the intervention process, they share data verbally or nonverbally through action taken or not taken. The community health nurse must analyze these new data carefully to determine if care plans need to be revised. Nursing care plans should never be static. Rather, they should be continuously open to renegotiation as the client's situation changes or new data are discovered.

The community health nurse must be *flexible* when implementing intervention strategies, since new data are often generated which alter original nursing diagnoses and client goals. Some clients are unable to identify the nature of their problems until they attempt to change their behavior and find that change does not relieve their discomfort. This was illustrated in Chapter 7, when Mrs. Lehi discovered that her headaches were related to guilt feelings about being a working mother rather than to excessive demands on her time. In this situation the nurse and Mrs. Lehi revised their original goal, "Mrs. Lehi will discover ways to adjust her daily schedule to reduce stress," to "Mrs. Lehi will identify ways to achieve her self-fulfillment needs without distress." Intervention strategies were altered accordingly. Instead of discussing Mrs. Lehi's daily activities and support systems, the nurse and Mrs. Lehi explored issues such as Mrs. Lehi's feelings about motherhood, the needs of school-age children, and an individual's need for self-fulfillment.

Both the client and the nurse should have responsibilities to meet when interventions are planned and mutually agreed upon. If either the client or nurse is unable to meet these responsibilities, this must be discussed and interventions revised as necessary. The family-centered nursing process is a collaborative process, and the client must be involved in its implementation. A nurse who assumes responsibilities for the client when he or she can independently handle them instead of talking about why planned interventions are not being implemented is not helping the client to move toward goal achievement.

During the implementation phase, it is not unusual to discover that clients do not wish to pursue a particular goal, even though they expressed a desire to do so during the planning phase. Sometimes clients verbalize an *awareness* that a problem exists but are not ready to change their behavior in the way that is necessary to resolve that problem. Clients may not recognize the difference between awareness and readiness until concrete plans have been made to alter their current situation. If this happens, it can be difficult for these clients to verbally convey to the nurse that they are not ready for change. Frequently they share this message nonverbally by not taking action. That is why it is so important for the community health nurse to find out why clients are not meeting commitments which had been mutually agreed upon. Goals and plans should be modified if clients are not ready to alter their behavior.

Some clients are resistant to change because all their alternatives for change have negative consequences. A woman, for example, who has limited financial resources, no preparation for a job, and few support systems may be very hesitant to divorce her husband, even though their marital relationship is destructive to her emotional health. The fear of not being able to support herself and being alone might be far more stressful to her than the emotional pain she is experiencing in the marital relationship. When community health nurses encounter such a situation, they must remain *empathic* and guard against feeling that the woman has no options. Community health nurses do find it difficult to handle situations when all the alternatives for change have some negative consequences, and they may find that feelings of sympathy rather than empathy evolve. If such feelings emerge, nurses should seek assistance from their peers and nursing supervisor in order to objectively evaluate what is happening in the therapeutic process.

Evaluating

Evaluation is the continuous critiquing of each aspect of the nursing process. Although it is discussed as a separate phase, it must take place concurrently with all phases of the nursing process. Ongoing feedback should be elicited from the client to determine whether goals, plans, and intervention strategies are appropriately focused. When objectives are established, defining how they will be evaluated is a necessity. A well-written objective will contain the potential for evaluation. For example, "John will learn how to give his own insulin injection by the end of the month" is a concise statement which can be used to determine whether John has or has not achieved a desired goal.

Although evaluation is one of the most significant aspects of the nursing process, it is the one most frequently neglected or haphazardly done. When developing the nursing care plan, intervals should be established for the systematic review of all aspects of the nursing process. Some community health agencies have a policy which states that all records should be summarized and analyzed after a given number of visits have been made or when the family case is being transferred to another nurse. Even if such a policy does not exist, summarization of records must be done on a regular basis because it facilitates evaluation of client services and outcomes. A well-written summary helps the community health nurse to synthesize data and to vividly identify what has or has not been accomplished in a specified period of time.

Summarizing records is one way to ensure that a systematic evaluation of family progress is done. Consulting with peers, supervisors, and other health care professionals can also help a community health nurse to review progress or lack of progress in family situations. Evaluation is absolutely essential and it must be carefully planned; lack of evaluation often prolongs the therapeutic process.

When evaluating the effectiveness of intervention strategies implemented by the client, the nurse, and other health care professionals, it is not sufficient just to identify that the family is participating in the therapeutic process. The *outcome* of actions taken by the family and health care professionals must also be examined. Noting only that the family has kept an appointment at a clinic provides very little data about the effectiveness of this intervention strategy. Identifying what happened when the family went to the clinic and what motivated them to do so is far more significant. This type of data provides the key for future interventions. Finding out, for instance, if the family was satisfied with the care they received or if the family understood the recommendations for follow-up can help the nurse to identify barriers to the utilization of health care services. Data obtained from these types of questions can also assist the nurse in planning interventions *specific* to the current needs of the family.

When evaluating the effectiveness of intervention strategies, the nurse may find that clients are not reaching their goals. This happens for a variety of reasons that are not always obvious to either the client or the nurse. Outlined below are some factors for the nurse to consider as guidelines when examining why client goals have not been achieved:

1. Data base inadequate to identify the actual needs of the family
2. Goals and objectives too broad and general
3. Goals and objectives not mutually established; nurse's goals being imposed on the family
4. Family priorities in relation to goals and objectives not ascertained
5. Family attempting to deal with too many problems at once
6. Family energies depleted as a result of maturational and situational crises
7. Barriers to care not identified because follow-up on client and nurse actions is neglected
8. Nursing diagnoses, goals, and objectives not revised as the family situation changes

9. Intervention strategies inappropriate
10. Family lacks the support they need to reduce anxiety during the change process
11. Coordination of care among all health professionals is being neglected; family receiving inconsistent messages about appropriate intervention actions; gaps in services

The coordination of services among all professionals is crucial. It should not be assumed that particular services will be provided by an agency when a client is referred to that agency. When multiple agencies are working with a family, clearly defined mechanisms for deciding who will do what and for evaluating the quality of the care being delivered by the health team should be established. The client must be involved in determining how interdisciplinary collaboration and coordination will evolve. Generally clients are more than willing to consent to an interdisciplinary approach to the delivery of health care when they understand why it is important and how it will help them.

When an interdisciplinary approach is used to provide services for clients, the community health nurse must carefully evaluate when nursing services are and are not needed. Referring a client to another community agency does not necessarily mean that all of the client's needs will be met by that agency. The community health nurse still has a responsibility to evaluate the effectiveness of the referrals that have been made (refer to Chapter 9) and to discern if the client has other needs that are amenable to nursing interventions. After the referral has been implemented successfully, it may be found that nursing services are no longer needed; the client is prepared for termination and the family case is closed to service.

Use of the evaluation process helps the community health nurse to provide care to clients more effectively. It assists the nurse in determining which goals have been accomplished, either completely or partially, and helps the nurse to modify intervention strategies if goals are not being reached. It also aids the nurse in making sound decisions about when to terminate nursing services.

Terminating

Terminating is seldom identified as a separate phase in the nursing process. It is alluded to during the evaluation phase but very little attention is devoted to discussing what impact termination has on the nurse and the client in the community health setting. Frequently, feelings associated with the separation process are not handled by the client or the nurse. To effectively intervene with clients in the community health setting, a nurse must become *involved.* The inability to deal with feelings associated with the termination process can stifle the development of close, caring professional relationships. It is for this reason that the authors label terminating as a separate phase in the family-centered nursing process.

Terminating is the period when the client and nurse deal with feelings associated with separation and when they distance themselves (Kelly, 1969, p. 2381). Ending a meaningful relationship with a client should be carefully planned. Clients, as well as nurses, need time to deal with the strong emotions that are often evoked by separation. Anger, sadness, denial, and rejection are some normal feelings experienced by both the client and the nurse during the termination phase. The type of reaction which occurs depends, to a great extent, on how the nurse and the client have dealt with separation in the past. In social situations the sense of sadness is verbalized when friends are leaving, but "denial, suppression and repression of feelings are encouraged." Because of this type of socialization process, clients and nurses alike have not learned how to talk freely about what separation means to them (Sene, 1969, p. 39).

In the community health setting, the nurse encounters termination issues frequently. Some clients are seen on a short-term basis, in three or four visits, whereas long-term relationships are established with other clients who have multiple problems to resolve. It is not uncommon to have a client move abruptly or to have a staff nurse's district changed. Clients who have experienced frequent changes in the nurse assigned to their case may have trouble becoming closely involved with any nurse. Talking about what these changes mean to the client and the nurse can be a learning process for both. A nurse who uses denial to cope with feelings associated with termination will be unable to help the client deal with these feelings.

The authors' clinical experiences have demonstrated that the issue of termination is too often neglected in the community health setting. Family case situations are closed without prior notice to the family, or a nurse's district is changed without providing sufficient time for the nurse to handle the termination process with clients. At times, cases are not closed because the client regresses when it is discovered that the nurse believes her or his services are no longer needed. The client may verbalize the same belief but still regress because he or she is not given the opportunity to explore feelings associated with loss. One 40-year-old client who had multiple sclerosis abruptly stopped doing his exercises when the nurse remarked how well he was progressing. He finally verbalized that he was afraid the nurse would no longer visit when he was able to care for himself. At other times, the nurse does not close a family case to service because of difficulty in ending the relationship with the family. The nurse may only visit monthly "just to see how they are doing," not recognizing that she or he is having difficulty ending a meaningful relationship.

The need to handle separation issues when terminating a nurse-client relationship is essential. Termination may not be an easy process, especially when the nurse and the client have had a long-term relationship. Clients need a supportive atmosphere which encourages them to express feelings and emotions. Often the nurse must initiate discussion about termination before the client will feel free to share feelings about this issue. This was dramatically illustrated when one of the authors ended a long-term relationship with a family because they were moving.

The Grostics had been visited weekly for approximately a year because they were dealing with both developmental and situational crises. Child neglect had been evident when the family case was first opened, but a year later both children were happy, thriving youngsters. Upon moving, Mrs. G. felt that the family still needed nursing services, so plans were made to refer the family for community health nursing follow-up in their new community. Both the client and nurse had shared positive feelings throughout their relationship, but neither verbalized these feelings when plans for referral were discussed. Mrs. G.'s mother altered this situation. She saw the nurse in the immunization clinic prior to the nurse's last visit to the family and stated that Mrs. G. was very upset about having a new nurse. "No one could be like you." Finally, during the last visit both the nurse and Mrs. G. hugged each other and openly discussed what they were feeling. The nurse felt even better when she heard that the family was doing well in their new location.

A client helped the nurse in the above situation see the value of dealing with feelings associated with termination and the rewards of involvement. Although termination may be difficult, it is a learning and growing experience for both nurse and client. When properly implemented, both are able to see what has and has not been accomplished in the therapeutic process and the reason(s) for the termination. Often termination occurs because all the goals established for the relationship have been reached and there is no further need for nursing service. The client should be informed that if health needs arise in the future, the community health nurse can be contacted again. Keeping records open just for the sake of keeping them open when no health goals are being actively worked on is not a good use of nursing time, nor does it project a realistic picture to the client of what nursing services are about.

SUMMARY

The family-centered nursing process is a systematic approach to scientific problem solving, involving a series of circular, dynamic actions—assessing, analyzing, planning, implementing, evaluating, and terminating—for the purpose of facilitating optimum client functioning. Nurses in all settings use this process in order to practice in an orderly, logical manner. It enables the nurse to individualize care for each client.

The principles of individualization, active participation, self-determination, and confidentiality must be applied in all phases of the nursing process. Contracting is increasingly used with clients because health care professionals experience more positive results when they encourage it. *Contracting* is a term used to denote a process that involves the establishment of mutually defined goals and intervention strategies. It is a working agreement between client and nurse, explicitly stated, in which all parties involved are working together to achieve a common goal.

Use of the family-centered nursing process is rewarding and challenging. The family-centered nursing process assists the nurse in helping the client to mobilize personal strengths that will enhance the client's self-care capabilities. It provides the nurse with a framework for facilitating client decision making about health care matters. It also enables the nurse to become truly involved with other human beings in a supportive, therapeutic way.

APPENDIX 8-1

King County Health Department, Seattle, Washington, Nursing Assessment Guide: Antepartum

Patient's name _____

EDC _____ GRAV _____ PARA _____ ABORT _____ DATE MED. CARE STARTED _____

M.D. _____ HOSP. _____SIGNIFICANT MEDICAL HISTORY OF PREGNANCIES _____

Mother's opinion of previous pregnancy, delivery, and newborn (NB) _____

Current pregnancy	Yes	No	*First assessment, comments* *Trimester 1 2 3 Date* _____	Yes	No	*Second assessment, comments* *Trimester 1 2 3 Date* _____
MEDICAL SUPERVISION						
Medical appointments made						
Plans to keep						
Dental appointments made						
Plans to keep						
M&I dental care completed						

Pt understanding of doctor's orders is:

SIGNS AND SYMPTOMS						
Nausea						
Vomiting						
Heartburn						
Spotting						
Bleeding						
Edema						
Leg cramps						
Varicosities						
Backache						
Dyspnea						
Constipation						
Hemorrhoids						
Dysuria						
Frequency						

King County Health Department, Seattle, Washington, Nursing Assessment Guide: Antepartum—cont'd

Current pregnancy	Yes	No	First assessment, comments Trimester 1 2 3 Date _____	Yes	No	Second assessment, comments Trimester 1 2 3 Date _____
Fetal Movements						
Braxton Hicks						
Other						

PERSONAL MANAGEMENT
Weight gain

	Yes	No		Yes	No	
Normal						

Diet—type _____
  Breakfast
  Lunch
  Dinner
  Snacks
  Dislikes
  Fluid intake pattern
  Comments

	Yes	No		Yes	No	
Sleep—No. of hours						
Naps						
Physical activity						
Very active						
Moderately active						
Limited activity						
Clothing						
Supportive						

Nursing assessment—Antepartum—Page 2
Current pregnancy
Emotional (complete with patient's feelings towards)

Patient's name _____

	First assessment Trimester 1 2 3 Date _____	Second assessment Trimester 1 2 3 Date _____
Pregnancy		
Motherhood		

	First assessment Trimester 1 2 3 Date____	Second assessment Trimester 1 2 3 Date____
Changes in self-image		
Mood swings		
Pregnancy and parenthood affecting personal family goals		
Husband-wife social and sexual relationships		
Stresses created by emotional and physical changes of this pregnancy		
Anxiety re: labor and delivery		
Social and financial family stability re: future plans for NB		
Past and present personality difficulties		
Fetus		
Father's awareness of, interest and attitude		

Nursing assessment—Antepartum—Page 3　　　　　　Patient's name _____

	Yes	No	Trimester 1 2 3 Date ____	Yes	No	Trimester 1 2 3 Date ____
PLANS FOR DELIVERY						
Made plans for hospitalization						
Make arrangements for care of family at home						
Knows what to expect of hospital routine						
Knows signs of labor						
Knows what to expect during labor and delivery						
Knows what to expect PP						

Continued.

APPENDIX 8-1

King County Health Department, Seattle, Washington, Nursing Assessment Guide: Antepartum—cont'd

	Yes	No	Trimester 1 2 3	Date ____	Yes	No	Trimester 1 2 3	Date ____
PLANS FOR NEWBORN								
Plans to breast feed								
Plans to bottle feed								
Adequate layette and equipment								
Plans to have help PP								
Knows what to expect of NB								
FAMILY PLANNING								
Knows methods of birth control								
Wants information on family planning								

What kind of help does family want from CHN?

_____

_____

_____

What kind of help does family want from CHN?

_____

_____

_____

Printed with permission from the Nursing Division, King County Health Department, 1000 Public Safety Building, Seattle, Washington.

APPENDIX 8-2

King County Health Department, Seattle, Washington, Nursing Assessment Guide: Postpartum

Patient's name _____

GRAV ____ PARA ____ M.D. _____

HOSPITAL ____ SIGNIFICANT MEDICAL HISTORY OF PREGNANCIES _____

Check items which best describe patient or complete with notation.

Postpartum exam	First assessment date ____		Second assessment date ____	
	Yes	No	Yes	No
Temp ____				
BREASTS				
Physical appearance:				
Normal				
Engorgement				
Soreness				
Soft				

APPENDIX 8-2

King County Health Department, Seattle, Washington, Nursing Assessment Guide: Postpartum—cont'd

Check items which best describe patient or complete with notation.

Postpartum exam	First assessment date _____				Second assessment date _____	
	Yes	No			Yes	No
Cracked						
Redness						
Caked						
Inverted						
Lactation: Leaking						
Filling						
Nursing						
Not nursing						
"Dry up" pills						
ABDOMEN Fundus (firmness, position)						
C-section (incision)						
RECTOVAGINAL Laceration						
Episiotomy:						
None						
Clean						
Healing						
Painful						
Hemorrhoids						
Other						
LOCHIA Rubra						
Serosa						
Alba						

APPENDIX 8-2

King County Health Department, Seattle, Washington, Nursing Assessment Guide: Postpartum—cont'd

Check items which best describe patient or complete with notation.

| | First assessment date _____ | | Second assessment date _____ | |
Postpartum exam	Yes	No	Yes	No
Clots				
No. pads per day				
VOIDING No difficulty				
Anuria				
Dysuria				
Frequency				
Burning				
BOWELS				
Constipated				
No difficulty				
Other				

First assessment date _____ Second assessment date _____

PERSONAL HEALTH PRACTICES (Describe what the patient is doing about the following.)

A. Care

    Bathing _____

    Peri-care _____

    Breast care _____

B. Rest _____

    Sleep _____

    Recreation _____

    Exercise and activity _____

C. Foundation garment _____

D. Diet—Type _____

    Breakfast _____

    Lunch _____

    Dinner _____

    Snacks _____

    Dislikes _____

    Fluid intake _____

APPENDIX 8-2

King County Health Department, Seattle, Washington, Nursing Assessment Guide: Postpartum—cont'd

Comments _____

_____

E. Sexual relations _____

PSYCHOSOCIAL (Describe mother's feeling or reaction to the following.)

Pregnancy _____

_____

Labor _____

_____

Delivery _____

_____

Newborn _____

_____

Motherhood _____

_____

Family's reaction to labor, delivery, NB _____

_____

Other _____

MEDICAL SUPERVISION	Yes	No		Yes	No
Medical appointments made					
Plan to keep					
Dental care up to date					

Patient's understanding of
doctor's orders is _____

FAMILY PLANNING

Future family plans (method, problems) _____

What kind of help does family want from CHN? _____

_____

_____

_____

APPENDIX 8-3

King County Health Department, Seattle, Washington, Nursing Assessment Guide: Newborn Assessment

(Name of infant)	(Number)	(Birth weight)	(Birthdate)

Significant history of pregnancy _____

(Name of doctor)	(Apgar score—time)	(Hospital)

Underline significant	Date *SU check and make comments*			Date *SU check and make comments*		
GENERAL APPEARANCE Length _____ cm Cry, color, spontaneous activity, body symmetry, subcutaneous fat, skin tumor						
SKIN Jaundice, edema, rashes, petechiae, transparent, unusual pigmentation, bruises, desquamation, forcep mark, hematoma, hemangioma, milia						
HEAD Circumference _____ cm Bulging or nonpalpable fontanels, caput succedaneum, cephalhematoma, overriding suture, enlarged head						
EENT Low-set ears, cleft lip and palate, eye opacities, sunset eyes, epicanthus folds, thrush, nevus, asymmetry, discharge, patency of nose and ears, gross reaction to light and sound						
CHEST AND NECK Chest retracted, respiratory patterns, webbing or swelling of neck, engorged breasts, mastitis						
ABDOMEN AND NAVEL Distention, drainage from cord, umbilical hernia						

APPENDIX 8-3

King County Health Department, Seattle, Washington, Nursing Assessment Guide: Newborn Assessment—cont'd

Underline significant	Date			Date		
	SU check and make comments			*SU check and make comments*		
GENITALIA AND RECTUM						
Hydrocele, hypospadius, anal stenosis, phimosis, undescended testicle, clitoris enlargement, genital size, tags, milky or bloody vaginal discharge, pilonidal dimple, circumcision						
BACK						
Contour of spine, hip abduction, skin folds, dermal sinus						
EXTREMITIES						
Paralysis, symmetric creases, club feet, metatarsus varus, webbed toes, extra digits						
REFLEXES						
State quality of reflexes assessed: Moro Tonic Grasp Root and suck						
STOOLS AND VOIDING (Including caliber of urinary stream)						

_____   _____
(Name of infant)   (Number)

History and observation of family care of infant

Date _____

FAMILY INTERACTION

FEEDING

Breast and supplement

Formula (amount, frequency, total 24-hr intake and preparation)

Solids

Continued.

APPENDIX 8-3

King County Health Department, Seattle, Washington, Nursing Assessment Guide: Newborn Assessment—cont'd

---

SKIN CARE

SLEEP PATTERN

CRYING PATTERN

MEDICAL SUPERVISION

Medical directions:
Appointment planned:
Appointment kept:

UNDERSTANDING OF DOCTOR'S ORDERS (Nurse's perception)

Printed with permission from the Nursing Division, King County Health Department, 1000 Public Safety Building, Seattle, Washington.

REFERENCES

American Nurses' Association: Standards of community health nursing practice, Kansas City, Mo, 1986, The Association.

Beall L: The corrupt contract: problems in conjoint therapy with parents and children, Am J Orthopsychiatry 42(1):77-81, 1972.

Beavers WR: Psychotherapy and growth: a family systems perspective, New York, 1977, Brunner/Mazel.

Beitler B, Tkachuck B, and Aamodt D: The Neuman model applied to mental health, community health, and medical-surgical nursing. In Riehl JP and Roy C, eds: Conceptual models for nursing practice, ed 2, New York, 1980, Appleton-Century-Crofts.

Benedict MB and Sproles JB: Application of the Neuman model to public health nursing practice. In Neuman B, ed: The Neuman systems model: application to nursing education and practice, New York, 1982, Appleton-Century-Crofts, pp 223-240.

Bigbee J: The changing role of rural women: nursing and health implications, Health Care Women Int 5:307-322, 1984.

Blazek B and McCaellen M: The effects of self-care instruction on locus of control in children, J School Health 53:554-556, 1983.

Bliss-Holtz UJ: Primiparas' prenatal concern for learning infant care, Nurs Res 37:20-24, 1988.

Bowers AC and Thompson JN: Clinical manual of health assessment, ed 3, St Louis, 1988, CV Mosby Co.

Boyd C: Toward an understanding of mother-daughter identification using concept analysis, Adv Nurs Sci 7(3):78-86, 1985.

Buchanan BF: Human-environment interaction: a modification of Neuman Systems Model for aggregates, families, and the community, Public Health Nurs 4:52-64, 1987.

Campbell JC: Nursing assessment for risk of homicide with battered women, Adv Nurs Sci 8(4):36-51, 1986.

Chang BL, Uman GC, Linn LS, Ware JE, and Kane RL: Adherence to health care regimens among elderly women, Nurs Res 34(1):27-31, 1985.

Clements IW and Roberts FB, eds: Family health: a theoretical approach to nursing care, New York, 1983, Wiley.

Curran D: Traits of a healthy family, Minneapolis, Mn, 1983, Winston Press.

Dunn H: High level wellness, Washington, DC, 1961, Mount Vernon Publishing.

Fawcett J: The relationship between identification and patterns of change in spouses' body images during and after pregnancy, Int J Nurs Stud 14:199-213, 1977.

Fawcett J: A framework for analysis and evaluation of conceptual models of nursing, Nurse Educator 5(6):10-14, 1980.

Fawcett J: Needs of Cesarean birthparents, J Obstet Gynecol Neonatal Nurs 10:371-376, 1981.

Fawcett J: Analysis and evaluation of conceptual models of nursing, Philadelphia, 1984, Davis.

Fawcett J: The metaparadigm of nursing: present status and future refinements, Image: J Nurs Scholarship 16(3):84-87, 1984.

Fawcett J and Carino C: Hallmarks of success in nursing practice, Adv Nurs Sci 11(4):1-8, 1989.

Flaskerudt JH and Halloran EJ: Areas of agreement in nursing theory development, Adv Nurs Sci 3:31-42, 1980.

Fox J: Primary health care of the young, New York, 1981, McGraw-Hill.

Freeman R and Lowe M, directors, Richmond-Hopkins Cooperative Nursing Study: The family coping index, Richmond, Va, 1964, Richmond Instructive Visiting Nurse Association and City Health Department and the Johns Hopkins School of Public Health.

Galli M: Promoting self-care in hypertensive clients through patient education, Home Healthcare Nurse March-April:43-45, 1984.

Gordon M: Manual of nursing diagnosis, 1988-1989, St Louis, 1989, CV Mosby Co.

Guzzetta CE, Bunton SD, Prinkey LA, Sherer AP, and Seifert PC: Assessment tools for clinical practice: designed for use with nursing diagnosis, St Louis, 1989, CV Mosby Co.

Haley J: Family therapy: a radical change. In Haley J, ed: Changing families: a family therapy reader, New York, 1971, Grune & Stratton.

Hanchett ES: Community health assessment: a conceptual tool kit, New York, 1979, Wiley.

Hanchett ES: Nursing frameworks and community as client: bridging the gap, Norwalk, Ct, 1988, Appleton-Lange.

Hanson J: The family. In Roy C, ed: Introduction to nursing: an adaptation model, ed 2, Englewood Cliffs, NJ, 1984, Prectice-Hall, pp 519-533.

Harper DC: Application of Orem's theoretical constructs to self-care medication behaviors in the elderly, Adv Nurs Sci 6(3):29-46, 1984.

Health Care Financing Administration (HCFA): Conditions of participation: home health agencies, 42CFR Part 484, Sections 484.1 through 484.52, Washington, DC, October 1989, US Department of Health and Human Services.

Hoch CC: Assessing delivery of nursing care, J Gerontal Nurs 13:10-17, 1987.

Kearney BY and Fleisher BJ: Development of an instrument to measure exercise of self-care agency, Res Nurs Health 2:25-34, 1979.

Kehoe CF: Identifying the nursing needs of the post partum Cesarean mother. In Kehoe CF, ed: The Cesarean experience: theoretical and clinical perspectives for nurses, New York, 1981, Appleton-Century-Crofts.

Kelly HS: The sense of an ending, Am J Nurs 69:2378-2381, 1969.

Kim MJ and Moritz DA: Classification of nursing diagnoses. Proceedings of the third and fourth national conferences, New York, 1982, McGraw-Hill.

Kruger S, Shawver M, and Jones L: Reactions of families to the child with cystic fibrosis, Image J Nurs Scholarship 12:67-72, 1980.

Laffrey SC: Health behavior choice as related to self-actualization and health conception, West J Nurs Res 7:279-295, 1985.

Levine NH: A conceptual model for obstetric nursing, J Obstet Gynecol Neonatal Nurs 5(2):9-15, 1976.

Lewis J, Beavers R, Gossett JT, and Phillips UA: No single thread: psychological health in family systems, New York, 1976, Brunner/Mazel.

Limandri BJ: Research and practice with abused women: use of the Roy adaptation model as an explanatory framework, Adv Nurs Sci 8(4):52-61, 1986.

Mahoney EA, Verdisco L, and Shortridge L: How to collect and record a health history, ed 2, Philadelphia, 1982, Lippincott.

Malasanos L, Barkauskas V, and Stoltenberg-Allen K: Health assessment, St Louis, 1989, CV Mosby Co.

Maluccio AN and Marlow W: The case for the contract, Social Work 19:28-36, 1974.

Maunz ER and Woods NF: Self-care practices among young adult women: influences of symptoms, employment and sex-role orientation, Health Care Women Int 9:29-41, 1988.

McCain F: Nursing by assessment—not intuition, Am J Nurs 65:82-84, 1965.

McPhetridge LM: Nursing history: one means to personalize care, Am J Nurs 68:68-75, 1968.

Michael MM and Sewall KS: Use of the adolescent peer group to increase the self-care agency of adolescent alcohol abusers, Nurs Clin North Am 15(1):157-176, 1980.

National Association for Home Care (NAHC): Code of ethics, Washington, DC, 1982, The Association.

National Commission to Prevent Infant Mortality: Home visiting: opening doors for America's pregnant women and children, Washington, DC, 1989, The Association.

Neuman B: The Betty Neuman model: a total person approach to viewing patient problems, Nurs Res 21(3):264-269, 1972.

Neuman B: The Betty Neuman health-care systems model: a total person approach to patient problems. In Riehl J and Roy C, eds: Conceptual models for nursing practice, ed 2, New York, 1980, Appleton-Century-Crofts.

Neuman B, ed: The Neuman systems model, New York, 1982, Appleton-Century-Crofts.

Neuman B: The Neuman systems model, application to education and practice, ed 2, Norwalk, Ct, 1989, Appleton-Lange.

Nunn D and Marriner-Tomey A: Applying Orem's model in nursing administration. In Henry B, Arndt O, Di Vincenti M, and Marriner-Tomey A, eds: Dimensions of nursing administration: theory, research, education, practice, Boston, 1989, Blackwell Scientific, pp 63-67.

Orem DE: Nursing: concepts of practice, New York, 1971, McGraw-Hill.

Orem DE: Nursing: concepts of practice, ed 2, New York, 1980, McGraw-Hill.

Orem DE: Nursing: concepts of practice, ed 3, New York, 1985, McGraw-Hill.

Orem DE and Taylor SG: Orem's general theory of nursing. In Winstead-Fry P, ed: Case studies in nursing, New York, 1986, National League for Nursing, pp 37-71.

Otto H: Criteria for assessing family strength, Family Process 2:329-338, 1963.

Pinkerton A: Use of the Neuman model in a home health-care agency. In Riehl JP and Roy C, eds: Conceptual models for nursing practice, New York, 1974, Appleton-Century-Crofts.

Pratt L: Family structure and effective health behavior: the energized family, Boston, 1976, Houghton Mifflin.

Price S and Wilson L: Pathophysiology, ed 3, New York, 1986, McGraw-Hill.

Pridham KF: Instruction of a school-age child with chronic illness for increased responsibility in self-care, using diabetes mellitus as an example, Int J Nursing Stud 8:237-246, 1971.

Rawnsley MM: Perceptions of the speed of time in aging and in dying: an empirical investigation of the holistic theory of nursing proposed by Martha Rogers, doctoral dissertation, Boston, 1977, Boston University.

Riehl-Sisca J, ed: The science and art of self-care, Norwalk, Ct, 1985, Appleton-Century-Crofts.

Rogers ME: An introduction to the theoretical basis of nursing, Philadelphia, 1970, FA Davis.

Rogers ME: Nursing: a science of unitary man. In Riehl JP and Roy C, eds: Conceptual models for nursing practice, ed 2, New York, 1980, Appleton-Century-Crofts, pp 329-337.

Rogers ME: Science of unitary human beings: a paradigm for nursing. In Clements IW and Roberts FB, eds: Family health: a theoretical approach to nursing care, New York, 1983, Wiley, pp 219-228.

Rogers ME: Science of unitary human beings. In Malinski UM, ed: Explorations on Martha Rogers' science of unitary human beings, Norwalk, Ct, 1986, Appleton-Century-Crofts, pp 3-8.

Rogers ME: Rogers' science of unitary human beings. In Parse RR, ed: Nursing science. Major metaparadigms, theories, and critique, Philadelphia, 1989, Saunders, pp 139-146.

Roy C: Adaptation: a conceptual framework for nursing, Nurs Outlook 18(3):42-45, 1970.

Roy C: Introduction to nursing: an adaptation model, Englewood Cliffs, NJ, 1976, Prentice-Hall.

Roy C: Family in primary care: analysis and application of the Roy adaptation model. In Clements IW and Roberts FB, eds: Family health: a theoretical approach to nursing care, New York, 1983, Wiley, pp 375-378.

Roy C: Introduction to nursing: an adaptation model, ed 2, Englewood Cliffs, NJ, 1984, Prentice-Hall.

Roy C: Roy adaptation model. In Parse RR, ed: Nursing science. Major metaparadigms, theories and critique, Philadelphia, 1987, Saunders, pp 35-44.

Roy C: An explication of the philosophical assumptions of the Roy adaptation model, Nurs Sci Quart 1(1):26-34, 1988.

Roy C and Roberts SL: Theory construction in nursing: an adaptation model, Englewood Cliffs, NJ, 1981, Prentice Hall.

Schmitz M: The Roy adaptation model: application in a community setting. In Riehl JP and Roy C, eds: Conceptual models for nursing practice, ed 2, New York, 1980, Appleton-Century-Crofts.

Seabury BA: The contract: uses, abuses and limitations, Social Work 21(8):39-45, 1976.

Sene B: Termination in the student-patient relationship, Perspect Psychiat Care 8:39-45, 1969.

Sills G: Bias of therapists in family therapy. In Smoyak S, ed: The psychiatric nurse as a family therapist, New York, 1975, Wiley.

Simmons DA: A classification scheme for client problems in community health nursing, DHHS Pub No HRA 80-16, Hyattsville, Md, 1980, US Public Health Service.

Simmons DA, Martin KS, Crews CC, and Scheet NJ:

Client management information system for community health nursing agencies, NTIS Accession No HRP-0907023, Springfield, Va, 1986, National Technical Information Service.

Story EL and Ross MM: Family centered community health nursing and the Betty Neuman systems model, Nurs Papers 18(2):77-88, 1986.

Tripp-Reimer T, Brink PJ, and Saunders JN: Cultural assessment: content and process, Nurs Outlook 32:78-82, 1984.

Wagner P: Testing the adaptation model in practice, Nurs Outlook 24:682-685, 1976.

Walborn KA: A nursing model for the hospice: hospice primary and self care nursing, Nurs Clin North Am 15(1):205-217, 1980.

West M: Patterns of health in mothers of developmentally disabled children, Unpublished master's thesis, University Park, 1984, Pennsylvania State University.

Whall AL: Nursing theory and the assessment of families, J Psychiatr Nurs Mental Health Serv 19(1):30-36, 1981.

Whall AL, ed: Family therapy theory for nursing: four approaches, Norwalk, Ct, 1987, Appleton-Century-Crofts.

Wood R and Kekahbah J, eds: Examining the cultural implications of Martha E. Rogers' science of unitary human beings, Lecompton, Ka, 1985, Wood-Kekahbah Associates.

World Health Organization: Constitution of the World Health Organization, WHO Chron 1:29-43, 1947.

SELECTED BIBLIOGRAPHY

Aukamp U and Shaw R: Nursing care plans for adult health clients: nursing diagnosis and interventions, Norwalk, Ct, 1990, Appleton-Lange.

Berg CL and Helgeson DM: That first home visit, Community Health Nurs 1:207-216, 1984.

Carey R: How values affect the mutual goal setting process, Community Health Nurs 6:7-14, 1989.

Dossey BM, Keegan L, Guzzetta CE, and Kolkmeier, LG: Holistic nursing: a handbook for practice. Rockville, Md, 1988, Aspen.

Fitzpatrick JJ and Whall AL, eds: Conceptual models of nursing: analysis and application, ed 2, Norwalk, Ct, 1989, Appleton-Lange.

Gulino C and LaMonica G: Public health nursing: a study of role implementation, Public Health Nurs 3:80-91, 1986.

Henderson V: The nursing process . . . is the title right? J Adv Nurs 7:103-109, 1982.

Houldin AD, Saltstein SW, and Ganley KM: Nursing diagnoses for wellness: supporting strengths, Philadelphia, 1987, Lippincott.

Martin ME and Henry M: Cultural relativity and poverty, Public Health Nurs 6:28-34, 1989.

Muecke MA: Community health diagnosis in nursing, Public Health Nurs 1:23-35, 1984.

Nettle C, Jones W, and Pifer P: Community nursing diagnosis, J Community Health Nurs 6:135-145, 1989.

Porter EJ: Critical analysis of NANDA nursing diagnosis taxonomy I, Image: J Nurs Scholarship 13:136-139, 1986.

Tapia JA: The nursing process in family health. In Spradley BW, ed: Readings in community health nursing, ed 2, Boston, 1982, Little, Brown.

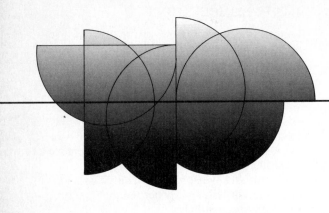

9

Continuity of Care through Discharge Planning and the Referral Process

Upon completion of this chapter, the reader will be able to:

1. Discuss the history of discharge planning.

2. Discuss the characteristics of discharge planning.

3. Explain the rationale for considering referral as a process and summarize basic principles that should be considered when making a referral.

4. Describe client and resource information needed in order for the community health nurse to implement discharge planning and referral effectively.

5. Summarize the steps of the referral process.

6. Distinguish between the levels of nursing intervention in the referral process.

7. Discuss barriers to the utilization of the referral process.

8. Describe the role of the home care coordinator in relation to discharge planning and referral.

Continuity of care is a process through which a client's ongoing health care needs are assessed, planned for, and met. It promotes coordination of health care services, and aids in the transition of the client to different settings and levels of care. Continuity of care demands thorough assessment of client needs, multidisciplinary planning and intervention, client and family participation and education, anticipatory guidance, case management, resource utilization, and follow-up and evaluation. The nurse is often put in the position of client advocate in providing for continuity of care.

The significant role of the community health nurse in maintaining continuity of care for clients was emphasized by the American Nurses' Association (ANA) in 1986 when its standards for home health nursing practice were published (refer to Chapter 19 for a complete list of these standards). A separate standard for "continuity of care" was identified in the ANA home care document. It read (ANA, 1986, p. 14):

Standard VIII. Continuity of Care

The nurse is responsible for the client's appropriate and uninterrupted care along the health care continuum, and therefore uses discharge planning, care management and coordination of community resources.

When continuity of care is not planned for the results can be disastrous to the client and costly to the health care system. An example of such a situation is given in Appendix 9-1. This example illustrates how an ineffectively planned hospital discharge for a ventilator-dependent child resulted in family stress, burnout, and hospital readmission.

Every client should have the opportunity to reach his or her potential for health and recovery, and planning for continuity of care helps to ensure this optimum. Integral components of continuity of care are *discharge planning*, the *referral process,* and care management. The concept of care management is discussed in Chapters 8 and 19.

DISCHARGE PLANNING

Discharge planning is an essential part of the nursing process and plays a major role in ensuring continuity of care. It has been defined by McKeehan (1981) as "That part of the continuity of care process which is designed to prepare the patient or client for the next phase of care and to assist in making any necessary arrangements for that phase of care, whether it be self-care, care by family members or care by an organized health care provider." The National League for Nursing (NLN) views discharge planning as the vehicle that moves the patient to the proper level of care and/or facility (Bristow, Stickney, and Thompson, 1976, p. 5). It facilitates continuity of care by consolidating the gains made at one level or setting while arranging for the resources necessary to meet the needs of another level or setting. It assists in ensuring quality health care. Written discharge planning policies and procedures and defined responsibilities greatly facilitate discharge planning efforts. The success of discharge planning activities is largely dependent on how accurately discharge needs are assessed and the extent to which the client and family participate in the process (Arenth and Mamon, 1985, p. 20).

Discharge planning takes into account the setting which the client is entering, the needs evidenced by the client, and the resources necessary to meet these needs. It is usually thought of in terms of a client being discharged from a hospital. In this text, the term *discharge planning* is used in the broader sense of a client leaving other health care settings such as long-term mental health facilities, nursing homes, outpatient settings, group health education experiences, and home care.

History of Discharge Planning

Discharge planning efforts are not new. There is evidence of discharge planning efforts in the late 1800s and early 1900s (Shamansky, Boase, and Horn, 1984, p. 15; O'Hare and Terry, 1988, p. 6). Lillian Wald was one of the first to recognize the need for such planning. In 1906 Bellevue Hospital in New York City referred to a nurse whose entire time and care was given to befriending those about to be discharged (O'Hare and Terry, 1988, p. 6).

The 1960s saw the first official use of the term *discharge planning* (Shamansky, Boase, and Horn, 1984, p. 16), and discharge planning became a part of many hospital programs. Edith Wensley's (1963) *Nursing Service Without Walls* urged hospitals to emphasize planning for home care services and referral to community services upon discharge. The National League for Nursing has strongly urged hospitals, nursing homes, and home nursing care agencies to have a designated staff person to develop plans for the next stage of nursing care, to carry out continuity of care activities, and to develop well-defined, clearly written procedures for client referral (O'Hare and Terry, 1988, p. 7). During the 1970s discharge planning became linked with quality control programs. This link between discharge planning and quality assurance has now become a mandate under Medicare and Medicaid.

Recent prospective payment system (PPS) and diagnostic related groups (DRGs) legislation has been instrumental in development of discharge planning activities. PPS and DRGs gave discharge planning a firm foothold by providing hospitals a financial incentive to discharge patients as early and efficiently as possible, and discharge planning became a method of cost containment (Feather, 1989). This legislation has made it essential to move the client through the health care system at the lowest appropriate level of care, in the shortest period of time, while maintaining quality and ensuring continuity of care (Willihnganz, 1984). Because of this legislation many patients at discharge need linkages with community resources, and an increased need for coordination between hospitals and community agencies has resulted.

The Omnibus Budget Reconciliation Act of 1986 influenced discharge planning by mandating the development of a standardized, uniform needs assessment instrument to evaluate the post-hospital needs of Medicare patients (McBroom, 1989, p. 1; Burlenski, 1989, p. 2). The Medicare Catastrophic Coverage Act of 1988 showed increased legislative interest in discharge planning (Burlenski, 1989, p. 2), and future legislation will undoubtedly focus on it.

Characteristics of Discharge Planning

Certain aspects of discharge planning are applicable to all discharge planning situations. Major aspects characterizing discharge planning are discussed here.

Discharge planning is based on a thorough assessment of client needs. Nurses carry out discharge planning activities early in the health care process, often commencing the day the client begins using a health care resource. A thorough assessment begins the discharge planning process. Comprehensive assessment leads to early recognition of client needs and resources, and facilitates planning and intervention efforts that will aid the client and family in adapting to the current situation. Areas to assess in discharge planning include health status (including previous hospitalizations, present plan of care, previous home health care experience, health resource utilization); psychosocial status (including educational status, physical environment, financial and occupational status, support systems, religious affiliation, culture, values, client/family knowledge and perceptions of the situation, and client/family preferences); and functional status (McBroom, 1989, p. 3; Kitto and Dale, 1985, p. 28; Siegel, 1988, p. 39). The client/family perceptions of health status and the health care delivery system must not be overlooked, since compliance with discharge planning activities is directly related to these perceptions (Strauss, Orr, and Charney, 1983). The nurse needs to assess client and family perceptions of expected discharge outcomes to see if they are feasible and realistic.

Discharge planning is multidisciplinary in nature. The key words here are *planning* and *multidisciplinary.* After a thorough assessment has been done it is time to plan for discharge needs. The holistic, comprehensive approach taken in discharge planning necessitates multidisciplinary planning efforts. In the early days of discharge planning these multidisciplinary efforts often involved the cooperative work of the nurse, social worker, and physician. Today, specialized discharge planners, home care coordinators, nutritionists, physical therapists, speech therapists, occupational therapists, exercise and fitness counselors, psychologists, and rehabilitation specialists are just some of those that may be involved in discharge planning. In order for discharge planning to work effectively, team members of the involved disciplines must understand it, realize that it facilitates their work, believe in it, take part in it, and be rewarded for their efforts (Chisholm, 1983).

Many health care resources, especially hospitals, are instituting multidisciplinary discharge planning teams, departments, and procedures. In a recent survey, 58 percent of the hospitals polled had an officially designated discharge planning department (Feather, 1989, p. 3). The same study showed that 38 percent of discharge planners report to the social work department, 19 percent report to nursing, 18 percent report to hospital administration, and 3 percent report to finance (Feather, 1989, p. 3).

Discharge planning involves intervention strategies and activities. Assessment and planning efforts become translated into intervention strategies that are appropriate and responsive to client needs. These interventions can be educative, preventive, therapeutic, or rehabilitative in nature. They might include health education in the home setting, rehabilitation services, home nursing services, home health aide services, or referral to any of a number of community service agencies. Discharge planning takes into consideration the services that will help clients to function effectively in their environment. Take, for example, Donnie's case (Appendix 9-1). Donnie was a ventilator-dependent child who spent his first 3 years of life in an acute intensive care unit. Donnie's first hospital discharge was ineffectively planned and implemented, and resulted in his readmission to the hospital 2 months later. Donnie's second hospital discharge was successful because the health care team assessed carefully the services and resources needed by the family in order to handle Donnie's medical problems in the home environment. Donnie's parents were trained to handle his ventilator equipment and were helped to obtain financial assistance and supportive community services.

This example illustrates how educating and involving the family, appropriately assessing discharge needs, and coordinating community resources is crucial to successful implementation of discharge goals. Interventions that fail to address the family unit may result in failure (Pratt, Koval, and Lloyd, 1983; McCubbin and Patterson, 1983).

When implementing discharge planning activities the nurse needs to be cognizant of the fact that clients may respond negatively to the accelerated rate of hospital discharge and departure and may even resist discharge planning efforts. Clients and their families may find it difficult to discuss discharge needs when they are in the middle of an acute care episode. The nurse will need to work cooperatively and emphatically with the client. Also, the nurse should be aware that as the client moves from one level of care to another or one setting to another change occurs, which may result in physical or mental stress, and gains that had been made may be lost or curtailed (Reichelt and Newcomb, 1980).

Discharge planning involves utilization of community resources. Discharge planning focuses on matching client and family needs with community resources (Arenth and Mamon, 1985, p. 20). It is important to discern with which community agencies the client is already involved so that duplication of efforts, and uncoordinated plans of action, can be minimized or avoided.

The nurse needs to be knowledgeable about community resources. Developing this familiarity with community resources, utilizing community resources, and the referral process are discussed later in this chapter.

Discharge planning needs to take into consideration the setting in which the client is being placed. The setting will have a major impact on the health care needs evidenced by the client. The case of 70-year-old Mrs. Flowers is an example.

Mrs. Flowers' cooking, cleaning, laundry, medical, and personal needs were taken care of while she was in the hospital. Now she is ready to return home, where she is responsible for these activities of daily living but unable to handle all of them by herself. Options to assist her, such as homemaker services, transportation, friendly visitors, Meals-on-Wheels, the local Visiting Nurse Association, the help of a friend or relative, or a more supervised living situation, should be explored and planned for before Mrs. Flowers leaves the hospital setting. Mrs. Flowers' support systems, financial resources, perceptions, and goals should be evaluated. The length of time that she will need care should also be considered. She must be involved in establishing and carrying out her plan of care.

Different settings necessitate different intervention strategies. The resources necessary to maintain clients independently in their homes will be very different from those needed by clients going to a nursing home setting.

Discharge planning efforts need to be evaluated. As with all parts of the nursing process, discharge planning needs to be evaluated. However, evaluation of discharge planning efforts is frequently neglected. Evaluations need to be carried out to demonstrate the effectiveness of discharge planning efforts and evaluate client satsifaction with the process (Kromminga and Ostwald, 1987, p. 224; Shamansky, Boase, and Horn, 1984, p. 20). Some agencies use feedback information from other agencies to which they have referred clients for follow-up, to evaluate discharge planning efforts (refer to Oakland County Health Department Referral Form, Figure 9-5).

The Discharge Planning Questionnaire

Many agencies have developed discharge planning questionnaires or guides to facilitate discharge planning efforts. These questionnaires often focus on the client's level of functioning, health care follow-up needs, home adaptation, financial resources, counseling and health education needs, support systems available, and necessary community resources (Kromminga and Ostwald, 1987, p. 224). The discharge questionnaire in Figure 9-1 is designed to facilitate assessment of clients' needs before their departure from

a formal health care setting, but it could be used in various settings. The information assists the nurse in identifying multiple client needs. It examines the psychosocial as well as the biological aspects of functioning and emphasizes preventive health care practices, in addition to needs for curative care. From the data obtained, hospital personnel and community health nurses have baseline information essential for determining further nursing interventions.

It must be remembered that the discharge planning needs evidenced by a client may be complex and long-term, as well as simplistic and short-term. Whatever the discharge planning needs, efforts should focus on facilitating continuity of care, family adaptation and growth, and matching the client with appropriate resources. The process through which the nurse helps clients to utilize resources is the *referral process.*

THE REFERRAL PROCESS DEFINED

The *referral process* is a systematic problem-solving approach involving a series of actions that help clients to utilize resources for the purpose of resolving needs. Clients may be either individuals or groups who require assistance from others in order to achieve their maximum level of functioning. The community health nurse's major goals for initiating a referral are to promote high-level wellness and to enhance self-care capabilities.

Referral is a unique and important process; completing a form or telling a client to contact a community agency is only one small aspect of this process. The referral process demands knowledge, skill, and experience to be implemented effectively. It demands knowledge of community resources, an ability to problem solve and set priorities, and the ability to collaborate and coordinate. It is an integral part of comprehensive, continuous client care and is essential to community health nursing practice (Combs, 1976, p. 122).

A *resource* is defined as an agency, group, or individual that assists a client in meeting a need. Resources provide multiple services and have varying requirements for usage. The community

Figure 9-1   Discharge questionnaire. (From Stone M: Discharge planning guide, Am J Nurs 66:1445-1447, 1979.)

The staff on (unit name) wants to make your return to the community as easy for you as possible. The nurse who is primarily responsible for helping you plan your discharge is _____. He or she will help you and your family reach any resources you may need for your health care at home. There are many agencies, including home care, which assist people in the community with health care problems.

   Please complete the following questions with your family as soon as you feel able. Your discharge nurse will be in contact with you within a few days of your admission.

Data #1
When you get home
1. With whom will you live? _____

2. Will they be able to help with your care if needed? _____

3. Will you have difficulty getting around your home—stairs, small bathroom, low bed, safety problems, to the telephone, to shower, or bathtub? _____

4. Will you have any problems in getting any of the following—transportation, food, medicine, heat, place to stay, child care, pet care, water supply? _____

5. Will you need any of these to function at home—wheelchair, brace, cane, walker, crutches, special equipment? _____

6. How much of the following will you be able to do? (Please mark appropriate column.)

	Independent	*With family*	*Unable to do*
Turning in bed			
Bathing			
Dressing			
Eating			
Sitting			
Standing			
Transfers to tub			
Transfers to toilet			
Walking			

Data #2
1. Have you had a problem with any of these areas recently?
   a. Eyes/ears
   b. Mouth/throat/teeth
   c. Skin
   d. Lungs/breathing
   e. Breasts
   f. Heart/blood vessels
   g. Stomach/bowel
   h. Bladder/kidneys/urine
   i. Genitals
   j. Mental status
   k. Nerves/muscles

2. Will you have difficulty getting to your physician, nurse, or therapist often enough to have these checked?_____

Data #3
Please mark any of the following areas that you would like to know more about:
1. Your disease/illness/accident
   a. What caused it
   b. What can be done to prevent a repeat
   c. How to recognize a repeat
   d. How it will affect you later

2. Your medication
   a. What it does
   b. How much to take
   c. When to take it
   d. What side effects to be aware of

3. Your treatments, procedures, or exercises
  a. What they do for you
  b. How to do them
  c. How often to do them
  d. What difficulties to be aware of

4. Supplies or equipment you'll use at home
  a. What it does
  b. When to use it
  c. How to get more or to get repairs

5. Your nutrition
  a. How it affects you
  b. Special diets—how much to eat, when to eat, what to avoid
  c. How much and what to drink

6. Preventive health practices
  a. How to examine your breasts
  b. Pap smears
  c. Birth control
  d. Effect of cigarettes
  e. Effect of alcohol and drugs
  f. Dental health
  g. Seat belts
  h. Immunizations (yourself or children)
  i. Exercise

7. Other _____

Data #4
1. Which of these agencies are you involved with?
  a. VNA/Home Health
  b. Senior Citizens
  c. Vocational Rehabilitation
  d. Social Welfare
  e. Planned Parenthood
  f. Mental Health Agency
  g. Diet Club
  h. Alcoholics Anonymous
  i. Cancer Society
  j. Ostomy Club
  k. Meals-on-Wheels
  l. Diabetes Association
  m. Dialysis Association
  n. MS Society
  o. MD Society
  p. Association for the Blind
  q. Other _____

2. Please mark any of the areas that you would especially like to discuss with your discharge nurse.
  a. Finances, jobs
  b. Drugs, alcohol
  c. Caring for children or elderly relatives
  d. Emotional or nerve problem
  e. Sexuality
  f. Family or marital relationships
  g. Grieving
  h. School or work
  i. Problem, retirement
  j. Spiritual needs
  k. Legal problems
  l. Other _____

STOP HERE. YOUR DISCHARGE NURSE WILL HELP YOU COMPLETE THE FORM. Ask to see him or her if you haven't met yet, especially if you think you might go home soon.

Assessments (To be done by RN and patient)
1. Will there be a need for help with physical care at home?

2. Will there be a need for a nurse or therapist at home to assess physical status, disease process, or exercise and therapy?

3. Will the patient or family need more health education about any of the areas above (Data #3), either during hospitalization or at home?

4. Will the patient or family need more information or assistance with any of the psychosocial areas listed in Data #4?

Plan (To be done by patient and nurse together)
Consider the four assessments above. If there are *no* yes responses, proceed to section B and complete. If there are any yes responses, you *must* select either part 1 or part 2 of section A before completing section B.
A. 1. No referral necessary, but must have further education before discharge regarding _____

   2. Refer to: (see above list of agencies)

B. 1. Equipment or supplies to leave with patient _____

   2. Transfer plan _____

   3. Medical follow-up _____

   4. Surgical follow-up _____

TABLE 9-1 Types of referral by initiator, extent of contact with resource, level of difficulty, and source and examples of each

	Type of referral	Example
Initiator	*Primary:* Referral initiated by client, often readily	Client suggesting marriage counseling
	Secondary: Referral initiated by someone other than client	Community health nurse suggesting marriage counseling
Extent of contact with resource	*Formal:* Contact made with a resource on behalf of a client; contact can be made by the client or someone on the client's behalf; contact generally made with client's permission; these referrals are often processed through a system of standardized forms and procedures	Client contacting a local department of social service (DSS) about obtaining food stamps
		Community health nurse talking about services a family member can provide, which the client subsequently uses
	Informal: Discussion of a resource between two or more persons without contact being made with the resource; often the initial step toward a formal referral	or
		Client and community health nurse discussing available DSS services (e.g., food stamps, general assistance, Aid for Families of Dependent Children, Medicaid)
Level of difficulty	*Simple:* Referral reaches need resolution on the initial attempt	On initial attempt, client goes to DSS and obtains food stamps
	Complex: Referral does not meet need resolution on the initial attempt; process needs to be reworked (refer to Figure 9-1 for steps in process)	Client goes to DSS seeking food stamps and finds out that she or he is not eligible, but the need for assistance with food budgeting still exists. Other community resources such as the Nutritional Extension Service may be more appropriate
Source	*Interresource:* Referrals made from one resource to another	Community health nurse referring client from the local health department to a neighborhood health clinic
	Intraresource: Referrals made within the resource itself	Community health nurse referring client to local health department sanitarian for water sampling
	Self: Client refers himself to a resource for service; some agencies will not accept these referrals—a form of a primary referral	Client calls local health department to arrange for community health nursing visits

health nurse needs to be knowledgeable about community resources, increase client awareness of resources, and assist the client in resource utilization.

Health care resources can be described as formal and informal. *Formal* health care resources exist primarily for the provision of health care services. They include, but are not limited to, hospitals, extended-care facilities, skilled nursing homes, health departments, outpatient facilities, and the offices of private health care practitioners.

Informal health care resources provide health services but do not exist primarily for this purpose. These resources can be relatives in the client's home, service organizations, and self-help groups. They are scattered throughout the community, are minimally coordinated, and are often more difficult to recognize than formal resources. An example of an informal health care resource is the local Lion's Club, which provides free ophthalmologic examinations and eyeglasses to children in the community who could not otherwise obtain them. It provides a health care service, but its primary function is not health related. There are many such resources within the community and they are important to the provision of health care for individuals, families, and populations at risk.

The community health nurse will make referrals to and receive referrals from health care resources. Referrals can be categorized according to referral initiator, the extent of client contact made with the resource, the level of difficulty of the process, and the source of the referral. Working through the referral process with a client can be an enriching and rewarding experience. Table 9-1 is a chart illustrating different types of referral.

Basic Principles of Referral

Wolff's (1962) classic article on referral delineated basic principles to take into consideration when helping clients to use the referral process. Others (Combs, 1976; Wheeler-Lachowycz, 1983; USDHHS, 1982) have reinforced the value of these principles and have expanded on them. These principles are listed below:

1. *There should be merit in the referral.* The referral should meet the needs and objectives of the client and should be necessary. Before referring the client to community resources, it is extremely important to assess what resources are available in the client's own environment. Often it will be found that family, friends, and neighbors can do as much as or more than formal community health resources.

2. *The referral should be practical.* The client should be able to utilize the referral in an efficient, effective manner. The referral should not be a waste of time, money, and effort on behalf of the client, the resource, or the referral facilitator.

3. *The referral should be individualized to the client.* A referral that meets the needs of one client may not meet the needs of another. It is essential to assess the individual needs and concerns of clients before decisions about the appropriateness of a referral are made.

For example, some clients can learn very well in a group setting whereas others cannot.

4. *The referral should be timely.* It should come at a time when the client is ready to work on the health care need and when it is the appropriate time to work on the need.

5. *The referral should be coordinated with other activities.* The referral should be congruent with other health care activities that are occurring. This aids in maximizing health care interventions, preventing duplication of service, and carrying out contradictory intervention strategies.

6. *The referral should incorporate the client and family into planning and implementation.* It has already been stressed that it is critical for the client and family to be involved in health planning and intervention and that without this involvement, interventions are likely to fail.

7. *The client should have the right to say no to the referral.* This principle acknowledges the client's right to self-determination. A competent client has the right to make decisions about health care (ANA, 1986, p. 3). The client has the right to refuse a referral, unless legal authority dictates otherwise. Cases of law are the exception and will vary from state to state. An example of a law that could require the community health nurse to refer a client without his or her consent is a child abuse law that mandates reporting suspected child abuse and neglect cases.

In order to protect this right of self-determination, the client must be aware of the referral. Referrals are sometimes made for clients without their consent, but this is not considered good referral practice. If the nurse makes contact with a client and learns that the client was not aware of the referral, and does not want it, the situation could be awkward. In such a case the nurse should explain the reason for the referral and the services the nurse can provide, and should apologize for any inconvenience to the client. This type of nursing intervention may help the client to see why the referral was made, and even to accept the referral.

At times, individuals are referred without their knowledge or consent because the referring agency considers them a threat to their own safety or the safety of others. The client still has the right to refuse a referral, unless legal authority dictates otherwise.

The refusal of a referral may be difficult for the nurse to accept, especially if the referral appears to be helpful to the client. However, the client's right to say no should be adhered to.

Confidentiality and Referral

Confidentiality of client information is an important professional ethic for the nurse to honor. As with self-determination, confidentiality is violated only if laws intervene. Nurses must receive the client's permission to share personal data and what information is shared should be carefully evaluated. Sharing of information should be in the client's best interest and for purposes of facilitating optimum care. Loosely sharing information about clients among staff members when it does not facilitate client care is not professional or ethical. Many agencies have release-of-information forms for sending and receiving data about clients. It is preferable to obtain written permission to share this data. Maintaining confidentiality is a professional responsibility.

Developing a Referral System

Before referral activities take place a referral system needs to be in place. Developing a referral system involves determining the types of resources necessary to carry out health care activities, locating these resources in the community, collecting information on the resources, developing a referral list, developing a referral protocol, developing a follow-up system, training people to make referrals, and periodically updating the referral and resource information (USDHHS, 1982, p. 27). These activities are discussed throughout this chapter.

Answering a Referral

Answering referrals is an important part of the referral process and helps to maintain effective communication networks between the client, staff, and resources (Reischelt and Newcomb, 1980). If referrals are not answered, or are answered incompletely or tardily, the referral source may become discouraged and not send further referrals. Prompt, complete, and courteous answering of a referral helps to establish and maintain good working relationships and facilitates follow-up and continuity of client care.

Referrals should be answered as soon as possible, ideally within a week after they have been received. The nurse should include in the communication with the referring agency comments on the needs that were recognized by the referring agency, as well as current assessment data, nursing diagnoses, and future actions and plans. If the client and nurse decide that nursing service should be continued, the referring agency should be given this information.

REFERRAL RESOURCES

Once the need for a referral has been established, the appropriate resources must be located in the community. The community health nurse needs to collect information on community resources and be familiar with them (Figure 9-2).

Health professionals and local health departments are excellent sources of information on community resources. Developing a network with helping professionals in the community can assist the nurse in compiling resource information and facilitate client care (Meisenhelder, 1982). Frequently, compilations of local resources are done by groups such as United Way Community Services, chambers of commerce, departments of social service, offices on aging, and health departments. Major service organizations, such as associations for retarded citizens, will compile resources specific to the groups they represent. City offices and planning commissions will also have local resource information as well as census data.

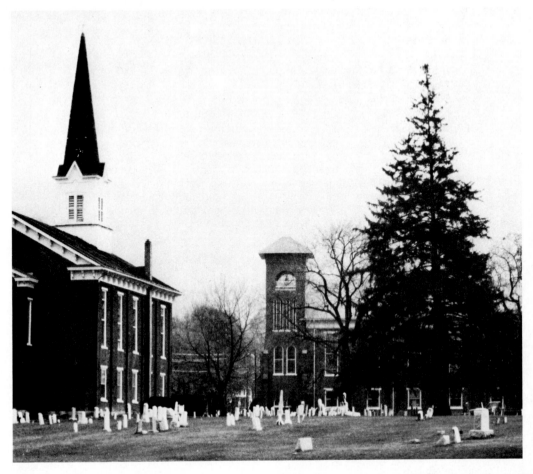

Figure 9-2 Churches are extremely valuable, informal community resources, which are often overlooked by health care professionals. Many churches provide numerous community services including home visiting to ill and disabled persons, home repair services for elderly church members, and monies to assist needy families who lack essentials of daily living. Community health nurses frequently find that churches in their districts will assist them to meet specific client needs, especially when there is no other community resource that can do so. (Courtesy of photographer, Henry Parks.)

Resource information should be sought out, and before referring a client, the nurse should independently explore the resource, and know whether the resource is appropriate for the client.

Collecting Information on Referral Resources

When collecting information on referral resources the nurse needs to develop a systematic way of recording and filing information (USDHHS, 1982, p. 28). Creating an ongoing file with a standard format, such as the one shown in Figure 9-3, can be helpful. Such a file should list resources both alphabetically and by service. In addition to the resource information on file the nurse can also keep resource brochures or other print materials to assist clients in resource selection. Resources that are frequently used, or used with success, may be colored-coded or tabbed for easy accessibility. It is necessary that resource information be clear, accurate, and concise.

National Foundation—March of Dimes
Payne County Office

Address: 20100 Maplewood, Mio, MI 47235
Phone: 811-2110 (Area 516)
Person in charge: Mrs. Nellie Scott, Director

Purpose and services: Through referral and direct aid, assistance is provided in the areas of prenatal care, genetic counseling, diagnosis, and treatment. Offers prevention and treatment services for clients who have congenital malformations or birth defects through research, direct patient services, and public education. Sponsors scholarships in related health fields.

Eligibility: No restrictions.

Application procedure: Referrals by private physicians, public health clinics, or health departments.

Individuals are encouraged to contact the office for further information.

Fees: None

Office hours: 9 A.M. to 3 P.M., Tuesday–Saturday

Geographic area served: Payne County

Compiled 6/90

Figure 9-3 Resource information.

The following information is essential for the nurse to know about a resource, and is readily kept on file cards or in a loose-leaf notebook: (1) name of resource (include address, phone number, and name and title of person in charge or contact person), (2) purpose and services, (3) eligibility (who may use the resource, including special requirements such as age and income), (4) application procedure, (5) fees, (6) office hours and days, and (7) geographic area served. Cards should be dated to aid in file updating (refer to Figure 9-3). Data on client response to utilization of the resource should also be kept.

The nurse should also be aware of specific information that a resource requests of a client when it provides service. Information frequently requested by resources includes the following:

1. Name, address, and telephone number of the client
2. Client age, sex, and marital status
3. Names and birthdates of family members and others living in the household
4. Medical care source and health history
5. Financial status and records
6. Resources with whom the client is presently working
7. Reason for seeking referral

A grid which shows frequently used resources can be a very valuable reference when one is visiting clients in the community setting. A grid that includes service areas and specific resources is especially helpful. An example of such a grid is presented in Table 9-2. It is not all-inclusive, and re-

TABLE 9-2   Resource grid

Service needed	Types	Resource
Food	1. Emergency	1. Department of Social Services, Salvation Army, local churches, American Red Cross, Goodfellows
	2. Low-cost or free foods	2. Food stamps, food coops, school lunch programs, WIC
	3. Counseling	3. Expanded nutrition program, Health Department
Financial assistance	1. Emergency and short-term	1. Department of Social Services, Salvation Army, Goodfellows, Lion's Club, Traveler's Aid, Volunteers of America, Kiwanis
	2. Long term	2. Department of Social Service, Social Security Administration, Veterans Administration
Housing	1. Emergency	1. Catholic Social Services, Jewish Action League, United Way Community Service, Department of Social Service, American Red Cross, Salvation Army, local churches, domestic violence facilities
	2. Public (low-cost)	2. Housing Commission, Department of Social Service

Adapted from the University of Michigan School of Nursing, Family and Community Health Nursing: Resource Grid, Ann Arbor, undated, University of Michigan School of Nursing.

sources will vary from area to area, but it does illustrate how a service resource grid can be organized.

STEPS OF THE REFERRAL PROCESS

The referral process is a systematic, problem-solving approach which involves a number of client and nurse actions (Atwood, 1971; USDHHS, 1982). Figure 9-4 depicts the steps involved in successfully implementing a referral. It will be found, when helping a client obtain needed assistance from community resources, that the process is circular. That is, as data are obtained in one step, other steps may need to be repeated. It is crucial to remember that these steps are interconnected and interrelated.

The following are the basic steps of the referral process:

1. Establish a working relationship with the client
2. Establish the need for a referral
3. Set objectives for the referral
4. Explore resource availability
5. Client decides to use or not use referral
6. Make referral to resource
7. Facilitate referral
8. Evaluate and follow-up

Client participation throughout the process is essential. The community health nurse guides the client through the process by facilitating informed decision making, assessing client needs and objectives, exploring alternatives for need resolution, assisting the client to utilize resources, and evaluating the results of the entire process. The client is encouraged to be independent whenever possible.

Establish a Working Relationship with the Client

The referral process usually evolves after a working relationship with the client has been established. This relationship involves the formation of trust between the nurse and the client. This trust facilitates cooperation; it may develop almost immediately, but more often evolves over a period of time. While establishing the relationship, the nurse is able to gather data necessary for helping the client to make health decisions. Clients in crisis often initially establish a working relationship more quickly than do other clients, because of the immediacy of their needs.

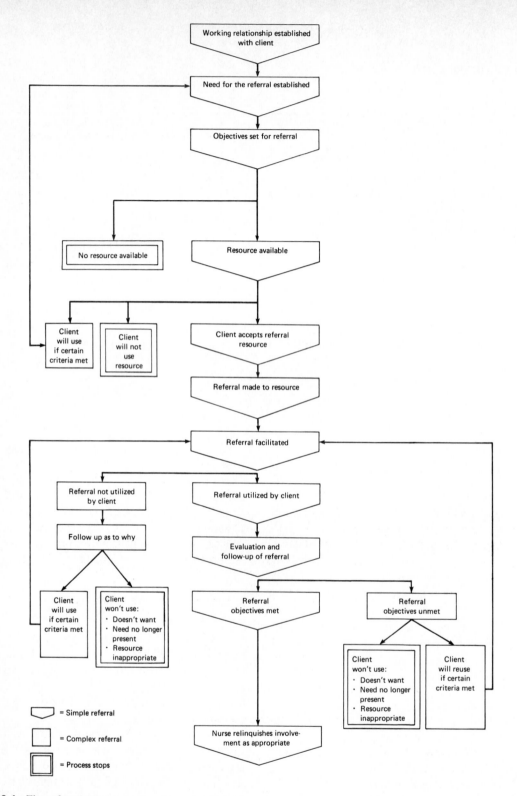

Figure 9-4   The referral process.

In establishing a working relationship, it is essential to give the client a fair and patient hearing, and start "where the client is at" in the therapeutic process (Goldstein, 1983). As a means of building this relationship, the helping professional needs to focus on the clients' feelings about their immediate life situation and to exhibit a willingness to perceive the world from the clients' frame of reference (Siporin, 1975; Goldstein, 1983).

In many cases, the referral process will commence as this relationship develops to its potential. If referrals are necessitated early in the relationship, the nurse should proceed with caution to be sure that sufficient data have been collected to determine if the referral is appropriate.

Establish the Need for a Referral

The community health nurse utilizes the nursing process to help the client to identify what health care needs necessitate referral. Clients often require assistance from the community health nurse to recognize referral needs. The nurse should aid the client in looking at referral alternatives. The client should be asked about preferences and special needs, and information on appropriate resources should be shared with the client (USDHHS, 1982, p. 31).

When establishing a need for referral, it is important to discriminate between problems the community health nurse can and cannot handle. For example, there are some budgeting problems that can be dealt with by a community health nurse and others that cannot. A community health nurse can help a family to analyze how its members can obtain the most for their food dollars by discussing such things as meal planning, low-cost meals, and inexpensive sources of protein. On the other hand, if the family is having difficulty with creditors, the family is usually referred to a credit-counseling resource.

The nurse needs to be honest with the client about the client's assessed health needs. The client may not be aware of a need, such as immunizations to prevent communicable disease, until the nurse raises his or her consciousness about it. There may be situations in which the nurse finds it difficult to share perceived client needs, especially when the client is using denial to cope or relieve anxiety. This is often the case when psychosocial problems such as marital crises exist. It often helps in these situations to assist the client in seeing that symptoms of stress are evident and that steps need to be taken to resolve the actual problem. Often, asking whether clients are aware of any changes that should be made in their life situation can facilitate discussion about real pressures being experienced. Clients must be ready to deal with their problems before they will continue to use a referral resource. Honest confrontation can be very motivating and necessary when clients have difficulty taking action. This is particularly true when a caring relationship has been established between the client and the community health nurse and when the client realizes that the nurse is acting in his or her best interests.

The community health nurse and client should thoroughly assess the need for referral. Unnecessary or unwanted referrals are costly, often strain relationships between referring agencies, and can adversely affect nurse-client relationships. Once the need for a referral has been established, the nurse and client should establish objectives for the services required and should look at which resources in the community can best meet the client's needs.

Set Objectives for the Referral

What the client would like to see accomplished, tempered with what is realistically feasible, combine to determine the objectives for the referral. The nurse can help the client to be realistic in resource expectations, but the decision about specific objectives to be achieved should be made by the client. It is often helpful to write out objectives with the client in behavioral terms such as "Mrs. Black will contact the Department of Social Services in regard to obtaining food stamps by March 30." An integral part of setting objectives for the referral is deciding on what services are necessary from the referral source, as well as on a time frame for obtaining these services. The nurse should be careful when setting objectives not to attempt more than what is reasonable to be accomplished within a specified time period.

In this phase of the referral process, one may find that the client expects more than an agency can offer. An agency does not solve the clients' problems, but it helps clients to help themselves. For example, Mrs. Quinn, a single mother, wanted counseling only for her 16-year-old daughter, who planned to drop out of school and marry her 21-year-old boyfriend. Mrs. Quinn thought a counseling agency could "talk some sense into her." The community health nurse assisted Mrs. Quinn in seeing that a family counseling agency helps a family to deal with its problems rather than assuming responsibility for them. Joint counseling sessions arranged through the local Family and Neighborhood Counseling Center helped both mother and daughter to communicate together more effectively and to understand each other's concerns and needs. These sessions also helped the family to develop a pattern of functioning that facilitated family problem solving and decision making.

Explore Resource Availability

A source of aid must be available before a referral can be made. An appropriate resource is one that can meet the client's needs and objectives and is available, acceptable, and accessible to the client. If more than one appropriate resource exists, the client should be allowed to choose between them. If no resource is available, the referral objectives may need to be redefined or a resource developed. Many times, resources in the community will reconsider the services they provide to clients, especially if the community health nurse acts as an advocate for certain services.

Client's Decision to Use or Not Use Referral

The client can say yes, no, or maybe when considering a referral. If the client says yes, the referral process continues. If the client says no or maybe, the nurse should explore with the client the reasons why. If the client does not want the referral under any condition, the right to self-determination must be respected.

The nurse should not become discouraged or believe he or she has failed if the client does not accept a referral. Imposing services on the client does not help; it only causes frustration for the nurse as well as the client, and may adversely affect the client's utilization and perception of the health care system.

If the client would utilize a referral if certain criteria were met, the nurse may be able to assist the client in meeting these criteria. For example, a client might say that she would utilize a referral to the health department immunization clinic for her 2-year-old if transportation to the clinic could be arranged. The nurse may be able to help this client obtain transportation services from other community resources. If a client continues to place conditions on referral utilization, the nurse and client should take a close look at the reasons behind these conditions. It is possible that the client really does not want the referral but fears saying no.

It may be found that clients do not want to use one resource to meet a health care need but are willing to utilize another resource. An example of this is Mrs. Schlosser.

Mrs. Schlosser was an elderly client who was eligible for food stamps but would not apply for them. She viewed food stamps as charity and stated, "I do not accept welfare." The community health nurse was frustrated because Mrs. Schlosser's diet was inadequate, largely for financial reasons. Discussing the food stamp program with Mrs. Schlosser did not change her mind about using food stamps. Thus, the nurse explored alternatives with her. Because she wanted to eat better, she was receptive to learning about how to prepare low-cost, nutritious meals at home and was also interested in applying for a reduced cost, Meal-on-Wheels program in which she would pay for her meals. Mrs. Schlosser had refused a referral for food stamps, but she and the nurse were able to develop alternatives that helped to meet her nutritional needs.

Timing influences how the client responds to the referral. Studies have shown that a referral should occur as soon as possible after detecting a risk; a rapid, well-handled referral often reinforces the importance of taking positive health action to the client (USDHHS, 1982, p. 27).

Referral Made to a Resource

When the nurse is referring a client to a resource, the referral content should be specific and comprehensive, and should reflect the client's objectives for the referral (Combs, 1976, p. 126). The appropriate forms should be filled out and procedures followed: referral information should be given out only with client consent, unless legally dictated otherwise. Clients usually do not hesitate to sign a release of information form when they have made a decision that they need a referral. The correct procedure for contacting the resource must also be followed. The referral is made formal at this point; if an appointment is necessary, it should be made. Either the client or nurse may be the contact person; however, the client should be encouraged to be as independent as possible in contacting the resource.

Many referrals can be made, at least initially, by telephone. Telephone referrals may be faster and more informative, since the agency can request any additional or specific information that is needed at the time (Wheeler-Lachowycz, 1983). A written referral can always follow. If the referral is written, it will include information such as client and family awareness of the diagnosis and prognosis; complete and detailed orders for medications and treatments; people living with the client; the client's religion; spoken language and diet; address and phone number; titles such as Doctor, Mrs., Mr.; goals for and estimated length of service; nursing diagnoses; and method of health care financing (Wheeler-Lachowycz, 1983).

An example of a referral form used by one local health department to refer clients to another resource is presented in Figure 9-5. This form includes essential referral information, such as data about the person making the referral, the individual or family being referred, the reason for the referral, summary of the client's situation, resources being used by the client, a statement on whether or not the client is aware of the referral, and a place for the receiving resource to share information with the referral agency to facilitate follow-up and evaluation..

Often, resources request that clients bring certain types of information with them to their first appointment. If clients are not aware of this requirement, they may have to return to the resource with the information or may be denied service. Returning to a resource takes additional time, effort, and money. It may present a barrier to the client in utilizing the referral.

Facilitate the Referral

Facilitating a referral involves preparing the client for the use of community services, as well as identifying and overcoming barriers to the utilization of these services. Throughout the process, the community health nurse evaluates the client's responses to the referral to determine if changes need to be made to effect client involvement. It is important to remember that client motivation is critical; if the client is not motivated to make the referral work, the referral process will probably not be successful. Barriers that decrease client motivation are discussed later in this chapter.

Evaluation and Follow-up

As with all aspects of the nursing process, referrals need to be evaluated. Ongoing evaluation and follow-up are probably of most importance in the referral process. Effective evaluation of the referral process encompasses reviewing how well client needs are being met as well as the client's reactions to the services being received.

Evaluation enhances the nurse's ability to develop competency in using the process and to make changes in the process when necessary. In evaluating, the nurse must realize that there are times when a referral is not or was not effective. However, this judgment should not be made quickly. It will be found that some clients need support and encouragement, especially if their problems are not resolved immediately. The case of Mr. Connant is an example.

Mr. Connant decided that he was not going back to the mental health clinic for counseling after his first visit because the clinic counselor "did nothing but talk." In evaluating this situation, the nurse realized that she

OAKLAND COUNTY DEPARTMENT OF HEALTH

1200 North Telegraph Road   27725 Greenfield
Pontiac, Michigan 48053   Southfield, Michigan 48075
Telephone 858-1280   Telephone 424-7000

REFERRAL FORM

TO _____   FROM: _____

ADDRESS _____   ☐ PONTIAC OFFICE

_____   ☐ SOUTHFIELD OFFICE

Attention: _____   Telephone # _____ Date _____

REGARDING _____   Aware of referral? ☐ Yes ☐ No

ADDRESS _____   Telephone # _____

FAMILY ROSTER (Names, birthdate, relationship)

REASON FOR REFERRAL

SITUATION

(over)

KNOWN MEDICAL, AGENCY, COMMUNITY RESOURCES

REPLY REQUESTED: ☐ No ☐ Yes   (see back)

Figure 9-5 Sample referral form. (Used by permission of the Nursing Division, Oakland County Health Division, Pontiac, Mi.)

Continuation of situation:

Agency reply to Oakland County Health Department

_____
(Signature)

Date _____

needed to discuss more specifically with Mr. Connant his expectations of counseling along with the need for him to share his feelings about his first session with the counselor at the clinic. Supportive assistance by the nurse facilitated Mr. Connant's return to the mental health center. Later, he expressed gratitude for the nurse's encouragement because counseling was helping him to work through many of the issues that had been troubling him.

During evaluation, the client should be helped to understand why the referral was necessary and anticipatory guidance should be used in preparing the client to handle similar situations in the future. If it is seen that a client evidences the same problem over and over, the nurse and client should thoroughly assess why this is happening. Usually in these situations it is found that client problems are not being diagnosed completely. For example, repeated need for emergency food orders should be a clue that the client is having difficulty managing his or her budget. This could be a result of having a too-limited income or of not knowing how to allocate funds that are available. Emergency food orders will not solve either of these problems on a long-term basis. If the client is not helped to explore other options, he or she may experience a crisis in the future which is difficult to resolve.

Probably the hardest part of the evaluation phase is realizing when it is time for the nurse to relinquish involvement with the client. This is an especially difficult task when the client and nurse have developed a strong, positive working relationship, and termination in these situations can provoke uneasy feelings within both the nurse and the client (refer to Chapter 8). Usually it is the case that clients are ready to function independently when they can identify personal health care needs, take initiative to contact health care resources, and take action to resolve health care problems. If a client does not demonstrate these behaviors or demonstrates them only when the community health nurse is not available, the nurse-client relationship should be closely examined, as it may be fostering an unhealthy dependency.

BARRIERS TO UTILIZATION OF THE REFERRAL PROCESS

For each resource and each client, the nurse must identify the barriers that adversely affect the utilization of referral services. Barriers involve individual and resource components. For example, an agency may have high fees for services (a resource barrier), which the client is unable to afford (a client barrier). In this case, fees are both a resource barrier and a client barrier. Some common resource and client barriers are briefly described below.

Resource Barriers
Attitudes of Health Care Professionals

The attitudes and biases of health care professionals have a great impact on whether clients utilize resource services (Goldstein, 1983). Clients are quick to sense the attitudes of health care personnel, and if they are not treated with respect and courtesy, they are hesitant to return. Short, nonspecific answers given to a client's questions, minimal interchange with the client on an informal level, and conveying frustration when clients ask questions are a few examples of behaviors that foster negative reactions when clients are using community resources.

The helping professional must be open to the opinions of others and must maintain a nonjudgmental attitude. People are inclined to pay attention to those events in life that confirm what they already believe and disregard those that are contradictory. This is defined as selective reality (Bruner, 1973). By falling into this trap, the helping professional may reinforce biases and attitudes not conducive to developing a therapeutic relationship with clients. Helping professionals' attitudes must blend with clients' beliefs and flow with the energy and direction of the challenge present in clients' various situations (Saposnek, 1980). A therapeutic relationship can be maintained while affirming that clients are the ultimate authority over their personal values and lifestyle, making the worker and the client both teachers and learners. Such a situation is a state conducive to establishing a helping relationship and building trust (Goldstein, 1983).

Physical Accessibility of Resource

Clients are less likely to use resources that are not readily accessible. Once a resource is beyond walking distance, other means of transportation must be found. Public transportation is sparse in this country. Even if the family has a car, the car may not be available at the time of the resource appointment. The problem is greatly magnified if the resource is at such a distance that the client must make arrangements for overnight stays in order to utilize the services it offers. Overnight stays often necessitate making arrangements for the care of small children or other members of the family, and they can be very costly to the client. Community resources such as a Ronald McDonald House have helped to meet this accessibility need.

Cost of Resource Services

How much a client can or is willing to pay for a health service is an individual matter. Any cost at all may be more than clients can pay if their income is minimal. If the service is not absolutely necessary or critical to the client's activities of daily living, the cost may be viewed as too high even when the client has money available for the service. On the other hand, if the client places a high priority on receiving a given service, he or she may not object to paying even high fees.

Client Barriers

Priorities

If the need is not of high priority for the client, he or she may not become actively involved in utilizing the referral services. If other needs are considered to be of higher priority, the nurse should assist the client in meeting these needs first. It may be more important for the family to care for an ill family member than to take a child to the well-baby clinic for immunizations; or if the family is having difficulty meeting its basic needs of food, clothing, and shelter, preventive health care services may not be viewed as a priority.

Motivation

If the client is not highly motivated to work on a need, it is not likely that much will be done by the client toward meeting that need. An integral part of client motivation is the concept of *awareness vs. readiness.* The fact that the client is aware of a need does not mean that he or she is ready to act on the need. If a differentiation is not made between awareness and readiness, the nurse may feel responsible for the failure of the client to follow through on a referral. Once it is established that the client is not ready to act on a need and the resultant referral, the nurse can help the client to prioritize the needs upon which he or she is ready to act. A good example of awareness vs. readiness is a client who acknowledges that his house needs to be cleaned, but after numerous nursing visits, much discussion, and ample time, the house is still not cleaned. The client is aware of the need but is not ready to act on it.

Previous Experience with Resources

If a client has not had a positive experience in utilizing a resource in the past, she or he may be hesitant to use this resource again or to utilize other community resources. In these situations, it is important to acknowledge the client's feelings as well as to explain ways to make further contacts with community services more meaningful. *Complaints about resources can be entirely justified.* However, it will be found that some clients were not ready to make changes when they used a community service the first time; hence, they have a negative view of the service because of the fact that their problems were not resolved. This is frequently the case when clients have psychosocial difficulties.

Lack of Knowledge about Available Resources

Clients need to know about resources before they will use them. A key role of the community health nurse is to help clients learn about health care services in the community (Combs, 1976; Gillespie, 1980). Lack of knowledge about resources is a major barrier to the utilization of health care services.

Lack of Understanding of the Need for a Referral

Clients who do not understand the need for a referral frequently do not take action to obtain referral services. This is often true of families who neglect to have their children immunized. Many people know that children need "baby shots" but do not understand why. These people will be more likely to follow through on a consistent basis in obtaining immunizations if they know the purpose for receiving immunizations and the consequences of not obtaining adequate protection against communicable diseases.

Client Self-Image

If clients do not have a positive self-image, they may be hesitant to seek care, and they may view themselves as unworthy of such care. The nurse should acknowledge these feelings and develop intervention strategies which will help clients to increase self-esteem.

Cultural Factors

Cultural differences can be a barrier to therapeutic interaction (Goldstein, 1983). Every culture has definite beliefs regarding health care practices. Resources may not be used if they violate these practices and beliefs. In Arab cultures, for example, women are generally not allowed to leave their homes or immediate neighborhoods without a male escort. Thus, health care services are better utilized by these women if they are located in a neighborhood facility.

Within any culture, it will also be found that there is individual variation in how persons respond to the utilization of health care services. That is why it is so important to comprehensively assess strengths, needs, and concerns of each family unit. Lindstrom (1975, pp. 757 and 759), studying 30 Mexican-American families, demonstrated that even though the families had a number of shared characteristics, there were also differences which influenced use or nonuse of child health services. Characteristics in common centered on family relationships; these relationships were strong, male-dominated, and extended, with an emphasis on maintaining privacy. In addition, all the families in her study had a minimal income, lived in poor neighborhoods, and many had had little formal education. Mothers who kept appointments, however, did differ from those who did not. These mothers had more responsibility and independence than mothers who were poor users of child health services and were likely to be or to have been the head of the household. These mothers also reported that they had transportation available and that they utilized either prenatal or child health services, because they wanted to be sure that everything was all right. Nonuser mothers tended to live in a nuclear family, and to see a doctor only when their children were ill.

Financial

Many clients do not use community resources, because they cannot afford the services offered by these resources. The near-poor client—one who does not qualify for welfare assistance but may be medically indigent—has difficulty paying for the high cost of health care (USDHHS, 1986). With today's high rates of unemployment, many families are finding themselves without health insurance, and often they may not qualify for the health assistance program of Medicaid. Increasing numbers of families with health insurance do not have major medical coverage that offsets the cost of physician and other health care services. It is a real challenge for the community health nurse not only to find resources that will assist these clients but also to locate these at-risk individuals. Often, they are unknown to the health care delivery system and receive needed health care only when services are brought to them.

Transportation

Lack of transportation is a major barrier to the utilization of health care services. Increasingly, it is being documented that clients often do not seek assistance from health care professionals because they have problems getting to health care facilities (Lindstrom, 1975; Rossman and Burnside, 1975; Keith, 1976). If low-cost transportation is not available in the community you are serving, car pooling or establishing clinic services in the neighborhood may reduce the number of transportation barriers.

LEVELS OF NURSING INTERVENTION WITH REFERRAL

Clients are at varying stages of ability to assume independent functioning when utilizing health care resources, and this necessitates different levels of professional intervention by the community health nurse. Identifying at what level the client is functioning helps the community health nurse to focus intervention strategies when utilizing the referral process.

Level I: At this level, the client is largely dependent on the nurse and will need assistance with all aspects of the referral process. Frequently, these clients have not had life experiences which have prepared them to deal adequately with systems external to their family unit. Or, their energies are depleted by crisis. These clients need considerable support and encouragement and, often, concrete help from the community health nurse before they can follow through on a needed referral. Frequently they assume a passive role. They may sincerely want assistance from others but fail to take action because they lack the energy or knowledge to do so, and basically feel inadequate to handle the referral by themselves. Community health nursing intervention with these clients involves health teaching and counseling so that they can identify health needs that necessitate referral. In addition, supportive assistance is necessary while they are learning how to use health care resources. A major goal when working with these clients is to help them to become more actively involved in taking responsibility for meeting their own health needs. At first, the community health nurse may have to assist these clients with making all the arrangements for warranted health care; just keeping an appointment can be a major accomplishment for them. Sometimes it is easier to do for the cli-

ent than to work with him or her, especially if the client follows through when the nurse makes all the necessary arrangements and decisions. It is important, however, for the community health nurse to work toward helping clients to utilize health resources independently.

Level II: At this level, mutual participation is evident. The client does not wait for the community health nurse to initiate discussion about health care needs. Rather, the client actively seeks information to determine what health actions are needed to resolve current health problems or to enhance wellness in the future. Clients at this level may need health teaching to understand the value of preventive health practices, to locate community resources that they can afford, or to learn about community services such as low-cost or free transportation, which will help them to use needed resources. They are more likely, however, to raise challenging questions and to identify when health care resources are inappropriate to meet their needs. At times, it may be difficult to recognize when these clients need assistance because they are functioning so well in most aspects of their lives.

Level III: At this level, the client can utilize the referral process independently. The nurse may be used as a resource person, but otherwise she or he assumes a passive participant role.

THE COMMUNITY HEALTH NURSE AS A HOME CARE COORDINATOR: DISCHARGE PLANNING AND THE REFERRAL PROCESS IN ACTION

The community health nurse working as a home care coordinator is often part of a hospital or acute care setting discharge planning team. The nurse may also be employed by a local health department to assist in meeting the home care needs of clients as they are discharged from a health care setting. Hospitals that employ home care coordinators on the staff have often found that the presence of such a position has a positive effect on the interaction of the hospital with community agencies (Reichelt and Newcomb, 1980). Such a position demonstrates to community agencies that the hospital is responsive to clients' community needs and gives community agencies a person to communicate with when they have questions about a client's condition. The home care coordinator is actively involved in discharge planning activities and the referral process, and adheres to the principles and practices of each. The objectives of the home care coordinator are as follows (Gonnerman, 1968; Gillespie, 1980):

1. To facilitate quality and continuous care between levels of health care
2. To receive community referrals from hospital staff
3. To evaluate clients for home health care or other community care
4. To coordinate a multidisciplinary plan of care with the client, family, and community resources
5. To help health care and other professionals recognize and plan for the discharge needs of clients
6. To promote multidisciplinary working relationships with discharge planning
7. To be knowledgeable about and maximize the use of health care resources and interpret these resources to client, family, and staff
8. To alleviate client and family anxiety about discharge needs
9. To make discharge planning referrals, as appropriate
10. To evaluate discharge planning

The multidisciplinary aspects of this role are very important. The job of a home care coordinator will involve planning with other disciplines including social workers, doctors, occupational therapists, physical therapists, and nutritionists. It will also involve working with other nurses, the client, and the client's family.

The home care coordinator must realize that not all nurses have a complete or adequate understanding of the role of the nurse in the com-

munity and that many hospital nurses have not worked in the community (Chisholm, 1983; Combs, 1976). Collaborative relationships among hospital and community health nurses are essential to successful discharge planning efforts, and open communication between these nurses should be facilitated. A major role of the home care coordinator is to increase staff awareness about these needs and the community resources that will assist clients in dealing with them (Gillespie, 1980).

In assessing client discharge needs, the home care coordinator must be aware that clients with illnesses that are not self-limiting and that involve a residual disability are most apt to need home care services (Gonnerman, 1968, p. 4). These clients may need such things as homemaker services; home health care; assistance with transportation; health teaching in relation to disease processes, medical regimens, and environmental modifications which can increase self-care capabilities; and counseling relative to career planning, financial management, and structural and process changes needed within the family system as a result of the client's illness. One single community agency often cannot ameliorate all of a client's discharge needs (Pratt, Koval, and Lloyd, 1983). The home care coordinator must maintain open channels of communication with community resources.

With the mandated emphasis on early discharge from hospital settings, it will become increasingly important for the home care coordinator to act quickly and efficiently when assessing and planning for discharge needs. As discharge is accelerated, the home care coordinator can expect to meet with at least some resistance on the part of clients, families, and community resources (Willihnganz, 1984). The client and family may not wish to think about the future until the needs of the present are met (e.g., surgery, radical treatment), and they may not be receptive to the concentrated efforts directed toward discharge (Willihnganz, 1984). They will likely need much help and support.

The home care coordinator should not wait for referrals, but should seek out prospective home

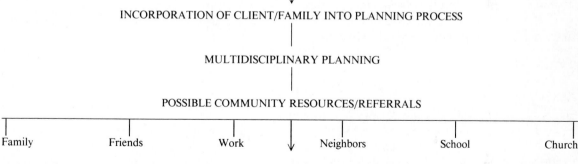

GOALS: Successful transition of client to home/community setting; healthy growth and development of mother and infant; successful adjustment to parenting

Psychosocial Factors	Health Status	Functional Status	Assessed Discharge Planning Needs
17-year-old unmarried primipara	Uneventful postpartum period	Independent in activities of daily living	Lack of knowledge of infant care
Resides with mother	No known medical/health problems		Lack of knowledge of community resources
No means of financial support	Breastfeeding infant		Potential lack of social/emotional support systems
Unfamiliar with community resources	No source of regular medical follow-up		Need for regular medical follow-up
No means of transportation	Infant healthy, Apgar 9		Disruption in normal growth and development processes (e.g., education and other normal developmental tasks)
11th grade education—plans to return to school			
Has never cared for an infant and requesting help with infant care			
Bonding well with infant			
No recent contact with infant's father			
Requesting home follow-up			

INCORPORATION OF CLIENT/FAMILY INTO PLANNING PROCESS

MULTIDISCIPLINARY PLANNING

POSSIBLE COMMUNITY RESOURCES/REFERRALS

Family   Friends   Work   Neighbors   School   Church

OTHER

(Local Health Department: Nurses, WIC, Clinics; LaLeche League; Young Mothers Support Group; DHHS: AFDC, Medicaid; Child and Family Services; Mom's Day Out Programs; Dial-A-Ride)

Figure 9-6 The home healthcare coordinator: assessing and analyzing discharge planning needs. (Adapted from Siegel H: Nurses improve hospital efficiency through a risk assessment model at admission, Nurs Management 19[10]:42, 1988, with permission.)

care clients. Planning regular visits to the different units within the institution, reviewing client records, and conducting in-service sessions for staff are examples of strategies used by home care coordinators to assess discharge planning needs.

As more and more clients receive early discharges from health care facilities, the community health nurse will become more and more in-

volved in coordinating home care needs. Some of these needs may have been overlooked during discharge efforts and some may be needs that evolved after discharge occurred.

An example of the community health nurse as a home care coordinator putting discharge planning and the referral process into action is given in Figure 9-6. This figure illustrates the goals of discharge planning, assessment parameters, diagnosed discharge planning needs, client/family participation, and potential community resources.

Discharge planning efforts do not cease if clients return to their home environment and have been referred to a community health nurse for follow-up services. Before community health nurses close a case to service, they develop discharge plans with clients. These plans address how clients will deal independently with health needs; what resources, if any, are needed to maintain clients in their home environment; and how clients will reenter the formal health care system if they cannot independently handle health care demands.

SUMMARY

Community health nurses provide general, comprehensive, and continuous care to clients in the community setting. Through the use of discharge planning and the referral process, they ensure continuity of care by coordinating services with other health care providers and by linking clients

to health care resources. Several key concepts are inherent in these processes: (1) clients have the basic responsibility for maintaining their health; (2) clients have the right to accept or refuse health care services; (3) planned intervention by professionals can promote full use of resources by community citizens; (4) interdisciplinary collaboration and coordination are essential to ensure continuity of care; and (5) clients can learn to independently utilize health care services. Effective utilization of discharge planning and the referral process not only helps clients to resolve their current health needs, but also prepares them to make decisions about how to handle health needs in the future.

As discharge planning becomes more and more an integral part of client plans of care, hospitals will need to work with existing ocmmunity agencies to maintain better tracking and follow-up of discharged clients, and expand on networking activities. There are limitless opportunities for the community health nurse to facilitate continuity of care through discharge planning and the referral process.

APPENDIX 9-1

The Child at Home with a Chronic Illness

I am Donnie's mother. I am here to present the parents' view. I will describe the implications of a child's chronic illness on the family, the financial issues, and the complex problems encountered by my family. In addition, I will compare experiences reported by other parents in our parents' group.

Donnie, my sixth child, was born with defects that involved the left side of his body including his left lung, which later on had to be removed. At the time of his birth, we were told that Donnie had to undergo immediate surgery because of what is called an omphalocele, which means that his navel and stomach had evolved outside his abdomen. Within 4 hours of birth, he was transported from Joliet Hospital to Children's Memorial Hospital in Chicago, where the first stage of surgery was performed immediately.

For us as parents, the first shock in the delivery room was knowing that our child had multiple birth defects. We were overpowered by fear of losing our child. Later, the fear was intensified by observing our child in the ICU, when his heart stopped 18 times and he had to be resuscitated. Only because

of the prompt response from health care personnel, Donnie survived all this without brain damage.

During his first 3 years in an acute intensive care unit, Donnie underwent a total of 20 operations. Most of the time he was breathing with the help of a machine—a ventilator—receiving numerous intravenous infusions and treatments while we were watching as helpless bystanders. We often did not understand what was done, the reason why, and we had no knowledge of the alternatives.

Our main social contacts were other parents of critically ill children in the ICU waiting area who, over a period of months, became like close friends to us. Some were the unlucky ones; their children died. We grieved with them, always thinking that we could be next. After years of this, we shut ourselves off and avoided contacts with those parents—even to the point of being abrupt.

We did not receive professional help to deal with the psychological stress we were under. My husband dealt with it by talking constantly about it, while I tried not to think or talk about it, which caused great problems between us. We lost a lot of our friends. They did not know what to say, so it was easier for them not to see us. Besides, we were no fun to be with, because we were constantly talking about our problem.

During his years in the ICU, attempts were made to wean Donnie off the ventilator. A pediatrician forcefully suggested that we take Donnie home, that is, to die. We took Donnie home. He had a tracheostomy; that is, a hole in his trachea. He was breathing poorly by himself; we thought he would not live much longer. We were not prepared to properly take care of him at home. We did not even know how to regulate oxygen flow. He was home for two months, only to return to the Children's Memorial ICU because of pneumonia and failure to thrive. By then, we had lived through two months of a nightmare with no help, no medical caregivers, no sleep—only worry. We were exhausted and burned out.

We shared this experience years later with other parents who at the time were sent home unprepared, with a child who could not breathe by himself without a mechanical aid. This couple had ventilated their child by hand 24 hours a day, taking turns day and night for months, until the decision was made that the child needed a mechanical ventilator at home.

Our home is in Joliet, Illinois, 60 miles from Children's Memorial Hospital in Chicago. Rather than spend 2 to 4 hours on the road a day, we chose to move into the waiting rooms at Children's Memorial Hospital, where we lived for over a year. We slept on the couch, showered in the basement locker rooms, ate hospital food, and paid parking fees. Our 5 children, ranging in age from 17 to 12 years, were left unattended most of the time. They learned to take care of themselves. After about a year, my husband and I decided that one of us had to stay at home in Joliet because our other children were beginning to feel the effects of our absence. I went to Joliet, returning to the hospital occasionally, and my husband stayed with Donnie. Consequently, he lost his business and to live we had to borrow money from family members. Besides dealing with this stress, there was no money or time to go on vacations with the other children. We haven't had a family vacation for 10 years!

Our insurance covered $100,000 of Donnie's care. After a few months, we were told to apply for financial assistance to Illinois Public Aid and the Division of Services for Crippled Children. Children's Memorial Hospital was very helpful in helping us apply. We qualified because Donnie was born with multiple deformities.

Why is it much easier to get aid if a child is born with defects than if some illness or accident causes defects at a later date? Others in our parent-group had children who had problems getting financial help. One parent was called into the hospital billing department and was presented with an astronomical hospital bill and was asked "How are you going to pay for this?" Some parents were advised to go on unemployment, go on public aid, and even get a divorce.

After spending the better part of 3½ years in an Acute ICU, Donnie was transferred into an intermediate care unit for his long-term care. Repeated attempts to wean him from his

breathing machine caused him to be lethargic, puffy, and turn blue. He ceased to grow. The only time he was well was when he was on his ventilator. Then he became a very active, happy child. His many arrests had apparently not damaged his brain. He had become a very precocious child, even inventing his own sign language!

Even though we were at his bedside as much as possible, many of the functions of a parent were taken over by nurses and other health caretakers. Correcting bad behavior or eating habits is hard to accomplish outside of a family setting.

Since Donnie was confined to this unit by being on the ventilator, he lacked opportunity for an education appropriate for a 4-year old. At this time, he got ½ hour of tutoring a day. Children's Memorial Hospital, being an acute care hospital, was unable to provide additional education for a chronically disabled child.

Then in 1978 a new idea was presented to us by a new staff physician. Give Donnie optimal ventilation so he can grow. Prepare him to go home safely with his ventilator. With our memories of the past experience, the idea horrified us. But after meeting with qualified medical personnel, we were assured that we would be trained and would have medical help to support us. Donnie needed to go home in order not to become socially handicapped. Once while I was talking to him on the phone, I told him I was sitting at the kitchen table. After he hung up, he asked his nurse "What is a kitchen table?" My other children were delighted when we told them that Donnie could come home, and they were anxiously awaiting his arrival.

In 1978 no money was allocated by Federal or State law to care for ventilator-dependent children at home. The State knew how to pay the high costs of intensive care but had no experience in providing funding for less expensive care at home. A long period of negotiation took place. The state officials finally found the solution to pay 100% for ⅔ less expensive medical care at home. We were luckier than others in the parents' group who were faced with the spend-down money (money to be paid according to income by the family to the state).

Some parents in our group had private insurance. The insurance company refused to change their reimbursement policy for home care. The insurance company was willing to pay everything in hospital, but refused payment for home care. As a result, the insurance company rapidly spent the $500,000 in the hospital. This money could have lasted for years at home. They had no incentive to change. Therefore, public funds were needed sooner, because the private insurance money was gone so quickly while the patient remained in the ICU. So the burden was transferred to the State and ultimately to the taxpayer.

Transition

It took nine months from the time the decision was made to send Donnie home before it really happened. During that time we built a specially adapted addition to our house. Regular meetings with the health care team were held. These meetings clearly defined goals acceptable to all, and provided clear objectives and specific plans for action. Each team member had accountability. The home discharge team included the dedicated clinical staff who had cared for Donnie over the years. The coordinator was his nurse; the educator was his respiratory therapist. Both were caregivers who had received him in the ICU shortly after his birth. The team also involved physical and child-life therapists, special service staff, social workers, etc. Initially, several members had to overcome their own fear and negative thinking, but the more educated they became, the more they were able to overcome this barrier.

My husband and I were trained to handle Donnie's ventilator equipment by both classroom teaching and "hands-on" experience. We passed a test and were certified. Nurses we recruited, selected, and hired to provide 24-hour home care were trained with us at the hospital, in the classroom, and at the bedside. Community support services, including a primary physician and emergency room staff in Joliet, were well-informed about their responsibility prior to their consent. Nursing, physical therapy, and respiratory therapy plans and exact procedures were clearly written, and local suppliers of medical equipment were found, motivated, and well-prepared. Funding was finally approved because of highly motivated and responsible actions of the leaders and staff of the Division of Services for Crippled Children, the Illinois Department of Public Health and SSI Disabled Children's Program.

The team work of all these individuals made the home program a reality.

Home

On September 19, 1979, our son came home to stay. It has been a difficult task. We are dealing with a lack of privacy, the ventilator breaking down, lack of service for equipment, and difficulties in getting medical supplies.

However, the benefits of having Donnie at home far outweigh the difficulties.

We are now a normal family, maybe different in some ways, but we are all together, sharing all the experiences of life. We no longer divide our time among our children. Donnie's health has improved; he has grown several inches. His oxygen need has decreased. His social life is no longer limited to the ICU where he never knew the difference between day and night. He is now getting an education, doing average-to-above-average work. He no longer has to regard cardiac arrests in the bed next to him as his only occasion for "social-get-together." Instead he goes to weddings; he was a ring bearer at his brother's wedding where he never missed a dance. Donnie is a joy to be with. He loves his religion. He celebrated his Holy Communion last month. He tolerates being off the ventilator with oxygen longer. He races his race car (recently he placed first in competition), climbs trees, and he even fell and broke his arm at a birthday party. Donnie worries right now whether he will get married one day. He is concerned that it is not much fun to go trick or treating, because no matter how he dresses up, everybody recognizes him by his tracheostomy. His nightly prayer includes: "Dear God, if you are listening, please get rid of my trach so I can play football."

We know we can go back to Children's Memorial Hospital any time we have any problems with Donnie. He will be well taken care of by loving people who know him and care for him and us.

We are deeply grateful to the staff of Children's Memorial Hospital. They never gave up hope. And thank God nobody pulled the plug in the ICU. Thank you.

From USDHHS: Report of the Surgeon General's Workshop on Children with Handicaps and Their Families, DHHS Publication No. PHS 83-50194 Washington, DC: 1982, US Government Printing Office, pp. 27-30.

REFERENCES

American Nurses' Association: Standards of home health nursing practice, Kansas City, 1986, The Association.

Arenth LM and Mamon JA: Determining patient needs after discharge, Nurs Management 16(9):20-24, 1985.

Atwood J: Principles of the nursing referral process, unpublished research project, Ann Arbor, 1971, University of Michigan.

Bristow O, Stickney C, and Thompson S: Discharge planning for continuity of care, New York, 1976, National League for Nursing.

Brunner JS: Beyond the information given. Studies in the psychology of knowing, New York, 1973, Norton.

Burlenski M: President's message, Access 7(1):2, 4, 1989.

Chisholm MM: Promise and pitfalls of discharge planning, Nurs Management 14(11):26-29, 1983.

Combs PA: A study of the effectiveness of nursing referrals, Public Health Rep 91:122-126, 1976.

Feather J: Hospital discharge planning: how has it changed since DRG's? Next Step VI(3):1-3, 8, 1989.

Garrard J, Dowd BE, Dorsey B, and Shapiro J: A checklist to assess the need for home health care: instrument development and validation, Public Health Nurs 4:212-218, 1987.

Gillespie ML: Coordination of services: hospital to home, New York, 1980, National League for Nursing.

Goldstein H: Starting where the client is, Social Casework 64:267-275, 1983.

Gonnerman AM: Introduction of planned discharge coordinators, Hosp Forum 10:4-6, 1968.

Keith PM: A preliminary investigation of the role of the

public health nurse in evaluation of services of the aged, Am J Public Health 66:379-381, 1976.

Kitto J and Dale B: Designing a brief discharge planning screen, Nurs Management 16(9):28-30, 1985.

Kromminga DK and Ostwald, SK: The public health nurse as a discharge planner: patient's perceptions of the process, Public Health Nurs 4:224-229, 1987.

Lindstrom CJ: No shows: a problem in health care, Nurs Outlook 23:755-759, 1975.

McBroom A: Uniform needs assessment instrument nearing completion, Access 7(1):1, 3-4, 1989.

McCubbin HI and Patterson J: Family transitions: adaptation to stress. In Figley CR and McCubbin HI, eds: Stress in the family, vol 1, New York, 1983, Brunner/Mazel.

McKeehan KM: Continuing care: a multidisciplinary approach for discharge planning, St Louis, 1981, CV Mosby Co.

Meisenhelder JB: Networking and nursing, Image: J Nurs Scholarship 14: 77-80, 1982.

Mitch AD and Kaczala S: The public health nurse coordinator in a general hospital, Nurs Outlook 16:34-36, 1968.

Oakland County Health Department, Nursing Division: Referral form, Pontiac, Mi, Oakland County Health Department, undated.

O'Hare P and Terry M: Discharge planning: strategies for assuring continuity of care, Rockville, Md, 1988, Aspen.

Pratt CC, Koval J, and Lloyd S: Services workers responses to abuse of the elderly, Social Casework 64: 147-153, 1983.

Reischelt PA and Newcomb J: Organizational factors in discharge planning, J Nurs Adm 10(10):36-42, 1980.

Rossman I and Burnside IM: The United States of America. In Brocklehurse JE, ed: Geriatric care in advanced societies, Baltimore, 1975, University Park Press.

Saposnek DT: A model for brief strategies therapy, Family Process 19:227-237, 1980.

Shamansky SL, Boase JC, and Horn BM: Discharge planning yesterday, today and tomorrow, Home Health Care Nurse 2(13):14-21, 1984.

Siegel H: Nurses improve hospital efficiency through a risk assessment model at admission, Nurs Management 19(10):38-40, 42, 44-45, 1988.

Siporin M: Introduction to social work practice, New York, 1975, Macmillan.

Stone M: Discharge planning guide, Am J Nurs 79:1445-1447, 1979.

Strauss JH, Orr ST, and Charney E: Referrals from an emergency room to primary care practices at an urban hospital, Am J Public Health 73:57-61, 1983.

United States Department of Health and Human Services (USDHHS): Source book for health education materials and community resources, Washington, DC, 1982, US Government Printing Office.

USDHHS: Report of the Surgeon General's Workshop on children with handicaps and their families, Washington, DC, 1982, US Government Printing Office.

USDHHS: Health status of the disadvantaged chartbook 1986, Washington, DC, 1986, US Government Printing Office.

University of Michigan, School of Nursing, Family and Community Health Nursing: Resource grid, Ann Arbor, University of Michigan School of Nursing, undated.

Wensley E: Nursing service without walls, New York, 1963, National League for Nursing.

Wheeler-Lachowycz J: How to use your VNA, Am J Nurs 83:1164-1167, 1983.

Willihnganz G: The next step: pre-admission planning for discharge needs, Coordinator 3:20-21, 1984.

Wolff I: Referral—a process and a skill, Nurs Outlook 10:253-256, 1962.

SELECTED BIBLIOGRAPHY

Beaudry ML: Effective discharge planning matches patient need and community resources, Hospital Prog 56(12):29-30, 1975.

Danis DM: Discharge referrals, J Emerg Nurs 9:44-45, 1983.

Ford M and Wasilewicz C: Bridging the gap between hospital and home, Canad Nurse 77:44-46, 1981.

Gikow F, Anderson E, Bigelow B, Bossi L, Hanford J, and Kisielius J: The continuing care nurse, Nurs Outlook 33:195-197, 1985.

Hochbaum M and Galkin F: Discharge planning: no deposit, no return, Society 19:58-61, 1982.

Marinker M, Wilkin D, and Metcalfe DH: Referral to hospital, can we do better? Brit Med J 646 (297):460-464, 1988.

Oleske D, Hauch WW and Heide E: Characteristics of cancer patient referrals to home care: a regional perspective, Am J Public Health 73:678-682, 1983.

Wahlstrom ED: Initiating referrals: a hospital based system, Am J Nurs 67:332-335, 1967.

Westchester Patient Assessment Program: Patient assessment for continuing care, Battle Creek, Mi, 1987, WK Kellogg Foundation.

Will M: Referral: a process not a form, Nursing 77 77(12):44-45, 1977.

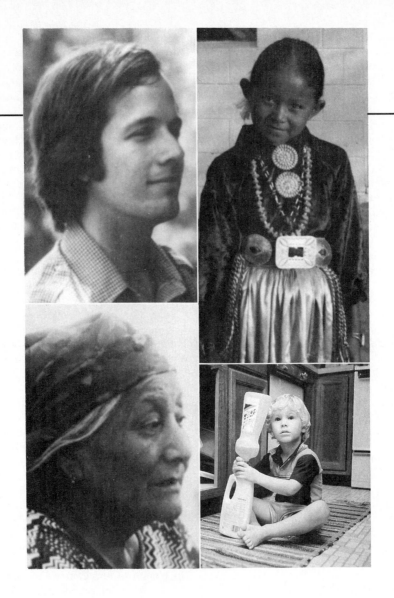

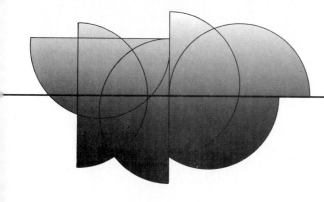

PART THREE

Planning Health Services for Populations at Risk

The uniqueness of community health nursing practice lies in the nurse's ability to assess the health needs of a community, to identify populations at risk, and to plan, implement, and evaluate intervention strategies that promote community wellness. A variety of approaches can be used to analyze the state of wellness in a community. Since community health nurses work with individuals, families, and populations across the life-span, a developmental, age-correlated approach to determining populations at risk can be extremely useful. The increasing number of clients across the life-span who have long-term care needs is a growing concern of all health care professionals.

Community health nurses utilize knowledge from public health and nursing practice in order to fulfill their responsibility to the population as a whole. Part 3 explores how knowledge from these two fields of practice is synthesized by nurses in the community when they plan health programs for groups at risk across the life-span. Emphasis is placed on analyzing how nurses utilize epidemiology, community assessment and diagnosis, health planning, management, quality assurance, and nursing principles to deliver high-quality services in various community settings.

Community health professionals are currently facing several significant challenges. To deal with these challenges, they must become politically active and more deeply involved in research activities. They must also develop skills in handling management information systems and in addressing the ethical dimension of their practice.

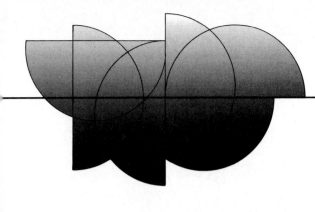

UNIT FOUR

Foundations for Community Assessment, Diagnosis, and Health-Planning Activities

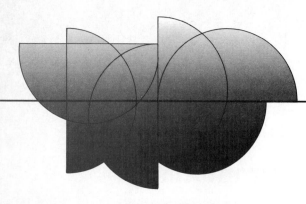

10

Basic Concepts and Strategies of Epidemiology

A *hound it was, an enormous coal black hound, but not such a hound as mortal eyes have ever seen. Fire burst from its open mouth, its eyes glowed with a smoldering glare, its muzzle and hackles and dewlap were outlined in flickering flames.*

SIR ARTHUR CONAN DOYLE

OBJECTIVES

Upon completion of this chapter, the reader will be able to:

1. *Define the term "epidemiology" and describe how the science of epidemiology has evolved over time.*
2. *Discuss the basic epidemiological concepts of populations at risk, natural life history of disease, levels of prevention, host-agent-environment relationships, multiple causation, and person-place-time relationships.*
3. *Summarize the steps of the epidemiological process.*
4. *Describe how the epidemiological process parallels the nursing process.*
5. *Discuss barriers to the epidemiological control of disease.*
6. *Differentiate between the common communicable diseases encountered by community health nurses in the practice setting.*
7. *Discuss epidemiology as it relates to chronic disease control.*
8. *Discuss the use of epidemiological concepts in community health nursing practice.*

Refer to p. 336 for a description of the hound of the Baskervilles, the object of Sir Arthur Conan Doyle's story which was based on an actual Devonshire legend and which was considered to be the greatest of all Holmesian tales. Sherlock Holmes used his brilliant powers of deduction and keen insight to find out why the demonic howl of this hound had brought fear to the Baskerville family. He was able, with his unique problem-solving abilities, to deduce that the howling of the hound was calculated to cause the death of the rightful heirs of the Baskerville fortune. The inheritance would thus fall into the hand of the bastard son of the villainous Hugo Baskerville.

Professionals in community health function very much like the great detective Sherlock Holmes to promote and protect the health of the community. They use an investigative problem-solving process to study the determinants of health and disease frequencies in populations and to plan and implement health promotion and disease control programs. These persons use knowledge, concepts, and methods of epidemiology to relate causative events (howl of the hound) to given occurrences (death) in order to identify at-risk populations (Baskerville heirs).

EPIDEMIOLOGY DEFINED

The word *epidemiology* derives from the Greek word *epidemic*. Literally translated this means *epi*, "upon," *demos*, "people" (collectively). Historically, the major focus of the epidemiologist was on analyzing major disease outbreaks (epidemics) so that ways to control and prevent *disease* occurrence in populations (people, collectively) could be determined. Today, the definition of epidemiology has been expanded to include the study of variables that affect *health*, as well as

The authors are indebted to Associate Professor Elizabeth Keller Beach and to Edna Jennings, friends and colleagues who helped both faculty and students to increase their understanding of the basic concepts of epidemiology and to recognize the value of applying these concepts in the clinical setting. Their support, assistance, and encouragement facilitated learning. Content and illustrations in this chapter reflect many of the ideas shared by them.

those that influence disease and condition occurrence.

There are many variations in the definition of the term *epidemiology,* but the meanings are essentially the same. Throughout this chapter, the following definition adapted from MacMahon and Pugh (1970, p. 1) is used:

Epidemiology is the systematic, scientific study of the distribution patterns and determinants of health, disease and condition frequencies in populations, for the purpose of promoting wellness and preventing disease/conditions.

Implicit in this definition are two basic assumptions. The first is that patterns and frequencies of health, disease, and conditions in populations can be identified. The second is that factors which either determine or contribute to the occurrence of health, disease, or conditions can be discovered through systematic investigation.

Community health nurses use the epidemiological process to carry out their systematic investigation of health, disease, and conditions in populations. This process is graphically depicted in Figure 10-1 and is discussed in detail later in this chapter. When examining Figure 10-1, note that the epidemiological process is similar to the nursing process. The steps are labeled differently but, in essence, they both involve a series of circular, dynamic problem-solving actions. Table 10-1 illustrates this point. Learning the language of epidemiology gives one a distinct advantage, however, because the terminology of epidemiology is used by all community health professionals; the terminology of the nursing process is not.

History and Scope of Epidemiology

Originally, the major focus and scope of epidemiology and public health involved the control of epidemics caused by communicable diseases such as smallpox, plague, diphtheria, whooping cough, cholera, and scarlet fever. The primary goal was to limit the spread of disease and to prevent its recurrence. Although the scope of epidemiology has changed dramatically over time, communicable disease control remains a major priority worldwide. Communicable diseases are still not

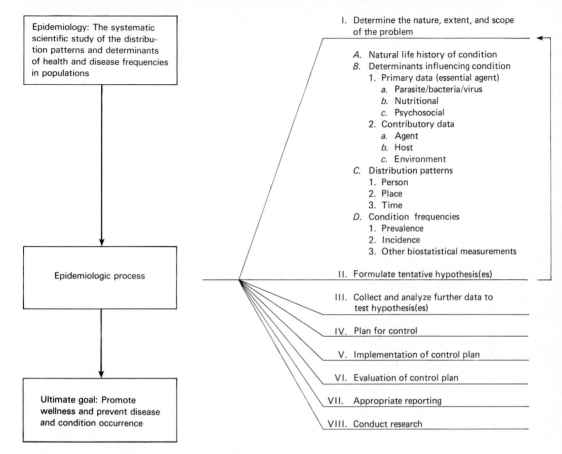

Figure 10-1   Graphic explanation of epidemiology.

conquered, and the new ones such as AIDS are emerging.

Some of the most dramatic examples of communicable disease occurrence in epidemiological history happened when people who had not acquired natural or passive immunity came in contact with the disease. For example, scholars and scientists believe that the small band of Spaniards that conquered the Aztecs would not have been able to do so without the help of smallpox, which, when introduced into the Aztec community, reduced the community's ability to defend itself during war; that Captain Cook was able to make his Hawaiian conquests through the accidental transmission of measles; and that the introduction of diseases such as smallpox, scarlet fever and tuberculosis made the American Indians vulnerable to conquest. The "Lost Colony," the Roa-

noke Island settlement founded in 1587 by Sir Walter Raleigh, mysteriously disappeared and many historians believe it succumbed to communicable disease. Lost in the mysterious disappearance was Virginia Dare, the first English child born in North America (Prescott, 1936; Woodward, 1932).

The 19th century brought about innovations that helped control communicable diseases such as the discoveries of Joseph Lister, a British surgeon who pioneered antiseptic surgery; Louis Pasteur, a French microbiologist who originated the germ theory of disease and developed pasteurization; and Robert Koch, a German medical scientist recognized as the father of microbiology. Koch developed pure cultures and discovered the tuberculosis, anthrax, and cholera bacilli, and in 1905 won a Nobel Peace Prize for his work in

TABLE 10-1   Comparison of the nursing process and the epidemiological process

Nursing process	Epidemiological process

Assessing (data collection to determine nature of client problems)	I. Determine the nature, extent, and scope of the problem
	   A. Natural life history of condition
	   B. Determinants influencing condition
	      1. Primary data (essential agent)
	         a. Parasite/bacterium/virus
	         b. Nutrition
	         c. Psychosocial factors
	      2. Contributory data
	         a. Agent
	         b. Host
	         c. Environment
	   C. Distribution patterns
	      1. Person
	      2. Place
	      3. Time
	   D. Condition frequencies
	      1. Prevalence
	      2. Incidence
	      3. Other biostatistical measurements

Analyzing (formulation of nursing diagnosis or hypothesis)	II. Formulate tentative hypothesis(es) III. Collect and analyze further data to test hypothesis(es)
Planning	IV. Plan for control
Implementing	V. Implement control plan
Evaluating	VI. Evaluate control plan
Revising or terminating	VII. Make appropriate report
Research	VIII. Conduct research

physiology. In the 20th century, the development of elaborate health care techology, along with the discovery of "sulfa" drugs, penicillin, and vaccines did much to aid in the prevention, control, and treatment of communicable disease.

In 1917, the American Public Health Association (APHA) published *Control of Communicable Diseases in Man.* That handbook is now in its 15th edition and is a worldwide classic on communicable disease. It should be included in every nurse's library.

Today, the scope of epidemiology has broadened to include the study of chronic diseases and conditions as well as psychosocial concerns and communicable diseases. In 1928, for example, New York City sent out "healthmobiles" to rid the city of one of its most dreaded diseases—diph-

theria (refer to Figure 10-2). Today, healthmobiles are still being used in many U.S. cities, but they are screening people for chronic conditions such as hypertension, glaucoma, cancer, and diabetes, rather than for controlling communicable disease.

Contemporary epidemiologists examine variables that keep people healthy. They analyze the etiology of chronic conditions, accidents, and other health-related phenomena such as child abuse, abortion, domestic violence, and communicable diseases including hepatitis B and AIDS. Epidemiologists are emphasizing the importance of studying *social* as well as physical factors which affect distributions of disease. Social epidemiologists investigate ways in which social conditions influence the likelihood that disease will develop.

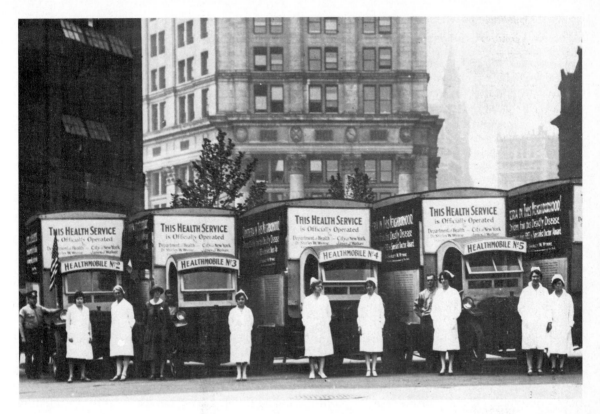

Figure 10-2 Death to diphtheria! With the able help of the visiting nurses, Mayor Jimmy Walker and Health Commissioner Hirley T. Wynne waged war on one of America's most dreaded diseases. This 1926 fleet of "healthmobiles" brought trained diphtheria detection teams to every hidden pocket of the city. (Visiting Nurse Service of New York.)

They focus attention on studying diseases and conditions—such as ulcers, heart disease, and alcoholism—which are influenced by social variables.

EPIDEMIOLOGY AND THE COMMUNITY HEALTH NURSE

Effective implementation of the epidemiological process requires a multidisciplinary approach. Nurses, environmental engineers, physicians, laboratory technicians, statisticians, health officers, social workers, lay persons, and others all carry out necessary and essential roles in the investigation and control of disease and the promotion of wellness. Any health professional can and should function as a member of the epidemiological team.

Community health nurses participate on the epidemiological team in a variety of ways. Their contacts with families in the home and with groups in various settings (clinics, schools, and industry) put them in a unique position to carry out many epidemiological activities. They regularly become involved in case finding, health teaching, counseling, and follow-up essential to the prevention of communicable diseases, chronic conditions, and other health-related phenomena. Illustrative of this are the actions taken by the community health nurse, in the following case situation, to prevent the spread of a streptococcal infection and the occurrence of chronic complications.

While visiting the Wills family, the community health nurse learned that Bobbie had a severe sore throat. Because Bobbie's symptoms were indicative of a streptococcal infection, the nurse stressed the significance of a proper medical evaluation to rule out or confirm a diagnosis of strep throat. The family followed through immediately. Bobbie's throat culture came back positive for streptococcal disease and he was treated with penicillin. The community health nurse, on a follow-up visit, taught the parents about the necessity of continuing the medication for 10 days even if Bobbie had no symptoms; she knew that a 10-day course of penicillin was needed to eliminate the streptococcal organisms. She also knew from theory and experience that if the organisms were not eliminated Bobbie could have serious chronic complications. By using her epidemiological knowledge, this nurse was able to effectively abort rheumatic fever, which can lead to a chronic heart condition or other chronic problems such as kidney disease.

In addition to the activities described above, community health nurses also utilize epidemiological concepts to carry out research in the community setting. A research team may carry out a study to survey major community needs (refer to Chapter 11) or to identify gaps in knowledge relative to disease causation, prevention, and control. A community health nurse's ongoing, comprehensive contact with the community and its resources allows her or him to make key contributions during these types of studies.

A community health nurse must apply the principles of epidemiology in order to provide preventive health services to *populations* in the community (refer to Chapter 2). The nurse must understand the significance of expanding epidemiological study to investigate health and disease in populations, as well as with individuals. Only in this way will the community health nurse effectively meet the health needs of the community as a whole.

BASIC CONCEPTS OF EPIDEMIOLOGY

To use the epidemiological process effectively, community health nurses need to have an understanding of the basic concepts, tools, and terms of epidemiology. Since epidemiology is operationally defined in terms of disease measurements, an understanding of the biostatistical concepts presented in Chapter 11 is essential. Biostatistics helps to describe the extent and distribution of health, illness, and conditions in the community and aids in the identification of specific health problems and community strengths. Biostatistics also facilitates the setting of priorities for program planning.

In addition to biostatistics, there are several basic concepts that guide epidemiological study. These are populations at risk, the natural life history of a disease, levels of prevention, host-agent-environment relationships, multiple causation, and person-place-time relationships. In general, these concepts provide a foundation for explaining how disease develops and how health is maintained, who is most susceptible to disease, and how disease can be prevented and health promoted.

Study of Populations at Risk

A key concept of epidemiology is that the study of disease in populations is more significant than the study of individual cases of disease. Epidemiological research has demonstrated that using large sampling groups is essential for formulating valid conclusions about the distribution patterns and determinants of health, disease, and condition frequencies in populations. It is by observing large groups that commonalities and differences among people who have or do not have a particular disease or condition can be identified.

The identification of commonalities and differences among groups focuses attention on the essential or contributory factors that produce illness or promote health. For example, it has been found repeatedly, through sampling of large groups, that people who smoke are more likely to develop coronary disease than people who do not smoke. This fact may never have been established if only individual cases had been examined, because some people who develop coronary disease do not smoke.

A preventive health philosophy has led professionals in community health to emphasize the study of groups. The goal of epidemiological study is to identify *populations at risk,* so that preventive health measures, such as those presented

TABLE 10-2 Epidemiology in action: health measures needed to improve the health of at-risk groups at each life stage

Infants	Children	Adolescents and young adults	Adults	Elderly
Education for parenthood	Early comprehensive childhood development programs	Roadway safety programs	Public education about smoking, alcohol, good nutrition, and adequate exercise, including how poor health habits increase risk of disease	Work and social activity for retired persons
Genetic counseling	Special support services to aid families under stress (e.g., child-abuse, low income, etc.)	Educational programs about smoking, alcohol, and drug use		Education about adequate exercise and nutrition
Good prenatal care	Injury reduction education	Nutrition and exercise guidance	Protection from environmental health habits	Preventive multiphasic screening programs
Sound prenatal nutritional guidance and services	Comprehensive pediatric care	Family planning services	Worksite health and safety programs	Education about proper use of medications
Counseling services to decrease adverse maternal habits which effect fetal development (e.g., smoking, drinking, drugs, exposure to radiation)	Immunizations	Sexually transmissible disease services including education, screening, and treatment	Hypertension prevention, screening, and control programs	Immunizations for influenza
Amniocentesis	Fluoridation of water supplies	Immunizations	Pap smears	Home safety programs
Breast feeding	Dental care	Mental health	Regular self-breast examination	Community and home services which facilitate independent living
Regular comprehensive care	Nutritional and exercise guidance	Actions to reduce the availability of firearms	Education about cancer signs	
Immunizations	Education to prevent and eliminate dysfunctional health habits (smoking, alcohol use, drug use, and unprotected sexual activity)		Mental health services	
Social services including financial assistance, day care, improved foster and adoption programs, and counseling for families under stress			Dental care	

Surgeon General: Healthy people: the Surgeon General's report on health promotion and disease prevention, vol II. Washington, DC, 1979, US Government Printing Office, pp 149-155.

in Table 10-2, can be used to stop the progression of disease or health-related phenomena. As previously defined in Chapter 2, populations at high risk are those who engage in certain activities or who have certain characteristics that increase their potential for contracting an illness, injury, or a health problem. For example, parents who were abused as children are at risk for abusing their own children. These activities or characteristics are known as risk factors.

Risk Factors

Risk factors are determined by a risk estimate process. Risk estimates are derived by comparing the frequency of deaths, illnesses, or injuries from a specific cause in a group having some specific trait or risk factor, with the frequency in another group not having that trait, or in the population as a whole (Surgeon General, 1979, volume I, p. 2). Risk factors fall under three major categories: (1) inherited biological characteristics; (2) physical, social, family, economic, and environmental factors; and (3) behavioral or lifestyle patterns. These risk factors increase susceptibility to death, illnesses, injuries, or psychosocial conditions. It has been shown, for instance, that "inherited biologic characteristics can increase one's risk for some mental disorders, infectious diseases, and common chronic diseases such as certain cancers, heart disease, lung disease, and diabetes. Inherited characteristics also predispose individuals to conditions generally recognized as inherited, like sickle cell anemia and hemophilia" (Surgeon General, 1979, volume I, p. 13).

Although heredity can increase one's risk for the occurrence of disease or adverse health conditions, health problems usually result from multiple interacting factors. When these multiple risk factors come together, they form an interrelated web of forces which increase their potential for causing harm.

Increasingly, it is recognized that *environmental factors* and *lifestyle patterns* are crucial variables in the development of disease and adverse conditions. Many of the leading causes of death could be substantially reduced if persons at risk improved their lifestyle patterns of diet, smoking, exercise, alcohol consumption, and use of antihypertensive medication. It has been stated that approximately 20 percent of all premature deaths could be eliminated if environmental hazards were controlled (Surgeon General, volume I, 1979). Anticipatory guidance at each stage across the lifespan can help individuals, families, and aggregates to develop lifestyle patterns which promote health and reduce the risk of disease and adverse health conditions. Table 10-2 summarizes the measures which assist clients at various life stages to improve their state of well-being.

In recent years, the importance of *socioeconomic and family environmental factors* in the development of poor health and disease has been particularly stressed. It has been shown that these factors play critical roles in the development of many serious infectious diseases as well as chronic health problems, injuries, and social conditions. For example, it is known that disadvantaged population groups are at risk for more health problems than are affluent aggregates. The disadvantaged experience more health risk because they often have inadequate income for good nutrition, safe housing, and adequate acute and preventive health care and are frequently exposed to more physical hazards in the environment (USDHHS, 1986; Michigan Department of Public Health, 1987, 1988).

Chapters 13 through 18 discuss many health problems related to socioeconomic and family environmental factors such as accidents, child abuse, suicide, domestic violence, alcoholism, and nutritional problems. Appendix 10-3 discusses information about thirteen most commonly acquired sexually transmitted diseases (STDs). STDs present major health risks for several segments of the population in the United States. Although we know the agents for STDs, we have been unable to control these diseases, and many are reaching epidemic proportions. The spread of STDs dramatically demonstrates that social determinants of disease cannot be ignored. Social situations and behavior patterns promote host exposure to STD agents.

Identifying populations at risk assists community health professionals to utilize available health

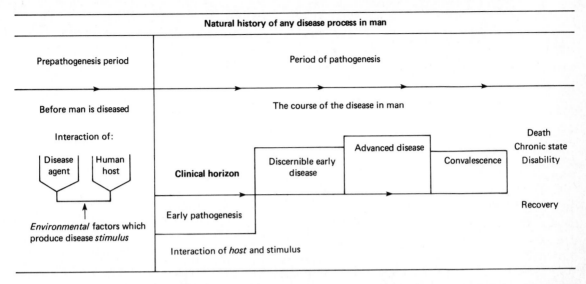

Figure 10-3   Prepathogenesis and pathogenesis periods of natural history. (Leavell HR and Clark EG: Preventive medicine for the doctor in his community: an epidemiologic approach, New York, 1965, McGraw-Hill, p 18.)

resources effectively. It also aids in establishing priorities for the allocation of funds and the use of health work force time. In Table 21-1, "Priorities in Community Health Nursing," guidelines for determining priorities for community health nursing services are presented. These guidelines are based on the at-risk concept and the philosophy of prevention.

Natural Life History of Disease

In the search for commonalities that may produce disease and health-related phenomena in specific populations, epidemiological study focuses on determining the natural life history of these conditions. Observing the natural life history of disease and health-related phenomena aids in identifying agent-host-environmental factors that influence their development, characteristic signs and symptoms during their different periods of progression, and approaches to preventing and controlling their effects on humans.

In their classic textbook, Leavell and Clark (1965, pp. 17-18) identified two distinct periods in the natural life history of any disease: *prepathogenesis* and *pathogenesis*. The combination of the processes involved in both of these stages is termed the *natural life history* of a disease or a

condition. In the prepathogenesis period, disease has not developed but interactions are occurring between the host, agent, and environment which produce disease stimulus and increase the host's potential for disease. The combination of high serum cholesterol levels and smoking, for example, increases the host's potential for developing coronary heart disease.

The pathogenesis period in the natural life history of disease begins when disease-producing stimuli (smoking or elevated serum cholesterol levels) start to produce changes in the tissues of humans (arteriosclerosis in the coronary vessels). Figure 10-3 shows the interrelationship between the prepathogenesis period and the pathogenesis period and how the latter progresses from the pre-symptomatic stage to advanced, overt disease. It also shows that disease occurs as a result of processes that happen in the *environment*—prepathogenesis—and processes that happen in *humans*—pathogenesis (Leavell and Clark, 1965, p. 18).

Levels of Prevention

The study of the natural life history of disease facilitates the achievement of the ultimate goal of epidemiology—the development of effective

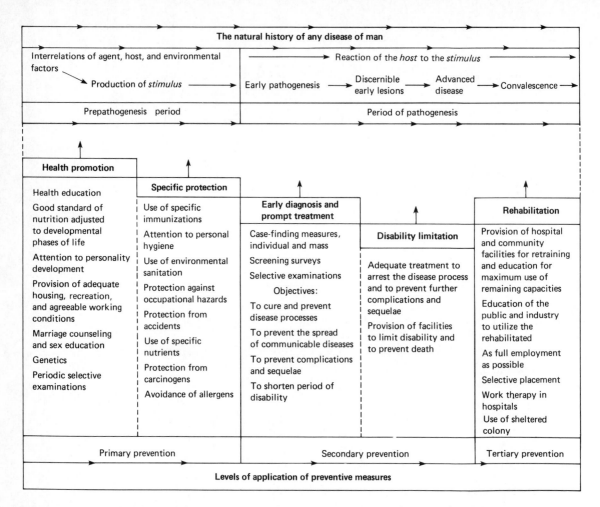

Figure 10-4 Levels of application of preventive measures in the natural history of disease. (Leavell HF and Clark EG: Preventive medicine for the doctor in his community: an epidemiologic approach, New York, 1965, McGraw-Hill, p 21.)

methods of *preventing* and controlling disease or conditions in populations. By identifying significant host-agent-environment relationships which influence the progression of the natural life history of a condition, the epidemiologist can identify populations at risk and develop ways to prevent disease occurrence among them.

A continuum of preventive activities is essential for the promotion of health in any community. As previously discussed in Chapter 2, preventive activities can be grouped under three levels: *primary* (health promotion and specific protection), *secondary* (early diagnosis, prompt treatment, and disability limitation), and *tertiary*

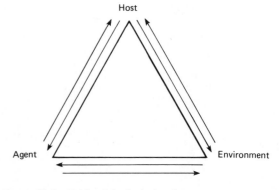

Figure 10-5 Epidemiological triangle.

(rehabilitation). Figure 10-4 presents a schema illustrating how to apply these levels of prevention in relation to the natural history of any disease. It implies that carrying out preventive activities during both the prepathogenesis and pathogenesis periods can alter the progression of a disease or a health problem. The degree to which preventive activities can be implemented will vary depending on the completeness of knowledge one has about the disease or health problem in question (Leavell and Clark, 1965, p. 20).

Host-Agent-Environment Relationships

When analyzing the natural life history of a disease or a condition and how to apply the three levels of prevention, epidemiological study focuses on the relationship of three variables: host, agent, and environment. These variables are defined as follows:

Agent: An animate or inanimate factor which must be present or lacking for a disease or a condition to occur

Host: Living species (humans or other animals) capable of being infected or affected by an agent

Environment: Everything external to a specific agent and host, including humans and animals

The interaction between host-agent-environment is frequently referred to as the *epidemiological triangle* (Figure 10-5). This triangle illustrates that it is the interactions (depicted by arrows in the model) among these variables that determine whether there is health or disease/conditions in a community. Health is maintained when the host-agent-environment variables are in a state of equilibrium. Disease or conditions occur when there is a change in any one of the three variables that disturbs the state of equilibrium.

Agents are biological, chemical, or physical and include such things as bacteria, viruses, fungi, pesticides, food additives, ionizing-radiation, and speeding objects. The normal habitat in which an infectious (biological) agent lives, multiples, and/or grows is called a *reservoir*. These habitats include humans, animals, and the environment.

The capacity of an infectious agent to infect *(infectivity)* and to produce subsequent disease *(pathogenicity)* is variable. The *virulence* or degree of pathogenicity of an infectious agent also varies (Centers for Disease Control, 1987, Principles of epidemiology: disease, pp. 5-7).

A wide variety of characteristics are classified as host factors. Examples of these factors are age, sex, ethnic group, socioeconomic status, lifestyle, and heredity (Centers for Disease Control, 1987, Principles of epidemiology: agent, p. 5). Four types of environment factors—physical, social, economic, and family—are elaborated on in a later section of this chapter.

Multiple Causation

The theory of multiple causation of disease illustrates and confirms that it is the interactions and relationships between host-agent-environment that actually cause a disease or condition—*not* host, agent, or environmental factors alone. The theory of multiple causation is critical to epidemiology. It is only natural to assume that the introduction of a disease agent (e.g., influenza virus) into a community is enough to cause illness among its members. However, in addition to this causative agent there must be a susceptible host, and an environment conducive to the interaction of agent and host. Factors such as the level of immunity in the population, individual susceptibility, availability of vectors, and the amount of contact between members of the population will affect disease/condition occurrence. The following example of an influenza outbreak illustrates how these factors influence disease occurrence.

An influenza outbreak that occurred in the United States demonstrates the concept of multiple causation. The agent, the influenza virus A/USSR, was introduced into the population. Outbreaks of this disease occurred in groups of young adults and children in environments of close contact: schools, colleges, and military training camps. Attack rates in these areas were high, ranging from 40 to 70 percent in most cases. The disease did not usually appear in adults over 25 years of age.

An analysis of this situation illustrates that the

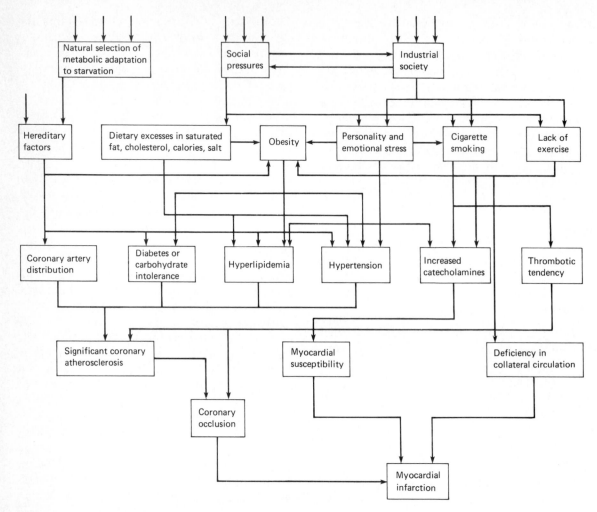

Figure 10-6 The web of causation for myocardial infarction: a current view. (Friedman GE: Primer of epidemiology, New York, 1974, McGraw-Hill, p 5.)

proper combination of multiple factors is necessary before disease will result. Outbreaks occurred in young adults and children because there was a virulent agent, susceptible hosts who lacked immunity, and crowded environmental conditions that supported the spread of the agent. The disease usually did not occur in those over 25 because they had been exposed to this virus earlier and had developed acquired immunity to the organism. This acquired immunity allowed them to maintain a balance in host-agent-environment factors and to escape the disease. If only one vari-

able, such as a virulent agent, was necessary to cause illness, individuals 25 years and older would also have had high attack rates in 1978.

The concept of multiple causation becomes even more apparent when one studies the natural life history of noninfectious diseases, chronic conditions, and health-related phenomena. Friedman's (1974, p. 5) diagram of the web of causation for myocardial infarction (Figure 10-6) clearly demonstrates that it is the interplay between multiple host-agent-environment characteristics that causes a chronic condition.

Person-Place-Time Relationships

It has been emphasized that the study of relationships is necessary for the community health professional to formulate valid hypotheses about disease or condition causation. Identification of measurable variables that can facilitate rapid and efficient data collection is essential to this study. In epidemiological study, the variables that have been found to be most useful are *person* (who is affected), *place* (where affected), and *time* (when affected). Some of the most frequently analyzed characteristics of these variables are the following (MacMahon and Pugh, 1970, pp. 31-32; Surgeon General, 1979, pp. 13-14):

1. *Person:* delineation of group involved
   a. Age, sex, race distribution
   b. Socioeconomic status, occupation, education
   c. Health habits and behaviors or lifestyle
   d. Acquired resistance and susceptibility
   e. Health history—natural resistance, hereditary characteristics
2. *Place:* geographic distribution in subdivisions of the area affected
   a. *Physical environment:* weather, climate, geography, radiation, vibration, noise, pressure, animal reservoirs, pollutants, housing facilities, workplace hazards, and sources of air, water, and food contamination
   b. *Social environment:* population density and mobility, community groups, occupations and other roles, beliefs and attitudes, technological developments, transportation, educational practices, and health care delivery system
   c. *Economic environment:* source of income; income level; employment status; job frustrations; and income for nutrition, housing, and other basic needs
   d. *Family environment:* family history; family dynamics; strategies utilized to handle stress; type, number, and timing of major life changes; home atmosphere; and family health and cultural patterns (refer to Chapters 6 and 7)
3. *Time:* chronological distribution of onsets of cases by days, weeks, months
   a. Incubation period: determine life cycle; factors affecting multiplication and virulence of organism
   b. Seasonal trends
   c. Onset of event
   d. Duration of event

Timing is a critical factor in disease diagnosis and control. Immediate reporting of a disease outbreak is crucial since the validity of data is often directly proportional to the time lapse incurred in obtaining the information. If a significant amount of time is lost in reporting, the ability to formulate valid hypotheses is decreased.

When monitoring incidence of infectious disease, the terms used to distinguish relative frequency in time and space include the following:

Sporadic: Presence of occasional cases of the event apparently unrelated in time or space

Endemic: Constant long-term presence of an event at about the *frequency expected* from the past history of the community

Epidemic: Presence of the event *at a much higher frequency than expected* from the past history of the community, usually over a short period of time (for example, one case of cholera would be labeled epidemic in a U.S. community; on the other hand, in some foreign countries, several cases of cholera would be considered an endemic occurrence).

Pandemic: Presence of an event in *epidemic proportions, involving many communities and countries* in a relatively short period of time.

When monitoring any disease or condition, it is important to remember that there are wide variations in the degree of symptoms. These variations range from inapparent infection to severe, pronounced symptomatology. It is the *inapparent, or subclinical, symptoms* that are the most significant in terms of disease transmission or occurrence. If efforts to prevent transmission or progression of a disease or a condition are limited to

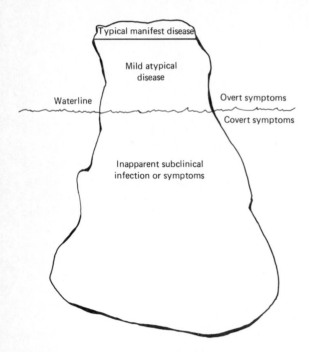

Figure 10-7   Comparison of inapparent infection to an iceberg. (Adapted from Beach EK: Environmental health and communicable disease module, Ann Arbor, 1974, University of Michigan, School of Nursing—Community Health Nursing, p 183.)

people with clinical manifestations, a very large proportion of the problem will be missed.

The iceberg analogy is frequently used to illustrate the importance of identifying individuals with subclinical symptoms during an epidemiological study. Most of the iceberg, as illustrated in Figure 10-7, is submerged. This unseen section is the most insidious and potentially dangerous portion to the seafarer because often no action is taken to avoid it. Individuals with subclinical infections or symptoms, like the submerged portion of the iceberg, present the most danger, because they do not have obvious symptoms, and are less likely to use preventive measures. An example of this is a female client who has asymptomatic gonorrhea. This person frequently transmits gonorrhea for a considerable length of time before it is known that she has the disease.

Psychosocial phenomena, such as substance abuse, domestic violence, child abuse, and mental illness tend to remain submerged much longer than infectious diseases. Increasingly, it is being recognized that these problems are far more prevalent than statistics reflect. Communities are beginning to conduct epidemiological investigations in order to determine the real magnitude of these problems.

EPIDEMIOLOGICAL PROCESS AND INVESTIGATION

Basic concepts in epidemiology have been discussed to lay a foundation for epidemiological investigation of community health problems. These concepts aid in identifying variables to consider when describing the distribution patterns and determinants of health, disease, and condition frequencies in populations. They help to analyze causal relationships in disease or condition outbreaks. To establish these causal relationships, health professionals use a scientific process known as the *epidemiological process.*

The epidemiological process is a systematic course of action taken to identify (1) who is affected (persons); (2) where the affected persons reside (place); (3) when the persons were affected (time); (4) causal factors of health and disease occurrence (host-agent-environment determinants); (5) prevalence and incidence of health and disease (frequencies); and (6) prevention and control measures (levels of prevention) in relation to the natural life history of a disease or a condition.

The epidemiological process has eight basic steps, which are graphically illustrated in Figure 10-1. Although each step is discussed separately, it is important to remember that these steps may overlap and may not always follow a sequential pattern. They are interrelated and dependent upon each other. For example, data collected in the initial step provide a foundation for all subsequent steps.

Step I: Determine the Nature, Extent, and Possible Significance of the Problem

The primary responsibilities during this initial step are twofold: (1) to verify the diagnosis by data collection from multiple sources; and (2) to determine the extent and possible significance of the verified problem. Data gathering begins when an index case is reported or when there is a noticeable change in the incidence rate for a particular disease or condition. The *index case* is the case which brings a household or other group to the attention of community health personnel. Once this case is known to health professionals, data are collected from a variety of sources in order to determine if a problem really exists.

Clinical observations, laboratory studies, and lay reporting assist the epidemiological team in confirming the homogeneity of the current events. If, for instance, four hospital emergency rooms have reported that several individuals were treated for food poisoning in the last 24 hours, health personnel would want to immediately take the following actions:

1. Interview the affected persons to determine the nature of their symptoms and to identify loci of origin according to person, place, and time.
2. Review laboratory studies to confirm a common causative organism. This process could establish that there are several events occurring at the same time.
3. Interview friends, relatives, and lay acquaintances to discern their description of the events which led up to the reported illness and to determine if other individuals have symptoms.

It is important to remember that *time* and *accurate* and *thorough* data collection are critical factors in Step I. Significant data may be destroyed if the data collection process is too slow. In addition, if only the "tip of the iceberg" or the most obvious events are observed, the extent of the problem will not be identified. The health professional needs to be like a detective, starting out with interviewing the affected individual and then branching out into this individual's environment to track down the host-agent-environment factors which influence disease occurrence. As previously discussed, the measurable variables which facilitate rapid and efficient data collection about host-agent-environment factors are person, place, and time.

Analyzing data in terms of person, place, and time helps to establish the magnitude of the problem. Data tell the health professional the proportion of the people affected, the seriousness of the effects on the host and the community, improvement or regression over time, and geographic distribution of the disease or condition. They also help in identifying potential sources of infection and causal relationships.

The use of spot maps (refer to "Analysis of All Available Data in Chapter 11) facilitates pinpointing the exact geographic location of the disease or condition. This type of map vividly and visually portrays an epidemiological problem very rapidly. If it is used on a regular basis, health personnel can compare current prevalence and incidence with the expected rates and can identify significant departures from normal. *Incidence* is the number of *new* cases of a disease in a population over a period of time (cases just starting). *Prevalence* is the number of *old* and *new* cases of a specific disease at a given time (refer to Chapter 11).

When comparing prevalence and incidence rates, one word of caution is necessary. If there is a distinct departure from normal, it must be ascertained if a problem really exists. It may be found that there is only an improvement in reporting, not an actual increase in disease occurrence.

If there has been an actual increase in the incidence of a particular disease or condition, the health professional makes an *educated guess* as to the nature of the causative agent, based upon the data collected. This formulation of a tentative diagnosis or hypothesis is done in order to enhance further data collection.

Step II: Formulate Tentative Hypothesis(es)

When dealing with infectious diseases, a rapid preliminary analysis of data is imperative. This is essential because infectious diseases can spread quickly, can affect a large number of people in a short period of time, and can have great ranges in severity. Usually this analysis results in the formulation of several hypotheses. Explanation of the most probable source of infection is made in terms of (1) the agent causing the problem; (2) the source of infection, including the chain of events leading to the outbreak of the problem; and (3) environmental conditions that allowed it to occur. Tentative hypotheses must be tested and may be found to be inappropriate. Laboratory tests are invaluable in validating hypotheses. An example of how tentative hypotheses are established is provided in the following situation.

From September 5 through 8, 1974, the "World's Largest American Indian Fair" was held near Gallup, New Mexico (Horwitz, Pollard, Merson, and Martin, 1977, pp. 1071-1076). An estimated 80,000 persons attended the fair. Beginning on September 6, 1974, and during the next few days, several hundred people with gastrointestinal symptoms sought attention at two hospitals near Gallup. Over 130 of them had stool cultures positive for a *Salmonella* group C organism, *Salmonella newport*. The hospitals immediately reported the apparent outbreak to the health department. Preliminary tentative hypotheses indicated that either the community water supply of the area or food served at a free barbeque which attracted thousands on September 5, 1974, was the vehicle of transmission for the agent *Salmonella newport*. Evidence favoring a water source included a broken water pipe at the fair grounds in an area soiled with animal feces. The barbeque was suspected because food preparation practices were reportedly improper and those who attended the barbeque appeared to have a high attack rate of illness.

Since two possible sources of infection were favored in this situation, health personnel took immediate steps to correct both problem situations and collected and analyzed further data to determine the exact cause of the *Salmonella* outbreak.

Waiting until all data are collected before instituting control measures can amplify the magnitude of the problem. A health professional must be willing to take risks while carrying out an epidemiological investigation.

Step III: Collect and Analyze Further Data to Test Hypothesis(es)

A basic starting point in this step is to identify the group selected for attack by the disease or problem under investigation. Individual epidemiological health histories should be done to classify persons according to their exposure to suspected or causative agents and to identify the clinical data and bacteriologic findings needed to substantiate the diagnosis. Significant variation of incidence in contrasted population groups should then be noted. These variations can be identified through study of attack rates.

An *attack rate* is an incidence rate which identifies the number of people at risk who became ill. In studying an outbreak of food-borne disease such as the one at the American Indian Fair, the attack rate for persons who ate certain foods would be compared with the attack rate for persons who did not eat certain foods. This is done in an attempt to identify which food was infected by the causative agent.

Attack rates are calculated in the following manner:

$$\frac{\text{No. of persons affected}}{\text{No. of persons eating food item}} \times 100$$

$$\frac{\text{No. of persons affected}}{\text{No. of persons } not \text{ eating food item}} \times 100$$

Table 10-3 illustrates how attack rates are graphically summarized. The attack rates in this table were calculated when people became ill after a banquet. They show that one food item, custard, was probably the infected food (note the differences between the two attack rate percentages). *Generally, the vulnerable food which shows the greatest differences between the two attack rate percentages is the infected food.*

It is essential to remember that attack rates do not positively confirm an infective food. Maxcy and Rosenau (1965, p. 18) have identified the following five reasons why the association of illness with a particular food is often difficult:

1. Some individuals are resistant to the agent and do not become ill even though exposed.
2. The definition of an ill person employed may include some who have unrelated illnesses, unless there is a specific test; and even then, if the illness is one which is prevalent, the ill subjects may include some cases not due to the ingestion of the common vehicle.

TABLE 10-3   Attack rate table

Vulnerable food	Persons who did eat vulnerable food				Persons who did not eat vulnerable food			
	Sick	Well	Total	Attack rate (%)	Sick	Well	Total	Attack rate (%)
Baked ham	19	56	75	25	30	5	35	86
Custard	45	15	60	**75**	4	46	50	**8**
Jello	20	35	55	36	29	26	55	53
Cole slaw	48	58	106	45	1	3	4	25
Baked beans	45	55	100	45	4	6	10	40
Potato salad	25	45	70	36	24	16	40	60

From Communicable Disease Center: Food-borne disease investigation: analysis of field data, Atlanta, Ga, 1964, US Public Health Service, p 8.

3. Contamination of one food by traces of another may take place during serving or before.
4. Errors in history taking may occur. These may be unbiased errors, due to memory lapses or misunderstanding; or they may be due to biases, either on the part of the questioner or the subject. Several kinds of biases are possible; the questioner may have a preconceived notion of what food was responsible and press his questions more vigorously with respect to that food in the case of ill persons than non-ill persons; or the subject may have preconceived notions, leading to the same result. The subject may have reasons for wishing either to claim or disclaim illness. Biases may affect the accuracy either of food histories or illness histories and produce spurious association.
5. Finally, biased sampling may also lead to spurious results.

All the above factors can affect the validity of an attack rate and thereby the choice of the appropriate infective food. Laboratory studies are necessary to identify the etiologic agent and its vector. A *vector* is an animate or inanimate vehicle such as food, clothing, or insects which transports disease from an infected host to a new host. However, identifying the causative agent is not the only step in preventing further spread of disease. It assists in treating infected individuals who seek medical care but does not tell how the disease is being transmitted. If the chain of transmission is not broken, disease will continue to occur.

Since one factor alone never causes a disease or condition, it is not sufficient to identify only a causative agent and the infective food. After the possible agents and the attack group have been identified, the common source(s) to which affected individuals were exposed should be investigated. With foodborne disease, the origin, method, and preparation of suspected foods would be primary factors to examine. Concurrently, environmental conditions should be evaluated. These conditions would include such things as the sanitary status of the restaurant, the area where food was served, and the water and dairy supply. Figure 10-8 depicts the type of data that one state collects when enteric infections such as *Salmonella newport* are suspected. Community health nurses are frequently responsible for completing this form during an epidemiological investigation. In some health departments, nurses are also responsible for collecting specimens for laboratory analysis. The epidemiological division of the state or local health department will provide information on how to properly collect, preserve, and ship specimens for epidemiological analysis.

Completing an epidemiological case history form provides an opportunity for health teaching and case finding. Often, the community health nurse identifies new cases during this process and helps clients to learn about the nature of the disease and how to prevent its spread.

It is important to use a variety of data-collection methods in determining the extent and source of an epidemiological problem because in-

ENTERIC INFECTIONS _____ CASE HISTORY
(Insert type)

DIVISION OF EPIDEMIOLOGY
Michigan Department of Public Health   No. _____

Name _____ Birth date _____ Birthplace _____

Address _____

Occupational address _____

Physician _____ Address _____

Health officer _____ Address _____

CLINICAL HISTORY: Date of onset _____ Diarrhea _____

Vomiting _____ Temp. _____ Weight loss _____ Other symptoms _____

_____ Duration of symptoms _____

Present condition _____

Previous pertinent history, if any _____

Source of water: ___ Well   ___ Municipal   ___ Other (specify) _____

Source of milk: ___ Pasteurized (name dairy) _____

                        ___ Unpasteurized (source) _____

Source of food: ___ Restaurant (name) _____

                        ___ Private home, other then given _____

                        ___ Other (specify) _____

Sewage disposal   ___ Privy   ___ Septic tank   ___ Municipal

Additional epidemiological data pertaining to this case:

Figure 10-8   Enteric infections case history. (Michigan Department of Public Health, Lansing, Mi, undated, Division of Epidemiology.)

All other persons in household

	Name	Age	Relation	History of recent illness	Laboratory data
1.					
2.					
3.					
4.					
5.					
6.					
7.					
8.					
9.					
10.					

Visitors to household during past month

	Name	Age	Relation	Address	Laboratory data
1.					
2.					
3.					
4.					
5.					
6.					

Case laboratory data

Specimens				Date	Positive	Negative	Laboratory
Blood	Feces	Urine	Bile				

Informant _____

Investigation by _____

Health Dept. _____

Please use ink in making out histories   Date _____

Figure 10-8, cont'd

dividuals who have only minor symptoms of illness often do not seek treatment. In the Gallup, New Mexico, outbreak, the extent of the problem was determined by a large questionnaire survey conducted from September 19 to 25, 1974. Using recently made maps of dwellings in the area, 500 dwellings, housing 2000 persons, were randomly selected for a visit by an interviewer who completed a questionnaire. The interviewer inquired about the occurrence and characteristics of diarrheal illnesses, the types and location of the household water supply, the amount of water consumed at the fair, the time of eating at the barbeque, and the types of food eaten. This survey revealed that attendance at the barbeque was highly associated with illness and confirmed laboratory studies which eliminated water as a vehicle of transmission. It also showed that eating potato salad at the barbeque was strongly associated with illness (Horwitz, Pollard, Merson, and Martin, 1977, pp. 1072, 1074).

Tentative hypothesis(es) must be tested. The survey conducted at Gallup, New Mexico, helped to confirm one of the original hypotheses on the source of contamination, the food served at the barbeque, and eliminated another, the contaminated water. At times, however, it will be found that none of the original hypotheses is appropriate.

Testing hypothesis(es) helps to determine if the initial control measures were sufficient to resolve the current outbreak. It also aids in identifying the natural life history of the disease and where further action is needed.

Step IV: Plan for Control

When planning for control, it is essential to identify preventive activities, based on the knowledge of the natural history of the disease in question, which can be used to control the further spread of disease occurrence. Host-agent-environment factors should be analyzed to determine the following:

1. Populations at risk
2. Primary, secondary, and tertiary preventive measures available (refer to Table 10-2) that would

a. Alter the behavior or susceptibility of the host (health education, case finding, immunization, treatment, or rehabilitation)
b. Destroy the agent (heat, drug treatment, or spraying with insecticides)
c. Eliminate the transmission of the agent (changes in host's health habits or environmental conditions)
3. Feasibility of implementing the control plan, considering such factors as available community resources, time required, cost of control vs. partial or no control, facilities, supplies, and personnel needed
4. Priorities in relation to legal mandates, significance of the problem relative to other community needs, and the feasibility of implementing the control plan

Public Opinion

Public opinion can have a significant impact on the effectiveness of any control plan. In the Gallup outbreak of salmonellosis, one control measure could have been to ban future food preparation and consumption for groups of persons numbering over 100 so that careful attention could be given to details. It is highly unlikely that this plan would be well received, since fairs are a major form of recreation on the Navajo Nation Indian Reservation and the Indians travel considerable distances to attend them. Clearly stating regulations for food preparation, with the mandatory attendance of one environmentalist per 1000 persons to oversee food preparation, would probably be a more realistic control measure for this situation.

Breaking the Chain of Transmission

Control measures are generally directed toward breaking the chain of transmission. This includes destroying or treating the reservoir of infection, interrupting the transmission of the agent from the reservoir to the new host, and decreasing the ability of the agent to adapt and multiply within the host. A *reservoir* is a living species or an inanimate object such as soil in which an infectious agent lives and multiplies and upon which it depends for survival and reproduction. When attempting to break the chain of transmission, the concept of multiple causation must be applied.

Referring again to the Gallup outbreak, the major cause of the disease was error in food preparation. There was prolonged storage of precooked ingredients for potato salad, within the 44° to 114° F range in which *Salmonella* have been demonstrated to multiply. The initial source of the *Salmonella* is unknown (Horwitz, Pollard, Merson, and Martin, 1977, p. 1074). As is often the case, the food handlers at this large gathering were lay persons, and their work was unsupervised. Large gatherings of people at which food is served should be considered high-risk settings for foodborne disease outbreak. It is advisable to have an epidemiologically trained person monitoring food preparation, storage, and serving at such occasions.

Herd Immunity

When one is dealing with infectious diseases, the concept of *herd immunity* is also important to consider while establishing a control plan. Herd immunity is the immunity level of a specific group. If, in a given group, 100 percent of the group had received measles vaccine, the herd immunity would be 100 percent. If 80 percent had received measles vaccine, the herd immunity would be at least 80 percent. Some people in the group have acquired immunity, raising the percentage higher.

Herd immunity does not have to be 100 percent to prevent an epidemic or to control a disease, but it is not known just what percentage is safe. Communities usually strive to achieve at least an 85 percent to 90 percent herd immunity level. It is important to realize that as herd immunity decreases, the chances for epidemics rise. In the United States, a major concern is that periodically, many school-age children are not receiving immunizations for communicable disease. This greatly decreases the level of herd immunity and is a major barrier to maintaining community health.

Community health nurses are instrumental in helping the public to see the need for effective control of disease by active immunization. This will continue to be a major function of the community health nurse, because immunizing populations at risk is the most effective way to control many of our childhood communicable diseases (refer to Chapter 13 for immunization schedules).

Casefinding

Casefinding is a major function of an epidemiologist and community health nurses. This process focuses on early diagnosis and treatment by discovery of new cases of a disease or condition. It may evolve through clinical observation or laboratory tests and may involve mass or individual testing. Opportunities for casefinding are limitless and come through home visits, clinic nursing, school visits, and prenatal classes, to name only a few. Community health nurses in these settings can pick up casefinding clues such as a tired young mother who seems unable to handle her three preschool children, possible scoliosis in a preadolescent girl, or a developmental delay in a toddler. By being alert to such clues many situations will be identified in which to use nursing skills to prevent disease and promote health. In some instances of casefinding, such as child abuse, a perceptive nurse may observe tendencies of abusive behavior in a parent and be able to assist the parent in working through these tendencies. This could prevent the abuse.

Step V: Implement Control Plan

An active effort should be made to elicit and coordinate the cooperation of the lay public, as well as private and official agencies, when putting control measures into operation. A control program that takes into consideration the beliefs, attitudes, and customs of the community is more likely to be accepted by the public than one that ignores community norms. Health education programs can help to "sell" a control program in the community, especially if they deal with current community attitudes and beliefs.

To evaluate the effectiveness of a control program, broad goals and specific objectives for the program must be identified before the program begins. Defining broad goals and specific outcome objectives such as the ones below makes it easier to determine if control efforts are successful.

> *Broad Goal:* To increase the herd immunity level for DPT to 85 percent in Centerville.

> *Objectives:* To increase the herd immunity level for DPT in census tracts 4 and 5 by 25 percent in 4 months by immunizing kindergarten and first-, fifth-, and tenth-grade students.
>
> To increase the herd immunity level for DPT in census tracts 8 and 9 by 17 percent in 4 months, by immunizing kindergarten and first-, fifth-, and tenth-grade students.

Control measures involve primary, secondary, and/or tertiary preventive activities. They include things such as disease reporting, quarantine, environmental control, human carrier control, health education, activities to decrease host susceptibility (e.g., immunizations), and technological advances.

Barriers to Control Programs

There are many barriers to the successful implementation of a control program for both infectious disease and noncommunicable conditions. Barriers to control involve factors such as unknown etiology, no known treatment, unavailable community resources, multifactorial etiology, long latency periods, and lack of reporting.

Low levels of immunity in an exposed population group increase the likelihood of disease occurrence. Mass and individual immunization programs are effective in raising immunity levels for some diseases. For many diseases, however, there are no specific prophylactic immunizations. Examples of such diseases are impetigo and STDs.

Individuals without overt disease symptoms, but who harbor the disease organism, can be a major vehicle in disease transmission. These individuals are known as *carriers.* Typhoid and salmonellosis are examples of diseases that are often transmitted by carriers.

With any disease and for a variety of reasons, some individuals will delay or not seek treatment. Whatever the reason, a delay in confirmation and treatment of the disease can enhance its spread and continuation and impede control plan implementation.

Individuals for whom the diagnosis is not suspected or confirmed are also barriers to the control of disease. Disease may not be confirmed for several reasons. Some people will evidence atypical symptoms of the disease in question. If clinical symptoms do not fit a disease model, the disease may be missed completely or misdiagnosed. Other individuals are seen too early or too late in the course of the disease process to either suspect or confirm the disease. In these situations, laboratory tests may be falsely negative or they may not be done at all because the clinical symptoms do not reflect a need. There are other times when a diagnosis cannot be confirmed because specimens (stools, emesis, or sputum) have inadvertently been destroyed or handled improperly. When working in the home or in other health care settings, it is vitally important to recognize that laboratory tests are needed to confirm most infectious disease diagnoses.

Lack of reporting, often reflecting nonacceptance of a diagnosis, is one of the key barriers in a control program. This can result from clerical error, indifference, fear, shame, or any of a number of variables. In some instances, professionals may not want to get involved or do not feel it appropriate to become involved. This is especially true when a social problem such as gonorrhea or child abuse is the disease or condition in question.

Community health nurses need to be acutely aware of these barriers because they are frequently in a position to help individuals, families, or health care professionals overcome them. Through the use of the referral process, knowledge of community resources, interviewing skills, and the ability to understand both health and disease processes, the community health nurse is uniquely able to assist in resolving these barriers.

Step VI: Evaluate Control Plan

An important part of the epidemiological process is evaluation. This ensures that the next time the process is repeated, it can be improved. It also ensures, through the problem-solving approach, that all elements of a problem have been reviewed. The first step in evaluation is to determine how well the objectives of the process were met. This implies that before carrying out the process, objectives were clearly and behaviorally written. The next question to be answered is how the current situation compares to the situation prior to the investigation. Finally, the practicality of the control measures should be determined. Feasibility and cost in terms of money, time, staff, facilities, and community support should be analyzed.

Step VII: Make Appropriate Report

Prompt, accurate, and concise epidemiological reporting will provide a basis for future investigations and control measures. Appropriate reporting demonstrates to the community the health professionals' accountability and clarifies the epidemiological situation. Reporting should include what was involved in the epidemiological process: diagnosis, factors leading to the epidemic, control measures, process evaluation, and recommendations for preventing similar situations.

Underreporting of many epidemiological investigations occurs. This happens for many reasons. Completion of necessary forms can be tedious and time-comsuming and, therefore, neglected. Frequently there is no one person assigned the responsibility for seeing that reports are completed and the responsibility is overlooked. Usually more effective reporting occurs when one person is designated to coordinate the reporting activities of others.

Societal and individual values and attitudes also contribute to underreporting. At times, conditions such as STDs, alcoholism, or mental illness are not discussed or reported because health care professionals are afraid to disturb the status quo in the community.

Accurate reporting is essential for the identification of major community health problems and preventive health action which would correct these problems. Treating only individuals with overt symptoms, rather than collecting and reporting data on populations at risk, does very little to prevent future health problems.

Step VIII: Conduct Research

If health services to populations are to be improved, epidemiological research is essential. Health professionals must be prepared to collect and analyze data systematically so that the gaps in

knowledge relative to disease causation, prevention, and control are eliminated. The ultimate goal of epidemiology—the prevention and control of infectious diseases, chronic conditions, and other health-related phenomena in populations—is far from being realized. Infectious diseases such as gonorrhea, syphilis, hepatitis, enteric disorders, and tuberculosis are still major health problems. In spite of scientific advances in the development of immunizations that prevent communicable diseases, epidemic outbreaks of childhood conditions, especially measles and diphtheria, continue to occur. Noninfectious conditions such as accidents and substance abuse and chronic diseases including cancer and heart conditions are fast-growing problems. Because of their complex nature, very little is known regarding their etiology or ways to prevent and control them. It is unfortunate that research in the practice setting is often lacking. Research can be exciting and challenging, especially when one discovers significant data that will aid a community to better its health status.

EPIDEMIOLOGICAL CHALLENGES OF THE FUTURE

Many contemporary challenges for epidemiologists exist. These challenges include the control of communicable and chronic diseases as well as selected psychosocial health phenomena. A major challenge on the epidemiological frontier is the control of acquired immunodeficiency syndrome (AIDS) which is at epidemic proportions in the United States today.

Communicable Disease: A Neglected Public Health Mandate

According to the Institute of Medicine's Committee for the Study of the Future of Public Health (1988), communicable disease has become a neglected mandate in the U.S. public health system. On a national level, the U.S. Public Health Service, Centers for Disease Control (CDC) in Atlanta, Georgia, is the major agency responsible for communicable disease control in this country (refer to Chapter 5). It maintains a national morbidity reporting system that collects, compiles, and publishes demographic, clinical, and laboratory data on many communicable and chronic diseases and conditions from each state. A department of each state has designated responsibility for control of communicable disease. This department maintains a morbidity reporting system based upon regulations adopted by the state board of health, which derives its authority to issue regulations from acts of the state legislature. These regulations usually specify *which* diseases or conditions are reportable (Appendix 10-1 identifies reportable diseases and conditions); *who* is responsible for reporting; *what* information is required for each case reported; *what* manner of reporting is needed; and to *whom* the information is reported. State regulations also commonly require reporting of any outbreak of unusually high prevalence of any disease and the occurrence of any unusual disease. Diseases which become important from a public health standpoint (e.g., AIDS) are usually promptly added to the list of reportable diseases (CDC, 1987, Principles of epidemiology: disease, pp. 2-3)

Diseases reported by the states to the CDC are determined by the Association of State and Territorial Health Officers. The CDC compiles state data and distributes a summary of this information to the states through its publication, *Morbidity and Mortality Weekly Report* (MMWR). The MMWR provides current statistics on communicable diseases as well as information on public health issues and conditions. The CDC provides an annual summary of disease reports from the states to the World Health Organization (WHO). However, CDC notifies WHO promptly of any reported cases of the internationally quarantinable diseases—smallpox, plague, cholera, and yellow fever—and influenza virus isolates (CDC, 1987, Principles of epidemiology: disease, p. 6).

Unfortunately, in the United States, the past strides made in communicable disease control and eradication have come to be taken for granted. We have become increasingly lax in many of our communicable disease practices. Although state health authorities document investigations of disease epidemics and outbreaks, there is *no* national system for surveillance of epidemics (CDC, 1989, Surveillance, p. 694). Many children

and adults in the United States are not completely immunized, and there has been an increase in the incidence of immunizable diseases such as measles and rubella (CDC, 1989, Mumps, p. 392). Measles eradication in the United States had been targeted for 1977, but that goal has not been met. Tuberculosis is on the rise in the United States (CDC, 1989, A strategic plan, p. 2), as are syphilis and hepatitis A (CDC, 1989, Mumps, p. 392). Many new sexually transmitted diseases are emerging, we have still not controlled or eradicated the old ones, and some are increasing in incidence. Appendix 10-2 provides information on some of the common communicable diseases that the community health nurse may have contact with in clinical practice. Information about commonly acquired sexually transmitted disease is given in Appendix 10-3. AIDS is discussed extensively in Chapters 13 and 15.

The American public needs to recognize communicable disease as a contemporary public health concern. The challenge to public health is to control the communicable diseases that already exist while meeting the demands of new communicable diseases—such as AIDS—as they develop.

Epidemiological Precautions to Prevent AIDS Transmission

AIDS is a contemporary public health challenge. Although it is discussed in greater depth in Chapters 13 and 15, the epidemiologically based precautions for minimizing transmission of the human immunodeficiency virus (HIV) are presented here.

In 1987, the CDC recommended that blood and body fluid precautions be consistently used for *all* patients to minimize transmission of the HIV and hepatitis B virus (HBV). This extension of blood and body fluid precautions to all patients is called "Universal Blood and Body Fluid Precautions" or "Universal Precautions" (CDC, 1988, p. 377). Universal precautions as well as additional precautions for invasive procedures, dialysis, and laboratories, with abbreviated environmental considerations for HIV transmission, are given in Appendix 10-4.

Under universal precautions, blood and certain

Body Fluids to Which Universal Precautions Apply and Do Not Apply	
APPLY	DO NOT APPLY*
Blood	Feces
Semen	Nasal secretions
Vaginal secretions	Sputum/Saliva
Cerebrospinal fluid (CSF)	Sweat
Synovial fluid	Tears
Pleural fluid	Urine
Peritoneal fluid	Vomitus
Pericardial fluid	Breast milk
Amniotic fluid	

*Universal precautions would apply to the above body fluids if they contained visible blood. The presence of human immunodeficiency virus and hepatitis B virus has been demonstrated in some of these fluids, but the risk of transmission is extremely low or nonexistent. Epidemiological studies have not implicated these fluids in the transmission of HIV and HBV infections.

From Centers for Disease Control (CDC): Update: universal precautions for prevention of transmission of human immunodeficiency virus, hepatitis B virus, and other bloodborne pathogens, MMWR 37:377-387, June 24, 1988; and CDC: Recommendations for prevention of HIV transmissions in health care settings, MMWR 36(Suppl S2), August 21, 1987.

body fluids are considered potentially infectious for human immunodeficiency virus (HIV) and hepatitis B virus (HBV). The body fluids to which universal precautions apply or do not apply are listed in the box above.

The box in the next column lists significant CDC publications about HIV transmission and precautions. The reader is encouraged to review these publications and to review upcoming issues of the CDC's *Morbidity and Mortality Weekly Report* (MMWR) periodically for further content, revisions, and related HIV and HBV information. The most recent publication noted in this box is intended for a technically informed, professional audience, and provides an overview of the modes of transmission of HIV and HBV in the workplace, an assessment of the risk for transmission, principles underlying the control of risk, specific risk-control recommendations for employers and workers, and information on medical management of persons who have sustained exposure at

the workplace (CDC, 1989, Publication of, p. 446). A separate document based on principles and practices discussed in this technical document is being developed for health education of the lay public.

Implementation of universal precautions does not eliminate the need for other category or disease-specific isolation precautions such as those for infectious diarrhea or pulmonary tuberculosis. Special precautions are strongly recommended for oral examinations and treatments in the dental setting and during phlebotomy. In addition to universal precautions, detailed precautions have been developed for the following procedures and/or settings in which prolonged or intensive exposures to blood occur: invasive procedures, dentistry, autopsies or morticians' services, dialysis, and the clinical laboratory. These detailed precautions are found in *Morbidity and Mortality Weekly Report:* Recommendations for prevention of HIV transmission in health-care settings, (Suppl 2S), August 21, 1987.

Chronic Disease and Conditions: An Increasing Challenge

Chapter 17 deals extensively with chronic and handicapping conditions. Chronic disease and conditions are of great concern to health professionals because they are long-term and often limit a person's ability to carry out major activities of daily living. Major activity refers to ability to

---

Selected CDC Publications on HIV Transmission and Precautions
CDC: Recommendations for prevention of HIV transmission in health-care settings, MMWR 36(Suppl 2S), August 21, 1987.
CDC: Universal precautions for prevention of transmission of human immunodeficiency virus, hepatitis B virus, and other bloodborne pathogens in health-care settings, MMWR 37:377-387, June 24, 1988.
CDC: Guidelines for prevention of transmission of human immunodeficiency virus and hepatitis B virus to health-care and public-safety workers, MMWR 38(Suppl S6), June 23, 1989.

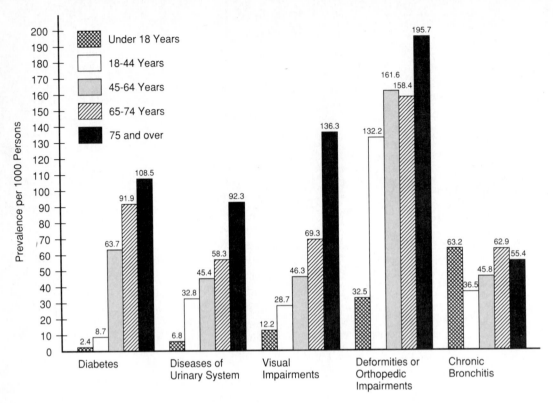

Figure 10-9 Prevalence of selected chronic conditions/1000 persons, by age, in the United States, 1986. (US Bureau of the Census: Statistical abstract of the United States, ed 109, Washington, DC, 1989, US Department of Commerce, p 114.)

work, keep house, or engage in school or preschool activities (Collins, 1986, p. 55). Chronic diseases and conditions have been studied extensively in the United States since the late 1940s. The prevalence of the diseases and conditions is increasing worldwide. Individuals experiencing chronic health problems require ongoing and comprehensive community health nursing and other health services.

The Commission on Chronic Illness, a national voluntary group, examined the extent of chronic disease and illness in the United States from 1949 to 1956. This commission defined chronic diseases as impairments or deviations from normal that have at least one of the following characteristics: permanency, residual disability, irreversible pathological causation and alteration, need for special rehabilitation training, and need for a long period of supervision, observation,

or care (Commission on Chronic Illness, 1957, p. 4). These concepts still guide practice related to chronic disease prevention and control.

Currently, data about the prevalence of selected chronic conditions are collected regularly by the National Center for Health Statistics by means of the National Health Interview Survey. In this survey, a condition is considered chronic if (1) the condition is described by the respondent as having been first noticed more than 3 months before the week of the interview, or (2) it is one of the conditions always classified as chronic regardless of time of onset. Examples of conditions always viewed as chronic are ulcers, emphysema, diabetes, arthritis, neoplasms, all congenital anomalies, and psychoses and other mental disorders (Collins, 1986, p. 54). The National Health Interview Survey also examines the concepts of impairment and disability related to chronic disease and conditions. These concepts are discussed in Chapter 17.

People of any age can evidence chronic conditions; these conditions are not synonymous with old age. It should be remembered that aging is the normal process of biological, psychological, and sociological change over time. However, because aging involves a gradual lessening in levels of efficiency and functioning in the various body systems, elderly people are more likely than young people to have chronic conditions. They also are likely to have more of them.

The Scope of Chronic Disease

Figure 10-9 illustrates that chronic conditions are evidenced across the age spectrum. People of all ages are affected by chronic disease. It should be noted, however, that the predominance of many chronic conditions is in the later years, from age 45 and on.

Chronic illness is a significant health problem in the United States. More than 31.5 million Americans have some degree of chronic activity limitation. A National Health Interview Survey published by the National Center for Health Statistics showed that 10.9 percent of all U.S. citizens had a chronic condition that placed a limitation on a major activity (Strauss, Corbin, Fagerhaugh, Glaser, Mainos, Suezek, and Weiner, 1984, p. 4). Chronic conditions also influence health services utilization and have an impact on disability days. For example, it has been found that each year heart conditions caused an average of 147.4 million bed disability days, arthritis caused 132.7 million bed disability days, and deformities or orthopedic impairments caused 101.4 million bed disability days (Collins, 1986, p. 15).

The 10 leading causes of chronic health conditions for the U.S. population as a whole are presented in Figure 10-10. Some other major causes of chronic health problems are dermatitis, migraine, visual impairments, diseases of the urinary tract, diabetes, and tinnitus. There are tremendous age-related variations relative to these chronic conditions. For example, statistical data show that the prevalence rate for hypertension is 409.2 per 1000 persons 75 years of age and over

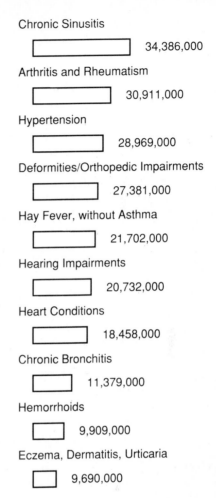

Chronic Sinusitis
34,386,000

Arthritis and Rheumatism
30,911,000

Hypertension
28,969,000

Deformities/Orthopedic Impairments
27,381,000

Hay Fever, without Asthma
21,702,000

Hearing Impairments
20,732,000

Heart Conditions
18,458,000

Chronic Bronchitis
11,379,000

Hemorrhoids
9,909,000

Eczema, Dermatitis, Urticaria
9,690,000

Figure 10-10   Ten major causes of chronic health conditions in the United States by number of persons, 1986. (US Bureau of the Census: Statistical abstract of the United States, ed 109, Washington, DC, 1989, US Department of Commerce, p. 114.)

and only 1.9 per 1000 persons under 18 years of age (U.S. Bureau of the Census, 1989, p. 114). Chapters 13 through 18 identify age-related health risks across the lifespan. When examining data about age-related risks, it is important to remember, however, that many chronic conditions found in later life have their roots in childhood or young adulthood and continue throughout the lifespan.

Why so much chronic disease? Strauss states that without question a major reason for the high rate of chronic disease in the United States is the elimination or control of infectious and parasitic diseases (Strauss, 1975, p. 3). The industrialized nations of the world are no longer greatly affected by preventable and controllable conditions. Instead, persons in these countries die from cancer, heart disease, stroke, and other long-term conditions such as diabetes.

The relatively low social value given to older people by our culture, as well as the acute care and cure orientation of health personnel, helps to explain why so little attention has been given to the care of persons with chronic conditions. This is unfortunate since there are many physical, social, and psychological components of long-term disease which require organized health care services and long-term conditions will undoubtedly play a major role in U.S. health care for years to come.

Levels of Prevention for Chronic Disease

The first of a four-volume series, based on the work of the Commission on Chronic Illness, was appropriately titled *Prevention of Chronic Illness.* Prevention must be the underlying approach to chronic conditions or these problems will only increase with time. Prevention on all three levels—primary, secondary, and tertiary—is essential for effective management and control of chronic conditions.

Primary prevention of many serious chronic illnesses is frequently impossible because health professionals are unable to determine the exact point in time when a condition begins. When, for example, does schizophrenia or asbestosis begin? Each of these diseases goes through a long latent period before symptoms are seen. They may stem from such variables as hereditary characteristics, occupational conditions, environmental stresses, or nutritional factors. Some chronic conditions can be prevented. Primary preventive efforts that control communicable disease, reduce accidents, emphasize adequate care during pregnancy, and suggest ways to cope with emotional stress all contribute to the prevention of certain chronic conditions. Primary prevention is an important task of the community health nurse.

Detection and treatment of chronic conditions

(secondary prevention) are often possible. For many conditions such as diabetes, hypertension, breast cancer, and glaucoma, large-scale national programs for early detection represent a profitable and economical approach to secondary prevention. Early diagnosis plays a significant role in the control of chronic disease and conditions.

A major secondary prevention effort relative to chronic illness occurred in the United States when the National Health Survey was authorized and conducted in 1956 to secure information about health conditions in the general population. This survey was enacted under the National Health Survey Act, which was proposed in 1955 by the U.S. Department of Health, Education, and Welfare (USDHEW). Under this act, the Surgeon General of the Public Health Service was authorized to conduct a survey in order to produce uniform, national statistics on disease, injury, impairment, disability, and related topics.

In 1972, a new survey mechanism initiated by USDHEW, the Health and Nutrition Examination Survey (HANES), began. Persons 1 to 74 years of age were examined, with emphasis on their nutritional status. Statistical data were collected on health records, fertility patterns, morbidity, and mortality. Today, HANES is the primary source of nationwide data on illnesses, disabilities, and physiological measurements.

Tertiary prevention activities, as well as primary and secondary ones, should be planned when working with people who have chronic conditions. Tertiary prevention involves rehabilitation, with the ultimate goal being cure or full restoration of the client's level of functioning. For some chronic conditions, this may be impossible; hence, the ideal goal must be replaced by more limited objectives, such as maximizing remaining functional potential or minimizing further deterioration. Another option would be to learn to live within the limitations that the chronic disease has imposed. A more detailed discussion of the concept of rehabilitation is presented in Chapter 17.

Approaches to the Study of Chronic Conditions

Two basic approaches to the study of chronic conditions and other diseases are *retrospective* and *prospective* studies. Retrospective and prospective studies are designed to determine if there is a relationship between a factor and a disease, as well as the intensity of that relationship. Mausner and Kramer (1985, pp. 159-174) discuss extensively the principles involved in these types of studies. Since only a brief summary of their thoughts is presented below, the reader should refer to Mausner and Kramer's text to obtain a better understanding of these approaches.

Retrospective studies look at people who are diagnosed as having a disease and compare them with those who do not have disease. The persons who do not have the disease are called *controls.* The controls come from the same general population segment as the individuals who have the condition and have the same characteristics as the study group except for the disease condition. A retrospective study examines factors in the person's past experience. One of the disadvantages of retrospective studies is that detailed information may not be available or accurate. The greatest problem, however, is finding a control group that is alike in all respects except for the condition under study. The advantages of this type of study are cost and the number of subjects needed. Retrospective studies are relatively inexpensive and require a small sampling size, because cases are identified at the onset.

Prospective studies start with a group of people (a cohort), all presumed to be free from a condition but who differ in their exposure to a supposedly harmful factor. This cohort is followed over a period of time to discover differences in the rate at which disease develops in relation to exposure to the harmful factor. A major advantage of this type of study is that the cohort is chosen for study before the disease develops. The cohort is, therefore, not influenced by knowledge that disease exists, as in retrospective studies.

Prospective studies allow calculation of incidence rates among those exposed and those not exposed. Thus, absolute difference in incidence rates and the true relative risk can be measured. The major disadvantage is that a prospective study is a long, expensive project. A large cohort must be used, especially if the disease has low incidence. Also, the larger the number of factors to

be studied, the larger the cohort must be. The loss of people from the cohort as a result of death, lack of interest, or job mobility is a major problem when a study lasts over an extended period of time. Changes in diagnostic criteria, administrative problems, loss of staff or funding, and the high cost of record keeping can all contribute to make this a study that should not be undertaken without careful planning.

Retrospective and prospective studies assist in identifying causes of disease as well as effective disease control mechanisms. It is not intended that this brief description of retrospective and prospective studies will prepare community health nurses to do them. The purpose is to familiarize readers with the basic concepts involved in the study of chronic conditions.

The community health nurse does, however, play an active role in the control of chronic conditions. Case finding through screening programs is a significant aspect of this part of the community health nurse's role.

Screening as a Method for Detection and Control of Chronic Conditions

Screening programs can be an efficient way to identify individuals in a community who may unknowingly have a chronic condition, as well as an infectious disease.

There are two types of screening programs whereby chronic and infectious disease is sought in apparently healthy individuals: the *single screening test* where only one condition is being identified, such as giving a group of teachers a TB tine test, and the *multiphasic screening test* where a battery of tests is used at one time to detect several disease conditions. Doing height and weight measurements, audiometry, and vision screening of all persons at a county fair is an example of multiphasic screening.

Screening tests do not provide a conclusive diagnosis of a disease, but rather are used to identify asymptomatic individuals who may unknowingly have a problem. Anyone who evidences symptoms of a disease through a screening program should have further medical diagnostic testing. This is essential since early diagnosis and treatment are the primary goals of a screening program. Early diagnosis and treatment are particularly beneficial for conditions such as hypertension and cancer, for which there are treatment measures available to prevent progression of the condition.

Advantages of screening programs are that often they are relatively inexpensive; take little time; need few professionals to administer them; provide opportunity for prevention, early diagnosis, and treatment; and present statistics on the prevalence of disease when there is adequate follow-up. Major disadvantages of screening programs are that people tend to substitute them for medical examination, findings of screening programs are presumptive and further testing should be done to confirm a diagnosis, screening programs often do not reach vulnerable groups of people, and conditions may be missed during screening, resulting in persons receiving a false impression of their health status.

Not all chronic conditions lend themselves to screening. Many authors have discussed criteria to consider when establishing screening programs. The following principles are seen as essential to good screening practices (Wilson and Jungner, 1968; Mausner and Kramer, 1985):

1. The condition sought should be an important health problem (affect a significant percentage of people).
2. There should be an accepted treatment for clients with recognized disease.
3. Facilities for diagnosis and treatment should be available.
4. There should be a recognizable latent or early symptomatic stage.
5. There should be a suitable test or examination (to detect the disease).
6. The test should be acceptable to the population.
7. The natural history of the condition, including development from latent to declared disease, should be adequately understood.
8. The cost of casefinding (including diagnosis and treatment) should be economically balanced in relation to possible expenditure for medical care as a whole.
9. Casefinding should be thought of as a continuing process and not a "once and for all" project.

It should be clear from reviewing these principles that although screening can be one method for early discovery of asymptomatic disease, it should be used judiciously and discriminately. Screening results need to be thoroughly evaluated and the conditions found must be treated.

SUMMARY

The epidemiological process helps community health nurses to identify the health status of the community in which they are working, and to prevent disease, chronic conditions, and other health-related phenomena such as child abuse, mental illness, and domestic violence. This process places emphasis on analyzing the needs of populations rather than the needs of individual clients. Like the nursing process, it is a scientific, systematic problem-solving approach to the study of health needs.

There are several key concepts inherent in the understanding and utilization of the epidemiological process. These are study of populations at risk, natural life history of disease, levels of prevention, host-agent-environment relationships, multiple causation of disease, and person-place-time relationships. In addition to these concepts, a community health nurse must understand biostatistics in order to effectively use the epidemiological process.

By applying the concepts and methods of epidemiology, community health nurses play a vital role in the prevention of disease, injuries, and social problems in a community. Through their contacts in a variety of settings, they are in a key position to do case finding, to eliminate barriers to the control of disease, and to promote health through teaching and counseling.

APPENDIX 10-1

Reportable Diseases and Conditions

Diseases reportable in most states

AIDS
Amebiasis*
Anthrax
Aseptic meningitis
Botulism
Brucellosis
Chickenpox
Cholera†
Diphtheria
Encephalitis, primary infectious
Encephalitis, postinfectious
Food-poisoning (outbreaks)*
Hepatitis A
Hepatitis B
Leprosy
Leptospirosis
Malaria
Meningococcal infections
Mumps
Pertussis*
Plague†

Poliomyelitis, total and paralytic
Psittacosis-Ornithosis
Rabies in man and animals
Rubella
Rubella congenital syndrome
Salmonellosis, excluding typhoid fever
Shigellosis
Smallpox†
Tetanus
Trichinosis
Tuberculosis (new active cases)
Tularemia
Typhoid fever
Typhus, fleaborne (murine)
Typhus, tickborne (Rocky Mountain spotted fever)
Venereal diseases
    Syphilis (primary and secondary)
    Gonorrhea
    Other specified venereal diseases*: chancroid,
        granuloma inguinale, and lymphogranuloma venereum
Yellow fever†

Diseases and conditions reportable in some states only

Abortions
Adverse drug reactions
Animal bites
Cancer
Cat-scratch fever
Congenital defects
Conjunctivitis
Echinococcosis
Epilepsy
Erysipelas
Erythema
Fungal infections
Glanders
Glomerulonephritis
Impetigo
Industrial and occupational diseases
Influenza
Keratoconjunctivitis
Lead poisoning
Listeriosis
Melioidosis
Meningitis, bacterial (except meningococcal)

Mycobacteriosis
Ophthalmia neonatorum
Otitis media
Parasitic diseases and infestations
Pneumonia
Poisoning
Q fever
Rat-bite fever
Reye's syndrome
Rheumatic fever, acute
Rickettsialpox
Septicemia
Staphylococcal infection
Steptococcal sore throat and scarlet fever
Tickborne diseases
Toxoplasmosis
Trachoma
Vaccinia
Vincent's angina
Viral infections
Yaws

*Diseases not routinely reported to CDC on a weekly basis.

†Diseases covered by International Quarantine Agreement.

From Centers for Disease Control, Training and Laboratory Program Office: Principles of epidemiology; disease surveillance, self-study course 3030-G, manual 5, Atlanta, Ga, 1987, CDC, pp 4-5; CDC: Personal communication, August 1990.

APPENDIX 10-2

Some Common Communicable Diseases Encountered by Community Health Nurses

Disease	Etiologic agent	Primary reservoir	Incubation period	Mode of transmission	Period of communicability	Symptoms	Treatment
Hepatitis A (infectious)	Virus	Humans	15–50 days (30 days average)	Person-to-person by fecal oral route	Maximum infectivity during the incubation period and continuing for a few days after onset of jaundice; no carrier state	Abrupt and "flu-like" with loss of appetite, nausea and vomiting, abdominal discomfort, jaundice, dark brown urine, light brown stool (may be asymptomatic)	No specific treatment (bedrest, increased fluids, no alcoholic beverages, no fried or fatty foods)
Hepatitis B (serum)	Virus	Humans	2 weeks–9 months (60–90 day average)	Percutaneous or permucosal exposure to infected body fluids (blood, saliva, semen, and vaginal fluids)	Weeks before onset of symptoms and infective for entire clinical course; carrier state can exist	Onset is gradual with symptoms similar to those of hepatitis A	Same as hepatitis A
Rubella (German measles)	Virus	Humans	14–21 days	Usually person-to-person (direct contact or droplet spread)	At least 4 days before rash and at least 4 days after onset of rash; very contagious	Mild febrile illness with a macular rash (adults may experience more serious illness); rash on scalp, body, and limbs; usually lasts 1–3 days	No specific treatment (bedrest, increase fluids)
Measles	Virus	Humans	7–21 days (10 days average)	Usually person-to-person (direct or contact or droplet spread)	At least 4 days before rash and at least 4 days after onset of rash; very contagious	Resembles a bad cold with eyes and nose running, red blotchy rash beginning usually on face (often behind ears) and then becoming generalized, cough, Koplik spots, more severe symptoms than in rubella; lasts about 4 days	No specific treatment (bedrest, increase fluids, place in darkened room if eyes hurt)
Mumps	Virus	Humans	14–26 days (18 days average)	Person-to-person (direct contact with saliva or droplet spread)	At least 6 days before parotitis and up to 9 days after; very infective about 2 days prior to symptoms	Pain and swelling in one or both parotid glands, fever, pain on opening and shutting mouth (may need to use a straw to drink)	No specific treatment (bedrest, increase fluids)

Disease	Causative agent	Reservoir	Incubation period	Transmission	Period of communicability	Symptoms	Treatment
Chickenpox	Virus	Humans	12-21 days (14 days average)	Person-to-person (direct contact; droplet or airborne spread)	2 days before vesicles and 6 days after vesicles appear; very contagious	Sudden onset; maculopapular rash that becomes vesicular and leaves a crusty scalp; generalized rash, itchy	No specific treatment (topical applications for itching, bedrest, encourage fluids, dress in loose clothing and caution person not to become overheated)
Pink eye	Multiple agents	Humans	24-72 hours	Person-to-person by direct contact, also through contaminated clothing, fomites	Entire course of disease, until redness and discharge have disappeared	Lacrimation, eye irritation, and redness of lids; photophobia and mucopurulent discharge	Treatment dependent on causative agent
Ringworm	Fungi	Humans	4-14 days (variable)	Direct skin-to-skin or indirect contact from items such as chairs, barber clippers	As long as lesions are present	Scalp: scaly patches of temporary baldness, crusty lesions, hair may become brittle. Body: Flat, spreading ring-shaped lesions that are red on the periphery and vesicular or pustular in center. Feet: "athlete's foot" characterized by scaling or cracking of the skin between the toes, itching	Topical fungicide; oral medication as prescribed
Scabies	Mite (*Sarcoptes scabiei*)	Humans	2-6 weeks for initial infestation; 1-4 days for reinfection	Direct skin-to-skin contact; transfer may occur from clothing	As long as condition is present—until mites and eggs are destroyed by treatment	Papular or vesicular; may evidence "burrows" on skin like grayish-white threads; lesions prominent around webs of fingers, wrists, elbows, belt line, intense itching	Kwell lotion
Pediculosis	Louse	Humans	2 weeks (8-10 days average)	Direct person-to-person or indirect contact with infected personal belongings	As long as eggs or lice are alive	Scalp: itching swollen lymph nodes can often see nits; or lice in hair. Pubic: itching; swollen glands	Kwell lotion or shampoo

Continued.

Some Common Communicable Diseases Encountered by Community Health Nurses—cont'd

Disease	Etiologic agent	Primary reservoir	Incubation period	Mode of transmission	Period of communicability	Symptoms	Treatment
Giardiasis	*Giardia lamblia,* a flagellate protozoan	Humans	5-25 days or longer (7-10 days average)	Ingestion of cysts in fecally contaminated water or food; person-to-person by hand-to-mouth transfer of cysts from feces	Entire period of infection	Chronic diarrhea, steatorrhea, abdominal cramps, bloating, frequent loose and pale greasy stools, fatigue, weight loss	Atabrine is drug of choice; metronidazole (Flagyl) is also effective; furazolidone pediatric suspension for young children and infants; enteric precautions should be used
Salmonellosis	Numerous serotypes of salmonella (bacterial); *S. typhimurium* is the most common	Humans and domestic and wild animals, including poultry, swine, cattle, rodents, and pets (e.g., dogs, cats, turtles, chickens)	6-72 hours (12-36 hours average)	Ingestion of organisms in food contaminated by feces; person-to-person by fecal-oral route	Entire period of infection, sometimes over 1 year; antibiotics can prolong this period	Acute enterocolitis, with *sudden* onset of headache, abdominal pain, diarrhea, nausea and sometimes vomiting; dehydration; fever nearly always present; anorexia and loose bowels persist for days	Rehydration and electrolyte replacement with oral glucose-electrolyte solution; antibiotics (ampicillin or amoxicillin) for infants under 2 months, the elderly and the debilitated, or patients with prolonged symptoms (antibiotics may prolong carrier state)

Shigellosis	Shigella (Group A., *S. dysenteriae*; Group B. *S. flexneri*; Group C. *S. boydii*; Group D, *S. sonnei*); bacterial	Humans	1-7 days (1-3 days average)	Person-to-person by fecal-oral route	During acute infection and until infectious agent is no longer present (usually within 4 weeks)	Diarrhea accompanied by fever, nausea, and sometimes toxemia, vomiting, cramps, and tenesmus; blood, mucus, pus in stool	Fluid and electrolyte replacement; antimotility agents contraindicated; antibiotic therapy (e.g., ampicillin, tetracyclines), based on antibiogram of isolated strain, for patients with severe symptoms
Impetigo	Bacteria (often *streptococci* or *staphylococci*)	Humans	Variable, but commonly 4-10 days	Person-to-person contact with lesions or secretions and mildly infectious through fomites	As long as purulent lesions continue	Draining, crusty skin lesions that may resemble ringworm or dry scales; often accompanied by fever, malaise, headache and loss of appetite	Antibiotics such as penicillin and erythromycin and antibiotic creams and lotions

From Vaughan G: Mummy, I don't feel well, London, 1970, Causton and Sons, Ltd.; Tennessee Department of Health and Environment: Protect them from harm, Murfreesboro, Tenn, 1983, Lancer; Benenson AS: Control of communicable diseases in man, ed 15, Washington, DC, 1990, American Public Health Association.

APPENDIX 10-3

Information about Thirteen Most Commonly Acquired Sexually Transmitted Diseases (STDs)

Disease	Usual symptoms	Diagnosis
Gonorrhea (clap, dose, drip)* Cause: *Neisseria gonorrhoeae* bacterium	Appear in 2-10 days or up to 30 days *Women:* 80% have no symptoms; may have puslike vaginal discharge; lower abdominal pain; painful urination *Men:* Thick, milky discharge from penis and/or painful urination; 10%-20% *have no symptoms* *Men and women:* Sore throat, pain and mucus when defecating; often no anal symptoms	*Women:* Culture from vagina, cervix, throat and/or rectum *Men:* Smear or culture from penis, rectum, and/or throat
Nongonococcal urethritis/cervicitis (NGU, NGC)* Common cause: *Chlamydia trachomatis.* Other causes: *Ureaplasma urealtyticum; Trichomonas vaginalis; Candida albicans and herpes simplex virus*	Appear in 1-3 weeks *Women* (NGC): Usually have no symptoms: may have frequent uncomfortable urination: vaginal discharge *Men* (NGU): Mild to moderate discomfort on urination; thin, clear or white morning discharge from penis	*Women:* No highly definitive diagnostic tool is currently available for chlamydial infection; culture (to rule out gonorrhea) and a vaginal smear (to rule out trichomonas and yeast) *Men:* Culture (to rule our gonorrhea) and a smear
Pelvic inflammatory disease (PID)† *Affects only women* Usual causes: *Neisseria gonorrhoeae; Chlamydia trachomatis;* enteric bacteria	Onset of symptoms varies; abnormal vaginal discharge; severe pain and tenderness in lower abdominal/pelvic area; painful intercourse and/or menstruation; irregular bleeding; chills and fever; nausea, vomiting	History, culture, and examination to rule out other problems (ectopic pregnancy, appendicitis, etc.); pelvic ultrasound; laparoscopy
Human papilloma virus infection/ Condylomata acuminata *(HPV, genital/venereal warts)* Cause: human papilloma virus	Appear in 1-6 months; firm, flesh-colored or grayish-white warts on vulva, anus, lower vagina, penis, scrotum, mouth, throat; lesions on cervix usually not visible to the naked eye; itching	Clinical examination and Pap smear of colposcopy for lesions on cervix

Possible complications	*Treatment*	*Special considerations*
Women: Pelvic inflammatory disease (10%-20% of cases) (see PID above) *Men:* Narrowing of urethra; sterility; swelling of testicles *Men and women:* Arthritis, blood infections, dermatitis, meningitis, and endocarditis *Newborns:* Eye, nose, lung, and/or rectal infections	Ceftriazone plus doxycycline or tetracycline or spectinomycin Ceftriazone	3-10 days after treatment and again in 4-6 weeks a culture test should be done (to show cure)
Women: Pelvic inflammatory disease (see PID above), cervical dysplasia (currently under study) *Men:* Prostatitis, epididymitis *Newborns:* Eye infections, pneumonia	Doxycycline or tetracycline (erythromycin for pregnant women and those resistant to tetracycline)	
Sterility; chronic abdominal pain; chronic infection (of the fallopian tubes, uterus and/or ovaries); ectopic pregnancy, death	*Inpatient:* Cefoxitin IV in combination with doxycycline or clindamycin and gentamicin IV. *Ambulatory:* Cefoxitin IM in combination with ceftiaxone and doxycycline or tetracycline; bedrest and no sex for at least 2 weeks	Usually the result of untreated gonorrhea or chlamydial infection Scarring of fallopian tubes may increase risk of future ectopic pregnancies IUD, if present, should be removed and replaced by another form of birth control *Careful medical follow-up is essential*
Blockage of vaginal, rectal, or throat openings; cervical dysplasia; cancer (currently under study)	Cryotherapy with liquid nitrogen or cryoprobe; podophyllin benzoin (contraindicated in pregnancy) or trichloroacetic acid; electrocautery.	Warts and invisible lesions are *highly* contagious; both will continue to multiply until completely removed

Continued.

APPENDIX 10-3

Information about Thirteen Most Commonly Acquired Sexually Transmitted Diseases (STDs)—cont'd

Disease	Usual symptoms	Diagnosis
Herpes, genital or oral (cold sores; fever blisters on mouth) Causes: herpes simplex virus I (HSV I; oral); herpes simplex Virus II (HSV II; genital)	May occur immediately or as late as 1 year after contact or not at all; some people exhibit few or no symptoms Itching, tingling sensation followed by painful blister-like lesions that appear in clusters at the site of infection (i.e., lips, nose, inner and outer vaginal lips, clitoris, rectum, thighs, buttocks); blisters dry up and disappear generally leaving no scar tissue HSV II symptoms in women may include increased vaginal discharge, painful intercourse and urination; painless lesions on cervix may go undetected *Primary episodes:* HSV II—some experience fever, body aches, flulike symptoms, swollen lymph nodes near infected areas *Recurrent episodes:* HSV I and HSV II—generally lessen in frequency and severity over time	Culture from sore, clinical examination or Tzanck smear Definitive diagnosis only possible when lesions are present
Syphilis‡ (syph, lues, pox, bad blood) Cause: *Treponema pallidum* (spirochete bacterium)	First stage—(appears in 10-90 days, average 3 weeks): painless sores (chancres) where bacteria entered body (genitals, rectum, lips, breasts, etc.) Second state—(1 week to 6 months after stage 1): rash; flulike symptoms; mouth sores; genital/anal sores (condylomata lata); inflamed eyes; patchy balding Latent stage—(10-20 years after state 2): None Final stage—See possible complications	Blood test; clinical examination
Vulvovaginitis Causes: *Trichomonas vaginalis* (protozoa)§; *Candida albicans* (fungus)‖; *Gardnerella/Haemophilus vaginalis* (bacteria)**	A. *Trichomoniasis* (Trich, TV, A, B, C Vaginitis) appear in 1-6 weeks *Women:* Thin, foamy yellow-green or gray vaginal discharge with foul odor; burning, redness, itching and/or frequent urination *Men: Usually no symptoms* May have slight, clear morning discharge from penis; itching after urination	*Women:* Vaginal smear; microscopic identification; urinalysis; culture (to rule out gonorrhea); clinical examination *Men:* Hard to diagnose

Possible complications	Treatment	Special considerations
Oral: Autoinoculation to skin or eyes *Genital:* Possible increased risk of cervical cancer; disturbance of bladder or bowel functioning (neuralgia); meningitis (nonfatal) *Newborns:* Blindness, brain damage, and/or death to baby passing through birth canal of mother with active lesions	*No known cure at present* The following may be helpful in reducing symptoms and/or recurrences: oral acyclovir; stress reduction techniques (yoga, meditation, etc.); keep sores dry/clean; healthy diet and exercise; inpatient therapy in severe cases: acyclovir I.V.	HSV I can be found genitally and HSV II can be found orally due to oral-genital sex or autoinoculation Recurrent attacks are unpredictable but often appear at times of high stress, when fatigued, after vigorous intercourse, around menstruation, at times of other illnesses, etc. Research is inconclusive regarding whether or not herpes is occasionally contagious when there are no active lesions Many experience difficult, but not insurmountable, adjustments in self-image and sexual behavior *Women:* Should have Pap smears twice yearly and if pregnant, inform their health care provider (of their herpes); cesarean delivery is indicated if mother has active lesions at the time of delivery; *cervical lesions may go undetected because they are not painful*
Adult: Blindness, deafness (usually reversible); brain damage; paralysis, heart disease, death *Newborns:* Damage to skin, bones, eyes, teeth, and/or liver; death	Penicillin, (tetracycline or doxycycline for penicillin-allergic patients; doxycycline used in nonpregnant patients only)	Many women will not notice chancre because it is painless and may be deep inside vagina Complications can be prevented if treated at 1st or 2nd stage Return for blood test 1 month after treatment and once every 3 months for 1 year
A. None	A. Metronidazole (Flagyl)	A. *All partners should be treated even if they have no symptoms* Cautions about Flagyl: very high doses have been shown to cause cancer in laboratory animals Should not be taken by

Continued.

Information about Thirteen Most Commonly Acquired Sexually Transmitted Diseases (STDs)—cont'd

Disease	Usual symptoms	Diagnosis
	B. *Candida infections* (yeast, monilia); onset of symptoms varies *Women:* Thick, white cottage cheese-like, foul smelling discharge which adheres to the vaginal walls; intense itching and irritation of genitals *Men: usually no symptoms;* dermatitis on penis C. *Gardnerella infections;* onset of symptoms varies *Women:* Thin, foul-smelling yellow-gray discharge; may have some vaginal burning	
Hepatitis B Cause: hepatitis B virus	Appear in 1-6 months, but often no clear symptoms General flulike symptoms; liver deterioration marked by darkened urine, lightened stool, yellowed eyes and skin, skin eruptions, enlarged and tender liver	Blood tests; clinical examination
Pediculosis pubis†† (crabs, cooties, lice) Cause: *Phthirus pubis* (crab louse)	Appear in 4-5 weeks Intense itching in hairy areas (usually begins in pubic hair)	Clinical examination; self-examination may reveal blood spots on underwear, eggs or nits
Scabies‡‡ (the itch) Cause: *Sarcoptes scabiei* (parasite mite)	Appear in 4-6 weeks Severe itching and raised reddish tracts; may appear anywhere on body and are caused by the mite burrowing under the skin	Clinical examination; microscopic observation

Symbols indicate that a particular STD may also be contracted in the following ways:

*Infants: while in birth canal of an infected mother.

†Increased risk through use of the intrauterine device (IUD) as a method of contraception.

‡Fluid from chancre coming in contact with cuts in the skin; infants: while in infected mother's womb.

§Sharing wet towels with an infected person.

‖Change in pH balance of vagina from pregnancy, diabetes, birth control pills, antibiotics, stress, douching.

**Puncture of skin with contaminated needle; using toothbrush, razor, etc., of an infected person.

††May be spread by fingers from one hairy area to another; sharing linen or clothing of an infected person.

‡‡Close physical contact (sexual or nonsexual).

From Venereal Disease Action Coalition. Sexually transmitted diseases: a community information and resource guide, Detroit, 1983, United Community Services of Metropolitan Detroit, pp 9-11; Centers for Disease Control: 1989 sexually transmitted diseases treatment guidelines, MMWR 38(No. S-8), 4-40, 1989.

Possible complications	Treatment	Special considerations
		pregnant or breastfeeding women Alcohol should be avoided when taking Flagyl as it may cause severe headaches and nausea
B. *Newborns:* Mouth and throat infections C. None	B. Miconazole nitrate, clotrimazole, butaconazole or teraconazole intravaginally C. Metronidazole (Flagyl) or clindamycin (effective in 50%-60% of cases)	A, B, and C. Recurrent infections are common and can be prevented: tub bathing during menstruation, loose clothing and cotton panties; also avoid use of bubble bath, deodorant, tampons, scented soaps, vaginal sprays and douches (as these may irritate the vagina and/or change the pH balance)
Chronic hepatitis; chronic acute hepatitis; cirrhosis; liver cancer; death	Bed rest; lots of fluids; a light, healthy diet and no alcohol; no specific drug therapy	Often confused with flu or a bad cold and thus not treated early Recovery usually 2-3 months Will not recur once cured Hepatitis B vaccine will provide immunity
None	Lindane (Kwell) cream, lotion, or shampoo (not recommended for pregnant or breastfeeding women); Pyrethrins and piperonyl butoxide applications	Common soap will not kill crabs All clothes and linen must be washed in hot water *or* dry-cleaned *or* removed from human contact for 1-2 weeks
Secondary bacterial infection (from scratching)	Lindane (Kwell) cream, lotion, or shampoo (not recommended for pregnant or breastfeeding women) or crotamiton (Eurox) cream or lotion	Common soap will not kill the mites All clothing and linen must be washed in hot water *or* dry-cleaned *or* removed from human contact for 1-2 weeks

APPENDIX 10-4

Precautions to Prevent Transmission of HIV: Universal Precautions, Precautions for Invasive Procedures, Precautions for Dialysis, Precautions for Laboratories, and Environmental Considerations for HIV Transmission

UNIVERSAL PRECAUTIONS (for prevention of transmission of human immunodeficiency virus, hepatitis B virus, and other bloodborne pathogens in health care settings)

Since medical history and examination cannot reliably identify all patients infected with HIV or other bloodborne pathogens, blood and body-fluid precautions should be consistently used for **all** patients. This approach, previously recommended by CDC and referred to as "universal blood and body-fluid precautions" or "universal precautions," should be used in the care of *all* patients, especially including those in emergency-care settings in which the risk of blood exposure is increased and the infection status of the patient is usually unknown.

1. All health-care workers should routinely use appropriate barrier precautions to prevent skin and mucous-membrane exposure when contact with blood or other body fluids of any patient is anticipated. Gloves should be worn for touching blood and body fluids, mucous membranes, or non-intact skin of all patients, for handling items or surfaces soiled with blood or body fluids, and for performing venipuncture and other vascular access procedures. Gloves should be changed after contact with each patient. Masks and protective eyewear or face shields should be worn during procedures that are likely to generate droplets of blood or other body fluids to prevent exposure of mucous membranes of the mouth, nose, and eyes. Gowns or aprons should be worn during procedures that are likely to generate splashes of blood or other body fluids.
2. Hands and other skin surfaces should be washed immediately and thoroughly if contaminated with blood or other body fluids. Hands should be washed immediately after gloves are removed.
3. All health-care workers should take precautions to prevent injuries caused by needles, scalpels, and other sharp instruments or devices during procedures; when cleaning used instruments; during disposal of used needles; and when handling sharp instruments after procedures. To prevent needlestick injuries, needles should not be recapped, purposely bent or broken by hand, removed from disposable syringes, or otherwise manipulated by hand. After they are used, disposable syringes and needles, scalpel blades, and other sharp items should be placed in puncture-resistant containers for disposal; the puncture-resistant containers should be located as close as practical to the use area. Large-bore reusable needles should be placed in a puncture-resistant container for transport to the reprocessing area.
4. Although saliva has not been implicated in HIV transmission, to minimize the need for emergency mouth-to-mouth resuscitation, mouthpieces, resuscitation bags, or other ventilation devices should be available for use in areas in which the need for resuscitation is predictable.
5. Health-care workers who have exudative lesions or weeping dermatitis should refrain from all direct patient care and from handling patient-care equipment until the condition resolves.
6. Pregnant health-care workers are not known to be at greater risk of contracting HIV infection than health-care workers who are not pregnant; however, if a health-care worker develops HIV infection during pregnancy, the infant is at risk of infection resulting from perinatal transmission. Because of this risk, pregnant health-care workers should be especially familiar with and strictly adhere to precautions to minimize the risk of HIV transmission.

Implementation of universal blood and body-fluid precautions for *all* patients eliminates the need for use of the isolation category of "Blood and Body Fluid Precautions" previously recommended by CDC for patients known or suspected to be infected with bloodborne pathogens. Isolation precautions (e.g., enteric, "AFB") should be used as necessary if associated conditions, such as infectious diarrhea or tuberculosis, are diagnosed or suspected.

In addition to Universal Precautions, the following precautions should be taken in invasive procedures, dialysis, and laboratories and laboratory procedures.

Precautions for Invasive Procedures   In this document, an invasive procedure is defined as surgical entry into tissues, cavities, or organs or repair of major traumatic injuries 1) in an operating or delivery room, emergency department, or outpatient setting, including both physicians' and dentists' offices; 2) cardiac catheterization and angiographic procedures; 3) a vaginal or Cesarean delivery or other invasive obstetric procedure during which bleeding may occur; or 4) the manipulation, cutting, or removal of any oral or perioral tissues, including tooth structure, during which bleeding occurs or the potential for bleeding exists. The universal blood and body-fluid precautions listed above, combined with the precautions listed below, should be the minimum precautions for *all* such invasive procedures.

1. All health-care workers who participate in invasive procedures must routinely use appropriate barrier precautions to prevent skin and mucous-membrane contact with blood and other body fluids of all patients. Gloves and surgical masks must be worn for all invasive procedures. Protective eyewear or face shields should be worn for procedures that commonly result in the generation of droplets, splashing of blood or other body fluids, or the generation of bone chips. Gowns or aprons made of materials that provide an effective barrier should be worn during invasive procedures that are likely to result in the splashing of blood or other body fluids. All health-care workers who perform or assist in vaginal or Cesarean deliveries should wear gloves and gowns when handling the placenta or the infant until blood and amniotic fluid have been removed from the infant's skin and should wear gloves during post-delivery care of the umbilical cord.
2. If a glove is torn or a needlestick or other injury occurs, the glove should be removed and a new glove used as promptly as patient safety permits; the needle or instrument involved in the incident should also be removed from the sterile field.

Precautions for Dialysis   Patients with end-stage renal disease who are undergoing maintenance dialysis and who have HIV infection can be dialyzed in hospital-based or free-standing dialysis units using conventional infection-control precautions. Universal blood and body-fluid precautions should be used when dialyzing *all* patients.

Precautions to Prevent Transmission of HIV: Universal Precautions, Precautions for Invasive Procedures, Precautions for Dialysis, Precautions for Laboratories, and Environmental Considerations for HIV Transmission—cont'd

Strategies for disinfecting the dialysis fluid pathways of the hemodialysis machine are targeted to control bacterial contamination and generally consist of using 500-750 parts per million (ppm) of sodium hypochlorite (household bleach) for 30-40 minutes or 1.5%-2.0% formaldehyde overnight. In addition, several chemical germicides formulated to disinfect dialysis machines are commercially available. None of these protocols or procedures need to be changed for dialyzing patients infected with HIV.

Patients infected with HIV can be dialyzed by either hemodialysis or peritoneal dialysis and do not need to be isolated from other patients. The type of dialysis treatment (i.e., hemodialysis or peritoneal dialysis) should be based on the needs of the patient. The dialyzer may be discarded after each use. Alternatively, centers that reuse dialyzers—i.e., a specific single-use dialyzer is issued to a specific patient, removed, cleaned, disinfected, and reused several times on the same patient only—may include HIV-infected patients in the dialyzer-reuse program. An individual dialyzer must never be used on more than one patient.

Precautions for Laboratories Blood and other body fluids from *all* patients should be considered infective. To supplement the universal blood and body-fluid precautions listed above, the following precautions are recommended for health-care workers in clinical laboratories.

1. All specimens of blood and body fluids should be put in a well-constructed container with a secure lid to prevent leaking during transport. Care should be taken when collecting each specimen to avoid contaminating the outside of the container and of the laboratory form accompanying the specimen.
2. All persons processing blood and body-fluid specimens (e.g., removing tops from vacuum tubes) should wear gloves. Masks and protective eyewear should be worn if mucous-membrane contact with blood or body fluids is anticipated. Gloves should be changed and hands washed after completion of specimen processing.
3. For routine procedures, such as histologic and pathologic studies or microbiologic culturing, a biological safety cabinet is not necessary. However, biological safety cabinets (Class I or II) should be used whenever procedures are conducted that have a high potential for generating droplets. These include activities such as blending, sonicating, and vigorous mixing.
4. Mechanical pipetting devices should be used for manipulating all liquids in the laboratory. Mouth pipetting must not be done.
5. Use of needles and syringes should be limited to situations in which there is no alternative, and the recommendations for preventing injuries with needles outlined under universal precautions should be followed.
6. Laboratory work surfaces should be decontaminated with an appropriate chemical germicide after a spill of blood or other body fluids and when work activities are completed.
7. Contaminated materials used in laboratory tests should be decontaminated before reprocessing or be placed in bags and disposed of in accordance with institutional policies for disposal of infective waste.
8. Scientific equipment that has been contaminated with blood or other body fluids should be decontaminated and cleaned before being repaired in the laboratory or transported to the manufacturer.
9. All persons should wash their hands after completing laboratory activities and should remove protective clothing before leaving the laboratory.

Implementation of universal blood and body-fluid precautions for *all* patients eliminates the need for warning labels on specimens since blood and other body fluids from all patients should be considered infective.

ENVIRONMENTAL CONSIDERATIONS FOR HIV TRANSMISSION

It should be noted that no environmentally mediated mode of HIV transmission has been documented.

Sterilization and Disinfection Standard sterilization and disinfection procedures for patient-care equipment are adequate to sterilize bloodborne pathogens including HIV. This equipment should be thoroughly cleansed before sterilization or disinfection. Contact lenses used in trial fitting should be disinfected after each fitting by using a contact lens disinfecting system or if the lens is heat resistant heat at 78-80C, 172.4-176F for ten minutes.

Housekeeping Environmental surfaces such as walls and floors are not associated with transmission of infections. Chemical germicides that are approved for use as hospital disinfectants and are tuberculocidal can be used to decontaminate spills of blood and other body fluids—gloves should be worn during cleaning and decontaminating. With large spills of cultured or concentrated infectious agents in the laboratory, the contaminated area should be flooded with a liquid germicide before cleaning, then decontaminated with fresh germicidal chemical(s)—gloves should be worn during cleaning and decontaminating.

Soiled Linen Soiled linen should be handled as little as possible and bagged at the location where it was used. It should not be sorted and rinsed in patient care areas. Linen soiled with blood or body fluids should be transported in bags that prevent leakage and washed in detergent water at least 71C (160F) for 25 minutes.

Infective Waste There is no epidemiological evidence to suggest that most hospital waste is more infectious than residential waste. Infective hospital waste should be incinerated or autoclaved before disposal in a sanitary landfill. Bulk blood, suctioned fluids, excretions, and secretions should be carefully poured down a drain that is connected to a sanitary sewer.

From Centers for Disease Control (CDC): Recommendations for prevention of HIV transmission in health care settings, MMWR 36(Suppl 2S), August 21, 1987.

REFERENCES

Beach EK: Environmental health and communicable disease module, Ann Arbor, 1974, University of Michigan, School of Nursing—Community Health Nursing.

Benenson AS: Control of communicable diseases in man, ed 15, Washington, DC, 1990, American Public Health Association.

Centers for Disease Control (CDC) Training and Laboratory Program Office: Principles of epidemiology: agent, host, environment (self-study course 3030-G, manual 1), Atlanta, Ga, 1987, CDC.

CDC Training and Laboratory Program Office: Principles of epidemiology: disease surveillance (self-study course 3030-G, manual 5), Atlanta, Ga, 1987, CDC.

CDC: Recommendations for prevention of HIV transmission in health-care settings, MMWR 36(Suppl 2S), August 21, 1987.

CDC: Universal precautions for prevention of transmission of human immunodeficiency virus, hepatitis B virus, and other bloodborne pathogens in health-care settings, MMWR 37:377-387, June 24, 1988.

CDC: Guidelines for prevention of transmission of human immunodeficiency virus and hepatitis B virus to health-care and public safety workers, MMWR 38(Suppl S6), June 23, 1989.

CDC: Publication of MMWR recommendations and reports on HIV and hepatitis B virus in health-care and public-safety workers, MMWR 38:446, 1989.

CDC: Surveillance for epidemics—United States, MMWR 38:694-696, 1989.

CDC: A strategic plan for the elimination of tuberculosis in the United States, MMWR 38(Suppl S3), April 21, 1989.

CDC: ACIP: mumps prevention, MMWR 38:388-400, 1989.

CDC: 1989 sexually transmitted diseases treatment guidelines, MMWR 38(S-8):4-40, 1989.

CDC: Personal communication, August 1990.

Collins JG: Prevalence of selected chronic conditions, United States, 1979-81 (DHHS Pub No [PHS] 86-1583), Hyattsville, Md, 1986, National Center for Health Statistics.

Commission on Chronic Illness: Chronic illness in the United States, vol 1: Prevention of chronic illness, Cambridge, Ma., 1957, Harvard University Press.

Communicable Disease Center: Food-borne disease investigation: analysis of field data, Atlanta, Ga, 1964, US Public Health Service.

Conan Doyle A: The hound of the Baskervilles, New York, 1971, Berkley.

Friedman GE: Primer of epidemiology, New York, 1974, McGraw-Hill.

Horwitz M, Pollard R, Merson M, and Martin SA: A large outbreak of foodborne salmonellosis on the Navajo Nation Indian Reservation: epidemiology and transmission, Am J Public Health 67:1071-1076, 1977.

Institute of Medicine—Committee for the Study of the Future of Public Health: The future of public health, Washington, DC, 1988, National Academy Press.

Leavell H and Clark EG: Preventive medicine for the doctor in his community: an epidemiologic approach, New York, 1965, McGraw-Hill.

MacMahon B and Pugh T: Epidemiology principles and methods, Boston, 1970, Little, Brown.

Mausner J and Bahn A: Epidemiology: an introductory text, Philadelphia, 1974, Saunders.

Mausner JS and Kramer S: Mausner and Bahn epidemiology: an introductory text, ed 2, Philadelphia, 1985, Saunders.

Maxcy RF and Rosenau MJ: Preventive medicine and public health, New York, 1965, Appleton-Century-Crofts.

Michigan Department of Public Health: Enteric infections case history, Lansing, Mi, undated, Division of Epidemiology.

Michigan Department of Public Health: Infant mortality in Michigan, Lansing, Mi, 1987, Task Force on Infant Mortality.

Michigan Department of Public Health: Minority health in Michigan: closing the gap, Lansing, Mi, 1988, The Department.

Prescott WH: History of the conquest of Mexico, New York, 1936, Random House, Inc.

Strauss A: Chronic illness and the quality of life, St Louis, 1975, CV Mosby Co.

Strauss A, Corbin J, Fagerhaugh S, Glaser BG, Maines D, Suezek B, & Weiner CL: Chronic illness and the quality of life, ed 2, St Louis, 1984, CV Mosby Co.

Surgeon General: Healthy people: the Surgeon General's report on health promotion and disease prevention, vol I and II, Washington, DC, 1979, US-DHEW.

Tennessee Department of Health and Environment: Protect them from harm, Murfreesboro, TN, 1983, Lancer.

US Bureau of the Census: Statistical abstract of the United States, ed 109, Washington, DC, 1989, US Department of Commerce.

US Department of Health and Human Services–Public Health Service: Health status of the disadvantaged, Chartbook 1986, Washington, DC, 1986, US Government Printing Office.

Vaughan G: Mummy, I don't feel well, London, 1970, Causton and Sons, Ltd.

Venereal Disease Action Coalition: Sexually transmitted diseases: a community information and resource guide, Detroit, 1983, United Community Services of Metropolitan Detroit.

Wilson JMG and Jungner F: Principles and practice of screening for disease, Public Health Papers No 34, Geneva, 1968, WHO.

Woodward SB: The story of smallpox in Massachusetts, N Engl J Med 206:1181, 1932.

SELECTED BIBLIOGRAPHY

Breslow L: Risk factor intervention for health maintenance, Science, 200:908-912, 1978.

Centers for Disease Control (CDC): Year 2000 national health objectives, MMWR 38:629-633, 1989.

CDC: First 100,000 cases of acquired immunodeficiency syndrome—United States, MMWR 38:561-563, 1989.

CDC: Mumps prevention, MMWR 38:388-400, 1989.

CDC: Common-source outbreak of giardiasis—New Mexico, MMWR 38:405-406, 1989.

CDC: Prevention and control of influenza: part I, vaccines, MMWR 38:297-312, 1989.

Christiansen EE: Family epidemiology: an approach to assessment and intervention. In Hymovich DP and Barnard MU, eds: Family health care, vol I: General perspectives, New York, 1979, McGraw Hill.

Dean AG: Population-based spot maps: an epidemiologic technique, Am J Public Health 66:988-989, 1976.

Donabedian D: Computer-taught epidemiology, Nurs Outlook 24:749-751,1976

Duncan DF: Epidemiology: basis for disease prevention and health promotion, New York, 1988, Macmillan.

Graham S: The sociological approach to epidemiology, Am J Public Health 64:1046-1049, 1974.

Greenberg BG: The future of epidemiology, J Chron Dis 36:353-359, 1983.

Haynes S and Feinleib M, eds: Second conference on the epidemiology of aging, NIH Pub No 80-969, Washington, DC, 1980, National Institutes of Health.

Richards IDG, and Baker MR: The epidemiology and prevention of important diseases, New York, 1988, Churchill Livingstone.

Tervis M: Approaches to an epidemiology of health, Am J Public Health 65:1037-1045, 1975.

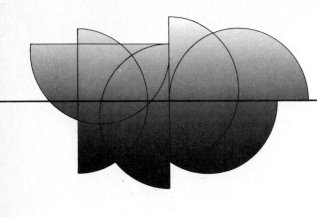

11

Community Assessment and Diagnosis for Health Planning

OBJECTIVES

Upon completion of this chapter, the reader will be able to:

1. Describe the relevance of community assessment and diagnostic activities to community health nursing practice.

2. Discuss the application of the nursing process to community-oriented practice.

3. Identify parameters for assessing a community's level of functioning.

4. Summarize methods for assessing a community's health status.

5. Explain the relevance of public health statistics to community health nursing practice.

6. Summarize federal, state, and local sources for obtaining community data.

7. Formulate guidelines for implementing community assessment and diagnostic activities in the practice setting.

Chapter 2 explored the ANA's and the APHA's definitions of community health nursing practice, which state that the dominant responsibility of nurses in community health is to the community or the population as a whole (ANA, 1986 and APHA, 1981). In order to fulfill this responsibility, community health nurses must "see," "smell," and "hear" the community and describe its people, its environment, its health status, and its health resources. Further, they must systematically analyze all facets of community dynamics (described in Chapter 3) so that populations at risk are determined and ways to meet their needs are identified.

Community health nurses at both administrative and staff levels must become involved in community assessment, diagnostic, and health planning activities in order to maintain appropriate health services for all citizens. Nursing directors and supervisors should assume leadership in establishing mechanisms for the ongoing survey of community needs and for maintaining collaborative relationships with consumers and other health care resources. They should encourage staff nurses to assess the characteristics of their work community (neighborhood, census tract, or district), so that staff understand how to effect change when resources are lacking as well as how to mobilize resources when they exist. Nursing administrators must provide an atmosphere within their agency which supports staff involvement in community activities; otherwise staff efforts will be focused on individual and family services.

Staff nurses must also take the initiative to expand their thinking to the community as a whole. When handling a family caseload and managing other professional responsibilities, such as clinic and school activities, it is easy for community health nurses to become narrow in their scope of practice. These activities are time-consuming and very important. Thus, the value of taking time to study the community in which the nurse practices and to implement community-focused activities is not always readily evident when work demands are heavy. Community-focused practice includes such elements as participation in health screening programs and epidemiological study, education of the community through the media, community advocacy, and outreach activities with disadvantaged populations (Anderson, 1983; Storfjell and Cruise, 1984).

WHY ASSESS THE COMMUNITY?

It is essential for the community health nurse to have an understanding of community dynamics, because health action occurs in the community. Every community has *patterns* of functioning or community dynamics, which either contribute to or detract from its state of health. The community health nurse must have a knowledge of these patterns in order to anticipate community responses to health action and to influence the direction of health programming. Without this knowledge, it is difficult to effect change.

Knowledge of community dynamics is obtained through systematic community assessment. Community assessment helps the nurse and other health care professionals to identify cultural differences in relation to consumer interests, strengths, concerns, and motivations. This assessment also assists health care professionals in analyzing processes through which community beliefs, values, and attitudes are transmitted. Having this information allows health professionals to individualize health planning activities for their community.

It is important for the community health nurse to recognize that the traditions in each community vary; hence, the type of programs designed to meet consumer needs should also vary. Programs appropriate for one community or for a group within a community may be ineffective in meeting the needs of other community populations. Walker (1979, pp. 667-671) substantiated this when he studied the utilization of health care ser-

The authors are indebted to A. Josephine Brown, friend and colleague, who encouraged both faculty and students to expand their thinking beyond individual client casework to the community as a whole. Through her efforts, community health nurses have learned how to use the nursing process to plan, implement, and evaluate community health programming. Content and case illustrations in this chapter reflect many of the concepts shared by her.

vices by migrant labor families in Laredo, Texas. The purpose of his study was to determine the relationship between economic barriers and the utilization of ambulatory health care services by migrant workers in Laredo. A system of prepaid health insurance was established for families enrolled in a special demonstration project. Three years of study demonstrated that even when economic barriers were removed, the migrant workers in Laredo used ambulatory health care services less often than other impoverished groups in the United States. In addition, the Laredo migrant workers showed lower usage rates than those of other migrant workers in Texas who were covered by the prepaid health insurance project. The conclusion was that further research and community assessment was needed to determine what unique characteristics of this migrant community influenced use or nonuse of health care services.

Studies such as those conducted by Walker reinforce the need to study the characteristics of the community in which one is working. They demonstrate that assumptions cannot be made about community response to health care delivery efforts, and they point out the relevance of identifying factors that facilitate or inhibit health action. Such studies also provide data that support the need for collaborative relationships between the consumer and the health care provider to enhance the delivery of health care services.

Assessment of the community is essential if the community health nurse plans to meet the needs of all populations in a given community. Experiences from one community setting cannot always be generalized to another, because health needs and resources are not consistent from one community to another. Data about a specific community are needed if the nature and origin of health problems and the responses to health matters are to be identified.

With the curtailment of federal monies for health care programs, it is even more imperative that community needs and priorities be documented. Funds are appropriated on the basis of documented evidence that a planned health program actually reflects a need within the community. Health programs will no longer be federally funded without data that support their need.

Purpose of Community Assessment for the Community Health Nurse

Within any community setting, there will be professionals from many disciplines and concerned citizens interested in community assessment, diagnostic, and health planning activities. Since it would be impossible for any one group to handle all the health care needs of a community, efforts by many should be encouraged and supported. Equally important is the need for each discipline to define its responsibilities in relation to community-focused activities so that overlapping and uncoordinated efforts will be avoided. Unfortunately, it is not uncommon to find that the linkages between various community agencies are weak and that health services are planned without the contributions that other health care professionals are making being taken into consideration (see Chapter 5). At times, cooperative efforts are not fostered because community agencies are more interested in supporting their own self-interests than in determining how consumer needs can best be met. This practice will not change until health disciplines subscribe to the belief that the community is their "client" and that interdisciplinary efforts are needed to achieve wellness for the population as a whole.

When assessing the community, community health nurses must recognize that they are members of an interdisciplinary team whose activities should not be carried out in isolation. Implicit in the concept of interdisciplinary functioning are several major premises: (1) there is a common endeavor or goal that all professionals are working toward; (2) interdisciplinary teams are established to meet client needs, thus, the client is the key member on the team; (3) professionals will share knowledge and information across disciplinary boundaries so that team goals can be reached; and (4) all disciplines will delineate and share the unique talents they have, so that the team can delegate responsibilities to appropriate team members (Kane, 1975).

The unique perspective that the community health nurse brings to an interdisciplinary community team is a holistic philosophy derived from a synthesis of nursing and public health knowledge. The community health nurse's professional experience, educational preparation, value system, and relationships with consumers provide the skills that allow her or him to integrate biopsychosocial data into a meaningful whole. Since it is known that all parameters of human functioning and all aspects of community dynamics have an impact on the client's (community) health status, the whole must be analyzed. Only when this is done will health programs truly reflect the needs of the consumer.

Prevention is often the one aspect of wholeness that is overlooked when community problems are analyzed and health services developed. This happens because many health care professionals have a curative rather than a preventive health philosophy. Because community health nurses, as well as other health department personnel, have educational preparation which enhances their ability to examine the preventive aspects of health behavior, they are delegated the major responsibility for monitoring preventive health practices in the community.

The community health nurse's primary purpose when assessing the community is to identify strengths and deficiencies in relation to preventive health practices. She or he places emphasis on examining the health care delivery system to determine if there are structural or process characteristics within this system that impede preventive health programming. In addition, the community health nurse works with consumers and other health care professionals to improve the quality of preventive health activities when deficiencies are identified.

DIAGNOSING PREVENTIVE HEALTH NEEDS IN THE COMMUNITY

When participating in community diagnostic activities, the community health nurse uses the nursing process as described in Chapter 8, but shifts emphasis from the family to the community as a whole. Data are collected from multiple sources (assessing) and analyzed in order to formulate nursing diagnoses about community health problems. Nursing diagnoses about health needs that exist, about health needs that are and are not being met, about community dynamics that either positively or negatively influence health action, and about deficiencies in the existing health care delivery system are generated for the purpose of facilitating health planning. In addition, nursing diagnoses about community strengths are made, because it is through its strengths that a community is able to resolve its health problems. Some examples of nursing diagnoses that might be made after the community health nurse has analyzed community assessment data are listed below:

- Children in census tracts 10 and 11 are at risk for lead poisoning because most homes were built before 1950, homes are poorly repaired, and housing regulations are inadequately enforced.
- Thirty-five percent of the aging persons in the community are experiencing social isolation because recreational activities and transportation for these persons are lacking.
- Teenagers are at risk for unwanted pregnancies because health care resources in the community refuse to provide birth control information for teenagers without parental consent.
- Community health nursing services need to be increased in census tract 5, because the number of new referrals from this area exceeds the time the current nurse has available for home visiting.
- Local churches within the community readily support health education efforts.
- Service clubs within the community respond very favorably when health care professionals request financial assistance for meeting unresolved health problems.

Nursing diagnoses describe the individual's, family's, or the community's health problem/condition/(strength) and the primary etiological or related factor(s) contributing to the problem/condition that is the focus of nursing treatment (Gordon, 1989, p. xiii). Community-focused nursing diagnoses are derived from a synthesis of assessment data, are based on the concept of risk relative to population groups (discussed extensively in Chapter 10), and are situations primarily resolved by nursing intervention. For example, note the above nursing diagnosis related to teenagers in the community. It is known that teenagers who find it difficult to obtain contraceptive services are at risk for unwanted pregnancies. Community health nurses are often in a key position to assist teenagers with their family planning needs through health education and program planning interventions and nursing treatment. Community health nurses are also frequently in a position to prevent or diagnose lead poisoning among children. Since many families are unaware of the dangers of this condition and its causes (etiology), community health nurses often plan health education programs designed to inform the public about lead poisoning. They also assess the environment during home visits and travel through their district to ascertain the extent of homes still having lead-painted surfaces (children at high risk for lead poisoning live in homes built before 1950 because lead was included in paint before this date).

Once nursing diagnoses are established, the community health nurse uses the principles of planning (refer to Chapter 12) to prioritize health needs, to determine alternative ways to resolve these needs, to develop specific objectives for health programming, and to identify ways to accomplish the stated objectives (planning). The following are a few examples of objectives that might be developed when planning a health program to meet the social needs of aging citizens in the community:

- The county commissioners will appropriate funds for a senior citizens project in census tract 2.
- St. Francis Catholic Church will donate space in their facilities once a week for recreational activities for the aging.
- Community volunteers will plan and implement recreational activities for the aging at St. Francis Church.
- The local chapter of the American Red Cross will provide transportation for aging citizens once a week, so that these persons can participate in the social activities planned at St. Francis Church.

The above objectives can be met in several ways. For example, the community health nurse might make all the necessary contacts personally or delegate responsibilities to others, perhaps by obtaining volunteers. Church groups, service clubs, and social workers from community agencies, for instance, often know of individuals who are interested in volunteering their time and energies for worthy community projects. Community health nurses usually seek help from others when planning a health program because they know that active participation by consumers and other professionals promotes long-term support and involvement.

Planning must result in action (implementing), and action must be evaluated; otherwise time and effort are wasted and community needs go unresolved. When one is evaluating action, it may be found that new problems emerge because insufficient data or data that are no longer valid were collected during the assessment phase (evaluating). If this is the case, objectives and intervention strategies should be altered so that they reflect ways to resolve existing needs.

Diagnosing community health problems and planning action to correct these problems are far more difficult than was just indicated. The point being made above is that the community health nurse uses the nursing process—assessing, analyzing, planning, implementing, and evaluating—when intervening into affairs of the population as a whole, as well as when working with individual families. How community health nurses assess the health status of populations and how they analyze community data is further elaborated on in this chapter. An overview of health planning is presented in Chapter 12.

METHODS FOR ASSESSING A COMMUNITY'S HEALTH STATUS

There are a variety of strategies a community health nurse can use to obtain data about community strengths and needs. Before selecting any method for data collection, the community health nurse must first define what needs to be assessed. Establishing guidelines for assessment helps the nurse to organize the data-collection process and

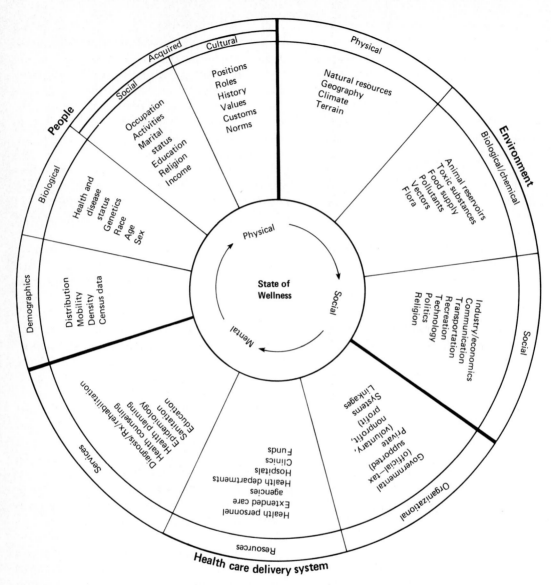

Figure 11-1 The community: its people, its environment, and its health care delivery system.

to identify significant factors that have an influence on a community's state of wellness.

Figure 11-1 summarizes the various parameters the community health nurse should examine when analyzing the health status of any community. It points out that the physical, social, and mental aspects of wellness are interrelated and that people, environmental, and health resource characteristics make an impact on a community's state of wellness. If there are changes in any one of these components, the balance of health is altered in the community setting. When diagnosing community needs, it is important to examine all components of wellness and to identify community dynamics that detract from or enhance community growth. Chapter 3 presents the knowledge needed to analyze community dynamics.

After determining the information needed to

establish appropriate nursing diagnoses about community problems, the community health nurse uses both subjective and objective data-collection methods to obtain this information. These methods are discussed below. It is important to keep in mind that no one method is sufficient for obtaining a comprehensive view of how a community is functioning. In evaluating community assessment methodology, it needs to be verified that adequate sampling and faithful description and interpretation have taken place (Ruffing-Rahal, 1985, p. 135).

Use an Assessment Tool

A systematic approach to data collection is needed in order to obtain a comprehensive profile of a community's level of functioning or competence. Use of a community assessment tool is one way to obtain information about community dynamics and health status data systematically. A community assessment tool helps community health nurses to identify assessment parameters, organize data in a meaningful manner, formulate diagnoses about community strengths and needs, and identify needed community intervention activities.

Increasingly, state and local health departments are developing community assessment tools to facilitate collection of essential community data needed for health planning. This is so because the demographics of the population are changing rapidly, significant health problems such as homelessness are emerging, and dramatic changes are occurring in the health care delivery system. A method for systematically monitoring these changes is needed. Changes in the way funding agencies support state and local health programs have also promoted the development of community assessment tools. For example, federal health block grant monies (refer to Chapter 12 for further discussion) are allocated to the states in a lump sum. States have the freedom to use these monies to support state and local health activities within the block grant functional areas of maternal child health, prevention, community health services, and alcohol, drug abuse, and mental health. Local health departments must submit a grant proposal to the state, which includes data to support a community need to obtain monies from the block grant allocations.

A community assessment tool to assist the beginning practitioner in obtaining community data very quickly was presented in Appendix 3-1. The assessment tool in Appendix 11-1 is systematically organized around the components of a community and community dynamics. This tool aids the practitioner in doing a comprehensive community assessment over an extended period of time.

Analyze Available Statistics

Many people immediately associate the term *statistics* with a long list of numbers, boring to read and difficult to use. If used effectively, however, statistical data can be exciting and intriguing. These data can quickly reveal facts about a community, including clues about why citizens do or do not become involved in health projects, as well as concrete information about the characteristics of the population being served. For example, one community health nurse was concerned because parents in one of the schools she serviced were not participating in health activities designed to promote child safety. When this nurse looked at census tract data, she found that 64 percent of the households in her district were headed by single-parent, working mothers who had a marginal income. This information suggested to the nurse that in order to reach these women she would have to plan activities outside the traditional 8 to 5 working hours. It also pointed out to her that she was dealing with families who were at risk for financial, social, and psychological crises. These data stimulated the nurse to design health programs that were relevant to mothers' as well as children's needs. One program, "How to Meet Your Social Needs While Caring for Small Children," was particularly well received. This program was planned because the nurse on several home visits heard mothers complain about the lack of time for leisure activities. The expressed concerns of these mothers, coupled with knowledge obtained from census tract data, led the nurse to believe that there were other mothers in the area who had the same concern. Her nursing diagnosis was valid and resulted in a meaningful health program that was well attended. Because this one program was so well received, an ongoing activity and discussion group for these mothers was established, with equally positive results. The processes this nurse used to develop her mother's group and to maintain it are presented in Chapter 20.

Use of statistical data can be very beneficial in community health nursing practice. The nurse in the above illustration found that statistical data provided her with clues about why families were not responding to school health activities. Statistical data also helped this nurse to identify some of the possible concerns of the population she was serving; and, thus she was able to predict health interests and plan health programs accordingly.

Statistical data often provide the basis for decision making in the face of uncertainty. The community health nurse frequently finds that there are several requests for nursing service and it is necessary to plan time to benefit the greatest number of people. Using census tract data, vital statistics, and health statistics can help community health nurses to determine where to focus their efforts. Take, for instance, the community health nurse who has several requests for the establishment of a well-baby clinic in various locations. If only one clinic can be funded, this nurse may use statistical data to document a need for a clinic in one location rather than another. The concentration of preschool children in a given area, the illness and death rates of these children, and the level of immunization protection can all be obtained from statistical data. These data provide information about where the greatest need exists and can be used to substantiate a decision a nurse might make about clinic location.

The importance of understanding and using statistical data becomes increasingly apparent to the community health nurse when decisions such as those described above must be made. Statistical data help the community health nurse to carry out many daily responsibilities more effectively. These data help the nurse to:

- Predict health needs of individuals, families, and populations
- Identify groups at risk
- Determine priorities when needs are greater than staff time available
- Evaluate the outcomes of nursing services
- Document accountability
- Support the need for increased funding for nursing services

Statistics Defined

The term *statistics* is generally used to describe two different phenomena: (1) numerical data that reveal actual counts of a given occurrence, such as the number of cases of reported hepatitis in a given community; and (2) methods or procedures developed to analyze and interpret numerical data. These methods are labeled either *descriptive* or *inferential.* The descriptive methods are emphasized in this chapter because they are used more frequently by the practitioner than are the inferential methods.

Descriptive methods involve relatively simple mathematical procedures, including such things as the construction of tables, graphs, or frequency distributions and the calculation of rates, percentages, or averages. These methods are used to organize and synthesize a mass of data. They help to describe and communicate to others such facts about a given population as age, height, weight, or causes of disease and death. *Inferential* methods are more sophisticated, mathematical tools (analysis of variance or t-tests) used by researchers and statisticians to draw generalizations from data obtained from a sample population. The term *population,* as it is used here, does not necessarily imply individuals living in the same geographic area. Rather, it means a set of individuals who have some characteristics in common. Sample populations are studied in order to make inferences about individuals who are at risk for developing health or health-related problems.

In community health, several terms are used to describe health or health-related data. These are *biostatistics, vital statistics, demographic statistics,* and *morbidity and mortality statistics. Bio-*

statistics is the overall broad term used to identify any data that delineate health or health-related events. Health statistics that describe birth, adoption, death, marriage, divorce, separation, and annulment patterns are labeled *vital statistics.* Because these events must be registered in each state, trends can be ascertained within each state and the country as a whole. Usually at least 5 years' data should be examined to see if significant patterns are occurring over time. Monitoring these significant changes helps the community health nurse to identify health promotion activities needed across the lifespan. For example, major causes of death for each developmental age group (refer to Chapters 13 through 18) are calculated from death registries each year. These death rates assist the health professional in determining key community health problems and in substantiating a need for specific health programs. The development of programs to prevent accidents and the establishment of screening clinics to identify at-risk persons for hypertension are examples of health activities that have been initiated to reduce the number of preventable deaths in the United States. Data related to the analysis of death trends are classified as *mortality statistics.*

Infant and maternal death rates or *mortality statistics* have traditionally been used in community health to make judgments about the health status of a community. Deaths in these two population groups are considered to be preventable and they are often associated with poor environmental conditions and inadequate health care. Thus, they may reflect not only unmet health needs but also deficiencies in the health care delivery system which need to be corrected.

Demographic statistics also aid the practitioner in identifying significant characteristics of a population, such as socioeconomic status, which influence the delivery of health care services in a community. Demographic data describe the number, characteristics, and distribution of people in a given area as well as changes in the population over time. These data are collected by censuses, special surveys, and registration systems (Duncan, 1988). Vital statistics are collected by

state registration systems. Special surveys are conducted by local, state, and federal government agencies, voluntary organizations, and private agencies and institutions. Special surveys are carried out to monitor current health problems, attitudes about health issues, or the health status of specific population groups. For example, on an annual basis, the University of Michigan's Institute for Social Research surveys high school seniors and young adults to determine the prevalence, trends, and attitudes about drug use in this population group.

Census data provide a wealth of information about a community's population characteristics. Census tracts and census blocks have been established and maintained throughout the country, so that social and economic changes can be easily identified from one census to another. For the 1990 census, the census tract was a key geographic statistical unit (Robey, 1989). Census tracts are small areas in large cities, having a population between 3000 to 6000, with fairly homogeneous characteristics with respect to ethnic origin and socioeconomic composition (Mausner and Kramer, 1985). Census blocks are similar to census tracts but are located almost exclusively in nonmetropolitan areas (Robey, 1989). Census tracts and census blocks boundaries are preserved from one national census to another so that variations in population characteristics can be studied over time.

The first national census was conducted in August 1790; a census has been completed every decade since, for several reasons. Census data are used to establish the number of representatives per state in the House of Representatives. These data are also used when revenue-sharing and other federal and state funds are allocated. In addition, census data assist marketing studies; academic research; federal, state, and local planning; affirmative action programs; and many other demographic and statistical activities (Robey, 1989).

Similar types of data are collected from one census to another so that trends over time can be analyzed. Some data (e.g., sex, race, age, name, address, marital status, and relationship to head of household) are collected from 100 percent of the enumerated population. More extensive information such as income, education, housing, and occupation are collected from a sample of the population (National Center for Health Statistics, 1989, p. 194). Although no census has been 100 percent accurate, extensive efforts are made to reach the greater proportion of the nation's population, including disadvantaged populations such as the homeless. It is, however, more difficult to reach the poor and alienated because they are harder to locate (Robey, 1989). In spite of this limitation, census data are extremely valuable.

Health professionals analyze census data because it has been documented that there is a significant relationship between educational background, economic status, and living conditions and the number of health needs in specified populations (USDHHS, 1986). This information can be obtained at a nominal cost from the United States Bureau of the Census, Washington, D.C.

In addition to vital and demographic statistics, the community health nurse uses morbidity statistics to assess the health status of the community. *Morbidity data* describe the extent and distribution of illness in a community. These data assist the nurse in identifying specific health problems and in setting priorities for program planning. One midwestern community, for example, used morbidity statistics to support the need for a neighborhood health clinic in one of their inner-city districts. A comprehensive analysis of these statistics revealed that 52 percent of all new tuberculosis cases, 61 percent of all new syphilis cases, 72 percent of all new gonorrhea cases, and 37 percent of all accidental poisoning cases occurred in one particular section of the city in a given time period. It was evident from this information that the health needs in this district were much greater than in other sections of the city. Special funds were allocated to determine if a new approach to delivering health services could alter the disease trends in this area; significant positive changes were noted within a 3-year time frame. Because morbidity statistics were collected before and during the time the clinic was in existence, state legislators responded favorably to a request

for additional funds to keep the clinic open. Health professionals in this situation had documented the need for and the effectiveness of their pilot health clinic. The use of statistics helped these health professionals to establish a neighborhood health center, as well as to keep the center functioning after the trial period.

How to Use Statistical Data*

Usually community health professionals express absolute numbers or actual counts in terms of relative numbers. This is done because relative numbers make it easier to compare results in populations of differing sizes or to visualize what proportion of a given population is affected by a given phenomenon. A *relative number* is one which shows a relationship between two absolute numbers; this relationship is expressed in terms of a round number. A *percentage* is an example of a relative number; 100 is the round number used to show relationships when percentages are calculated.

The value of using relative numbers becomes clearer when the nurse actually works with raw data. For example, stating that 45 teenagers in a mental health institution need foster home placement has very little meaning until this number is related to the total number of teenagers in the institution. If there are only 100 teenagers in this setting, then 45 is a significant proportion (45 percent) of this given population. If, on the other hand, there are 1000 teenagers in this environment, 45 is a relatively small proportion (4.5 percent) of the total population. The percentages are identified by relating 45 (absolute number) to 100 or 1000 (absolute numbers) and then multiplying the results by 100 (round number).

Raw data from populations of differing sizes cannot be compared unless absolute numbers are converted to relative numbers. For instance, knowing the number of students who received free lunches in 1990 in each school in the county becomes relevant only when one summarizes the

*Handout materials distributed by the community health nursing faculty at Michigan State University, East Lansing, Michigan, provided the framework for this section.

percentage of children in each school who received free lunches. The following figures illustrate how deceptive absolute numbers can be when making comparisons from one population to another; even though the number of children (250 vs. 75) receiving free lunches is much higher in the Burns Park High School, the proportion of children needing free lunches in Kent Elementary School is two times greater than the proportion of children needing free lunches in Burns Park High School:

$$\frac{75}{150} \times 100 = 50\% \text{ of the children in Kent Elementary School received free lunches in 1990}$$

$$\frac{250}{1000} \times 100 = 25\% \text{ of the children in Burns Park High School received free lunches in 1990}$$

Besides percentages, two other relative numbers—ratios and rates—are commonly used to analyze health or health-related events. A *ratio* expresses the size of one number in relation to the size of another number. The number of females to males (sex ratio), and per capita expenditure for health care in a given state are examples of ratios. Per capita ratios are obtained by dividing the amount of money spent for health care (event) by the population in a given state (population).

A *rate* is actually a ratio but with the additional features of expressing what has happened in terms of a certain unit of *time* and the *population at risk* for a given event. It delineates the relationship between the number of times an event has occurred to the size of the population at risk. *In demographic study, the unit of time for a rate is usually a year unless otherwise stated.*

The formula for a rate is given as follows:

$$\frac{\text{Event in a given time}}{\text{Pop. at risk in same time period}} \times \text{Round no.}$$

The *event* in this formula is the number of times a phenomenon (births, deaths, or disease) has occurred. The *population* is usually the number of persons at risk for a given event. The round

number is one which makes the rate above the value of 1. If, for instance, an event such as polio occurs infrequently within a large population at risk, the round number used would be 100,000. On the other hand, when an event such as death occurs frequently within a population at risk, the round number used would be 1000.

Following are examples of how to apply the rate formula. Note particularly the population at risk, which varies depending on the nature of the event. When morbidity rates (incidence and prevalence) are calculated, the total population of the community may be at risk. In determining infant mortality rates, only infants born within a certain time period are at risk.

Incidence rate. This is the number of *new* cases of a disease in a population over a period of time.

Incidence rate = number of "new" cases of a specified disease or condition occurring during a given time period (as during a year) ÷ population at risk during a given time period × 100,000

Bay City, January through December 1990, 50 new cases of diabetes in a population of 75,000.

$$\text{Incidence rate} = \frac{50}{75,000} \times 100,000 = 66.66$$

Incidence rate for diabetes in Bay City 1990: 66.66 new cases of diabetes per 100,000 population.

Prevalence rate. This is the number of *old* and *new* cases of a specified disease existing at a given time.

Prevalence rate = number of "old" and "new" cases of a specified disease or condition existing at a "point" in time ÷ total population at a point in time × 100,000

Bay City, December 1990, 1200 cases of diabetes in a population of 75,000.

$$\text{Prevalence rate} = \frac{1200}{75,000} \times 100,000 = 1600$$

Prevalence rate for diabetes in Bay City, December 1990: 1600 cases of diabetes per 100,000 population.

TABLE 11-1 Formulas for rates and ratios frequently calculated in community health nursing practice

Rate or ratio	Formula	Commonly used round number
Mortality statistics		
Crude death rate	Number of deaths from all causes during a given year ÷ population estimated at midyear	× 1000 population
Age-specific death rate	Number of deaths for a specified age group during a given year ÷ population estimated at midyear for the specified age group	× 1000 population
Cause specific death rate	Number of deaths from a specific condition during a given year ÷ population estimated at midyear	× 100,000 population
Maternal mortality rate	Number of deaths from puerperal complications during a given year ÷ number of live births during the same year	× 100,000 live births
Infant mortality rate	Number of deaths under 1 year of age during a given year ÷ number of live births during the same year	× 1000 live births
Neonatal mortality rate	Number of deaths under 28 days of age during a given year ÷ number of live births during the same year	× 1000 live births
Fetal mortality rate	Number of fetal deaths 20 weeks gestation or more during a given year ÷ number of live births and fetal deaths during the same year	× 1000 live births and fetal deaths
Birth-death ratio	Number of live births in a specified population ÷ number of deaths in a specified population	× 100
Case fatality ratio	Number of deaths from specified disease or condition ÷ number of reported cases of the specified disease or condition	× 100
Morbidity statistics		
Incidence rate	Number of "new" cases of a specified disease or condition occurring during a given time period ÷ population at risk during the same time period	× 100,000 population
Prevalence rate	Number of "old" and "new" cases of specified disease or condition existing at a "point" in time ÷ total population at a point in time	× 100,000 population
Vital and demographic statistics other than mortality		
Crude birth rate	Number of live births during a given year ÷ population estimated at midyear	× 1000 population
General fertility rate	Number of live births during a given year ÷ population estimated at midyear for females ages 15-44 during the same year	× 1000 female population (15-44 years old)
General marriage rate	Number of marriages during a given year ÷ number of persons 15 years of age and over in the population in the same year	× 1000 persons 15 years of age and over
General divorce rate	Number of divorces during a given year ÷ persons 15 years of age and over in the population in the same year	× 1000 persons 15 years of age and over
Dependency ratio	Persons under 20 years of age and persons 65 years and over ÷ total population ages 20-64	× 100

Infant mortality rate. This is the number of deaths of infants under 1 year of age per 1000 live births during a given year.

Infant mortality rate = number of deaths under 1 year of age during a given year ÷ number of live births during a given year × 1000 live births

Bay City, 1990: 25 infant deaths.

Infant mortality rate $= \dfrac{25}{1275} \times 1000 = 19.6$

Infant mortality rate Bay City 1990: 19.6 infant deaths per 1000 live births.

Frequently Calculated Rates and Ratios

In addition to the above examples, there are several other rates and ratios that are used to measure the state of health in a community. The formulas for calculating rates and ratios frequently used in community health nursing practices are presented in Table 11-1. Besides helping to identify the major health problems in a community, these statistics aid in projecting future health service and personnel needs. For example, examining the crude birth rate assists health care professionals in determining the demand for childhood health services over the next 20 years.

Rates, ratios, or percentages are the types of descriptive statistics most commonly used in community health nursing practice. At times, however, there is a need to use other descriptive measures, such as averages, in order to organize and characterize data. This is so when a series of measurements or quantitative data is being analyzed. Generally, in any series of data, characteristic values tend to cluster near the center of the distribution. Thus, averages are often labeled measures of central tendency.

Measures of Central Tendency

Averages help to identify a value which is most characteristic of a set of raw data. There are several kinds of averages used to summarize quantitative measurements; the most frequently used ones in community health nursing practice are the arithmetic mean, the median, and the mode.

The *mean* is the arithmetic average of a set of observations. It is the value in a series of data equivalent to the sum of the measurements divided by the number of measurements. The formula for calculating the mean is:

$$\text{Arithmetic mean} = \frac{\text{sum of measurements}}{\text{no. of measurements}}$$

A community health nurse who wanted to determine the average weight of children in a second-grade classroom would compute the average or mean as follows:

Weight of children in pounds: 51.2, 53.1, 55, 54, 53, 47.5, 48.8, 52.9, 50.5, 51.5, 53, 49.5, 53, 55.1, 49.9

Sum of measurement = 778.3 or 778
Number of measurements = 15
Mean weight = 51.9
Arithmetic mean $= \dfrac{778}{15} = 51.86$ or 51.9

Knowing the mean or "average" value of a series of measurements helps the community health nurse to identify quickly persons who may have health needs or who are at risk for health problems in the future. Persons who fall far below or far above the average should be comprehensively assessed to determine why this is happening.

The *median* is the "middle" value in a series of quantitative data which divides the measurements into two equal parts. That is, 50 percent of the measurements are less than and 50 percent are greater than the median value. To calculate the median, the measurements in the distribution must be arranged in order of size. Referring again to the children in the second-grade classroom, the median weight of these children would be determined by putting all of their weights in numerical order so that the middle value can be identified. This is illustrated below:

47.5, 48.8, 49.5, 49.9, 50.5, 51.2, 51.5, **52.9** 53, 53, 53 (mode), 53.1, 54, 55, 55.1 (median)

The median is *52.9,* or the eighth measurement, because 50 percent of the measurements are less than this value and 50 percent are greater than this value. If there had been an even number of measurements, the median would be found by dividing the sum of the two middle measurements by two, which is illustrated below.

48.8, 49.5, 49.9, 50.5, 51.2, 51.5, **52.9, 53**, 53, 53, 53.1, 54, 55, 55.1

Middle measurements = (52.9 + 53.0) ÷ 2 = 52.95 (median)

The median is usually computed when there are very high or very low extremes in a series of measurements because the mean is distorted by very high or low values but the median is not. When census tract data are reported, for instance, median income is usually given because there is such a great variation in family income, ranging from below poverty level to over $50,000. Generally, however, the mean is the most frequently used measure of central tendency in community health practice because it takes into account all measurements in a series and is the most stable.

The *mode* is the measurement that appears most frequently in a series of quantitative data. It is identified by counting the number of times a particular value appears. The measurements do not have to be ordered. Fifty-three points is the mode or typical value of the weights of our second-grade classroom children because it occurred more frequently than any other weight. The mode is helpful when one wants to identify an average value very quickly. It is only an estimate, however, and not too reliable; other measurements of central tendencies should be used when refining data analysis.

Relative numbers, including rates, ratios, percentages, and measures of central tendency are computed so that comparisons between sets of absolute numbers can be made. When a series of relative numbers is being studied, it is helpful to present the data graphically.

Graphic Presentation of Data

Graphic presentation of data is an efficient way to show large numbers of observations at one time.

TABLE 11-2 Demographic and clinical distribution of pediatric AIDS patients <13 years as of February 1, 1988: United States and Michigan

| | *Horizontal axes* | |
Characteristic	*United States* *(N = 789)*	*Michigan* *(N = 10)*
Vertical axes:		
Age		
<5 years	86%	80%
>5 years	14%	20%
Race		
Black	54%	80%
Hispanic	23%	0
White	22%	20%
Etiologic risk factors		
Parent with AIDS virus or in high risk category	76%	80%
Blood transfusion	14%	0
Coagulation disorders	5%	20%
Not known	4%	0
Clinical diagnosis		
Pneumocystis carinii pneumonia	52%	30%
Other opportunistic infection	47%	70%
Kaposi's sarcoma	1%	0

From Maternal and Infant Task Force on AIDS: Perinatal AIDS in Michigan, Lansing, Mi, 1988, Michigan Department of Public Health, p 3.

Numerical figures are more easily remembered when presented graphically because data are organized and relationships are demonstrated. Tables, graphs, and charts are some of the instruments used to present statistical information symbolically. Guidelines for presenting data in this form include the following:

- Illustrate only the amount of data which are appealing to the sight.
- Number a table, graph, or chart if more than one is used (Table 11-1 or Table 11-2).
- Title each table, graph, or chart, including in the title information identifying *what, where,* and *when.*

- Label both the horizontal and vertical axes of the graphic presentation.
- Identify the source of the data at the bottom of the chart, including author, title of publication, publisher, date of publication, and reference page number.

When these guidelines are used, a table would look like the example that is presented in Table 11-2.

Graphic presentation of data has popular appeal and is frequently used to portray quickly a large number of facts. Graphs, charts, and tables can be misused or misunderstood, however, especially if one attempts to relate data that are unrelated. Also, attempting to present too many facts in one table defeats the purpose for using visual presentations of data; when this is done, it confuses rather than clarifies the events being illustrated.

Available data on a community should be used in the most effective way possible to get across the significance of a community's health problems. These data should not, however, be misrepresented on tables, graphs, and charts. If available data are not sufficient to reach decisions about a community's state of health, do not try to make them be so by graphically presenting incomplete or inaccurate findings. Rather, use other methods to collect the data needed to analyze what is happening in the community.

Carry out Surveys

Surveys are commonly conducted in community health nursing practice because existing data from census, vital statistics, and morbidity records are inadequate to substantiate a need for the development of a particular health program. Standard sources of data, such as those mentioned above, may show that suicide is one of the leading causes of death for older adolescents. This information is significant in that it focuses attention on a major health problem of this developmental age group. It is not sufficient, however, to identify health action needed in a particular community for reducing adolescent mortality as a result of suicide. Other types of information must be collected before a health project is initiated in a local community. Data about such things as the use of available mental health resources by teenagers, attitudes of professionals and consumers in relation to the needs of the adolescent, and reasons for teenage suicidal actions must be ascertained before health planning can be effective. A survey is frequently conducted to obtain this type of information.

A community survey is a systematic study designed to collect data about a community's functioning. Data about a specific segment of the population, about a particular component of the health care delivery system, or about health needs of the entire community may be collected when conducting a survey. The scope varies depending on the purpose and the financial and work force resources available. It is important to define specifically the reason for doing a survey because this process can be costly and time consuming. On the other hand, this process can provide essential data for health programming and may save time and monies if it is planned carefully (refer to Figure 11-2).

Sometimes health care professionals become enthusiastic and attempt to speed up the survey process by decreasing planning time. This practice is not wise because planning can actually decrease the time it takes to effectively implement a survey. For example, conducting a pilot study or a small-scale survey during the planning phase can help to eliminate major problems in the survey process before an extensive study is initiated. This, in turn, could significantly reduce the amount of time that is needed to obtain appropriate data.

There are a variety of ways in which a community can survey its needs. Personal interviews, telephone interviews, or written questionnaires are a few examples of the methods that can be used to collect data about community health problems and strengths. It is important to select carefully survey methods and tools because resources and needs vary from one community to another. Reviewing the literature about what other professionals are discovering in their work is useful.

Siemiatycki (1979, p. 238), examined the cost and quality of data collection when utilizing three

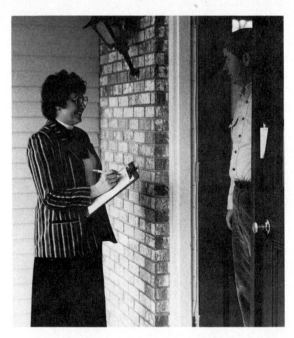

Figure 11-2 House-to-house surveys assist health care professionals in obtaining a comprehensive understanding of their local communities. A *well-planned* survey can provide data about such things as resource utilization patterns, social concerns, and specific health needs of a particular community. The public health professional pictured was a member of an epidemiological team which was conducting a city-wide family health study. Higher-than-average infant deaths prompted the local health department to initiate this study. The results of the survey helped the health department to focus its maternal-child health (MCH) efforts. Ten years after the survey was completed, this local community no longer qualified for special state MCH funds, because of its low-infant mortality rate. (Courtesy of photographer, Henry Parks.)

different survey strategies: mail, telephone, and home interview. It was found "that telephone and mail strategies with intensive follow-up achieved response rates comparable to those achieved by the home interview strategy and for between 45 and 56 percent of the cost." It was also discovered in this study that home interviews did not improve the quality of data collected. In fact, respondents answered questions about sensitive topics more readily by mail than during a home interview (Siemiatycki, 1979, pp. 243-244).

Aneshensel, Fredrichs, Clark, and Yokopenic (1982, pp. 1018, 1020) also found that telephone interviews appear to be an acceptable, low-cost method for conducting community health surveys. However, in their study, they did note that disability days were more likely reported during in-person interviews than during telephone interviews.

Studies like the one conducted by Siemiatycki

and Aneshensel and colleagues can provide data that help a community to make a more knowledgeable decision about fact-finding methods. They support the value of investigating the literature before initiating a costly project to determine community needs. If a community can obtain information at less cost and still preserve the quality of data that are collected, considering the use of the less costly method is warranted. If time is not taken to review what others have done, a less costly method may never be considered. It must be remembered, though, that research studies do not provide all of the answers for a particular community. A more costly method might be selected if that is the only way to obtain certain types of data. Home interviews should be used, for instance, if environmental conditions need to be observed or if obtaining data about disability days is of high priority.

Surveys should be used to obtain data that are

not available from other sources. Generally, accurate data can be obtained about vital events (births, deaths, or marriages), but morbidity data are often incomplete. Disease rates and data about health-related phenomena (alcoholism, mental disorders, child abuse) are usually only estimates, because of the lack of adequate reporting. It is frequently unknown how many individuals are affected by these conditions or how many who are affected are receiving adequate care. Surveys may be able to elicit such data. In addition, a survey can help to determine comprehensive needs of a particular segment of a population. Census information provides data about a census tract in relation to income, housing, education, and transportation. It does not provide data about specific health problems, social needs, or health care resources.

Data obtained from a survey provide the foundation for more extensive investigation of health needs in a community. Research is frequently conducted after surveys are completed to explore the potential cause-and-effect relationships between differing community phenomena. Surveys do not provide sufficient evidence to substantiate cause-and-effect conclusions because generally there are very few controls built into a survey design (Polit and Hungler, 1987).

Conduct Research

Research to document the effectiveness of nursing services and to identify cause-and-effect relationships is critically needed in the community health nursing setting. Funders of health care services are demanding concrete data that support the need for nursing personnel, the need for certain health programs, and the value of using one intervention strategy rather than another. If qualitative data are not available, funders evaluate effectiveness only on the basis of quantitative counts, such as the numbers of home, school, or clinic visits. When this happens, the quality of nursing care can suffer.

Research can help the health care professional to document effectiveness of quality, as well as to identify community needs and to propose intervention strategies that best meet these needs. Illustrative of this is the study conducted by Skinner, German, Shapiro, Chase, and Zauber (1978, pp. 1195, 1201), which demonstrated that the near-poor population—those families who did not qualify for Medicaid benefits but who had inadequate financial resources to meet health care costs—were a special population at risk within a community. This study showed that the near-poor in East Baltimore were using fewer health care services than were Medicaid recipients. When financial barriers were removed by enrolling the East Baltimore near-poor in a prepaid health plan, this difference in use was minimized.

Time must be provided so that practitioners can investigate clinical practice issues and concerns. It is only in this way that a profession can remain viable. Collaborative relationships established between service settings and academic environments can facilitate practitioners' involvement in research. Research can be stimulating and challenging to practitioners, especially if they have support and encouragement from individuals who are involved in clinical research on a regular basis.

Lindeman (1975, p. 697) conducted a nationwide survey among nurses to determine priorities for clinical nursing research. Among the top 15 priorities identified were items related to the improved use of the nursing process, evaluation of quality care, and the role of nursing in the provision of preventive health services. These priorities reflect concerns experienced daily by the community health nurse.

In 1981, the ANA also examined priorities for nursing research and reaffirmed the need to focus attention on preventive health services as well as nursing care needs of vulnerable groups and the population as a whole (ANA, 1981). Currently, the National Center for Nursing Research (NCNR) supports research in three categories: health promotion/disease prevention, acute and chronic illness, and nursing systems. NCNR is collaborating with the National Advisory Council on Nursing Research and the nursing scientific community to develop priority areas under these categories. Priority areas under consideration are 1) low birthweight—mothers and infants; 2) HIV infection—prevention and care; 3) long-term care for the elderly; 4) symptom management; 5) information systems; 6) health promotion; and 7) technology dependency across the lifespan (Office of Information and Legislative Affairs, NCNR, 1989, p. 1).

It is clear that a major thrust in nursing research, on the national level, is aimed at community-based practice (refer to Chapter 23).

Contact Consumers and Community Leaders

Research and surveys tend to focus on the present. Since a community's current characteristics are an outgrowth of its historical development, it is beneficial to interview consumers and community leaders to identify what has gone on in the past and how the past is affecting the present. The values, attitudes, and interests of previous community leaders often subtly influence the current direction of health planning. Contact with key community persons or *informants* can help community health nurses to understand why there is resistance to certain health programs, how to reduce resistance to change, and whom nurses might work with to enhance their productivity in the community setting.

Directors of housing projects, clergy, professionals in other health care agencies, local politicians, owners of long-established businesses, and unofficial community spokespersons are some of the individuals a nurse might contact to obtain information about community dynamics. These individuals can help the nurse to gain knowledge about the power relationships within a local area, community values and attitudes, and environmental factors which enhance or detract from a community's state of health. Unofficial spokespersons often provide the most candid opinion of how the consumer views health and the health care delivery system. Clergy, agency clients, and cultural organizations, such as International Neighbors or the Polish club, can frequently assist a community health nurse in identifying these spokespersons.

A community health nurse should use every opportunity available to relate to community people outside and within the agency. The oppor-

tunities are limitless and require only motivation on the part of the nurse and supervisory support to take advantage of them. A visit to the local library can provide very valuable information about a community's history. On the other hand, talking with people the nurse meets while carrying out regular caseload responsibilities can be just as valuable. Spontaneous interchange often provides an atmosphere for free, honest communication. This type of dialogue also helps to create a positive image in relation to what health care professionals are doing to improve the health of people. The ability to relate to others in the community, such as school principals, physicians, administrators in mental health agencies, secretaries, and clergy, is essential if one wants to diagnose community needs accurately.

Observe, Listen, and Analyze

Data about a community can be obtained daily by observing, listening, and analyzing. What the environment looks like when the nurse drives in the district, how families are dressed when they are seen in the clinic setting, and who relates to whom during community meetings all provide the community health nurse with clues about a community's state of health. Community health nurses who are really interested in the welfare of their community will take time to analyze what has been observed and heard. They will be alert to environmental conditions that adversely affect the state of a community's health. If, when driving through the district, a nurse finds older homes in poor repair, he or she can raise questions about the potential for lead poisoning and the need for enforcement of housing legislation. An astute nurse will not ignore observations or accept them as a matter of fact without trying to effect change.

Analysis of community observations must focus on strengths as well as needs, because it is through a community's strengths that health problems are resolved. One community health nurse, for example, was able to effect environmental changes in her district because she had identified that the parents in the area were genuinely concerned about the welfare of their children. Rat-infested vacant lots in the neighborhood presented a serious threat to the children who played in them. This nurse, with the assistance of a minister, was able to mobilize parents' energies so that the garbage from these lots was removed and rats were killed. Maintaining the lots as suitable play areas became a major community project.

A community health nurse who views the community as the unit of service is more likely to meet the needs of individual families than the nurse who focuses only on family health care needs. Family problems are interrelated with community problems and often cannot be resolved until changes occur within the community system. A nurse needs to collect data on the community in order to determine the extent to which family health problems are influenced by community values, attitudes, and beliefs. Frequently, families from differing ethnic backgrounds are labeled "social" problems because they do not relate to social systems as do middle-class Americans. When this is the case, change will not occur if the community health nurse works only with individual families. In these situations, the community health nurse needs to help social systems gain an appreciation of different cultural values and attitudes and must help families learn how to interact with social systems unfamiliar to them.

SOURCES OF COMMUNITY DATA

There are numerous federal, state, and local agencies and individuals that a community health nurse can contact in order to obtain data about the community. Some have been mentioned previously in this chapter and are summarized here to give a composite picture of the multiple sources of data one can use when diagnosing community needs.

The only federal agency specifically established for the collection and dissemination of health data is the National Center for Health Statistics. This agency conducts the National Health Survey, which provides valuable information on the health and illness status of U.S. residents (refer to Chapter 10). In addition, this agency provides official information on vital statistics and data about the supply and use of health resources (Office of the Federal Register, 1988).

Several other federal agencies will supply health data on request. The Alcohol, Drug Abuse, and Mental Health Administration, the Health Resources and Services Administration, and the Centers for Disease Control are a few examples of such agencies. Appendix 11-2 presents selected sources of data on the health of the U.S. population, the availability and use of health sources, and health care expenditures. The *United States Government Manual,* which can be purchased from the Superintendent of Documents, U.S. Government Printing Office, Washington, D.C., is a valuable reference for identifying other government agencies that disseminate health data. This manual describes the purposes and programs of most federal agencies.

The importance of obtaining data from the Bureau of the Census on the size, distribution, structure, and change of populations in the United States cannot be overemphasized. These data demonstrate patterns over time and provide general characteristics of a community's total population. Knowing that there is a high concentration of individuals 65 years and over, or of children ages 1 through 5 in a community, assists health care professionals in predicting the types of health problems and health care services needed in a particular community. For example, a community health nurse who knows from census tract data that 30 percent of the people in his or her census tract are 65 years or older should become concerned if limited or no geriatric families are in the caseload and then investigate why referrals for this age group are not being received.

In addition to helping individual staff nurses, census tract data help nursing administrators to determine where nursing services are most needed. Knowledge about the concentration of people, the economic status, and housing conditions in an area assists administrators in predicting populations at risk in segments of their community. Often, state health departments will help local health departments to use census tract data to identify at-risk groups. State health departments have statistical divisions that provide consultation in relation to data collection and analysis.

State health departments are a major source of data for identifying the health status of citizens in a particular state. Vital statistics, morbidity data, health work force, and resource information are usually collected and disseminated by this agency. The department of education, the bureau of mental health, and the office of services to the aging are some other state agencies that supply health and health-related information. Obtaining a state directory of social agencies will help each reader to determine which agencies in her or his state furnish information about specific health needs in local communities. The number of state agencies that supply health and health-related data are too numerous to list here.

On the local level, some key sources for obtaining community data are the chamber of commerce, city planner's office, health department, county extension office, intermediate school districts, libraries, health and welfare professionals, hospital records, clergy, community leaders, and consumers. Again, sources are too numerous for all of them to be listed here. Most cities and counties have social services directories which provide information on the major health and welfare resources in their community. Experienced practitioners can also help new community health nurses to identify the most appropriate source for obtaining specific data about the area in which they are functioning.

Legislators and public officials on all three levels of government are usually more than willing to assist the health care professional in analyzing social and health care legislation. Laws and ordinances related to community health reflect the values and priorities of a community, the state, and the federal government. Every health care professional should be familiar with legislation that influences the health of his or her community. Specific laws and ordinances are discussed throughout this text. Here it is sufficient to emphasize the importance of studying legislative trends in order to gain an understanding of a community's priorities in relation to health care issues.

ANALYSIS OF ALL AVAILABLE DATA

Data should not be collected merely for the sake of having data. Unfortunately, this is often the case. Daily activity reports, vital statistics, and census data are frequently collected, but just as frequently filed in a drawer without being used. This benefits no one. Once community data are assembled, they should be organized in a meaningful way so that patterns of functioning and trends can be ascertained. Many techniques can be used to synthesize community data. Charts, figures, and tables are often used for this purpose. Graphic presentation of such things as population distributions, morbidity data, or vital statistics for several decades can be very effective in pinpointing significant community problems. Growth or lack of growth in a community, for instance, can be identified when population distributions are graphically visualized. Lack of growth in a community can be a very serious problem, because many federal and state health funds are allocated on a per capita basis, that is, a given amount of money is allocated for each person residing in the area.

Mapping is another technique that facilitates data analysis. Dotted scatter maps can be used to determine at a glance such things as high-risk populations, poor environmental conditions, the distribution of illness, disease, and health, and the accessibility of health care services. When this technique is used, school districts or political jurisdictions are usually outlined on a county map. Point symbols or spots are then distributed within these divisions as specified events happen (disease, death, health-related phenomena, or condemned housing), at the exact locations where the events occurred. Figure 11-3, Reported Cases of Hepatitis in Howard County, illustrates the mapping technique. The clustering of hepatitis cases in census tracts 12, 13, and 9 was related to an outbreak of hepatitis that occurred in a trailer camp in census tract 12. Relatives and friends from census tracts 9 and 13 had contact with family and friends in census tract 12 while they were in a communicable state. An epidemiological investigation provided evidence which supported that a

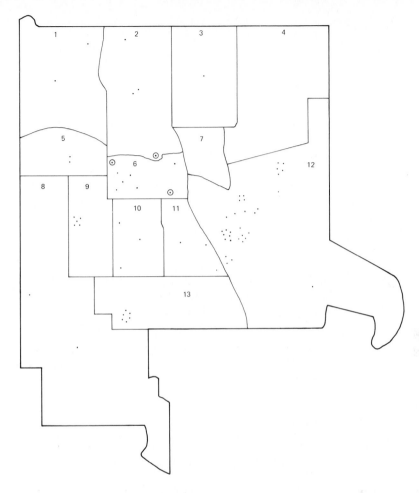

Figure 11-3 The mapping technique: reported cases of hepatitis in Howard County, January through June 1990. ● = cases of hepatitis; ⊙ = drug suppliers; 1-13 = census tracts.

major outbreak of hepatitis had occurred in a very short time period. The clustering of hepatitis cases in census tract 6 was a result of drug problems.

Dotted scatter maps can be very impressive and useful, but they can also be misleading if the population base is not analyzed. A geographic area may have far fewer cases than another because there are far fewer people in that area. Calculating rates, ratios, and percentages aids in making comparisons between census tracts. These descriptive statistics also help to compare the occurrence of significant events with other communities and with state and national rates.

Comparing community rates with state and national rates is very beneficial. It can highlight specific health problems as well as community strengths. It helps a community to determine priorities for program planning. If a community's infant and maternal mortality rates, for instance, are much higher than state and national rates, a community would want to examine carefully its maternal-child health programming. On the other hand, a community may find, when making these comparisons, that its maternal-child health statistics are far superior to those of other areas. This, in turn, could demonstrate to the community the value of maintaining adequate health programs for these two age groups in the population.

Analysis of data often supports the need for further data collection. This is illustrated in the following case situation:

In one census tract of a large urban area, the health department became aware of a maternal infant health problem. This census tract was a residential rental area with basement efficiency apartments renting for $240.00 or higher per month. The population was 75 percent students and young working people, referred to as the "swinging singles." Of the remaining 25 percent, 20 percent were elderly first-generation Jewish merchants, and 5 percent were young black families living in the city housing project. The area had a high reported incidence of mugging, purse snatching, and apartment thefts, with rumors of drug manufacturing, pushing, and usage.

Few referrals were made to the health agencies in the area; case finding was negligible; records of nursing services showed few home visits to individuals in this district. The explanation given for this situation was that the majority of the population in this census tract was either at school or working and, therefore, inaccessible to agency personnel during the working day. Evening office hours were scheduled by private physicians as well as by several health clinics in the area. The health department became particularly concerned about the lack of referrals from this census tract when they analyzed the infant and maternal death rates for the entire county. It was discovered that only in this census tract did these rates significantly vary from national statistics.

Infant and maternal mortality rates for the specified census tract were:

23.4 infant deaths per 1000 live births
7.2 maternal deaths per 1000 live births

Infant and maternal mortality rates in the United States during the same time period were:

12.1 infant deaths per 1000 live births
3.1 maternal deaths per 1000 live births

It was obvious from the vital statistics that something had to be done to improve the health status of mothers and children in this area. However, more specific data were needed to determine causes of death, health status of area residents, and use of health care services, as well as related health problems, including socioeconomic difficulties, drug use, and attitudes about the "establishment." Personnel from a drug clinic and the student organization at a local college assisted the health department in collecting the data they

needed. Lack of transportation, extremely limited incomes, lack of knowledge, inadequate nutrition, and resistance to normal channels of health care were some of the major problems identified. The establishment of a neighborhood health clinic, staffed mostly by college students and area residents, produced positive results. Data analysis at the end of 3 years reflected a significant decrease in both the infant and maternal mortality rates for this area.

The above situation dramatically illustrates the importance of analyzing data once they are compiled. Community diagnostic activities are carried out so that appropriate decisions about health planning can be made. If data are not analyzed, health action probably will not occur.

PRACTICAL TIPS FOR IMPLEMENTING COMMUNITY ASSESSMENT AND DIAGNOSTIC ACTIVITIES

Community assessment and diagnostic activities are exciting and challenging. It should be apparent, however, that they cannot be left to chance. If these activities are to be implemented effectively, time for planning, assessing, and analyzing must be set aside and administrative support must be available. Equally important is the need to always keep the framework of the "community" in clear perspective when providing nursing care. Community dynamics that adversely affect the health status of individuals, families, and populations at risk should not be ignored. Nursing intervention strategies should be planned to resolve community problems as well as to resolve needs of individual clients.

New practitioners often experience feelings of frustration and disillusionment when first entering the practice setting because there are tremendous gaps between reality and the ideal. Presented below are suggestions for bridging some of these gaps in relation to community organizational activities.

Do Preliminary Community Assessment during Orientation Period

It is only natural for newly employed nurses to want immediate involvement in client casework.

Reading policy and procedure manuals and attending orientation meetings can be tiring and less than rewarding. It is important, however, to remind oneself that orientation periods are designed to facilitate functioning in all aspects of one's job responsibilities. Do not overplan family visits during this time period. Rather, balance family and community activities so that time is available to learn about community dynamics and population characteristics. Allowing time in your schedule to engage in the following activities during the orientation period will help you to function more effectively in the community health setting.

- Analyze census tract and vital statistics data to learn about population characteristics in your district.
- Attend case conferences and community meetings (PTA, social service council, citizen group activities) with an experienced employee.
- Attend a board of health meeting to identify the values and attitudes of those responsible for policy making in the health department.
- Drive through your district, observing environmental conditions, interactions between people, and the location of health care and welfare resources, recreational facilities, local churches, school systems, and shopping areas.
- Shop in your district to determine cost of essentials, such as food and clothing.
- Make field visits with personnel from other departments in your agency (environmental health, mental health, or nutrition).
- Observe in clinic settings (well-baby, STD, adult screening, or prenatal).
- *Ask questions.*

Most agencies allow new employees to help design their own orientation. The above activities should be planned for, even if similar experiences were available during one's course of study in the academic environment. In the educational setting, these types of experiences are planned so that students have the opportunity to apply theoretical concepts in the practice setting. Educational experiences cannot, however, provide the practitioner with the specific information needed to understand the unique characteristics of the population being served.

Discuss Community Problems during Supervisory Conferences

In community health nursing practice, the practitioner is frequently unable to meet client needs because of deficiencies in the health and welfare systems. There may also be insufficient time to work comprehensively with all the families referred to the nurse. These difficulties should be discussed with the nursing supervisor because the supervisor is in a favorable position for initiating major change in community systems. In addition, the supervisor can provide support and assistance in relation to caseload management activities as well as give suggestions about innovative intervention strategies for dealing with community problems. For example, it is not uncommon for the nursing supervisor to help the staff develop a new well-baby clinic when child health services are lacking. It is also not uncommon for the nursing supervisor to provide support and assistance when a staff member wants to establish group activities in order to expand her or his services to a larger number of clients.

Include Community-Focused Activities in Evaluation Tools

Staff-level community-focused activities are seldom evaluated or rewarded. As a result, very little priority is placed on these types of activities and the focus of service shifts from the community as a whole to individual clients. To alter this pattern, the practitioner must take time to revise evaluation tools and procedures so that community activities are assessed during the evaluation process. Only if this is done will time be allocated for community work. Listed below are a few examples of items one might want to include under a community service category on a staff evaluation tool:

- Assesses health needs and strengths of specific populations (school, clinic, industry) in assigned district
- Works with nursing supervisor to discern

health action needed for at-risk populations in assigned district
- Works with the nursing supervisor to develop intervention strategies (group work, clinic services) for populations at risk in assigned district
- Collaborates with other professionals on health-planning projects for populations at risk in the community

SUMMARY

Meeting the health needs of at-risk populations is a major function of the community health nurse. A nurse must know the community before this responsibility can be effectively carried out. A variety of strategies must be used to assess the health status, the health capability, and the health action potential of the nurse's community. Data must be analyzed as well as collected so that target groups for nursing service can be identified. Use of the nursing process facilitates implementation of these activities.

There are numerous professionals and consumers who will assist the community health nurse in identifying community health problems and strengths. Interdisciplinary collaboration and consumer participation must be fostered during the community assessment and diagnostic processes, because no one person alone can appropriately diagnose community needs.

Exploring the community, its organization, and its activities is extremely rewarding because it gives one a clearer picture of community health action. It provides the foundation for health-planning activities which are designed to improve the health status of high-risk groups. It further helps the community health nurse to assist individual families more effectively because often family health problems cannot be resolved until changes occur in the health care delivery system. It may be difficult for the community health nurse to integrate community-focused activities into an already busy schedule, but it is essential to do so in order to meet the needs of individuals, families, and populations at risk.

APPENDIX 11-1

Community Assessment Tool: Overview of Its People, Environment, and Systems

Community _____   Date _____

Check (✓) appropriate column*	Strength	Potential need	Problem	Description-Comments
I. *People*				
A. Vital and demographic statistics				
1. Population density				
2. Population composition a. Sex ratio				
b. Age distribution				

*Place check in only one column—strength, potential need, or problem.

Community Assessment Tool: Overview of Its People, Environment, and Systems—cont'd

Check (√) appropriate column*	Strength	Potential need	Problem	Description-Comments
c. Race distribution				
d. Ethnic origin				
3. Population characteristics a. Mobility				
b. Socioeconomic status				
c. Level of unemployment				
d. Educational level				
e. Marriage rate				
f. Divorce rate				
g. Dependency ratio				
h. Fertility rate				
i. Head of household				
4. Mortality characteristics a. Crude death rate				
b. Infant mortality rate				
c. Maternal mortality rate				
d. Age-specific death rate				
e. Leading causes of death				
5. Morbidity characteristics a. Incidence rate (specific diseases)				
b. Prevalence rate (specific diseases)				

Continued.

Community Assessment Tool: Overview of Its People, Environment, and Systems—cont'd

Check (√) appropriate column*	Strength	Potential need	Problem	Description-Comments
B. History of community (i.e., founding, growth)				
C. Values, attitudes, and norms				
D. Individual and family living practices				
1. Types of families				
2. Number of children per family				
3. Leisure activities				
II. *Environmental*				
A. Physical 1. Natural resources				
2. Geography, climate, terrain				
3. Roads/ transportation				
4. Boundaries				
5. Housing (types available by percent, condition, percent rented, percent owned)				
6. Other major structures				
B. Biological and chemical 1. Water supply				
2. Air (color, odor, particulates)				
3. Food supply (sources, preparation)				
4. Pollutants, toxic substances, animal reservoirs or vectors				

Community Assessment Tool: Overview of Its People, Environment, and Systems—cont'd

Check (√) appropriate column*	Strength	Potential need	Problem	Description-Comments
5. Flora and fauna				
6. Is this a predominantly urban, suburban, or rural community? (How is land used?)				
III. *Systems*				
A. Health 1. Preventive health care practices and facilities (list)				
2. Treatment health care facilities (e.g., acute care, medical, and surgical hospitals) (list)				
3. Rehabilitation health care facilities (e.g., alcoholism) (list)				
4. Long-term health care facilities (e.g., nursing homes) (list)				
5. Respite care services for special population groups (list)				
6. Hospice care services (list)				
7. Catastrophic health care facilities and services (list)				
8. Special health services for population groups (what and how provided) a. Preschool				

Continued.

Community Assessment Tool: Overview of Its People, Environment, and Systems—cont'd

Check (√) appropriate column*	Strength	Potential need	Problem	Description-Comments
b. School age				
c. Adult or young adult				
d. Occupational health				
e. Adults and children with handicapping conditions				
9. Voluntary health care resources				
10. Sanitation services				
11. Health work force (population ratios)				
12. Health education activities				
13. Methods of health care financing (approximate percent) a. Private pay				
b. Health insurance				
c. HMO				
d. Medicaid/ Medicare				
e. Worker's Compensation				
14. Prevalent diseases and conditions (list)				
15. Linkages with other systems				
16. Health care resource overall availability				

APPENDIX 11-1

Community Assessment Tool: Overview of Its People, Environment, and Systems—cont'd

Check (√) appropriate column*	Strength	Potential need	Problem	Description-Comments
17. Health care resource overall utilization				
B. Welfare				
1. Official (public) welfare resources a. General (list; e.g., Department of Social Services)				
b. Safety and protection (list; e.g., fire department)				
2. Voluntary welfare resources (list)				
3. Transportation resources (public and private)				
4. Facilities to meet needs (e.g., shopping areas, public housing)				
5. Special services for population groups (list)				
6. Resource accessibility				
7. Resource utilization				
C. Education				
1. Public educational facilities (list)				
2. Private educational facilities (list)				
3. Libraries (list)				
4. Educational services for special populations a. Pregnant teens				
b. Adults				

Continued.

Community Assessment Tool: Overview of Its People, Environment, and Systems—cont'd

Check (√) appropriate column*	Strength	Potential need	Problem	Description-Comments
c. Developmentally disabled children and adults				
d. Other				
5. Resource accessibility				
6. Resource utilization				
D. Economic				
1. Major industry and business (list)				
2. Banks, savings and loans, credit unions (list)				
3. Major occupations (list)				
4. General socioeconomic status of population				
5. Median income				
6. Percent of population below poverty level				
7. Percent of population who are retired				
E. Government and leadership				
1. Elected official leadership (list with title)				
2. Nonofficial leadership (list with title affiliations)				
3. City offices (location, hours, services)				

APPENDIX 11-1

Community Assessment Tool: Overview of Its People, Environment, and Systems—cont'd

Check (√) appropriate column*	Strength	Potential need	Problem	Description-Comments
4. Accessibility to constituents				
5. Support of community resources				
F. Recreation 1. Public facilities (list)				
2. Private facilities (list)				
3. Recreational activities frequently utilized (list)				
4. Leisure activities frequently utilized (list)				
5. Coordination with educational recreation facilities and programs				
6. Programs for special population groups a. Elderly				
b. People who are handicapped				
c. Others				
7. Resource accessibility				
8. Resource utilization				
G. Religion 1. Facilities by denomination (list)				

Continued.

Community Assessment Tool: Overview of Its People, Environment, and Systems—cont'd

Check (√) appropriate column*	Strength	Potential need	Problem	Description-Comments
2. Religious leaders (list)				
3. Community programs and services				
4. Resource accessibility				
5. Resource utilization				
IV. *Community dynamics* (describe) A. Communication (diagram and describe)				
1. Vertical (community to larger society)				
2. Horizontal (community to itself)				
3. Specific resources (e.g., television, radio, newspapers)				
V. *Major sources of community data* A. Government (list, e.g., local health department, city planning office)				
B. Private (list, e.g., chamber of commerce)				

Questions for the community health nurse

1. In general, are resources readily available and accessible?
2. What does the community see as its major strengths and needs?
3. How self-sufficient is the community in meeting its perceived needs?
4. What does the community health nurse see as the community's major strengths and needs?

5. Health care
   a. How does the community view and utilize the health care system?
   b. What does the community see as its health care needs?
   c. What are the goals and major activities of the health system?
   d. How self-sufficient is the community in meeting its health needs?

Community health care goals and activities to implement them

Date	Goals	Activities to implement

Assessor _____ Date _____
Assessor _____ Date _____
Assessor _____ Date _____

NOTE: The material presented in Chapters 3, 4, 5, 11, and 12 is especially helpful to the nurse when utilizing this assessment tool. The nurse initially collects available data and then adds to this assessment on an ongoing basis.

APPENDIX 11-2

Selected Sources of Data on the Health of the United States Population, the Availability and Use of Health Sources, and Health Care Expenditures

Source of data	Type of data
Department of Health and Human Services	
National Center for Health Statistics (NCHS)	Only federal agency specifically established for the collection and dissemination of health data.
National Vital Statistics System	Collects and publishes data on births, deaths, marriages, and divorces in the United States: The recording of births and deaths has been complete since 1933.
National Natality Survey	Conducted by NCHS periodically since 1963; latest survey was 1980. This survey is designed to collect data about the nature of live births in the United States. The 1980 survey data came from information obtained on birth certificates and from questionnaires sent to *married* mothers, hospitals, attendants at delivery, and other medical providers. The low-birth-weight infant was oversampled in 1980, in order to do special studies on high-risk infants.

Continued.

Selected Sources of Data on the Health of the United States Population, the Availability and Use of Health Sources, and Health Care Expenditures—cont'd

Source of data	Type of data
National Health Interview Survey (NHIS)	A nationwide, continuing, sample survey; data are collected through personal household interviews on personal and demographic characteristics, illnesses, injuries, impairments, chronic conditions, utilization of health resources, and other health topics.
National Health Examination Survey (NHES)	A nationwide, continuing sample survey, established in 1960-1962. Data were collected through direct standardized physical examinations, clinical and laboratory tests, and measurements on the total prevalence of certain chronic diseases and the distributions of various physical and physiological measures including blood pressure and serum cholesterol levels. In 1971, the survey name was changed to the *National Health and Nutrition Examination Survey.*
National Health and Nutrition Examination Survey (NHANES)	A nationwide, continuing, sample survey where health-related data are obtained by direct physical examinations, clinical and laboratory tests, and related measurement procedures. A major purpose of this survey is to measure and monitor indicators of the nutritional status of the American people. The first NHANES was conducted from 1971 through 1974 and obtained detailed examination data on cardiovascular, respiratory, arthritic, and hearing conditions. The second NHANES was conducted from 1976 through 1980, and obtained detailed data on diabetes, kidney and liver functions, allergy and speech pathology, as well as the nutritional status of U.S. residents.
National Master Facility Inventory (NMFI)	NMFI is a comprehensive file of inpatient health facilities (hospitals, nursing and related care homes, and other custodial or remedial care facilities) in the United States.
National Hospital Discharge Survey (NHDS)	A continuing, nationwide sample survey which collects data about discharges from short stay hospitals.
National Nursing Home Survey (NNHS)	Two sample surveys (August 1973 through April 1974 and May through December 1977) done to obtain data about nursing homes, their expenditures, residents, staff, and discharged patients (1977 survey only).
National Ambulatory Medical Care Survey (NAMCS)	NAMCS is a continuing national probability sample of ambulatory medical encounters in the offices of nonfederally employed physicians.
National Medical Care Utilization and Expenditure Survey (NMCUES)	NMCUES is a national sample survey which examined health expenditures for and use of personal health services and individual and family insurance coverage during 1980. It also checked, through an administrative records survey, the eligibility status of the household survey respondents for the Medicare and Medicaid programs.
Health Resources and Services Administration	
Bureau of Health Professions	This bureau evaluates both the current and future supply of health manpower in the various occupations. It also designates Health Manpower Shortage Areas for three federal programs: the National Health Service Corps and the Loan Repayment and Scholarship programs. These shortage area designations are also used to determine funding priorities for other programs.
Centers for Disease Control (CDC)	
Center for Infectious Diseases	This center maintains a national morbidity reporting system, which collects demographic, clinical, and laboratory data on conditions such as rabies, aseptic meningitis, diphtheria, tetanus, encephalitis, foodborne outbreaks, and others. One of its primary purposes is to maintain national surveillance of infectious diseases. Currently, a

APPENDIX 11-2

Selected Sources of Data on the Health of the United States Population, the Availability and Use of Health Sources, and Health Care Expenditures—cont'd

Source of data	Type of data
	major surveillance system has been established by this center to deter epidemiological trends relative to AIDS. The *AIDS Surveillance* is conducted by health departments in each state, territory, and the District of Columbia. Using a standard confidential case report form, the health departments collect information on each identified AIDS case. The pamphlet, *Morbidity and Mortality Weekly Report (MMWR),* published by CDC provides extremely valuable, up-to-date information on a broad base of public health concerns and issues, as well as current statistics on infectious diseases.
Epidemiology Program Office (EPO)	EPO, in partnership with the Council of State and Territorial Epidemiologists (CSTE), operates the *National Notifiable Diseases Surveillance System.* The purpose of this system is primarily to provide weekly provisional information on the occurrence of diseases defined as notifiable by CSTE.
Center for Chronic Disease Prevention and Health Promotion	This center maintains an *Abortion Surveillance* system which provides epidemiological data on abortions in all states in the United States.
Center for Prevention Services	This center conducts a U.S. Immunization Survey which is used to estimate the immunization level of the nation's child population against the vaccine preventable diseases. Periodically, immunization level data are also collected on the adult population.
Alcohol, Drug Abuse, and Mental Health Administration	
National Institute on Alcohol Abuse and Alcoholism	Funds national surveys of drinking habits, which provide data on trends in alcohol consumption.
National Institute on Drug Abuse	This institute conducts *National Household Surveys on Drug Abuse* to obtain data on trends in use of marijuana, cigarette, and alcohol among youths 12-17 years of age and young adults 18-25 years of age
National Institute of Mental Health	The Institute conducts surveys of inpatient and outpatient psychiatric facilities and studies to determine characteristics of patients served by these facilities.
Health Care Financing Administration	
Bureau of Data Management and Strategy	This bureau compiles annual estimates of public and private expenditures for health by type of expenditure and source of funds. It also maintains a Medicare statistical program which tracks the eligibility of employees and the benefits they use, the certification status of institutional providers, and the payments made for covered services.
Department of Commerce	
Bureau of the Census	This bureau has taken a census of the United States population every ten years since 1790. It also conducts a monthly Current Population Survey (CPS) to provide estimates of employment, unemployment, and other characteristics of the general labor force, the population as a whole, and various subgroups of the population.
Department of Labor	
Bureau of Labor Statistics	This bureau prepares monthly the *Consumer Price Index* (CPI) which is a measure of the changes in average prices of the goods and

Continued.

APPENDIX 11-2

Selected Sources of Data on the Health of the United States Population, the Availability and Use of Health Sources, and Health Care Expenditures—cont'd

Source of data	Type of data
	services purchased by urban wage earners and by clerical workers and their families. The CPI shows trends in medical care prices based on specific indicators of hospital, medical, dental, and drug prices. This bureau also publishes data on employment and earnings.
Environmental Protection Agency	This agency collects data on the five pollutants for which National Ambient Air Quality Standards have been set (refer to Chapter 16) and maintains a National Aerometric Data Bank (NADB).
National Institutes of Health (NIH)	NIH through its National Cancer Institute maintains 11 population-based cancer registries known as the Surveillance, Epidemiology and End Results (SEER) Program. This program provides data on all residents diagnosed with cancer during the year and follow-up information on previously diagnosed patients.
National Institute for Occupational Safety and Health (NIOSH)	NIOSH conducted the *National Occupational Hazard Survey* (NOHS) between February 1972 through June 1974 to obtain data on employee exposure to particular chemicals and physical agents in various industries. Beginning in 1981, NIOSH began a second national survey of worksites patterned after NOHS, known as the *National Occupational Exposure Survey (NOES)*.
United Nations	The statistical office of this organization prepares the *Demographic Yearbook*, which is a comprehensive collection of international demographic statistics.
Alan Guttmacher Institute	This institute is the research and development division of the Planned Parenthood Federation of America, Inc. It conducts, on an annual basis, a survey of abortion providers. This institute also prepares educational documents related to other fertility issues such as teenage pregnancy.
American Hospital Association (AHA)	AHA annually surveys hospitals in the United States to obtain data about characteristics of clients served by the hospital, services provided, demographic and geographic characteristics (e.g., bed size and location), length of hospital stays, and the like.
American Medical Association (AMA)	AMA has maintained a master file of physicians since 1906. From 1920 to 1957 AMA also conducted annual censuses of all hospitals registered by the Association.
Public Health Foundation	The Association of State and Territorial Health Officials (ASTHO) Reporting System, operated by the Public Health Foundation, is a statistical system that provides comprehensive information about the public health programs of state and local health departments. This system was established in 1970.

From National Center for Health Statistics: Health and prevention profile, United States, 1983, DHHS Pub No PHS 84-1232, Public Health Service, Washington, DC, December 1983, US Government Printing Office, pp 207-216. National Center for Health Statistics: Health, United States, 1988, DHHS Pub No PHS 89-1232, Washington, DC, 1989, US Government Printing Office, pp 185-197.

REFERENCES

American Nurses' Association, Commission on Nursing Research: Research priorities for the 1980s: generating a scientific basis for nursing practice (D-682M), Kansas City, Mo, 1981, The Association.

American Nurses' Association Community Health Nursing Division: Standards of community health nursing practices (Pub No CH-10), Kansas City, Mo, 1986, The Association.

American Public Health Association, Public Health Nursing Section: The definition and role of public health nursing in the delivery of health care, Washington, DC, 1981, The Association.

Anderson EJ: Community focus in public health nursing: whose responsibility? Nurs Outlook 31:44-48, 1983.

Aneshensel CS, Fredrichs RR, Clark VA, and Yokopenic PA: Telephone versus in-person surveys of community health status, Am J Public Health 72:1017-1021, 1982.

Community Health Nursing Faculty: Public health statistics notes, East Lansing, Mi, 1968, Michigan State University.

Duncan DF: Epidemiology: basis for disease prevention and health promotion, New York, 1988, Macmillan.

Gordon M: Manual of nursing diagnosis, 1988-1989, St Louis, 1989, CV Mosby Co.

Kane RA: Interprofessional teamwork, Syracuse, NY, 1975, Syracuse University School of Social Work.

Lindeman CA: Priorities in clinical nursing research, Nurs Outlook 23:693-698, 1975.

Maternal and Infant Task Force on AIDS: Perinatal AIDS in Michigan, Lansing, Mi, 1988, Michigan Department of Public Health.

Mausner JS and Kramer S: Mausner and Bahn Epidemiology—an introductory text, ed 2, Philadelphia, 1985, Saunders.

National Center for Health Statistics: Health and prevention profile, United States, 1983, DHHS Pub No PHS 84-1232, Public Health Service, Washington, DC, December 1983, US Government Printing Office.

National Center for Health Statistics: Health, United States, 1988, DHHS Pub No (PHS)89-1232, Washington, DC, 1989, US Government Printing Office.

Office of the Federal Register: United States government manual, 1988/89, Washington, DC, 1988, The Office.

Office of Information and Legislative Affairs, NCNR: National Center for Nursing Research: facts about funding, Bethesda, Md, 1989, National Center for Nursing Research.

Polit DF and Hungler BP: Nursing research: principles and methods, ed 3, Philadelphia, 1987, Lippincott.

Robey B: Two hundred years and counting: the 1990 census, Pop Bull 44(1), Washington, DC, 1989, Population Reference Bureau, Inc.

Ruffing-Rahal MA: Qualitative methods in community analysis, Public Health Nurs 2:130-137, 1985.

Siemiatycki J: A comparison of mail, telephone and home interview strategies for household health surveys, Am J Public Health 69:238-245, 1979.

Skinner EA, German PS, Shapiro S, Chase GA, and Zauber AG: Use of ambulatory health services by the near poor, Am J Public Health 68:1195-1201, 1978.

Storfjell JL and Cruise PA: A model of community-focused nursing, Public Health Nurs 1:85-96, 1984.

United States Department of Health and Human Services (USDHHS): Health status of the disadvantaged chartbook, 1986, Washington, DC, 1986, US Government Printing Office.

Walker GM: Utilization of health care: the Laredo migrant experience, Am J Public Health 60:667-671, 1979.

SELECTED BIBLIOGRAPHY

Allor MT: The "community profile," J Nurs Educ 22:12-17, 1983.

Burchell RW and Sternlieb G, eds: Planning theory in the 1980s: a search for future directions, New Brunswick, NJ, 1978, Center for Urban Policy Research.

Finnegan L and Ervin NE: An epidemiological approach to community assessment, Public Health Nurs 6:147-151, 1989.

Hamilton P: Community nursing diagnosis, Adv Nurs Sci 5(3):21-36, 1983.

Hanchett E: Community health assessment: a conceptual tool kit, New York, 1979, Wiley.

Klein DC: Assessing community characteristics. In Spradley BW, ed: Readings in community health nursing, ed 2, Boston, 1982, Little, Brown.

Ludke RL, Curry JP, and Saywell RM: The community survey and the health services provider, J Health Care Market 3(3):39-52, 1983.

McLaughlin JS: Toward a theoretical model for community health programs, Adv Nurs Sci 5(1):7-28, 1982.

Muecke MA: Community health diagnosis in nursing, Public Health Nurs 1:23-35, 1984.

Reinhardt AM and Chatlin ED: Assessment of health needs in a community: the basis for program planning. In Reinhardt AM and Quinn MD, eds: Current practice in family-centered community nursing, St Louis, 1977, CV Mosby Co., pp. 138-185.

Training and Laboratory Program Office: Principles of epidemiology: statistical measures used in epidemiology, self-study course 3030-G, manual 3, Atlanta, Ga, 1987, Public Health Service, CDC.

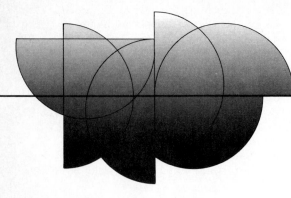

12

Community Health Planning for Populations at Risk

There was a little girl who had a little curl
Right in the middle of her forehead;
When she was good she was very very good
And when she was bad she was horrid.

Upon completion of this chapter, the reader will be able to:

1. Describe the concept of health planning.
2. Compare the nursing, epidemiological, and health care planning processes.
3. Analyze the steps of the health care planning process.
4. Summarize key principles involved in health planning.

5. Identify significant legislation that has influenced health planning activities.
6. Describe barriers to health planning.
7. Discuss the use of health planning concepts in community health nursing practice.

This nursery rhyme at the beginning of this chapter describes the state of health care services in the United States: some of them are very, very good and some of them are appalling. One can say with certainty that the overall picture of health care services is not orderly, equitable, or logical. Failure to reach certain at-risk segments of the population, notably low-income and rural people, is a reflection on health planning activities. Other problems include the rapid escalation of health care costs, concerns about the distribution and use of technology, and inappropriate distribution of both health care facilities and personnel around the country. Further, the services that are available are often institutional in nature, and health promotion and disease prevention efforts are not maximized.

Nursing has often not been assertive in health-planning activities for population groups. This has historical roots in nursing practice. In 1903 Lavinia Dock, a nurse, wrote that "nursing has not made itself a moral force; is not a public conscience, takes no position in large public questions, is not feared by those of low standards; allows all manner of new conditions and developments in nursing affairs to arise, flourish, succeed, or fail" (Ashley, 1975, p. 1466). Nursing has come a long way from those nonassertive days but still has significant strides to make.

Today the professional nurse is beginning to assume assertive leadership roles in meeting the health needs of consumers. She or he is becoming increasingly involved in health planning and political activities and is realizing the importance of understanding health legislation and financing. Unfortunately, nurses have often thought that the subjects of health planning, politics, legislation, and financing were dull or "not nursing." Yet, nursing involves all these things.

Health planning is one of the primary functions of a community health nurse. The ANA and the APHA believe that the dominant responsibil-

The authors are indebted to Assistant Professor Nancy Watson, who helped faculty and students at the University of Rochester to understand basic concepts of population-based health planning. Content and illustrations in this chapter reflect many of her ideas.

ity of nurses in community health is to the community or the population as a whole and that the nurse must acknowledge the need for comprehensive health planning to implement this responsibility (ANA, 1980, 1986; APHA, 1981). This chapter emphasizes the role of the community health nurse in health planning for population groups.

DEFINING HEALTH PLANNING

Health planning is an ongoing process whereby information about a community is systematically collected and used to structure a usable community health plan. It is a process based upon scientific principles and methods and the goal is to maximize the health of the community as a whole.

Health planning is a problem-solving approach which helps a community to evaluate and bring about specific changes in its health care delivery system. The problem-solving approach is the basis for planning nursing care with individuals and families, and it can be expanded to population groups. The health planning process for population groups involves the same steps used in the nursing process: assessing, analyzing, planning, implementing, and evaluating. Basic concepts of epidemiology (Chapter 10), biostatistics (Chapter 11), and management (Chapter 21) are used to refine decision-making and diagnostic skills and to expand intervention options during the health planning process.

Table 12-1 illustrates how the steps in the problem-solving approach can be utilized in various situations. This chapter discusses in detail each step of the population-based health planning process, utilizing the scientific problem-solving approach.

Many people do health planning: individuals, groups within organizations, organizations, groups of organizations, communities, and regions. Within institutions, there are individual planners as well as groups who carry out these functions. These groups include governing boards, committees, and staff planning groups.

However, not everyone does *population-based*

TABLE 12-1   Comparison of the nursing, epidemiological, and health care planning processes

Nursing process	Epidemiological process	Health planning process

Assessing
  Data collection to determine nature of
  client problems
	I. Determine the nature, extent, and
	    scope of the problem
	    A. Natural life history of condition
	    B. Determinants influencing
	       condition
	       1. Primary data (essential agent)
	          a. Parasite, bacterium, or virus
	          b. Nutrition
	          c. Psychosocial factors
	       2. Contributory data
	          a. Agent
	          b. Host
	          c. Environment
	    C. Distribution patterns
	       1. Person
	       2. Place
	       3. Time
	    D. Condition frequencies
	       1. Prevalence
	       2. Incidence
	       3. Other biostatistical
	          measurements
		Preplanning
		Assessment

Analyzing	II. Formulate tentative hypothesis(es)	
Formulation of nursing diagnoses or hypotheses	III. Collect and analyze further data to test hypothesis(es)	Policy development
Planning	IV. Plan for control	
Implementing	V. Implement control plan	Implementation
Evaluating	VI. Evaluate control plan	Evaluation
Revising or terminating	VII. Make appropriate report	
	VIII. Conduct research	

health planning. Those groups who have this as their goal include health systems agencies (described later in this chapter) and community organizations such as the health department, Red Cross, Visiting Nurse Associations, and school and occupational health teams.

For these people, the emphasis in health planning is on the health of population groups within the community, and problems, solutions, and actions are defined on this level. By comparison, in clinical nursing, the emphasis is on the individual as the unit of service (Williams, 1977, p. 251). In community health nursing, the family is the unit of service and the client is the community.

It is important to remember that another distinguishing feature of population-based health

planning is its focus on the prevention of existing health problems in the population being served, as well as on the promotion of health and well-being. Chapters 13 through 19 will focus on population groups, utilizing a developmental framework. For each age group, existing health problems are presented, at-risk populations identified, and preventive intervention strategies discussed.

Major Health Problems

As previously discussed, several recent documents have reviewed the health of Americans in the last decade. These include: *Healthy People. The Surgeon General's Report on Health Promotion and Disease Prevention (1979); Promoting Health, Preventing Disease. Objectives for the Nation,*

(1980); Health United States (1987); Prevention '86/'87: Federal Programs and Progress (1987); and The 1990 Health Objectives for the Nation: A Midcourse Review (1986). A draft of *Promoting Health/Preventing Disease: Year 2000 Objectives for the Nation (1989)* is being circulated for review and comment among health professionals and representatives of consumer groups. This report will replace the 1979 Surgeon General's report on the health of our nation and will guide health planning efforts for the coming decade. Other re-

ports which address the needs of specific aggregates such as children (U.S. Congress, Office of Technology Assessment, 1988) and the aged (Commonwealth Fund Commission, 1987) are available and assist health planners in obtaining an in-depth understanding of the health problems of these groups. In addition, *The Future of Public Health* (Institute of Medicine, 1988) report will assist planners in making recommendations about how to improve the delivery of official public health services. This report and the health sta-

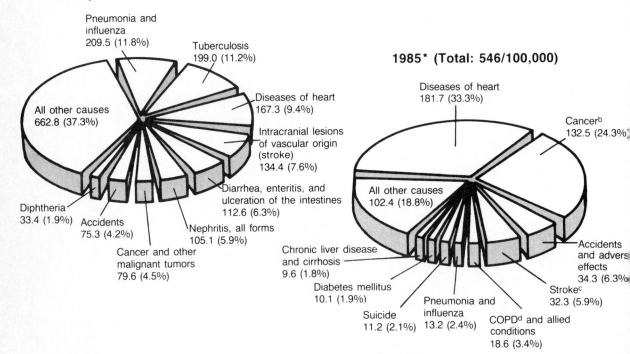

*Provisional data.

aData for 1900 are for the 10 death-registration States and the District of Columbia. This area accounted for only 26 percent of the population of the continental United States.

bCancer = malignant neoplasms, including neoplasms of lymphatic and hematopoietic tissues.

cStroke = cerebrovascular diseases and allied conditions.

dCOPD = chronic obstructive pulmonary diseases.

Notes: These charts display death rates per 100,000 population, age adjusted to the 1940 U.S. population. Numbers in parentheses indicate percentages of total age-adjusted death rate. The sum of data for the 10 causes may not equal the total because of rounding.

Figure 12-1   Age-adjusted rates for major causes of death in the United States in 1900 and for leading causes of death in 1985. (From National Center for Health Statistics, cited in Public Health Service: Prevention '86/'87: federal programs and progress, Washington, DC, 1987, US Government Printing Office, p 18.)

tus documents on the population as a whole were discussed extensively in Chapter 4.

A striking fact in these documents is that many improvements in the health of our citizens are traceable to activities that people themselves carry out and that promoting health through risk reduction is essential in order to combat contemporary health problems. Figure 12-1 presents age-adjusted rates for major causes of death in the United States in 1900 and for leading causes of death in 1985. The age-adjusted death rate of 545.9 in both 1984 and 1985 is the lowest ever recorded. At the same time, a record number of deaths occurred in 1985, an expected figure given the increase in the population and the increasing proportion of older people. Life expectancy at birth was 74.7 in both 1984 and 1985. The 10 leading causes of death and their ranked order did not change from 1984 to 1985. Of the 10 leading causes of death, the first four continue to account for three of every four deaths: diseases of the heart, cancer, strokes, and accidents (USDHHS,

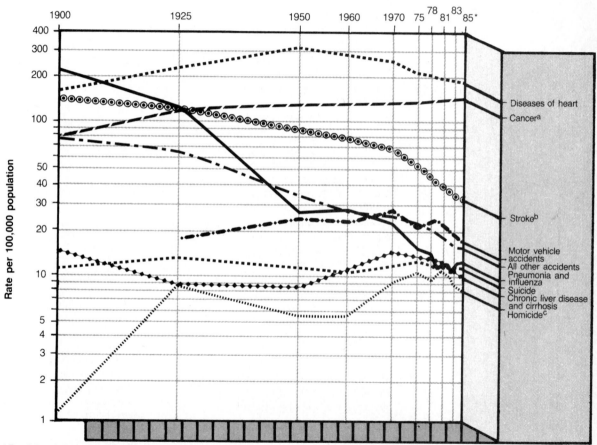

*Provisional data.

aCancer = malignant neoplasms, including neoplasms of lymphatic and hematopoietic tissues.

bStroke = cerebrovascular diseases.

cHomicide = homicide and legal intervention.

Note: Age adjusted to the 1940 U.S. population.

Figure 12-2   Trends in age-adjusted death rates from selected causes: selected years, 1900-1985. (From National Center for Health Statistics, cited in Public Health Service: Prevention '86/'87: federal programs and progress, Washington, DC, 1987, US Government Printing Office, p 19.)

TABLE 12-2 Examples of health promotion activities in various settings for major age groups

Settings	Infants	Children
Schools	Support programs for adolescent parents Parenting education in school curricula (for both boys and girls)	Comprehensive health education curricula with emphasis on positive health behaviors Physical fitness testing, training, and awards programs Health screening and immunization programs Healthful snacks in vending machines
Worksites	Employer-sponsored day care programs, including parent education and support groups Maternity/paternity leave and related programs that facilitate family formulation Policies that facilitate breastfeeding Notification of employees about reproductive risks associated with work environments Flexible work schedules for parents	Family health and safety topics in health promotion programs
Health care settings	Nutrition counseling and guidance in risk reduction for pregnant women and parents of infants Information and support for breastfeeding Parent counseling on infant screening to identify high-risk families Poisoning prevention programs Community outreach and education	Counseling for parents on normal childhood growth and development Education for parents on health habit formation and child safety Classes for parents about home care of minor acute illness and injuries Involvement of children in decisions about their health care
Communities	Nutrition programs for pregnant and lactating women Media campaigns such as "Healthy Mothers, Healthy Babies" Support and education for parents Injury control programs and ordinances	Public service announcements countering advertisements directed at children Assistance for parents in educating their children about sex and family life After-school recreation programs

From USDHHS, Public Health Service: Prevention '82, DHHS Pub No PHS 82-50157, Washington, DC, 1982, Government Printing Office, pp 4-5.

Adolescents and young adults	Adults	Other adults
Development of overall school climate of discipline and achievement	Health education programs through community colleges and high school evening programs	Extension of school meal programs to older adults
School health education curricula with emphasis on positive health behaviors	Extension of high school exercise facilities for adult use	Volunteer service opportunities to promote interaction between older adults and children
Establishment of peer group counseling efforts	Health education classes through colleges and universities	
Family use of worksite exercise facilities	Health promotion and employee counseling programs	Expansion of worksite health promotion programs to retirees
Flexible work policies to maximize opportunities for adolescents	High blood pressure detection and treatment programs	Lifting mandatory retirement age
	Provision of exercise facilities	Flexible work schedules to ease retirement transition
	Organization-wide policies designating nonsmoking areas	
	Cafeteria programs to promote good nutrition	
	Policies and programs to help ensure a safe and healthy work environment	
	Reduction of excessive stress in the work environment	
Adolescent health counseling programs	Education and counseling programs to reduce risk and maintain therapeutic regimens	Improved training of health care providers for geriatric practice
	Education about unnecessary surgery and procedures; second opinion programs	Development of home care alternatives to institutionalization
	Self-care education	
Volunteer service opportunities	National Health Promotion Training Network, e.g., health education and support programs sponsored by coalitions of local organizations	Meals-on-Wheels and other nutrition support programs
Targeted media programs, such as the 1982 Alcohol Abuse Prevention campaign		Education on hypothermia and heat stress
Adolescent health education programs sponsored by youth-serving agencies	Media campaigns such as "HealthStyle"	Walking groups and exercise programs designed for older adults
	Improved nutrition information through food labeling, print and electronic media, and advertising	Promotion of positive attitudes toward aging and the elderly
	Community intervention programs for specific health risks, such as the Trilateral High Blood Pressure Education Program	Bereavement counseling
		Senior health promotion volunteer programs
		Promotion of drug profile records

1987, Prevention '86/'87, p. 18). Figure 12-2 shows trends in age-adjusted death rates from selected causes: selected years, 1900-1985. Over half of the leading causes of deaths—diseases of the heart, cancer, stroke, accidents, suicide, and chronic liver disease—showed slightly lower rates of death in 1984 than in 1985 (USDHHS, 1987, Prevention '86/'87, p. 19).

To control the predominant health problems of the 1990s we need to change our belief systems as well as our definitions of health. Contemporary health planners write about the need to approach health care planning by defining health as having four major dimensions: environment, lifestyle, the system of health care, and human biology (Blum, 1981; Dever, 1980; and Lalonde, 1974). The epidemiological model used with infectious disease which looks at simple cause and effect will no longer work when we grapple with the health problems of today. Health planners must focus on the epidemiological model which emphasizes the multiple causation of conditions and diseases (refer to Chapter 10).

There is substantial evidence that community and individual measures can be taken to foster the development of lifestyles that not only prevent many contemporary health problems, but also enhance the state of health and well-being of individuals, families, and communities. Table 12-2, gives illustrations of population-based health planning programs in which community health nurses have been involved in various community settings. These programs help individuals and groups to examine and deal with health risks and to establish a lifestyle which promotes healthy living. Chapters 13 through 19 discuss the role of the community health nurse in relation to these programs for groups across the life span.

The Community Health Nurse and Health Planning

The community health nurse is particularly well qualified to carry out population-based health planning. Each day the nurse sees the needs of population groups within the community through home visits, clinics, classes, schools, and other nursing activities. She or he is able to obtain a composite picture of the health needs of a population group such as lack of prenatal care, family-planning services, or public transportation. The nurse's continual, comprehensive contact with the community makes her or him knowledgeable about available resources and gaps in service provision. The staff nurse should share these assessed health needs with supervisory personnel, and together they can discuss the alternatives to the situation. The agency's philosophy of service, policies, priorities, and staff variables will affect the alternatives offered. By sharing assessed needs with people in an agency who are in a position to assist in implementing change, the nurse is taking a beginning step in health planning for the needs of the community.

Nurses usually see only the "tip of the iceberg" when diagnosing problems common to families in their caseloads. What has been assessed, however, can become the basis for an epidemiological investigation of community needs, because the family is the smallest epidemiological group (Taylor and Knowelden, 1964, p. 303). Epidemiological studies examine groups of families in an agency's geographical area. They frequently involve investigation of needs in census tracts or specific political boundaries such as cities, towns, or counties.

Health needs of population groups can also be dealt with by building upon research studies and known problems and solutions. How this is done was illustrated by community health nurses in a southern city who served schools as well as provided general nursing service to the community. The school intervention program included only hearing and vision screening and episodic encounters with children who were referred by others or themselves. The community health nurses were aware that such a program did not involve continuous problem solving or comprehensive services. A decision was made to continue the usual nursing services to the school and to begin a pilot program that was preventive and directed to a defined group.

The pilot program was based upon research that demonstrated that (1) a small proportion of persons have the greatest number of illnesses in a group, (2) a good predictor of a student's absence is the past attendance record, and (3) at least 80 percent of school absences are for health reasons.

Using these data, personnel decided that children with a record of many absences and their families could benefit from nursing service. The major objectives for the study were "1) to consider the utility of directing nursing services to a defined risk group and 2) to document the results of the experience in terms of patient outcomes, specifically, change in absence experience" (Long, Whitman, Johansson, Williams, and Tuthill, 1975, p. 389). The study validated that "it is possible to incorporate a prevention-oriented service directed to a defined risk group into an on-going school health program" (p. 392).

The primary goal of health planning activities such as those described above is to develop comprehensive health care options for all citizens in the community. Working with one community subgroup, school-age children, helps health planners in developing comprehensive services for all.

THE HEALTH CARE PLANNING PROCESS*

As was illustrated in Table 12-1, the phases of the health care planning process have different labels, but in essence, they are the same problem-solving phases utilized in both the epidemiological process and the nursing process. Professionals from all disciplines use the health planning process. Thus, learning the terminology related to their problem-solving approach is important, because it unites scientific thinking across disciplines. Since health planning most often requires interdisciplinary team effort, it is crucial that team members have a common framework from which to work. The health planning process provides this framework.

The health care planning process is orderly and logical; it is a tool that helps those using it to organize large amounts of community data which describe community problems and strengths, as well as health planning solutions. For purposes of discussion, the health care planning process is di-

---

*Christine DeGregorio, M.S.P., University of Rochester doctoral student in political science, first wrote the phases and steps of the community planning process as outlined here. Much of the content and many of the illustrations in this section reflect her thinking and creativity. It is used with her permission.

vided into five phases: preplanning, assessment, policy development, implementation, and evaluation. Each of these phases is separately developed, but in reality, they are overlapping and inseparable.

The Preplanning Phase

Into this phase is built the foundation for the rest of the process. Prior to developing policies for health planning, it is crucial that planners test their ideas and validate that what they perceive as a problem is also seen by others as a problem severe enough to warrant changes. The planning organization and environment needs to be "tested" to ascertain whether there are sufficient resources as well as commitment to devote to the work required to bring about the change. Preliminary expectations as well as skeleton organizational plans need to be outlined. These sound like simple commonsense comments; in reality these very basic parts to the process are often skipped and positive results are then difficult to achieve.

The preplanning phase has five steps: (1) development of a broadly defined problem statement, (2) statement of a goal, (3) delineation of a timetable that accounts for the remaining four phases of the process, (4) assessment of resources for the task that needs to be done, and (5) planning for data collection strategies to be utilized. Each of these steps helps to build the framework needed for future planning activities.

Development of a Broadly Defined Problem Statement

A problem is a condition that is sufficiently distressing that change to bring relief is desired or sought. Everyone involved in the planning needs to be clear about the problem under consideration. An example of a broadly defined problem statement from which policy development could begin might be the following: "Deaths from motor vehicle accidents for people 15 to 24 years of age in Jones County have substantially increased over the past year." This statement has a broad, yet clear, focus. All involved in the planning process would know that the concern is increased motor vehicle accidents for a certain age group in a specific area in a given year.

Statement of a Goal

A goal is a general statement of intent or purpose that provides guidance for the activities that are to take place. A goal emanating from the above problem statement might be: "The Jones County Health Department will work toward reducing the rate of fatalities from motor vehicle accidents among people 15 to 24 years of age by 10 percent in 3 years."

Delineation of a Timetable That Accounts for the Remaining Four Phases of the Process

In order to develop a realistic timetable, planners must have a general idea of what they plan to accomplish in the months ahead. After a specific goal is delineated, health planners have a preliminary discussion about what needs to be done to achieve the stated goal. This discussion focuses on examining the nature of the tasks to be accomplished and what is feasible for the agency or community to do, considering other priorities.

Figure 12-3 presents a sample health planning timetable. As discussed earlier, this figure illustrates that the phases do overlap as well as build upon one another.

Assessment of Resources for the Task That Needs to Be Accomplished

Resources can be positive as well as negative, and they can be both internal (part of the organization) and external to an organization. Positive resources include money, enthusiasm for the goal, space in which to work, time, technical expertise (such as ability to work on a computer or knowledge of the planning process), and experienced workers who have popularity, esteem and charisma, and commitment to the goal. Negative resources can include a deficit of all the above.

Resources may be found within the organization or elsewhere. Space and money, for example, may need to be obtained from voluntary community agencies and technical expertise requested from a university. Knowing the community in which one works helps the community health nurse to quickly identify valuable resources during the planning process (refer to Chapter 11).

One of the most valuable health planning resources is a committee which works toward the goal and which has power and authority to make decisions. To be viable, the committee must have tasks assigned to it which are crucial to the goal; the committee must also have an audience which expects results. Health planning committee members should be chosen on the basis of their interpersonal skills, their knowledge of the planning process, their commitment to the goals, and their power and authority within the agency. Not every committee member will likely have all of these ingredients for successful planning; however, these ingredients must be present in some degree if successful planning is to take place. Inexperienced planners should be part of the group so that learning can take place for future planning activities. The planning committee may need to be trained in the planning process if this is an entirely new activity for committee members. Help with the process may be obtained from a variety of community resources such as the United Way, the county health planning council, and local university faculty members.

Planning That Delineates the Data Collection Strategies to Be Used

A plan needs to be developed to assess the problem of concern. When developing this plan, the

Phases	Time in months										
	Dec	Jan	Feb	Mar	April	May	June	July	Aug	Sept	Oct
Preplanning	———										
Assessment		————————————									
Policy development				————————————————							
Implementation								————————————————			
Evaluation									———————		

Figure 12-3   Timetable for Jones County Health Department's motor vehicle accident project.

planning group needs to focus on *what* type of data is needed, from *whom* they need input, *how* they should obtain data, *who* will be responsible for collecting the data, and *when* the data collection process will be completed. For example, the Jones County Health Department planning group may want input from parents, teachers, legislators, and police officers when they examine vehicle fatalities.

The plan for data collection should be written in sufficient detail, so that all involved parties are clear about what needs to be accomplished. A worksheet such as the one presented in Table 12-3 facilitates the planning process.

At the conclusion of these five steps, the planning group should have a good grasp of the problem, should be aware of the power and authority they have, should know their strengths and weaknesses, and should have delineated the time frame for the process. The group is then ready to move to the next phase of the planning process: *assessment*.

The Assessment Phase

In population-based planning,

A specific population is analyzed to determine its health problems. The health system is then studied to determine how it must function if those problems are to be addressed. Population-based planning can be contrasted with demand or resource-based planning, which begins by examining the capabilities and/or utilization

TABLE 12-3   Jones County Health Department Motor Vehicle Accident Project: worksheet for planning data collection strategies

Goal: Reduce the rate of motor vehicle accidents among 15- to 24-year-old youths in Jones County.

Rationale for Goal: The rate of fatal motor vehicle accidents (MVA) among 15- to 24-year-old youths has increased 5 percent in the past year.

Type of data	Data source	Collection method	Time for completion	Responsibility of
Data Collection Plan for Organizational Assessment:				
Characteristics of accident victims	Clients	Personal interview	April 30, 1992	Staff CHN
Epidemiological data	Accident reports & interview data	Review of reports	April 30, 1992	Planning committee
Data Collection Plan for Community Assessment:				
Causes of accidents	Law enforcement officers	Mail survey	April 30, 1992	Planning committee
Content covered in driver education courses	Driver education staff	Telephone interview	April 30, 1992	Planning committee

of the health population (USDHEW, 1979, Guidelines, p. 5).

In population-based planning, three steps in the assessment phase of the health care planning process must be completed. These are (1) conducting a needs assessment, (2) setting priorities upon which the planning committee can focus, and (3) specifying objectives to which organizational and community resources can be applied. Each of these steps assists planners to become more specific as they progress through the planning process.

Conducting a Needs Assessment

A needs assessment is a systematic method of gathering information about populations. This assessment helps to detect and measure problems and determine the relevance, adequacy, and appropriateness of services designed to combat them. It analyzes the need for human services through multiple measurement approaches. It also delineates population strengths, such as concerned citizen groups, which can be tapped when developing policies and implementation strategies.

Defining the parameters of the population to be studied is an area of concern to the planning committee. Will it be the county? Will it be a school district? Will it be a town or a city or a metropolitan area? Chapter 11, in the section entitled "Methods for Assessing a Community's Status," presents guidelines for defining these parameters.

Assessing a population's needs is a complex matter that goes beyond defining who the population actually is. Needs are relative, and they are based on values, culture, history, and the experiences of the individual, the family, and the community. Human needs are not easily identified, but are diffuse and related. For example, motor vehicle deaths may be related to poor roads that are the result of a low-level tax base for road construction, due to high unemployment. Human needs often change, because communities which influence human need are dynamic and their needs are in a constant state of flux: a need today may not be a need next year. Most importantly,

translating assessed needs into community programs is greatly influenced by the availability of human and financial resources as well as the availability of technology. Thus, a needs assessment must analyze community resources in addition to the characteristics of the population and the nature of the problem being encountered by the population.

Community resources should be identified when the nature of the problem is examined. When examining the nature and extent of the problem, planners discern trends over a certain period of years, and cite the problem's significance, implications, and comparisons with norms or other standards. The following assessment tool, designed to collect data about motor vehicle accidents in Jones County, can be utilized as a guide when collecting data about other health problems in a community:

1. Community assessment of the problem of fatalities from motor vehicle accidents
   a. Mortality data
   b. Morbidity data (incidence and prevalence) trends in recent years
   c. Demographic characteristics associated with mortality and morbidity (at-risk groups) in the defined community
   d. Local factors, such as road conditions, thought to influence trends
   e. Lifestyle of population groups
      (1) Environmental characteristics promotive of health or illness
      (2) Economic base of population, income, and occupation
      (3) Health behaviors, such as drinking patterns, that influence health states
   f. Local perception of needs, problems, or priorities
2. Community resources
   a. Health services, strengths, and limitations
   b. Utilization rates for health services
   c. Population coverage
3. Extent of knowledge related to the problem under consideration
   a. Magnitude of the problem in other populations: national data
   b. Etiologic factors (*results* of case-control

and cohort studies or theories)

c. Physiological, sociological, and psychological processes related to pathology

d. Inferences for *primary* prevention and early detection of problems

e. Treatment potential

   (1) Inferences for therapeutic strategies at the individual, family, or aggregate level

   (2) Inferences for *secondary* and *tertiary* prevention (both of above are based on *results* of clinical trials and other types of evaluative studies or theories)

How and where health planners obtain the above data are presented in the section "Sources of Community Data" in Chapter 11.

Setting Priorities

The next step in the assessment phase of the planning process is to set priorities in relation to the problem that the planning committee should concentrate on during the planning process. A priority is a designation given to one problem over another. Problem areas are usually put into rank order of significance; this promotes focused sequential action. Illustrative of priority setting is the emphasis of this area contained in the legislation of Public Law 92-641, the National Health Planning and Resources Development Act. This law established 10 national priorities which are presented later in this chapter. These 10 priorities were ranked relative to other national health problems and needs.

There are three approaches to setting priorities in the planning process (MacStravic, 1978). The first and most common one is to set priorities based on the *severity of the problem* or the desirability of some objective. Utilizing the mortality problem in Jones County, the first priority might be to reduce the fatalities for the group under study to at least the rate of 2 years past, since it increased by 5 percent in the past year. Another method of setting priorities is to focus on a measure of the *problem's susceptibility to solution.* In order to utilize this kind of approach, planners need to know the kinds of solutions that are available. The assumption is that besides knowing the

severity of the problem, planners must also know if anything can be done about it and then give highest priority to problems for which the solutions are known. The continuing example of motor vehicle accidents in Jones County provides another priority based on solution-oriented methods: prevent alcohol intake among teenagers, since assessment has demonstrated that there is a causal relationship between drinking and teenage car accidents. The final method of setting priorities is to utilize outcome-oriented methods which focus primarily on the *cost benefit of specific interventions.* The logic of this method is that planners should give highest priority to the action that will yield the best return. Given the information that the planning committee likely has about the problem of fatalities among teenagers in Jones County, its priority when utilizing the outcome-oriented method might be to raise the drinking age in Jones County to 21.

Whatever method is used by the planning committee, the chosen priority will affect the timing and the amount of resources allocated to that priority.

Specify Objectives

The last step in this assessment phase is to specify objectives to which organizational and community resources can be applied over a specified period of time. Objectives are specific, concrete, measurable statements of outcomes that need to be accomplished in order to eventually reach a broad goal. They are intended to guide the operations of the agency to reach the goal.

Objectives focus on the what and when. They specify *results,* not strategies, for getting results. For example, two objectives that help to reach the goal, reduce the rate of fatalities from motor vehicle accidents might be (1) define who is at risk for motor vehicle accidents among people aged 15 to 24 years in Jones County by March 1992, and (2) lower the fatality rate for people aged 15 to 24 years in Jones County by 5 percent in the next year.

Spiegel and Hyman (1978, pp. 16-18) designed criteria for testing the feasibility of objectives. As planners write their objectives, they need to keep these criteria in mind:

- The organization should have the authority to undertake the objectives.
- Objectives should be within the capabilities of the agency in terms of organization, personnel, equipment, facilities, and techniques.
- Objectives should fall within budget restrictions
- Objectives should fit into the available timetable.
- Objectives should be legal and consistent with the ethical and moral values of the community affected.
- Objectives should be practical and must be implementable.
- Objectives must be acceptable to those who are responsible for carrying them out.
- Minimum negative side effects should result from the achievement of the objectives.
- Objectives should be measurable in concrete terms

At the conclusion of the three steps of the assessment phase, planners will know the details of the problem under consideration. They will also know the resources that are available both within and outside the organization and the community, which can help deal with the problem. When this information is known, health planners concentrate on the third step in the planning process, *policy development.*

The Policy Development Phase

Policy development involves the determination of strategies to achieve the objectives that emerge as the result of the assessment done in phase two of the planning process. These strategies include methods for allocating resources such as money, personnel, and equipment. The strategies also clarify relationships that affect rights, status, and resources. In this phase, planners need to pay attention to social and political parameters: where are the greatest resources? Where is there resistance to the objectives? What methods or strategies could best achieve the objectives? Will one of the strategies be a modification of what already exists or will it be even better communication than what exists? Will the strategies to meet the objectives

involve contracts with other organizations and/or support for these organizations so that they can better meet the objective? Answers to these questions will result in an allocation of resources, the identification of responsibilities, and, finally, the establishment of an action plan that has tasks, responsibilities, and a time frame clearly delineated.

Sound social policy and value considerations provide the guidelines for the allocation of community resources, program development, and coordination. Policy development is frequently a process of negotiation among the different groups involved in the planning process: consumers, service providers, decision makers, and resource persons. Further, during the policy development phase, planners must anticipate expected changes in services, legislation, and general trends, and then must foresee what impact these changes will have on the local community. A balance must be achieved which will most effectively utilize community resources that meet the needs perceived by ordinary citizens, as well as needs perceived by professionals with expertise.

The need for sound public policies cannot be overemphasized. A renowned community health nurse has described how the health of people in the United States is the result of the environments in which they live and the patterns which they follow (Milio, 1981). She further writes about how these patterns and environments are shaped by public policy that is, in turn, shaped by available information. For example, Milio (1988) suggests that the United States adopt public policy measures already utilized in other countries, such as the one in Norway, where a comprehensive farm, food, and nutrition policy has the goal of improving national dietary policies, improving poor rural areas, and offering support to farm families. Its 10-member steering committee is multidisciplinary and includes government officials as well as food cooperatives, retailers, educators, and researchers. Although change is not occurring rapidly, it is taking place.

Health care planners should develop this kind of mind-set as they think about solutions to problems: that policy decisions are constantly being made that affect the health of Americans—

through management of the ecology, the economy, and farm and factory production, distribution, and consumption.

In order to discuss the policy development phase of the planning process, it is divided into four steps: (1) assess various strategies to achieve objectives, (2) match tasks with resources, (3) negotiate new organizational liaisons as needed, and, finally, (4) establish contracts as needed. The result will be an action plan as presented below, as the steps of the policy development phase are discussed.

Assess Various Strategies to Achieve Objectives

Generating alternatives to meet the objectives that have been written in phase two is one of the most exhilarating steps in the process. It is a time to be creative and innovative, to exercise a flair for originality.

Certain methods for generating various strategies have proved to be the most efficient and effective way to meet the objectives. Simple idea generation, or writing down ideas in a group is one. Another well-known one is *brainstorming*— throwing caution to the wind and citing any idea that comes to mind. *Think tanks* (getting together to talk over the problem with people who are involved in it) and *forced association* (exploring relationships between words) are two more methods of generating strategies. Spiegel and Hyman (1978) describe in detail how to generate various alternatives. The strategies that are chosen to reach the objectives will be based on their cost. They are also affected by accountability (whom does the public associate with the outcomes of the strategy) as well as whether the decisions about the strategy are attributed to the decision maker.

Match Tasks with Resources

After several strategies have been chosen for each objective, resources need to be assigned to make certain that the task or strategy is accomplished. This results in an action plan which specifies the work activities needed to achieve the objective. It includes what is to be done, who is responsible, and by what date each step should be completed. It should be possible to accomplish action steps in 1 to 12 months; each objective may have many action steps. For example, if one objective is "To raise the drinking age to 21 in Kentucky by 1992," the action plan that matches strategies with resources to achieve that objective might look like the one presented in Table 12-4.

Step two of the policy development phase results in an action plan that delineates specific action steps with responsible individuals, along with a realistic time frame. This type of plan facilitates the completion of necessary health planning activities.

Negotiate New Organizational Liaisons As Needed, and Establish Contracts As Needed

These steps of planning help planners to complete action steps. For example, if Ms. Alexander is responsible for a monthly newspaper article regarding the need to raise the drinking age to 21, she will need to have a firm commitment from the editor that the paper will print it. This may involve a visit by administrative personnel in the health

TABLE 12-4   Jones County Health Department: one action plan for the motor vehicle accident project

Objective: To raise the drinking age to 21 in Kentucky by 1992

Action steps	*Date*	*Person responsible*
Get support of the 15 Jones County PTAs	March 15, 1991	Eigsti
Get support of all district legislators	March 15, 1991	Clemen and Jones
Put one article each month of the year in the "Democrat and Chronicle"	Monthly	Alexander
Get support of grocery association	August 1, 1991	McGuire

department to the editorial director of the newspaper and a written or verbal agreement that such a plan is feasible. This may also be the situation if support from legislators is desired; liaison activities with community organizations interested in causes of motor vehicle accidents among youth and the health department who then, together, ask for political support may likely be necessary. These two steps may be the most difficult, and yet the most important, aspects needed to achieve positive outcomes from program planning activities.

Table 12-5, showing the planning sequence, summarizes the differences between goals, plans, objectives, and action steps, as well as the following parameters of each of these: functions, leadership, data base, time-span, and accountability.

Having an awareness of these differences is important, because each level of planning must be completed to ensure effective and efficient community health planning.

The Implementation Phase

The fourth phase of the health care planning process is implementation. All the work of the other phases finally leads to achievement of concrete outcomes in the real world. Implementation is, to a great extent, a political process which requires that those seeking to bring about change be very aware of the various forces present in the community. Will these forces help the changes to take place or can they be mobilized to provide support for the changes? Implementation involves incentives for people to change, public hearings, and

TABLE 12-5   The planning sequence

Planning level	Function	Primary leadership	Data base	Time-span	Accountability
Goals	To provide broad purpose and general direction for the organization	Board	Ideology, values, role, mission	Infinite	Everyone
Plans	To provide definitive direction and a plan for the organization	Chief executive Planning chairman Planning committee Adopted by board	Operational Societal (issues & trends) Opinions of community leaders, key internal lay & staff leaders	2-5 years	President, planning chairman, executive director
Objectives	To provide measurable specification of attainable outcomes within operational goals	Unit executives Unit boards and committees	Operational Clients Community Opinions of key internal lay and staff leaders of operating units	1 year	Executive director, specific staff
Action steps	To provide specification of steps to be taken and activities to be conducted to achieve objectives; persons responsible; completion dates	Unit Executives Staff	Operational Available resources	1-12 months	Individual staff

Developed by Christine DeGregorio, MSP, doctoral student in political science, University of Rochester, Rochester, NY.

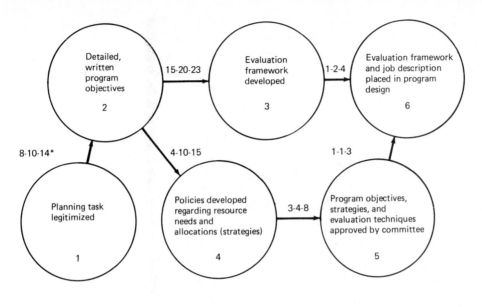

*Time in weeks

Figure 12-4 PERT chart sample sheet. (Developed by Christine De Gregorio, MSP, Graduate Student in Political Science, University of Rochester.)

advocacy for change. This phase calls for trust, rapport, and patience to work out new and difficult relationships and to respond to the unanticipated ramifications of the change.

In short, implementation is carrying out the plan. It involves organizing, delegating, and managing work so that the action steps prepared in the last phase are completed and objectives are accomplished within the specified time. These are the questions that planners need to answer in the implementation phase: What is to be done? How will it be done? Who will do it? What are the deadlines for each step? Who will monitor progress? How and when will the solution be evaluated?

A flowchart of activity that anticipates management problems is utilized throughout this phase. Two common methods of plotting this activity are program evaluation and review technique (PERT) charts and Gantt or Milestone charts.

A PERT chart (Figure 12-4) is designed to show the varied components that make up a planning system and the sequence and relationships among these components. It helps to evaluate progress toward planning objectives, aids in finding potential and actual problems, and predicts the likelihood of reaching objectives.

The first step in developing a PERT network is to specify the program objective(s) clearly and to visualize all the individual tasks needed to complete the program in a clear manner. In the following diagram, *event* (shown within the circles) represents the start or completion of a specified step in the program. Since it is an event, it does not consume time. An *activity* takes time and resources to progress from one event to the next; therefore the activity is represented by lines connecting circles or the events. An activity needed to accomplish event 1 on Figure 12-4, "Planning Task Legitimized," might be to meet with the executive director of the agency to gain the director's support for the program.

Events are typically represented by numbers that are not necessarily in sequential order. Numbering makes the identification and location of events and activities possible, since each event becomes known by its number and each activity by the numbers of the events at its start and completion. Since PERT is primarily concerned with control over time, three estimates for time are assigned to each activity. These help to measure the uncertainty and are estimated by people most familiar with the activity involved. The type of time estimates used in a PERT chart are:

1. *Optimistic time:* an estimate of the minimum time an activity will take, based on "everything going right the first time"
2. *Most likely time:* an estimate of the normal

time an activity will take if you were to repeat the activity over and over
3. *Pessimistic time:* an estimate of the maximum time an activity will take should a string of bad luck occur. (If one goes beyond this length of time, the program will not be completed.)

The three time estimates are usually written over the arrows that represent the activities in the PERT with "optimistic time" first, "pessimistic

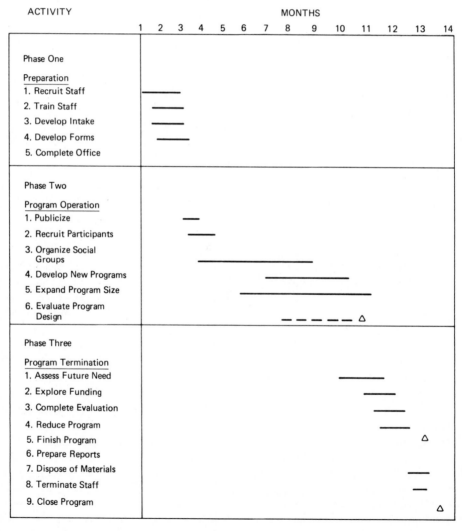

Figure 12-5   Gantt or Milestone chart. (Developed by Christine De Gregorio, MSP, Graduate Student in Political Science, University of Rochester.)

time" last, and "most likely time" in the middle. For example, in Figure 12-4, it is projected that event 1, "Planning Task Legitimized," could optimistically be completed in 8 weeks. However, it is most likely that this event will be done in 10 weeks or even in 14 weeks maximum. Thus, the time estimates would be written like this: 8-10-14.

Gantt is the name of the person who first promoted the second type of program time line. In a simple Gantt Timeline (Figure 12-5), the project is indicated by major events rather than a breakdown of the elements of that event. For example, "Train staff" may be the item noted on the chart. The event may have several major elements that will not be indicated on a simple Gantt. These might include needs assessment of staff, internal training resources, needed external resources, development of training materials, actual training, and evaluation of future training. On the chart, this process would be indicated by a line or arrow. If planners wanted to explain what occurred in that time frame, they would have to provide an additional explanation narrative to accompany the Gantt Timeline.

In a Gantt Milestone grid, one might use a small triangle to indicate the actual event. In combining these two types of charting, the process and the actual event on the chart, planners might use a dotted line to indicate a pre- or post-planning evaluation process and a triangle to indicate the event.

The Gantt Milestone is a good tool to use when there are many complex areas of program development that would require a very complex PERT chart. Planners use the Gantt Milestone approach to program development as a backup to needs assessment, program planning, and budget development. When one of these techniques is used, the best procedure is to list what must be done, who will do it, and when it must be done. Through such planning charts, many program or project directors have been able to avoid planning too many tasks for the same time period or tackling less urgent tasks until all essential tasks have been completed.

It is important to monitor the implementation plan to make certain that the correct sequence of

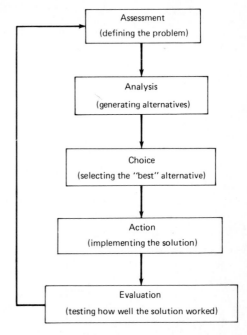

Figure 12-6 Summary of the planning process. (Developed by Christine De Gregorio, MSP, Graduate Student in Political Science, University of Rochester.)

activities needed to reach the program objectives is being carried out. This monitoring also enables the organization to identify successful and unsuccessful strategies and helps to monitor the progress being made in the achievement of objectives. While monitoring the implementation phase, the emphasis among planners is on the next phase of the health planning process—*evaluation*.

The Evaluation Phase

The fifth phase of the health care planning process, evaluation, is best seen as a continuous feedback process; it looks back upon actions to determine their effectiveness in order to make decisions regarding future actions. Figure 12-6 illustrates the feedback nature of the evaluation process.

There are three steps in the evaluation phase: document progress, compare achievements against a performance standard, and prepare for needed modifications. If any one of these steps is ignored, the evaluation process will be incomplete.

Document Progress

Keeping accurate and complete records of successes and problems in the process is a key activity to a productive evaluation. The following critique can be made of the planning document:

1. Are problems clearly defined?
2. Are the problems documented?
3. Are the solutions appropriate?
4. Do the solutions have many associated risks?
5. Is the scope of change envisioned satisfactory?
6. What impacts will the change have on rights, resources, and structures?
7. Are the risks worth the gains?
8. Are the objectives feasible?
9. Is the evaluation plan appropriate?

With the information obtained by asking the above questions, planners can move to the next step in the evaluation phase.

Compare Achievements against a Performance Standard

Performance standards are based on the objectives which were written in the assessment phase of the process. For each action step written to reach each objective, criteria or standards should be established prior to implementation. For example, if the objective is "to raise the drinking age to 21 years of age by 1992," and one of the action steps is to get support of the 15 Jones County Parent Teacher Associations, standards to evaluate this action step might be:

1. High achievement—support of all 15 PTAs
2. Adequate achievement—support of 10 PTAs
3. Inadequate progress—less than 10 PTAs support

Standards for evaluation should be established prior to the implementation of action steps. In addition, ways to determine if the standards were met should be developed. The method to obtain data about PTA support might involve a verbal report from the coordination PTA group. This method would be delineated on an action plan (refer to Table 12-4) as follows:

1. Source of data: verbal report from coordination PTA group
2. Time: May 1990
3. Responsibility: Mary Cox, CHN

For each action step, this kind of information should be collected so that there are objective data about the manner in which each objective is accomplished. Collecting objective data helps planners to more effectively evaluate progress or lack of progress. Objective data are usually more accurate than are subjective data. For example, "knowing you have support" of the PTA groups is far more significant than "thinking you have support." In addition, funders of health programs respond more favorably to objective data than they do to subjective information.

Prepare for Needed Modifications

The information obtained in the final step of the evaluation phase is used by planners to make decisions about the changes that need to be made in the objectives and associated action plans. The following questions need to be asked about the planning process:

1. Have any key informants been left out of the community planning process—citizens, professionals, leaders?
2. Was an adequate decision-making process used?
3. Have responsibilities and tasks been allocated appropriately?
4. Has there been negative feedback or a destructive impact (lost trust or commitment or heightened resistance) thus far?
5. What positive community responses (improved cooperation, trust, problem solving, heightened commitment, or greater resources) have occurred thus far?

As Figure 12-6 demonstrates, evaluation is a cycling process. "Although evaluation looks to past performance as planning looks to future performance, both are dependent upon skilled use of information in making decisions . . . to build in evaluation means to build into our thinking an analytic approach to what we are doing . . . it means continually asking the simple but pertinent question about every program action: Why should this be done?" (Arnold, Blankenship, and Hess, 1971, p. 282).

All five phases of the planning process—preplanning, assessment, policy development, implementation, and evaluation—are interrelated and are, in reality, not carried out separately in the manner that they have been presented. When the basic elements included in each phase are followed, planners have a much greater likelihood of success than when they are passed over. The health care planning process is a valuable tool for planners who wish to bring about change to solve a difficult problem.

Planners need to consider a number of other broad principles when planning for population groups. These broad principles assist planners to make knowledgeable decisions when progressing through all phases of the planning process.

KEY PRINCIPLES INVOLVED IN HEALTH PLANNING

When studying the subject of comprehensive health planning for developmental population groups, a number of principles emerge.

Community Diagnosis

Understanding the concepts presented in Chapter 11 relative to community diagnosis, along with the epidemiological variables of person, place, and time is essential to answer the key questions that health planners must ask as they assess health planning needs. *People* involve the "who" of community diagnosis. The cultural, ethnic, psychosocial, spiritual, and biological characteristics of the person variable must be considered when planning health services. These characteristics influence how persons define health and illness. Since these terms do not have a common meaning to all people, it is crucial to identify how the population being served views these concepts. If, for instance, a population narrowly defines health as the absence of disease, this population would probably respond more favorably to the provision of curative care than to the provision of preventive care.

Place describes the setting where services are planned. It may be rural or urban, the inner city or suburbia. When examining the characteristics of place, the availability, accessibility, and cost of present services should be analyzed. Size is also a factor to consider when looking at place. A community with 1000 residents will have different needs from a community which has a population of 1 million. The cost to deliver health services, the kinds of personnel and financial resources that are available, and the complexity involved in planning and implementing services are some factors that vary among populations of different sizes.

The basic unit of service in health planning is the population to be served and their distribution. Any planning that is done should take into consideration population size and distribution and needs as reflected by health statistics. Population size and mortality and morbidity rates for the future should be estimated. Future demands on the health care delivery system are determined in this way.

Time, in relation to urgency, needs to be considered when doing health planning. If the problem under consideration, for example, is an emergency such as influenza among aging citizens, immediate action must be taken. Other health problems such as accident prevention may not require immediate action but can necessitate action over time.

Long-term action presents more complex demands on the health planner. When long-term intervention is needed, mechanisms must be established to ensure that evaluation occurs periodically during the intervention phase, that coordination of all persons involved in the process is supported, and that public awareness of the problem and the health program is maintained.

It is extremely important to determine when the time is appropriate to initiate the health program under consideration. Analyzing such things as community values and attitudes, availability of resources, and cost-benefit factors helps the health planner to determine the appropriate time to begin health-planning intervention.

Examining a community's developmental history is another significant factor to consider when looking at the time variable. An older, inner-city ethnic community would probably have more set values and attitudes about health and illness than would a newer community, such as a prospering subdivision. Analyzing how values and attitudes have evolved over time in an older community assists the health planner identify key community leaders who can influence value and attitude changes and intervention strategies which have facilitated health behavior change in the past.

Planning for Comprehensive Care

A comprehensive health care system should plan for preventive, episodic, and catastrophic health care services for the entire population. Preventive services focus on the prevention of condition occurrence. Episodic services are diagnostic, curative, and restorative. Catastrophic services are designed to handle emergency and disaster situations and to help families who incur health situations beyond the scope of their financial resources.

Within the health care system there are various patterns for providing comprehensive services to populations. Generalized and specialized school health services, as well as generalized and specialized medical care offices, are examples of the types of patterns used to deliver health care. However, within each of these patterns, comprehensive care needs to be built into the program. How the nurse in the school setting plans for the delivery of comprehensive services to the school-age population is discussed in depth in Chapter 14. Planning preventive focused immunization programs against measles, rubella, and diphtheria, developing protocols for the handling of episodic health care needs, such as outbreaks of "nuisance" diseases, and establishing guidelines for handling emergency or catastrophic incidents are examples of some of the activities a nurse in the school setting would carry out to ensure that comprehensive care is available for the entire school-age population.

Communication

To function in a health-planning group, the nurse must be able to communicate well, openly, and assertively. The nurse must understand the contributions nursing can bring to the health of people and be able to explain these contributions to others. This skill develops with time and experience. Because functioning in a health-planning group with other professionals is an expected activity of every nurse working in community health, supervision must be available until the nurse learns the process and becomes more confident about his or her skills.

Communicating effectively in a health-planning group requires a firm understanding of group dynamics and a knowledge of population needs. A change in mindset is frequently necessary when beginning to plan for groups because nurses are often prepared to work only with individual clients. A concern for the problems of a community and planning for a group of people with similar characteristics means that the nurse must deal with problem defining and solving on a group level, involving other health care professionals. Nurses cannot, by themselves, resolve all the health care needs of a community.

Integration of Health Care Services

The integration of health care services for clients should be a high priority. In our present health care system, clients are seen by numerous caregivers and gaps in services and duplication of services are evident. Settings such as well-child clinics and school health services have often fostered the inefficient separation of routine physical examinations from diagnostic and treatment services. It is possible to establish protocols or standards of care within health care settings so that one health professional is able to take care of most client needs. At this time, a concentrated effort to integrate health care services and to develop standards for care is needed.

Total Health Care Programs

The concept of a total health program is basic to comprehensive health care. Rather than thinking of a nursing program offering health services, planners should identify the role of nursing in a health care program as well as the role of other disciplines, such as physicians, occupational therapists, nutritionists, and social workers.

No single discipline has all the answers in health planning. Team members need to acknowledge and respect each other's contributions. Team members may include ministers, priests, rabbis, pharmacists, health educators, school personnel, architects, physicians, psychiatrists, social workers, and environmentalists. Each of these professions brings a skill that aids clients with specific problems: the rabbi deals with spiritual affairs, the pharmacist deals with medicine regimens, and the nutritionist deals with nutritional concerns. The nurse's unique role is to be able to collate all of the information gathered by other professionals and to synthesize it when analyzing health care situations (Kinlein, 1977, p. 10). In addition, the nurse is in a key position to collect data that provide a foundation for understanding the health care needs of groups. For example, as the nurse visits homes, where and how families obtain food, prepare it, and eat it becomes known. The nurse may also learn where and how people buy medications, how well they do or do not follow prescribed therapy, and where health care services are or are not available.

The community health nurse is skilled in forming health care plans based on clients' lifestyles and the cultural and socioeconomic factors of the community. This knowledge, as well as data collected during home visiting, should be transmitted to other members of the health team when health planning for groups within the community takes place.

Consumer Participation

Consumer participation during the health-planning process is an absolute necessity for several reasons. The consumer is the recipient of care and can help to ensure that the provided services will be of high quality and at a reasonable cost. Consumers can also ascertain whether or not the services are responsive to the needs of those for whom they are intended. In addition, they can help to evaluate whether or not health-planning action has been effective. Finally, involving the consumer in the planning process helps to raise the consciousness of those participating about what constitutes good health and how to reach optimal health.

Lip service is more often given to the concept of consumer input than effort to effect actual consumer involvement. Consumers need to feel wanted and their efforts utilized. They need to be well informed about the health needs of the community and reasons for various health programs. They need the opportunity to share their concerns and needs and to influence community health action. Community planning must be truly community oriented.

SIGNIFICANT HEALTH LEGISLATION

Health planning does not have a long history in the United States. It began with the establishment of area-wide councils in the 1930s, which were formed to raise and allocate money for hospital construction and modernization. The members on these hospital councils were lay people involved in philanthropic and civic affairs as well as professionals such as hospital administrators (National Academy of Sciences, 1980, p. 13). For a long period of time, health planning was primarily reactive. Only after a health problem that affected a large number of people had been found was there an attempt to solve it. Beginning with some of President Johnson's Great Society programs in the 1960s, however, health planning was emphasized at the federal level. As described in Chapter 4, the Heart Disease, Cancer, and Stroke Amendment (Public Law 89-239), known as the Regional Medical Program, actively involved professionals in health planning. In 1966, the Comprehensive Health Planning and Public Health Service Amendment (Public Law 89-749) was passed. This was a significant document written to enable states and communities to plan for better use of health resources. There were many problems with this law, one being that no new plans could interfere with existing patterns of private practice of medicine and dentistry. The law was also inadequately funded. Because of these problems, other legislative action was taken in the mid-70s.

The National Health Planning and Resources Development Act of 1974 (Public Law 93-641) was signed by President Gerald Ford on January 4, 1975. Its purpose was to provide funding for program development activities and services which would improve the delivery of health care in local communities. It was hoped that this legislation would improve accessibility of health care services, curtail rising costs, and monitor the quality of care being provided.

The goals of the National Health Planning and Resources Development Act were clearly delineated in the preamble. The preamble stated that this law was passed "to facilitate the development of recommendations for a national health planning policy, to augment area wide and state planning for health services, manpower and facilities, and to authorize financial assistance for the development of resources to further that policy" (Rubel, 1976, p. 3).

The terms of Public Law 93-641 ended the existing Hill-Burton Act (1947-1974), Regional Medical Programs (1966-1974), and the Comprehensive Health Planning Programs (1966-1974). All of these programs were designed to correct health care delivery problems but none had the power to be comprehensive.

There were two new titles in Public Law 93-641: title XV and title XVI. Title XVI provided federal financial assistance for construction and modernization of health care facilities. Title XV created a national network of local health systems agencies (HSAs), state health planning and development agencies (SHPDAs), and statewide health coordinating councils (SHCCs). These agencies were regulatory and were responsible for health planning and the development of resources under the law. The HSAs were very important elements of Public Law 93-641. They were geographically located in designated regions where effective planning and development of resources could be implemented at the community level. Their purpose was to improve the health of residents in the area by increasing the availability, continuity, and quality of health services while simultaneously limiting the costs of health care. Decreasing duplication of services was also a major goal of these HSAs.

Public Law 93-641 also created a new National Council for Health Policy (NCHP). This council was located within the Department of Health and Human Services, and made recommendations to the secretary of DHHS on national health policy planning.

There were several major elements in the law that represented a new approach to planning for health services (Rubel, 1976, p. 4). First, there was an emphasis on strong local planning as well as local control over the development of services. All segments of the health care system, including providers of care, consumers, and third-party payers, must be part of health-planning boards. Second, the *certificate of need* (CON) program was to ensure that states did not develop health services that were not needed. Last, there were incentives to states to hold the cost of health care down.

The Demise of Public Law 93-641

The system of federally mandated health planning continued for 7 years. During this time, HSAs were taken seriously as planning agencies. This is evidenced by the fact that there was extensive investment of time and energy by volunteers in the activities of HSAs; newspapers regularly carried stories of their work; and the field of health law developed as hospitals and consumers hired attorneys to aid them in deliberations with the HSAs.

However, there were also problems. Political conservatives did not like government regulation of health care and many resented what they perceived to be the interference of the federal government in local government. Some critics felt that the program did not save enough money, and others felt that there was not sufficient concern for quality care.

By 1981, the Reagan administration proposed the goal of eliminating federal health planning requirements by 1982. Its arguments for this goal were that Public Law 93-641 had not controlled cost and that states should be making their own planning decisions. Further, regulation of supply was counter to free market competition.

The Omnibus Budget Reconciliation Act, passed in 1981 (discussed in Chapter 19), ended the federal mandate for planning under Public Law 93-641. Under the Reconciliation Act, states could request that all funding for HSAs be eliminated. Further, this act stipulated that HSAs were no longer required to collect data or review existing facilities and proposed federal grants. Appropriations for funding HSAs were reduced from their high of $167 million in 1980 to $64 million for 1981. The result was that there was not enough money to support HSAs at the staffing levels required by law. Finally, in 1987, HSA legislation was repealed.

The Development of Health Block Grants

Another piece of legislation passed during the Reagan administration which had a tremendous impact upon health care planning in the 1980s was the development of health block grants. Block grants were part of the Federal Omnibus Budget Reconciliation Act (Public Law 97-35), which reorganized the amount and type of federal health care expenditures. The act had two effects: traditional federal categorical grant programs and the funding for these programs was reduced by 25 percent. This legislation affected four areas of health care: maternal and child health; prevention; community health services (primary care); and alcohol, drug abuse, and mental health.

A block grant is a funding mechanism through which the federal government supports a state or local health program. Normally, a block grant is a lump sum given by the federal government to a state unit such as a health department; the state unit has the freedom (under some broad restrictions) to finance various activities within the block grant functional area. Categorical grants also make federal money available to state and local units for health care programs. However, categorical grants can be used only for specifically designated programs and are usually limited to activities narrowly defined by federal laws. Thus, categorical grants allow much less flexibility in the use of funds than do block grants.

The reasoning of the Reagan administration for establishing health block grants was that state-controlled block grants would result in improved, less costly service by allowing the development of health care programs that are more responsive to local needs. It was believed that states would accomplish this by consolidating programs which address similar needs and by having fewer restrictive federal requirements on how money was spent in a given community. Unfortunately, the result is that block grant programs can also "harm local health programs that already exist by terminating federally established program allocation criteria, decreasing program evaluation and monitoring, setting up unclear new state administrative procedures, and using the funds for political rather than public health concerns" (Massachusetts Public Health Association, 1982, p. 4). Further complicating these problems is the major reduction in overall funding for the four programs mentioned above at a loss of about 25 percent of the previous federal monies spent on health care.

Community health nurses need to be aware of the significance of health block grants, because they affect four vital areas of concern to professionals who care about the health and well-being of population groups. In particular, mothers and children are one of the most vulnerable populations affected by this new legislation. Planners need to ask what critical services will be or have been cut under this legislation.

INTERDISCIPLINARY FUNCTIONING

Nursing's role in the formulation of health policy remains to be developed almost from the ground floor. Collaboration with other members of the health team in this formulation is an exciting, evolving responsibility of nurses in all settings. It is a responsibility that provides challenging opportunities for expanding one's awareness of community needs and for influencing community health action.

A team is a group of persons who have a set of tasks that need to be accomplished. A cooperative and collaborative effort is essential if tasks are going to be completed. To be truly effective, the energy of the group should be spent on accomplishing its tasks as well as developing team cohesiveness and satisfaction. Defining team tasks is not an easy process, but if it is not done, confusion and lack of direction in decision making results.

Defining tasks for an interdisciplinary team in the community setting presents special planning

TABLE 12-6 Comparison of effectiveness of two different teams

Condition	Surgical team	Community primary care team
Purpose	Specific: to operate and heal	General: comprehensive care
Task	Very clear	Somewhat unclear: probably many tasks
Who does what?	Roles and functions very clear	Roles ambiguous: several members may perform same functions for different patients
Where work is performed	In one location	In a number of locations
Decision making	Clear hierarchy: surgeon, first assistant, scrub nurse	Unclear: group of colleagues with different information and skills; group decisions sometimes required
Communication	One-way command system	May be discussion and problem solving
Goal priorities	Same for all members	May vary among members

From Beckhard R: Organizational issues in the team delivery of comprehensive health care, Milbank Q 1:293, 1972.

challenges for the community health nurse and other health care professionals. This is so because professionals in the community setting have a much broader health focus than do professionals in other settings. Identifying specific tasks to be accomplished when one has a broad focus can be difficult and more time-consuming. Beckhard (1972) substantiated this fact when he compared the effectiveness of a surgical team and a community primary care team. Both were defined as teams, and yet the amount of time to maintain the community care team was lengthy compared with the surgical team. Table 12-6 presents some of the reasons why the community team was less effective in this particular study. Beckhard's findings are not atypical, however. Handling role ambiguity concerns, resolving priority issues, defining specific tasks when goals are very broad, and facilitating group decision making are common activities that all interdisciplinary community health teams need to address.

Every interdisciplinary team needs to openly discuss, very early in the planning phase, the problems identified by Beckhard. Group members need to state what contributions they can make during the health-planning process and the role of their discipline in the community setting. The group's end goals must be defined so that each team member is working toward the same goal. Mechanisms for enhancing decision making

must be established, otherwise goals will never be reached. Communication should be open so that differences of opinion can be questioned and ambiguities can be addressed.

Communicating effectively takes time, is never perfect, and requires the leadership of a person who is skilled in helping each person to contribute. Individuals on the health-planning team will communicate in a group as they communicate in other settings: some are aggressive and others will withdraw. The seasoned leader can aid the group in functioning effectively. This leader may be part of the administration of the agency or may be a state-level or university consultant.

There is a wealth of information written for those who are interested in perfecting the state of working collaboratively with other disciplines (Wise, Beckhard, Rubin, and Kyte, 1974; Kane, 1975). The reader may wish to refer to these writings to obtain a more in-depth view of interdisciplinary team functioning.

BARRIERS TO HEALTH PLANNING

Each step in the process of health planning goes down neatly on paper. Carrying out the process in "real life" is a different and challenging activity. There are several barriers to health planning that need to be acknowledged. Some of these, such as unavailability and inaccessibility of resources, inadequate knowledge, and lack of commitment to health planning, were addressed previously. Others are presented below.

A major barrier to effective health planning is a lack of understanding of the term *health*. Health is an elusive state that is difficult to define. What causes health is not easy to enumerate. It is possible to list healthy behaviors, but no one can guarantee health because both health and disease are affected by multiple, interrelated variables (multiple causation principle). Epidemiological research has not yet been sufficient to document what these multiple causes are for many conditions or what health actions most effectively promote health and prevent disease. Thus, it is difficult for health planners to develop health action strategies for many situations. As more epidemiological research is conducted, this barrier should become less acute.

The disease-oriented focus in our present health care delivery system presents another key barrier to health planning. Health promotion and prevention concepts are very often not accepted by lay and professional people alike in this system. Skyrocketing health costs have severely disrupted the health care system of the country, and thus community health prevention programs have been badly neglected. Basically what has happened is that persons spend so much money curing illness that there is little money left for preventive health care.

Lack of sufficient money and personnel is a constant barrier. Health may not be a priority for communities so that energy and money are spent in other directions. Health planning is often a political rather than a technical or analytical exercise, and it is possible to see an ongoing contest between local, state, and federal governments for control of planning agencies and money.

Noncompliance with health-planning activities is also a barrier. In the United States, freedom of choice is a highly prized right. Safety belts save lives, but one may choose whether or not to use them. Healthy behaviors can be presented as options but that is all. Differing values promote different priorities. If an individual is not motivated to seek preventive care, preventive health-planning action will be ineffective.

The health care system in the United States is an enormous industry that has unbelievable growth each year. Health care is a basic part of the American economy; it is inevitable that it should not function perfectly. Efforts are being made, however, to improve the quality of health care in our country.

TRENDS IN COMMUNITY HEALTH PLANNING

Several trends are emerging in the health care planning sector (Sofarer, 1988). They include the growth of institutional strategic planning as can be seen in such facilities as hospitals, which have added planners to their staff. These planners are challenged to define goals and strategies that will ensure the competitive economic advantage of that institution; community needs are important but only when they generate market driven demands for service. Another trend is the development of consumer coalitions such as businesses and labor unions, which understand that they have substantial purchasing power in the health care market and can demand sophisticated health care. These consumers understand that they do not need to take on the increasing costs; they challenge insurers to manage their risks within a cost-constrained environment. The most recent trend is the emergence of ad hoc groups to deal with problems that the health care system cannot effectively address. Community forums are emerging to deal with the problems of the indigent, the homeless, and the uninsured. These trends reflect our continuing failure to create and maintain effective planning for the community's health.

SUMMARY

Health planning for population groups is a major function of the community health nurse. In any community setting, there are groups at risk for specific health problems. The developmental framework helps the community health nurse to identify groups at risk across the life span.

Community health nurses provide unique contributions during the health planning process. Educational experiences prepare nurses to comprehensively analyze needs of families as well as populations. Clinical practice brings them in touch daily with consumer concerns and helps in identifying gaps or duplication in the health care delivery system.

Currently, there are obvious deficiencies in the health care delivery system which warrant health planning action. Health care services are frequently fragmented, extremely costly, and often lacking for specific segments of the population. However, there has been a positive trend evolving which places emphasis on developing new ways to meet the health care needs of all citizens.

Involvement in health-planning activities can be exciting and rewarding. Nurses are increasingly recognizing the importance of actively participating on health-planning teams and engaging in political activities aimed at changing health policy.

REFERENCES

American Nurses' Association, Division on Community Health Nursing: A conceptual model of community health nursing (CH-10 2M), Kansas City, Mo, 1980, The Association.

American Nurses' Association, Community Health Nursing Division: Standards of community health nursing practice (Pub No CH-10), Kansas City, Mo, 1986, The Association.

American Public Health Association, Public Health Nursing Section: The definition and role of public health nursing in the delivery of health care, Washington, DC, 1981, The Association.

Arnold M, Blankenship L, and Hess J: Administering health systems. Issues and perspectives, Chicago, 1971, Aldine & Atherton.

Ashley JA: Nursing and early feminism, Am J Nurs 75:1465-1467, 1975. Reprinted with the permission of the American Journal of Nursing Company. Copyright by the American Journal of Nursing Company.

Beckhard R: Organizational issues in the team delivery of comprehensive health care, Milbank Q 1:287-316, 1972.

Blum HL: Planning for health—generics for the eighties, ed 2, New York, 1981, Human Sciences Press.

Commonwealth Fund Commission: Medicare's poor: filling the gaps in medical coverage for low-income elderly Americans, Baltimore, Md, 1987, The Commission.

Dever GE: Community health analysis. A holistic approach, Germantown, Md, 1980, Aspen Systems.

Institute of Medicine: The future of public health, Washington, DC, 1988, National Academy Press.

Kane RA: Interprofessional teamwork, Syracuse, NY, 1975, Syracuse University School of Social Work.

Kinlein ML: Independent nursing practice with clients, Philadelphia, 1977, Lippincott.

Lalonde M: A new perspective on the health of Canadians, Ottawa, 1974, Office of the Canadian Minister of National Health and Welfare.

Long GV, Whitman C, Johansson M, Williams C, and Tuthill RW: Evaluation of a school health program directed to children with a history of high absence, Am J Public Health 65:388-393, 1975.

MacStravic R: Setting priorities in health planning: what does it all mean? Inquiry 15:20-24, 1978.

Massachusetts Public Health Association: Block grants in Massachusetts: recommendations and issues, Boston, 1982, The Association.

Milio N: Promoting health through public policy, Philadelphia, 1981, FA Davis.

Milio N: Public policy as the cornerstone for a new public health: local and global beginnings, Fam Community Health 10(2):57-64, 1988.

National Academy of Sciences, Institute of Medicine: Health planning in the United States: issues in guideline development, Washington, DC, 1980, The National Academy.

National League for Nursing, Public Affairs Advisory: The purposes and politics of HSA's, New York, 1979, The League.

Rubel EJ: Implementing the National Health Planning and Resources Development Act of 1974, Public Health Rep 91:3-8, 1976.

Ruybal SE: Community health planning, Fam Community Health 1:9-18, 1978.

Sofarer S: Community health planning in the United States: a postmortem, Fam Community Health 10(4):1-12, 1988.

Spiegel AD and Hyman HH: Basic health planning methods, Germantown, Md, 1978, Aspen Systems.

Taylor I and Knowelden J: Principles of epidemiology, ed 2, Boston, 1964, Little, Brown.

US Congress, Office of Technology Assessment: Healthy children: investing in the future (OTA-H-345), Washington, DC, 1988, US Government Printing Office.

US Department of Health and Human Services (USDHHS): Promoting health/preventing disease. Objectives for the nation, Washington, DC, 1980, US Government Printing Office.

USDHHS: Prevention '82 (DHHS Pub No PHS 82-50157), Washington, DC, 1982, US Government Printing Office.

USDHHS: The 1990 health objective for the nation: a midcourse review, Washington, DC, 1986, US Government Printing Offfice.

USDHHS: Health United States, Washington, DC, 1987, US Government Printing Office.

USDHHS: Prevention '86/'87: federal programs and progress, Washington, DC, 1987, US Government Printing Office.

USDHHS: Public Health Service: Promoting health preventing disease: year 2000 objectives for the nation, Washington, DC, 1989, US Government Printing Office.

US Department of Health, Education, and Welfare (USDHEW): Healthy people: the Surgeon General's report on health promotion and disease prevention (DHEW Pub No PHS 79-55071A), Washington, DC, 1979, US Government Printing Office.

USDHEW: Guidelines for the development of health systems plans and annual implementation plans, Hyattsville, Md, 1979, Bureau of Health Planning.

Williams CA: Community health nursing—what is it? Nurs Outlook 25:250-254, 1977.

Wise H, Beckhard R, Rubin I, and Kyte A: Making health teams work, Cambridge, Ma, 1974, Ballinger.

SELECTED BIBLIOGRAPHY

American Nurses' Association: Community-based nursing services: innovative models, Kansas City, Mo, 1986, The Association.

Bagwell M and Clements S: A political handbook for health professionals, Boston, 1985, Little, Brown.

Battista RN and Lawrence RS, eds: Implementing preventive services, New York, 1988, Oxford University Press.

DeBella S, Martin L, and Siddall F: Nurses' role in health care planning, New York, 1986, Appleton-Century-Crofts.

Emery KR: Developing a new or modified service: analysis for decision making, Health Care Super 4(2):30-38, 1986.

Navarro U: Why some countries have national health insurance, others have national health services, and the United States has neither, Int J Health Services 19:384-404, 1989.

Oda DS: The imperative of a national health strategy for children: is there a political will? Nurs Outlook 37:206-208, 1989.

Rosenbaum S and Johnson KA: Providing health care for low-income children: reconciling child health goals with child health financing realities, Milbank Q 64:442-478, 1986.

Salem DA and Levine IS: Enhancing mental health services for homeless persons: state proposals under the MHSH block grant program, Public Health Rep 104:241-246, 1989.

Spotts H and Schewe C: Communicating with the elderly consumer: the growing health care challenge, J Health Care Market 9(3):36-44, 1989.

Wheelan TL and Hunger JD: Strategic management and business policy, ed 3, Reading, Ma, 1989, Addison-Wesley.

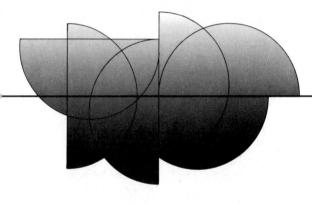

UNIT FIVE

Meeting the Needs of Populations at Risk across the Lifespan

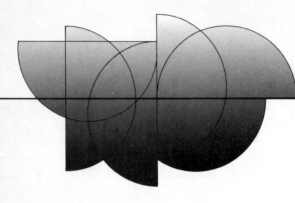

13

The Needs and Services of Children from Birth to 5 Years and the Care and Nurture of Their Parents

Train up a child in the way he should go, and when he is old he will not depart from it.

Common Health Risks

    Risks before Birth

    Risks after Birth

    Problems of Children Ages 1 to 5

Health Promotion Needs

    Health Promotion before Birth

    Health Promotion during Pregnancy

    Health Promotion after Birth

    Single Parents

    Preventive Health Care

    Accident Prevention

    Prevention of Child Maltreatment

    Preschool Assessments

Day Care for Children

General Concepts of Health Promotion

Infants with Long-Term Physical/Neurological Handicaps

Significant Health Legislation

    Medicaid

    Child Maltreatment

    Maternal-Child Health Program

    Developmental Disabilities

Barriers to Health Care

The Roles of the Community Health Nurse

Summary

OBJECTIVES

Upon completion of this chapter, the reader will be able to:

1. *Describe U.S. trends in infant and maternal mortality and why health care professionals are concerned about these trends.*
2. *Discuss the 1990 Federal Program Objectives for Pregnancy and Infant Health.*
3. *Discuss the leading causes of mortality among infants and children 1 through 5 years of age.*
4. *Analyze factors associated with high-risk pregnancies and births.*
5. *Discuss common health problems for infants and children aged 1 through 5.*

6. *Analyze health promotion needs of families with children in the 0- to 5-year age group and community health nursing interventions to address these needs.*
7. *Discuss significant legislation that has influenced maternal and child health care delivery.*
8. *Describe barriers to the delivery of services to the 0- to 5-year old population and their parents.*
9. *Identify the roles assumed by the community health nurse to promote maternal, infant, and child health.*

The wise King Solomon wrote the proverb found at the beginning of this chapter 3000 years ago. Today, parents are still struggling to find out what it means to "train up a child in the way he should go," although a modern version would certainly translate the end result to be the maximizing of the child's potential and helping him or her maintain balance and direction in the environment (Dunn, 1973, p. 4). Maximizing the potential and maintaining balance is not easy. Children and their parents form an important team in reaching developmental milestones. It is difficult to separate the health of one from the health of the other. Although parents struggle with all of the child's developmental age levels, the first 5 years in a child's life are the most important for the simple reason that they come first. They are the formative years and their influence upon the years that follow are beyond calculation.

Federal, state, and local health professionals have had concern for maternal-infant health that can be traced to the turn of the century. The concern for maternal-infant health stems from the fact that the health of the infant cannot be separated from the health of the parents, and particularly the mother. In 1900 deaths of mothers and children were major contributors to mortality figures: approximately 60 mothers died for every 10,000 pregnancies that produced live-born infants; of every 1000 live births, 100 infants did not survive the first year of life (Pickett and Hanlon, 1990, p. 400).

Statistics such as these motivated concerned individuals to develop community maternal-child health programs; nursing assumed a major leadership role in this effort (refer to Figure 13-1). Lillian Wald, the pioneer community health nurse and feminist, helped establish milk stations in 1903 at the Henry Street Settlement House in New York City to ensure the safety of milk for babies. Diarrhea caused by contaminated milk in the summer months was the cause of many deaths. The City of New York followed this example and in 1911 authorized the establishment of 15 milk stations:

A nurse is attached to each station to follow into the homes and there lay the foundation, through education, for hygienic living. A marked reduction in infant mortality has been brought about and moreover, a realization, on the part of the city, of the immeasurable social and economic value of keeping the babies alive. (Wald, 1915, p. 57)

Traditionally, childbearing women, infants, and children are considered to be the most dependent and vulnerable members in a society. As the society develops, there is a trend toward greater concern for this segment of the population. The health of a society's children ensures that society's future, so this concern for infants and children is justified on economic as well as other grounds.

The mortality rates for mothers and children are frequently used to assess the health of populations. Since the turn of the century, significant progress has been made in the United States in reducing maternal and infant mortality. During the past 50 years, maternal mortality decreased approximately 99 percent and infant mortality declined about 89 percent (Pickett and Hanlon, 1990, p. 393). This progress was due to factors such as improved medical care, better housing, sanitation, and nutrition, as well as the decline of infectious diseases because of immunizing agents and the introduction of antibiotics and other therapeutic medicines.

During the period 1970 to 1987, the infant mortality rate declined from 20 to 10.1 deaths per 1000 live births (USDHHS, Office of Maternal and Child Health, 1989, p. 16). Explanations for this decline include the falling birth rate and the advent of better maternity and infant care services for high-risk mothers and babies. The outcome is that more mothers and babies are surviving.

Although dramatic progress has been made in reducing infant mortality throughout this century, it continues to be of great concern to health professionals. Our country, which had one of the lowest infant mortality rates 30 years ago, ranked last among 20 industrialized nations in 1986 (Brecht, 1989, p. 18). The rapid decline in the infant mortality rate experienced during the 1960s and 1970s slowed for both blacks and whites in the 1980s.

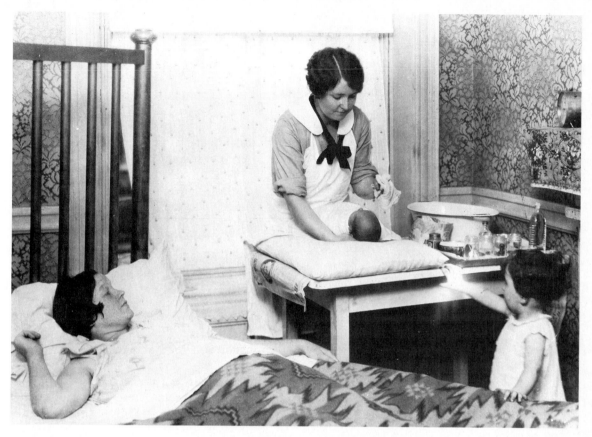

Figure 13-1 A community health nurse from the Visiting Nurse Service of New York City visits a mother with a new baby at home in the early 1930s. (Visiting Nurse Service of New York City.)

The increasing complexity and cost to the public of meeting the needs of those 0 to 5 years old, as well as the numbers of deaths and handicapping conditions that are present, make it essential that efforts to fulfill the health needs of this age group and their parents be organized on all levels of society. Everyone, regardless of race or economic level, has the right to health care and health education. All persons also need assistance in altering unhealthy behaviors.

The national "priority objectives" for pregnancy and infant health are displayed in the box on p. 456. These objectives were set by the Surgeon General of the United States in 1979 in an effort to improve the status of maternal and infant health by 1990. Current projections for 1990 reflect that the majority of these objectives will not

be met (Centers for Disease Control, 1988, p. 405). Thus, maternal and child health will continue to be a major focus in the *Year 2000 Objectives for the Nation.* These objectives reflect emphases similar to those in the 1979 federal priorities and target special population groups, namely low-income, black, American Indian/Alaska natives and Hispanic women, and black and American Indian/Alaska native infants (USDHHS, Public Health Service, 1989, pp. 11-3 and 11-5).

Both public and private efforts were initiated in the 1980s to combat infant and maternal mortality. The Healthy Mothers, Healthy Babies Coalition was started in December 1980 by six national organizations, one of which was the American Nurses' Association, following the Surgeon Gen-

---

1990 Federal Priority Objectives for Pregnancy and Infant Health

IMPROVED HEALTH STATUS

1. National infant mortality rate (IMR) should be reduced to no more than 9 deaths per 1,000 live births.
2. The neonatal death rate should be reduced to no more than 6.5 deaths per 1,000.
3. The perinatal death rate should be reduced to no more than 5.5 deaths per 1,000.
4. No county, racial, or ethnic group should have an IMR in excess of 12 deaths per 1,000.
5. No county, racial, or ethnic group should have a maternal mortality rate of more than 5 deaths per 100,000 live births.

REDUCED RISK FACTORS

6. Low birthweight (LBW) babies (less than 2,500 grams) should constitute not more than 5% of live births.
7. No county, racial, or ethnic group should have an LBW rate that exceeds 9%.
8. The majority of infants should leave hospitals in car safety seats.

INCREASED PUBLIC AWARENESS

9. Eighty-five percent of women of childbearing age should be able to choose foods wisely and should understand the hazards of smoking, alcohol, and drugs during pregnancy and lactation.

IMPROVED SERVICES AND PROTECTION

10. All women and infants should be served at a level appropriate to their need by a regionalized system of perinatal care.
11. The proportion of women in any county, racial, or ethnic group who obtain no prenatal care during the first trimester of pregnancy should not exceed 10%.
12. All newborns should be screened for metabolic disorders for which effective tests and treatments are available.
13. All infants should be able to participate in comprehensive primary health care.

From Centers for Disease Control: Progress toward achieving the 1990 objectives for pregnancy and infant health. MMWR 37:406, July 8, 1988.

---

eral's Workshop on Maternal and Infant Health. This coalition is now a cooperative venture of 80 national voluntary, health professional, and government organizations. It is focusing on high-level prenatal, obstetric, and neonatal care; preventive

services during the first year of life; education of health professionals; and broad public information activities aimed at pregnant women and their families (Arkin, 1986).

The National Commission to Prevent Infant Mortality was created by Congress (Public Law 99-660) in 1986 to establish a national strategic plan for the United States, designed to reduce infant mortality and morbidity (National Commission to Prevent Infant Mortality, 1989, Home visiting). The Commission's plan for action was presented to Congress in August, 1988, in its report entitled, "Death Before Life: The Tragedy of Infant Mortality." The commission focused on practical solutions for improving maternal and child health and identified two major goals: a) that every pregnant woman and infant receive adequate care, the woman as soon as she knows she is pregnant and the infant from the moment of birth; and b) that maternal and child health and well-being become a national priority (National Commission to Prevent Infant Mortality, 1988, August).

Infant mortality is a critical problem; each year about 40,000 babies die before their first birthday (National Commission to Prevent Infant Mortality, 1988, May, Infant Mortality and the Media). All sectors of society—government, communities, health professionals, business, and industry—must focus attention on this problem. Infant mortality is very costly to society, in both human and economic terms (National Commission to Prevent Infant Mortality, 1988, May, 1985 Indirect Costs).

Figure 13-2, which presents infant mortality rates for the United States from 1950 through 1987 by specified race, graphically illustrates that the color of an infant's skin is a measure of the chances of that infant's survival. Although infant mortality in the United States has declined over the years, and though the disparity between white and minority infant death rates has narrowed, black infant death rates continue to be twice as high as those for whites (USDHHS, Office of Maternal and Child Health, 1989).

Morbidity among the 0- to 5-year-old population, as well as mortality, presents a major public

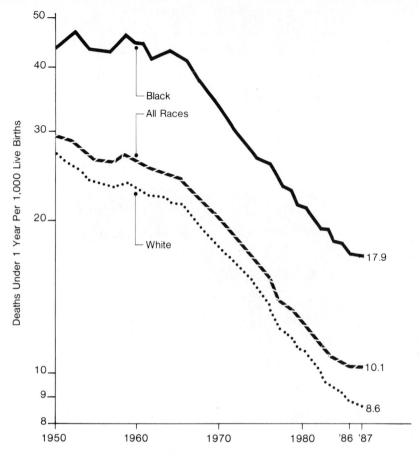

Figure 13-2   U.S. infant mortality rates by race, 1950-1987. (From National Center for Health Statistics cited in USDHHS, Office of Maternal and Child Health: Child health USA '89, Washington, DC, 1989, US Government Printing Office, p 16.)

health concern. In the process of growing up, children encounter injuries and illnesses that interfere with normal functioning. Jack and Jill's broken crown and Humpty Dumpty's fall off the wall are common experiences known to every child.

There are health problems common to the 0- to 5-year age group that can be prevented as well as problems that necessitate secondary and tertiary prevention. In order to plan health services for this group, the community health nurse should be familiar with factors that increase children's risk for morbidity and mortality. Having this knowledge facilitates application of the three levels of prevention as well as case finding.

COMMON HEALTH RISKS

Figures 13-3 and 13-4 show the leading causes of death for children under 1 year as well as children 1 to 14 years. About two thirds of all infant deaths occur in the neonatal period or the first 28 days of life (U.S. Congress, Office of Technology Assessment, 1988, p. 4). Infants most at risk during this period are low-birth-weight babies or those weighing less than 5½ pounds. These babies are 40 times more likely than normal-weight infants to die during the neonatal period (Institute of Medicine, 1985). Congenital anomalies cause a significant number of infant deaths during both the neonatal

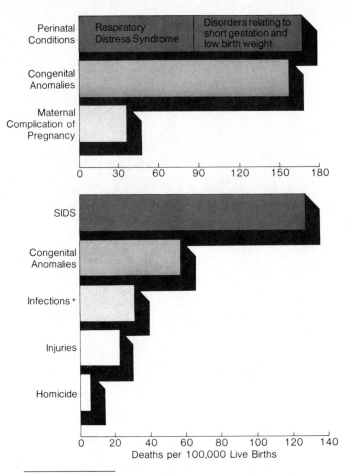

*The category entitled infection includes pneumonia, influenza, septicemia, meningitis, bronchitis, and viral diseases.

Figure 13-3 Neonatal (*top*) and postneonatal (*bottom*) mortality, 1987. (From National Center for Health Statistics cited in USDHHS, Office of Maternal and Child Health: Child health USA '89, Washington, DC, 1987, US Government Printing Office, p 17.)

and postneonatal (28 days to 1 year) periods. In 1985, 45 percent of all deaths among infants under 1 year of age were attributable to this cause (National Safety Council, 1988, p. 8). The most important cause of death during the postnatal period is sudden infant death syndrome (SIDS). SIDS accounts for more than one third of all postnatal deaths. Economic and educational deprivation, the continuing high rate of teenage pregnancy, and barriers impeding access to prenatal, perinatal, and infant care, particularly for disadvantaged groups, are other factors known to have a negative impact on infant survival (Task Force

on Infant Mortality, 1987; USDHHS, Office of Disease Prevention and Health Promotion, 1986). As children become mobile, accidental injuries become the major cause of death.

Risks before Birth

Factors associated with high-risk pregnancies (refer to the box on p. 460) have been known for a considerable length of time, and have not changed significantly in recent years. These factors are important to know because they provide the basis for the high mortality and morbidity rates during the first year of life and contribute to

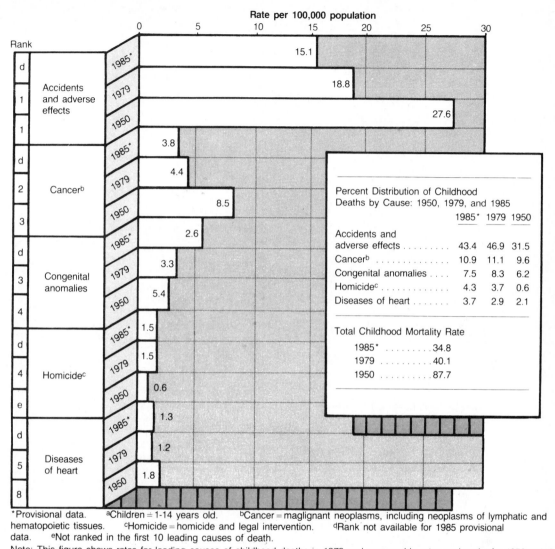

Rate per 100,000 population

Rank	Cause	Year	Rate
d	Accidents and adverse effects	1985*	15.1
1		1979	18.8
1		1950	27.6
d	Cancer[b]	1985*	3.8
2		1979	4.4
3		1950	8.5
d	Congenital anomalies	1985*	2.6
3		1979	3.3
4		1950	5.4
d	Homicide[c]	1985*	1.5
4		1979	1.5
e		1950	0.6
d	Diseases of heart	1985*	1.3
5		1979	1.2
8		1950	1.8

Percent Distribution of Childhood
Deaths by Cause: 1950, 1979, and 1985

	1985*	1979	1950
Accidents and adverse effects	43.4	46.9	31.5
Cancer[b]	10.9	11.1	9.6
Congenital anomalies	7.5	8.3	6.2
Homicide[c]	4.3	3.7	0.6
Diseases of heart	3.7	2.9	2.1

Total Childhood Mortality Rate

1985*	34.8
1979	40.1
1950	87.7

*Provisional data.   [a]Children = 1-14 years old.   [b]Cancer = maglignant neoplasms, including neoplasms of lymphatic and hematopoietic tissues.   [c]Homicide = homicide and legal intervention.   [d]Rank not available for 1985 provisional data.   [e]Not ranked in the first 10 leading causes of death.
Note: This figure shows rates for leading causes of childhood deaths in 1979 and comparable rates and ranks for 1950 and 1985.

Figure 13-4 Leading causes of childhood deaths: 1950, 1979, and 1985. (From National Center for Health Statistics cited in USDHHS: Prevention '86/87, federal programs and progress, Washington, DC, 1987, US Government Printing Office, p 24.)

the high maternal mortality rates. They are danger signs, signaling threat to the newborn and the mother. Those caring for the pregnant mother can effectively use these high risk indicators to identify mothers and infants who have special care needs and can benefit from preventive interventions.

Many of the same elements that influence infant mortality have an effect on maternal mortality. Among the most important of these are the continuing high rate of teenage pregnancy; late entry into prenatal care; barriers impeding access to maternity care; inadequate "systems" of care for high-risk women; and the continuing high rate of unintended births (USDHHS, Office of Disease Prevention and Health Promotion, 1986, pp. 41-42). As is demonstrated in the box on p. 460, socially and economically deprived persons are

---

Factors Associated with High-Risk Pregnancy

1. DEMOGRAPHIC FACTORS

 a. Lower socioeconomic status
 b. Disadvantaged ethnic groups
 c. Marital status: unwed mothers
 d. Maternal age
   (1) Gravida less than 16 years of age
   (2) Primigravida 35 years of age or older
   (3) Gravida 40 years of age or older
 e. Maternal weight: nonpregnant weight less than 100 lb or more than 200 lb
 f. Stature: height less than 62 in (1.57 m)
 g. Malnutrition
 h. Poor physical fitness

2. PAST PREGNANCY HISTORY

 a. Grand multiparity: six previous pregnancies terminating beyond 20 weeks' gestation
 b. Antepartum bleeding after 12 weeks of gestation
 c. Premature rupture of membranes, premature onset of labor, premature delivery
 d. Previous cesarean section or mid- or high-forceps delivery
 e. Prolonged labor
 f. Infant with cerebral palsy, mental retardation, birth trauma, central nervous system disorder, or congenital anomaly
 g. Reproductive failure: infertility, repetitive abortion, fetal loss, stillbirth, or neonatal death
 h. Delivery of preterm (less than 37 weeks) or postterm (more than 42 weeks) infant

3. PAST OR PRESENT MEDICAL HISTORY

 a. Hypertension or renal disease or both
 b. Diabetes mellitus (overt or gestational)
 c. Cardiovascular disease (rheumatic, congenital, or peripheral vascular)
 d. Pulmonary disease producing hypoxemia and hypercapnia
 e. Thyroid, parathyroid, and endocrine disorders
 f. Idiopathic thrombocytopenic purpura
 g. Neoplastic disease
 h. Hereditary disorders
 i. Collagen diseases
 j. Epilepsy

4. ADDITIONAL OBSTETRIC AND MEDICAL CONDITIONS

 a. Toxemia
 b. Asymptomatic bacteriuria
 c. Anemia or hemoglobinopathy
 d. Rh sensitization
 e. Habitual smoking
 f. Drug addiction or habituation
 g. Chronic exposure to any pharmacologic or chemical agent
 h. Multiple pregnancy
 i. Rubella or other viral infection
 j. Intercurrent surgery and anesthesia
 k. Placental abnormalities and uterine bleeding
 l. Abnormal fetal lie or presentation, fetal anomalies, oligohydramnios, polyhydramnios
 m. Abnormalities of fetal or uterine growth or both
 n. Maternal trauma during pregnancy
 o. Maternal emotional crisis during pregnancy

Adapted from Vaughn VC, McKay RJ, and Behrman RE, eds, and Nelson WE, senior ed, Textbook of Pediatrics, ed 11, Philadelphia, 1979, Saunders.

more likely than others to have high-risk pregnancies. This is at least partially explained by the lack of adequate prenatal care, which is unavailable to many population groups, including the inner city and rural poor, teenage mothers, and disadvantaged ethnic groups (e.g., black, Hispanic, and Native American women).

Early, regular prenatal care results in improved pregnancy outcomes: numerous studies have demonstrated that prematurity and infant mortality rates are lowest when prenatal care begins before the fourth month of pregnancy and continues with at least eight prenatal visits (USDHHS, 1985). However, in spite of the effectiveness of timely prenatal care, almost one fourth of all pregnant women receive late or no care (National Center for Health Statistics, 1988). Trends in the use of prenatal care are disturbing. Since 1980, the percentage of all births in women who have had late or no prenatal care has risen among all races, and this trend is most pronounced among black women (Brown, 1989).

Numerous personal and system barriers limit participation in prenatal care (refer to box on p. 461). Economic status and health insurance coverage play large roles in determining whether or not a woman obtains prenatal care (Brown, 1989). Nevertheless, the number of women of

Barriers to Use of Prenatal Care

I. SOCIODEMOGRAPHIC

Poverty
Residence: inner-city or rural
Minority status
Age: <18 or >39
High parity
Non–English-speaking
Unmarried
Less than high school education

II. SYSTEM-RELATED

Inadequacies in private insurance policies (waiting
periods, coverage limitations, coinsurance and
deductibles, requirements for up-front payments)
Absence of either Medicaid or private insurance
coverage of maternity services
Inadequate or no maternity care providers for
Medicaid-enrolled, uninsured, and other low-
income women (long wait to get appointment)
Complicated, time-consuming process to enroll in
Medicaid
Availability of Medicaid poorly advertised
Inadequate transportation services, long travel time to
service sites, or both
Difficulty obtaining child care
Weak links between prenatal services and pregnancy
testing
Inadequate coordination among such services as WIC
and prenatal care

Inconvenient clinic hours, especially for working
women
Long waits to see physician
Language and cultural incompatibility between
providers and clients
Poor communication between clients and providers
exacerbated by short interactions with providers
Negative attributes of clinics, including rude
personnel, uncomfortable surroundings, and
complicated registration procedures
Limited informtion on exactly where to get care
(phone numbers and addresses)

III. ATTITUDINAL

Pregnancy unplanned, viewed negatively, or both
Ambivalence
Signs of pregnancy not known or recognized
Prenatal care not valued or understood
Fear of doctors, hospitals, procedures
Fear of parental discovery
Fear of deportation or problems with the immigration
and Naturalization Service
Fear that certain health habits will be discovered and
criticized (smoking, eating disorders, drug or alcohol
abuse)
Selected lifestyles (drug abuse, homelessness)
Inadequate social supports and personal resources
Excessive stress
Denial or apathy
Concealment

From Brown S: Drawing women into prenatal care, Family Planning Perspectives 21(2):75, March/April 1989. © The Alan Guttmacher Institute.

childbearing age without insurance is increasing, while at the same time the cost of maternity care is rising: some 15 million women have no insurance to cover maternity care; 10 million of these women have no insurance of any sort (Alan Guttmacher Institute, 1987).

Although financial factors significantly affect a woman's decision to obtain prenatal care, other sociodemographic, system-related, and attitudinal barriers must be addressed by health care professions (refer to box above). Women who have insurance also delay or receive no prenatal care. Reasons for lack of participation in prenatal care vary among high-risk groups. For example, adolescents frequently cite fear as a reason for not seeking health care services. Women who are experiencing stressful life situations, characterized by daily problems and struggles, often attach a low value to prenatal care. More recently, it is believed that drug abuse could be a prominent reason for insufficient use of prenatal services (Brown, 1989).

Community wide, well-coordinated initiatives are needed to address problems related to pregnancy and insufficient prenatal care. Since needs vary among different segments of the population, a comprehensive array of programs must be developed (Alan Guttmacher Institute, 1989; Chamberlin, 1988; National Commission to Prevent Infant Mortality, 1989, Home visiting). As previously discussed, coalition or constituency building among all sectors of society is a must to enhance service delivery to mothers and children. There is renewed interest in the importance of home visiting to reach geographically isolated and/or other disadvantaged groups (Chamberlin, 1988; National Commission to Prevent Infant Mortality, 1989, Home visiting). Home visiting activities can improve many health outcomes including increasing attendance in cost-effective prenatal care, encouraging healthy behaviors, and discouraging harmful activities during pregnancy such as smoking and drug use (National Commission to Prevent Infant Mortality, 1989, Home visiting).

Risks after Birth

Once a baby is born, gestational age, birth weight, and environment are significant factors in the chances for survival. The newborn period (birth to 1 month) is particularly important since the majority of all infant deaths occur within the first 28 days of life (USDHHS, 1985, p. 53). Most of these deaths are associated with prematurity. Premature infants are usually of low birth weight, that is, less than 5½ lb (2500 g). Prematurity also can have an adverse effect on maternal-infant bonding. Low-birth-weight infants are not necessarily premature. All low-birth-weight infants, whether premature or not, are highly vulnerable to disease and death. The incidence of neurological and psychological abnormalities occurring during the first year of life is four times as high for low-birth-weight infants as others. Very low-birth-weight babies experience the highest risk: 16 percent of these infants are moderately or severely handicapped (U.S. Congress, Office of Technology Assessment, 1988). Low-birth-weight infants represent a major public health problem.

Problems developing before the infant reaches 1 month of age are usually related to gestational age and birth weight and in utero problems. Problems after 1 month are more often related to environmental factors. Here the community health nurse plays a significant role in prevention, especially in relation to morbidity.

Parent-Child Bonding

Parent-child bonding can be adversely affected when an infant is separated from its primary care giver for a period of time. This separation can occur when an infant is premature or otherwise at risk and must have long-term health care away from parents. Even with normal hospital deliveries, mothers may not see their infants for 12 to 24 hours following delivery. Studies have shown that this period is crucial for the formation of attachment bonds between mothers and their babies and is important for establishing mothering behavior (Klaus and Kennell, 1976). Klaus and Kennell hypothesize that all disorders of mothering, ranging from a persisting concern about a minor abnormality, to abusing and neglecting children, are in part the end result of separation in the early newborn period (Klaus and Kennell, 1976, p. 124).

Another problem associated with high-risk infants—those who are small, or have other physical, familial, and psychological problems—can be their failure to thrive. A child who fails to thrive is one in whom no clear organic etiology can be demonstrated for the growth failure. Instead, the problem seems to arise from situations of environmental, sensory, or parental deprivation. Placement of a child in a nurturing atmosphere often brings improvement.

In one study of 39 infants who failed to thrive, 41 percent were below 5 lb 8 oz at birth and 57 percent were born of complicated pregnancies (Shaheen, Alexander, and Barbero, 1977, pp. 205-206). Other areas of stress that contributed to failure to thrive in this study were the family constellation, socioeconomic status, and disruption in the infant's immediate and extended family. Sixty-two percent of the families had involvement with community agencies prior to the child's hospitalization.

Whaley and Wong (1987) have suggested that nursing care with families who have children that fail to thrive must include support that encourages adaptive mothering behaviors and promotes mother-child attachment. The nursing care should also include teaching specific nurturing techniques, including adequate feeding and interaction with the environment. Assistance to the family in resolving problems that interfere with their ability to provide a nurturing environment is another important element of nursing care. Several tools assist the community health nurse to analyze the mothering behaviors, infant behaviors, and the nursing intervention with these families (Bray, Brosnan, and Erkel, 1989).

Child Maltreatment

Child maltreatment involves direct harm or intent to injure, including intentionality without physical injury. Different types of child maltreatment occur, including physical and/or psychological abuse and neglect and sexual abuse. In general, abuse refers to acts of commission such as beating or excessive chastisement. Neglect refers to acts of omission such as failure to provide adequate food, clothing, or emotional care. However, the line separating the two is a very thin one (U.S. Congress, Office of Technology Assessment, 1988, p. 167).

The problem of child maltreatment is growing. Between 1976 and 1987, the number of reports of child abuse and neglect increased 225 percent. An estimated 2.2 million child maltreatment reports were made in 1987 (USDHHS, Office of Maternal and Child Health, 1989, p. 28). Research by Straus and Gelles (1986) on parent-to-child violence in 1985 revealed that a significant percentage of children are dealing with a high level of violence: it was estimated that 10.7 percent of children were the objects of severe acts of violence, and 1.9 percent of extremely severe acts of violence. These percentages are probably underestimates since some high-risk groups were excluded in Straus and Gelles' study.

Child abuse or neglect is a cumulative problem since the scars which result from such behavior have long-term effects. The most damaging aspect of child abuse and neglect is on the developmental process and emotional growth of the child. Abused children do not feel safe and are unable to trust others—Erikson's first stage in development.

"The most important parental risk factors for child maltreatment are those related to poverty and unemployment and a history of abuse as a child" (U.S. Congress, Office of Technology Assessment, 1988, p. 176). Parents may follow *their* parents' method of child rearing: if it was char-

acterized by abuse and neglect, their own child-rearing style may duplicate their own experience. At the same time, it is possible that intergenerational violence could be related in part to the perpetuation of poverty from one generation to the next (U.S. Congress, Office of Technology Assessment, 1988, p. 175).

Parents of abused children often do not understand normal growth and development patterns and expect too much of their children. As a result, the child is criticized and physically and emotionally punished. A sense of failure, lack of confidence and faith in one's own abilities often results in abused and neglected children who in turn may abuse and neglect others.

Family functioning patterns in households experiencing parent-child violence reflect a disturbance in parental nurturing skills as a result of many factors (Garbarino, 1977). These include blocks to the role transition of parent because of not having been able to develop the role of care giver. The parents may also have had inadequate role models. Such parents lack knowledge about what is involved in parenting, both physically and emotionally, and thus do not know what to expect realistically of themselves or their children. Abusing parents often consider their own needs more important than their children's needs: they have an inappropriate concept of the legitimacy and value of their own needs when ranked with their children's needs. Expecting children to fulfill parents' needs is another problem. Abusing parents feel that they are unable to have any effect and control over events inside and outside the family. Unfortunately, these same families are often characterized by great demands for adjustment to stresses such as moves, job changes, and illnesses. Difficulties may also arise when children begin demanding independence, pushing away from families, or when they are negativistic.

Garbarino also suggests that abusing families are socially isolated from support systems. This isolation may be a result of mobility patterns, characteristics that alienate others, social stresses that cut families off from potential and actual supports, as well as social service agencies that are unable to identify and care for high-risk families.

Community health nurses need to be alert to situations where abuse and neglect have the possibility of occurring, and intervene before this happens. Marital strain, poverty, isolation, and overwhelmed parents are signals to be heeded. Premature births or having children with developmental disabilities are stressful situations that need to be noted. Parents who expect infants to be responsible for their acts and who respond with physical punishment also bear watching.

Mental retardation, emotional disorders, and learning disorders can be other evidences of a less-than-positive nurturing environment for infants. Organic pathologic factors are contributors to these disorders, but there are also psychosocial and other factors which influence the development of these disorders. A summary of physical and behavioral indicators that can assist nurses in identifying child abuse and neglect can be found in Chapter 14, Table 14-4.

Presently there are no states with enough resources and personnel to deal adequately with the increasing number of reported cases of abuse and neglect, not to mention working with families who have already been identified as needing care.

Sudden Infant Death Syndrome

Another sequel to high-risk pregnancy may be the sudden infant death syndrome (SIDS). In the United States, 2 of every 1000 live-born infants die annually from SIDS. It is the number one cause of death in infants between the ages of 1 month and 1 year. Although SIDS was identified as early as in the writings of the New Testament, no single cause for this condition has been discovered. It is suspected that SIDS is caused by a combination of events and some type of biochemical, anatomical, or developmental defect or deficiency (National SIDS Clearinghouse, 1989). Helping parents handle grief and guilt feelings is the major role of the community health nurse in these situations. The impact of death on siblings is another area where the nurse must intervene.

Increasingly, communities are setting up crisis teams to assist families who have experienced a child's death from SIDS. One health department in a northern city employs a pediatric nurse practitioner who works full time with such families.

She facilitates family adjustment as they work through the grief process after death has come to a seemingly healthy infant. Helping families to deal with their feelings about future parenting is very important (Chan, 1987).

Recently, it has been found that public health professionals have a significant preventive intervention role as well as a therapeutic role when dealing with SIDS. A 7-year study of unexpected infant deaths in England suggested that home visiting by health visitors was directly related to a reduction in mortality of infants scored to be at risk for unexpected infant death (Carpenter, 1983, p. 724). The scoring system for ascertaining who was at risk included factors such as the mother's age, her previous pregnancies, duration of the second stage of labor, mother's blood group, birth weight, single or multiple birth, breast- or bottle-fed, and presence of urinary infection of mother during pregnancy.

Home visits by health visitors were made for SIDS preventive follow-up, every 2 weeks for 3 months and every month for up to 6 months, to those infants scoring at high risk. "The reduction in mortality attributed directly to the effect of increased visiting of high-risk infants is numerically similar to the number of lives saved by treating cancers in children. This suggests that home visiting by health visitors is highly cost-effective" (Carpenter, 1983, p. 723).

Acute Illnesses

Respiratory diseases and other conditions such as diarrhea result in short-term disability and account for many doctor visits to infants. These diseases caused much death in the past. Today, there is less mortality from these conditions but a tremendous amount of professional time is spent in controlling acute illnesses. The nurse in the pediatric clinic or the nurse who makes home visits will see these kinds of problems and will need the expertise to explain their origin and treatment to parents.

Problems of Children Ages 1 to 5

Children do change in their capacities. As developmental growth occurs, infants and children's needs and problems become different.

Accidental Injuries

As Figure 13-3 demonstrates, accidental injuries are among the five leading causes of infant deaths. They become a leading cause of death in children 1 to 14 years of age. In 1985, 44 percent of all deaths among children ages 1 through 4 were caused by injuries (National Committee for Injury Prevention and Control, 1989). In 1985 vehicle-related accidents caused the greatest number of accidental fatalities (36 percent) among children in this age group. Fires/burns and drowning also cause a significant number of accidental deaths in this population group (National Safety Council, 1988).

Accidental injuries disproportionately strike the young which is costly to society from many perspectives. Accidental injuries can cause tremendous social and emotional stress, significant activity limitation, and financial burdens. "More than half of the impairments caused by injuries result in activity limitations: seventy percent of impairments due to injuries are deformities or orthopedic impairments" (National Institute on Disability and Rehabilitation Research, 1989, p. 26). It is not difficult to see that accidents are a major health problem and that present education and legislation are not as effective as they should be in combating a problem that is preventable.

Respiratory and Gastrointestinal Problems

Upper respiratory infections become a common cause of illness in the 1- to 5-year age group, especially when these children begin to play in groups. Upper respiratory infections can be minor and cause only minimal interference to living. Others can be life-threatening, especially when no treatment is obtained. Lower respiratory tract infections result generally from infections of the upper respiratory tract.

Minor gastrointestinal problems are almost as common as respiratory infections. The use of epidemiology in examining the numbers of cases in a family and a community helps to determine whether the causative agent is or is not communicable. Epidemiological investigation also helps to identify significant environmental conditions that need changing, especially when a child has repeated infections. In one day-care center, for ex-

ample, repeated episodes of diarrhea among a number of the children led the supervisor to look for a cause. It was discovered that feeding bottles were left in tote bags until the noon feedings and that spoiled milk was the result. After its epidemiological investigation, the day-care center began to refrigerate bottles immediately upon the arrival of infants and parents.

Prompt treatment of acute conditions, ongoing medical care, educating parents regarding good health care practices, and early detection of illness can help to prevent or curtail respiratory and gastrointestinal problems.

Chronic Conditions

Chronic diseases are important because of their long-term effects. They can significantly limit a child's normal activities and increase health care utilization. In 1987 over three million, or 5 percent of all children 1 through 19 years of age, had some limitation of activities due to chronic illnesses and impairments. Children with activity limitations have 2½ times as many physician contacts and spend over 11 times as many days in the hospital as do other children; they account for 40 percent of all hospital days among children ages 1 through 19 years (USDHHS, Office of Maternal and Child Health, 1989, pp. 45-46).

A death rate of 6 of every 100,000 of the 1- to 5-year population results from cancer. The types of cancers that are seen in children differ from those seen in adults. Those affecting children are the leukemias, embryonal tumors, and sarcomas. Regular medical follow-up can aid in early diagnosis of such conditions.

Under the category of chronic problems come children with developmental disabilities such as phenylketonuria, Down's syndrome, cerebral palsy, blindness, mental retardation, or deafness. Also included are children with physical health problems such as diabetes, rheumatoid arthritis, and kidney disease. These children present problems to their families that demand special attention, study, and creative problem solving.

Between 100,000 and 200,000 babies born each year in the United States are mentally retarded. The causes of the retardation can be identified in only one fourth of the cases. In the other three fourths, inadequacies in prenatal and perinatal care, nutrition, child rearing, and social and environmental opportunities are suspected as causes (USDHHS, 1985). Many of these suspected causes can be dealt with in some manner by the community health nurse.

Communicable and Preventable Diseases

Preventable communicable diseases are still a major community health problem. The seven major childhood diseases—poliomyelitis, mumps, tetanus, diphtheria, rubella, pertussis, and measles—can cause permanent disability and death. In spite of the fact that effective immunizations have been available for several decades to protect children from these diseases, a significant number of preschool children are not adequately immunized. Over one third of children aged 1 to 4 years were not properly immunized in 1985 (USDHHS, Office of Maternal and Child Health, 1989). Community health nurses are working in local communities across the country to increase the herd immunity level. By 1990, public health professionals wanted at least 90 percent of children to have had their immunization series completed by age 2. It appears that this objective will not be met; data from the latest U.S. Immunization Survey in 1985 revealed that only 77 percent of 2-year-old children, whose parents had immunization records, had completed their basic immunization series (Centers for Disease Control, 1988, October). The National Childhood Immunization Initiative of 1977 has greatly influenced the immunization levels of school-age children. Almost 98 percent of all children entering kindergarten/first grade were fully immunized in 1987 (USDHHS, Office of Maternal and Child Health, 1989, p. 32). However, immunization levels of preschool children are much harder to control. Of particular concern is the low immunization level among minority children and those from low-income families. The percentage of these children fully immunized is far lower than that of children in the general population. Those not fully immunized are considered target populations for community health nursing interventions.

Table 13-1, relating complications from child-hood diseases, summarizes the problems that can result from the preventable childhood diseases. The contributing factors that allow children, especially preschoolers, to remain unimmunized include the lack of consumer awareness, understanding, and responsibility; the complicated vaccine schedule which can be easily misunderstood; the increased mobility of families, which can lead to fragmented health care; inadequate funding for immunization research at the federal level; resistance by public school systems to compliance with state immunization requirements; and apathy because the evidences of childhood disease are no longer obvious.

Pediatric AIDS

Pediatric acquired immunodeficiency syndrome (AIDS) is a major public health problem in the United States. "The fastest growing group of reported AIDS patients is children" (Hopp and Rogers, 1989, p. 13). Between April 1987 and December 1989, there was a 423 percent increase in the reported cases of pediatric AIDS. As of December 1989, there were 1995 reported cases of AIDS among children under 13 years of age and the number rises daily. These data become especially significant when one considers that pediatric AIDS is seriously underreported (Centers for Disease Control, 1990, January).

The majority of pediatric AIDS cases are the result of transmission from infected mothers (USDHHS, Office of Maternal and Child Health, 1989, p. 20). In 1989, 81 percent of the pediatric HIV-infected cases to date were acquired from HIV-risk mothers, 11 percent were associated with transmission of blood or blood products, and 5 percent were of children who had hemophilia or other coagulation disorders (refer to Figure 13-5) (Centers for Disease Control, 1990, January). Approximately 65 percent of infants born to infected mothers will contract the disease (Koop, 1987, p. 4).

The epidemiological characteristics of AIDS victims are discussed in Chapter 15. Children with AIDS have characteristics similar to those of heterosexual adults with AIDS, particularly women: the majority of perinatally acquired pe-

TABLE 13-1   Some complications from selected childhood diseases for which immunizations are available

Complications	Mumps	Measles (rubeola)	Rubella	Rubella (in utero)	Polio	Tetanus	Pertussis	Diphtheria
Mental retardation		X	X	X			X	
Brain damage		X	X	X			X	
Meningoencephalitis	X	X	X	X				
Paralysis					X			X
Blindness		X	X	X				
Deafness	X	X	X	X				X
Pancreatitis	X							
Juvenile-type diabetes	X							
Orchitis (postpubertal)	X							
Oophoritis (postpubertal)	X							
Sterility (males)	X							
Pneumonia	X	X				X	X	X
Heart damage, pericarditis	X							X
Polyarthritis			X					
Hepatitis	X							
Nephritis	X							X
Cerebral hemorrhage							X	
Muscle spasm						X		
Death	X	X	X	X	X	X	X	X

Adapted from Garner MK: Our values are showing: inadequate childhood immunization, Health Values: Achieving High Level Wellness 2:130, 1978; Hoekelman RA, Blatman S, Brunell PA, Friedman SB, and Seidel HM: Principles of pediatrics health care of the young, New York, 1978, McGraw-Hill; Scipien GM, Barnard MU, Chard MA, Howe J, and Phillips PJ: Comprehensive pediatric nursing, ed 3, New York, 1986, McGraw-Hill.

diatric AIDS cases are related to intravenous (IV) drug abuse or sexual contact with IV drug abusers; the geographic areas most heavily affected by perinatal transmission of AIDS are the New York City metropolitan area, northern New Jersey, and southern Florida; and the majority of children with perinatally acquired HIV infection are black or Hispanic and are inner-city residents of low socioeconomic status (Rogers, 1987, p. 17). Perinatally acquired AIDS is usually seen in children under the age of 2 (Berry, 1988, p. 341).

Professionals working with families who have children with AIDS must address an array of complex medical, social, and emotional problems. The children must be kept comfortable, well nourished, and protected from opportunistic infections, and must receive nurturing parenting (Berry, 1988). Families need supportive assistance to help them to handle the physical care needs of their children, obtain adequate financial and

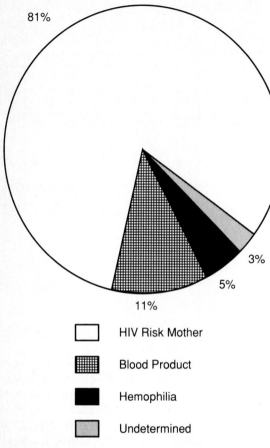

HIV Risk Mother

Blood Product

Hemophilia

Undetermined

Notes: 81% children of HIV risk mother (mother with/at risk for AIDS HIV infection); 11% recipient of transfusion blood, blood components, or tissue; 5% children who have hemophilia or other coagulation disorder; and 3% cases undetermined.

Figure 13-5 Pediatric AIDS by exposure category December, 1989. (Centers for Disease Control: HIV/AIDS surveillance, year end edition, MMWR, Special report, p 9, 1990.)

health care resources, and cope with the stresses related to the progression of the disease. These families frequently need an advocate in the health care delivery system and the community and help in coordinating health care services. "Emotional support is an absolute necessity for these families because each family member is experiencing stress" (Berry, 1988, p. 344). Family members can experience social isolation, fear, guilt, financial burdens, grief, and physical stress. The community health nurse assumes a major role in helping families to deal with these emotions and experiences. The community health nurse also plays a significant role in educating families, professionals, and communities about AIDS prevention. Pediatric AIDS must be prevented! It cannot be cured!

Lead Poisoning

At present, lead poisoning is one of the most common preventable *environmental* diseases of childhood in the United States. Mental retardation, learning disabilities, and other neurological handicaps are the needless results of this condition. Infants and young children are at highest risk for complications of lead toxicity (Centers for Disease Control, 1988, Childhood lead poisoning; Coppens, Hunter, Bain, Gatewood, Gordon, and Mailloux, 1990).

There are two principal routes of exposure to lead—ingestion and inhalation (Chadzynski, 1986). Some important sources of lead are described in Table 13-2. Lead-containing paint is the major source for children in the United States; approximately 12 million children are exposed to leaded paint in older homes. However, a significant number of children are also exposed to lead from contaminated drinking water (10.4 million children), gasoline (5.6 million children), dust/soil (5.9-11.0 million children), and food (1.0 million children) (Centers for Disease Control, 1988, Childhood lead poisoning).

Lead poisoning is not confined to poor children in deteriorated neighborhoods; no economic or racial subgrouping of children is exempt from the risk of adverse health effects from lead toxicity (Centers for Disease Control, 1988, Childhood lead poisoning). It has been identified that children from some ethnic groups (e.g., Hmong, Chinese, and Hispanic) are exposed to lead through folk remedies used to treat minor ailments. Chinese herbal medicines, Pay-loo-ah, an Asian folk medicine used for treating fever in children, and Azarcon, a Mexican folk remedy for "empacho" or chronic indigestion have been identified as sources of lead poisoning among children (Chadzynski, 1986).

TABLE 13-2   Environmental sources of lead potentially harmful to children

Lead-based paint chips or flakes	Many small children habitually eat chips or flakes of peeling paint
Dust from lead-based wall and ceiling paints	Inhaled by persons in the rooms
Airborne lead (about 1 kg per person per year)	About 5 percent from industrial sources and 90 percent from burning leaded gasoline
Cigarette smoke	Nonsmokers, too, ingest lead when inhaling cigarette smoke
Drinking water	Especially in cities where water pipes are old or known to contain lead, or both
Vegetables cooked in lead-containing water	Vegetables can concentrate lead from cooking water by a factor of five or more
Food	Especially vegetables grown in urban plots, where both soil and air are often heavily contaminated
Snow and ice contaminated by automotive exhaust fumes, especially in urban areas	Children who eat snow and lick icicles ingest significant amounts of lead
Paper coated with pigments containing lead	Children may chew or swallow pieces of such papers; the papers may be burned in fireplaces or incinerators, releasing lead into the air; lead in the pigments may leach into groundwater from dumps or landfills

From Drummond AH: Lead poisoning in children, J School Health 51:44, 1981. Copyright 1981, American School Health Association, Kent, Ohio.

Yearly lead screening is recommended for all high-risk children aged 9 months to 6 years. Children who live in or frequently visit older housing that is dilapidated or undergoing renovation and poor black children are especially at risk for lead toxicity (U.S. Preventive Services Task Force, 1989, p. 177). Children with elevated blood lead levels of 25 μg or more of lead per tenth liter of blood (≥ 25 μg/dl) and an erythrocyte protoporphyrin (EP) level ≥ 35 μg/dl should be referred for medical evaluation (Centers for Disease Control, 1985). Since there is growing evidence that the toxic effects of lead in children can occur at blood levels previously considered noninjurious (WHO, 1987), it is important for community health professionals to observe for other symptoms of lead toxicity: black lines along the gums; gastrointestinal symptoms of anorexia, nausea, vomiting, abdominal pain, and constipation; hematological findings of anemia or pallor; and neurological signs of stupor, lethargy, or convulsions are some other characteristics of lead poisoning.

Although knowledge about its etiology, pathophysiology, and epidemiology has increased significantly in the past two decades, childhood lead poisoning continues to remain a major public health problem. Each year this condition causes death, mental retardation, and other problems in thousands of children. The long-term effects of lead poisoning can be subtle; the neurological defects may not be discovered until a child enters school and the teacher notes a slight deficiency in the child's performance. The increasing number of children being observed with long-term effects of lead toxicity, with blood lead levels much lower than previously believed harmful, is an area of major concern. It is estimated that several million children are exposed to low-dose levels of lead (Centers for Disease Control, 1988, Childhood lead poisoning).

Eliminating pediatric lead poisoning will require substantial effort and expense. This condition will not be eradicated until lead hazards are identified and removed from the environment. The likelihood of this occurring in the near future is doubtful because of the extensive prevalence of lead in the environment; it is estimated that lead paint remains on 30 to 40 million dwellings in the United States (Chadzynski, 1986).

A comprehensive, community-wide approach is essential in order to control lead poisoning among children. To be successful, a lead toxicity prevention program must include environmental management as well as screening and diagnostic and treatment approaches. These approaches should focus on controlling lead exposure in high-risk areas, epidemiological investigation of environmental hazards, case finding, early diagnosis and treatment, dissemination of educational materials to professionals and the public, and the passage of effective legal regulations. Community health nurses assume responsibility for many of these activities.

Several problems need to be addressed to achieve successful control of lead poisoning. Physicians and other health professionals, as well as the public, are often not aware of the magnitude of this problem. As a result, there is a high rate of recurrence of lead toxicity among children as a result of the lack of epidemiological follow-up of reported cases. Children are treated and then sent back into the same environment that produced the poisoning; the cycle then repeats itself.

Some other problems that need to be addressed are weak and ineffective housing laws, lack of enforcement of existing laws, the cost of eliminating lead from the environment, limited housing for low-income families, inability to reach many high-risk children, and access to care issues for disadvantaged populations. To resolve many of these problems, priority must be placed on public education about environmental hazard identification and elimination.

Nutritional Inadequacies

Another condition seen by the community health nurse when working with children aged 1 to 5 is nutritional inadequacy and anemia. Inadequate diets can cause growth retardation. Data from the 1983 CDC Nutrition Surveillance reflected that growth retardation existed at levels ranging from 10.9 to 23.6 percent in a selected group of low-income children (those participating in the WIC and EPSDT programs in 29 states and the District of Columbia), 3 to 23 months old. Children screened in the 1983 CDC survey were from white, black, Hispanic, Native American, and Asian ethnic groups (USDHHS, Office of Disease Prevention and Health Promotion, 1986, p. 213).

Two feeding problems seen by the nurse are overfeeding of infants and young children and too early an introduction of foods other than milk or formula. Feeding solid foods at an early age is viewed by parents as a developmental milestone and thus they push the infant before he or she is ready. There appears to be little evidence to support giving solids before the age of 3 to 4 months, because the result of this practice is the replacement by solids of the milk the infant needs for growth. Another result is that the child may be overfed if the amount of milk given is not decreased when solids are given. Solids are not digested well by young children because of their immature gastrointestinal systems. Spoon feeding begun too early can result in frustration for both parent and child.

The most prevalent form of anemia in the United States is dietary iron deficiency (USDHHS, the Surgeon General's Report, Public Health Service, 1988, p. 16). Infants and children particularly at risk are those who are born prematurely, have perinatal blood loss, have congenital heart disease, are irritable and anorexic, have pica or disturbed sleep patterns, and are fed homogenized cow's milk before the age of 9 months. Cow's milk induces enteric blood loss and significantly influences the occurrence of iron-deficiency anemia. Breastfeeding is being advocated to reduce the prevalence of nutritional deficiencies among infants. However, current trends are not encouraging. Since 1982, there has been a slight but continuing decline in breastfeeding. Women least likely to breastfeed are those who are low-income, black, under 20 years of age, and/or who live in the southeastern region (USDHHS, Office of Maternal and Child Health, 1989, p. 19).

Another problem, overnutrition, results from the popular notion that to be healthy is to be fat and the equating of rewards for good behavior with food. Obesity is not condoned for adults, but fat children are often considered cute. Unfortunately, childhood fat may not disappear in adulthood. Plotting body weight in comparison with body height helps parents and nurses to determine whether obesity is a problem.

While nutritional inadequacies can and do affect children from all socioeconomic groups, they are found more frequently among low-income children. A major nutrition study conducted in Massachusetts provided evidence to support this fact. It also demonstrated that nutritional inadequacies continue to plague many of our children.

The 1983 Massachusetts Nutrition Survey (MNS) was a cross-sectional study designed to estimate the prevalence of nutritional deficiencies among a sample of 129 low-income children, 5 through 12 years of age. The survey was a point prevalence study which described the nutritional status of the sampled population at a single point in time (Massachusetts Department of Public Health, 1983). The survey targeted those individuals who were most likely to develop nutritional deficiencies. The following were major findings of the study (pp. ii and iii):

- *Chronic malnutrition is a significant public health problem in low-income preschool children in Massachusetts.* In the population sampled, 9.8 percent were identified as having low height-for-age levels, a measure of chronic undernutrition. This result is significantly higher than U.S. standards. It is estimated that there may be between 10,000 and 17,500 chronically undernourished low-income preschool children in the Commonwealth of Massachusetts. The implications of this level of undernutrition include retarded growth, impaired learning ability, and increased health problems.
- *Anemia and obesity were identified as nutritional problems among this group of Massachusetts children. However, acute undernutrition does not appear to be a widespread problem.* Anemia is a clinical condition which in children generally results from iron deficiency. Of those children who had hematocrits measured within 6 months prior to the survey, 12.2 percent were anemic. The prevalence of childhood obesity, a major predictor of adult obesity and its related diseases, was 8.1 percent in the sampled population. This is significantly higher than the national standards for this indicator of poor nutrition. The

prevalence of low weight-for-height levels (i.e., severe, short-term undernutrition) identified by the 1983 MNS is 3.0 percent. This suggests that, at least for this health-care user sample, the problem is not a major public health concern. Not including obesity, the percentage of survey children who had at least one indicator of malnutrition was *18.1 percent.*

- *Three groups were identified by the 1983 MNS as being at particularly high risk for malnutrition: (1) all children below the poverty level, (2) poor white children, and (3) southeast Asian children.* For all racial groups, children living below poverty were more likely to be chronically undernourished than higher-income groups; however, in the white children studied, this relationship within the low-income group was statistically significant. It may be that poor white families have special characteristics that increase the likelihood of chronic undernutrition in their young children. Further analysis of these data is needed to explain this finding. The southeast Asian children sampled had levels of low height-for-age and low weight-for-height which were significantly higher than the other racial groups. This survey was not designed to establish the causal links between nutritional status and sociodemographic variables such as income and race.
- *Children whose source of payment for their health-care visit was Medicaid had a higher prevalence of low height-for-age levels than children whose medical visit was covered by another source.* Twelve percent of children then receiving Medicaid benefits had low height-for-age levels. This suggests that Medicaid, while providing low-income children with access to health care, does not appear to guarantee adequate nutritional status. The importance of this finding is that the children on Medicaid are an identifiable target group for nutritional assessment and intervention.
- *The WIC program achieved a high saturation level in this health center user population. However, a population was identified who*

were income-eligible and nutritionally eligible but who were not receiving benefits at the time of the survey. While numerous other studies have established the efficacy of the WIC Program, this survey was not designed to do so. However, it can be used to describe the sample population's characteristics with regard to this program. Of those children in the survey population who were income-eligible, 45.8 percent were participating in the WIC program as of June 1983. However, the survey also identified a population that was income-eligible and had documented nutritional deficits who were not receiving WIC benefits.

Community health nurses play a significant role in preventing nutritional deficiencies. Many children experience inadequate diets related to knowledge deficits of parents, cultural food patterns, and financial difficulties. Community health nurses are often in a unique position to identify these problems, to instruct regarding needed alterations in eating habits, to provide information about food preparation on a low-income budget, and to make appropriate referrals to community resources which deal with nutritional problems.

Dental Problems

Poor dental hygiene is another significant problem that begins in the preschool years. Although the prevalence of dental caries increases with age, children 5 through 9 years of age in 1987 had an average of four baby teeth affected by decay. It is estimated that 5 percent of children aged 2 through 4 years have "bottle-mouth caries," a condition caused by sucking at bedtime on a bottle containing milk or juice. Prevalence of baby bottle tooth decay increases dramatically among low-income children; 53 percent of children from low-income families and Native American children have this condition (USDHHS, Office of Maternal and Child Health, 1989, p. 26). Other causes of dental caries among preschool children include, but are not limited to, eating foods high in sugars, eating frequent between-meal snacks without brushing teeth, and the cariogenicity of

some liquid medications such as Pen-Vee-K and phenytoin (Dilantin) (Whaley and Wong, 1987).

Unfortunately, it is often only after children reach school age that parents become concerned with dental hygiene, and by then much damage may have been done to the teeth. The appearance of their mouth contributes to the way people feel physically and emotionally, and the financial cost of dental repair can be very high.

Behavioral Problems

Disturbance of sleep patterns, toilet training, eating, and relationships with strangers and continual whining and crying are some behavioral problems seen by the nurse who works with children. Parents will often have questions about problems in these areas that seem minor but can cause daily discomfort to a family and develop into more major problems.

HEALTH PROMOTION NEEDS

Identifying areas where families and larger groups can increase the state of their health, where they are working toward maximizing their potential, is one of the most exciting and challenging aspects of family and community health nursing.

Health promotion in the 0- to 5-year age group is particularly important because this period provides the foundation for the physical, intellectual, and emotional health for the rest of the child's life.

The nurse needs to remember the concept that behavior changes with age in a patterned, predictable manner. Behavior has form and shape just as physical patterns do. All growth, whether physical or emotional, implies organization.

Norms for various ages can be dangerous if they are used as absolute standards because each child develops with a different rhythm. Making diagnoses from the behavior a child exhibits takes knowledge, skill, and experience. However, norms for various ages can be guides for planning health promotion programs. The Denver Developmental Screening Test and the Washington Guide, which are discussed later, provide normal growth and development ranges.

Health professionals across the nation recognize the value of health promotion services for the 0- to 5-year age population group. They also recognize that there is still much to be accomplished in order to protect our nation's most precious resources—our children.

The monitoring of children's health status is a prime priority (Miller, Fine, Adams-Taylor, and Schorr, 1986). The box on p. 456 presents the priority maternal/child health objectives the United States focused on during the past decade.

Health Promotion before Birth

Good health begins before a child is conceived. Children need to be wanted and planned, and people need to learn how to be parents. Becoming pregnant does not confer readiness for children because an individual does not automatically put aside all personal needs to prepare for a child's world, which is in itself not a rational world. Thus, parent education needs to start early. It needs to become a part of school curricula, community organizations, and church groups. Parenting programs need to include information regarding the physical aspects of child care; nutrition for the mother and the child; the physical, intellectual, and emotional development of children; and the stresses of role changes for parents. Some schools use the team approach, with the teacher, the school nurse, the social worker, and the nutritionist all working together to promote nurturing parenting skills.

The nurse in the school setting can help teachers and administrators plan parenting classes at the junior- and senior-high level. Accompanying information on parenting must include courses on responsible sexuality, the physiology of sexual development, the part optional parenthood and contraception play in teenagers' sexuality, and the consequences of poor health practices during adolescent years.

State teenage pregnancy initiatives to reduce unintended pregnancy among adolescents have increased significantly since 1985 and include actions such as programs to enhance life options, school-based clinics which provide contraceptives and a broad range of physical and mental health services, and family life education (Alan Guttmacher Institute, 1989).

The nutrition of the female throughout her life plays a role in the health of the children she delivers. As girls become responsible for their own nutrition and can make choices about what they eat, they need to know what proper nutrition is. They also need to be aware that their choices are affecting the health of their future children. The school setting is an appropriate place to teach this kind of information. Health professionals must include adolescents' preferences for fast foods (those prepared with minimum time in franchise restaurants) when planning lunch meals and doing nutritional counseling. Fast foods are eaten as meals and as snacks and, for many people, they provide a significant proportion of their daily caloric intake. Hanson and Wyse (1979) have developed "nutrient profiles" of fast foods, some of which contain significant quantities of nutrients. The community health nurse can utilize these profiles to make eating of fast foods more positive.

Fathers-to-be are often neglected in family life and parenting programs. Males can play a major role in preventing unintentional pregnancies and sexually transmitted diseases, both of which cause significant problems related to conception and pregnancy. However, males need appropriate information to develop responsible decision making about sexuality. They also need an opportunity to obtain information necessary to develop nurturing parenting skills.

Health Promotion during Pregnancy

Pregnancy is a developmental task for both parents. Parents need support throughout pregnancy because this is a time of change and of strong emotions, some positive, some negative, and most ambivalent. How people feel about pregnancy varies widely and depends upon whether or not the parents are married, whether they have other children, whether the mother is working, whether memories of their childhood are positive or negative, and how they feel about their parents. Lack of support can cause the parents to feel stress, can delay preparation for the infant, and can retard bond formation. Supportive intervention efforts during pregnancy and the few months following the birth can improve maternal and child health outcomes (National Commission to Prevent Infant Mortality, 1989).

Prenatal classes, groups such as La Leche League, and visits by the community health nurse can help with this kind of support. The nuclear family system of the United States as well as the mobility of many Americans often means that the parents do not have other family members, family physicians, close friends, or neighbors who can be helpful in this period.

Concerns that parents have during the time of pregnancy, which should be addressed during prenatal classes, involve preparing for labor and delivery, how to physically prepare the home environment for the new baby, whether or not to breast-feed, whether or not the new mother should work outside the home, and how to prepare other siblings for the additional family member. Moreover, the mother needs to know that alcohol, smoking, and other drugs can adversely affect the fetus; she should, of course, begin seeing her obstetrician or family doctor as soon as she suspects she is pregnant.

Parents should know that their genetic backgrounds can play a crucial role in their child's health. Ideally, this concern would occur prior to marriage, but often it does not. Down's syndrome, Tay-Sachs disease, sickle-cell anemia, cystic fibrosis, hemophilia, and Huntington's disease are some diseases which have a genetic origin. When parents know that these diseases are in their family constellations, they have several choices. They can have genetic testing prior to conception, they can adopt, or they can choose not to bear a child. They can also choose to conceive and then have genetic testing to ascertain whether or not the fetus carries the disease. Another alternative is to conceive and deliver without having genetic tests. If couples know about genetic problems before they marry, they may also make the decision not to marry. The community health nurse needs to be able to help people look at alternatives and provide sources of genetic counseling. There are an increasing number of genetic counseling centers throughout the country.

Expectant parents need more than knowledge to make the transition to parenthood successfully. They need the chance to review the various situations that arise in parenting, compare different ways of dealing with them, and develop their own style of parenting. Nurses have used prenatal class settings to provide clarification about the role of the parent, to do actual role modeling by actively discussing problems and exploring alternatives, and to provide opportunities for role rehearsal. Role rehearsal can be done by using case studies and situations with the opportunity for parents to react and respond. Case studies and sharing of personal experiences to stimulate problem solving can be used with parents throughout any of the developmental and maturational crisis periods they may experience with their children.

Home births have had a mild resurgence of popularity. The rise in home deliveries is not great, from 0.87 percent of all deliveries in 1975 to 0.97 percent in 1980. Of the 35,888 out-of-hospital births reported in 1980, physicians, midwives, and "others" (friends, relatives, and "quacks" of various sorts) delivered equal proportions (Editorial, 1983, pp. 635-636). However, the cries for home births are a "healthy adaptation to the public's depersonalization of medical practice" (Editorial, 1983, p. 637). Hospitals have created birth centers that involve the family in the birth process and facilitate early discharge to home. This discharge can take place as early as 4 hours postdelivery in some cases. The importance of this resurgence in home births for community health nurses is that they need to be skilled in handling nursing care needs of mothers and babies during the immediate postdelivery period. The nurse shown in Figure 13-6 is visiting a family with an infant only 24 hours old. Insurance benefits for this family include coverage for nursing visits, laboratory tests, and homemaking services.

Health Promotion after Birth

The community health nurse should be cognizant that sometimes health services are not offered to new parents between the postpartum hospital discharge and the sixth-week checkup. The mother

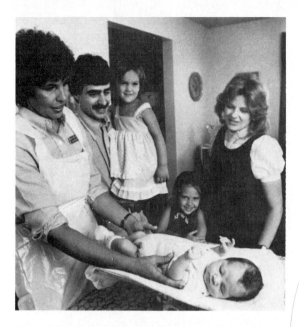

Figure 13-6 A community health nurse whose services are financed under the auspices of the Genesee Region Home Care Association visits an infant only 24 hours old. (Genesee Region Home Care Association, Rochester, NY.)

is often not in optimum physical condition after experiencing a loss in blood volume, rapid weight loss, and displacement of internal organs during the birth process. Yet she needs to meet the needs of a dependent infant whose respirations are not well established, who is undergoing massive blood changes, and who may be weak, dehydrated, and irritable. In addition, when the mother goes from the protected hospital environment to the home setting, she needs to adjust to role changes and the responsibility of infant care. Nurses in the hospital who work with parents postpartum should make selective referrals of those families needing the services that a community health nurse can offer. The nurse, with observation, is able to "pick up" stresses and provide needed help.

The community health nurse has an important role in the referral process from hospital to home with families who have newborns. The community health nurse can discuss with the hospital nurse the types of families who need referrals. The hospital nurse should assess the entire family situation, assess the parent-child bonding, and make appropriate referrals based upon this information. The referral process is based upon the hospital nurse's assessment, and it is vital that she or he understand what an appropriate referral is and what the community health nurse can do with families who have newborns.

Table 13-3 is a compilation of concerns with which new parents may desire help during the puerperium. The puerperium is a short period of time, but it can be a highly troubled one if needed help is not present. These concerns should be taken into consideration when a nurse is identifying parents for referral or when a community health nurse is making a home visit.

Parenting

Parenting is a developmental stage in the life cycle, and growth and development should continue for the parent as well as for the child. Ideally, this stage is fairly free of anxiety and guilt, but that is not always the case. Most parents, in fact, experience some stress. The huge numbers of best sellers written over the years for parents on how to do the job well testify to the insecurity that many parents feel (Biller and Meredith, 1974; Comer and Poussaint, 1975; Illingsworth and Illingsworth, 1977; Samuels and Samuels, 1979; Kiester and Kiester, 1980; Spock & Rothenberg, 1985; Sammons, 1989).

Each of the sources listed above proclaims the "right" way to parent. Which one should parents choose? How can parents do the "right" things for their children?

If they are interested in promoting moral and social maturity in later life, the answer is simple: they should love them, enjoy them, and want them around. They should not use their power to maintain a home that is only designed for the self-expression and pleasure of adults. They should not regard their children as disturbances to be controlled at all cost. (McClelland, Constantian, Regalado, and Stone, 1978, p. 53)

In the study cited above, which investigated child rearing, it was the easygoing, loving parents whose children turned out to be the most mature (this is basically common sense) and what

TABLE 13-3   Percentages of mothers noting specific concerns during the puerperium

Area of concern	Percent of mothers concerned			Area of concern	Percent of mothers concerned		
	Minor concern	Major concern	Total		Minor concern	Major concern	Total
Return of figure to normal	30	65	95	Discomfort of stitches	33	20	53
Regulating demands of husband, housework, children	42	48	90	Breast care	40	10	50
				Constipation	35	15	50
Emotional tension	48	40	88	Setting limits for visitors	27	23	50
Fatigue	28	55	83	Interpreting infant's behavior	27	23	50
Infant behavior	47	33	80				
Finding time for self	45	33	78	Breast soreness	35	13	48
Sexual relations	53	20	73	Hemorrhoids	25	23	48
Diet	33	40	73	Labor and delivery experience	28	20	48
Feelings of isolation, being tied down	42	28	70	Father's role with baby	22	23	45
Infant's growth and development	45	25	70	Lochia	35	5	40
				Other children jealous of baby	27	13	40
Family planning	25	43	68	Other children's behavior	25	15	40
Exercise	23	45	68	Infant's appearance	18	20	38
Infant feeding	43	25	68	Traveling with baby	27	8	35
Changes in relationship with husband	35	25	60	Clothing for baby	20	10	30
Physical care of infant	45	13	58	Feeling comfortable handling baby	15	8	23
Infant safety	33	25	58				

From Gruis M: Beyond maternity: post partum concerns of mothers, Am J Maternal Child Health 2:185, 1977.

counted most among the different methods of child rearing that were studied was the child's feeling that he or she was loved and wanted.

Parenting also involves the father; his important role in the child-rearing process has long been neglected, but this is changing. Fatherhood begins when the woman first finds out that she is pregnant. As she goes through many physical and emotional changes, so does he. Even though his body is not physically altered, he may experience body-image changes, such as gastrointestinal disorders, backaches, toothache, leg ache, and syncope, that can have a profound effect on the pregnancy experience (Fawcett, 1978). The nurse can help reduce the father's anxiety and confusion resulting from these changes by providing information about them and encouraging him to share

them with others in group situations. The nurse can help parents to understand that although the changes are a concern, they are normal and learning to adapt to them is part of the process that occurs as the pregnant family takes on the parent role.

Fathers have to learn how to be fathers just as mothers need to learn how to be mothers. Our society has often given males the message that being an involved father is not a major goal for a man. The result has been that fathers and babies are often deprived of a warm relationship. Fathers can offer different stimulation, handling, and voice qualities from mothers, which enlarges the infant's environment. A positive relationship between baby and father benefits the entire family.

Teaching people how to parent became popular during the 1960s; such programs focused on low-income families and were aimed at preventing educational failure. However, during the 1970s, parenting became a major concern for the country. At the Fifth National Conference on Child Abuse and Neglect (National Center for Child Abuse and Neglect, 1981), the following rationale for parent education was developed:

Parent education programs are effective in and of themselves. They are also effective in the prevention and treatment of child abuse and neglect. There is no longer any doubt that in our society, being a good parent requires knowledge, understanding, the ability to empathize with one's children, and a nurturing support system. There is also no longer any doubt that imparting the needed factual knowledge and skills and the needed support and nurturing to parents (people who are not parents, people who will be parents, or people who have made mistakes in parenting) is the key to prevention and treatment of child abuse and neglect. It is also clear that good parenting saves money through alleviating violence and keeping it from occurring in the first place. Good parenting also alleviates and prevents from occurring a range of other pressures on our nation's overburdened and underfunded social, medical, and law enforcement services, and the taxpayers who support these services.

Several issues emanated from this conference. These were:

- *Who can be taught?* The history of parenting programs did begin with a focus on deficits and with efforts directed at disadvantaged populations. Today, with the increasing recognition that parenting can present problems for all parents and that parental self-esteem does affect children, not only is there an extension of programs to all classes of people but also an eager reaction by parents of all classes who do want to become better parents.
- *What should or can be taught?* More than cognitive knowledge, *modeling of positive parent-child interaction* and *nurturing support systems* for parents seem to be two key ingredients of successful parent education programs. Among the needed programs are (1) education for parenting, including direct firsthand experiences working with children; (2) par-

enting programs geared toward cultural minorities, which would build on natural support systems and cultural strengths; (3) programs for parents-to-be, including techniques for human nurturing and improvement of interpersonal skills; and (4) programs for those who are already parents, which would provide parent drop-in centers, self-help support groups, health home visitors, and warmlines.
- *Who should support the necessary programs?* In the current economic crisis, the challenge for the future is funding and carrying the message of success to the public. A significant trend appears to be localization. This can be found not only in utilization of local sources, but also in relying on parents themselves, both as teachers and organizers of others and as contributors of time, efforts, and funds.
- *When should parent education occur?* Two family events give logical occasion to parent education, namely (1) the birth of a child and (2) the start of a child in school. Both these times signal a change in family dynamics and patterns, an increase in expectation and vulnerability, and parental contact with a system.

The nurse should realize that an increasing number of children are being parented completely by divorced, widowed, and single fathers and mothers. Health programs need to specifically address the needs of parents and children in these situations.

Single Parents

Adolescent single parents and their infants are at high risk both emotionally and physically. Help with parenting skills for this age group is a high priority for the community health nurse. Adolescents usually have not completed their own physical, mental, and emotional growth, and becoming responsible for another human being presents both a maturational and a situational crisis for them. Pre- and postnatal clinics set up for intensive and personal care for this group, as well as alternative education classes within the school system, have been ways in which this has been accomplished. Chapter 14 discusses adolescent parenthood further.

Divorced, single, or separated parents often find themselves fulfilling the roles of individual, father, mother, breadwinner, homemaker, and citizen. This can be an overwhelming situation unless appropriate resources are available and utilized. The community health nurse is able to help single parents look at the reality of their situation and at the options and resources available to them. Community groups, such as Parents Without Partners and local family counseling centers, may be helpful. Many times these parents are functioning quite well in relation to the responsibilities they encounter. The positive aspects and actions evidenced should be reinforced.

The single father can be at a greater disadvantage for receiving societal supports than the single mother. Many programs have been designed and implemented for maternal-child health, since this is considered the natural occurrence. The father, whose involvement with his children has only recently received societal sanction, often finds himself less prepared and with fewer supports in his dual-parent role.

Another dilemma of the single parent is that of the "weekend parent." Many divorced fathers are put in the role of seeing their children on a limited basis. They are unsure of their role with their children and have many concerns about how to facilitate their children's developmental growth. Again, the nurse, with counseling and referral to appropriate resources, can be helpful and can facilitate adjustment to the weekend parent role.

Preventive Health Care

Newborn Assessment

Assessment of the newborn is viewed as a decisive foundation for early case finding and preventive care. The kinds of observations that are made help to determine the nursing and medical care that the infant will receive as well as the kind of parenting that is given.

During the assessment, the nurse should get baseline data about the infant's surface features, movement patterns, and general health for comparisons with future examinations. Since health promotion is the concern, systematic periodic assessment over a period of time is important. The developmental approach, rather than the traditional disease-oriented model, should be the focus. Parental involvement in the assessment process helps the nurse to see how the family interacts. It also provides the opportunity to begin anticipatory guidance and problem solving.

The Neonatal Behavioral Assessment Scale developed by T. Berry Brazelton (Brazelton, 1973) is a valid and useful method for observing, making judgments, and scoring selected reflexes, motor responses, and interactive behavioral responses of newborns. The main focus of the scale is on the observation and rating of the infant's interactive behavior. It measures a total of 27 behavioral responses of the infant organized into the following six categories:

1. Habituation—how soon the infant diminishes responses to specific stimuli
2. Orientation—when and how often the infant attends to auditory and visual stimuli
3. Motor maturity—how well the infant coordinates and controls motor activities
4. Variation—how often the infant coordinates and controls motor activities
5. Self-quieting abilities—how often, how soon, and how effectively the infant uses personal resources to console himself or herself
6. Social behaviors—smiling and cuddling behaviors

Using the Brazelton scale points out vividly that newborns are able to control their responses to external stimuli. Generally, the abilities of newborns have been underestimated by both parents and health professionals. Erickson (1976) has described how child care professionals can best utilize the Neonatal Assessment Scale.

Appendix 13-3 presents other possible screening tools available to the community health nurse for gathering baseline data about infants and children.

Anticipatory Guidance

Anticipatory guidance in helping parents to know what to expect of their children at different stages is one of the *most basic and significant* health promotion needs of parents. Through anticipatory guidance, parents can gain knowledge about average development, and thus they will not expect too much or too little from their children. They can also learn that, although there are patterns, each child is unique within a pattern. Parents readily acquire literature on growth and development from the hospital or pediatrician. The community health nurse should be familiar with this material and explain to parents that it is to be used a guide.

Parents are able to assess quite accurately their children's problems when they are given adequate information. This is logical because their proximity makes them frequent observers. Parents' assessment is important because how they define health or behavior as a problem influences interaction in the home and the child's further development.

Since an infant's growth and development is so rapid during the first 2 years, it is imperative that periodic and systematic screening be done. An illustration of this is the infant's reflexes which are present during the first weeks and then develop into purposeful movements as the central nervous system develops. Periodic comprehensive assessment and use of the developmental model facilitates the study of an infant's growth, early behavior patterns, and general development. If, for example, the infant's reflexes are questionable in symmetry, equality, or movement, this might be a sign of immaturity or a lack of integration in the central nervous system. These might also be signals of serious impairment of the central nervous system. Periodic screening and evaluation helps parents and professionals to evaluate more carefully the questionable status of the reflexes and to plan stimulation that enhances sensory development.

Baseline information compiled through periodic assessment is the key to planning early intervention. It allows for objectivity in conclusions that can be made about an infant's early development and can aid in planning interventions. The baseline data also serve as a basis for self-comparison of an infant or child over a period of time. It is imperative that the nurse know "normal" expectations for development so that what

TABLE 13-4   Recommended immunization schedule for infants and children*

Recommended age	Vaccine(s)†‡
2 months	DTP-1, OPV-1
4 months	DTP-2, OPV-2
6 months	DTP-3
15 months	DTP-4, OPV-3, MMR
18 months	Hib
4-6 years	DTP-5, OPV-4
11-12 years‡	MMR
14-16 years and every 10 years thereafter	Td

*Vaccines work best when they are given at the recommended time and on a regular schedule. Measles vaccine, for example, is not usually given to infants before the age of 15 months. When given earlier than that, it may not be as effective. Oral polio and DTP vaccines must be given over a period of time, in a series of properly spaced doses and shots.

†DTP = diphtheria and tetanus toxoids combined with pertussis vaccine; OPV = oral poliovirus vaccine with three types (Types 1, 2, and 3) of attenuated poliovirus; MMR = a combined vaccine with live measles, mumps, and rubella; Hib = Haemophilus b conjugate vaccine; and Td = full dose adult tetanus toxoid combined with a reduced dose of diphtheria toxoid developed for adult use.

‡The American Academy of Pediatrics, Committee on Infectious Diseases recommended, in December 1989, that a second dose of MMR be given to children between the age of 11 to 12 years. (Refer to American Academy of Pediatrics, Committee on Infectious Diseases: Measles: reassessment of the current policy, Pediatrics 84[6]:1110-1113, 1989.)

From USDHHS, Public Health Service: Parents guide to childhood immunization, Atlanta, Ga, 1988, Centers for Disease Control, p 18.

is unusual, abnormal, or delayed can be quickly recognized.

There are numerous schedules available for preventive child health care. Appendix 13-1 presents a summary of the health care which should be provided at specified intervals. Table 13-4 presents the recommended immunization schedule for infants and children. Children whose immunization program has been delayed will have a different schedule (refer to Tables 13-5 and 13-6). Providing parents a written immunization schedule can help to prevent confusion. Effective anticipatory guidance helps parents to determine when children should have immunizations and the value of them.

Immunizations are important, but they are not without their problems. If a child has a fever, im-

TABLE 13-5 Recommended immunization schedule for infants and children up to their 7th birthday, delayed in beginning immunizations

Timing	Vaccine(s)
Age at first visit	
2-14 months of age	DTP-1, OPV-1
15-24 months of age	DTP-1, OPV-1 and MMR*
18 months of age or older	DTP-1, OPV-1, MMR, and Hib†
2 months after DTP-1, OPV-1	DTP-2, OPV-2
2 months after DTP-2	DTP-3
6-12 months after DTP-3	DTP-4, OPV-3
Preschool (4-6 years of age)‡	DTP-5, OPV-4

*MMR—should be given on first visit after child reaches 15 months of age.

†Hib—should be given at 18 months of age or as soon as possible thereafter. Hib is not generally recommended for children 5 years (60 months) of age or older.

‡The preschool dose is not necessary if the fourth dose of DTP and the third dose of OPV are given after the fourth birthday.

From USDHHS, Public Health Service: Parents guide to childhood immunization, Atlanta, Ga, 1988, Centers for Disease Control, p 19.

TABLE 13-6 Recommended immunization schedule for persons 7 years of age or older who have not received any vaccines previously*

Timing	Vaccine(s)
First visit	Td-1, OPV-1†, and MMR
2 months after Td-1, OPV-1	Td-2, OPV-2
6-12 months after Td-2, OPV-2	Td-3, OPV-3
10 years after Td-3 and every 10 years thereafter	Td

*If a series of these immunizations has been started, then interrupted, it need not be restarted but simply completed at proper intervals.

†OPV not routinely given to those 18 years of age or older.

From USDHHS, Public Health Service: Parents guide to childhood immunization, Atlanta, Ga, 1988, Centers for Disease Control, p 19.

munizations are not to be given since they cause increased fever. Usually a child with a chronic illness, especially allergies and a central nervous system disorder, should have a physician's order for an immunization. Allergy to the substance any vaccine was grown on is an indication that the im-

munization should not be given. Another consideration is that at least 1 month should elapse between injections of live vaccine because live organisms can reduce the immunity potential of other live organisms. In general, problems of immunologic deficiency and immunosuppressive therapy, such as the use of corticosteroids, are contraindications for vaccines without a physician's specific order.

The Immunization Practices Advisory Committee has published information about the risks of pertussis disease and pertussis vaccine to infants and children with a personal or family history of convulsions (Centers for Disease Control, 1984, p. 170). Figure 13-7 provides general guidelines, developed by this committee, to follow when immunizing infants and children who are at risk for experiencing a convulsion after receiving a dose of DTP.

Though vaccines are available to prevent measles, mumps, rubella, whooping cough, diphtheria, and polio there is none to prevent chicken pox. Chicken pox, or varicella, strikes about 85 percent of all the children in the United States. However, a preventive vaccine may be available soon.

Also included in the preventive child health care schedule are the history to be obtained from parents and physical measurements to be done. The Denver Developmental Screening Test (Erickson, 1976, pp. 173-192) and the Washington Guide (Barnard and Erickson, 1976, pp. 75-95) are valuable tools that assist the nurse in checking for developmental landmarks, giving norms for their attainment. Areas of concern to parents about infants include nutrition, frequency and amounts of feedings, weaning, sleeping patterns, teething, handling of the genitals, and dealing with common illnesses. After the first year of life, the child matures and new behavior patterns develop. Parents thus have additional areas of concern after a child is a year old, such as how to provide adequate nutrition when appetite decreases. This is normal, because the child is also having a decrease in growth. Other concerns during this period include sleep disturbances and nightmares, nocturnal enuresis, bowel and bladder training, thumbsucking, temper tantrums, masturbation,

The following general guidelines cannot cover every situation. Individualized medical judgment in specific cases may indicate a different course of action.

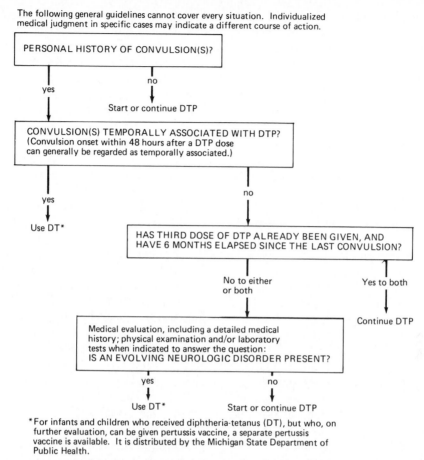

*For infants and children who received diphtheria-tetanus (DT), but who, on further evaluation, can be given pertussis vaccine, a separate pertussis vaccine is available. It is distributed by the Michigan State Department of Public Health.

Figure 13-7   Guidelines for diphtheria-tetanus-pertussis (DTP) immunization of infants and young children with histories of convulsion(s). (Michigan State Department of Public Health, Lansing, Mi, 1985, unpaginated.)

stuttering, negativism, and the increased need for independence and exploration. A thoughtful hearing of questions in relation to these concerns gives the nurse an idea of how the parents perceive the problem. Answers based on the child's development are supportive and help to eliminate some major concerns and problems.

Helping parents to know when a child is ill enough to call a doctor is important. This action can help to prevent minor upper respiratory infections (URIs) and gastrointestinal (GI) upsets from becoming major problems. Fever of 101° F for over for 24 hours is a signal to parents to call the doctor.

The possibilities for preventive health care are varied and almost endless when helping parents to learn to handle childhood illness. Questions such

as the following help a community health nurse to determine what information parents need in order to prevent serious illness: Do the parents have a thermometer and do they know how to use it? Do they understand the meaning of dehydration? Do they know basic first aid and when to call a physician?

Accident Prevention

Since accidents are the major cause of death after the age of 1 year, prevention of them is critical. Appendix 13-2 summarizes typical actions that cause accidents and lists precautions to take at varying age levels to avoid accidents.

It has long been recognized that a child's environment significantly influences his or her state of health. The most common site of accidental injuries to children under the age of 15 is the home (USDHHS, Office of Maternal and Child Health, 1989, p. 27). Human as well as physical factors in the home can lead to accidents. For example, parents' lack of knowledge about childhood growth and development can contribute to accidents. Parents who lack this understanding often neglect to "safety proof" the child's environment. Infants and toddlers need to be protected from hazards in the environment. They lack the cognitive development needed to understand what things or activities could lead to injury. Developmental characteristics which place young children at risk for specific types of accidents are identified in Appendix 13-2. Providing parents with this type of information can help them to identify potential hazards in a child's environment.

Parents cannot remove all environmental hazards and they *cannot* and *should not* control their children 24 hours a day. However, with a combination of child supervision, education of parents, and legislative and environmental changes to get rid of hazards, accidents can be reduced. Families need an understanding of the philosophy of accident prevention. As specified by the National Safety Council, it is not a barrage of dos and don'ts but rather it is doing things the right way in the interest of the welfare of others.

One method the nurse can use to improve the family approach to accident prevention is accident analysis after an accident occurs. What, how, to whom, where, when, and why did the accident happen? Families must understand that the purpose of this is not to fix blame but rather to prevent a recurrence. Often, teaching the parent who is the primary care provider for the child will have an impact on accident prevention. The nurse can help this parent to be alert to hazards in the environment when home visits are made.

Automobiles are also killers of children. Safety belts or safety car seats should always be worn by children in the car since children can become flying missiles against the dashboard or window. Children can fall from moving cars if they are able to manipulate the locks. Obviously, seatbelts prevent such an accident. Children should never be left alone in parked cars. The cigarette lighter, gear shift, steering wheel, and clutch are all very dangerous playthings.

Booklets with simple pictures about traffic safety can form the basis for real world child and parent experiences. They can help children assume pedestrian responsibility safety. Such booklets can be found in local bookstores and are also available from many state and local health departments.

There are community approaches to the problem of accident prevention as well as individual ones. "Children Can't Fly" was a program developed by the New York City Department of Health to combat the high incidence of child morbidity and mortality due to falls from windows. As a result of the community education approach, including counseling, referral, data collecting, media campaign, community education for prevention, and the provision of free window guards, falls were reduced by 50 percent from 1973 to 1975 (Spiegel and Lindaman, 1977). The program continues as a result of its success, and is a strategy being advocated nationwide to reduce accidental injuries among children.

Child-resistant caps have dramatically decreased the accidental ingestion of prescription drugs and household poisons. In 1972, accidental poisoning deaths of children were listed at 216. By 1980, this number had dropped to 12. Child-resistant closures are credited with saving these lives (Child resistant caps, 1984, p. D4).

Prevention of Child Maltreatment

As previously mentioned in this chapter, abuse and neglect are symptoms of stress in a family. The conditions of poverty, undernutrition, unemployment, overcrowding, restricted physical surroundings, and inadequate education support this problem. Knowledge currently available tells us that antenatal poverty and nutritional deficits produce a high-risk infant; at the same time, high-quality medical care is least available to the very people who are at highest risk. The high-risk infant and ill-prepared parents have the fewest resources for achieving the best health possible. Communities can deal with these poverty problems at a local level. However, the nation needs to deal with them at a federal level to make the fullest impact.

To save a child from the serious effects of abuse and neglect, nurses need to be alert when they notice that families are having children very quickly with no relief between pregnancies (Robarge, Reynolds, and Groothuis, 1982, p. 199). The danger signs of marital stress, isolation, and overwhelmed parents need to be seen also. Premature births, where questionable bonding has taken place, indicate a need for priority service, as do families where there are children with developmental disabilities and chronic disease.

Every parent needs to know how children grow and develop; the concept that babies are responsible for their acts and can think and reason like an adult is all too commonly believed and must be corrected.

Education of personnel, including judges, attorneys, social workers and doctors, is necessary so that abused children are found and identified as such, and then given treatment. Parents must not be treated as criminals but rather given help so that their stress is alleviated. Equally important are the rights of children.

Social institutions such as churches and schools need to be utilized to help support families. In our mobile society where people move frequently, families can feel isolated and alone and uncared for. Homemaker services, big brothers and sisters, and parent aides, as well as community volunteers, could fill some of the gaps experienced by families who are isolated.

Preschool Assessments

Kindergarten and preschool health assessments are excellent developmental points at which to look at the physical, intellectual, and emotional growth of children. At this time, parents are increasingly aware of and concerned about the learning and thought competency of their children. They want to know that their children are ready to begin school. A child's ability to learn, see, perform appropriate gross and fine motor tasks, follow instruction, speak, communicate, and relate socially with others are all indicators of readiness for school (refer to Figure 13-8). The Denver Developmental Screening Test is one method used by community health nurses to look at these areas.

Preschool assessments also provide an excellent opportunity to enforce state immunization laws so that all children receive immunizations before they are in school. Evidence suggests that a sizable number of preschoolers are not fully immunized. "In the most recent U.S. Immunization Survey in 1985, only 77% of 2-year-olds whose parents had records at home had received their basic series" (Centers for Disease Control, 1988, October, p. 614). Recent outbreaks of measles and mumps among preschoolers suggest that the population of children fully immunized may be declining (USDHHS, Office of Maternal and Child Health, 1989, p. 37).

Day Care for Children

Societal attitudes about raising normal healthy children are changing. At one time, parents were criticized if the mother was not in the home 24 hours a day with the children. However, today, many mothers want to work and many of them must work. In 1988, the participation of mothers in the labor force aged 18 to 44 years with newborn children reached 51 percent (Bureau of the Census, Fertility of American Women, 1989, p. 4). The number of single-parent situations more than doubled between 1970 and 1988 (Bureau of the Census, 1989, Studies in Marriage and the Family, p. 14). In the future, the majority of preschoolers will very likely have mothers who are in the labor force. Day care can help parents who want to work or have to work to deal with the stress associated with parenting and full-time employment. It may also help children from these families to obtain emotional, intellectual, and physical stimulation, as well as positive human relationships that will lay the foundation for growth in these areas. However, day care does not eliminate all the problems families must adapt to when both parents are working. Day care, for instance, does not take care of a child who is acutely ill. Thus, if a child is sick, parents need to find other resources for child care. As previously discussed, illness is common among preschool children.

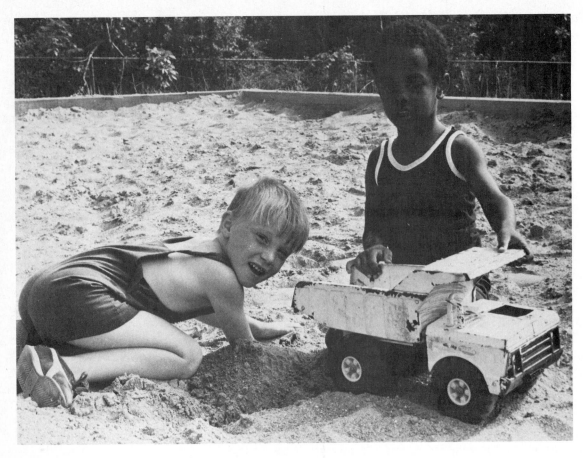

Figure 13-8   Healthy 5-year-old children.

In the near future, there will be a growing demand for day-care services for preschool children. However, disadvantaged populations may find it increasingly difficult to obtain such services. Since 1981, federal funds under Title XX have been significantly cut. Day care was one of the three highest funded services under this legislation (Kamerman, 1983, p. 38). Hopefully, health planners will focus on day-care services as one of their major priorities for program development in the coming years.

GENERAL CONCEPTS OF HEALTH PROMOTION

Health promotion needs are based on the developmental tasks and common health problems of the specific population group. For the 0- to 5-year-old and parenting population, the following factors should be considered when developing a health promotion program:

1. A monitoring system to identify high-risk infants and parents
2. An organized community program to combat problems such as accidents and child abuse
3. An organized system for provision of preventive health services, such as physical examinations and immunizations
4. Health education program to meet anticipatory guidance needs of parents and children
5. A well-established procedure for follow-up

care of clients with identified health care needs.

6. Passage and revision of significant legislation, such as the enforcement of immunization laws

INFANTS WITH LONG-TERM PHYSICAL/ NEUROLOGICAL HANDICAPS

Over the past two decades, it has become increasingly possible to save smaller and sicker newborns. Twenty years ago, nine of every 10 babies born weighing less than 1000 grams (2.2 lb) died. Today, with the median birth weight at 7 lb 8 oz, up to 75 percent of the babies who weigh between 1.7 and 2.2 lb survive.

It is the rare low-birth-weight infant, however, who does not suffer serious complications such as brain or pulmonary hemorrhages, heart failure, or infections—among others. Further, the number of babies born each year with multiple defects totals about 30,000.

An increasing number of these babies receive sophisticated treatment at birth and are growing into young children whose lives are regulated by technology. One such group of children are infants who are ventilator-dependent.

Increasing numbers of parents are opting to care for such children at home and, with adequate support, are able to do so. Community health nurses need expert technical skills to care for the nursing problems inherent in their care. They also need the ability to give support to families who struggle with overwhelming financial, emotional, familial, and other problems.

To consider the questions and issues that arise when meeting the health care needs of children with disabilities, the Surgeon General's Workshop on Children with Handicaps and Their Families was convened on December 13, 1982. More than 150 people participated in the workshop, including patients, families, and experts in health care. The ventilator-dependent child was used as a model to discuss the question: Can quality care for children with several medical problems be provided in a home and community setting, rather than in a high-technology medical center?

The following recommendations were generated by the workshop (USDHHS, Public Health Service, 1982):

1. *Define the scope of the problem.* More definitive information is needed about the numbers and types of disabilities experienced by infants, children, and young adults in this country, as is a better assessment of the impact of these statistics on social, health, educational, and family-related needs. Considerable progress has been made in some areas, but a system integrating functional, social, health, and family concerns remains to be defined, accepted, and consistently used by all service personnel and agencies.

2. *Develop model standards for care.* Model guidelines and standards must be developed for identifying, evaluating, and providing coordinated care at all levels for persons with disabilities. Care standards for cohorts of disabled children with special needs must be superimposed on generic care standards for all children with disabilities. *All standards must focus on family needs,* with an eye to innovation and with compassion and concern for the quality of life of each disabled child. Careful consideration must be given to identifying methods of care that conserve and effectively use scarce fiscal and human resources.

3. *Develop systems of regionalized care.* Matching the needs of disabled children with available resources will demand a system of care that reflects concern for social, educational, health, and family issues and that can focus on times of transition in disabled children's lives. Targets for concentration of resources will be determined by such factors as incidence, prevalence, and severity of the disability; location of the needed service; and other geographic and demographic considerations. Traditional methods will suffice for providing community-based health care for infants, children, and young adults with relatively uncomplicated disabling conditions; however, regionalized care will be required

for disabled children who have life-threatening conditions or who require highly specialized tertiary care.

4. *Improve financing of care.* The service system must reward providers and consumers using out-of-hospital facilities that are close to patients' home communities and that meet established standards of care. Funding mechanisms must also be made available for expensive out-of-hospital technical equipment that reduces the length of hospital stays. Planning and coordination of services for patients with complicated and serious disabilities must be recognized as a legitimate, reimbursable expense.

5. *Identify areas that have potential for abuse.* Both actions and inactions can contribute to abuse of the care system for the disabled child. Elimination of unnecessary, duplicative, or inappropriate services promotes quality care and controls costs. Standards and regulations must be developed and monitored by qualified professionals familiar with service delivery issues.

6. *Incorporate principles of care for disabled children in training curriculums for health professionals.* There is a need for incorporation of clinical experiences relating to the care of disabled infants, children, and young adults into all levels of preservice and inservice education for health professionals. Teaching models should enhance professional satisfaction in caring for disabled children. Methods to improve communication by professionals with patients, patients' families, and coworkers must be components of the training program.

7. *Support research on the care of children with disabilities.* Although our scientific understanding of many disabling diseases and conditions is sophisticated, we need to learn much more about optimal methods of health care delivery for disabled children. Among the subjects research should address are ways to provide better training for health professionals in evaluative methods and treatment techniques, methods for improving communication and coordination of skills among professionals, techniques for immediate dissemination of new information concerning the care of disabled children, and ways to improve financial reimbursement procedures. Increasing concern for fiscal responsibility and accountability will point up the wisdom of devoting significant portions of available resources to expand research and development endeavors.

Appendix 9-1 reveals one mother's graphic story of her struggles to keep her ventilator-dependent child at home and the strengths and weaknesses of the health care team who aided the family in its struggle. She was present at the Surgeon General's Workshop on Children with Handicaps and Their Families and presented this material there.

Families who have children with special needs, like ventilator-dependent children, need coordinated, comprehensive health care services which ensure continuity of care. They also need to have a clear understanding of the referral process and community resources which can promote family stability and concrete assistance during times of stress. Chapters 7, 9, and 17 are helpful to review when visiting families in the community who have "special" children.

SIGNIFICANT HEALTH LEGISLATION

During the past 70 years there has been much federal legislation and many demonstration projects concerned with the health of infants and mothers in America. The Children's Bureau was established in 1912. White House Conferences on Children and Youth have been held every 10 years since 1910. The Shepherd-Towner Act of 1921 created maternal and child health services at the state level, supported by the federal government. Title V of the Social Security Act of 1935 provided for grants to states for maternal and child health services and services to crippled children. The Emergency Maternity and Infant Care Program existed during the 1930s. The need for community mental health programs was recognized in the 1960s. The Eighty-ninth Congress, during President Johnson's time in office (1963–1968), brought huge changes in child health legislation with the establishment of the Office of Economic Opportunity and its Headstart Program, Medicaid, and the National Institutes of Child Health and Human Development. Some of the significant current legislation follows.

Medicaid

The largest current public medical program for children is Medicaid. Title XIX of the Social Security Act mandated Medicaid, which was enacted to reach high-risk, high-priority children and youth in needy families. Those eligible for Medicaid coverage include children who are members of families receiving Aid to Families of Dependent Children or who are covered by a state's medically needy program. Medicaid benefits are covered in Chapter 4 under Governmental Health Assistance Programs.

The Early Periodic Screening, Diagnosis, and Treatment program (EPSDT) was designed to periodically assess all children under 21 in the Medicaid program (Health Care Financing Administration, 1988). Federal regulations are established by the Department of Health and Human Services for this screening, and the suggested schedule is at the time of hospital discharge for a new infant, 2 to 6 weeks, 2 to 4 months, 5 to 7 months, 8 to 10 months, 11 to 14 months, 17 to 19 months, 21 to 25 months, 3 to 4 years, and 5 to 6 years. The EPSDT has the following five stages:

1. Outreach and case finding, which include all of the services necessary to find, identify, inform, and assist eligible persons to utilize the EPSDT program. Federal regulations state that recipients of welfare must be informed about the program and its benefits and efforts must be made to bring eligible children into the program
2. Screening, administering, coordinating, and developing new resources as needed, as well as evaluating and monitoring the existing screening resources
3. Testing of children done by a trained nurse

which includes an unclothed physical examination, developmental appraisal, growth measurements, anemia screening, lead-poisoning screening, tuberculosis testing, vision and hearing testing, dental screening, and the evaluation of nutritional status
4. Compilation and reporting of results which composes a health profile for each screened individual from the findings of the testing
5. Follow-through and treatment which ensures follow-up and treatment indicated by the testing and health profile

The Consolidated Omnibus Budget Reconciliation Act of 1985 (COBRA), the Omnibus Budget Reconciliation Act of 1986 (OBRA), and the Omnibus Budget Reconciliation Act of 1989 (OBRA-89) contained Medicaid amendments of significance to the health of mothers and children (refer to Chapter 4). All three of these acts expanded Medicaid coverage to low-income pregnant women who previously would not have qualified for this coverage. OBRA legislation also expanded Medicaid to low-income infants under 1 year of age, and children up to 8 years old in families below a state-established income level, which may be as high as 100 percent of the federal poverty level. OBRA-89 requires states to extend Medicaid coverage to all children born after September 30, 1990, up to age 6, in families with incomes below 133 percent of the federal poverty level (National Association for Home Care, 1989, p. 3). ORBA legislation needs to be monitored carefully by health care professionals because amendments to this act significantly influence the type of maternal and child health and other health care services funded by the federal government.

Child Maltreatment

The Child Abuse, Prevention and Treatment Act (Public Law 93-247) was signed into law in 1974 in response to the need for a nationwide effort to solve this complex problem. This act created the National Center on Child Abuse and Neglect as the primary place where the federal government can focus its efforts on identifying, treating, and preventing child abuse and neglect (Combating child abuse, 1988, p. 369). To carry out the mandates of the act, the National Center has begun programs in four areas: demonstration and research, information gathering and dissemination, training and technical assistance, and assistance to states. In 1962, the Children's Bureau developed and promoted a model state child abuse mandatory reporting law which, in effect, states that professionals or child-care workers must report suspected child abuse to the appropriate officials. Public Law 93-247 reinforced this mandate.

The Child Abuse, Prevention and Treatment Act of 1974 has been amended several times in the past decade and a half. In 1988, Congress passed legislation to reauthorize three programs designed to prevent and treat child abuse and domestic violence and to encourage the adoption of hard-to-place children. This legislative act was entitled "The Child Abuse, Prevention, Adoption, and Family Services Act of 1988" (Public Law 100-294). It consolidated into one act the Child Abuse Prevention and Treatment Act of 1974, the Child Abuse Prevention and Treatment and Adoption Reform Act of 1978, and the Family Violence Prevention and Services Act of 1984.

Public Law 100-294 mandates funding to support state and local efforts designed to prevent abuse and family violence and to identify and treat the victims. It also ensures funding of the National Center on Child Abuse and Neglect, a national commission on child and youth deaths, a project to study the nationwide incidence of family violence, and initiatives to eliminate barriers to the adoption of older children, minority children, and children with physical and mental handicaps. Additionally, it mandates support of professional training and research activities (USDHHS, Administration for Children, Youth, and Families, 1988).

The states have acted upon Public Law 100-294 in various ways and community health nurses must know the laws that are in effect in the states in which they are working. Health care professionals are directly affected by this law and by state child protection laws that require the reporting of child abuse and neglect.

Maternal-Child Health Program

Title V of the Social Security Act has authorized the Maternal and Child Health Program since 1935 and has mandated categorical and discretionary funding to the states to reduce infant mortality, to promote maternal and child health, and to treat crippled children. Title V was continued with significant amendments by the 1981 Omnibus Budget Reconciliation Act (OBRA), Public Law 97-35. OBRA combined seven categorical programs into a maternal and child health block grant, provided funding for special projects, genetic disease testing and counseling programs, and hemophilia diagnostic and treatment centers, and reauthorized selected maternal and child health categorical programs, including the childhood immunization, venereal disease control, tuberculosis prevention and control, migrant health centers, family planning, and adolescent pregnancy programs.

Within Title V, there are two major funding components: MCH block grants to states, and discretionary grants, known as Special Projects of Regional and National Significance (SPRANS). MCH block grant funds are allocated to state health agencies on the basis of specified formulas. SPRANS grants are awarded on a competitive basis to a variety of nonprofit and for-profit organizations (Information Sciences Research Institute, 1989).

Maternal and Child Health (MCH) Block Grant

MCH block grants are provided to states to ensure access to quality maternal and child health services; to reduce infant mortality and the incidence of preventable diseases and handicapping conditions among children; to promote the health of mothers and children; to provide rehabilitation services for blind and disabled individuals under age 16; and to provide assistance to children who are in need of special health care services (known as *crippled children services* in many states). States must apply for block grant monies each year and supply to the federal government needs assessment data and a proposal describing how these funds will be used (Information Sciences Research Institute, 1989).

Many services can be covered under the MCH block grants including services dealing with, but not limited to, maternal and child health; crippled children; disabled children receiving Supplemental Security Income; prevention of lead poisoning; sudden infant death syndrome; hemophilia; genetic diseases; and adolescent pregnancy. In 1989, MCH service projects proposed under the Healthy Birth Act of 1989 were attached to the MCH block grant. New community-based comprehensive service delivery projects authorized were *maternal-child health home visiting programs* aimed at improving poor pregnancy and infant health outcomes; *"one-step shopping"* projects designed to provide integrated and co-location human service delivery models; and a *maternal and child health handbook.* Funding was provided only for the MCH handbook (The National Commission to Prevent Infant Mortality, 1990).

Special Projects of Regional and National Significance (SPRANS)

The OBRA of 1981 included a stipulation that allowed the federal government to retain 10 to 15 percent of the MCH block grant appropriation each fiscal year to support discretionary programs or Special Projects of Regional and National Significance (SPRANS). The SPRANS grant categories are MCH research; MCH training; genetic disease testing, counseling, and information dissemination; hemophilia diagnostic and treatment centers; and other special projects. The "other special projects" category includes a wide range of demonstration and innovative initiatives designed to improve maternal, infant, adolescent, and family health (Information Sciences Research Institute, 1989). Some of the well-known SPRANS projects are the Maternity and Infant Care Projects, Projects for Intensive Care of Infants, Children and Youth Projects, and Dental Health for Children Programs. SPRANS grants offer professionals the opportunity to experiment with new systems of care or new approaches to the delivery of MCH services. They also provide funding for the training of specialized health professionals and continuing education for state and local MCH personnel. Heavy emphasis is placed on research in SPRANS projects.

Women, Infants, and Children Program (WIC)

As discussed in Chapter 4, WIC is a federal nutrition and health assistance program administered by the U.S. Department of Agriculture. This program makes food available to nutritional at risk pregnant and lactating women, and infants and children up to the age of 5 years. Some factors that place women and children at risk are anemia, poor diet, chronic disease, developmental disabilities, too much or too little weight gain during pregnancy, age (under 17 years or over 34 years), history of problems during pregnancy, and a pregnancy within the preceding 6 months. WIC participants receive coupons which they may redeem for food at retail stores authorized to accept food coupons. Women and children may receive milk, cheese, eggs, juices rich in vitamin C, cereals rich in iron, dried peas or beans, or peanut butter. Infants may receive infant formula, cereal, or juice; infants less than 3 months of age receive only formula (Michigan Department of Public Health, 1986).

The WIC program helps to correct or prevent malnutrition and also helps participants to receive necessary health care. This program provides nutrition and health screening, health education services, food, and referral to needed community resources. Amendments to WIC legislation in 1986 require states to develop plans for outreach to pregnant women for the purpose of encouraging early enrollment in the program (Child Nutrition Amendments of 1986). WIC regulations also provide incentives for breast feeding. Breastfeeding women are allowed to receive benefits for up to 1 year postpartum while non-breastfeeding women are eligible for only 6 months of benefits. Breastfeeding participants also can receive a greater variety and quantity of food than non-breastfeeding participants and receive a higher priority for WIC services when waiting lists are in effect (Food and Nutrition Service Research, 1989).

The WIC program can positively influence the health outcomes of pregnancy and the utilization of health services during pregnancy. Research suggests that participation in the WIC program during pregnancy is associated with higher birth weight, reduced fetal deaths, and reduced health care costs (Kotelchuck, 1984; Rush, 1986; Schramm, 1986). WIC participation has also been shown to increase the likelihood that a woman will receive adequate prenatal care (Bowling and Riley, 1987). Community health nurses play a significant role in encouraging at-risk mothers and children to utilize WIC services.

Fertility Related State Laws

In recent years, several states have enacted fertility related laws: in 1982 alone, 45 such laws were passed. These new laws cover such issues as sterilization, abortion, insurance benefits for pregnancy-related health care, family planning services and information, and maternal and infant health. Much of the legislation reflected a growing concern about the health problems of low-income women, infants, and children.

Legislative developments generally reflect the issues of major concern to the public and to policy-makers. Although the 1982 laws indicate a declining interest in regulation of abortion, legislators probably will continue to pass laws to limit Medicaid funding of abortions as well as insurance coverage. The Supreme Court rulings on waiting period of informed consent requirements, hospitalization for second-trimester abortions and parental consent may generate considerable legislative activity later this year.

In general, though, states can be expected to pass laws aimed at broadening pregnancy benefits and improving pregnancy outcome and access to family planning services. Concerns over high teenage pregnancy rates may result in legislation relating to sex education as well as fertility-related services (Bush, 1983, p. 111). These concerns continue into the 1990s. As previously discussed, OBRA legislation has broadened pregnancy benefits. However, issues related to abortion and family planning are becoming increasingly controversial.

Developmental Disabilities

Scientific advances in recent decades have made it possible to save infants who previously would have died at birth. However, this phenomenon has created special challenges for health care professionals. The number of infants and children with developmental disabilities is increasing significantly. These children need assistance to help them to achieve their maximum potential. Because this assistance was often very costly and not available for many children with developmental disabilities, the Congress has passed, in the past decade and a half, two significant pieces of legislation that were designed to promote early intervention with handicapped and at-risk young children.

The Education for All Handicapped Children Act (Public Law 94-142) was enacted in November 1975. This act entitles all handicapped children between the ages of 6 and 18 years a free and appropriate education regardless of the type of handicap or the degree of impairment. It also allows incentive monies for providing services to children beginning at age 3 and for young adults between 18 and 21. This act is discussed more extensively in Chapter 14.

The Education of the Handicapped Act Amendments of 1986 (Public Law 99-457) significantly expanded services to preschool children 3 to 5 years old and at-risk infants and toddlers up to age 3 years. This law created two new federal programs—the preschool grant program and the handicapped infants and toddlers program. By 1990-1991, state educational agencies must provide a free and appropriate education for all handicapped children beginning at the age of 3 years. Significant federal funding was allocated to support the preschool grant program. The handicapped infants and toddlers program was established to reduce the potential for developmental delays, help families to meet the special needs of their handicapped children and toddlers, minimize institutionalization of handicapped individuals, and reduce educational costs to our society. Incentive funding for this program will help states to develop and implement quality early intervention programs and to coordinate early intervention services. Community health nurses are active participants on the multidisciplinary teams that are providing services to infants and toddlers under this program.

BARRIERS TO HEALTH CARE

Major barriers to the delivery of services to the 0- to 5-year-old population and their parents have been discussed earlier in this chapter and in Chapter 12. The following case situations illustrate some specific problems parents have in obtaining care for themselves and their children, ages 0 to 5 years:

Sue was 17 years old when she became pregnant. Her husband, Tom, age 18, worked as a gas station attendant. His income provided only the basic necessities of food and rent but was too high to allow them any public assistance. Sue decided to "save" money by waiting for antepartum care until near her EDC. Upon her first antepartum visit to the doctor 1 month before delivery, she was found to be severely hypertensive as well as diabetic. Her infant weighed 10 lb at birth and required 1 month's hospitalization. Sue and Tom felt that they were severely criticized by the health personnel for not receiving adequate antepartum care.

Diane and Jim Jones have four children under 5 years of age. Jim has a job-related back injury and is unemployed. The Joneses have a Medicaid card and they utilize the outpatient department of a large teaching hospital in their city for medical care. They go there only when they absolutely must. The family has no car and utilizes the city bus line, which involves three transfers for the 4-mile trip. With four children, Mrs. Jones finds this most difficult, especially in cold weather. When she does arrive at the hospital, she must wait several hours and then sees a different physician each time so that she must repeatedly give her family's health histories. Mrs. Jones feels that "the people in that hospital don't care about or understand me and my kids."

As part of the *Healthy Mothers, Healthy Babies campaign* initiated by the U.S. Department of Health and Human Services to help achieve the maternal and infant health objectives for the nation (Bratic, 1982), a study was carried out to document the perceived barriers to seeking health care and information among women of a lower socioeconomic status. Three major barriers were identified ("Healthy Mothers" Market Research: How to Reach Black and Mexican American Women, 1982): (1) *low priority of preventive health care,* because it takes considerable energy for many of these mothers to meet basic needs and because government funding sources do not adequately finance preventive health services, (2) *difficulties encountered within the health care system,* including communication barriers, perceived negative attitudes of staff, and the unavailability or inappropriateness of educational materials, and (3) *low motivation to adopt good health practices,* because many clients generally have a day-to-day orientation, multiple life problems, and a support group which does not understand or support certain health habits or practices.

THE ROLES OF THE COMMUNITY HEALTH NURSE

The community health nurse plays a number of roles in providing service to the 0-to-5 age group. The following paragraphs describe some of these roles.

Advocate-Planner

Since the children in the 0- to 5-year-old age group cannot speak for themselves, the nurse becomes an advocate. This can involve pointing out to caregivers the safety hazards in the environment and urging necessary changes. On a broader level, the nurse is an advocate for the development of day-care centers in a community and publicizes the inadequacy of health and medical care for economically disadvantaged families. This role of advocate means that the nurse must be involved in the political process to correct issues such as unemployment, lack of adequate income, overcrowding, and the cycle of poverty, which can ultimately be solved only with legislative changes. Attitudes of assertiveness, a knowledge of the political process, and a willingness to take risks are necessary tools for this role.

Teacher

The community health nurse needs to be a teacher. This includes demonstrating information about child care to families and involving parents in the learning process. Helping parents to understand good nutrition for this age group, or why safety seats and belts are necessary in cars, means involvement of all concerned in the process of teaching and learning and changing values and attitudes. The community health nurse is well versed in the developmental tasks of this age group. Teaching parents about these tasks is a form of anticipatory guidance and assists in task accomplishment.

Group Worker

In order to meet the needs of the 0- to 5-year-old population, the community health nurse needs to be attuned to opportunities for group teaching and counseling. Working with the LaLeche League or Parents Anonymous, a crisis intervention program set up to help or prevent damaging relationships between parents and their children are possibilities. Other possibilities are numerous. One community health nurse, for example, had in his caseload area a large mobile park. Within the park, he found five families who had children in special school classes because of developmental disabilities, each of whom expressed a need for help with their child. This staff nurse helped the parents form a weekly discussion group and the results were that isolated families received mutual supportive help in the form of baby sitting, shared meals, and problem solving about how to deal with difficult situations.

Coordinator

Coordinating community resources is another significant role of the community health nurse. There are numerous services available to families, and this is positive. However, families can feel uncared for and torn apart when the department of social services, Medicaid screening clinic, the community health nurse, the school nurse, and the child guidance center all request the same information in detail, or when these same health professionals do not communicate with each other and plan different goals. Professionals need to be careful to ask the permission of a family before they share information they have regarding that family with another professional or agency. They should seek this permission as soon as they identify that families are working with multiple agencies.

Closely tied to this role is the facilitating role of the nurse. Helping families and the larger community to understand their rights as people and to understand services offered in the community all facilitate the better utilization of these services. The nurse helps families work toward desired change. In every community there are persons with ideas and skills, and all that needs to be done is to give them direction and reinforcement. Milio's *9226 Kercheval: The Storefront That Did Not Burn* is the story of how one community health nurse helped an inner-city area establish its own day-care center (Milio, 1970). This nurse found that people saw a great problem with children who were not cared for while mothers worked. She acted as a catalyst to assist in solving the problem and was a facilitator and enabler as well.

Case Finder

Because of the nurse's proximity to infants and children, case finding has been a strategic role for many years. At-risk children are identified and followed periodically as they develop. Disabilities are lessened when treatment is begun early, and some can be prevented by primary intervention. A system needs to be established in each community to periodically screen all children for problems. The Early Periodic Screening, Diagnosis, and Treatment Program (EPSDT) of Medicaid is one schedule that can be followed.

In 1988, the North American Nursing Diagnosis Association accepted "alterations in parenting," "potential alteration in parenting," and "weak mother-infant or parent-infant attachment" as appropriate diagnostic terms in nursing and acceptable nursing diagnoses for clinical testing (Gordon, 1989). These diagnoses are presented in Tables 13-7, 13-8, and 13-9. The defining characteristics developed by the association provide practitioners with useful parameters for case finding when working with families with children.

Epidemiologist

Collecting data on health problems and care is an important epidemiological role. Nurses are concerned about why parents do not use available health services and what motivates those who do.

TABLE 13-7   The North American Nursing Diagnosis Association: Nursing diagnosis for altered parenting

Nursing diagnosis: Altered parenting

Definition: Inability of nurturing figure(s) to create an environment which promotes optimum growth and development of another human being. (Adjustment to parenting, in general, is a normal maturation process following birth of a child.)

Etiological or related factors	Defining characteristics
Knowledge or skill deficit (specify: parenting skills, developmental guidelines, etc.)	Inattentive to infant/child needs*
Fear (specify focus)	Inappropriate caretaking behaviors, (toilet training, feeding, sleep/rest, etc.)*
Social isolation	History of child abuse or abandonment by primary caretaker*
Physical impairment (blindness, etc.)	Actual alteration:
Mental or physical illness	Verbalization cannot control child
Support system deficit (between/from significant other[s])	Abandoment of infant/child
Interrupted parent-infant bonding (e.g., illness of newborn)	Runaway
Family or personal stress (financial, legal, recent crisis, cultural change, multiple pregnancies)	Incidence of physical and psychological trauma
Unmet social, emotional, or developmental needs (of parenting figures)	Lack of parental attachment behaviors
Interruption in bonding process (i.e., maternal, paternal, other)	Inappropriate visual, tactile, auditory stimulation
	Negative identification of infant's/child's characteristics
Unrealistic expectations (self, infant, partner)	Negative attachment of meanings to infant's/child's characteristics; verbalization of resentment toward infant/child
Perceived threat to own survival (physical and emotional)	
Lack of role identity	Verbalization cannot control child
Lack of, or inappropriate, response of child	Evidence of physical and psychological trauma to infant/child
Physical or psychosocial abuse (of nurturing figure)	Constant verbalization of disappointment in gender or physical characteristics of the infant/child
Limited cognitive functioning	Verbalization of role inadequacy
	Verbal disgust at body functions of infant/child
	Noncompliance with health appointments for infant/child or self
	Inappropriate or inconsistent discipline practices
	Frequent accidents (infant/child); frequent illness (infant/child)
	Growth and development lag of infant/child
	Verbalizes desire to have child call parent by first name versus traditional, cultural tendencies
	Child receives care from multiple caretakers without consideration for the needs of the infant/child
	Compulsively seeks role approval from others

*Denotes critical, or major, defining characteristics.
From Gordon M: Manual of nursing diagnosis 1988-1989, St Louis, 1989, CV Mosby Co, pp 240, 242.

TABLE 13-8 The North American Nursing Diagnosis Association: Nursing diagnosis for potential altered parenting

Nursing diagnosis: Potential for altered parenting

Definition: Presence of risk factors during prenatal or child-bearing period which may interfere with process of adjustment to parenting.

Defining characteristics (risk factors)

Unavailable or ineffective role model

History of physical and psychosocial abuse (of nurturing figure)

Support system deficit (between/from significant others)

Unmet social, emotional, developmental needs (of parenting figures)

Interruption in bonding process (maternal, paternal, other)

Unrealistic expectation (self, infant, partner)

Perceived threat to own survival (physical, emotional)

Physical impairment (blindness, etc.)

Physical or mental illness

Presence of stress (financial, legal, recent personal crisis, cultural change, multiple pregnancies)

Knowledge or skill deficit (specify: parenting skills, developmental progression, etc.)

Limited cognitive functioning

Lack of role identity

Lack of, or inappropriate, response of child to relationship

Social isolation

Fear (specify focus)

From Gordon M: Manual of nursing diagnosis 1988-1989, St Louis, 1989, CV Mosby Co, p. 238.

A community health nurse carried out a study to determine answers to these concerns and found that users of child health services had access to free medical care, were younger, and had more children than nonusers (Selwyn, 1978, p. 231). Reasons why people do and do not utilize health care are important elements in planning health services.

When the community health nurse visits parents after accidental poisoning incidents, the nurse can add to the epidemiological understanding of the predisposing and immediate causes of the accident and make recommendations to prevent them from occurring again. If it were the case that 75 percent of the families who have poisoning accidents have other health problems, there is evidence that this kind of stress leads to poisoning accidents.

A good record system in the health agency will help nurses to collect data on health problems, to plan interventions, and to evaluate care given. These data can provide information on changing health needs and necessary health services.

A good record system will collect data on the 0- to 5-year-old child that provide the basis for a health history upon which later events in the family system can be compared and built.

Clinic Nurse

Community health nurses have long worked in well-baby clinics where, at regular intervals, the health of children up to the age of 5 is assessed, immunizations are given, and parents have the opportunity to discuss concerns of growth and development. This role has been expanded to an assessment and treatment role. Nurses deal with problem behavior such as delayed play, immature social behavior, and temper tantrums. With the nurse's knowledge of child development, behavior modification, and management techniques, the roles of observer, consultant, and counselor to parents, preschool teachers, and day-care workers are valuable in dealing with minor problems that can develop into major ones.

Home Visitor

A well-known role of the nurse caring for the needs of the 0- to 5-year-old age group is that of the community health nurse who visits parents and babies in their homes. Each health department sets its own priorities and standards for the care of parents and children. This ranges from the pre- and postnatal referral of each pregnancy, in some areas, to the referral of only those mothers and infants at high risk. The broad background of community health nurses equips them with skills to help establish the standards as to which newborns and parents will be visited. The nurse who

TABLE 13-9   The North American Nursing Diagnosis Association: Nursing diagnosis for weak mother-infant attachment or parent-infant attachment

---

Nursing diagnosis: Weak mother-infant attachment or parent-infant attachment

Definition: Pattern of unreciprocal bonding relationship between parent and infant or primary caretaker and infant

Etiological or related factors	Defining characteristics
Parental anxiety	Minimal smiling, close contact, enfolding, talking to baby
Fear (specify)	Does not assume "en face" position, eye-to-eye contact
Parent-infant separation	Minimal touching, stroking, patting, rocking, holding, kissing of infant except when
Perceived low parenting competency (infant care)	necessary to feed or change diapers
	Does not attempt comforting responses to crying or continues unsuccessful methods
Low (infant) social responsiveness	Low reciprocal interaction pattern (e.g., minimal smiling, babbling response to
Support system deficit	touching, kissing, etc.)
Family stress	Irritable infant or low responsiveness to parent
	Few positive comments about infant; expressions of disappointment
	Bottle propped or tense posture during breastfeeding
	Infrequent visitation of hospitalized infant (e.g., less than twice a week)
	Prenatal history of ambivalence, negative feelings regarding pregnancy
	High-risk adolescent parent, physically or mentally ill parent

From Gordon M: Manual of nursing diagnosis 1988-1989, St Louis, 1989, CV Mosby Co, pp 246, 248.

visits in the home, especially when both parents are present, is in a privileged position to closely and periodically assess the baby's, the parents', and the family's development. The nurse can also identify stress, help parents deal with problems of poor bonding, provide role modeling for bonding and parenting, give anticipatory guidance, and help reinforce positive behavior. The nurse aids families in utilizing community resources as necessary. For example, when parents and a new baby with a diagnosis of spina bifida, Down's syndrome, or cleft palate come home from the hospital, it is most often the community health nurse who introduces the family to the resources of Crippled Children's Services for financial aid, to the physical therapy offered by the intermediate school program, or to the interdisciplinary diagnostic services of university-affiliated centers. This same nurse will likely be one of the persons to help parents as they go through the grief process related to having a baby who is less than "perfect." The nurse can also be alert to signs of stress

within the family in this situation; living 24 hours a day with a helpless infant who has additional problems can be an overwhelming problem for some families. Homemakers, parent's aides, and parent-support groups are useful when families are in such a situational crisis.

One of the major characteristics of handicapped children, and particularly the mentally retarded, is some delay in reaching developmental milestones in self-help skills. It is sometimes assumed that these skills will develop without intervention as a result of physical growth and maturation. Often this is not the case and the child is unable to function independently. This leads to institutionalization, enormous financial and personal expenditures, and waste of human potential. With the use of behavior modification technology, most self-help skills can be attained by handicapped persons, including those who are profoundly retarded. The community health nurse is in a unique position to help families with these skills. Beginning immediately after birth with early infant stimulation is essential. The goal is that each person attain his or her own potential. The nurse can aid the family in recognizing this potential and give guidance in the process of reaching it. Time needed to exercise and teach the young child with developmental disabilities can lead to the neglect of other children. Parents and nurse must be cognizant of this situation.

SUMMARY

The years from birth to age 5 provide the foundation for a child's lifelong physical, mental, and social development. The child's health and that of the parents is inextricably interwoven; and both have health care needs that the community health nurse can help to fill.

Utilization of the developmental health promotion model to assess the needs of young children and their parents provides a positive way of involving this group in their own health care. It can also help to prevent many of the major health problems of those 0- to 5-years of age, or at least weaken their impact. This is the challenge for community health nurses!

Children are our nation's greatest resource. Decreasing infant and maternal mortality rates reflect this value as does legislation such as Medicaid, which provides health care for at least a segment of the 0- to 5-year-old population.

APPENDIX 13-1

Suggested Schedule for Preventive Child Health Care

Age	History*	Measurement†	Physical examination	Developmental landmarks*‡	Discussion and guidance*	Procedures†, §	Attending
1 month	Initial Eating Sleeping Elimination Crying At every visit mother should be asked for questions	Height Weight Head circumference Temperature Evaluation of hearing	Complete¶	Eyes follow to midline Baby regards face *While prone, lifts head off table*	Vitamins Sneezing Hiccoughs Straining, with bowel movements Irregular respiration Startle reflex Ease and force of urination Night bottle Colic "Spoiling" Accidents	PKU Urinalysis	MD and assistant

*May be accomplished in part by assistant if physician desires. Much of this may be accomplished in part by appropriate pamphlets or leaflets where deemed desirable.

†Usually accomplished by assistant.

‡Age given for landmarks indicates approximate age at which 90 percent of children have accomplished test. Adapted from Denver Developmental Screening Test.

§Immunization schedules updated from USDHHS, Public Health Service: Parents guide to childhood immunization, Atlanta, Ga., 1988, Centers for Disease Control, p. 18.

¶By physician. Observation of child, completely undressed, by assistant trained to observe respiration, skin, musculature, motor activities, and so forth.

**Obvious deviations from normal must be checked by physician.

NOTE: Italicized items indicate report of parent and may be accepted as proof of accomplishment. May be obtained by assistant.

Suggested Schedule for Preventive Child Health Care—cont'd

Age	History*	Measurement†	Physical examination	Developmental landmarks*‡	Discussion and guidance*	Procedures†, §	Attending
2 months	Health Sensory-motor development Eating Sleeping Elimination Happiness	Height Weight Head circumference Temperature	Complete or observation**	*Vocalizes* *Smiles responsively*	Solid foods Immunizations Thumbsucking	DTP-1 tOPV-1 Urine screening	MD and/or assistant
3 months	Health Eating Sleeping Elimination Crying Other behavior	Height Weight	Complete or observation**	Holds head and chest up to make 90 degree angle with table Laughs	Feeding Accidents Sleeping without rocking Coping with frustrations		
4 months	Health Eating Sleeping Elimination Other behavior Sensory-motor development Current living situation Parent-child interaction	Height Weight Head circumference Temperature	Complete§	Holds head erect and steady when held in sitting position *Squeals* Grasps rattle Eyes follow object for 180 degrees	Feeding Schedule to fit in with family Attitude of father Respiratory infections	DTP-2 tOPV-2	MD and/or assistant
5 months	Health Eating Sleeping Elimination Sensory-motor development	Height Weight Temperature	Complete or observation¶	*Smiles spontaneously* *Rolls from back to stomach or vice versa* Reaches for object on table	Feeding Vitamins (if not previously mentioned)		MD and/or assistant
6 months	Health Eating Sleeping Elimination Other behavior	Height Weight Head circumference Temperature Evaluation of hearing	Complete or observation¶	No head lag if baby is pulled to sitting position by hands	Feeding Accidents Night crying Fear of strangers Separation anxiety	DTP-3	MD and/or assistant

Continued.

Age	History*	Measurement†	Physical examination	Developmental landmarks*‡	Discussion and guidance*	Procedures†, §	Attending
	Sensory-motor development				Description of normal micturition		
8-9 months	Health Eating Sleeping Elimination Sensory motor development Behavior	Height Weight Temperature	Complete or screening¶	Sits alone for seconds after support is released Bears weight momentarily if held with feet on table Looks after fallen object Transfers block from one hand to the other Feeds self cracker	Use of cup Eating with fingers Fear of strangers Accidents Need for affection Normal unpleasant behavior Discipline		MD and/ or assistant
10 months if last exam at 8 months	Health Eating Sleeping Elimination Behavior Sensory-motor development Speech development Current living situation Parent-child interaction	Height Weight Temperature	Complete or observation**	*Pulls self to standing position* *Stands holding on to solid object (not human)* Pincer grasp; picks up small object using any part of thumb and fingers in opposition *Says Da-da or Ma-ma* Resists toy being pulled away *Plays peek-a-boo* Makes attempt to get toy just out of reach *Initial anxiety toward strangers*	Toilet training: when to start Normal drop in appetite Independence vs. dependency Discipline Instructions for use of syrup of ipecac	Hemoglobin or hematocrit	MD and/ or assistant
12 months	As for 10 months	Height Weight Head circumference Temperature	Complete¶	*Cruises: walks around holding onto furniture* *Stands alone 2-3 seconds if outside support is removed*	Negativism Likelihood of respiratory infections "Getting into things"	Tuberculin test (intradermal preferred) Urinalysis	MD and assistant

Suggested Schedule for Preventive Child Health Care—cont'd

Age	History*	Measurement†	Physical examination	Developmental landmarks*‡	Discussion and guidance*	Procedures †, §	Attending
				Bangs together two blocks held one in each hand	Weaning from bottle		
				Imitates vocalization heard within preceding minute	Proper dose of vitamins		
					Control of drugs and poisons		
				Plays pat-a-cake			
15 months	As for 10 months	Height Weight Temperature	Complete or observation**	*Walks well*	Temper tantrums	DTP-4	MD and/or assistant
				Stoops to recover toys on floor	Obedience	OPV-3	
				Uses Da-da and Ma-ma specifically for correct parent		MMR	
				Rolls or tosses ball back to examiner			
				Indicates wants by pulling, pointing, or appropriate verbalization (not crying)			
				Drinks from cup without spilling much			
18 months	As for 10 months	Height Weight Temperature	Complete¶	Puts one block on another without its falling off	Reaction toward and of siblings	Hib	MD and assistant
				Mimics household chores like dusting or sweeping	Toilet training Speech development		
21 months	As for 10 months Peer reaction	Height Weight Temperature	Complete or observation**	Walks backward and upstairs	Manners "Poor appetite"		MD and/or assistant
				Feeds self with spoon			
				Removes article of clothing other than hat			
				Says three specific words besides Da-da and Ma-ma			

Continued.

Age	History*	Measurement†	Physical examination	Developmental landmarks*‡	Discussion and guidance*	Procedures†, §	Attending
2 years	Health Eating Sleeping Elimination Toilet training Sensory-motor development Speech Current living situation Peer and social adjustment	Height Weight Temperature Hearing	Complete¶	Kicks a ball in front of him with foot without support *Scribbles spontaneously—purposeful marking of more than one stroke on paper* Balances four blocks on top of one another *Points correctly to one body part* Dumps small objects out of bottle after demonstration *Does simple tasks in house*	Need for peer companionship Immaturity: inability to share or take turns Care of teeth From this point on, guidance may be indicated by the mother's answers to a questionnaire about behavior and emotional problems	Hemoglobin and/or hematocrit Urinalysis	MD and assistant
2½ years	As for 2 years	Height Weight Temperature	Complete¶	*Throws overhand after demonstration* Names correctly one picture in book, e.g., cat or apple Combines two words meaningfully	Guidance for questionnaire answers Dental referral Perversity and decisiveness		MD and/or assistant
3 years	As for 2 years	As for 2 years Blood pressure	Complete¶	Jumps in place *Pedals tricycle* Dumps small article out of bottle without demonstration *Uses plurals* *Washes and dries hands*	*Guidance from questionnaire answers* Sex education Nursery schools: qualifications of a good one Obedience and discipline	As for 2 years	MD and assistant
4 years	As for 2 years	As for 2 years Vision ("E" chart) Blood pressure	Complete¶ Fundus examination	Builds bridge of three blocks after demonstration Copies circle and cross *Identifies longer of two lines*	*Guidance from questionnaire answers* Kindergarten Use of money Dental care	As for 2 years	MD and assistant

Suggested Schedule for Preventive Child Health Care—cont'd

Age	History*	Measurement†	Physical examination	Developmental landmarks*‡	Discussion and guidance*	Procedures†, §	Attending
				Knows first and last names			
				Understands what to do when "tired"			
				Plays with other children so they interact—tag			
				Dresses with supervision			
5 years	As for 2 years (omit toilet training) Kindergarten	As for 2 years Vision ("E" chart) Color blindness Audiometer Blood pressure	Complete¶	Hops two or more times Catches ball thrown 3 feet Dresses without supervision *Can tolerate separation from mother for a few minutes without anxiety*	Guidance from questionnaire answers Readiness for school Span of attention: how to increase it	As for 2 years DTP-5 tOPV-4	MD and assistant

Reprinted with permission from Committee on Standards of Child Health Care, Council on Pediatric Practice, American Academy of Pediatrics, 1972. Copyright American Academy of Pediatrics 1972 and 1977.

APPENDIX 13-2

Accident Prevention at Various Age Levels

Typical accidents	Normal behavior characteristics	Precautions
First year		
Falls	After several months of age can squirm and roll, and later creep and pulls self erect	Do not leave alone on tables, etc., from where falls can occur
Inhalation of foreign objects		Keep crib sides up
Poisoning	Places anything and everything in mouth	Keep small objects and harmful substances out of reach
Burns	Helpless in water	Use infant car seat
Drowning		Have syrup of ipecac at home
Second year		
Falls	Able to roam about in erect posture	Keep screens in windows
Drowning	Goes up and down stairs	Place gate at top of stairs
Motor vehicles	Has great curiosity	Cover unused electrical outlets; keep electric cords out of easy reach
Ingestion of poisonous substances	Puts almost everything in mouth	Keep in enclosed space when outdoors; not in company of an adult
Burns	Helpless in water	Keep medicines, household poisons, and small sharp objects out of sight
		Keep handles of pots and pans on stove out of reach and containers of hot food from edge of table
		Protect from water in tub and in pools
		Use safety belts and car seats
2-4 Years		
Falls	Able to open doors	Keep doors locked when there is danger of falls
Drowning	Runs and climbs	Place screen or guards in windows
Motor vehicles	Can ride tricycle	Teach about watching for automobiles in driveways and in streets
Ingestion of poisonous substances	Investigates closets and drawers	Keep firearms locked up
Burns	Plays with mechanical gadgets	Keep knives, electrical equipment out of reach
	Can throw ball and other objects	Teach about risks of throwing sharp objects and about danger of following balls into street
5-9 Years		
Motor vehicles	Daring and adventurous	Use seat belts
Bicycle accidents	Control over large muscles more advanced than control over small muscles	Teach techniques and traffic rules for cycling
Drowning		Encourage skills in swimming
Burns	Has increasing interest in group play; loyalty to group makes him willing to follow suggestions of leaders	Keep firearms locked up except when you can supervise their use
Firearms		

From Vaughn VC, McKay RJ, Behrman RE, eds, and Nelson WE (senior ed): Textbook of pediatrics, ed 11, Philadelphia, 1979, Saunders, p 264.
Adapted from: T. E. Shaffer: Pediatr Clin North Am 1:426-427, May 1954.

APPENDIX 13-3

Screening Tests for Gathering Baseline Data about Infants and Children

Type of test	Name of screening test procedure	Author	Age span	Method of administration	Where to obtain test
General development (social-emotional, cognitive, coordination)	1. Home Observation for Measurement of the Environment (HOME)	Bettye M. Caldwell	Birth-3 years; 3-6 years	Interview	Dr. Bettye Caldwell, Center for Early Development and Education, University of Arkansas, 814 Sherman Street, Little Rock, Ark. 72202
	2. Valett Developmental Survey of Basic Learning Abilities	Robert E. Valett	2-7 years	Observation of individual performance	Consulting Psychologists Press, 577 College Avenue, Palo Alto, Calif. 94306
	3. Columbia Mental Maturity Scale	Bessie B. Burgemeister, Lucille H. Blum, Irving Lorge	3 years 6 months-9 years 11 months	Observation of individual performance	Harcourt Brace Jovanovich, Inc., Health Care Publications Division, 737 Third Avenue, New York, N.Y. 10017
	4. Quick Test (QT)	R.B. Ammons, C.H. Ammons	2 years-adult	Observation of individual performance	Psychological Test Specialists, Box 1441, Missoula, Mont. 59801
	5. Slosson Intelligence Test (SIT)	Richard L. Slosson	Birth-adult	Observation of individual performance	Western Psychological Services, Publishers and Distributors, 12031 Wilshire Boulevard, Los Angeles, Calif. 90025
	6. Carey Infant Temperament Questionnaire	William B. Carey	4-8 months	Interview	Dr. William B. Carey, M.D., 319 West Front Street, Media, Pa. 19063
	7. California Preschool Social Competency Scale	Samuel Levine, Freeman F. Elzey, Mary Lewis	2 years 6 months-5 years 6 months	Observation of individual performance	Consulting Psychologists Press, Inc., 577 College Avenue, Palo Alto, Calif. 94306
	8. Vineland Social Maturity Scale	Edgar A. Doll	Birth-adult	Interview	American Guidance Service, Inc., Circle Pines, Minn. 55014
	9. Behavior Questionnaire	J.A. Willoughby, R.J. Haggerty	18 months-6 years	Interview	Department of Pediatrics, University of Rochester Medical School, 260 Crittenden Boulevard, Rochester, N.Y. 14603 (Printed in Pediatrics, 34:798-806, 1964.)

Continued.

APPENDIX 13-3

Screening Tests for Gathering Baseline Data about Infants and Children—cont'd

Type of test	Name of screening test procedure	Author	Age span	Method of administration	Where to obtain test
	10. Animal Crackers (a test of motivation to achieve)	D.C. Adkins, B.L. Ballif	Preschool, kindergarten, 1st grade	Observation of individual performance	CTB/McGraw-Hill, Del Monte Research Park, Monterey, Calif. 93940
	11. Developmental Test of Visual-Motor Integration (VMI)	Keith E. Beery, Norman A. Bucktenica	2-15 years	Observation of individual performance	Follett Publishing Company, Customer Service Center, Box 5705, Chicago, Ill. 60680
	12. Comprehensive Identification Process (CIP)	R.R. Zehrback	2 years 6 months-5 years 6 months	Observation of individual performance	Scholastic Testing Service, 480 Meyer Road, Bensenville, Ill. 60106
	13. Primary Self-Concept Inventory	D.G. Muller, R. Leonetti	Kindergarten-6th grade	May be administered to individual children or to small groups	Learning Concepts, 2501 West Lamar, Austin, Tex. 78705
	14. Neonatal Perception Inventories	E. Broussard	Newborns	Checklist	(Information contained in Hellmuth J, editor: Exceptional Infant, vol. 2, New York, 1971, Brunner/Mazel)
Vision	1. STYCAR Vision Tests	Mary D. Sheridan	6 months-7 years (mental ages)	Observation of individual performance	NFER Publishing Company, Ltd., 2 Jennings Buildings, Thames Avenue, Windsor, Berks, England SL4 1QS
Hearing	1. STYCAR Hearing Tests	Mary D. Sheridan	6 months-7 years (mental ages)	Observation of individual performance	NFER Publishing Company, Ltd., 2 Jennings Buildings, Thames Avenue, Windsor, Berks, England SL4 1QS
	2. Kindergarten Auditory Screening Test	Jack Katz	Kindergarten and 1st grade	Observation of individual performance	Follett Publishing Company, Customer Service Center, Box 5705, Chicago, Ill. 60680
Speech and language	1. Verbal Language Development Scale—1971	Merlin J. Mecham	0-15 years	Interview	American Guidance Service, Inc., Circle Pines, Minn. 55014

	Test	Author	Age	Method	Source
2.	Language Facility Test	John T. Dailey	3-15 years	Interview	Allington Corporation, 801 North Pitt Street #701, Alexandria, Va. 22314
3.	Screening Test for Auditory Comprehension of Language	Elizabeth Carrow	3-6 years	Observation of individual performance	Learning Concepts, 2501 North Lamar, Austin, Tex. 78705
4.	Peabody Picture Vocabulary Test	Lloyd M. Dunn	2½-18 years	Interview	American Guidance Service, Inc., Circle Pines, Minn. 55014
5.	Predictive Screening Test of Articulation	Charles Van Riper, Robert L. Erickson	Primary school-age children in the 1st grade	Observation of individual performance	Continuing Education Office, Western Michigan University, Kalamazoo, Mich. 49001

School readiness and academic achievement

	Test	Author	Age	Method	Source
1.	Test of Basic Experience (TOBE)	Margaret H. Moss	Preschool, kindergarten and 1st grade	Observation of individual performance	CTB/McGraw-Hill, Del Monte Research Park, Monterey, Calif. 92940
2.	Sprigle School Readiness Screening Test (SSRST)	Herbert A. Sprigle, James Lanier	4 years 6 months-6 years 9 months	Interview	Psychological Clinic and Research Center, San Marco Boulevard, Jacksonville, Fla. 32207
3.	First Grade Screening Test	John E. Pate, Warren W. Webb	End of kindergarten to early 1st grade	Observation of individual performance	American Guidance Service, Inc., Circle Pines, Minn. 55014
4.	Peabody Individual Achievement Test (PIAT)	Lloyd D. Dunn, Frederick C. Markwardt	2 years 6 months-18 years	Interview	American Guidance Service, Inc., Circle Pines, Minn. 55014
5.	Cooperative Preschool Inventory (rev. ed. 1970)	Bettye M. Caldwell	3-6 years	Observation of individual performance	Educational Testing Service, 1947 Center Street, Berkeley, Calif. 94704
6.	SCREEN	Gerald M. Senf, Andrew L. Comrey	Kindergarten and 1st grade	Observation of individual performance	Computer Psychometric, Affiliates Inc., Chicago, Ill. 60607
7.	School Readiness Survey	F.L. Jordan, James Massey	4-6 years	Observation of individual performance	Consulting Psychologists Press, 577 College Avenue, Palo Alto, Calif. 94306
8.	ABC Inventory	Normand Adair, George Blesch	4 years 9 months-4 years 11 months	Observation of individual performance	Educational Studies and Development, Division of Test Maker, Inc., 1368 East Airport Road, Muskegon, Mich. 49444
9.	Preschool Readiness Experimental Screening Scale (PRESS)	W.B. Rogers, Jr., Robert A. Rogers	5 years (prekindergarten)	Observation of individual performance	Clin Pediatr 2(10):253-256), 1972.

Continued.

APPENDIX 13-3

Screening Tests for Gathering Baseline Data about Infants and Children—cont'd

Type of test	Name of screening test procedure	Author	Age span	Method of administration	Where to obtain test
	10. Ready or Not? Handbook for School Readiness Checklist	John J. Auston, J. Clayton Lafferty	4, 5, 6 years	Checklist	Research Concepts, Division of Test Maker, Inc., 1368 Airport Road, Muskegon, Mich. 49444
	11. Riley Preschool Developmental Screening Inventory	Clara M.D. Riley	3-5 years	Observation of individual performance	Western Psychological Services, 12031 Wilshire Boulevard, Los Angeles, Calif. 90025
	12. Screening Test of Academic Readiness (STAR)	A. Edward Ahr	4 years-6 years 5 months	Observation of individual performance	Priority Innovations, Inc., P.O. Box 792, Skokie, Ill. 60076
	13. Parent Readiness Evaluation of Preschoolers (PREP)	A. Edward Ahr	3 years 9 months-5 years 8 months	Observation of individual performance	Priority Innovations, Inc., P.O. Box 792, Skokie, Ill. 60076
	14. Primary Academic Sentiment Scale (PASS)	Glenn Robbins Thompson	4 years 4 months-7 years 3 months	Observation of individual performance	Priority Innovations, Inc., P.O. Box 792, Skokie, Ill. 60076
	15. Preschool Attainment Record (PAR)	Edgar A. Doll	6 months-7 years	Observation of individual performance	American Guidance Service, Inc., Circle Pines, Minn. 55014
	16. Meeting Street School Screening Test (early identification of children with learning disabilities)	Peter K. Hainsworth, Marian L. Siqueland	5 years-7 years 6 months	Observation of individual performance	Crippled Children and Adults of Rhode Island, Inc., Meeting Street School, 333 Grotto Avenue, Providence, R.I. 02906
	17. SEARCH	A.A. Silver, R.H. Hagin	5-7 years	Observation of individual performance	Walker Educational Book Corporation, 720 Fifth Avenue, New York, N.Y. 10019
	18. Wide Range Achievement Test	J.F. Jastak, S.W. Bijou, S.R. Jastak	5 years-adult	Observation of individual performance	The Psychologist Corporation, 1372 Peachtree Street N.W., Atlanta, Ga. 30309

From Stangler S, Huber C, and Routh D: Screening growth and development of preschool children. A guide for test selection, New York, 1980, McGraw-Hill, pp 304-309.

REFERENCES

Alan Guttmacher Institute: Blessed events and the bottom line: the financing of maternity care in the United States, New York, 1987, The Institute.

Alan Guttmacher Institute: Teenage pregnancy in the United States: the scope of the problem and state responses, New York, 1989, The Institute.

American Academy of Pediatrics, Committee on Infectious Diseases: Measles: reassessment of the current immunization policy, Pediatrics 84(6):110-113.

Arkin EB: The Healthy Mothers, Healthy Babies Coalition: four years of progress, Public Health Rep, 101:147-156, 1986.

Barnard KE and Erickson ML: Teaching children with developmental problems, St. Louis, 1976, CV Mosby Co.

Berry RK: Home care of the child with AIDS, Pediatr Nurs 14:341-344, 1988.

Biller H and Meredith D: Father power, New York, 1974, McKay.

Bowling JM and Riley P: Access to prenatal care in North Carolina, Raleigh, NC, 1987, North Carolina State Center for Health Statistics.

Bratic E: Healthy mothers, healthy babies coalition—a joint private-public initiative, Public Health Rep 97:503-509, 1982.

Bray C, Brosnan C, and Erkel E: Failure to thrive: a dilemma for the community health nurse, Community Health Nurs 6(17):31-36, 1989.

Brazelton TB: The neonatal behavioral assessment scale, Philadelphia, 1973, JB Lippincott.

Brecht M: The tragedy of infant mortality, Nurs Outlook 37:18-22, 1989.

Brown S: Drawing women into prenatal care, Family Planning Perspect 21(2):73-80, 88, 1989.

Bureau of the Census: Fertility of American women: June 1988, Current Population Reports, Series P-20, No 436, Washington, DC, 1989, US Government Printing Office.

Bureau of the Census: Studies in marriage and the family, Current Population Reports, Series P-23, No 162, Washington, DC, 1989, US Government Printing Office.

Bush D: Fertility related laws enacted in 1982, Family Planning Perspect 15(3):111-116, 1983.

Carpenter RG: Prevention of unexpected infant death, Lancet i:723-727, 1983.

Centers for Disease Control (CDC): Supplementary statement of contraindications to receipt of pertussis vaccine, MMWR 33:169-171, 1984.

CDC: Preventing lead poisoning in young children: a statement by the Centers for Disease Control, Atlanta, Ga, 1985, USDHHS.

CDC: Progress toward achieving the 1990 objectives for pregnancy and infant health, MMWR 37:405-408, July 8, 1988.

CDC: Progress toward achieving the national 1990 objectives for immunization, MMWR 37:613-617, October, 1988.

CDC: Childhood lead poisoning—United States: report to the Congress by the Agency for Toxic Substances and Disease Registry, MMWR 37(32):481-485, August 19, 1988.

CDC: HIV/AIDS surveillance, year end edition, MMWR special report, January, 1990.

Chadzynski L: Manual for the identification and abatement of environment lead hazards, Washington, DC, 1986, Division of Maternal and Child Health.

Chamberlin RW, ed: Beyond individual risk assessment: community wide approaches to promoting the health and development of families and children, Washington, DC, 1988, The National Center for Education in Maternal and Child Health.

Chan MM: Sudden infant death syndrome and families at risk, Pediatr Nurs 13(3):166-168, 1987.

Child Nutrition Amendments of 1986, National Defense Authorization Act, Public Law 99-661.

Child resistant caps saving lives. Ann Arbor News, Ann Arbor, MI, January 24, 1984, p D4.

Combating child abuse, Congressional Q Almanac 44:369, 1988.

Comer JP and Poussaint AF: Black child care, New York, 1975, Simon & Shuster.

Committee on Labor and Public Welfare, Subcommittee on Health, United States Congress (hearing): School-age mothers and child health act, 1975, Washington, DC, November 4, 1975, US Government Printing Office.

Coppens NM, Hunter PN, Bain JA, Gatewood AK, Gordon DA, and Mailloux MS: The relationship between elevated lead levels and enrollment in special education, Family Commun Health 12(4):39-46, 1990.

Drummond AH: Lead poisoning in children, J School Health 51:43-47, 1981.

Dunn HL: High level wellness, Arlington, Va, 1973, RN Beatty.

Editorial: The valley of the shadow of birth, Am J Public Health 73(6):635-637, 1983.

Erickson ML: Assessment and management of developmental changes in children, St Louis, 1976, CV Mosby Co.

Fawcett J: Body image and the pregnant couple, Am J Maternal Child Nurs 3:227-233, 1978.

Food and nutrition service research and support encourage breast feeding, Public Health Rep 104:310-311, 1989.

Garbarino J: The human ecology method of child maltreatment: a conceptual model for research, J Marriage Family 39:721-735, 1977.

Garner MK: Our values are showing: inadequate childhood immunization, Health Values: Achieving High Level Wellness 2:129-133, 1978.

Gordon M: Manual of nursing diagnosis 1988-1989, St Louis, 1989, CV Mosby Co.

Gruis M: Beyond maternity: post partum concerns of mothers, Am J Maternal Child Health 2:182-188, 1977.

Hanson RG and Wyse BW: Planning for the inevitable: snack foods in the diet, Family Commun Health 1:31-39, 1979.

Health Care Financing Administration (HCFA): State Medicaid manual, Part 5. Early and periodic screening, diagnosis, and treatment (EPSDT), HCFA Pub No 45-4, Baltimore, Md, 1988, Printing and Publications Branch, Office of Management and Budget.

"Healthy mothers" market research: how to reach black and Mexican American women, Contract No 232-81-0082. Submitted to USDHHS, PHS, September 14, 1982, by Juarez and Associates, Inc, 12139 National Blvd, Los Angeles, Ca.

Helfer RE and Kempe CH, eds: Child abuse and neglect, Cambridge, Ma, 1976, Ballinger.

Hoekelman RA, Blatman S, Brunell PA, Friedman SB, and Seidel HM: Principles of pediatrics: health care of the young, New York, 1978, McGraw-Hill.

Hopp JW and Rogers EA: AIDS and the allied health professions, Philadelphia, 1989, FA Davis.

Illingsworth R and Illingsworth C: Babies and young children, New York, 1977, Churchill Livingstone.

Information Sciences Research Institute: Understanding Title V of the Social Security Act: a guide to the provisions of federal maternal and child health services legislation, Vienna, Va, 1989, The Institute.

Institute of Medicine: Preventing low birthweight, Washington, DC, 1985, National Academy Press.

Kamerman SB: Child-care services: a national picture, Monthly Labor Rev 106:35-59, December 1983.

Kennell J, Voos D, and Klaus M: Parent infant bonding. In Helfer RE and Kempe CH, eds: Child abuse and neglect. The family and the community, Cambridge, Ma, 1976, Ballinger.

Kiester E and Kiester SV: Better Homes and Garden's new baby book, New York, 1980, Bantam.

Klaus MH and Kennell JH: Maternal-infant bonding, St Louis, 1976, CV Mosby Co.

Klaus MH and Kennell JH: Mothers separated from their newborn infants. In Schwartz JL and Schwartz LH, eds: Vulnerable infants, a psychosocial dilemma, New York, 1977, McGraw-Hill.

Kleinman J: Perinatal and Infant Mortality, recent trends in the United States, Proceedings of the international collaborative effort perinatal and infant mortality, vol 1, DHHS Pub No, (PHS) 85-1252, Hyattsville, Md, 1985, National Center for Health Statistics.

Koop CE: Excerpt from keynote address. In Silverman BK, ed: Report of the Surgeon General's workshop on children with HIV infection and their families, DHHS Pub No HRS-D-MO 87-1, 1987, pp 3-5.

Kotelchuck M: WIC participation and pregnancy outcomes: Massachusetts statewide evaluation project, Am J Public Health 74:1086-1092, 1984.

Massachusetts Department of Public Health: Massachusetts nutrition survey, Boston, Ma, 1983, Division of Family Health Services.

McClelland DC, Constantian CA, Regalado D, and Stone C: Making it to maturity, Psychology Today 12:42-53, 114, June 1978.

Michigan Department of Public Health: Facts about the WIC program, Lansing, Mi, 1986, The Department.

Milio N: 9226 Kercheval: the storefront that did not burn, Ann Arbor, 1970, University of Michigan Press.

Miller CA, Fine A, Adams-Taylor S, and Schorr LB: Monitoring children's health: key indicators, Washington, DC, 1986, American Public Health Association.

National Association for Home Care: Home care and hospice provisions contained in the Omnibus Budget Reconciliation Act of 1989, HR 3299, Washington, DC, December 8, 1989, The Association.

National Center for Health Statistics: Advance report of final natality statistics, 1986, Monthly Vital Stat Rep 37(3), Hyattsville, Md, 1988, The Center.

National Commission to Prevent Infant Mortality: Infant mortality and the media, Washington, DC, May 1988, The Commission.

National Commission to Prevent Infant Mortality: 1985 indirect costs of infant mortality and low birthweight, Washington, DC, May 1988, The Commission.

National Commission to Prevent Infant Mortality: Death before life: the tragedy of infant mortality, Washington, DC, August 1988, The Commission.

National Commission to Prevent Infant Mortality: Home visiting: opening doors for America's pregnant women and children, Washington, DC, 1989, The Commission.

National Commission to Prevent Infant Mortality: Personal communication, February 1990.

National Committee for Injury Prevention and Control: Injury prevention: meeting the challenge, a summary, Newton, Ma, 1989, Education Development Center.

National Institute on Disability and Rehabilitation Research: Chartbook on disability in the United States, An InfoUse report, Washington, DC, 1989, The Institute.

National Safety Council: Accident facts, 1988 edition, Chicago, 1988, The Council.

National SIDS Clearinghouse: Fact sheet: what is SIDS? McLean, Va, 1989, The Clearinghouse.

Pickett G and Hanlon JJ: Public health administration and practice, St Louis, 1990, Times Mirror/Mosby College Publishing.

Prevention Briefs: Lead poisoning threat to 1 in 25 preschoolers, Public Health Rep 98(1):51, 1983.

Robarge JP, Reynolds ZB, and Groothuis JR: Increased child abuse in families with twins, Res Nurs Health 5:199-203, December 1982.

Rogers MF: Transmission of human immunodeficiency virus infection in the United States. In Silverman BK, ed: Report of the Surgeon General's workshop on children with HIV infection and their families, DHHS Pub No HRS-D-MC 87-1, Rockville, Md, 1987, USDHHS, Division of Maternal and Child Health, pp 17-19.

Rush D: National WIC evaluation, vol 1 summary, report to the US Department of Agriculture, Research Triangle Park, NC, 1986, Research Triangle Institute.

Sammons WAH: The self-calmed baby: a revolutionary new approach to parenting your child, Boston, 1989, Little, Brown.

Samuels M and Samuels N: The well baby book, New York, 1979, Summit.

Schneider J, Aurori B, Armenti L, and Soltanoff D: Impact of community screening on diagnosis, treatment and medical findings of lead poisoning in children, Public Health Rep 96:143-149, March-April 1981.

Schramm W: Prenatal participation in WIC related to

Medicaid costs for Missouri newborns: 1982 update, Public Health Rep 101:607-614, 1986.

Scipien GM, Barnard MU, Chard MA, Howe J, and Phillips PJ: Comprehensive pediatric nursing, ed 3, New York, 1986, McGraw-Hill.

Select Panel for the Promotion of Child Health: Better health for our children: a national strategy: the report of the select panel for the promotion of child health to the United States Congress and the Secretary of Health and Human Services, vol 1, DHHS Pub No PHS 79-55071, Washington, DC, 1981, Department of Health and Human Services.

Selwyn BJ: An epidemiological approach to the study of users and nonusers of child health services, Am J Public Health 68:231-235, 1978.

Shaheen E, Alexander D, and Barbero GJ: Failure to thrive: a retrospective profile. In Schwartz JL and Schwartz LH, eds: Vulnerable infants. A psychosocial dilemma, New York, 1977, McGraw-Hill.

Spiegel CN and Lindaman FC: Children can't fly, Am J Public Health 67:1143-1147, 1977.

Spock B and Rothenberg M: Dr. Spock's baby and child care, New York, 1985, Pocket Books.

Stangler S, Huber C, and Routh D: Screening growth and development of preschool children: a guide for test selection, New York, 1980, McGraw-Hill.

Steele BF: Violence within the family. In Helfer RE and Kempe CH, eds: Child abuse and neglect. The family and the community, Cambridge, Ma, 1976, Ballinger.

Straus MA, and Gelles RJ: Societal change and change in family violence from 1975 to 1985 as revealed by two national surveys, J Marriage Family 48:465-479, 1986.

Subcommittee on Child and Human Development, Committee on Human Resources: United States Senate (hearing), Extension of the Child Abuse Prevention and Treatment Act, 1977 Washington, DC, April 6-7, 1977, US Government Printing Office.

Task Force on Infant Mortality: Infant mortality in Michigan, Lansing, Mi, 1987, Michigan Department of Public Health.

US Bureau of the Census: Fertility of American women: June 1988, Current Population Reports, Series P-20, No 436, Washington, DC, 1989, US Government Printing Office.

US Congress, Office of Technology Assessment: Healthy children: investing in the future, OTA-H-345, Washington, DC, 1988, US Government Printing Office.

US Department of Health Education and Welfare

(USDHEW): Healthy people, the Surgeon General's report on health promotion and disease prevention, DHEW Pub No PHS 79-55071, Washington, DC, 1979, US Government Printing Office.

US Department of Health and Human Services (USDHHS), Public Health Service: Health of the disadvantaged chart book-II, DHHS Pub No (HRA) 80-633, Washington, DC, 1980, Health Resources and Services Administration.

USDHHS: Promoting health, preventing disease: objectives for the nation, Washington, DC, 1980, US Government Printing Office.

USDHHS, Public Health Service: Report of the Surgeon General's workshop on children with handicaps and their families, DHHS Pub No PHS 83-50194, Washington, DC, 1982, US Government Printing Office.

USDHHS, Public Health Service: Prevention '84/'85, Washington, DC, 1985, US Government Printing Office.

USDHHS, Office of Disease Prevention and Health Promotion: The 1990 health objectives for the nation: a midcourse review, Washington, DC, 1986, US Government Printing Office.

USDHHS: Health status of minorities and low income groups, DHHS Pub No (HRSA) HRS-P-DV 85-1, Washington, DC, 1986, Health Resources and Services Administration.

USDHHS: Prevention '86/'87: federal programs and progress, Washington, DC, 1987, US Government Printing Office.

USDHHS, Public Health Service: Parents guide to childhood immunization, Atlanta, Ga, 1988, Centers for Disease Control.

USDHHS, Administration for Children, Youth and Families: Child Abuse Prevention, Adoption and Services Act of 1988, Washington, DC, 1988, US Government Printing Office.

USDHHS, Public Health Service: The Surgeon General's report on nutrition and health, DHHS (PHS) Pub No 88-5021, Washington, DC, 1988, US Government Printing Office.

USDHHS, Public Health Service: Promoting health/preventing disease: year 2000 objectives for the nation (draft for public review and comment), Washington, DC, 1989, US Government Printing Office.

USDHHS, Office of Maternal and Child Health: Child health USA '89, Washington, DC, 1989, US Government Printing Office.

US Preventive Services Task Force: Guide to clinical preventive services: an assessment of the effectiveness of 169 interventions, Baltimore, 1989, Williams & Wilkins.

United States Statutes at Large—Public Law 97-35, 1982.

Vaughn VC, McKay RJ, and Behrman RE, eds, and Nelson WE, senior ed: Textbook of pediatrics, ed 11, Philadelphia, 1979, Saunders.

Wald L: The house on Henry Street, New York, 1915, Holt.

Whaley LF and Wong DL: Essentials of pediatric nursing, ed 3, St Louis, 1987, CV Mosby Co.

World Health Organization (WHO): Air quality guidelines for Europe, Copenhagen, 1987, WHO Regional Office for Europe, pp 242-261.

SELECTED BIBLIOGRAPHY

Ahmann E: Home care for the high risk infant: a holistic guide to using technology, Rockville, Md, 1986, Aspen.

Bausell RB: A national survey assessing pediatric preventive behaviors, Pediatr Nurs 11:438-442, 1985.

Bomar PJ: Perspectives on family health promotion, Family Commun Health 12(4):1-11, 1990.

Children's Defense Fund: The nation's investment in children: an analysis of the president's FY 1990 budget proposals, Washington, DC, 1989, The Fund.

Flage L: Changing household structure, child-care availability, and employment among mothers of preschool children, J Marriage Family 51:51-63, 1989.

Institute of Medicine: Prenatal care: reaching mothers, reaching infants, Washington, DC, 1988, National Academy Press.

Kamerman SB: Toward a child policy decade, Child Welfare 68:371-390, 1989.

Kodadek S: When a child is handicapped: parents' perspectives on the experience. In Family Nursing Continuing Education Project, Nursing of families' acute or chronic illness, Portland, Or, 1988, Oregon Health Sciences University.

McBride AB: Transitions during the intense years of parenting. In Family Nursing Continuing Education Project, Nursing of families in transition, Portland, Or, 1988, Oregon Health Sciences University.

Olds DL, Henderson CR, Chamberlain R, and Tatelbaum R: Preventing child abuse and neglect: a randomized trial of nurse home visitation, Pediatrics 78(1):65-68, 1986.

Olds DL, Henderson CR, and Tatelbaum R: Improving

the delivery of prenatal care and outcomes of pregnancy: a randomized trial of nurse home visitation, Pediatrics 77(1):16-28, 1986.

Regional Task Force on Quality Assurance: Enhancing quality: standards and indicators of quality care for children with special health care needs, Boston, 1989, New England Serve.

Wilson D: An overview of sexually transmissible diseases in the perinatal period, J Nurse Midwifery 33(3):115-128, 1988.

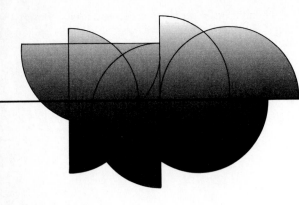

14

Planning Health Services for the School-Age Child

Children are one-third of our population and all of our future.

SELECT PANEL FOR THE PROMOTION OF CHILD HEALTH (1981).

OBJECTIVES

Upon completion of this chapter, the reader will be able to:

1. Identify the rights of children as delineated in the Children's Charter.

2. Explain how fluctuations in the birth rates since post–World War II have affected health planning for the school-age population.

3. Describe the major childhood mortality and morbidity risks and the community health nurse's role in decreasing these risks.

4. Discuss the role of the community health nurse when working with families who have children with chronic handicapping conditions.

5. Analyze select psychosocial problems of childhood and adolescence and discuss community health nursing interventions for addressing these problems.

6. Discuss the components of a comprehensive school health program.

7. Describe the role of the community health nurse in the school setting.

8. Summarize how health and educational legislation affect the delivery of health care services to the school-age population.

9. Compare and contrast role responsibilities of select disciplines on the school health team.

10. Formulate guidelines for implementing community health nursing role responsibilities in the school setting.

During the twentieth century, a concerted effort has been made to improve the health status of all children. However, the goals of the 1930 Children's Charter (see box on p. 515) which emphasized that children, regardless of their race, color, or creed (Figure 14-1), should have an environment and life experiences allowing them to develop to their fullest potential, are still far from realized.

Since the turn of the century, there have been major achievements in relation to the health status of school-age children and the services provided for them. In the early sixties Wallace noted three particularly noteworthy advances: (1) a decrease in mortality in this age category; (2) the expansion of organized school health services; and (3) the recognition that adolescents have special problems and needs (Wallace, 1962, p. 25). Despite these accomplishments, there remain a sizable number of children who will never reach their fullest potential. Although health care in the United States is considered a right rather than a privilege, there is still failure to meet the health needs of specific segments of the population. Children of racial minorities, children from poor, central-city, and rural families, and children with handicapping conditions continue to have a higher incidence of mortality and morbidity. They also use health care services less frequently than the population as a whole (Director's Task Force on Minority Health, 1988; U.S. Congress, Office of Technology Assessment, 1988; USDHHS, Office of Disease Prevention and Health Promotion, 1986; USDHHS, Office of Maternal and Child Health, 1989). Evidence exists that indicates that children are increasingly being underserved by the U.S. health care system (Alan Guttmacher Institute, 1987; National Commission to Prevent Infant Mortality, 1989; U.S. Congress, Office of Technology Assessment, 1988). Improving children's access to health care will be a major challenge for health professionals in the 1990s.

Providing effective and efficient health and welfare services for all segments of the school-age population is no easy task. Demographic, vital, and morbidity statistics reveal that professionals need to deal with an array of health risks when

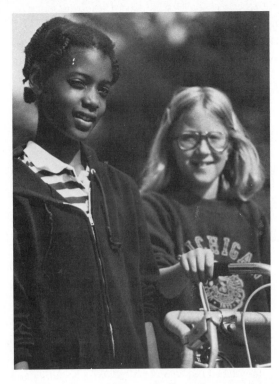

Figure 14-1 All children, regardless of race, color, or creed, need positive life experiences in order to develop to their fullest potential.

planning health and welfare services for this population group. The following review of these risks clearly illustrates the complex nature of the difficulties encountered when health care professionals work with school-age children.

Historically, community health nurses have assumed a major role in developing child health services. Lillian Wald initiated a special project in New York City schools in 1902 to demonstrate to city officials the value of preventive health counseling in relation to the needs of school-age children (Kalisch and Kalisch, 1986). Since that time, nursing services to meet the needs of our youth have grown steadily. Community health nurses are now working with children in a variety of settings including their homes, schools, clinics, and residential settings for special populations at risk. In order to plan nursing services for children in a variety of settings, the community health nurse must have knowledge about their needs and an

The Children's Charter

President Hoover's White House Conference on Child Health and Protection, recognizing the rights of the child as the first rights of citizenship, pledges itself to these aims for the children of America.

I For every child spiritual and moral training to help him to stand firm under the pressure of life

II For every child understanding and the guarding of his personality as his most precious right

III For every child a home and that love and security which a home provides; and for that child who must receive foster care, the nearest substitute for his own home

IV For every child full preparation for his birth, his mother receiving prenatal, natal, and postnatal care; and the establishment of such protective measures as will make childbearing safer

V For every child health protection from birth through adolescence, including: periodical health examinations and, where needed, care of specialists and hospital treatment; regular dental examinations and care of the teeth; protective and preventive measures against communicable diseases; the insuring of pure food, pure milk, and pure water

VI For every child from birth through adolescence, promotion of health, including health instruction and a health program, wholesome physical and mental recreation, with teachers and leaders adequately trained

VII For every child a dwelling-place safe, sanitary, and wholesome, with reasonable provisions for privacy; free from conditions which tend to thwart his development; and a home environment harmonious and enriching

VIII For every child a school which is safe from hazards, sanitary, properly equipped, lighted, and ventilated. For younger children nursery schools and kindergartens to supplement home care

IX For every child a community which recognizes and plans for his needs, protects him against physical dangers, moral hazards, and disease; provides him with safe and wholesome places for play and recreation; and makes provision for his cultural and social needs

X For every child an education which, through the discovery and development of his individual abilities, prepares him for life; and through training and vocational guidance prepares him for living which will yield him the maximum of satisfaction

XI For every child such teaching and training as will prepare him for successful parenthood, homemaking, and the rights of citizenship; and, for parents, supplementary training to fit them to deal wisely with the problems of parenthood

XII For every child education for safety and protection against accidents to which modern conditions subject him—those to which he is directly exposed and those which, through loss or maiming of his parents, affect him indirectly

XIII For every child who is blind, deaf, crippled, or otherwise physically handicapped, and for the child who is mentally handicapped, such measures as will early discover and diagnose his handicap, provide care and treatment, and so train him that he may become an asset to society rather than a liability. Expenses of these services should be borne publicly where they cannot be privately met

XIV For every child who is in conflict with society the right to be dealt with intelligently as society's charge, not society's outcast; with the home, the school, the church, the court and the institution when needed, shaped to return him whenever possible to the normal stream of life

XV For every child the right to grow up in a family with an adequate standard of living and the security of a stable income as the surest safeguard against social handicaps

XVI For every child protection against labor that stunts growth, either physical or mental, that limits education, that deprives children of the right of comradeship, of play, and of joy

XVII For every rural child as satisfactory schooling and health services as for the city child, and an extension to rural families of social, recreational, and cultural facilities

XVIII To supplement the home and the school in the training of youth, and to return to them those interests of which modern life tends to cheat children, every stimulation and encouragement should be given to the extension and development of the voluntary youth organizations

XIX To make everywhere available these minimum protections of the health and welfare of children, there should be a district, county, or community organization for health, education, and welfare, with full-time officials, coordinating with a statewide program which will be responsive to a nationwide service of general information, statistics, and scientific research. This should include:

(a) Trained, full-time public health officials, with public health nurses, sanitary inspection, and laboratory workers

(b) Available hospital beds

(c) Full-time public welfare service for the relief, aid, and guidance of children in special need due to poverty, misfortune, or behavior difficulties, and for the protection of children from abuse, neglect, exploitation, or moral hazard

For every child these rights, regardless of race, or color, or situation, wherever he may live under the protection of the American Flag.

understanding of the range of services required to meet these needs.

DEMOGRAPHIC, VITAL, AND MORBIDITY STATISTICS

Knowledge and use of statistical data about this age group are essential for the nurse to carry out effective health planning and implementation activities. Statistical data help the community health nurse to identify how many people need nursing services and what type of services can best help the population to resolve its health problems (refer to Chapter 11). Since health needs and services differ with age, it is important to analyze the composition of the population and the mortality

and morbidity statistics specific to the particular age group under consideration.

Composition of the Population

One of the most significant characteristics of a country's population composition is age structure. It is important to examine this variable because health risks are frequently age-related, and the absolute number of people in a particular age category influences the amount of resources needed to provide adequate health care services.

The age structure of the population in the United States has been changing. Fluctuations in the birth rates since World War II and dramatic changes in life expectancy have significantly altered the age distribution in the nation over the

TABLE 14-1   Number of resident population by age, sex, and race, United States, 1960, 1970, 1975, 1980, 1985, 1987*

Sex, age, and race	Unit	Year					
		1960	1970	1975	1980	1985	1987
Total							
Both sexes, all ages	Million	180.7	203.3	215.5	226.5	241.1	243.4
Age distribution							
Under 5 years old	Million	20.3	17.2	16.1	16.3	18.0	18.3
5-17 years old	Million	44.2	52.5	51.0	47.4	45.0	45.3
18 years old and over	Million	116.1	133.5	148.3	162.8	175.7	179.8
25-34 years old	Million	22.9	24.9	31.3	37.1	42.0	43.3
35-44 years old	Million	24.2	23.1	22.8	25.6	31.8	34.3
45-64 years old	Million	36.2	41.8	43.8	44.5	44.9	45.3
65 years old and over	Million	16.6	20.0	22.7	25.5	28.5	29.8
Median age	Year	29.4	28.0	28.7	30.0	31.5	32.1
Racial distribution							
White	Million	160.0	178.1	187.2	194.8	202.8	205.8
Black	Million	19.0	22.6	24.7	26.6	28.9	29.7
Percent of resident population	Percent black	11.0	11.1	11.5	11.8	12.2	12.2
Persons of Spanish origin	Million	NA†	9.1	NA	14.6	16.9	18.8

*Resident population as of July 1.

†NA, not available.

From 1960 Data from U.S. Bureau of the Census. Current population reports, Series P-25, Nos. 311, 519, and 917; 1970 through 1987 data from U.S. Bureau of the Census, U.S.A. statistics in brief, 1988: a statistical abstract supplement, Washington, D.C., 1988, U.S. Department of Commerce, unnumbered pages.

past three decades. Table 14-1 illustrates the changes that have occurred since 1960. Overall, aging of the population is evident. In 1987, the median age reached its all-time high of 32.1 years. Since the Baby Boom generation will be over the age of 35 by the year 2000, a sharp increase in the median age will occur during the rest of the century (U.S. Bureau of the Census, 1989, Population Profile of the United States).

Changing birth rates have greatly influenced the distribution of the school-age population in the past 30 years. The decrease in the number of preschool children from 11.2 percent in 1960 to 7.4 percent in 1975 and the increase in the 18- to 65-year-old population during the same time period are the direct result of these changes. The baby boom immediately following World War II expanded the preschool population in the 1960s and the 18-and-above population group in the 1970s. The declining birth rate of the 1970s is reflected in the decline of the 1975 preschool percent distribution. The decline in the overall U.S. fertility rate has, however, leveled off since 1976. This is due to the higher fertility rates for women between 18 and 39 years of age and especially for women in their thirties. Since 1985, the recent rise in births has brought about an increase in the preschool age group (Select Panel, 1981, Vol. IV; U.S. Bureau of the Census, 1989, Fertility of American Women; U.S. Bureau of the Census, 1989, Population Profile of the United States).

Shifts in the age distribution of a population in such a short time frame present special difficulties for health professionals. This is especially true when they are attempting to predict what health services are needed for a specific age group in the future. When birth rates fluctuate, it is easy to have either an overabundance or an underabundance of health personnel and services. Health professionals in the 1950s and 1960s, for example, were underequipped to handle the number of school-age children resulting from the postwar baby boom.

What the future holds is unknown. The fluctuations in fertility in the United States over the last four decades illustrate that family-size preference has varied in response to financial and so-cial conditions and may do so in the future (National Center for Health Statistics, 1988). A difference of only one additional child per family can have a tremendous impact on the range of services needed for our school-age population. It is projected that the elementary school-age population (5 to 13 years) will be approximately 3 million larger in 1995 than it was in 1987, and will then decline by 2 million between 1995 and 2005. Between 1987 and 1990, the high school age group will decline by 1.3 million but will return to its current size (14.5 million) by 1995. (U.S. Bureau of the Census, 1989, Population Profile of the United States, pp. 6-7).

A younger school population is evolving. The increasing demand for preprimary school enrollment presented real challenges for the health and educational systems in the 1980s and is projected to do so in the future. "From 1970 to 1986, preprimary enrollment increased from 4.3 to 6.5 million. Nursery school enrollment contributed two thirds of this increase as the enrollment rate of 3- and 4-year-olds increased from 21 to 39 percent" (U.S. Bureau of the Census, 1989, Population Profile of the United States, p. 20).

"In 1986, there were 60.1 million persons enrolled in school, including 12.4 million college students and 6.5 million children enrolled in preprimary school" (U.S. Bureau of the Census, 1988, School Enrollment, p. 1). This certainly is no small number, and it supports the need to examine carefully the common health problems of this age group and to plan *organized* health services to meet these needs. When planning for these health services, it is imperative that one analyze local as well as national statistics, because there are striking differences in the fertility rates in various segments of the population. In 1988, for example, significantly higher fertility rates were found among Hispanic women 18 to 44 years old and black women 18 to 24 years old than among their white counterparts (U.S. Bureau of the Census, 1989, Fertility of American women). Thus, in communities where there is a high percentage of women from these two minority groups, there may be a greater need for child health services.

Community health nurses who work with the school-age population encounter a variety of physical, psychosocial, cultural, environmental, and developmental health problems and concerns. Since in this chapter emphasis is placed on planning health services, only general morbidity and mortality statistics and growth and development data will be presented here. The reader can obtain a comprehensive understanding of childhood problems and specific growth and development characteristics by referring to *Comprehensive Pediatric Nursing* (Scipien, Barnard, Chard, Howe, and Phillips, 1986) and *Nursing Care of Infants and Children* (Whaley and Wong, 1987).

Childhood Mortality Risks

Accidents, cancer, congenital anomalies, diseases of the heart, and homicide are the leading causes of death for children ages 1 to 14 years old. For children ages 10 to 14 years, suicide is ahead of diseases of the heart as a leading cause of death. Suicide is also a major cause of death in adolescents 15 to 19 years old (USDHHS, Office of Maternal and Child Health, 1989, p. 23). Figure 14-2 presents the major causes of mortality for children ages 1 to 19 years of age. When one is reviewing statistical rates such as those presented in Figure 14-2, it is important to keep in mind that these rates may vary significantly within seg-

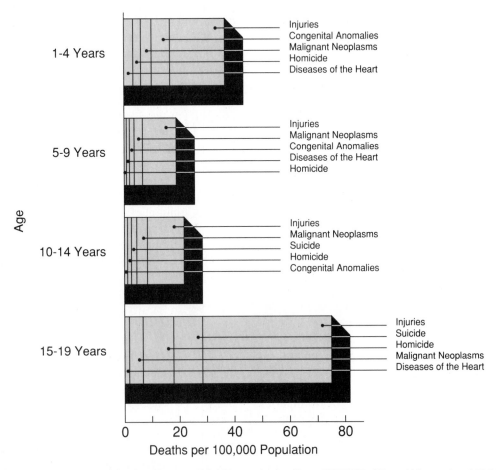

Figure 14-2 Leading causes of death, 1986, per 100,000 population. (From USDHHS, Office of Maternal and Child Health: Child Health USA '89, HRS-M-CH8915, Washington, DC, 1989, Bureau of Maternal and Child Health Resources Development, p 23.)

ments of the population and regions. For example, the homicide rate for black males (aged 15 to 24 years old) is five and a half times higher than the rate for white males (USDHHS, 1987, p. 28). In Michigan in 1984, homicide was the second highest cause of death among black children in the 1- to 14-year-old age group. Their death rate as a result of this cause was nearly eight times higher than the white rate for the same age group (Director's Task Force on Minority Health, 1988, p. 117).

It is striking to note when examining the statistics in Figure 14-2 that the majority of childhood deaths could be prevented; environmental, social, and behavioral factors greatly influence their occurrence. It is estimated that approximately "50 percent of our United States deaths are due to unhealthy behavior or lifestyle; 20 percent to environmental factors; 20 percent to human biological factors; and only 10 percent to inadequacies in health care" (USDHEW, 1979, p. 9).

Accidents/Injuries

Although deaths from accidents or injuries have declined 45 percent between 1950 and 1985, they continue to be the single largest cause of deaths among 1- to 14-year-old children (USDHHS, 1987, p. 27). Injuries are fatal nearly four times more often for children in this age category than the next leading cause of death—cancer. For adolescents and young adults between the ages of 15 and 24, accidents account for more than 50 percent of all fatalities, claiming about five times more lives than the next leading cause—homicide (USDHHS, Office of Disease Prevention and Health Promotion, 1986, p. 127). Some of the leading causes of premature deaths from accidents are motor vehicle injuries, drowning, fires (burns), firearms, falls, and poisoning (National Safety Council, 1988, pp. 8-9). Motor vehicle accidents account for just under half of all accidents.

A significant challenge for community health professionals for the next decade is to find ways to reduce fatalities from accidents/injuries (USDHHS, Office of Disease Prevention and Health Promotion, 1986, p. 25). An important role of the community health nurse is to promote driving safety among adolescents and young adults, including identifying at-risk individuals. Driving without wearing a seat belt or while under the influence of alcohol or other drugs increases an individual's risk for becoming a motor vehicle fatality. Data reflect that a significant number of adolescents engage in risk-taking behaviors. Fifty-six percent of the respondents to the National Adolescent Student Health Survey in 1987 reported not wearing a seat belt the last time they rode in a motor vehicle; 44 percent of the tenth-grade respondents and 32 percent of the eighth-grade students had ridden during the most recent month with a driver who was under the influence of alcohol or other drugs (Centers for Disease Control, 1989, p. 147).

The community health nurse can also assume a major role in preventing accidents and injuries in younger school-age children through health education activities designed to prevent poisonings, fires, falls, and other causes of accidents. The Consumer Product Safety Commission (1-800-638-CPSC) provides material on consumer product safety including product hazards, product defects, and injuries sustained in using products. This information can help the nurse to plan sound educational programs. The National Child Safety Council Childwatch (1-800-222-1464) answers questions and distributes literature on safety and sponsors the Missing Kids program (publicized through milk cartons).

Homicide

In 1974, for the first time in our country's history, homicide became a major killer of children and young adults. "The homicide rate for blacks ages 10 through 19 years is significantly greater than for whites" (USDHHS, Office of Maternal and Child Health, 1989, p. 30). Homicide is the leading cause of death for black males ages 15 to 44 (USDHHS, Office of Maternal and Child Health, 1986, p. 243).

Certainly no one factor accounts for the increase in homicide among children. Poverty, family breakup, the availability of handguns, and characteristics of adolescence which make a teenager prone to violence are some important factors that should be considered when planning strategies to reduce childhood mortality resulting from violence (USDHHS, Office of Disease Prevention and Health Promotion, 1986; USDHHS, Office of Maternal and Child Health, 1986). It is also crucial to examine societal attitudes, because violence is portrayed as an acceptable and often successful conflict resolution strategy (National Committee for Injury Prevention and Control and Education Development Center, Inc., 1989, p. 15).

Community health nurses can no longer deal only with physical health problems. They must work closely with all agencies in the community so that a concerted effort is made to *prevent* death from homicide in our school-age population.

Suicide

Since 1960, the incidence of suicide among our youth has been steadily increasing and is now the second leading cause of death for persons ages 15 to 19 and the third leading cause of death for children 10 to 14 years of age. Suicide is a large contributor to death in adolescents (USDHHS, Office of Maternal and Child Health, 1989). Although overall, the suicide rate of youths has been relatively stable since 1978, the rate for young Americans is now triple that of 30 years ago (USDHHS, Office of Disease Prevention and Health Promotion, 1986, p. 247). Health professionals view suicide as a problem of extreme importance in the adolescent population, because it is an indicator that social, emotional, and physical stress is great. Rapidly changing societal values, population mobility, and economic pressures have presented adolescents with decision-making conflicts that result in uncertainty and stress (refer to Figure 14-3).

The extent of the suicide problem is much greater than the recorded figures indicate. Because suicide is often viewed by our culture as a cowardly and disgraceful act, it is often concealed by families and medical personnel. Many suicides are not recorded as such on the death certificate, and it can be difficult to differentiate between suicide and death resulting from an accident. The result is that the recorded incidence reflects only a

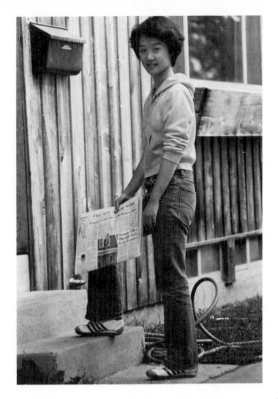

Figure 14-3 Accelerated societal changes have exposed American youth to increased opportunities as well as increased stresses. American youth are exposed much earlier than their previous counterparts to such things as human sexuality concerns, pressures from peers to use alcohol and drugs, and various lifestyles. Community health nurses are often in a favorable position to detect youth who are having difficulty coping with the demands of life.

proportion of the deaths caused by suicide. In addition, when one looks at the rate of attempted suicide, the problem becomes even more significant because suicide attempts far exceed actual suicides. Eighteen percent of the girls and 11 percent of the boys who participated in the National Adolescent Student Health Survey reported they had tried to injure themselves in a way that might have resulted in their death. Additionally, 25 percent of the boys and 42 percent of the girls reported that they had seriously considered committing suicide at some time during their lives (Centers for Disease Control, 1989, p. 148).

"Suicide clusters" and the possible "contagion" effect of adolescent suicide is a growing public concern. A suicide cluster is the occurrence of suicides or attempted suicides closer together in space and time than is considered usual for a given community. It is estimated that suicide clusters account for approximately 1 percent to 5 percent of all suicides among adolescents and young adults. In a cluster, suicides occurring later in the cluster often appear to have been influenced by earlier suicides. Thus, a community-wide intervention approach is needed to address this problem. Persons at risk need to be identified and interviewed, personal counseling services should be provided for close friends/relatives of the victims and potentially suicidal adolescents, and the community needs to be supported in a way that minimizes sensationalism (Centers for Disease Control, 1988, CDC recommendations).

Adolescence is normally a period of turmoil, frequently characterized by rebellious and impulsive behavior. During times of stress, thoughts of suicide are not abnormal. These thoughts usually do not, however, result in suicide. Studies have shown that adolescents who do commit suicide have greater problems than just the normal mood swings of adolescence. Suicidal adolescents often have a long-standing history of chronic childhood and family problems. Frequently they exhibit signs and symptoms of depression, with feelings of despair and hopelessness. Often they are crying out for help because they are dealing with overwhelming burdens such as divorce, illness, and lack of material resources to meet their basic needs, as well as changes in their social relationships (Hoekelman, Blatman, Brunell, Friedman, and Seidel, 1978, p. 667). Adolescents who are severely depressed rarely give evidence of suicidal intent (Whaley and Wong, 1987).

Problems of childhood can escalate during adolescence. Thus community health nurses should carefully observe teenagers who suddenly have difficulty coping with activities of daily living. Changes in behavior such as a drop in school attendance, decreased attention to personal hygiene, crying spells without specific cause, loss of appetite, and withdrawal from extracurricular activities should not be ignored. Adolescents who feel isolated are at risk for suicide. Look for the loners who lack initiative and who seemingly do not care how they relate to others. Individuals who are severely depressed or who are at odds with themselves and the people close to them are at highest risk for suicide (USDHEW, 1979; Whaley and Wong, 1987).

Community health nurses, especially those functioning in the school setting, are in a key position to detect troubled youth. When they work with adolescents who are potentially suicidal, nurses must demonstrate a caring attitude and a genuine interest in learning about their problems. Nurses should also encourage these adolescents to talk about their suicidal thoughts and plans and provide assistance so that they reach out for the help they need. Working with the troubled adolescent's family is also important. Families need supportive services and often assistance in determining how to obtain help for their children. The principles of crisis intervention (refer to Chapter 7) should be applied when working with these families. Prompt recognition of distressed youth may prevent suicidal behavior.

Congenital Anomalies

Many factors increase the risk for congenital anomalies, including congenital heart diseases. Poverty, poor housing, malnutrition, pregnancy at a young age, use of alcohol and cigarettes, and inadequate medical care increase the likelihood that illness, disability, or death will occur. It has been shown that mothers in all age categories who are disadvantaged are at risk for producing an unhealthy child (Binsacca, Ellis, Martin, and Petitti, 1987; National Center for Health Statistics, 1989; Stockwell, Swanson, and Wicks, 1988; Task Force on Infant Mortality, 1987). The risk of having an abnormal birth increases as a mother's consumption of alcohol and smoking increase (USDHEW, 1979, p. 316). Young mothers and mothers who have inadequate health care are more likely to have low-birth-weight babies than other mothers. Low-birth-weight infants have a high incidence of congenital malformations (Hutchins, Kessel, and Placek, 1984, p. 171). It is obvious from these facts that a preventive health program designed to reduce childhood mortality due to congenital malformations must include ways to eliminate poor environmental and social conditions, to expand the use of prenatal services by young and disadvantaged mothers, and to alter unhealthy behaviors (alcohol consumption and smoking) which increase the risk for abnormal births.

Malignant Neoplasms

Cancer is a significant contributor to the causes of death in children 1 through 14 years of age. It is the leading cause of death *from disease* in children in the 3- to 14-year-old age group. Leukemia is the most frequent cancer in children 9 years of age and under: lymphomas are the most common form of cancer in children 10 to 14 years of age. Leukemia accounts for almost half the deaths from cancer in childhood (American Cancer Society, 1989). It is estimated that 7167 new cases of cancer will be diagnosed in the United States every year among children aged 1 to 14 years (Fergusson, Ruccione, Waskerwitz, Perin, Diserens, Phil, Nesbit, and Hammond, 1987).

Cancer places a tremendous burden on families and society. The severe nature of this condition and the prolonged treatment needed cause pain and anguish for both the child and the family. Cancer in childhood also causes financial hardship for many families, because funding for catastrophic illness is frequently not available. Health planning efforts for cancer should focus on providing early detection, treatment, and supportive services, funding for research, and monies to eliminate individual financial hardships. Community health nurses can significantly assist families in coping with childhood cancer by providing hospice care services and by helping them to obtain needed resources from community agencies (Martinson, Armstrong, Geis, Anglim, Gronseth, Macinnis, Kersey, and Nesbit, 1978). The American Cancer Society, for instance, supplies dressings and equipment free of charge. Other community agencies such as the department of social services and Crippled Children's Association provide funds for medical treatment. Helping parents to establish and maintain support networks is an important role for nurses working with families who are coping with childhood cancer (Lynam, 1987).

Childhood Morbidity Risks—Acute Conditions

The incidence of acute conditions in childhood is difficult to ascertain because (1) many acute conditions are not reportable; (2) reportable acute conditions are often not reported; and (3) acute illness is frequently treated at home and as a result is not brought to the attention of health professionals. Data from the national health surveys since 1956 do give estimated patterns of incidence over time. According to this survey, acute conditions are illnesses and injuries that last no longer than 3 months and have either been treated by medical personnel or have resulted in restricted activity of 1 day or more (USDHHS, 1985, p. 89). The major types of acute illness for children, ages 6 through 16 years, fall into five major categories. In order of frequency, these are respiratory conditions, infective and parasitic diseases, injuries, digestive system conditions, and all other conditions. The number of days lost from school per year due to acute conditions is shown in Table 14-2. School-age children miss approximately 4.2 days of school per year due to these conditions. The number of school-loss days per year per 100 children has not changed significantly over the past two decades (U.S. Bureau of the Census, 1989, Statistical abstract, p. 133).

Respiratory conditions account for over 50 percent of the reported acute illnesses among school-age children. These conditions are frequently ignored because "everyone gets a cold or an earache;" colds and earaches are "a normal part of life." However, these seemingly minor illnesses must not be disregarded. They do interfere with activities of daily living and may often lead to serious, chronic disabilities. In a study by Heazlett and Whaley (1976, p. 146), it was noted that the common cold—the respiratory condition with the highest incidence rate—affected adversely to a significant degree the perceptual and learning performance of junior high students. Otitis media, the third leading reason for pediatrician contact, can, if untreated, result in permanent hearing loss and/or chronic ear infection. In 1988, about 25 percent of the children who responded to the National Health Interview Survey on Child Health reported they had had repeated ear infections during their lifetime (Hendershot, 1989). Diseases of

TABLE 14-2   School days lost associated with acute conditions: 1962 to 1986*

Condition	1962	1965	1970	1975	1980	1985	1986 Total†	Male	Female	White	Black
All acute conditions §	521	456	452	451	487	387	423	372	475	450	287
Infective and parasitic diseases	108	139	90	81	99	94	79	68	91	82	67
Respiratory conditions¶	342	238	264	261	282	216	247	209	288	269	149
Upper respiratory	174	147	147	121	118	91	73	69	78	75	60
Influenza and other	168	91	117	140	164	124	175	141	210	194	88
Digestive system conditions	14	13	24	21	22	13‡	12‡	12‡	12‡	10‡	18‡
Injuries	27	29	36	52	37	24	29	37	21‡	27	32‡
All other acute conditions	29	38	38	36	47	41	55	47	64	62	21‡

*Days lost per 100 children, ages 6 to 16 (beginning 1985, ages 5 to 17). Based on data collected during the period July of the previous year to June of the year shown through 1980; beginning 1985 is based on calendar year data.

†Includes other races not shown separately.

‡Figure does not meet standards of reliability or precision.

§Discrepancies exist between totals and column numbers because only whole numbers being used.

¶Respiratory conditions totals include upper respiratory and influenza and others.

From US National Center for Health Statistics, series 10, and unpublished data, US Bureau of the Census: Statistical Abstract of the United States, ed 109, Washington, DC, 1989, US Department of Commerce, p 133.

the respiratory system were the major cause of hospitalization of children 1 through 9 years of age in 1987 (USDHHS, Office of Maternal and Child Health, 1989, p. 24).

Infective and parasitic diseases are of concern to all health personnel because of their contagious nature. Many of them, such as scabies, impetigo, ringworm, and head lice, are still considered "diseases of the poor and unclean" even though this myth has been disproved. Children who have experienced these conditions are often socially isolated from their peers and labeled "dirty kids" even after treatment ceases. The reader will find the American Public Health Association Handbook, *Control of Communicable Diseases in Man* (Benenson, 1990), an extremely useful resource when identifying and recommending follow-up for any of these communicable conditions. It must be remembered, however, that physical care and treatment is not sufficient. The social stigma associated with these diseases is often more devastating than the disease itself. Epidemiological investigation (refer to Chapter 10) to determine

the source of infection is essential in order to prevent further disease incidence as well as the social stigma associated with infective and parasitic diseases.

Injuries disproportionately strike the young. Injuries are the leading cause of death and a major cause of morbidity and disability among children and youth (National Research Council, 1985). The most common single site of injuries to children under age 15 is the home. "Injuries occurring at school account for about 21 percent of all injuries among children aged 10 through 14 years" (USDHHS, Office of Maternal and Child Health, 1989, pp. 23, 27). Injuries present a significant burden on society. "One in every nine children is hospitalized for accidental or other injuries before age 15; 10 million emergency room visits per year are made for accidents or other injuries" (U.S. Congress, Office of Technology Assessment, 1988, p. 5). An estimated 60 million injuries occurred in 1986. Data from U.S. Consumer Product Safety Commission's National Electronic Injury Surveillance System

(NEISS) reveal that sports and recreation are responsible for more treatments in hospital emergency rooms than any other category of injuries (Verhalen, 1987, pp. 673-674).

Males have a significantly higher rate of nonfatal injuries than females, because of differences in activities and behavior such as participation in contact sports. Better-planned sports programs might substantially reduce the number of sports-related injuries. Monitoring environmental conditions in homes and schools and promoting highway safety and regulations such as child safety seat laws could also significantly decrease childhood injuries.

Diseases of the digestive system, such as stomach ache, vomiting, diarrhea, Hirschsprung disease, celiac disease, appendicitis, and colitis, were the third leading cause of hospitalization of children aged 1 through 14 years in 1987 (USDHHS, Office of Maternal and Child Health, 1989, p. 25). Some of these diseases have a psychosocial etiology or are aggravated by psychosocial stresses. An astute community health nurse will assess for stressors as well as physical causes when working with children who have digestive tract problems. This is especially important to do when a child has recurrent unexplained abdominal pains. Some key variables to consider when physical causes for digestive conditions have been ruled out are inadequate nutrition; family conflict; separation due to death, divorce, and illness; child abuse; tense classroom atmosphere; unfavorable teacher-student relationships; poor academic achievement; unrealistic expectations for performance; and lack of peer support.

Childhood Morbidity Risks—Chronic Conditions

Childhood chronic conditions are of special concern to health professionals for several reasons. First, these conditions may inhibit normal developmental processes and cause disability in later life. Second, the stress of chronic illness frequently affects significant others as well as the child who has the chronic condition. Last, prevention, treatment, and management services for chronic conditions are costly because of the long-term nature of these conditions and the number of persons affected by them.

The wars of our nation dramatically illustrated the need to focus attention on preventing chronic health problems in our youth. During both World War I and World War II, a significant number of men were rejected for military service because of existing chronic conditions such as dental problems, psychiatric difficulties, and orthopedic abnormalities. In spite of recognition since the early 1920s that the health status of our nation's youth was far from ideal, 15 percent of the 18-year-olds were rejected for military service in 1965 because they had chronic handicapping conditions. It was believed that two-thirds of these conditions could have been prevented if they had been detected before age 15 (Travis, 1976, p. 4).

It is estimated that approximately 10 percent to 15 percent of all children have some form of chronic health condition, many of which are mild. However, 2.8 million or 6.2 percent of all children 5 through 17 years of age are limited in their usual activities because of chronic illnesses and impairments, and 4.4 percent or 2 million of these children experience limitations at school (Prevalence of disability, 1988, p. 2). The percentage of children with limitation of activity has doubled since 1960. Disadvantaged children are consistently more limited in activity as a result of chronic conditions than their wealthier counterparts (USDHHS 1987, Surgeon General; USDHHS, Office of Maternal and Child Health, 1989).

Table 14-3 presents the types of chronic handicapping conditions of childhood. Among persons under 18 years of age, the leading causes of chronic conditions in 1986, in rank order, were chronic sinusitis, hay fever, chronic bronchitis, asthma, dermatitis including eczema, deformities or orthopedic impairments, and diseases of sebaceous glands (U.S. Bureau of the Census, 1989, Statistical abstract). Asthma tends to limit a child's activity more than other respiratory conditions and is a main cause of days lost from school in this age group. In 1988, 6 percent of the sample children in the National Health Interview Survey on Child Health had had asthma, about 7 percent had had hay fever, and about 8 percent had had eczema or skin allergies (Hendershot, 1989).

TABLE 14-3 Types of chronic childhood handicapping conditions

Categories of conditions	Types of conditions
A. Disorders of the central nervous system (CNS)	1. Poliomyelitis 2. Cerebral palsy 3. Epilepsy and other seizure disorders 4. Spina bifida 5. Spinal cord and cranial injury
B. Sensory disorders	1. Speech disorders: cleft lip, palate, articulation defects, stuttering, mutism 2. Hearing impairment, including deafness 3. Vision impairments
C. Cosmetic disorders	1. Facial deformities: severe acne, severe scarring 2. Burns 3. Scoliosis 4. Dwarfism 5. Cleft lip, palate 6. Many CNS disorders
D. Mobility disorders (muscular and skeletal systems)	1. Various orthopedic disorders 2. Thalidomide deformities 3. Osteogenesis imperfecta 4. Amputations 5. Muscular dystrophy 6. All the CNS disorders
E. Systemic disorders	1. Diabetes 2. Hemophilia, sickle cell anemia, and other blood dyscrasias 3. Cystic fibrosis 4. Asthma 5. Arthritis 6. Heart disease 7. Kidney disease
F. Malignancies	1. Leukemia 2. Other cancers
G. Mental retardation	1. Borderline 2. Severe 3. Many CNS disorders
H. Psychiatric disorders	1. Schizophrenia and psychosis 2. Severe affective disturbances 3. Personality disorders 4. Long-term behavior disorders
I. Severe developmental disorders	1. Failure-to-thrive syndrome 2. Autism
J. Persistent learning disability	

From Select Panel for the Promotion of Child Health: Better health for our children: a national strategy, vol IV, DHHS Pub No (PHS) 79-55071, Washington, DC, 1981, US Government Printing Office, p 324.

Community health nurses provide supportive assistance in a variety of ways to families whose children have chronic conditions. They assist these families in obtaining adequate health care, in making necessary adjustments in family lifestyle, and in obtaining community resources which will help them to promote their child's growth and development. *Compuplay* is one such resource. Compuplay Resource Centers serve families with children 2 to 14 years of age with physical, mental, sensory, or behavioral disabilities. These centers provide computer play classes, software lending libraries, and local in-service training for professionals. Families interested in this resource can obtain further information by writing to the INNOTEK Director, National Lekotek Center, 2100 Ridge Avenue, Evanston, IL., 60204 or by calling (312) 328-0001 (Compuplay Centers, 1988, p. 5). Other resources that may be helpful to families dealing with a chronic illness are listed in Chapter 17, Appendix 17-2.

Community health nurses also assume a significant role in assisting school-age children to accept peers who have a chronic condition. A program to help children adjust to other children with chronic, disabling conditions is *Kids on the Block*. This program is a puppet presentation showing puppets in wheelchairs, with assistive devices, and with various physical and mental conditions. This program stimulates discussion of childrens' feelings about peers who are different. Educational and health professionals can obtain more information about *Kids on the Block* by contacting 1-800-368-KIDS.

In addition to chronic diseases, school-age children may experience many chronic social problems which present serious difficulties for both them and their families. Homelessness, for example, is becoming increasingly prevalent among families with children. This problem is discussed extensively in Chapter 15. Four other social problems of particular concern to community health nurses who are working with school-age children are child maltreatment, teenage parenthood, sexually transmitted diseases (STDs), and drug abuse. None of these difficulties is unique to the school-age population. However, because a sizable proportion of our youth are experiencing these problems, a discussion of them is warranted.

Child Maltreatment

As a result of increased reporting requirements in recent years, it is now known that child maltreatment is reaching epidemic proportions among the school-age as well as the preschool population. Child maltreatment can involve physical and/or psychological abuse and neglect and/or sexual abuse. "In 1987, there were almost 2.2 million reports of abused or neglected children nationwide. This represents an increase of 225 percent since 1976" (USDHHS, Office of Maternal and Child Health, 1989, p. 28). A document prepared in 1984 by the American Association for Protecting Children (AAPC), dealing with reported child neglect and abuse, states that the average age for all maltreated children was 7.3 years. Children who experienced serious physical injuries were younger, with an average age of 5.3 years. Emotionally maltreated children were on average 8.1 years old (AAPC, 1986).

Several risk factors have been identified as the causes of child maltreatment. Substantial physical force is most likely to be used against children under 5 or against 15- to 17-year-old youths (AAPC, 1986, p. 173). The risk of being sexually abused for girls between 10 and 12 years of age is more than double the average rate for all girls between 1 and 18 years. Girls are more likely to be sexually victimized than boys (Finkelhor and Araji, 1986). Statistics also reveal that disabled children and youths, as well as those who are relatively unresponsive socially, have an increased risk of being abused (O'Day, 1983).

The average age of the abuser is 31 years, reflecting that maltreating parents range from young to old (AAPC, 1986; U.S. Congress, Office of Technology Assessment, 1988). As was previously discussed in Chapter 13, "the most important parental risk factors for maltreatment of children are poverty, unemployment, and a history of abuse as a child" (U.S. Congress, Office of Technology Assessment, 1988, p. 176). A relatively high number of parents who were abused as children abuse their children. Although abuse occurs in families of all socioeconomic levels, parents in poor families or those who are experiencing unemployment are most likely to maltreat their children. However, it is significant that in the majority of poor families children are not abused (U.S. Congress, Office of Technology Assessment, 1988).

Although reporting of child maltreatment has improved in the last decade, this problem continues to be underreported and is often not identified. All health care professionals, including the community health nurse, must expand their efforts to identify undetected abuse and neglect in school-age children. Presented in Table 14-4 is a summary of physical and behavioral indicators that can assist nurses in identifying child abuse

TABLE 14-4 Physical and behavioral indicators of child abuse and neglect

Type of CA/N*	Physical indicators	Behavioral indicators
Physical abuse	Unexplained bruises and welts:	Feels deserving of punishment
	On face, lips, mouth	Wary of adult contacts
	On torso, back, buttocks, thighs	Apprehensive when other children cry
	In various stages of healing	Behavioral extremes:
	Clustered, forming regular patterns	Aggressiveness
	Reflecting shape of article used to inflict (electric cord, belt buckle)	Withdrawal
	On several different surface areas	Frightened of parents
	Regularly appear after absence, weekend, or vacation	Afraid to go home
	Unexplained burns:	Reports injury by parents
	Cigar, cigarette burns, especially on soles, palms, back, or buttocks	Vacant or frozen stare
		Lies very still while surveying surroundings
	Immersion burns (socklike, glovelike, doughnut-shaped on buttocks or genitalia)	Will not cry when approached by examiner
	Patterned like electric burner, iron, etc.	Responds to questions in monosyllables
	Rope burns on arms, legs, neck, or torso	Inappropriate or precocious maturity
	Infected burns, indicating delay in seeking treatment	Manipulative behavior to get attention
	Unexplained fractures or dislocations:	Capable of only superficial relationships
	To skull, nose, facial structure	Indiscriminately seeks affection
	In various stages of healing	Poor self-concept
	Multiple or spiral fractures	
	Unexplained lacerations or abrasions:	
	To mouth, lips, gums, eyes	
	To external genitalia	
	In various stages of healing	
	Bald patches on the scalp	
Physical neglect	Underweight, poor growth pattern, failure to thrive	Begging, stealing food
	Consistent hunger, poor hygiene, inappropriate dress	Extended stays at school (early arrival and late departure)
	Consistent lack of supervision, especially in dangerous activities or long periods	Rare attendance at school
		Constant fatigue, listlessness, or falling asleep in class
	Wasting of subcutaneous tissue	Inappropriate seeking of affection
	Unattended physical problems or medical needs	Assuming adult responsibilities and concerns
	Abandonment	Alcohol or drug abuse
	Abdominal distention	Delinquency (e.g., thefts)
	Bald patches on the scalp	States there is no caretaker

*CA/N = child abuse and neglect.

Continued.

TABLE 14-4   Physical and behavioral indicators of child abuse and neglect—cont'd

Type of CA/N*	Physical indicators	Behavioral indicators
Sexual abuse	Difficulty in walking or sitting	Unwilling to change for gym or participate in physical education class
	Torn, stained, or bloody underclothing	Withdrawal, fantasy, or infantile behavior
	Pain, swelling, or itching in genital area	Bizarre, sophisticated, or unusual sexual behavior or knowledge
	Pain on urination	Poor peer relationships
	Bruises, bleeding, or lacerations in external genitalia, vaginal, or anal areas	Delinquent or runaway
	Vaginal or penile discharge	Reports sexual assault by caretaker
	Venereal disease, especially in preteens	Change in performance in school
	Poor sphincter tone	
	Pregnancy	
Emotional maltreatment	Speech disorders	Habit disorders (sucking, biting, rocking, etc.)
	Lags in physical development	Conduct and learning disorders (antisocial, destructive, etc.)
	Failure to thrive	Neurotic traits (sleep disorders, inhibition of play, unusual fearfulness)
	Hyperactive or disruptive behavior	Psychoneurotic reactions (hysteria, obsession, compulsion, phobias, hypochondria)
		Behavior extremes:
		Compliant, passive
		Aggressive, demanding
		Overly adaptive behavior:
		Inappropriately adult
		Inappropriately infant
		Developmental lags (mental, emotional)
		Attempted suicide

From Heindl C, Krall CA, Salus M, and Broadhurst DD: The nurse's role in the prevention and treatment of child abuse and neglect, Washington, DC, 1979, National Center on Child Abuse and Neglect, Children's Bureau, Administration for Children, Youth and Families, Office of Human Development Services, p 10.

and neglect. Using data such as those previously discussed relative to risk factors can help professionals to identify potential abusers and victims of maltreatment. Strategies aimed at preventing initial maltreatment or a recurrence should be focused on changing risk factors that have been demonstrated to have a major influence on child maltreatment. For example, strategies designed to reduce poverty-related stresses, such as referring families to community agencies for financial aid, are appropriately aimed at eliminating a significant risk factor of child maltreatment (U.S. Congress, Office of Technology Assessment, 1988).

The problems of child abuse and neglect are compounded for professionals who work with the school-age population, because often they must deal with the lasting effects of conditions which existed during infancy and the preschool years.

Longitudinal studies are beginning to report findings which indicate that there are long-term detrimental consequences of child abuse. Children who are abused during early childhood tend to have difficulty establishing trust, have more aggessive and behavioral problems than children who have not been abused, and frequently manifest a general air of depression, unhappiness, and sadness. Children who are sexually abused initially exhibit anger, hostility, and sexual problems, but long-term more serious problems such as diminished self-esteem, fear, and depression emerge (Dubowitz, 1986). In addition, data suggest that long-term effects of child maltreatment may include other problems such as juvenile delinquency, attempted suicide, substance abuse, truancy, and runaway behavior (Lindberg and Distad, 1985; McCord, 1983). There are an estimated 1 million runaways in the United States (National Center on Child Abuse and Neglect, 1986).

The effects of maltreatment can be devastating and the costs to society extremely high. Professionals and community citizens must join together to deal with this critical problem. To ensure that all children reach their optimal level of functioning, mechanisms must be established for early identification, reporting of actual or suspected abusing situations, and early and adequate intervention. Both health professionals and the public need educational opportunities that will increase their knowledge about child abuse and neglect and help them to intervene effectively with abusive families. The *Clearinghouse on Child Abuse and Neglect* (P.O. Box 1182, Washington, D.C., 20013, Phone: 1-703-821-2088) was established in 1975 by the federal government to assist communities with their educational needs relative to child maltreatment. This clearinghouse disseminates information and resource materials on all types of child maltreatment, responds to public inquiries, and has a computerized database which maintains updated statistics. Hotline services are also readily available to help communities and troubled families. The *National Child Abuse Hotline* (1-800-422-4453) provides information, professional counseling, and referrals for treatment.

The *Parents Anonymous Hotline* (1-800-421-0353; 1-800-352-0386 in California) provides information on self-help groups for parents involved in child maltreatment.

Teenage Parenthood

While the birth rate for adolescents aged 15 to 19 years declined between 1970 and 1986, the birth rate for young adolescents (under 15 years of age) remained essentially unchanged during this time period. There was also a substantial increase in births to percent adolescents, and the incidence of induced abortions increased steadily among this age group. Black adolescents are almost twice as likely to be single parents than white teens. However, the proportion of births increased significantly more for single white teenagers aged 15 to 19 years (181 percent increase) than for single black teens (43 percent) between 1970 and 1986 (National Center for Health Statistics, 1988).

Each year in the United States one adolescent in 10, aged 15 through 19, becomes pregnant. This figure is significantly higher than that of Canada, England, or France, where fewer than one teen in 20 becomes pregnant (USDHHS, Office of Maternal and Child Health, 1989, p. 31). The problem of teenage pregnancy has become extensive enough that the federal government has established the Office of Adolescent Pregnancy Programs in the Department of Health and Human Services (200 Independence Avenue, SW., Room 736E, 1-202-245-7473). The primary mission of the office is to prevent adolescent pregnancy and improve the quality of care for pregnant adolescents.

Over 1 million U.S. teenagers became pregnant in 1985; of these, 31,000 were under 15 years of age. Over 46 percent of these pregnancies ended in a live birth; over 40 percent ended in an induced abortion; and a spontaneous abortion occurred in over 13 percent. More than half of all pregnancies to teenagers under 15 years were reported to end in abortion (USDHHS, Office of Maternal and Child Health, 1989, p. 31).

Data suggest that the United States has a higher rate of teenage pregnancy than any other industrialized country because these teenagers are less likely to practice contraception. When they do, they are likely to practice it less effectively than do teenagers in European countries (Jones, Forrest, Goldman, Henshaw, Lincoln, Rosoff, Westoff, and Wulf, 1985). Teenagers account for about one third of all the unintended pregnancies in the United States; three-quarters of these pregnancies occur among adolescents who are not using any method of contraception (Westoff, 1988). Mosher and Horn (1988, p. 33) found that only 17 percent of young women aged 15 to 24 make their first family planning visit before they begin having intercourse, and 73 percent wait an average of 23 months after first intercourse to begin using services.

Several factors influence nonuse or inconsistent use of birth control among teenagers (Orr, 1984). Many are poorly informed about their sexual development, believing that they are too young to get pregnant or not knowing how women conceive. Others find it difficult to obtain contraceptive services, feel it is morally wrong to use birth control measures, or believe that contraceptive use interferes with the pleasures of sex, and can be dangerous to one's health. Some want to become pregnant to fulfill needs of love, attention, and belonging.

Van Dover (1985) has demonstrated that contracting (refer to Chapter 8) can positively influence both family planning knowledge and behavior with young, sexually active women. She found that clients with whom she contracted achieved significantly higher knowledge scores and showed significant increases in contraceptive consistency than did the routine clinic-care control group (pp. 53-54).

The multiplicity and complexity of needs manifested during teenage parenthood mandate close coordination among professionals from all disciplines. Pregnancy can pose serious physical and psychosocial health problems and concerns for the teenage parents, their families, and the community at large. The involved teenagers are dealing with two developmental crises, adolescence and parenthood, which may result in adverse, long-lasting psychosocial consequences if effective intervention is not available.

Medically, both the teenage mother and her baby are at high risk. Children born to teenage parents have a much higher neonatal, postnatal, and infant mortality rate. These babies have a higher incidence of prematurity, low birth weight, and respiratory distress. The mothers tend to have more physical problems throughout their pregnancy. Considering that adolescence is a period when marked physical changes and rapid growth occurs, it is understandable that the additional stress of pregnancy increases a teenage mother's susceptibility to health difficulties. Toxemia, hypertension, nutritional deficiencies, prolonged labor, pelvic disproportion, and cesarean sections are a few complications of pregnancy common to the teenage mother (Osofsky, 1985).

Parenthood in adolescence can present a number of special problems. Adolescent mothers face increased risks of single parenthood, incomplete education, poverty, unemployment, and welfare dependency. If these mothers marry, they are at increased risk of experiencing separation and divorce (National Academy of Sciences, 1987). Financially, teenagers are often not able to provide for such basic needs as food, clothing, and shelter. Frequently they need assistance from social service agencies to adequately care for themselves and their children. Because they are not prepared for a career, it is difficult for them to obtain productive employment. Often a pregnant teenager drops out of school, which increases the likelihood that future employment opportunities will be limited and that social isolation from peers will occur. In addition to peer isolation, teenage parents frequently feel rejected by their families. Dependence on welfare systems, school disruption, unstable home situations, and limited peer support often result in further pregnancies outside of marriage. Every effort should be made to ensure that teenage parents, both mother and father, are able to achieve the developmental tasks of adolescence. They need counseling which will help them to deal with the role of adolescence, as well as the role of parenthood. Their families need assistance with resolving their negative feelings so that they can help their children to handle successfully their new roles.

The Adolescent Family Life Bill of 1981 and the Adolescent Family Life Demonstration Projects Amendments of 1983 have assisted professionals in providing both physical and psychosocial services to teenage parents and their families. The goals of these legislative acts are as follows:

(1) find effective means, within the context of the family, of reaching adolescents before they become sexually active; (2) to promote adoption as an alternative for adolescent parents; (3) to establish innovative, comprehensive, and integrated approaches to the delivery of care services for pregnant adolescents; (4) to encourage and support research projects and demonstration projects concerning the societal causes and consequences of adolescent premarital sexual relations, contraceptive use, pregnancy, and child rearing; (5) to support evaluative research to identify services which alleviate, eliminate, or resolve any negative consequences of adolescent premarital sexual relations and adolescent childbearing for the parents, the child, and their families; and (6) to encourage and provide for the dissemination of results, findings, and information from programs and research projects relating to adolescent premarital sexual relations, pregnancy, and parenthood. (Perovich and Tipon, 1984, p. 186)

The Adolescent Family Life (AFL) program was incorporated into the Omnibus Budget Reconciliation Act of 1981 (Public Law 97-35, which is presented in Chapter 4). In 1988, 12 research projects and 88 care and prevention demonstration projects were funded under this program. The prevention projects target teens not yet sexually active and promote adolescent abstinence. The care projects provide comprehensive, integrated services to improve the immediate health outcomes for mother and child and their prospects for a productive future. The AFL program supports research which examines adolescent sexuality and pregnancy (USDHHS, Public Health Service, 1988).

Individual counseling with teenage parents is necessary but not sufficient to prevent unintended adolescent pregnancies. The Panel on Adolescent Pregnancy and Childbearing (1987) believes that "the responsibility for addressing adolescent pregnancy should be shared among individuals, families, voluntary organizations, communities, and governments, and that public policies should affirm the role and responsibility of families to teach human values" (p. 120). This panel further recommends that prevention of adolescent pregnancy have the highest priority and that needs of young adolescents and disadvantaged youth be given priority if resources are inadequate to address all the needs. Making contraceptive methods available and accessible to sexually active teens, addressing adolescent sexuality from the perspective of both sexes, and promoting strategies that help adolescents to develop the necessary capabilities to make and carry out responsible decisions about sexual and fertility behavior were also recommended by the Panel on Adolescent Pregnancy and Childbearing (1987).

Sexually Transmissible Diseases (STDs)

One alarming consequence of the increased sexual experimentation among youths is the dramatic rise in the incidence of sexually transmissible diseases in this age category. As with most social problems, hard data reflect only the tip of the iceberg. Professionals frequently do not accurately report the occurrence of sexually transmissible diseases, and many nonapparent subclinical infections go untreated. From estimated reports over time, however, it is apparent that sexually transmissible diseases, especially gonorrhea, chlamydial infections, and herpes have reached epidemic proportions in recent years (Venereal Disease Action Coalition, 1983, p. 3).

Sexually transmitted diseases (STDs) are among the most common infectious diseases in the United States today (National Institute for Allergy and Infectious Diseases, 1987, An introduction). During the 1980s public and professional interest in the STD problem escalated, because this problem expanded at an alarming rate, both in its scope and in its complexity. There is now a greater understanding of both the range of agents transmitted through sexual contact and the relationship of STD to reproductive and other health problems. Acquired immunodeficiency syndrome (AIDS) emerged as a major threat during the 1980s (USDHHS, Office of Disease Prevention and Health Promotion, 1986).

The most common STDs are AIDS, chlamydial infections, genital herpes, genital warts, gonorrhea, and syphilis. Appendix 10-1 presents information about these and some of the other commonly acquired sexually transmitted diseases which affect adolescents as well as adults. STDs affect both sexes from all backgrounds and economic levels. However, they are most prevalent among teenagers and young adults. About one third of all cases involve teenagers (National Institute for Allergy and Infectious Diseases, 1987, An introduction). STD Action Coalitions as well as local health departments are valuable resources for the nurse working with adolescents who suspect they may have a STD. Immediate treatment is essential. When diagnosed and treated early, almost all STDs can be treated effectively (National Institute for Allergy and Infectious Diseases, 1987, An introduction, p. 2). However, many young people suffer serious permanent complications from these infections. For example, every year an estimated 1 million women have an episode of pelvic inflammatory diseases (PID), the most serious and common complication of STDs among women. About one fifth of these PIDs are experienced by teenagers. PID can lead to infertility, tubal pregnancy, chronic pelvic pain, and other serious consequences. Over 100,000 women become infertile as a result of PID each year (National Institute for Allergy and Infectious Diseases, 1987, Pelvic inflammatory disease).

Any community health nurse working with the school-age population must realize that the occurrence of sexually transmitted diseases is a *major* health problem in this age category. Programs that provide preventive, curative, and educative services for all children in the population served by the nurse must be planned. Use of the epidemiological process (Chapter 10) and the principles of health planning (Chapter 12) will facilitate the accomplishment of such a task. For readily accessible STD information, the nurse or client may want to utilize the VD Hotline at 1-800-227-8922. This hotline provides information on all types of STDs and confidential referrals for diagnosis and treatment. The American School Health Association and United Way sponsor this service.

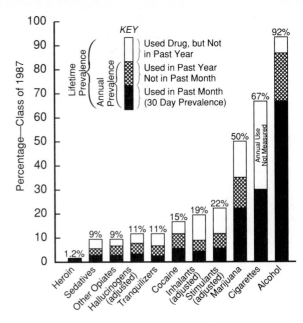

Note: The bracket near the top of a bar indicates the lower and upper limits of the 95% confidence interval.

Figure 14-4 Prevalence and recency of use of 11 types of drugs, class of 1980. (From Johnston LD, Bachman JG, and O'Malley PM: Illicit drug use, smoking, and drinking by America's highschool students, college students, and young adults 1975-1987, DHHS Pub. No. ADM 89-1602, Washington, DC, 1988, US Government Printing Office, p 31.)

Drug Abuse

Illegal use of drugs, like sexual experimentation and STDs, is a serious national health problem among youth. Since 1975, the Monitoring the Future Project of the University of Michigan Institute for Social Research has conducted a yearly survey to collect data on the range of substance use among American youth. Figure 14-4 presents data obtained by this project. It illustrates the prevalence and recency of use of 11 types of drugs among American high school seniors in 1987; alcohol, cigarettes, marijuana, and stimulants are the substances used most frequently by American adolescents (Johnston, Bachman, and O'Malley, 1988).

Data from the Monitoring the Future Project reveal that there was a marked increase in drug use by high school seniors from 1975 to 1978, but since that time this trend has slowed down. Recent survey findings are encouraging. In 1987, there was a sharp downturn in the use of cocaine among all three populations surveyed—high school seniors, young adults through age 29, and college students. There was also a significant decline in the use of other drugs; marijuana use among seniors fell to its lowest annual level since 1975; and use of stimulants, especially amphetamines, signficantly declined among all three populations (Johnston, Bachman, and O'Malley, 1988, pp. 5-6). These trends continued in 1988 and it was found that the number of seniors who had had one or more alcoholic drinks in the most recent 30 days declined significantly. One of the most important findings of the 1988 Monitoring the Future Survey was a decline in the use of crack cocaine among high school seniors (Gallagher, 1989, p. 3).

In spite of a recent decline in drug use by American youth, substance abuse continues to warrant considerable attention by public health professionals. Overall, drug use among high school students and young adults remains widespread. A staggering 60 percent of today's young adults have tried an illicit drug other than marijuana by their mid-20s. Our youth's level of involvement with illicit drugs is greater than that found in youth in any other industrialized nation. Heavy consumption of alcohol is also widespread (Johnston, Bachman, and O'Malley, 1988, p. 14). Of grave concern is the high percentage of young people who are cigarette smokers. Although the rate at which smoking begins has stabilized since 1984, a sizable number of youth smoke (Gallagher, 1989, p. 5).

Although there are regional and population density differences in the use of illicit drugs among our youth, no community is free of illegal drug use by this group (Johnston, Bachman, and O'Malley, 1988). As with other major health problems, it is important for health professionals to survey the extent of the problem in their local community. Hahn (1982) found, when conducting such a survey to determine the extent of alcohol and marijuana use among urban and rural seventh, ninth, tenth, and twelfth grade students, that the differences between urban and rural drug use were not as great in the population he surveyed as had been previously presented in other studies. Johnson, Backman, and O'Malley (1988, p. 44) had findings similar to Hahn's. These researchers found that overall illicit drug use is highest in the largest metropolitan areas and lowest in the rural areas, but that the differences across three different sizes of community were small. They concluded from their survey that illicit drug use has spread throughout the population.

Multiple factors contribute to illegal drug use among our youth. One key variable is availability. The more widely used drugs are those reported to be most available. Other significant variables are peer influence, community norms, personality factors such as low self-esteem, family dysfunction, lack of supervision, and child maltreatment (Goodstadt, 1989; Johnston, Bachman, and O'Malley, 1988; U.S. Congress, Office of Technology Assessment, 1988; Young, Werch, and Bakema, 1989). Children may resort to taking drugs to escape poor home environments and unhappy social situations and to mask such feelings as sadness, boredom, hopelessness, fear, and anger. Children from homes where there is a lack of affection and discipline need extra attention and support from adults so that their psychosocial developmental needs will be met through supportive relationships rather than through drug use.

Data suggest an urgent need for health care professionals to focus attention on the drug problem among our youth. Multiple health interventions are essential to successfully prevent and resolve drug abuse. Drug abuse prevention programs have traditionally employed one or both of two strategies: educational or social control through policy, and regulation or legislation (Goodstadt, 1989, p. 247). Goodstadt (1989), after reviewing the research and theory related to these strategies, promotes the joint development and implementation of educational and policy strategies to combat drug abuse in school settings. To be effective, a drug prevention program must have support from the school, family, peers, and community.

In order to provide the type of support needed

by youth who use illegal drugs, community health nurses must have an understanding of the dynamics associated with drug use as well as knowledge about the developmental characteristics of this age group. Having knowledge about effective drug prevention strategies is also essential. Professionals who specialize in working with clients who are drug abusers are valuable resource persons and should be consulted when one is having difficulty handling drug problems.

For the youth, parent, or professional interested in obtaining drug abuse information, several national hotlines are available. The National Cocaine Hotline (1-800-COCAINE) answers questions on the health risks of cocaine and provides referral services. The National Federation of Parents for Drug-Free Youth (1-800-554-KIDS) provides referrals for parents of children with drug and alcohol problems. The National Parents' Resource Institute for Drug Education (PRIDE: 1-800-241-7946) provides a broad range of educational and professional materials on drug-related issues and will refer families to appropriate organizations. The National Institute on Drug Abuse (NIDA) hotline (1-800-662-HELP) provides general information on drug abuse and AIDS (as it relates to intravenous drug users) and offers referrals to drug rehabilitation centers. The Target Resource Center (1-800-366-6667) is a service of the National Federation of State High School Associations, and provides information on school programs, publications, videotapes, and other drug education materials. It also makes referrals to organizations for alcohol and drug abuse information.

DEVELOPMENTAL TASKS OF SCHOOL-AGE CHILDREN

Stuffed rabbit
Seven years my nocturnal security
Now neglected worn and eyeless
Lying in the memory-choked attic
Stabbed by blunt dusty shafts of sunlight
Recalling to me
Evenings of forbidden play beneath giggle-muffling
　blankets
Recalling to me the day that I grew

Too big
Too old
To sleep with innocence while hugging security.
　I'll leave you here stuffed rabbit,
　You're dead
But God, what a long slow funeral we're having!

Gregory Smith, written at age 18

All school-age children must accomplish certain developmental tasks to achieve happiness and self-fulfillment. The author of "Stuffed Rabbit," above, was describing the overall task of adolescence: "relinquishing a child's life-style and attaining an adult life-style" (Nicholson, 1980, p. 11). He was giving up secure patterns of behavior to achieve emotional independence.

Social scientists such as Erikson, Havighurst, Freud, Piaget, and Sullivan have provided professionals with a variety of ways in which to explain human development. The manner and sequence of growth and development are universal and predictable features of childhood. However, children's behavioral responses do vary and are influenced by the culture and environment in which they live (Whaley and Wong, 1987).

To work effectively with all age groups, community health nurses must have knowledge of normal growth and development processes. They must also understand how these processes are influenced by psychosocial factors and how they affect families as well as individuals. As children, for example, become increasingly independent of parents and seek support and advice from others (peers, teachers, significant adults outside the home), parents can experience a great deal of anxiety. During these times they may need reassurance that they are not "losing" their children and an opportunity to express feelings of frustration and fear of failing as a parent. Supportive intervention can help parents to cope successfully with stresses associated with normal growth and development.

When working with children, it is critical for all health care professionals to observe for lags in normal growth and development. Early case finding and intervention can prevent permanent disability. A comprehensive biopsychosocial and cultural assessment should be done with every child and family when the child is not performing at the appropriate developmental age level. Chapters 6 and 13 present tools for facilitating this assessment. Intervention should be started immediately if a developmental disability is confirmed (refer to Figure 14-9).

Developmental Disabilities

Developmental disabilities are increasingly identified among school-age children and present significant stresses to those affected. Although estimates of the number of children handicapped by developmental disabilities vary significantly, it is known that several million children and their families are dealing with this problem. A diagnosis of a handicapping condition constitutes a crisis for a family and may require multiple adjustments in their lifestyle. Community health nurses frequently assume a significant role in promoting physical and psychosocial well-being among families by addressing the issues related to developmental disabilities.

As of 1978, the definition of developmental disabilities is found in Public Law 95-602 (Comprehensive Rehabilitation Service Amendments of 1978) and reads as follows:

"Developmental disability" means a severe, chronic disability of a person which—

a) Is attributable to a mental or physical impairment or a combination of mental and physical impairments;
b) Is manifested before the person attains age 22;
c) Is likely to continue indefinitely;
d) Results in substantial functional limitations in three or more of the following areas of major life activity;
  i. Self-care
  ii. Receptive and expressive language
  iii. Learning
  iv. Mobility
  v. Self-direction
  vi. Capacity for independent living, and
  vii. Economic sufficiency; and
e) Reflects the person's need for a combination and sequence of special, interdisciplinary, or generic care, treatment, or other services which are of lifelong or extended duration and are individually planned and coordinated.

The major life activity for preschool children is play and for school-age children is learning or school (Collins, 1986, p. 55). In 1987, more than 3 million of all children 1 through 19 years of age were limited in their usual activities because of chronic illnesses and impairments (USDHHS, Office of Maternal and Child Health, 1989, p. 46). Problems such as mental retardation, "learning disabilities," cerebral palsy, epilepsy, blindness, autism, and other emotional difficulties, speech and hearing impairments, and orthopedic difficulties can affect learning abilities. Environmental factors can also influence a child's progress along the growth and development continuum.

As with average children, the degree to which children with developmental disabilities adjust successfully as healthy individuals varies. The nature and quality of their previous and current life experiences and their physical, emotional, and cognitive status greatly influence how well children with developmental disabilities progress. Typically, these children have different life experiences from average children and these differences are weighted in a negative direction. Clinical experience reveals that often children with developmental disabilities have deficient socializing experiences, both in quantity and quality, during childhood (Clemen and Pattullo, 1980, p. 197).

Numerous variables affect the socioadaptive capacity of children with developmental disabilities. The interdependence of these variables is graphically shown in Figure 14-5. An overwhelming number of the factors are influenced by environmental conditions. Few of them are inherent in the child, immutable to change (Clemen and Pattullo, 1980, p. 226).

In spite of the passage on November 29, 1975, of Public Law 94-142, Education for All Handicapped Children Act, there are still many children who are not receiving the services they need to develop to their fullest potential. It is extremely important for health professionals to focus attention on case finding when working with school-age children so that developmental disabilities are identified early. It is also important for health professionals to assume an advocacy role when they

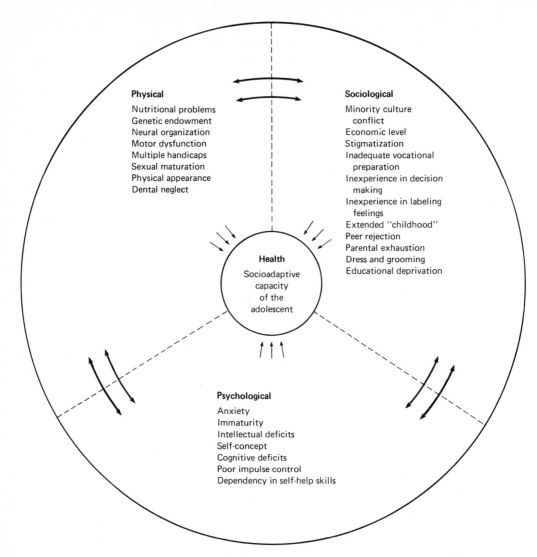

Figure 14-5   Factors influencing the health and socioadaptive capacity of the adolescent with mental retardation. (Adapted from Figure 12, Concept of multiple causation in mental retardation. In Gerrard SB: Mental retardation in adolescence, Pediatr Clin North Am 7(1):150, 1960; and Clemen S and Pattullo A: The adolescent with mental retardation. In Howe J, ed: Nursing care of the adolescent, New York, 1980, McGraw-Hill, p 226.)

identify that children with handicapping conditions are not receiving the health services they need. Parents should be assisted in obtaining necessary resources and should be informed of their rights, including the mandates of Public Law 94-142. The National Information System for Health Related Services (NIS) helps families who have developmentally disabled and chronically ill chil-dren up to age 12 to obtain needed services. This organization makes referrals to support groups and sources of financial, medical, and legal assistance and can be reached at 1-800-922-9234 or 1-800-922-1107 (South Carolina).

Public Law 94-142 mandates that every school system receiving special federal educational funds must provide a "free, appropriate education for all handicapped children between the ages of six and eighteen, regardless of the type of handicap or the degree of impairment." It also provides incentive monies to extend services to children beginning at age 3 and for young adults between 18 through 21. Public Law 99-457, passed in September, 1986 made some significant changes to Public Law 94-142. This law created a new Preschool Grant Program which mandates that children beginning at the age of 3 have the "right to education." It also created a new Handicapped Infants and Toddlers Program which dispenses incentive monies to provide educational services for handicapped and at-risk infant and toddlers. Public Law 99-457 is discussed more extensively in Chapter 13.

Under Public Law 94-142 school systems which do not have appropriate diagnostic and therapeutic facilities and personnel are legally bound to purchase whatever is required. In addition to full educational opportunities, the other rights covered by this law are as follows:

1. Due process safeguards which assist parents in challenging decisions regarding their children
2. Education in the mainstream to the fullest extent possible
3. Assurance that tests and other evaluation materials do not reflect cultural or racial bias
4. A "child-find" plan to identify all children within the state who have special needs

Many states have been more progressive than the federal government in planning services for handicapped children and have mandated services for a wider age range (e.g., birth to 25 years). The Developmental Disabilities Assistance and Bill of Rights Act (Public Law 95-602) and subsequent amendments to this act have assisted states in expanding services to persons with developmental disabilities in the 1980s. This act ensures availability of funds to help states provide comprehensive services to persons whose needs cannot be met under the Education for All Handicapped Children Act, the Rehabilitation Act of 1973, or other health, education, or welfare programs (Michigan State Planning Council for De-

velopmental Disabilities, 1983). A more extensive discussion of this legislative act and other acts that provide services for individuals with a handicapping condition can be found in Chapter 17.

Children with developmental disabilities, like all school-age children, need organized, comprehensive community health services designed to foster optimal growth. The coordination of services between professional disciplines cannot be overemphasized. No one community system can provide the entire spectrum of services needed by the school-age population. Lack of coordination results in duplication of efforts, inefficient use of time and energies, inconsistent messages, and deficiencies in services. One community health nurse, for example, visited a family who had a newborn infant with Down's syndrome. The nurse referred the family to the intermediate school district for diagnostic and follow-up services. The physical therapist, the occupational therapist, and the psychologist from this special service division of the educational system visited the family to assess their needs. Although each of these disciplines provided a valuable service, it was difficult for the family to work with all of them. Alert intervention on the part of the community health nurse kept the family from rejecting the offered services.

Since most children attend school, the school is a logical environment in which to promote the health of all children. The components of an effective school health program will be elaborated on below. The reader should remember, however, that health services rendered in the school environment must be viewed within the context of the broader community. School health cannot be separated from the ecological and social conditions of the home and the community.

SCHOOL HEALTH PROGRAM

As early as 1850, the importance of health promotion activities in the school environment was stressed. At that time, Lemuel Shattuck (1850, pp. 178-179) wrote the following:

Every child should be taught, early in life, that, to preserve his own life and his own health and the lives and health of others, is one of his most important and constantly abiding duties. Some measure is needed which shall compel children to make a sanitary examination of themselves and their associates, and thus elicit a practical application of the lessons of sanitary science in the everyday duties of life. The recommendation now under consideration is designed to furnish this measure. It is to be carried into operation in the use of a blank schedule, which is to be printed on a letter sheet, in the form prescribed in the appendix, and furnished to the teacher of each school. He is to appoint a sanitary committee of the scholars, at the commencement of school, and, on the first day of each month, to fill it out under his superintendence. . . . Such a measure is simple, would take a few minutes each day, and cannot operate otherwise than usefully upon the children, in forming habits of exact observation, and in making a personal application of the laws of health and life to themselves. This is education of an eminently practical character, and of the highest importance.

There are several key concepts delineated in Shattuck's writings which have relevancy for current school health practices. Specifically, the following ideas extracted from Shattuck's comments are important to consider when establishing a school health program:

1. All citizens have the responsibility to preserve life and promote health in the community. In order to assume this responsibility, lay persons as well as health professionals need *knowledge* (sanitary sciences) and an opportunity to *apply* health principles in daily living situations. It is both logical and useful to help children in the school setting to learn healthy habits of functioning, because children spend a considerable amount of time in this environment.

2. "Sanitary examination" can prevent spread of communicable disease. Even though there has been a drastic reduction in the incidence of communicable conditions, school-age children are still very susceptible to these conditions because they are constantly exposed to them and are in environmental situations that support the spread of agents (see Chapter 10). Whenever a large number of individuals are confined in a limited space,

such as a school environment, the likelihood of transmission of disease from one individual to another increases. The significance of sanitary examinations in the school setting should not be underestimated. It is also important to recognize that lay persons (children, parents, and school personnel) can learn how to observe for signs and symptoms of illness. Health care professionals do not have to routinely conduct sanitary examinations. Their time can be better spent in helping others to care for themselves.

3. Health education is an appropriate function for the school system because it provides children with skills that assist them to function effectively in society and to meet their individual health care needs. Educational curricula should be designed so that learners obtain the knowledge and skills necessary to cope adequately with the demands and stresses of situations they will be encountering after leaving the educational environment. Individuals must handle health matters constantly throughout life.

4. A "sanitary committee" or health council should be used to monitor the effectiveness of the school health program. Without such a committee, it is often found that the health component of school services is neglected.

Today, comprehensive school health programs incorporate Shattuck's ideas as well as several other activities aimed at promoting healthful living. Modern school health activities are divided into three basic interrelated categories: (1) health services, (2) health education, and (3) healthy school environment. In order to provide all the services discussed under these three categories, a school system must develop mechanisms that will facilitate interdisciplinary teamwork. Interdisciplinary coordination and collaboration is the key to successful implementation of a comprehensive school health program.

Health Services

School health services are designed to protect and promote the health of all students and all school personnel. The type of health services needed in a school setting will vary from community to community, depending on the availability of other community resources and the characteristics of the population being served. Prior to developing a school health program, health professionals, school personnel, and community citizens should jointly study the needs of their community in order to identify what specific health services must be provided in the school environment. School health services should not duplicate community services already available. Rather, they should augment community services so that the comprehensive health care needs of the school-age population are met. For example, if a community has a shortage of physicians or families cannot afford preventive health examinations for their children, physical examination services may be provided in the school setting. In some school settings, however, these services may not be needed because the community has an adequate number of physicians or sufficient clinic services or because families are financially stable.

Regardless of the resources available in the community, certain basic health services should be provided in all school systems. Procedures should be established to achieve the following objectives:

1. To appraise the health status of students and school personnel on a continual basis
2. To counsel students, parents, teachers, and others regarding appraisal findings
3. To encourage health care to correct remedial defects
4. To provide emergency care for injury or sudden illness
5. To prevent and control infectious diseases
6. To identify children with handicapping conditions and to arrange for educational programs that will enhance the maximum potential of these children

To accomplish these objectives health education, health promotion, and environmental inspection activities must be integrated. Having one person in the school system responsible for coordinating this integration is essential.

Health Education

Health education is a process that helps people to make sound decisions about personal health practices and about individual, family, and community well-being. Knowledge alone does not necessarily foster appropriate health habits. In order to facilitate effective decision making in health matters, the school system should provide every child with the opportunity to acquire *knowledge* essential for understanding healthy functioning, to develop *attitudes* that foster preventive health behaviors, and to establish health *practices* conducive to effective living (Anderson, 1972, p. 223; Stone and Rubinson, 1979, pp. 45, 48). To achieve these goals, the child, the family, and the community must be involved in the educational process. This is essential because the development of sound health habits is influenced by a variety of forces including such things as societal norms, beliefs and attitudes of significant others, and the internal motivations and beliefs of the individual.

Eberst (1984, p. 102) has developed a model (Figure 14-6) that depicts the multiple factors which exert an influence on health habits. He views health as a quality of life which encompasses at least six overlapping dimensions (mental, physical, vocational, emotional, social, and spiritual) that synergistically interact. He believes that the multiple factors identified in Figure 14-6 exert an influence on each dimension of health and that school health education can exert a greater influence on some of these factors than others.

A *planned* series of *integrated* health educational activities based on input received from students, parents, community citizens, health care professionals, and educators is needed to ensure that health education will become an integral component of a school's curriculum. Informal health counseling with individual students and special health projects such as "know your heart" and "maturational processes" are valuable but can never adequately prepare children to make sound decisions about all the personal, family, and community health needs they will encounter. Special health projects usually have a narrow focus. When only this instructional modality is

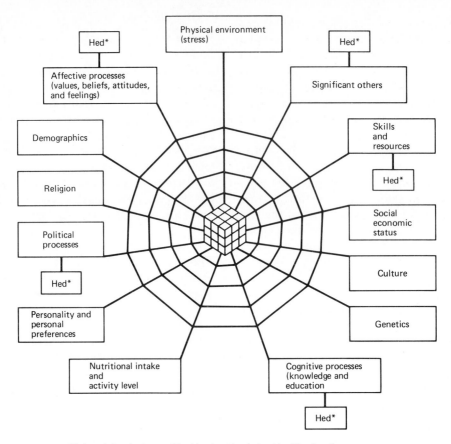

*Selected sites for input of health education (school health education,
community health education, patient education and community organization).

Figure 14-6 The "spider web" of factors exerting influence on health. (From Eberst RM: Defining health: a multidimensional model, J School Health 54:102, 1984. Copyright, 1984, American School Health Association, Kent, Ohio 44240.)

used to disseminate information about health and health-related phenomena, students become very knowledgeable about certain health needs, such as dental hygiene and nutritional requirements, but learn very little about other relevant health issues.

Unfortunately, too many school districts rely on uncoordinated, incidental methods when planning ways to handle health education in their curricula. Teachers are often requested to cover specific health topics throughout the year, but frequently they are unaware of the health content that has been presented to their students in previous years. When this happens, some concepts are repeated from one year to another and others

are not covered at all. Respondents to the 1987 National Adolescent Student Survey reported on the health instruction they received since the beginning of the seventh grade. While most had received instruction on the effects of drugs and alcohol (84 percent), nutrition and choosing healthy foods (74 percent), and how to prevent unintentional injuries (65 percent), fewer students received instruction on ways to avoid fighting and violence (43 percent); on AIDS (35 percent); on STDs (32 percent); on suicide prevention (28 percent); and on selecting health products and services (27 percent) (Centers for Disease Control, 1989, p. 148).

The School Health Education Evaluation (SHEE), conducted from 1982 through 1984, provides evidence that exposure to a school health education curriculum can result in substantial changes in health-related knowledge, practices, and attitudes, and that such changes increase with the amount of instruction. SHEE estimates that the potential impact of these changes is large and could greatly affect the nation's health. Data from the SHEE program suggest that school health education is an effective strategy for improving the health behaviors of youth (Centers for Disease Control, 1986, pp. 593, 595).

Curriculum planning for health instruction is the responsibility of all professionals in the school system. The school nurse is often asked to assume a major role in organizing health education activities. A school nurse's educational preparation and clinical experience and contact with the community puts her or him in a favorable position for understanding the essential concepts of health and illness and for coordinating activities between the school and the community. It is crucial to remember, however, that a school nurse alone cannot implement a sound health education program. Without administrative support and active involvement of all teachers, it would be impossible to achieve appropriate selection and sequencing of health content throughout the grade levels or to obtain sufficient time for health educational activities.

When planning a health education curriculum, it is beneficial to have a conceptual framework for organizing the selection and sequencing of all health education activities. Many states have developed models of comprehensive school health education that can be obtained from the department of education and/or the department of public health. These models provide a valuable framework for organizing curriculum-development activities. However, to be used effectively, teachers as well as health care professionals must understand the concepts being presented and must be prepared to adequately address them.

In addition to curriculum models, there are many excellent educational materials and audiovisual aids available to school nurses who are designing health programs for their specific school populations. Some companies, such as Lever Brothers, produce educational materials that address childhood health needs. Local and state health departments and departments of education often maintain information about where to obtain these materials.

Health educational activities in the school system should be aimed at promoting both physiological and psychosocial functioning. Students must be helped to analyze how normal growth and development progresses and to discuss their needs in relation to the maturational process. They should also be assisted in seeing how ineffective health practices can be altered and how they can prevent physical and psychosocial distress. In addition, it is important for children to learn how environmental forces affect the health status of all community citizens and to identify ways to promote healthy community functioning.

Healthy School Environment

Environmental factors that affect the health and well-being of children in the school setting are numerous. Psychosocial as well as physical aspects of the environment need to be monitored to ensure an optimal setting for student learning. A healthy school environment is one which promotes optimum psychosocial and physical growth and development among school-age children and school personnel. It provides an atmosphere which fosters sound mental health and favorable social conditions. It is organized in a way which reduces unhealthy stress and eliminates safety hazards for all students and school personnel.

A healthful school environment has the following features:

1. An architectural design which takes into consideration the developmental characteristics of the population being served and the needs of the instructional program
2. A comfortable environment that has adequate seating, lighting, heating, ventilation, toilet facilities, and drinking fountains
3. An organized safety program, including provisions for emergency care and adequate transportation

4. An established mechanism to ensure safe, sanitary conditions
5. A recreational program that allows all students to participate
6. A planned schedule of school activities which takes into account the physical and psychosocial needs of children at varying grade levels
7. An organized school lunch program which provides nutritious foods, adequate time for good personal hygiene, and sufficient facilities for comfortable eating
8. An established program that provides psychosocial counseling and consultation services for staff and students

No one professional discipline can plan and implement all the services described in the above three components—health services, health education, healthy school environment—of a total school health program. The role of nursing in the school setting is described below. The reader should keep in mind, however, that effective teamwork is essential for successful school health programming.

THE ROLE OF THE COMMUNITY HEALTH NURSE IN THE SCHOOL HEALTH PROGRAM

Since the turn of the century when Lillian Wald placed Lina Rogers, the first school nurse, in the New York City schools, the role of nursing in the school health program has been evolving. Control of communicable disease is no longer the primary focus of nursing service. It is now recognized that the school nurse has a significant contribution to make in all aspects of the total school health program. The American Nurses' Association, in 1966, identified 20 functions and 83 related activities for staff-level school nurses (ANA, 1966, pp. 4-14). These functions and activities were designed to enhance the educability of all school-age children and to improve the health of all citizens in the United States. They were developed to ensure that the ANA's philosophy of school nursing, which follows, would be implemented in the school setting.

Philosophy of School Nursing

School nursing is a highly specialized service contributing to the process of education. That it is a socially commendable, economically practical, and scientifically sound service can be well demonstrated. It must be diligently pursued through health and educational avenues to the end that positive health among all the citizenry of this country will be a reality.

The professional nurse with her experience and knowledge of the changing growth and behavioral patterns of children is in a unique position in the school setting to assist the children in acquiring health knowledge, in developing attitudes conducive to healthful living, and in meeting their needs resulting from disease, accidents, congenital defects, or psychosocial maladjustments.

Nursing provided as part of a school program for children is a direct, constructive, and effective approach to the building of a healthful and dynamic society. (ANA, 1966, p. 1. Reprinted by permission of ANA.)

School nursing is an exciting, rewarding field of nursing practice which provides numerous opportunities for creative, independent functioning. Needs of the population being served, community resources, and patterns for delivery of service influence how each of these nurses functions.

Patterns for Providing School Nursing Services

Two administrative patterns are being used to provide nursing services in the school setting: specialized and generalized. Specialized services are provided by school nurses who are employed by the board of education. These nurses are accountable to school administrators and work only with the school-age population. Some health departments are developing special school-health units within the health department. These specialized school nurses are accountable to the community health nursing director. Generalized services are provided by community health nurses hired by health departments or visiting nurse associations. These nurses function part time in the school setting as part of a generalized community health nursing program. They work with all at-risk populations in their assigned area.

There is a great deal of controversy about which pattern for delivering school nursing services is most appropriate. Clinical experience has shown both patterns can be effective. Mechanisms must be established, however, to ensure that:

- The school nurse is a sanctioned member of the school health team
- Health care for the school-age child is provided within the context of the family and the community
- The nurse serving the school-age population has an understanding of the health needs and the growth and development characteristics of the school-age child
- School health services are adequately financed by the community
- The school nurse has professional nursing supervision

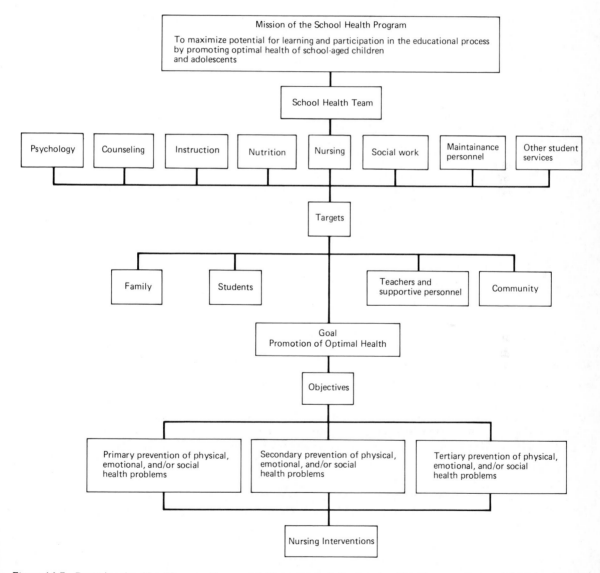

Figure 14-7   Rustia's school health promotion model. (From Rustia J: Rustia school health promotion model, J School Health 52(2):109, 1982. Copyright 1982, American School Health Association, Kent, Ohio 44240.)

The activities of generalized and specialized school nurses vary among school systems. Unfortunately, there are still many educational systems that use the nurse only to provide first aid and emergency care. A school nurse who is able to clearly articulate her or his role and functions and who demonstrates clinical expertise to all members of the school health team is more likely to be used appropriately than one who has trouble defining what it is a school nurse has to offer.

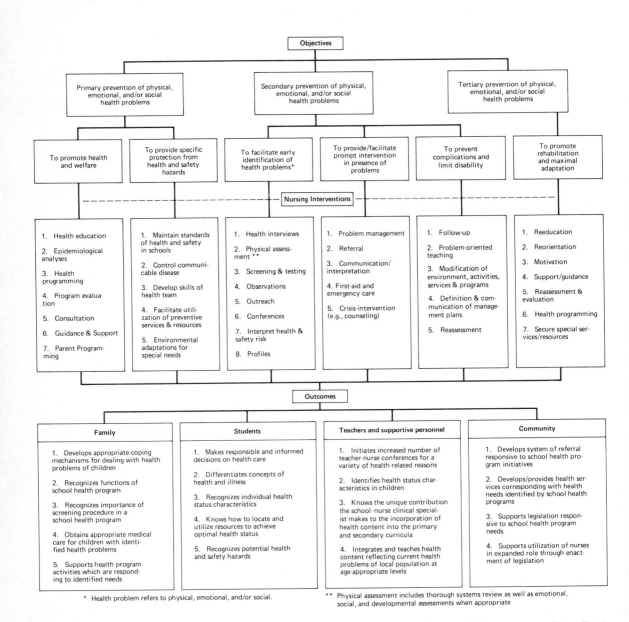

Figure 14-8 Rustia's school health promotion model: delineation of nursing interventions and client outcomes. (From Rustia J: Rustia school health promotion model, J School Health 52(2):109, 1982. Copyright 1982, American School Health Association, Kent, Ohio 44240.)

Functions of the Nurse on the School Health Team

School nurses frequently have difficulty defining what it is they have to contribute to the school health team and thus they are often used in a very narrow context. Traditionally, nurses are seen as the professionals who provide first aid, give injections, inspect for communicable disease, or counsel dirty children. In any school system, the nurse must sell what she or he has to offer by demonstrating that these traditional views of nursing are very limited and not an effective way to use a nurse's talents.

Rustia's school health promotion model (Figures 14-7, 14-8, and 14-9) clearly illustrates that nurses have multiple functions in the school setting and that these functions involve nursing interventions beyond traditional physical health care activities. Clinical experience has shown that professionals from other disciplines have a greater respect for school nurses who assume functions beyond the traditionally defined ones than for school nurses who limit their functioning to the provision of routine physical health care. Described below are the various functions a nurse should implement in the school setting.

Advocacy

There still are too many school-age children who are not receiving the health care they deserve. Outreach to assist families to more effectively enter the health care system and a reevaluation of the methods for delivering services to children are needed if this trend is to be changed. Every professional, including the school nurse, must speak out for our children.

The nurse in the school setting is in a prime position to identify children who have health needs and who need more effective health care services. The school nurse must take the initiative to help the families of these children to obtain medical, socioeconomic, and emotional counseling on a continuing basis. If services are lacking, the school nurse should become actively involved in influencing funders to allocate monies for such services. It is known, for instance, that develop-

Primary Prevention — To promote health and welfare	Secondary Prevention — To provide and/or facilitate prompt intervention in presence of health problem	Tertiary Prevention — To promote rehabilitation
1. Teacher conferences to determine special needs of teachers in working with handicapped/terminal children; provide support and guidance. Be involved in IEP development.*	1. Document student problems by direct observation techniques.	1. Identify inconsistent behaviors in teachers/staff and counsel accordingly.
2. Frequent parent/teacher/nurse conferences to assure consistency between home/school in management of behavior and learning, goal setting.	2. Consult with physician and render appropriate primary care, e.g., postural drainage programs.	2. Interpret physician and special therapy instructions.
3. Assess and record developmental progress and revise individual education plan accordingly.	3. Refer to school or other resources for additional psychoeducational testing and evaluation.	3. Coordinate services to assist families in their psychological adjustment to a chronically ill child and assess family coping periodically.
	4. Counsel directly with child and family about problems, feelings, behavior, etc.	4. Plan classroom and building adaptations to maximize ability to function.
	5. Participate on committees for admission, review, or dismissal of handicapped students in Special Education.	5. Assess home environment, identify needs, and suggest modifications.

* IEP = Individual education plan

Figure 14-9 Rustia's school health promotion model: selected nursing interventions for children and adolescents with handicapping conditions. (From Rustia J: Rustia school health promotion model, J School Health 52(2):109, 1982. Copyright, 1982, American School Health Association, Kent, Ohio 44240.)

mentally the adolescent has different needs from younger school-age children. Often, however, community services that specifically address the needs of the adolescent are lacking or inadequate. A concerned school nurse will have knowledge about the factors that affect an adolescent's use of health care and will take action to promote the development of programs designed to meet the unique needs of this developmental age group.

The school nurse should be an advocate for needed health services within the school system as well as within the community. It is not uncommon for the school nurse to identify environmental conditions that are unsafe, or gaps in health education programs, or deficiencies in the delivery of personal health services. These situations must not be ignored by the school nurse because they may prevent children from reaching their maximum potential.

In order for the school nurse to successfully carry out the advocacy function in the school setting, the legal issues involved in delivering care to children must be understood. The nurse must also be knowledgeable about legislative programs that finance health care services for our youth.

Since laws and health services vary from one state to another, every nurse functioning in the school setting should become familiar with those that exist in his or her state (Knecht, 1981, p. 606). There are, however, some basic issues which all nurses must deal with when working with school-age children. Specifically, issues related to parental consent for the health care of minors, confidentiality in relation to the health record, laws requiring the reporting of child abuse and neglect, and legislation which mandates that children with special needs have equal educational opportunities should be examined carefully.

School-age children are minors. Parental consent is generally necessary for minors to receive health care treatment for such things as immunizations, medical treatment by a physician, and special psychological testing for learning difficulties. Children may be treated by a physician in any emergency situation without parental consent. Since, however, it is very difficult to establish what constitutes an emergency, every school

should develop policies that deal with emergency situations. An emergency consent form which includes the following information should be on file for each child:

- Child's full name, address, and telephone number
- Where to reach the parents during school hours
- Whom to call if the parents cannot be reached
- The name, address, and telephone number of the child's family physician
- The family's preference for hospital care
- Insurance or Medicaid numbers
- Any known allergies or chronic health problems of the child
- Parent's consent for ambulance transportation

In addition to the emergency form, every school should have a teacher who is designated as the school's primary first-aid person. This is crucial because the school nurse is often responsible for serving many school buildings and thus is frequently not available when emergencies occur. The permanent staff member assigned the responsibility for handling emergency first aid should take refresher first-aid courses as needed.

The parental consent regulations were designed to protect the rights of minors. It is increasingly recognized that children, especially adolescents, have not had access to certain health care services because they could not or would not obtain parental consent. Thus, many states have changed their laws so that minors who are emancipated or sufficiently mature to understand the consequences of their decision can obtain certain types of health care treatment without parental consent. Age stipulations for when minors can seek help on their own vary from state to state.

Laws that allow minors to seek medical treatment without parental consent usually deal with human sexuality problems, drug abuse, and mental health services. Every state now allows minors to receive medical treatment for STDs on their own. Several states permit physicians to diagnose pregnancy and to provide prenatal care for minors without parental knowledge. Confidential contraceptive services are available to minors in many states. Only a few states, however, have laws which stipulate that minors can obtain assistance for drug abuse or mental health problems without parental consent (Hoekelman, Blatman, Brunell, Friedman, and Seidel, 1978, pp. 526-527).

Health laws and educational laws are not necessarily the same. Youth, for instance, may receive health education relative to contraceptive practices in a medical clinic but may not be allowed to receive this same information in the educational setting. Professionals providing health care services must learn how both health and educational laws influence their practice in a particular state. Health care professionals should be advocates for change if these laws do not agree with their philosophy of professional practice.

Confidentiality regarding a client's health record is a legal issue that concerns every health care provider in the school system. Indiscriminate sharing of school records has resulted in the passage of the Family Privacy and Education Act of 1974. This act mandates that "parents of students under 18 years of age, attending educational institutions receiving federal funds, may view their child's educational records on request and may seek expungement or correction of false or inaccurate entries. No information can be released outside of the school setting without proper parental authorization. This right devolves on students themselves once they become 18" (Hofmann, 1978, p. 531). Generalized school nurses are technically not official members of the school system, which could present a problem when they need to use the school records. Some school systems have coped with this dilemma by adopting a policy which makes the generalized school nurse an official member of the school staff.

Besides the Family Privacy and Education Act of 1974, there are several other pieces of federal legislation that influence the delivery of health care services to the school-age population. Most of these have already been described in Chapter 13 or other sections of this chapter: Medicaid, EPSDT, maternal child health, family planning, dental health, crippled children and child support laws, and the McKinney Homeless Assistance Act

all ensure funding for essential child health or health-related services. Legislation related to child nutrition programs (National School Lunch Programs, School Breakfast Program, Child Care Food Program, Summer Food Service Program, Special Milk Program, Supplemental Food Program for Women, Infants, and Children, and Commodity Supplemental Food Programs) is currently and has historically provided funds for child health services. The National School Lunch Program is the oldest and largest of the child nutrition programs. It was started in the 1930s to safeguard the health and well-being of American children and to encourage the consumption of nutritious foods. Most of the other child nutrition programs were initiated in the 1960s after passage of the Child Nutrition Act of 1966. The Omnibus Reconciliation Act of 1980, Public Law 96-499, included many changes in the child nutrition programs. These changes and the legislative history of child nutrition programs are summarized in the document *Child Nutrition Programs: Description, History, Issues, and Options* prepared by the Committee on Agriculture, Nutrition, and Forestry (1983). Frequently, youth who should be benefitting from child nutrition programs are not. A concerned school nurse should work to alter this situation if it exists in the school system in which she or he is functioning. By helping others to see the correlation between poor nutrition and illness, the community health nurse may influence people in power to support a process that facilitates rather than hinders use of federal school-lunch monies.

The Child Abuse Prevention, Adoption and Family Service Act, the Education for All Handicapped Children Act, the School Age Mother and Child Acts, and the Adolescent Family Life Bill, all of which were previously discussed, were passed to protect the rights of high-risk children. School personnel must report suspected abuse or neglect to the legal authorities. They must also provide educational services for all handicapped children and pregnant mothers if they desire to remain in school.

The Adoption Assistance and Child Welfare Act of 1980 (Public Law 96-272) was also passed to protect the rights of high-risk children. This piece of legislation is considered to be one of the most significant welfare bills of the past two decades. It was designed to encourage permanent placement of children, either with their natural families or through adoption, and to discourage foster care arrangements. It is hoped that through this legislation, children will no longer be allowed to drift in the legal system, being shifted from one foster home or institution to another. Public Law 96-272 is particularly significant for hard-to-place children. In the past, too many of these children never experienced a stable family life, because some families who were interested in adopting them could not afford to do so. Many hard-to-place children have special needs which require financial expenditures which a normal family budget cannot handle. Now, families can adopt special children and obtain federal assistance to help them pay for these expenses. In addition, services are available for children, especially adolescents, who cannot remain in their homes or live in a foster care setting (Calhoun, 1980, p. 2). Children who are hard to place are more likely to be found, because Public Law 96-272 requires states to conduct an inventory on such children.

State as well as federal legislation is written to promote and protect the health of school-age children. Compulsory school attendance acts, immunization requirements before school entry, legislation on health education in the school system, and laws that exclude ill children are some examples of state legislation that assist children to reach their optimal health status. One national health action, the enactment of the National Childhood Immunization Initiative of 1977, is assisting states to better enforce their immunization requirements. The National Childhood Vaccine Injury Act of 1988 promotes permanent access to immunization records and prevention of complications from certain vaccines and toxoids. This act requires that health care providers permanently record vaccinations and mandates the reporting of selected events after vaccination related to side effects from specific vaccines and toxoids (Centers for Disease Control, 1988, National Childhood Vaccine).

A knowledge of federal and state laws helps school nurses to speak out on behalf of children when services are not being provided. Laws also provide legal backing for encouraging parents to assume responsibility for acting in the best interest of their children. In addition, laws require health professionals to carry out an advocacy function when they identify that the rights of children are being abused.

Casefinding

"Every child has a right to have an education which will meet his individualized needs and to have care and treatment for handicapping conditions so that he can learn more effectively" (1930 Children's Charter). Casefinding is essential if these goals are to be accomplished. All personnel in the school system have a responsibility to identify as early as possible children at risk for physical, behavioral, social, or academic disabilities.

The school nurse uses a variety of methods for identifying at-risk children. Observing their appearance and behavior during their daily school activities is one way to quickly discern which students need more extensive follow-up. Many orthopedic problems, for example, have been picked up by an alert school nurse who has watched children in the school setting walk down the hall during recess. Eating lunch in the school cafeteria has helped other school nurses to identify children with poor dietary habits. Walking out on the playground during recess frequently assists school nurses in determining which children are having difficulty relating with their peers.

Incidental observations like those mentioned above are extremely valuable, but they do not replace the need for periodic, systematic health observations. The school nurse should meet with every teacher in the school system to encourage them to observe on a regular basis the health status of all students in the classroom. Teachers are the key persons in a health appraisal program. Their position in the classroom setting provides them with frequent opportunities to make significant observations of each child's health status. The school nurse can help to enhance a teacher's observational skills by discussing signs and symptoms of illness, by developing teacher health observational forms, and by responding to teachers' concerns about a particular child's health. In-service programs for all teachers in the school system can also sharpen teachers' observational skills. One school nurse, for instance, noted a significant increase in the number of student referrals from teachers after she showed the film *Looking at Children* to the faculty in one of her elementary schools. This film was developed by Metropolitan Life Insurance Company for the purpose of promoting improved observations of children by teachers. There is no rental charge for its use and a supplementary reference pamphlet, *Looking for Health,* is also provided at no cost by Metropolitan Life. Many local and state health departments have these Metropolitan Life materials available for loan to local school districts.

Teachers' concerns should be taken seriously, because they observe children daily and they are likely to identify abnormal behaviors more quickly than any other member of the school health team. The authors' clinical experiences have dramatically supported this statement. One of the authors, for example, received a referral from a kindergarten teacher because a pupil in her classroom looked anemic. The teacher was also concerned because it took this child longer than most children to get up after a fall on the playground. The child was seen by his family physician and found to have a congenital heart defect, a condition that had never been diagnosed before even though the child had been seen regularly by medical personnel.

Planned comprehensive screening sessions are another way to systematically observe a child's health status. School nurses should see that such programs are developed, but they do not necessarily need to conduct all screening tests themselves. Hearing and vision technicians, school aides, teachers, social workers, nutritionists, and all other members of the health team can play a vital role in a screening program. Height and weight measurements, hearing and vision tests, dental examinations, and immunization checks have traditionally been conducted in the school settings. In many school settings, a more comprehensive screening is being done to identify children at risk. In addition to the traditional procedures, screening for scoliosis, urinary tract infections, anemia, and psychosocial difficulties is being done. Identifying the characteristics of the population being served will help the community health nurse to determine what type of screening program to initiate in the school setting in which she or he is working. Remember, when analyzing population data, that children from all socioeconomic backgrounds have health problems which may not be obvious to them or their families. One middle-class mother was very appreciative of the school's vision screening program after her 6-year-old daughter was found to have serious visual difficulties. The mother reported to the school nurse after her daughter obtained glasses that for the first time her daughter was able to see leaves on the trees. Without glasses, this 6-year-old child could see only large masses in her environment. Her mother felt distraught that her daughter's eye problem had not been detected sooner.

Screening programs have identified many students in the school setting who have health problems. It is a waste of time and money to screen for defects, however, if follow-up health activities are neglected. Follow-up is a school nurse's most important function in a screening program. The school nurse can direct families to appropriate agencies for diagnostic, treatment, and rehabilitation services and can find funds for these services if necessary. The Lions' Club, for instance, frequently provides funds for glasses when the client is of school age.

Contact with students in the health clinic as well as reviewing of school records are other methods school nurses use to identify high-risk children. The school nurse should be alert to problems other than the stated concern when a child visits the health clinic. Orthopedic, visual, dental, and relationship difficulties are often identified while the nurse is putting on an adhesive bandage or comforting a crying child. Previously, in this chapter, the problems of teenage parents were discussed. Too often the needs of the father are neglected. When a pregnant, unwed teenage mother visits the health clinic, the school nurse should not forget that there is another person involved in this girl's situation: single teenage fathers do need help. The school nurse can frequently help a teenage father by discussing with the mother the feelings that he might be experiencing and the services available to him for verbalizing his concerns. The nurse can also meet with the father in the clinic or home setting to identify what type of assistance he needs or can provide. The Teen Father Collaboration project (Sander and Rosen, 1987) has demonstrated that some teenage fathers are interested in contributing to the well-being of their children and take advantage of social services available to them (Sander and Rosen, 1987).

Record reviews help the school nurse to discern those children who should be contacted in the school setting or families that should be visited in the home. Frequently school nurses identify significant health problems that should be discussed with both school personnel and families when they examine school entry physicals. One school nurse, for example, noted that a kindergarten child's blood pressure was extremely high. Follow-up revealed several interesting facts: (1) the physician thought that this child's blood pressure was elevated because he was anxious about seeing a physician; (2) the child's father had hypertension; and (3) the teacher had noted that the child's ears turned bright red with physical exertion. This child was indeed hypertensive and was placed under the care of a cardiac specialist, because the school nurse took the time to review health records and did not ignore health problems identified during this review.

Review of absenteeism records, along with health records, is another way of identifying high-risk children. Studies have shown that students who are frequently absent from school have a high prevalence of health problems and are at risk for future illnesses and absenteeism. Preventive intervention services may help families as well as children when a nurse intervenes with children at risk for high absenteeism. Helping families is probably the best way to help their children. Referring them to community resources, for in-

stance, may help these families to meet their basic human needs for clothing, shelter, and food, and could reduce the number of illnesses experienced by their children.

High-risk children are present in any school system. When school nurses discover that they are spending all of their time providing first-aid services, they should carefully evaluate their nursing practice. School nurses must regularly determine if steps have been taken to identify children in need. Sitting in the health clinic is not an effective way of delivering nursing services in the school setting.

Community Liaison Activities

Some of the most important factors that the school nurse must consider when working with school-age children are the beliefs, values, and resources of the community where these children reside. The health status of individuals is greatly affected by the beliefs and values which exist in the home and the community and by health resources which are available to meet their needs. The interrelationship among all of these variables cannot be ignored when health programs are being planned to resolve problems encountered by the school-age population. The problems of STDs and teenage pregnancies, for example, can be dealt with in the school setting only when the values and beliefs present in the home and the community allow this to happen.

School nurses have more opportunities than other school personnel to unite all of these variables. They have the freedom and flexibility to visit families in their homes and to coordinate services between the home, the school, and other community agencies. Viewing the health status of children at school often provides school nurses with data necessary for identifying health priorities and needs in the community. Health needs of school-age children tend to reflect needs of the community in general. When children lack dental care, for instance, this is frequently so because there are limited community services to meet their dental needs.

School nurses must engage in community liaison activities in order to meet the needs of all school-age children. No school system has adequate resources to handle all the health problems experienced by the children it serves. Cooperative planning and collaboration between the educational system and other community agencies who are assisting children can serve only to enhance the effectiveness of the school's health program.

Community involvement should be sought by the school nurse during all stages of the health-planning process. Health programs conducted at school which fulfill health needs as identified by the community are far more successful than programs that ignore community priorities. Perceptions of health problems differ from community to community. Thus, it is important for community health nurses working in the school setting to ascertain from their consumers what constitutes the communities' most pressing health problems.

Community liaison activities can be challenging and rewarding for several reasons. Working with others in parent-teacher organizations or community agencies can strengthen the school health program. This, in turn, can increase a nurse's satisfaction because children who need help are receiving it. Community liaison activities also expose school nurses to different viewpoints, which help nurses to expand their range of alternative solutions for health problems. In addition, these activities enhance creative thinking through stimulation by others, facilitate continuity of care, and increase community participation in health programming. Community interest groups are more motivated to implement a health program if they have participated in designing that health program. School nurses, through their involvement with groups, can gain a greater appreciation of community issues, demands, and needs.

Consultation

Nurses bring to the school setting a unique set of skills which allow them to become valuable, contributing members of the school health team. Specifically, there are three major areas where nursing differs from other disciplines in the school setting. First, nurses have been prepared to assess comprehensively all the variables which have an influence on a child's health status. Nurses' understanding of normal growth and development, as well as disease processes, provides them with the knowledge needed for identifying both physical and psychosocial health problems and for determining how to handle health concerns. Teachers frequently ask school nurses questions about disease conditions such as diabetes, epilepsy, hepatitis, or scabies. They may question if a child is ill, when to send a child home when he or she is not feeling well, or whether a child with a chronic condition should be allowed to participate in recreational activities. Children with heart problems or other chronic conditions are frequently overprotected by school personnel until medical recommendations are interpreted by the nurse. It is also not uncommon for the school nurse to encounter fear when infectious diseases are present in the school system and school personnel do not understand the etiology of communicable diseases or how to prevent the spread of these diseases. One teacher, for example, became so upset after she heard that one of her students had hepatitis that she moved the child's desk into the hall and immediately called the school nurse. She wanted the nurse to talk with her class about "what to do when they got hepatitis." The teacher was sure that everyone in the classroom would become ill, because all she knew about this condition was that it was contagious. Her anxiety was reduced once the nurse explained the etiology and the mode of transmission of this disease process and the treatment needs of the ill child. Appendix 10-2 summarizes some of the common communicable diseases encountered by community health nurses in the school settings.

The nurse's preparation for dealing with the family as the unit of service is a second major area of uniqueness. Family problems may affect a child's functioning in the school setting and often problems of all family members need to be addressed before a child's functioning in school changes. Problem behavior such as poor school attendance, aggressive behavior, use of drugs, or withdrawal from school activities often signals that a child's family is having difficulty. The adolescent depicted in the following case situation had a high absenteeism record until the school nurse helped her mother to obtain medical care for herself.

Pattie Lynne Babcock was a 14-year-old junior high school student who was missing an average of 2 days of school per week when the school social worker referred her to the generalized school nurse. Even though Pattie only had a functional heart murmur, her mother would relate any illness she had to her "bad heart." The school social worker felt that Pattie Lynne's mother needed help with understanding how her fears were affecting Pattie Lynne's perceptions of her health. Mrs. Babcock was very receptive to the nurse's visit. She had been widowed recently and wasn't sure how "to care for Pattie Lynne properly." During the nurse's first home visit, Mrs. Babcock related that she hadn't been feeling well lately. Her heart pounded so fast at times that she feared she might have a heart attack. She had trouble with her vision but felt it was because she was getting old. Mrs. Babcock had a history of hypertension but had stopped taking "her blood pressure medication because it made her feel worse." The nurse found her blood pressure to be 210/116 and stressed the need for immediate medical follow-up. Mrs. Babcock reluctantly made an appointment with her family physician while the nurse was in the home. She felt she had too many other things to take care of to worry about herself. Utilizing crisis intervention principles, the school nurse in this situation helped Mrs. Babcock to identify what it was she had to handle and then encouraged her to work on one thing at a time. The nurse's promise to return motivated Mrs. Babcock to seek medical care. During the nurse's second visit the following week, Mrs. Babcock reported that she was feeling better physically and was also able to verbalize that she thought she was going to die. She could identify that when she was afraid, "it was nice to have Pattie Lynne home with me." She also saw how her fear of having a heart attack altered her perceptions of Pattie Lynne's heart murmur. The school nurse continued to make home visits until Mrs. Babcock developed mechanisms to cope with the changes in her life. Like all school-age children, Pattie Lynne continued to miss a day of school periodically. Her attendance record improved dramatically, however, once the nurse assisted Mrs. Babcock in dealing with her problems.

Extensive knowledge of community resources and the referral process is the third unique skill the school nurse has to contribute in the school setting. There are many families within school systems who do not have a regular source of medical supervision. Other families have their own physician and dentist but cannot afford to use these services. One student community health nurse came back to the health department disturbed following her second visit to an inner-city junior high school. She was appalled at the number of children who had obvious dental caries and questioned why their parents did not care enough about them to obtain dental care. A staff nurse suggested to her that limited financial resources might be preventing many of these families from obtaining the dental supervision they needed. When the student contacted the parents of these children, she found that in fact this was the case. After she discussed the services available at the health department dental clinic, two families requested that all of their children be referred to this resource. School personnel were appreciative of these referrals and identified several other children who needed dental assistance.

Parents and school personnel do *care.* If school nurses demonstrate that they are willing to use the unique skills they have, both families and other members of the school health team will confer with them regularly. The opportunities are endless. School nurses who reflect a genuine interest in the welfare of children and their families, a nonthreatening, accepting attitude toward other professionals seeking advice, and competency in decision making based on sound scientific principles are more likely to be used effectively than school nurses who do not demonstrate these characteristics.

Epidemiological Investigation

Health services in a school setting should be designed to meet the needs of the total school population. Health counseling and instruction with individual students reaches only the tip of the iceberg in a given population. Nurses must use the epidemiological process to identify *groups at risk* and to plan and implement scientific health programming.

Effective school nurses organize the data they have to identify factors that influence the health status of school-age populations. The characteristics of populations are studied in order to determine the most appropriate intervention strategies to meet their needs. One school nurse utilized health records, data obtained during home visits, contact with students in the health clinic, and census tract information to substantiate the need for a breakfast program in the school system. These data revealed several significant facts. Children frequently came into the health clinic complaining of a stomach ache because they had not eaten breakfast. Fifty-five percent of the children came from one-parent homes where the income was minimal. Of the 167 children enrolled in this elementary school, 110 qualified for a free lunch program. During home visits, the school nurse made numerous community referrals because families did not have adequate financial resources to meet their basic needs. In addition, several children from this school district, who were screened through the Medicaid EPDST program at the health department, had been diagnosed as having nutritional anemia. All of these data were organized and shared with the school principal. Seeing the hard facts, he agreed with the nurse that federal funds should be sought to support a breakfast program in order to improve the nutritional status of students in the school district.

An epidemiological approach to school health is a prevention-oriented approach. In the above situation, the nurse worked to prevent nutritional problems such as anemia and to prevent learning difficulties in the future; children who are ill often do not learn well. Prevention is far less costly than treatment.

There are numerous situations in the school setting that require primary preventive intervention. Accidents, for example, are the leading cause of death in the school-age population. Astute school nurses may be able to identify factors that cause accidents in the school setting by analyzing their health records and by observing their school environments. Identifying commonalities among those children who receive care for accidents can result in eliminating environmental factors that increase the potential for hazardous accidents. Debris in the playground, unsupervised play, and playground equipment inappropriate to the developmental age level of children are some such factors which may need to be changed in the school setting to reduce frequent accidents.

Accurate and complete record keeping is essential if epidemiological studies are to be effective. Too often, nursing services are not well documented and it is impossible to retrieve data about what was done by the school nurse to solve a health problem. A record system must be designed to allow for complete and efficient recording of data. A cumulative record of each child's health status should be maintained and records of children with special health problems tagged. A tagging system allows for quick analysis of the needs of the population as a whole. If 50 children in a school system, for example, have problems with obesity, group counseling sessions and changes in curriculum planning may be warranted.

It is imperative for community health nurses in the school setting to evaluate the results of their interventions. When nurses work with aggregates, the epidemiological process is the tool that most appropriately helps them to examine the results of their group intervention strategies (refer to Chapter 10). *Until nurses begin to document what they have accomplished, they will not be used to their fullest potential.*

Health Counseling

Children and youth are currently facing difficult and complex health problems and concerns. They are exposed much earlier than their previous counterparts to such things as human sexuality issues, varying life-styles, pressures from peers to use alcohol and drugs, knowledge about health problems, decisions regarding future career planning, and family disruption and disorganization. Often they have knowledge about these issues but they do not understand how to deal with them. They have a need to discuss their feelings and emotions with a nonthreatening adult. Because the school nurse does not evaluate a student's academic performance, which helps students to view her or him as nonthreatening, and because students may have physical health complaints when experiencing emotional stress, the school nurse is frequently the first member of the school health team to identify a student's need for counseling. The school nurse should take advantage of these opportunities and assist these students in obtaining the help they need.

As in other settings, the nurse in the school utilizes the family-centered nursing process to determine appropriate management goals and intervention strategies. Too often in the school setting, however, data are hurriedly collected because other children are waiting to see the nurse. Problems are missed when this is done and intervention strategies are inappropriate to the child's needs. The case situation which follows illustrates the need to collect sufficient data to diagnose a child's actual health problems and to plan a variety of intervention strategies to resolve these problems.

Lindsey Elizabeth, a first-grader, was lying on the cot in the health clinic when the community health nurse arrived for her weekly visit. The school secretary reported to the nurse that Lindsey had just come into her office crying because she had a stomach ache. When asked by the school nurse how she was feeling, Lindsey sobbed and stated, "My stomach hurts." A physical examination revealed that no one spot hurt more than another and that with a little attention Lindsey stopped crying. When she was asked if her parents knew she did not feel well this morning, her answer was, "My mother doesn't love me anymore. She went away." The nurse helped Lindsey to verbalize her feelings of rejection and let her know that she understood how much it hurts to lose someone you love. A hug by the nurse assisted Lindsey in recognizing that others did care about her and so she was ready to go back to class that day. The nurse realized, however, that Lindsey had received only temporary relief from her distress. She had a conference with her teacher and ways to give Lindsey special attention were discussed. In addition, the nurse contacted Lindsey's father. He was very angry that his wife had left and found it extremely difficult to talk to his children about what was happening. Fortunately he was concerned about how his separation was affecting Lindsey and agreed to seek family counseling at a local mental health clinic. Lindsey's mother never did return home. Her father, however, learned how to deal with his anger and gradually was able to allow his children to talk

about their mother. This, coupled with support from an empathic teacher, helped Lindsey to function more effectively in the school setting.

Elementary school children often verbalize their feelings more readily than do older school-age children. Since one of the developmental tasks of adolescence is to achieve emotional independence from parents and other adults, students at the junior or senior high level may test the school nurse before they share their real concerns. One such case is described below:

Noel, a 14-year-old junior high student, wandered into the health clinic during class breaks 3 weeks in a row with minor physical complaints. Finally he asked the nurse if he could talk with her alone. He wanted to know "how a person could tell if he had VD." Further discussion revealed that Noel was having nocturnal emissions and thought he had gonorrhea because he had learned in a health class that a purulent discharge occurred with this disease. Noel had never heard about nocturnal emissions and was fearful that his wet discharges at night were due to gonorrhea. He was greatly relieved when he found out that he was normal. The nurse encouraged him to return to the clinic if he had other questions and suggested that his father might be able to talk with him about other developmental changes that occur during adolescence. The need to discuss normal developmental changes as well as to review how STDs are transmitted was also shared with the teacher responsible for the eighth-grade health class.

Health counseling opportunities such as the ones described above are numerous and present in all school settings. Nurses who are attuned to the developmental needs and the social characteristics of the population they are serving will not be "Band-Aid" pushers. Rather, they will take time to find out from other school personnel which students have health problems and will be alert for students who need to talk.

Health Education

The ultimate goal of nursing intervention is to help the client to help himself or herself. Through health education activities in the school setting, school nurses are preparing children and their families, school personnel, and the community to make sound health decisions. They recognize that the population they serve needs adequate knowledge as well as the opportunity to explore values and attitudes about health matters before they can assume responsibility for maintaining their personal health status.

The following examples demonstrate that the nurse in the school setting has both direct and indirect responsibilities in relation to health education. Nurses utilize the principles of teaching and learning to carry out effectively their health education responsibilities:

1. *Incidental health education with students.* A second-grader was advised to keep his hands clean to avoid infection after his nail was pulled away from the skin of the right forefinger during gym class. A 14-year-old junior high girl was helped to understand body changes during adolescence after frequent visits to the health clinic with menstrual cramps. Dental hygiene was discussed with a 10-year-old boy who had several dental caries. A tenth-grader was helped to see the relationship between her frequent headaches and her refusal to wear her glasses.

2. *Incidental health education with school personnel.* A seventh-grade teacher was advised to see his family physician after several spontaneous nose bleeds. The etiology and prevention of ringworm were discussed with a first-grade teacher when she informed the school nurse that three children were absent from school because of this condition.

3. *Incidental health education with parents.* A young mother of three children, ages 5 years, 3 years, and 1 month, was given a pamphlet on breast-feeding during a nurse-parent conference. She was breast-feeding for the first time and was late for the conference because of breast discomfort. A father of a second-grader was taught to watch for signs and symptoms of brain concussion after his son was hit on the head by a swing in the playground.

4. *Planned direct health teaching.* Child care, including such things as feeding, bathing, and dressing, was demonstrated to a group of school-age parents. Physical and emotional maturational changes were reviewed with a sixth-grade class the first time a new teacher was covering this topic with the students. What a school nurse does was discussed with first-graders. Opportunities in nursing were shared with senior high students during a career day.

5. *In-service health education.* Teachers in an elementary school were shown the film *Looking at Children* to help them identify common childhood health problems. Parents were shown the maturational films their fifth-graders were to see so that they could respond to their children's questions. A drug education workshop was conducted for junior high teachers after a sharp increase in the incidence of drug usage was noted in their school system.

6. *Curriculum planning.* Diet planning was integrated into the health class after the school nurse noted on student records that a sizable number of students had anemia or were obese. The school nurse was asked to serve on the school health committee after sharing with the school administrators several health concerns of parents she encountered while making home visits.

7. *Health instruction planning with teachers.* A resource file designed to help teachers understand common health problems was established after one school nurse received numerous requests for such information. A second-grade teacher was provided with information about dental health, was given dental models to demonstrate effective dental care, and was helped to obtain pamphlets on dental hygiene when she requested that the school nurse conduct a unit on dental care for her class. The nurse felt that the teacher knew her students better than she did and could more effectively develop teaching strategies appropriate to their needs.

The nurses in these situations all believed in the value of health education as an appropriate strategy to help clients help themselves. They involved all members of the school health team, including parents and students, so that health education would be an ongoing process, even when the nurse was not available. Health education is an essential component of any school health program. School nurses can play a very significant role in ensuring that this component is not neglected. They must, however, be careful not to assume the responsibilities of others when functioning in the school setting: health education should be *integrated* into the overall curriculum. This will never occur if the school nurse continually teaches sporadic health classes. Helping teachers to assume responsibility for health education activities is a much more beneficial approach. There may be times when a teacher is very uncomfortable with a particular topic. Demonstrating that sensitive issues can be handled effectively in the classroom setting often reduces a teacher's fears about covering this topic in the future. If, however, teachers continually ask to have the nurse present certain health topics, the need for in-service education with the teachers should be considered. It is impossible for nurses to carry out their other functions in the school setting if all their time is spent teaching in the classroom.

Home Visiting

Parents are vital members of the school health team. They are ultimately responsible for the health care of their children and they greatly influence their children's health practices. Contact with parents in the home environment is a most effective way of increasing their understanding and involvement with their child's health problems. Home visits also demonstrate that the school nurse cares about parents as individuals and respects their parental rights.

At times, home visiting is the only way to obtain a comprehensive picture of a child's health status. Family dynamics do have an impact on a child's functioning. Assessment of parent-child relationships is best obtained in the client's natural setting. Observations of how the child is physically handled, of environmental conditions, and of interactions between a child, the parents, and siblings is more easily assessed in the home environment. These observations provide a different type of data than a conference with a parent in the health clinic. Parents may not be aware of how they interact with their children so that what they verbalize may not always be what is actually occurring.

Most parents do care about their children, and they desire to do the very best they can to help them develop normally. Sometimes they do not take action when their child has a health problem because they do not understand why it is necessary to do so or know what they should do to resolve the problem. At other times, health care is not obtained because the family has multiple pressures they must deal with first. Fear, guilt, and not knowing that a problem exists are some other reasons why health action is not taken. A home visit by a concerned nurse can serve as a catalyst for motivating parents to seek help for their child's health needs.

The school nurse cannot possibly visit at home every child served in the school system. Children who manifest needs or difficulties such as the following should receive priority for home visits:

1. History of many absences due to illness
2. Behavioral problems which interfere with academic functioning or which adversely affect social relationships with peers
3. Adjustment difficulties related to a chronic condition such as diabetes, epilepsy, heart defects, or obesity
4. Suspected child abuse or neglect
5. Special programming needs in relation to a developmental disability
6. Lack of medical follow-up on an identified health problem
7. Pregnancy
8. Frequent exposure to infectious diseases

Home visiting can be rewarding and extremely beneficial. It frequently is the key which opens the door to a happier life for many children. The following case situation describes how a home visit helped one 8-year-old child to positively increase her interactions with her peers:

Tammie Baxter was referred to the school nurse because she had a pronounced body odor. Her peers shunned her, and she appeared to be a lonely child. Tammie's teacher had many questions about her home environment and the health status of her parents. She had heard that Tammie's father was ill as a result of complications of diabetes. A very receptive mother answered the door when the school nurse made her first home visit. The nurse discovered that a family of seven was living in a five-room home, including a living room, a kitchen, two bedrooms, and a bath. All five Baxter children, ages 8, 6, 4, 2, and 1, were sleeping on mattresses on the floor in one bedroom. Tammie smelled like urine, not because she was ill, but because three of her siblings wet the bed at night. She had limited clothes because the family was having severe financial problems. Tammie's difficulties with personal hygiene were resolved quickly once the mother discovered how the other children were treating her. A referral was made to a community clothes closet so that Tammie could be dressed like her peers. Tammie's teacher was amazed at how quickly her personal hygiene changed after this referral. A little extra attention from the teacher also helped to alter Tammie's relationships with her classmates.

A long-term helping relationship between the Baxter family and the school nurse evolved from this one simple teacher referral. Tammie was not, however, the focus of the conversation on subsequent visits. Her father was indeed in need of medical care. Mr. Baxter was laid off from work at an industrial plant because he was showing sugar in his urine; a telephone call between the community health nurse working in the school and the industrial nurse clarified that Mr. Baxter could return to work as soon as his diabetes was under control. Several community referrals helped this family to obtain medical care.

Team Participation

No one discipline can meet the needs of all the school-age children. Team cooperation and collaboration are essential if children are to receive the health services they deserve. The school nurse who has a "me" philosophy rather than a "we" philosophy will quickly become frustrated and will soon recognize that it is impossible to achieve goals without the help of others.

In order for school health nurses to carry out their functions effectively and efficiently, they must provide nursing services within the framework of the total health program, working cooperatively with other school personnel. Understanding the roles of each member of the school team (Table 14-5) can facilitate planning and implementation of nursing services. The role definitions presented in Table 14-5 are only guidelines. When entering a new school system, every nurse should spend time with all of these individuals to determine how they function in that given system.

Interdisciplinary functioning can be stimulating and rewarding. For this to happen, all team members must define how they can integrate their specific skills into an effective group effort which emphasizes a common endeavor. A philosophy of care must also be delineated and goals established which are acceptable to all.

No team effort with school-age children will be successful unless the central figures on the team are the child and involved family. Planning *for* others does not work. Rather, they must be *involved* in decision making before they can internalize health beliefs and attitudes and change health behavior.

Practical Tips for Role Implementation

Implementing multiple and varied functions is a formidable task. This is especially true for the nurse in the school setting because the school's primary goal is to educate students, not to provide health care services. School nurses must demonstrate that what they have to offer will enhance a child's learning. In addition, school nurses must often deal with diverse role expectations. School administrators, teachers, parents, and students frequently define the nurse's role differently from how the nurse defines it, because they have had various encounters with nurses in the past. It is important for school nurses to avoid panic or withdrawal when they do not initially accomplish what they have hoped to or when they experience role conflicts. It takes time to develop a meaningful role in any setting. Provided below are some suggestions for facilitating the role implementation process in the school setting:

Define Your Philosophy of Nursing Practice

If school nurses cannot articulate the role of the nurse in the school health program, they cannot

TABLE 14-5 Role descriptions for selected members of the school health team

Discipline	Role description
Principals	School administrators who are responsible for planning and providing direction for all activities carried out to meet the goals of the school, including nursing services.
Teachers	Staff members who are responsible for the educational aspects of the school program. Teachers enhance the total school health program by conducting health education activities in the classroom and by identifying children who have physical and emotional health problems that impede learning.
Teacher consultants	Pupil personnel specialists* who have advanced training for handling educational programming for children with special learning needs such as reading problems, mental retardation, and emotional disturbances.
Teachers, homebound	Pupil personnel teachers, specially trained, to deal with physical handicaps and the educational implications of these conditions. These persons work in the home with children who have been certified by a physician as being unable to physically attend school due to a noninfectious physical disability. These individuals provide both educational instruction and counseling services for homebound students.
School social workers	Pupil personnel specialists who provide direct counseling services for a child and family, if the child is demonstrating adjustment difficulties in the school setting. School social workers apply the principles and methods of social casework to help students to enhance their social and emotional adjustment and to adapt to change. The primary purpose of their intervention is to reduce impediments to learning. These individuals are often used as resource persons by all other members of the school health team.
Screening technicians	Pupil personnel staff trained to identify particular health problems, usually vision and hearing difficulties, through the use of screening tests.
Volunteers	Lay staff who receive in-service education to carry out defined tasks for other staff members. Responsibilities should relate to the in-service training they have received. Careful selection, training, and supervision by professional staff is a must if these individuals are to be utilized successfully in the school setting.
Therapists, physical	Pupil personnel specialists who treat muscular disabilities of children on a prescriptive order from the child's physician. Their services are designed to enable students to improve their physical health status so that their physical health problems do not impede learning.
Therapists, speech	Pupil personnel specialists who work with children who have difficulty producing and combining certain sounds in words, who are unable to speak with reasonable fluency, who speak with an abnormally pitched voice, or who have physical anomalies such as cerebral palsy. Speech therapists help children to develop normal speech patterns which help them to more effectively develop social relationships and to advance academically.
School psychologists	Pupil personnel specialists whose major responsibility is to determine the reasons for a child's inability to learn. These specialists are often known as the school diagnosticians because the primary purpose of their service is to identify or diagnose causes of learning problems. These individuals use psychological tests, such as IQ and personality tests, during the psychological assessment. Parental permission must be obtained before a child can be tested by these specialists. The amount of direct counseling a psychologist does with a child varies from one school to another. Usually, however, this person functions as a consultant to other school personnel. Psychologists in other settings are often more involved in direct counseling services.

*Pupil personnel division—a special service division of a local board of education. Personnel in this division are accountable to the superintendent of schools.

Adapted from Jackson County Intermediate School District, Special education services available to Jackson County, Jackson, Mi, undated.

expect other members of the health care team to use them as they would like to be used. Reviewing the literature devoted to school nursing and the school health policies developed by your agency will provide you with information needed to formulate a philosophy of practice with which you can feel comfortable.

Study Your Community

Understanding the needs of the population you are serving is essential. Children, families, and school personnel will respond more quickly to your suggestions if you demonstrate a sensitivity to their concerns and if you support your comments with data. Review the students' health records to identify their pressing health problems. Analyze census tract data to determine the characteristics of the families in the school district. Talk with students and teachers as you walk around the school building. Avoid sitting in the health clinic. Leave the school setting and drive through the area in which your school is located. Do a community analysis.

Contact Key People

A school nurse who takes the initiative to contact school personnel and community groups responsible for the implementation of the school health program is more likely to become quickly involved than one who functions in isolation. Meet with the school principal before school starts. Explain your role and determine a time when you can orient teachers to the nursing services you have to offer. Find out the name of the president of the PTA and the student health council. A telephone call to these individuals may open the doors to the community and the student body.

Demonstrate Your Skills

The best way to help others to understand what it is you do is to show them what you can do. Follow up quickly on the referrals sent to you by other school personnel. Share with them the results of your interventions. A nurse who too quickly states that an activity is not the nurse's responsibility is apt to make other members of the team hesitant to use her or him. Often the nurse is requested to provide first aid or to inspect for communicable disease because individuals making these requests are afraid to handle these situations. Respond to their concerns by first caring for the children and then providing school personnel with information so that they can handle these situations in the future.

Communicate with All Members of the School Health Team

Do not wait for others to come to you. Relate with teachers in their lounge and in their classroom. Ask questions about the students which will help you to determine where your services are most needed. Share in writing or in person when you have followed up on a referral. Use the bulletin board to provide health information to students. *Talk with the school secretary.* She or he probably knows the students and their families as well as any other person in the building.

Organize Your Activities

A school nurse who just lets things happen frequently does not accomplish goals. Establish a calendar of activities for the year. Be specific about the goals you want to accomplish. Know when you will orient the teachers to your services, when you will provide in-service education, when you will review student records, and when you will follow up on student health problems. A tickler system (refer to Chapter 20) can help you to monitor student follow-up needs. A *calendar is a must.* If you do not plan your time, others will plan it for you.

Set Priorities

A nurse cannot be all things to all people. Identify what needs to be done and then determine what you can handle, considering the time you have available. Request consultation from the school health team to establish priorities significant to the needs of the population being served.

Document Your Activities

People respond favorably to concrete data. Keep a daily record of your activities. Use these records with others to substantiate what you have done, to support the need to set priorities, and to document the need for a new health program or changes in the existing health program. *Remember, changes generally do not occur when concrete data are lacking.*

SUMMARY

Traditionally, community health nurses have assumed a major role in planning health services for school-age children. Currently they work with this population group in a variety of settings such as the home, the school, clinics, and residential settings for children with special needs. A family-centered, prevention-oriented, interdisciplinary approach is the most effective way to meet the needs of school-age children, regardless of the setting in which the nurse is functioning.

In 1986 in the United States there were approximately 60.1 million persons enrolled in school who needed health services. Community health nurses who work with these children encounter an array of physical, psychosocial, cultural, environmental, and developmental health problems and concerns. A well-organized comprehensive health care system which takes into consideration the developmental characteristics of children and adolescents is essential if youth are to reach their maximum potential.

Since most children attend school, the school is a logical environment in which to promote the health of all children. The role of the community health nurse in the school health program has been evolving since the turn of the century. Initially, a school nurse was seen as the professional who provided first aid, gave injections, inspected for communicable diseases, or counseled "dirty" children. Now, she or he is an advocate, a health counselor, a health educator, an epidemiologist, a consultant, a community health planner, and a coordinator. Teamwork is essential for successful implementation of these roles. The central figures on the team *must* be the school-age child and his or her family.

Working with school-age children and their families can be challenging and rewarding. A philosophy of nursing practice that stresses the need to help others help themselves and focuses on the client's strengths, reaps the nurse the most benefits.

REFERENCES

Alan Guttmacher Institute: Blessed events and the bottom line: financing maternity care in the United States, New York, 1987, The Institute.

American Association for Protecting Children: Highlights of official child neglect and abuse reporting—1984, Denver, Co, 1986, American Humane Association.

American Cancer Society: Cancer facts and figures, Atlanta, Ga, 1989, The Society.

American Nurses' Association: Functions and qualifications for school nurses, New York, 1966, The Association.

Anderson CL: School health practice, St Louis, 1972, CV Mosby Co.

Benenson A, ed: Control of communicable diseases in man, ed 15, Washington, DC, 1990, American Public Health Association.

Binsacca DB, Ellis J, Martin DG, and Petitti DB: Factors associated with low birthweight in an inner-city population: the role of financial problems, Am J Public Health 77:505-506, 1987.

Buscaglia LF and Williams EH, eds: Human advocacy and PL 94-142: the educator's roles, Thorofare, NJ, 1979, Slack.

Calhoun JA: The 1980 Child Welfare Act: a turning point for children and troubled families, Children Today 9:2-4, 1980.

Centers for Disease Control (CDC): The effectiveness of school health education, MMWR 35(38):593-595, 1986.

CDC: National Childhood Vaccine Injury Act: requirements for permanent vaccination records and for reporting of selected events after vaccination, MMWR 37:197-220, 1988.

CDC: CDC recommendations for a community plan for the prevention and containment of suicide clusters, MMWR 37(S-6):1-12, 1988.

CDC: Results from the National Adolescent Student Health Survey, MMWR 38(9):147-150, 1989.

Clemen S and Pattullo A: The adolescent with mental retardation. In Howe J, ed: Nursing care of the adolescent, New York, 1980, McGraw-Hill.

Collins JC: Prevalence of selected chronic conditions, United States, 1979-81, DHHS Pub No (PHS) 86-1583, Hyattsville, Md, 1986, National Center for Health Statistics.

Committee on Agriculture, Nutrition, and Forestry, United States Senate: Child nutrition programs: description, history, issues, and options, Legislative hearings of the 98th Congress, 1st Session, Washington, DC, 1983, US Government Printing Office.

Compuplay Centers provide computer resources: NARIC Q 1(3):5, 1988.

Directors' Task Force on Minority Health: Minority health in Michigan: closing the gap, Lansing, Mi, 1988, Michigan Department of Public Health.

Dubowitz H: Child maltreatment in the United States: etiology, impact and prevention, Washington, DC, 1986, US Congress, Office of Technology Assessment.

Eberst RM: Defining health: a multidimensional model, J School Health 54:99-103, 1984. Copyright 1984, American School Health Association, Kent, Ohio 44240.

Enos WF, Conrath TB, and Byer JC: Forensic evaluation of the sexually abused child, Pediatrics 78:385-398, 1986.

Fergusson J, Ruccione K, Waskerwitz M, Perin G, Diserens D, Phil M, Nesbit M, and Hammond GD: Time required to assess children for the late effects of treatment, Cancer Nurs 10:300-310, 1987.

Finkelhor D and Araji S: A source book on child sexual abuse, Beverly Hills, Ca, 1986, Sage.

Fisher B, Berdie J, Cook J, and Day N: Adolescent abuse and neglect: intervention strategies, DHHS Pub No (OHDS) 80-30266, Washington, DC, 1980, US Government Printing Office.

Gallagher T: Teen drug use continues decline, according to U-M survey, Ann Arbor, University of Michigan News and Information Services, February 24, 1989.

Garrard SD: Mental retardation in adolescence, Pediat Clin N Am 7:147-164, 1960.

Goodstadt MS: Substance abuse curricula vs. school drug policies, J School Health 59:246-250, 1989.

Hahn DB: A statewide comparison of student alcohol and marijuana use patterns at urban and rural public schools, J School Health 52:250-255, 1982.

Heazlett M and Whaley R: The common cold: its effects on perceptual ability and reading comprehension among pupils of seventh-grade class, J School Health 96:145-146, 1976.

Heindl C, Krall CA, Salus M, and Broadhurst DD: The nurse's role in the prevention and treatment of child abuse and neglect, Washington, DC, 1979, National Center on Child Abuse and Neglect, Children's Bureau, Administration for Children, Youth and Families, Office of Human Development Services.

Hendershot GE: The 1988 National Health Interview Survey on Child Health: new opportunities for research, Atlanta, Ga, 1989, National Center for Health Statistics.

Hoekelman RA, Blatman S, Brunell PA, Friedman SB, and Seidel HM, eds: Principles of pediatrics: health care of the young, New York, 1978, McGraw-Hill.

Hofmann AD: Legal issues of child health care. In Hoekelman R, Blatman S, Brunell P, Friedman SB, and Seidel H: Principles of pediatrics: health care of the young, New York, 1978, McGraw-Hill.

Hutchins U, Kessel S, and Placek P: Trends in maternal and infant health factors associated with low infant birth weight, United States, 1972 and 1980, Public Health Rep 99:162-172, 1984.

Johnston LD, Bachman JG, and O'Malley PM: Illicit drug use, smoking and drinking by America's high school students, college students, and young adults 1975-1987, DHHS Pub No ADM 89-1602, Washington, DC, 1988, US Government Printing Office.

Jones EF, Forrest JD, Goldman N, Henshaw SK, Lincoln R, Rosoff JI, Westoff CF, and Wulf D: Teenage pregnancy in developed countries: determinants and policy implications, Family Plan Perspect 17(2):53-63, 1985.

Kalisch PA and Kalisch BJ: The advance of American nursing, ed 2, Boston, 1986, Little, Brown.

Knecht LD: Consent and confidentiality: legal issues in adolescent health care for the school nurse, J School Health 51:606-609, 1981.

Lindberg FH and Distad LJ: Survival response to incest: adolescents in crisis, Child Abuse Neglect, 9:521-526, 1985.

Lynam MJ: The parent network in pediatric oncology, supportive or not? Cancer Nurs 10:207-216, 1987.

Martinson I, Armstrong G, Geis D, Anglim M, Gronseth E, Macinnis H, Kersey J, and Nesbit M: Home care for children dying of cancer, Pediatrics 62:106-113, 1978.

McCord J: A forty-year perspective of the effects of child abuse and neglect, Child Abuse and Neglect 1:265, 1983.

Metropolitan Life: Looking for health, New York, 1969, Metropolitan Life.

Michigan State Planning Council for Developmental Disabilities: Developmental disabilities three year state plan: Fy 1984-86, State of Michigan, Lansing, Mi, 1983, Michigan Department of Mental Health.

Mosher WD and Horn MC: First family planning visits by young women, Family Plan Perspect 20:33-40, 1988.

National Center for Child Abuse and Neglect: A report to the Congress: joining together to fight child abuse, Washington, DC, 1986, US Government Printing Office.

National Center for Health Statistics (NCHS): Advance report of final natality statistics, 1986, Monthly Vital Statistics Report, vol 37, no 3, suppl DHHS Pub No (PHS) 88-1120, Hyattsville, Md, 1988, US Public Health Service.

NCHS: Health, United States, 1988, DHHS Pub No (PHS) 89-1232 Public Health Service, Washington, DC, 1989, US Government Printing Office.

National Commission to Prevent Infant Mortality: Home visiting: opening doors for America's pregnant women and children, Washington, DC, 1989, The Commission.

National Committee for Injury Prevention and Control and Education Development Center, Inc: Injury prevention: meeting the challenge, Newton, Ma, 1989, Education Development Center, Inc.

National Institute for Allergy and Infectious Diseases: An introduction to sexually transmitted diseases, Bethesda, Md, 1987, The Institute.

National Institute for Allergy and Infectious Diseases: Pelvic inflammatory disease, Bethesda, Md, 1987, The Institute.

National Research Council, Institute of Medicine, Committee on Trauma Research: Injury in America, Washington, DC, 1985, National Academy Press.

National Safety Council: Accident facts, 1988 edition, Chicago, Il, 1988, The Council.

Nicholson SW: Growth and development. In Howe J, ed: Nursing care of adolescents, New York, 1980, McGraw-Hill.

O'Day, B: Preventing sexual abuse of persons with disabilities: a curriculum for hearing impaired, physically disabled, blind and mentally retarded students, Santa Cruz, Ca, 1983, Network Publications.

Olds DL, Henderson CR, Tatelbaum R, and Chamberlain, R: Improving the delivery of prenatal care and outcomes of pregnancy: a randomized trial of nurse home visitation, Pediatrics 77:16-28, 1986.

Orr MJ: Private physicians and the provision of contraceptive services to adolescents, Family Plan Perspect 16:83, 1984.

Osofsky HJ: Mitigating the adverse effects of early parenthood, Contemp Ob-Gyn 25(1):57-59,65,68,1985.

Panel on Adolescent Pregnancy and Childbearing, National Research Council: Risking the future: adolescent sexuality, pregnancy, and childbearing, Washington, DC, 1987, National Academy Press.

Perovich JD and Tipon ES, eds: United States code service: lawyers edition, 42USCS The Public Health and Welfare §§295f-300z-10, Rochester, NY, 1984, Lawyers Co-operative Publishing.

President's Commission for the Study of Ethical Problems in Medicine and Biomedical and Behavioral Research: Securing access to health care: the ethical implications of differences in the availability of health services: vol 3, Library of Congress No 83-

600501, Washington, DC, 1983, US Government Printing Office.

Prevalence of disability in childhood: Disability Stat Bull 1:2, Spring, 1988.

Rustia J: Rustia school health promotion model, J School Health 52: 108-115, 1982, Copyright, 1982, American School Health Association, Kent, Ohio 44240.

Sander JH and Rosen JL: Teenage fathers: working with the neglected partner in adolescent child bearing, Family Plan Perspect 19:107-110, 1987.

Scipien GM, Barnard MU, Chard MA, Howe J, and Phillips PJ: Comprehensive pediatric nursing, New York, 1986, McGraw-Hill.

Select Panel for the Promotion of Child Health: Better health for our children: a national strategy, vol IV, DHHS Pub No PHS 79-55071, Washington, DC, 1981, US Government Printing Office.

Shattuck L: Report of the Sanitary Commission of Massachusetts, Boston, 1850, Dutton and Wentworth.

Spencer MJ and Dunklee P: Sexual abuse of boys, Pediatrics 78:83, 1986.

Stockwell EG, Swanson DA, and Wicks JW: Economic status differences in infant mortality by cause of death, Public Health Rep 103:135-142, 1988.

Stone DB and Rubinson LG: Suicide among teenagers reflects troubled society, American Medical Association, 230-1246, December 2, 1979.

Task Force on Infant Mortality: Infant mortality in Michigan, East Lansing, Mi, 1987, Michigan Department of Public Health.

Travis G: Chronic illness in children: its impact on child and family, Stanford, Ca, 1976, Stanford University Press.

US Bureau of the Census: School enrollment: social and economic characteristics of students: October, 1986, Current Population Report, Series P-20, No 429, Washington, DC, 1988, US Government Printing Office.

US Bureau of the Census: USA statistics in brief, 1988: a statistical abstract supplement, Washington, DC, 1988, US Department of Commerce.

US Bureau of the Census: Population profile of the United States: 1989, Current Population Reports, Series P-23, No 159, Washington DC, 1989, US Government Printing Office.

US Bureau of the Census: Statistical abstract of the United States, ed 109, Washington, DC, 1989, US Department of Commerce.

US Bureau of the Census: Fertility of American women: June 1988, Current Population Reports, Series P-20, No 436, Washington, DC, 1989, US Government Printing Office.

US Congress, Office of Technology Assessment: Healthy children: investing in the future, OTA-H-345, Washington, DC, 1988, US Government Printing Office.

US Department of Health, Education and Welfare (USDHEW): Healthy people: the Surgeon General's report on health promotion and disease prevention, DHEW Pub No PHS 79-55071, Washington, DC, 1979, US Government Printing Office.

United States Department of Health and Human Services (USDHHS): Health status of minorities and low income groups, DHHS Pub No (HRSA) HRS-P-DU 85-1, Washington, DC, 1985, US Government Printing Office.

USDHHS: Health status of the disadvantaged chartbook, 1986, Washington, DC, 1986, US Government Printing Office.

USDHHS, Office of Disease Prevention and Health Promotion: The 1990 health objectives for the nation: a midcourse review, Washington, DC, 1986, US Government Printing Office.

USDHHS, Office of Maternal and Child Health: Surgeon General's workshop on violence and public health report, DHHS Pub No HRS-D-MC 86-1, Rockville, Md, 1986, The Office.

USDHHS: Prevention '86/'87: federal programs and progress, Washington, DC, 1987, US Government Printing Office.

USDHHS: Surgeon General's report: children with special health care needs, campaign '87, DHHS Pub No HRS/D/MC 87-2, Washington, DC, 1987, US Government Printing Office.

USDHHS, Public Health Service: Adolescent family life program: fact sheet, Washington, DC, 1988, The Service.

USDHHS, Office of Maternal and Child Health: Child health USA '89, HRS-M-CH 8915, Washington, DC, 1989, Bureau of Maternal and Child Health Resources Development.

Van Dover LJW: Influence of nurse-client contracting on family planning knowledge and behaviors in a university student population, Unpublished doctoral dissertation, Ann Arbor, 1985, University of Michigan School of Nursing.

Venereal Disease Action Coalition: Sexually transmitted diseases: a community information and resource guide, Detroit, Mi, 1983, United Community Services of Metropolitan Detroit.

Verhalen RD: Other unintentional injuries, Public Health Rep 102:673-675, 1987.

Wallace H: Health services for mothers and children, Philadelphia, 1962, Saunders.

Westoff CF: Contraceptive paths toward the reduction of unintended pregnancy and abortion, Family Plan Perspect 20(1):4-13, 1988.

Whaley LF and Wong DL: Nursing care of infants and children, ed 3, St Louis, 1987, CV Mosby Co.

Young M, Werch CE, and Bakema D: Area specific self-esteem scales and substance use among elementary and middle school children, J School Health 59:251-254, 1989.

SELECTED BIBLIOGRAPHY

Chen Shu-Pi C and Sullivan JA: School nursing. In Werley HH and Fitzpatrick JJ, eds: Annual review of nursing research, vol 3, New York, 1985, Springer, pp 25-48.

Glynn TJ: Essential elements of school-based smoking prevention programs, J School Health 59:181-188, 1989.

Henshaw SK, Kenney AM, Somberg D, and Van Vort J: Teenage pregnancy in the United States: the scope of the problem and state responses, Washington, DC, 1989, The Alan Guttmacher Institute.

Holt SJ and Robinson TM: The school nurse's family assessment tool, Am J Nurs 79:950-953, 1979.

Katz M, Gunn WJ, and Inverson DC: Design of the school health education evaluation, J School Health 55:301-304, 1985.

Mercer RT: Teenage pregnancy as a community problem. In Werley HH and Fitzpatrick JJ, eds: Annual review of nursing research, vol 4, New York, 1985, Springer, pp 49-76.

Natapoff JN and Essoka G: Handicapped and able-bodied children's ideas of health, J School Health 59:436-440, 1989.

Pletsoh PK and Leslie LA: Urban adolescents: what are their health needs? Public Health Nurs 5:170-176, 1988.

Ritter AM: Using a teacher's health observation form to evaluate school child health, J School Health 96:235-237, 1976.

Stark AJ and Siddons PJ: The public health nurses' school caseload: can we measure outcomes? One agency's experience, Can J Public Health 74:208-214, 1983.

US Preventive Services Task Force: Guide to clinical preventive services: an assessment of the effectiveness of 169 interventions, Baltimore, 1989, Williams & Wilkins.

Yudkin M: When kids think the unthinkable, Psychol Today 16(4):18-25, 1984.

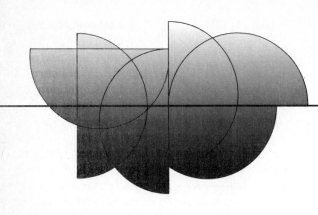

15

The Health Needs of the Adult: A Focus on Wellness

Upon completion of this chapter, the reader will be able to:

1. *Discuss the developmental stages and tasks of adulthood and how achievement of developmental milestones can enhance growth.*
2. *Discuss the roles of adults in relation to nursing interventions for wellness.*
3. *Summarize the national priorities for adult health promotion and protection and preventive health activities.*
4. *Rank and discuss the major causes of mortality and morbidity for the adult population group.*
5. *Discuss factors that increase adults' risk for mortality and morbidity.*
6. *Discuss the community health nurse's role in adult health promotion.*
7. *Describe common situational crises experienced during adulthood and nursing interventions which assist adults in coping with these crises.*

Adults are the pillars and the core of American society. They are the caretakers of the general population, and on them rests the survival of the nation. Adults are the leaders, teachers, and workers of our nation. They are expected to be economically solvent, emotionally sound, physically strong, self-sufficient, and committed to the welfare of others. Along with these roles and responsibilities, they are developing as people and have their own health to maintain. This chapter focuses on maintaining the health of the well adult. The adult who has a handicapping condition is discussed in Chapter 16, and occupational health as it relates to adult health is discussed in Chapter 17. It is not the intent of this chapter to focus on disease processes; the reader is referred to texts such as Thompson, McFarland, Hirsch, Tucker, and Bowers (1989), *Mosby's Manual of Clinical Nursing,* for information on specific health conditions that may affect the adult.

AN OVERVIEW OF ADULTHOOD

Consensus on the age boundaries for adulthood does not exist. In addition, adult roles, responsibilities, and criteria for adulthood vary significantly across ethnic groups, cultures, and history. In this text, the age range from 18 to 29 is used to designate young adults, and middlescence encompasses the age range from 30 to 65 years of age. These ranges should be viewed not as arbitrary, but, rather, in terms of individual variability.

Maintaining the health of the adult is a complex and important task. Community health nurses play a significant role in facilitating wellness among the adult population group. They work with adults in a variety of settings and carry out varying health promotion activities to deal with the health risks and needs of well adults.

Developmental Tasks of Adulthood

Research supports the statement that significant personality growth and development occurs during adulthood (Erikson, 1963, 1982; Havinghurst, 1972; Stevenson, 1977). Adults are changing and learning, and they pass through developmental stages which require achievement of predictable

tasks. Accomplishment of these tasks provides the adult with a foundation for growth. If tasks are not accomplished, future development can be jeopardized or altered. There are individual differences in how well adults achieve developmental tasks.

Adult development does not occur in a vacuum, and it is not simple. Adults have individual, family, and community responsibilities and their development is influenced by many variables including interpersonal relationships, established patterns for coping, available support systems and community resources, and societal mandates, norms, roles, and expectations. Table 15-1 presents the developmental stages and tasks of adulthood, they are expansive and complex.

Erikson's Intimacy, Generativity, and Ego Integrity

Adults go through developmental stages. Erik Erikson's (1963) classic work on developmental theory stressed the importance of psychosocial components in development. Erikson realized that development was a continuous process, and that delays or crisis at one developmental stage could diminish successful achievement of other stages. His psychosocial theories address stages of development, developmental goals and tasks, psychosocial crises, and coping processes (Newman and Newman, 1975; Taylor, Lillis, and LeMone, 1989, p. 155). Erikson described eight developmental stages from birth to death, three of which apply to the 18- to 65-year-old population. According to Erikson (1963, 1982) these stages are *intimacy* (young adult), *generativity* (middle adult), and *ego integrity* (older adult). A brief summarization of Erikson's (1963, 1982) theory of these developmental stages follows.

Young adults are involved in an intense search of self. At the same time they are at the developmental stage of *intimacy,* and need to begin to relate to others and become partners in friendships and in sexual, work, and community relationships. It is a time for development of close personal relationships based on commitment to others. In addition, they must develop the ethical strength to abide by these commitments, even

TABLE 15-1 Developmental tasks of the adult (ages 18-65): major goals—to develop intimacy, generativity, and ego integrity

Young adult	Middlescent	
	Middlescence I	Middlescence II
Age: 18-29 years	Age: 30-50 years	Age: 51-65 years*
1. Establishing autonomy from parents or parent surrogates	1. Developing socioeconomic consolidation	1. Maintaining flexible views in occupational, civic, political, religious, and social positions
2. Choosing and preparing for an occupation	2. Evaluating one's occupation or career in light of a personal value system	2. Keeping current on relevant scientific, political, and cultural changes
3. Developing a marital relationship or other form of companionship	3. Helping younger persons to become integrated human beings	3. Developing mutually supportive (interdependent) relationships with grown offspring and other members of the younger generation
4. Developing and initiating parenting behaviors for use with own, and other's, offspring	4. Enhancing or redeveloping intimacy with spouse or most significant other	4. Reevaluating and enhancing the relationship with spouse or most significant other or adjusting to his or her loss
5. Developing a personal life-style and philosophy of life	5. Developing a few deep friendships	5. Helping aged parents or other relatives progress through the last stage of life
6. Accepting one's role as a citizen and developing participatory citizen behaviors	6. Helping aging persons progress through the later years of life	6. Deriving satisfaction from increased availability of leisure time
	7. Assuming responsible positions in occupational, social, and civic activities, organizations, and communities	7. Preparing for retirement and planning another career when feasible
	8. Maintaining and improving the home and other forms of property	8. Adapting self and behavior to signals of the accelerated aging process
	9. Using leisure time in satisfying and creative ways	
	10. Adjusting to biological or personal system changes that occur	

*In her text, Stevenson assigns the age range for Middlescence II to be 50-70 years.

Material on middlescence from Stevenson JS: Issues and crises during middlescence, New York, 1977, Appleton-Century-Crofts, pp 18, 25.

when this may call for significant sacrifices and compromises. Frequently, young adults experience conflicting values and ideas as they try to sort out what life means to them, and what types of commitments they want to make. The young adult who is successful in achieving intimacy will develop the ability to love, whereas unsuccessful resolution can result in isolation and self-absorption.

As life continues into middlescence, it is expected that the adult will guide and care for the younger generation and will assist the older one. This involves an ability to care and do for others. When these attributes exist, the adult becomes *generative* in nature. Generativity is viewed in terms of procreativity, productivity, and creativity, and is cyclic in nature. Caring or generative adults help to promote these same qualities in children.

If generativity is not reached, stagnation can occur. Stagnated adults do not demonstrate the need or inclination to care for others. Instead, they are egocentric and self-absorbed. It is difficult for them to extend themselves to others.

Toward mid-to-late middlescence the adult establishes *ego integrity.* Establishing ego integrity involves reassessment of self. This is a contemplative process that involves looking at where one has been and where one is going. It also involves examining personal values, decisions, and lifestyles. One also strives to accomplish major educational, career, family, personal, and civic aspirations during this stage of life, and to become self-fulfilled. If life aspirations are not fulfilled, adulthood can be a time of disillusionment, disenchantment, and despair. However, the person who has achieved ego integrity knows and likes himself or herself and is able to accept individual strengths and weaknesses. The person is able to distinguish between the things over which she or he does and does not have control, and can accept those things that cannot be changed. Despair is likely to occur if ego integrity is not reached.

In order to promote wellness and to enhance an adult's self-care capabilities, the community health nurse needs to have an understanding of the processes involved in developing intimacy, generativity, and ego integrity. Adults should be moving toward accomplishment of these developmental tasks, if health is to be maintained. The community health nurse can facilitate accomplishment of adult developmental tasks through anticipatory guidance, stress and crisis intervention, health risk appraisal, teaching, referral to appropriate community resources, and health promotion activities.

The Roles of the Adult and Nursing Intervention

When one examines the developmental tasks of adulthood and the roles assumed by the adult in achieving these tasks, it can be seen that life for an adult is complex and changing. Major roles assumed by the adult are varied and include parent, grandparent, individual, spouse or companion,

son or daughter, citizen, friend, leisure-time user, and worker. A role assumed in one setting will often influence a role assumed in another. A person may not be developmentally ready to assume another role when chronological age requirements dictate change, or unexpected situations make the role assumption mandatory. Examples of role changes which people often are not prepared to make are mandatory retirement at age 65 years and parenthood when a pregnancy was unplanned.

Individual

The adult's role as an individual is an extremely important one. The adult is his or her own person with individual experiences, thoughts, and feelings: when working with adults, nurses should obtain information about their individual needs. Labeling and stereotyping must be avoided, and plans of care should be developed to meet the needs of the individual.

The community health nurse should always remember that all adults need to define what is personally important to them and set personal life goals. This concept can create conflict for the nurse, especially when the goals of clients differ from those of the nurse. The nurse who recognizes that accepting the client's right of self-determination generates trust, cooperation, and self-esteem finds it easier to handle this conflict.

An example of when a client's and nurse's values may differ can be seen in the contemporary issue of women's striving for equality. Today, for example, many women have a career outside the home. This can create feelings of anxiety and insecurity in some women who do not have outside work interests. These women may enjoy staying at home but also question if something is wrong with them because they do not have interests similar to "all" other women. A community health nurse working with such women should keep in mind that the goal is to help clients to learn what is self-fulfilling for them. Work outside the home is not the only way to achieve happiness and satisfaction. The nurse should assist women who are having these conflicts to determine why they are having them; is it because they want to change their style of living or because they feel society expects them to do so? The nurse can also help these women to explore the alternatives they have for achieving self-fulfillment. The nurse should guard against stressing career alternatives over others. At times, options which have been rewarding to the nurse are emphasized; *remember that various lifestyles are healthy, not abnormal.*

The individual needs to be prepared physically, mentally, and socially to take on the future in a manner which will promote personal growth and development. The changes that the adult experiences can produce frustration, confusion, and lack of direction. The nurse is able to help adults cope with these changes by providing supportive guidance. Familiarizing adults with the developmental tasks that they are facing, helping adults to explore how these tasks might be achieved, and emphasizing that stress is normal when one encounters new and different situations are a few examples of supportive activities which may enhance adaptation or promote growth when adults are experiencing stress.

Parent/Grandparent

The generative aspect of middlescence is explicit when the roles of parent and grandparent are discussed. One extends oneself to one's children and grandchildren. In the role of parent, the adult is expected to maintain the family physically and emotionally, take part in the allocation of family resources and the division of labor, and assist in the socialization process. In addition, the generative person also extends herself or himself to others outside the family. One does not have to be a biologic parent to be generative.

Parenting in the young adult years has been discussed in depth in Chapter 13. Parenting issues in the middle years often involve dealing with the developmental concerns of their adolescent children. This situation can be particularly stressful for middlescent adults because they must adapt to stresses associated with two developmental stages: adolescence and middlescence. It is helpful for the nurse to discuss the developmental tasks of adolescence with parents, which can help them to understand that some of what they thought was re-

bellious and abnormal is a part of normal adolescent development. Although this may not make living through the series of events easier, it helps to reassure and give hope. It also helps parents to see where normal growth and development may have gone astray and where professional help may be needed. Parents who have accomplished the developmental tasks of middlescence are more likely to foster independence in their children and relinquish control than those who have not. Middlescent parents who have not faced the developmental issues of their life period find it difficult to "let go." The community health nurse can assist parents in achieving this generational balance; helping each person progress along his or her developmental continuum should be the major goal.

A primary task of the parent in the middle years is launching children from the parental home. Launching is a time when the young adult becomes independent and autonomous, and the family maintains a state in which other members can successfully function. Launching can be a prolonged period. Many more different roles, responsibilities, and relationships occur in the early stages of launching than in the later stages. The permanence of the launching situation has much to do with the adjustment to it. Also, it is not just the launching activity but the surrounding psychosocial variables that will have a great effect on its success. The nurse can help parents through this process by discussing with them the tasks involved in launching, along with ways to accomplish them. Assisting parents in identifying ways, other than child rearing, to achieve satisfaction is one of the most significant activities a community health nurse performs when working with launching families. Adolescents and young adults have a greater chance of achieving healthy independence when their parents support their efforts.

Sons are often allowed more emancipation during the launching process than daughters. Knafl and Grace (1978, p. 514) note that parents provide sons with earlier and more frequent opportunities for independent action, give them more privacy in personal affairs, and hold them to less exacting filial and kinship obligations than daughters. This pattern of functioning can cause family conflict and stress, especially if daughters are about the same age as sons. Helping parents to identify the differences in their behavior when dealing with similar issues may help them to evaluate and change their behavior.

The community health nurse can help parents to be aware of how their involvement with their children should change during launching. Parents must become less directive and recognize that young adults need time to sort out what they want from life. Launching is often a time when parents reflect on how they have raised their children. They frequently evaluate their parenting on the basis of how their children have progressed toward financial independence and whether or not they have established a stable, happy home. Many parents do not consider a child fully launched until these two tasks have been achieved (Knafl and Grace, 1978, p. 311).

Duvall and Miller (1985, p. 276) have discussed the family developmental tasks involved in launching as follows:

1. Adapting physical facilities and resources for releasing young adults
2. Meeting launching-center families' costs
3. Reallocating responsibilities among grown and growing offspring and their parents
4. Developing increasingly mature roles within the family
5. Interacting, communicating, and appropriately expressing affection, aggression, disappointment, success, and sexuality
6. Releasing and incorporating family members satisfactorily
7. Establishing patterns for relating to in-laws, relatives, guests, friends, community pressures, and impinging world pressures
8. Setting attainable goals, rewarding achievement, and encouraging family loyalties within a context of personal freedom

It is important during the launching period that children recognize the stresses their parents may be experiencing. Too often, the focus of nursing intervention is only on the parent. Parents are frequently made to think that what they are doing is "all wrong." Adolescents and young adults need to understand that they are not the only ones experiencing stress and that they need to take responsibility for their own actions. The rights of the parents, as well as those of the children, should be protected. This is illustrated in the following case situation:

John Michael, age 22, decided to live with his parents because he wanted to save money to buy a condominium. He expected to live free of charge, to have no household responsibilities in his parents' home, and to come and go as he pleased. Conflicts arose when John's parents did not agree with his plans. His parents were experiencing financial stress. They had two other children in college and had just finished spending a considerable amount of money for John's education. John was making an adequate salary and they expected him to contribute financially toward family expenses, at least by paying for his groceries. They also felt that he should assume responsibility for some of the household chores, just as he would do if he were living independently. John became angry. He wanted the freedom of adulthood without having to assume the responsibilities that went along with this freedom.

The community health nurse was involved with John's family because Mrs. Michael was a newly diagnosed diabetic. It was during her third home visit that the nurse identified the stress between John and his parents. During the visit, John's mother was tense, almost to the point of being in tears. Observing her distressed state, the nurse encouraged her to verbalize her feelings and afterward made arrangements to meet jointly with John and his parents. During this conference, the nurse requested that each family member share his or her perceptions of what was happening. Emphasis was also placed on identifying alternative ways to resolve the family conflict and on assisting each family member to see his or her needs and responsibilities.

One issue that became apparent during this conference was that John realized his parents also had needs and were experiencing stress. Just as parents must examine the developmental needs of their children, adult children also must be capable of looking at the developmental needs of their parents. Children often fail to do this, especially when they are working toward establishing self-identity. The child at launching age is able to relate at least partially to the needs of his or her parents, but may need some help in recognizing this fact.

In addition to launching, grandparenting is also encountered in the middle years. Some middlescents experience significant anxiety when their first grandchild arrives, because they perceive this event as a sign that they are getting "old." Other middlescents are delighted and eagerly wait for grandchildren. Often grandparents find that they have more time to spend with their grandchildren than they did with their own children. A grandparent can greatly enhance the growth of younger generations. Duvall (1962, p. 409) states that

Children need grandparents who have come to terms with life and accept it philosophically as parents have not yet learned or have not had the time to do. When those who are at the beginning of the journey hold hands with those who have travelled a long way and know all the turns in the road, each gains the strength needed by both.

Adults who have achieved generativity, intimacy, and ego integrity are more likely to hold hands with their grandchildren than those who have not achieved these strengths. The birth of a grandchild to them is not viewed as a negative sign of aging, but rather it is seen as a process which extends and expands their lives.

Spouse or Companion

Adulthood is a time spent in developing and redeveloping relationships with spouse or significant others. A significant other can be anyone with whom the adult has a close, meaningful relationship. With today's many lifestyles, it is completely possible that there will be a significant other who is not a spouse. This significant other may be part of a heterosexual or homosexual relationship. Being nonjudgmental about various lifestyles is essential if the community health nurse is to help the adult achieve self-fulfillment.

Adulthood is a time to enjoy joint activities and to spend time in a companion relationship. Once the problems associated with the raising of a family have been significantly resolved, as in later middlescence, the adult can look in new directions for ways to use physical, mental, and social energies. It is important for the couple to maintain separate interests and activities while developing, maintaining, or redeveloping complementary relationships.

Establishing satisfying sexual relationships is a major task of adulthood. However, it is an area often overlooked during nursing assessment and nurse-client interactions. Clients frequently do not raise sexuality concerns unless encouraged by the health care professional to do so. Specific issues that might need to be addressed during a health interview with an adult include family planning concerns, sexual experimentation before marriage, incompatibility problems, prevention of sexually transmitted diseases, and cultural norms that inhibit the development of meaningful sexual interactions.

The human sexual and emotional responses to menopause and the climacteric can adversely affect spouse or companion relationships. The nurse can help partners to be aware of the changes that they and their mate are experiencing and encourage an emotionally supportive relationship. The adult experiencing these changes should be assisted in seeing that they are normal and do not necessarily have to interfere with sexual activities.

Son or Daughter

Adults are striving for independence from their parents while at the same time trying to maintain or establish meaningful relationships with them. During this time, adults can experience role reversal with their parents. As parents age, some become less able to carry out activities of daily living for themselves. Adult children may then be placed in the position of helping aging parents progress through these later years. Adults need to assist these aging persons without dominating their lives and without taking over decision making for them. They must achieve a balance without feeling guilty for doing too little or too much and must realize that it is only possible to do one's best with the resources that are available.

The community health nurse should encourage the adult who is caring for aging parents to verbalize feelings. This is especially important to do when the question of whether to place the parent in a nursing home or other extended-care facility arises. It is essential at this time to identify the needs of both the adult and the adult's parents and how the needs of each can be met.

During the middlescent period, it is also important to deal with the eventual death of aging parents and relatives. Burial arrangements and the handling of personal affairs should be discussed, and plans should be made. In a society that does not often deal openly with death, this is not an easy task. Health care professionals need to be comfortable talking about dying, death, and grief. Situations involving death and dying are inevitable, yet the American public has little involvement or teaching in death education. For many Americans, death education comes late in life, if it comes at all. Adults are often not equipped to deal with death in relation to themselves or others.

Certain life skills can enhance the individual's ability to cope with death and dying situations. These skills include: decision-making ability, successful coping behaviors, information sharing and processing ability, and values clarification. Knowledge of the grief process, coupled with these life skills, should assist the adult in resolving grief associated with death. A great number of middlescents experience death for the first time with the loss of a parent. The death of the remaining parent is a major crisis point in the adult's life. Death becomes more of a reality as one approaches middlescence, and there is often the urge to make more of one's life before it is too late. Death education and helping a family work through the grieving process are important community health nursing activities.

It is also crucial that adults realize that when aging parents talk about death they are not emotionally disturbed. This is a normal developmental occurrence which should not be denied simply because it arouses difficult feelings. Assisting aging parents to resolve their feelings about death can help adults in accepting their own eventual death, and other grief, dying, death, and loss situations.

Citizen

During the early adult years, persons are usually involved in civic memberships and responsibilities. These involvements often directly affect their families, such as membership in a parent-teacher organization, block clubs to improve their envi-

ronment, and political elections when school millage is an issue. During middlescence, the individual tends to become engaged to a greater degree in civic activities, because time is freed from family responsibilities and there is stability in occupational endeavors.

People in middlescence are accorded the highest positions in American society, including the presidency, company top executive jobs, and high military and civil positions. They are often also expected to take an active role in civic activities. Middlescents have much influence in the community and tend to run for federal, state, and local offices. They are sought as community leaders and often serve as community volunteers. Adults are valuable resources as volunteer staff and supporters for health projects in the community. However, the middlescent who does not experience a lessening in home and work responsibilities will have less time for such activities unless other adjustments are made. This is increasingly becoming a problem, because two-career families are frequently postponing the onset of parenthood.

The existence of people available to carry out civic activities is critical to the survival of the nation. Not having persons in leadership and volunteer positions would be a great loss for this country. Community health nurses can help make adults aware of their importance to the community. They can help adults to see the need for balancing citizen commitments with family and individual responsibilities.

Friend

Adulthood is a time of life when developing and maintaining a few deep friendships is beneficial and rewarding. It is also a time when one has decreased contact with members of the immediate family, due to mobility, death, or launching of children. Having friends that one can count on and enjoy being with helps to provide support and pleasure when family contacts are limited. Middlescent adults often find it satisfying to have friends with whom they can share their activities.

The community health nurse frequently encourages the adult to mobilize additional friendship support in times of stress. Sharing ways to meet other adults with similar interests is helpful. Volunteer work with health or other community agencies, social clubs in the community, church activities, or adult discussion groups are some of the options that the nurse could explore with the adult who has limited friendships. Some adults will prefer not to develop or maintain these friendships.

Leisure-Time User

Leisure is not an easy word to define; it means many things to many people. Leisure is antithetical to work as an economic pursuit. It is a planned activity that promotes growth and is pleasurable. Table 15-2 differentiates between work and leisure activities. *Internal motivation* is the key factor to consider when working with clients who do not plan leisure activities.

In our society, many adults do not seriously engage in leisure-time activity. We are work-oriented, and leisure activity is given a lower priority than other activities. When leisure activity does occur, it is largely in the environments of home and community. Some adults limit their leisure activities mainly to the home setting because they have a number of responsibilities that closely tie them to this environment. However, for the person with many responsibilities at home, leisure time may be more relaxing and fulfilling outside that setting.

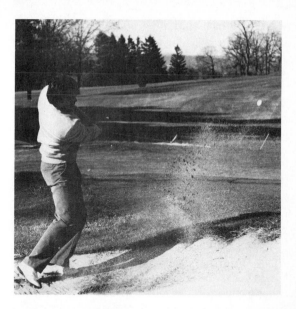

Figure 15-1   Using leisure time in satisfying and creative ways is a significant developmental task of middlescents, but one which is frequently neglected by career-oriented individuals. Effective use of leisure time can reduce stress, promote sound mental health, and provide satisfying outlets and relationships. This businessman finds that golfing on a regular basis helps him to better deal with the pressures of a busy work environment. While he enjoys his career activities very much, he also recognizes that work cannot fulfill all his needs. (Courtesy of photographer, Henry Parks.)

Using leisure time in satisfying and creative ways (Stevenson, 1977) is a developmental task for adulthood. The community health nurse should encourage the adult to make a conscious effort to devote time to these activities. Otherwise, an important developmental area is being overlooked (refer to Figure 15-1). People need time in which to enjoy themselves and relax. The great amount of free time that often accompanies later life will be better spent if individuals have developed leisure-time activities that are satisfying to them.

Frequently the adult needs help in examining why he or she does not engage in leisure activities. Often it will be found that many adults do not know how to use the free time they have and thus they devote all their time to work or other responsibilities. The nurse can assist these individuals by helping them to identify interests they have had

TABLE 15-2   Comparison of work and leisure

Dimension	Work	Leisure
Decision-making control	Relatively more external	Relatively more internal
Spatial parameter	Continuity of space	Freedom of space
Time parameter	Structured time	Nonstructured time
Social structure	Permanence of structure	Transiency of structure
Activity	Defined activity	Emerged activity

From Stevenson JS: Issues and crises during middlescence, New York, 1977, Appleton-Century-Crofts, p 72.

in the past or would like to develop now, as well as to explore ways in which they can meet their current interests. Take for example, the case of Sara Washington:

Sara Washington was a 40-year-old divorced woman with no children. She was referred to the community health nurse for health supervision visits by her family physician following hospitalization for severe hypertension. After her divorce, Sara devoted herself to work. She was an interior designer who was well respected in her field; promotion came very rapidly. Most of her social involvements were work-related.

Sara's recent hospitalization scared her. When the community health nurse took a social history on her first home visit, she replied, "I know I can't keep working like I have been, but I get bored when I don't have something to do. There is very little social life for a woman my age in this town. My peers are all married or divorced themselves. Those who are divorced are like me, they work all the time."

Community health nursing intervention helped Sara to discover how much she missed contact with people on a personal level, the types of social activities she might explore, her fears about getting involved, and the middlescent's need for leisure-time activities to achieve normal growth and development. Sara had enjoyed cooking, entertaining friends, art, and drama before her divorce. Supportive encouragement by the community health nurse facilitated her getting involved once again in these activities. She especially enjoyed dance lessons and found that they provided several opportunities for socializing. "You know, when one takes the time, it really isn't that difficult to find something fun to do," stated Sara during one of the nurse's home visits.

Adults who have experienced a stressful life event such as divorce frequently use work to reduce their tension and anxiety. Unfortunately, this develops into a regular pattern of functioning whereby work becomes the central focus of life and leisure activity is eliminated. An astute community health nurse might prevent this from happening by providing anticipatory guidance and supportive encouragement when encountering adults during times of heightened stress.

Worker

The health of the worker and the role of the occupational health nurse are discussed in Chapter 16. Work as a major adult role is discussed here. Working is generally essential to one's economic stability and has psychological implications for the individual as well.

The young adult is in a stage of training for, and deciding upon, a career. The middlescent is often at a career peak and derives much satisfaction from her or his job; this is usually the time of maximum power and influence. Americans in executive positions are often 40 to 65 years old and earn a large part of the nation's income.

By the time a person reaches middlescence, career patterns are usually well established. It will be found, however, that some adults are in the process of changing careers or are dissatisfied with their present jobs. The community health nurse must realize that both of these situations can be difficult for the adult and may require crisis intervention services. Through the use of the nursing process, the community health nurse can help these adults to identify why they are dissatisfied with their career choice, what options or alternatives are open, and the career planning resources available in the community, including agencies like career counseling centers, state employment security commissions, and departments of vocational rehabilitation.

Job dissatisfaction is often related to other personal difficulties; stresses at work can be compounded when an adult has home pressures to handle. This was the case with Ed Sorka.

Ed Sorka was a 29-year-old husband and father of two daughters, ages 3 and 5. He became disillusioned with his job because "his boss demanded too much and gave too few rewards." Ed's wife had multiple sclerosis which was getting progressively worse. She required help with activities of daily living and found it hard to participate in social events. Ed was a devoted husband and father. All his spare time was spent with his family. He found it difficult to talk about his wife's condition or his need for leisure activities; verbalizing stress encountered at work was much easier for him to handle. When the community health nurse helped him to examine both work and home stresses, Ed discovered that he really did not want to change jobs but that he did need time for himself. Arrangements were made for homemaker services to reduce the demands on Ed's time.

Some adults change jobs or careers out of necessity and not by choice, because of changes in the job market or personal health problems. These individuals and their families can experience intense stress, especially if the adult who is changing careers derived great satisfaction from the previous work. The McSweeney family, for instance, had an increased incidence of health problems when Mr. McSweeney returned to college to prepare for another career.

George McSweeney was a 38-year-old engineer, husband, and father of three school-age children. As a result of industrial noise, he lost 50 percent of his hearing. Unable to continue functioning at his job, he returned to college to prepare for another career. Financially, his family had few difficulties because Mr. McSweeney received workers' compensation and federal scholarship monies. The community health nurse encountered the McSweeney family after they had repeatedly taken Lisa, their 10-year-old daughter, into the emergency room for treatment of an asthmatic condition. The nurse was well received by the family because both parents were unsure of when to seek medical care for their daughter. The nurse discovered that Lisa's condition had been under good control until the family moved and she had to change schools. In addition, she found that Mr. McSweeney was having tension headaches regularly; a medical evaluation ruled out organic problems. Lisa had fewer asthma attacks and Mr. McSweeney had fewer headaches as the family began to verbalize the frustrations associated with the multiple changes they had recently experienced.

Stress on the family system can also occur when a wife returns to work during the middlescent years. Many wives stay home during the young adult years to raise a family and to tend the home. As home responsibilities decrease, there are an increasing number of women in middle years who seek employment. Both spouses' working brings up a number of considerations. Dual career family situations greatly affect the amount of time that either spouse has available for civic, leisure, or other activities outside the home and work. With the combined incomes, however, dual careers can give increased financial flexibility and allow families to purchase services, such as housekeeping and lawn maintenance, which they do not have time to do. This situation gives the family more choices in relation to recreational activities and plans for the future. The wife's working can also create changes in roles and role expectations which result in stress. The husband may now be expected to assume more responsibility for household chores, meal patterns may change, and the wife may develop interests outside the home that do not include her husband. Families who have a flexible division of labor before the wife goes back to work are more likely to adjust to these changes than families whose roles are rigidly allocated prior to this time (refer to Chapter 6).

As the adult approaches middlescence, retirement is another area for which planning is needed. Many people look forward to retirement and see it as an opportunity for doing things that they were previously unable to do. Others dread it because they either do not want to cease working or realize that they are not financially stable enough to enjoy it. Success in retirement depends on planning for it during this period of life. Chapter 18 discusses ways in which families can plan for aging and deal with issues associated with retirement.

The variety and diversity of the roles adults assume are only part of the complicated experience of being an adult. Being an adult is not an easy task, and, thus, individual health concerns are put aside for family or civic issues. Often, health care professionals do not focus on the health care needs of the well adult: Screening programs are overlooked, primary prevention activities are neglected, and mental health needs may be left unseen. It must not be forgotten that the well adult also has health needs.

The Human Body in Adulthood

Achieving health for the adult involves maintaining physical, mental, and social well-being. Most adults are considered healthy, but the well adult has many health care needs. These needs may be overlooked due to the self-sufficient nature of the adult and the caretaker role accorded to her or him by society. A combination of the two may put an adult in the position of being "too busy" or "too involved" to look after personal health. It can be difficult to persuade the well adult to obtain health care and to practice preventive health habits. The human body during adulthood is briefly discussed to help illustrate some of the physical and mental changes that the adult experiences.

The human body is constantly undergoing physical and mental changes. During adulthood the person begins to develop an acute awareness of growing older and is faced with adjusting to a changing body image as physical alterations occur. This adjustment is often difficult in American society, as the beauty and stamina of youth are prized. The incidence of chronic and handicapping conditions increases with age and these conditions can also affect how one views oneself.

Several physical changes occur in the human body during adulthood. The senses of taste and smell begin to diminish. Vision is usually well maintained in early adulthood, but presbyopia (farsightedness) is extremely common by middlescence. Presbyopia is caused by a decreased lens elasticity which reduces the power of accommodation. It hinders the ability of the individual to view objects at close range, and glasses may be necessary for reading or close work. After age 30, the cornea begins to lose transparency and the pupil decreases in size. These changes allow less light to be admitted to the eye and result in poor illumination.

Permanent sensorineural hearing loss as a result of aging (presbycusis) accelerates during middlescence. The person experiencing presbycusis has decreased auditory acuity for higher tones and may have difficulty engaging in normal conversation, including talking over the telephone. The duration and type of noise exposure that a person encounters during earlier life influences how soon presbycusis begins. For example, the person exposed to industrial noise and the avid hunter may experience presbycusis earlier than their counterparts because of more extensive sensorineural hearing damage during youth.

Metabolic function—the combining of food with oxygen to create energy—decreases during adulthood. This, coupled with the fact that the person is often becoming more sedentary, can mean increased weight. The basal metabolism rate gradually decreases by middle age with a resultant need for reduction in caloric intake of approximately 7.5 percent (Murray and Zentner, 1989, p. 471).

Decreasing elasticity of the blood vessels, especially the coronary arteries, predisposes the middlescent to cardiovascular disease. Many middlescents evidence the symptomatology of cardiac conditions, such as shortness of breath, chest pains, and dyspnea on exertion. Incidence of death from cardiovascular disease is on the rise in adulthood.

In middlescence the female's ovarian estrogen production and menstruation cease. This event is called *menopause* and usually occurs between the ages of 45 and 55 years. The symptoms that a woman experiences during menopause are an interplay of physiological, sociological, and psychological changes. The physiological changes are largely a result of decreased ovarian activity and the resultant estrogen deficiency. Menopause does not have to affect one's sexual enjoyment or pleasure. However, the capability to have children ceases. The point of cessation of childbearing ability is still somewhat in question. To be safe, it has been recommended that a woman continue to use a reliable method of birth control for at least 1 year after she has gone 12 consecutive months without a menstrual period (Caldwell, 1982).

Once the female passes through menopause, her childbearing capabilities cease. This often has greater psychological meaning than physical significance. Some of the physical symptomatology that may be evidenced during menopause are hot flashes, sweating, chills, dizziness, headaches, palpitations, and atrophic vaginitis. Psychological symptomatology includes depression, change in sexual drive, insomnia, fatigue, headache, irritability, and backache.

In middlescence, the male passes through a period called the *climacteric,* when the testes decrease, but do not cease, testosterone production. During this time, the testes atrophy slightly, sperm production decreases, and in about 20 percent of men, hypertrophy of the prostate begins

(Murray and Zentner, 1989, p. 468). The male usually goes through this period between ages 50 and 60. He may or may not experience any physical symptoms. Psychological symptoms such as irritability, easy frustration, depression, and change in sexual drives are sometimes evidenced. Many people are not aware that this period exists for men and are often bewildered by male behavior during the climacteric.

Decalcification of the bones, a condition called *osteoporosis,* begins in middlescence. When this happens, the bones become fragile and are easily broken. Vertebral compression can occur and result in backache, headache, and other problems.

As a person ages, the amount of skeletal muscle decreases and muscle cells are replaced by adipose and connective tissue. As a result of these changes, adults have decreased muscle tone, a flabbier appearance, and decreased muscle strength. Exercise will help to maintain muscle tone and strength. The adult can engage in a variety of activities and sports, but it is advised that individuals check with a physician before beginning any vigorous exercise routine. The adult should exercise consistently, gradually increasing the amount to avoid overexertion.

An example of how an adult undergoing the physical changes of middlescence can be affected by these changes is seen in the following case situation.

Marge, a 50-year-old widow and mother of three daughters, ages 24, 27, and 30, is a typical example of how many people react to body changes during middlescence. She sought help at a local adult screening clinic because she perceived that the physical changes she was undergoing were making her look older than her chronological age. She wanted to maintain a youthful look and stated, "I am having a hard time getting old. I fear the physical changes and the dependency associated with aging." These thoughts were triggered when Marge's oldest daughter celebrated her thirtieth birthday.

By the standards of her culture, Marge was doing well. She had an established career and had just recently developed an intimate relationship with a man that could lead to marriage. She was loved and respected by her children and had frequent contact with them without interfering in their lives. Friends enjoyed being with her and described her as intellectually stimulating and fun. Marge, however, could focus only on her physical changes and was experiencing anxiety in relation to them. She was questioning whether she should terminate her relationship with her male companion so that she would not be hurt in the future. "Men only marry beautiful women."

The community health nurse who saw Marge at the adult screening clinic made arrangements to visit her at home. This nurse utilized the principles of crisis intervention to help her sort out reality. Marge was helped to identify her strengths and to look more realistically at the changes in her physical appearance. She was assisted in seeing that she had several alternatives open to her regarding her life and that withdrawing from personal relationships could increase her social aging process. Marge gradually began to realize that if she focused on her physical appearance alone, she could lose the joys of life she had already achieved.

Marge is not atypical of the many adults with whom the community health nurse will work. The physical changes of the aging process can be difficult to handle. The development of generativity, intimacy, and ego integrity helps an individual to adapt to physical changes associated with the aging process, because these life goals give meaning and direction to one's future.

Even though physical functioning changes or decreases, mental function can be maintained or increased during adulthood. Cerebral capacity begins to weaken relatively slowly, unless other factors such as cerebrovascular occlusion or depression occur. At age 70, the person can be as intellectually capable as at age 30 and has a greater experiential base than in youth to draw from when making decisions (Division of Gerontology, 1957, p. 58). General intelligence of the middlescent is greater than at any other time of life.

NATIONAL HEALTH OBJECTIVES AND ADULT HEALTH

One of the major goals in the document that laid the groundwork for national health objectives for the past decade, *Healthy People: The Surgeon*

General's Report on Health Promotion and Disease Prevention, was to improve the health of American adults, and by 1990 to reduce deaths among people ages 25 to 64 by at least 25 percent (USDHEW, 1979). It listed the major causes of death for adults in this age group as heart disease, cancer, and stroke. Although good strides have been made in reducing deaths from these conditions, they are still prominent causes of adult mortality. The report also cited other notable threats to adult health such as accidents, alcohol abuse, and mental illness.

Healthy People discussed priority health activities in terms of preventive services, health protection, and health promotion. Table 15-3 lists the 15 priorities related to adult health. All these priorities have a significant effect on the health of the adult population group.

Minority Health in the United States

People in the United States are healthier now than ever before. In spite of this fact, there continues to be a greater proportion of deaths and illnesses experienced by U.S. racial and ethnic populations. In 1984 the Department of Health and Human Services organized the Secretary's Task Force on Black and Minority Health to analyze this disparity. The Task Force found that the gap between minority and majority health was most dramatic when measured in "excess deaths." Excess deaths are defined as deaths that would not have occurred if minorities had the same age and sex-specific death rate as the majority population. Approximately 40 percent of all minority deaths fall into this category (Office of Minority Health—Resource Center, 1989, Health and, p. 1). Over 80 percent of minority excess deaths fell into the six categories of heart disease/stroke, homicide/accidents, cancer, infant deaths, chemical dependency, and diabetes. The Task Force generated extensive recommendations meant to improve the health of minority populations.

As a result of Task Force efforts and findings the Office of Minority Health (OMH) was established to develop, coordinate, and monitor a national strategy to promote minority health, and implement Task Force recommendations. The OMH–Resource Center (OMH-RC) was estab-

TABLE 15-3   National priorities for adult health activity/service in the 1980s

Category	Activity/service
Preventive services	Family planning
	Pregnancy and infant care
	Immunizations
	Sexually transmissible diseases services
	High blood pressure control
Health protection	Toxic agent control
	Occupational safety and health
	Accidental injury control
	Fluoridation of community water supply
	Infectious agent control
Health promotion	Smoking cessation
	Reducing misuse of alcohol and drugs
	Improved nutrition
	Exercise and fitness
	Stress control

From US Department of Health, Education, and Welfare: Healthy people. The Surgeon General's report on health promotion and disease prevention, Washington, DC, 1979, US Government Printing Office, pp 81-138.

lished in 1987. This resource center maintains information on federal, state, and local minority health-related resources, serves as a minority health information center, stimulates the development of minority health resources, and publishes fact sheets on minority health. The OMH-RC can be contacted by calling 1-800-444-MHRC.

Efforts are being made to try to reduce the gap in the minority health status, but we still have a long way to go. Community health nurses can be instrumental in getting health education materials and programs to minority groups, ensuring that these materials are culturally sensitive, improving accessibility to services and serving as advocates for minority health and research.

HEALTH RISKS FOR THE ADULT: SELECTED CAUSES OF MORBIDITY AND MORTALITY

Although adults in the 18- to 65-year age range are generally considered to be physically and

TABLE 15-4 Deaths and death rates by age and sex, 1985

Cause	Number of deaths			Death rates*		
	Total	Male	Female	Total	Male	Female
15 to 24 Years						
All Causes†	**37,935**	**28,162**	**9,773**	**95.9**	**141.1**	**49.9**
Accidents†	**19,161**	**14,791**	**4,370**	**48.4**	**74.1**	**22.3**
Motor vehicle	14,277	10,680	3,597	36.1	53.5	18.4
Drowning	1,346	1,232	114	3.4	6.2	0.6
Firearms	479	430	49	1.2	2.2	0.3
Poison (solid, liquid)	427	308	119	1.1	1.5	0.6
Fires, burns	380	244	136	1.0	1.2	0.7
Suicide	5,121	4,267	854	12.9	21.4	4.4
Homicide	4,772	3,767	1,005	12.1	18.9	5.1
25 to 44 Years						
All Causes†	**117,667**	**80,848**	**36,819**	**159.5**	**220.8**	**99.0**
Accidents†	**25,940**	**20,438**	**5,502**	**35.2**	**55.8**	**14.8**
Motor vehicle	15,034	11,403	3,631	20.4	31.1	9.8
Poison (solid, liquid)	2,385	1,881	504	3.2	5.1	1.4
Drowning	1,547	1,384	163	2.1	3.8	0.4
Falls	1,057	906	151	1.4	2.5	0.4
Fires, burns	929	644	285	1.3	1.8	0.8
Cancer	20,026	9,344	10,682	27.1	25.5	28.7
Heart disease	15,539	11,538	4,001	21.1	31.5	10.8
45 to 64 Years						
All Causes†	**403,114**	**251,031**	**152,083**	**897.3**	**1,169.7**	**648.1**
Cancer	138,829	74,883	63,946	309.0	348.9	272.5
Heart disease	132,610	94,399	38,211	295.2	439.9	162.8
Stroke (cerebrovascular disease)	16,910	9,126	7,784	37.6	42.5	33.2
Accidents†	**15,251**	**10,915**	**4,336**	**33.9**	**50.9**	**18.5**
Motor vehicle	6,885	4,682	2,203	15.3	21.8	9.4
Falls	1,639	1,198	441	3.6	5.6	1.9
Fires, burns	965	662	303	2.1	3.1	1.3
Poison (solid, liquid)	678	389	289	1.5	1.8	1.2
Ingestion of food, object	658	426	232	1.5	2.0	1.0
Chronic obstructive pulmonary disease	12,901	7,541	5,360	28.7	35.1	22.8
Chronic liver disease cirrhosis	12,506	8,499	4,007	27.8	39.6	17.1

*Death per 100,000 population in each age group. Rates are averages for age groups, not individual ages.

†The all causes and accident totals for each age group include deaths not shown separately.

Deaths are for 1985, latest official figures from National Center for Health Statistics, Public Health Service, US Department of Health and Human Services. In National Safety Council: Accident Facts, 1988 edition, Chicago, 1988, The Council, p 9.

mentally healthy, many deaths do occur during this developmental period. Table 15-4 presents selected major causes of death for the adult and points out a need for health promotion activities that will aid in identifying adults at risk for premature death. It can readily be seen that accidents, heart disease and stroke, and cancer are major causes of death for adults. Many of these deaths are preventable.

Accidents

Accidents cause enormous loss of life in the United States and are the leading cause of death in the first four decades of life (USDHHS, 1986, p. 127). The true rate of accidental morbidity and mortality is likely underestimated, and only 15 percent of state health authorities have developed plans for uniform reporting of injuries (USDHHS, 1986, p. 144). Accidental deaths include deaths by such means as motor vehicles, falling, drowning, homicide, and suicide. Most accidental deaths are preventable. One area where deaths are being prevented is on American highways, likely the result of increased use of seat belts.

The community health nurse can play a major role through health education and health promotion activities to prevent premature deaths in the adult population. Health education activities geared to fire safety, home safety, water safety, seat belt use, general motor vehicle safety, CPR training, health risk information awareness, stress reduction, and poison control and treatment are just some of the activities that the nurse can use to help lower the adult mortality rate from accidents in this country.

Cardiovascular Disease

Cardiovascular diseases are the number one killer in America. These diseases kill almost one million Americans each year—close to one person every 32 seconds (American Heart Association [AHA], 1989, 1990 Heart, p. 1). If statistics hold true, close to one in two Americans will die of cardiovascular disease (AHA, 1989, 1990 Heart, p. 1). Deaths from cardiovascular diseases add up to almost as many deaths as from cancer, accidents, pneumonia, influenza, and all other causes com-

bined (AHA, 1989, 1990 Heart, p. 1). The majority of deaths from cardiovascular diseases are from *heart attacks, stroke, hypertensive disease, rheumatic heart disease, and congenital heart defects.* Cardiovascular disease is responsible for more days of hospitalization than any other single disorder (USDHEW, 1979, p. 56). Cardiovascular disease can be disabling. It is the greatest cause of permanent disability claims among workers under age 65 years in the United States, and is responsible for more days of hospitalization than any other single disorder (USDHEW, 1979, p. 56).

Heart attacks are the number one cause of death in America. Although the death rate from heart attack has dropped significantly in the last decade (Heart attacks, 1988, p. 50), more than 500,000 Americans die from heart attacks each year (AHA, 1989, 1990 Heart, p. 12). Over 1,500,000 Americans suffer heart attacks each year (AHA, 1989, 1990 Heart, p. 12). The nurse can be instrumental in reducing morbidity and mortality from heart attacks. The nurse can educate clients about risk factors such as dietary habits, smoking, alcohol use, stress, and family history. The nurse can also encourage families to be able to do cardiopulmonary resuscitation, be aware of the warning signals of a heart attack, and be acquainted with emergency community resources and telephone numbers. The American Heart Association (1989, 1990 Heart, p. 17) lists the warning signals of heart attack as 1) uncomfortable pressure, fullness, squeezing, or pain in the center of the chest lasting 2 minutes or longer, 2) severe pain spreading to the shoulders, neck, or arms, and 3) severe pain, lightheadedness, fainting, sweating, nausea, or shortness of breath. The association notes that not all these warning signs occur in every heart attack, and if any of these begin, the person should seek help immediately. About one half of all heart attack victims wait 2 hours or longer before deciding to get help, which greatly reduces their likelihood of survival because most heart attack victims who die do so within 2 hours of the first awareness of symptoms (AHA, 1989, 1990 Heart, p. 15). The nurse can help families understand the need for immediate action.

Strokes rank third among all causes of death in the United States, behind heart attacks and cancer. Annually more than 500,000 Americans suffer strokes, resulting in close to 150,000 deaths (AHA, 1989, 1990 Heart, pp. 2, 21). When direct medical expenses and community resource utilization are combined with lost income and productivity, the cost of stroke is estimated to be about $14 billion annually (National Institute on Disability and Rehabilitation Research [NIDRR], 1989, p. 1). No one can calculate the cost of stroke in terms of human suffering, lost income, and years of potential life lost.

Stroke is a major cause of long-term disability. Approximately 2 million people in the United States have been disabled by strokes (NIDRR, 1989, p. 1). Many victims are disabled by paralysis, and suffer resultant speech/language and memory deficits (AHA, 1988). Again, the nurse can do much to decrease morbidity and mortality through health education activities such as risk factor education. The long-term rehabilitation needs of persons with stroke can cause great emotional and psychological distress for both client and family. The nurse can be instrumental in helping the family work through the adaptation and rehabilitation process, and assist in resource coordination and utilization.

More than 60 million Americans have hypertension (AHA, 1989, 1990 Heart, p. 9). Hypertension is linked to the incidence of heart attack and stroke. The National Heart, Lung, and Blood Institute estimates that approximately 70 percent of the cases of hypertension are mild in severity (Hypertension, 1988, p. 60). However, more than 30,000 Americans die from hypertension annually (AHA, 1989, 1990 Heart, p. 9). Black Americans are at much higher risk for developing hypertension than white Americans. Controlling high blood pressure has been shown to be one of the most effective means available for reducing mortality in the adult population (U.S. Preventive Services Task Force, 1989).

The box at right lists the risk factors associated with heart disease and stroke. Americans are becoming increasingly aware of these risk factors (USDHHS, 1986, p. 19). People with more than one of these elevated risk factors are at especially

Risk Factors Associated with Heart Disease and Stroke
1. Smoking
2. Consistent hypertension
3. Elevated cholesterol
4. Diabetes
5. Overweight
6. Inactivity
7. Genetic predisposition
8. Personality patterns (such as patterns established to cope with stress)
9. Use of oral contraceptives or estrogen replacement

From US Department of Health, Education, and Welfare: Healthy people. The Surgeon General's report on health promotion and disease prevention, Washington, DC, 1979, US Government Printing Office, pp 57-59.

high risk of dying from heart disease (USDHHS, 1983, p. 16). Major risk factors that cannot be changed include heredity, age, and sex (presently American men are at greater risk of experiencing a heart attack than women). Risk factors that can be alleviated include cigarette smoking, high blood pressure, elevated blood cholesterol, nutrition, stress, and level of physical activity.

The death rate as a result of heart attacks is nearly twice as high among cigarette smokers (almost 47 million Americans) as among nonsmokers; heart attacks are approximately twice as frequent among diabetics as among nondiabetics; and diabetic women have five times the risk of arteriosclerotic heart disease as normal women (USDHEW, 1979, pp. 57-59). Coronary heart disease and heart attacks are twice as frequent in inactive Americans as in active Americans (Monmaney, 1988, p. 60). It has been known for more than 20 years that elevated serum cholesterol levels put one at risk for developing cardiovascular disease. It is estimated that about 60 million Americans over the age of 20 years are candidates for medical advice and intervention for high blood levels of cholesterol (Sempos, Fulwood, Haines, Carroll, Anda, Williamson, Remington, and Cleeman, 1989, p. 45).

An organization actively involved in cardiovascular education, treatment, and research is the American Heart Association. The association was founded in 1924 to promote the exchange of information about heart disease. It has more than 1850 affiliates in all 50 states; a main commitment is to research. This commitment involved an investment of almost $69,000,000 in 1989, and since 1949 the association has invested more than $820 million in cardiovascular research (AHA, 1989, 1990 Research; AHA, 1989, Research). The lifesaving efforts of this organization are to be applauded. The nurse should make the client aware of this excellent community resource.

As has been mentioned, the community health nurse should focus on primary prevention activities in relation to cardiovascular disease. The nurse can help to make clients aware of cardiovascular risk factors and what can be done to decrease them, encourage clients to have regular medical supervision, and make them aware of available community resources. The health education activities of the nurse in this area cannot be overestimated. Americans have remarkable knowledge gaps about how to protect themselves against the disease that is most likely to kill them

(Monmaney, Springen, Hager, and Shapiro, 1988, p. 57). The nurse can play a large role in educating people about cardiovascular conditions and risk factors, and reducing cardiovascular morbidity and mortality.

Cancer

Cancer is the second leading cause of death in the United States. The death rate has risen in recent years, largely the result of an increase in cancer of the lung. In 1989 about 1 million Americans were diagnosed as having cancer and more than 500,000 died of it (American Cancer Society [ACS], 1989, p. 3). Of those who died, an estimated 178,000 could have been saved if they had received early diagnosis and treatment (ACS, 1989, p. 3). About 30 percent of Americans now living will eventually have cancer (ACS, 1989, p. 3). Many advances in diagnosis and treatment have resulted in remarkably improved survival rates for many cancers.

Avoiding known carcinogens is an excellent way to prevent some forms of cancer. Most lung cancer is caused by cigarette smoking and most skin cancers are caused by frequent, prolonged exposure to direct sunlight. Many people develop cancer from occupational or environmental ex-

TABLE 15-5   Risk factors associated with cancer

Risk factor	Data about risk
1. Smoking	Smokers have 10 times the frequency of lung cancer as nonsmokers, 3-5 times the frequency of oral cavity cancer, 3 times the frequency of cancer of the larynx, and 2 times the frequency of urinary bladder cancer as nonsmokers.
2. Excessive alcohol intake	Heavy drinkers have higher rates of cancer of the larynx, oral cavity, liver, and esophagus.
3. Diet	The precise relationship between dietary differences and cancer is not known, but some striking international differences have been seen.
4. Radiation exposure	Is suspected of causing various forms of cancer such as leukemia.
5. Excessive sunlight exposure	Has been shown to cause skin cancer.
6. Occupational exposures	To materials with cancer-causing potential, such as radiation and asbestos; workers exposed to asbestos have 15 times the expected cancer rates of the respiratory tract.
7. Environmental pollution	Water pollution, air pollution.
8. Heredity	The precise relationship is unknown, but some cancers show familial tendencies (e.g., breast).

From US Department of Health, Education, and Welfare: Healthy People. The Surgeon General's report on health promotion and disease prevention, Washington, DC, 1979, US Government Printing Office, pp 62-65.

posure to known carcinogens. Some factors that put people at risk are listed in Table 15-5.

The warning signals of cancer, as established by the American Cancer Society (1989) are:

1. *C*hange in bowel or bladder habits
2. *A* sore that does not heal
3. *U*nusual bleeding or discharge
4. *T*hickening or a lump in the breast or elsewhere
5. *I*ndigestion or difficulty swallowing
6. *O*bvious change in a wart or mole
7. *N*agging cough or hoarseness

The first letters of those lines combine to spell: CAUTION. People should take caution when dealing with cancer. If the nurse notes any of the above warning signals, the client should be referred to a physician immediately!

A study by the National Center for Health Statistics (NCHS) puts yearly medical costs for cancer at $71.5 billion (ACS, 1989, p. 25). It accounts for 10 percent of the total cost of disease in the United States (ACS, 1989, p. 25). The immense toll that cancer takes in human pain, suffering, and death cannot be measured in dollars.

The National Cancer Institute is our chief source of cancer information, education, and research. The institute publishes pamphlets on different types of cancer that give a description of the cancer, its incidence, causes and prevention, detection and diagnosis, stages, treatment, and advances. The institute publishes *Taking time. Support for people with cancer and the people who care about them,* an excellent resource the nurse can share with families. *Taking time* covers such topics as sharing the diagnosis, sharing feelings, coping within the family, assistance, self-image, the world outside, living each day, and resources.

By dialing 1-800-4-CANCER (1-800-638-6070 in Alaska) one can access the Cancer Information Service of the National Cancer Institute (U.S. Department of Health and Human Services). This service provides information on community agencies and services, answers questions, and mails publications and a publication list. It also provides information about active treatment centers for specific types of cancer.

The National Cancer Institute has developed the PDQ (Physician Data Query), a computerized database designed to give doctors quick and easy access to the latest treatment information for most types of cancer, descriptions of clinical trials that are open for patient entry, and the names of organizations and physicians involved in cancer care (National Cancer Institute, 1989, p. 11). To gain access to PDQ a doctor can use an office computer with a telephone hookup and a PDQ access code or the services of a medical library with online searching capability. Patients can call 1-800-4-CANCER to get PDQ information.

The American Cancer Society is at the forefront of private sector cancer education and research in the United States. It traces its origins to 1913 when the American Society for the Control of Cancer was founded to disseminate knowledge concerning the symptoms, treatment, and prevention of cancer; to investigate conditions under which cancer occurs; and to compile statistics on cancer (ACS, 1989, p. 22). It is one of the oldest and largest voluntary health agencies in the United States today, with more than 3200 chapters (ACS, 1989, p. 22). American Cancer Society public education programs reached more than 50 million Americans in 1988 (ACS, 1989, p. 23). The society is actively involved in professional education, publishes *Cancer Nursing News* (sent to about 90,000 nurses around the country), supports professorships in clinical oncology, and offers clinical oncology awards. Society service and rehabilitation activities include but are not limited to resource and information services; *Can-Surmount*—a short-term home visitor program for patients and families of patients; *Reach to Recovery*—a patient visitor program that addresses the needs of women who have had breast cancer; laryngectomy rehabilitation volunteers in coordination with the International Association of Laryngectomees (IAL); and ostomy rehabilitation volunteers in coordination with the United Ostomy Association.

The nurse can play a central role in health education and in assisting families to locate available resources. The nurse can help the family with a member who has cancer to adjust to and cope

TABLE 15-6 Incidence, warning signs, risk factors, and survival rate for selected cancers, United States

	Lung cancer	Colon/rectum cancer	Breast cancer	Prostate cancer	Skin cancer
Incidence	155,000 new cases	151,000 new cases	142,900 new cases	103,000 new cases	500,000 new cases
Mortality	142,000 deaths	61,300 deaths	43,300 deaths	28,500 deaths	8,200 deaths
Risk factors	Heavy cigarette smoking History of smoking 20 or more years Exposure to certain occupational substances such as asbestos and radiation	Family history of colon/rectum cancer Personal or family history of rectal polyps Inflammatory bowel disease	Over age 50 Family history of breast cancer Never had children First child after age 30	Incidence increases with age Black Americans Exposure to certain occupational substances such as cadmium	Excessive exposure to the sun Fair complexion Occupational exposure to coal, tar, pitch, creosote, arsenic compounds, and radium Severe sunburn in children
Warning signs	Persistent cough Sputum streaked with blood Chest pain Recurring attacks of pneumonia or bronchitis	Bleeding from the rectum Blood in the stool Change in bowel habits	Breast changes such as: a lump, thickening, swelling, dimpling, skin irritation Retraction or scaliness of the nipple Nipple discharge Breast pain or tenderness	Weak or interrupted flow of the urine Need to urinate frequently, especially at night Blood in urine Painful urination	Any unusual skin condition A change in the size or color of a mole
Survival rate (5 yr)	33% if localized 13% all stages	87% colon 79% rectum } localized 40% colon 31% rectum } spread	Almost 100% if localized 60% if spread	84% if localized 71% all stages	89% malignant melanoma 95% basal and squamous cell } localized

From American Cancer Society: Cancer facts and figures 1989, Atlanta, Ga, 1989, pp 9-13.

584

with the situation. The nurse uses the principles of crisis intervention and grieving as discussed in Chapter 7. Hospice care is discussed in Chapter 19.

Scientists are searching for ways to trigger the body's own defenses against cancer. This search is leading to the discovery of hundreds of substances called *biological response modifiers* that boost, direct, or restore many of the normal defenses of the body (Antoine, 1988, p. 1). Advances such as this, along with new treatments and early diagnostic procedures, are helping in the war against cancer.

Table 15-6 presents the incidence rate, mortality rate, warning signs, risk factors, and survival rate for lung cancer, colon and rectum cancer, breast cancer, cancer of the prostate, and skin cancer. Table 15-7 portrays the trends in survival by site. It is encouraging to note that the survival rates for many cancers, with the exception of lung cancer, are increasing. Although skin cancer has the highest incidence it is amenable to treatment and does not carry a high mortality rate. Lung cancer and colon/rectum cancer carry relatively high mortality rates. Lung cancer is now equal to breast cancer as the leading cause of cancer death in American women (ACS, 1989). Unfortunately, diagnostic procedures such as chest x-ray films and sputum examinations usually do not reveal lung cancer until it has already spread. In adult men, 90 percent of all lung cancer deaths have a direct relationship to smoking (USDHHS, 1989). Fortunately, several effective screening procedures are now available to detect breast cancer and cancers of the colon or rectum. Women can do regular self-examination of the breasts, and can have a physical examination and mammography.

Cancer in Minorities

The health status of Americans as a whole has improved over the past generation. However, studies by the Secretary's Task Force on Black and Minority Health (U.S. Department of Health and Human Services Public Health Service) reflect that there continues to be a disparity in deaths and illnesses experienced by racial and ethnic groups (OMH-RC, 1989, Cancer and Minorities,

p. 1). A study by the Centers for Disease Control showed that the death rate for blacks is 2.5 times higher than for whites and that in 31 percent of the cases the difference cannot be explained on the basis of health risk factors and family income (Friend, 1990, p. 1D).

Cancer disproportionately strikes minority groups; a recent report by the Secretary's Task Force on Black and Minority Health found wide gaps in cancer death rates between minorities and whites (OMH-RC, 1989, Cancer hits, p. 1). Data from the Task Force, comparing mortality of minorities and whites, reveal the following: Japanese living in the United States have a higher incidence of stomach cancer; Chinese living in the United States have a higher incidence of cervical and stomach cancers; Hawaiians have a higher incidence of lung and stomach cancers and the highest rate of breast cancer; Native Americans have higher rates of gallbladder, stomach, cervical, and lung cancers; and blacks have a higher rate of lung cancer.

Cancer survival rates are higher today than ever before because of earlier diagnosis and better treatment. Almost half of all cancer patients now survive 5 years or more (OMH-RC, 1989, Minority survival, p. 3). However, minority survival rates are lower. Only 38 percent of blacks survive 5 years after diagnosis compared to 50 percent of whites (OMH-RC, 1989, Minority survival, p. 3). This may in part reflect health care access problems for the population group. Figure 15-2 illustrates the cancer survival gap between minority and white populations.

Smoking and Health

It has been more than 25 years since publication of *Smoking and Health. Report of the Advisory Committee to the Surgeon General of the Public Health Service* (USDHEW, 1964). This report, prepared by an independent body of scientists that had been approved by the Tobacco Institute and eight health organizations, reviewed more than 7000 studies (Warner, 1989, p. 141; USDHHS, 1989, p. viii). The document, often referred to as the first Surgeon General's Report on Smoking and Health, stated that there was a

TABLE 15-7 Trends in survival by site of cancer, by race. Cases diagnosed in 1960-63, 1970-73, 1974-76, 1977-78, 1979-84

	White					Black				
	Relative 5-yr survival					Relative 5-yr survival				
Site	1960-63*	1970-73*	1974-76*	1977-78†	1979-84†	1960-63*	1970-73*	1974-76*	1977-78†	1979-84†
All sites	39%	43%	50%	50%	50%	27%	31%	38%	38%	37%
Oral cavity and pharynx	45	43	54	53	54	—	4	35	35	31
Esophagus	4	4	5	6	7	1	4	4	2	5
Stomach	11	13	14	15	16‡	8	13	15	16	17
Colon	43	49	50	52	54‡	34	37	45	44	49
Rectum	38	45	48	50	52‡	27	30	40	40	34
Liver	2	3	4	3	3	1	—	1	1	5
Pancreas	1	2	3	2	3	—	2	2	3	5
Larynx	53	62	66	69	66	—	7	58	59	55
Lung and bronchus	8	10	12	13	13‡	5	7	11	10	11
Melanoma of skin	60	68	78	81	80‡	—	—	62§	—	61**
Breast (females)	63	68	74	75	75‡	46	51	62	62	62
Cervix uteri	58	64	69	69	67	47	61	61	63	59
Corpus uteri	73	81	89	87	83‡	31	44	61	58	52‡
Ovary	32	36	36	37	37‡	32	32	41	40	36
Prostate gland	50	63	67	70	73‡	35	55	56	64	60‡
Testis	63	72	78	86	91‡	—	—	77**	—	82**
Urinary bladder	53	61	73	75	77‡	24	36	47	53	57‡
Kidney and renal pelvis	37	46	51	50	51	38	44	49	54	53
Brain and nervous system	18	20	22	23	23	19	19	27	24	31
Thyroid gland	83	86	92	92	93	—	—	88	92	95
Hodgkin's disease	40	67	71	73	74‡	—	—	67**	79**	69
Non-Hodgkin's lymphoma	31	41	47	48	49‡	—	—	47	46	49
Multiple myeloma	12	19	24	24	24	—	—	28	30	29
Leukemia	14	22	34	37	32	—	—	30	31	27

*Rates are based on End Results Group data from a series of hospital registries and one population-based registry.

†Rates are from the SEER Program. They are based on data from population-based registries in Connecticut, New Mexico, Utah, Iowa, Hawaii, Atlanta, Detroit, Seattle-Puget Sound and San Francisco-Oakland. Rates are based on follow-up of patients through 1985.

‡The difference in rates between 1974-76 and 1979-84 is statistically significant (p < .05).

§The standard error of the survival rate is greater than 10 percentage points.

**The standard error of the survival rate is between 5 and 10 percentage points.

—Valid survival rate could not be calculated.

From Surveillance and Operations Research Branch, National Cancer Institute. As cited in American Cancer Society. Cancer facts and figures—1989, Atlanta Ga, 1989, The Society.

causal relationship between cigarette smoking, lung cancer, and other serious diseases, and that remedial action was necessary. It stirred a wave of controversy, unrest, opposition, and legislation on the issue of smoking and health.

As a result, Congress passed the Federal Cigarette Labeling and Advertising Act of 1965 and the Public Health Cigarette Smoking Act of 1969. These laws required that health warnings be printed on cigarette packages, banned cigarette advertising in the broadcast media, and increased public awareness of the hazards of smoking. In 1964 the U.S. Public Health Service established the National Clearinghouse for Smoking and Health that is now the Office on Smoking and Health. This office has published more than 20 reports on the health consequences of smoking. Since the 1964 report *every* Surgeon General of the United States has reinforced that smoking is one of the most significant causes of disease and death.

In 1979, *Healthy People* addressed smoking as a major national health problem, and in 1980, *Promoting Health. Preventing Disease Objectives for the Nation* set forth national health objectives about smoking cessation and proposed to reduce the proportion of adults in the United States who smoked to below 25 percent by 1990. Surgeon General C. Everett Koop championed the cause of a "Smoke-Free Society" by the year 2000. In continuing these efforts, in 1989 the U.S. Department of Health and Human Services published *The Surgeon General's 1989 Report on Reducing the Health Consequences of Smoking: 25 Years of Progress.* The report gave an overview of smoking since 1964. It stated that smoking is responsible for more than one of every six deaths in the United States today, and is the single most important preventable cause of death. While it lauded the progress that Americans have made, it also indicated that smoking continues to be a major health problem.

Since 1964 research has consistently shown that smoking increases the morbidity and mortality rates of many diseases and conditions. Smoking is responsible for 30 percent of all cancer deaths, 21 percent of all deaths from coronary

heart disease, 18 percent of stroke deaths, and 82 percent of deaths from chronic obstructive pulmonary disease (USDHHS, 1989, p. 2). More than 3800 chemicals are found in smoke (Byrd, Shapiro, and Schiedermayer, 1989, p. 209), and 43 substances in tobacco smoke have been determined to be carcinogens (USDHHS, 1989, p. 9).

At this writing nearly one half of all adults in the United States who have ever smoked have quit (USDHHS, 1989, p. 9). Yet, more than 50 million Americans continue to smoke. Had it not been for the efforts spearheaded by the federal government after publication of the 1964 report, the number of smokers would be some 90 million according to estimates. Decisions made to quit smoking or not to start are believed to have avoided or postponed 2.1 million smoking-related deaths between 1986 and the year 2000 (USDHHS, 1989, p. xi). Fortunately, an increasing number of Americans have become educated about the health effects of smoking. For example, at the time of the 1964 report less than 50 percent of American adults believed that cigarette smoking caused lung cancer, whereas that percentage has now increased to 92 percent (including 85 percent of current smokers) (USDHHS, 1989, p. 19).

At the time of the 1964 report it was estimated that approximately 50 percent of the adult male population and 32 percent of the female population smoked cigarettes. The percentages have now fallen to 31.7 percent for males and 26.8 percent for females (USDHHS, 1989, p. 20). Smoking among teenagers (aged 12 to 18 years) decreased steadily through 1987, but has now leveled off at about 20 percent. Each day more than 3000 American teenagers start to smoke (USDHHS, 1989, p. ix), and smoking among teenage girls has increased. Although most states ban tobacco sales to minors, many do not enforce the laws. There are fewer legal restrictions today on children's access to tobacco products than in 1964, in spite of what has been learned since then about the dangers of tobacco use (Smoking also, 1989, p. 6). Research has shown that although blacks are less likely to be heavy smokers than whites, they are significantly less likely to stop smoking once they

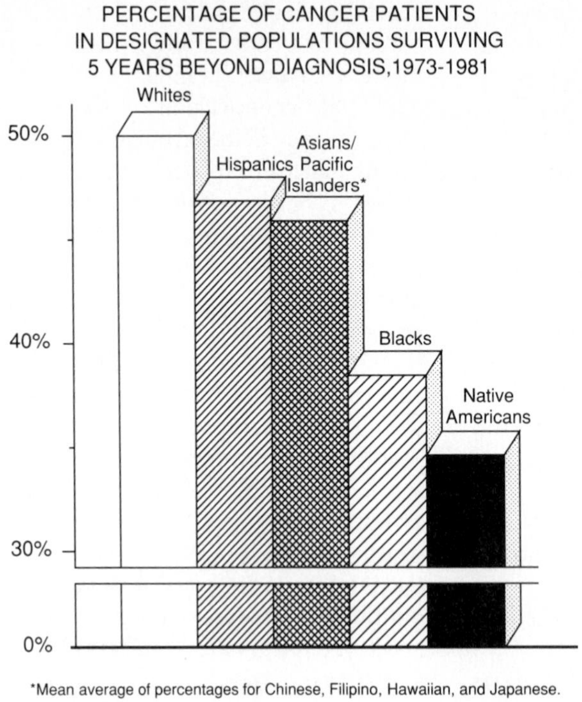

PERCENTAGE OF CANCER PATIENTS
IN DESIGNATED POPULATIONS SURVIVING
5 YEARS BEYOND DIAGNOSIS, 1973-1981

THE SURVIVAL GAP

Survival rates, the number of cancer patients living 5 or more years beyond diagnosis, differ markedly from one type of cancer to the next. Early diagnosis and effective treatments help to keep survival figures high for breast and prostate cancers, while numbers remain low for cancers of the lung, esophagus, and pancreas.

Within any type of cancer, survival rates also vary widely between populations. As the chart on the left demonstrates, when all cancer cases are considered together, serious gaps are revealed between minority and non-minority populations. (Source: SEER)

*Mean average of percentages for Chinese, Filipino, Hawaiian, and Japanese.

Figure 15-2   Minority cancer survival rates: the survival gap. (From Office of Minority Health–Resources Center: Cancer and minorities. In Cancer and minorities: closing the gap, Washington, DC, 1989, Department of Health and Human Resources, p 1.)

start (Novotny, Warner, Kendrick, and Remington, 1988, p. 1187). Cigarettes remain one of the most heavily advertised products in the United States (Cigarette advertising, 1990, p. 261). Cigarette advertising campaigns are increasingly aimed at women, youth, minorities, and blue-collar workers (Cigarette advertising, 1990, p. 261).

Radio and television advertisements for cigarettes are no longer allowed; programs and literature aimed at helping the smoker to stop smoking have been published; the rights of nonsmokers are being stressed; nonsmoking areas have been designated in many public places and on public transportation; and higher cigarette taxes have been levied. As of 1988 more than 320 communities had adopted laws or regulations restricting smoking in public places (USDHHS, 1989, p. 9). Many workplaces have banned smoking, limited it to specific areas, or are phasing it out. Some department stores are banning cigarette sales in

vending machines, and Congress is having second thoughts about the amount of tobacco the United States exports. Smoking is now banned on air flights of 6 hours or less in the United States, accounting for 99.8 percent of daily domestic flights.

Since 1964, attitudes toward smoking have changed drastically. Whereas in the 1940s, 1950s, and early 1960s smoking was glamorized and considered chic and stylish, smoking is becoming increasingly shunned and socially unacceptable. Unlike the movies of yesteryear, today's movies rarely show smokers. Though James Bond lights up in *License to Kill* the Surgeon General's warning appears in the credits. Actors, politicians, educators, health care professionals, and other notable people are infrequently seen smoking. These changing attitudes and policies are helping to shape the smoke-free America of tomorrow.

Cigarette smoking is the most important preventable cause of death in our country

(USDHHS, 1986, p. 177). Smoking is financially and socially costly; it is related to 390,000 deaths each year (ACS, 1989, p. 20; Smoking also, 1989, p. 6). Its estimated annual costs range from $52 to $65 billion (ACS, 1989, p. 20; Squitieri, 1990, A1). Approximately one third of this cost is spent directly for health care; two thirds is due to absenteeism, lost productivity, and lost wages. Smoking is also costly in terms of human life, suffering, and disability. Unless smoking habits change, as many as 10 percent of all persons now alive may die prematurely of heart disease attributable to their smoking behavior (Office on Smoking and Health, 1982).

The link of smoking to lung cancer has become firmly established over the past 25 years. The American Cancer Society estimates that cigarette smoking is responsible for 83 percent of all lung cancer deaths—85 percent among men and 75 percent among women (ACS, 1989, p. 20). The cancer death rate for male smokers is more than double that of nonsmokers (ACS, 1989, p. 20). Lung cancer has now surpassed breast cancer as a cause of death for women.

Smoking as a health problem is a major concern. Antismoking legislation is being introduced by many states, as well as on the national level, and nonsmokers are beginning to assert their right to live in a smoke-free environment. Antismoking action and legislative efforts, such as clean air bills and smoking bans, will continue. A health word to the wise is, If you smoke, STOP; if you don't smoke, don't start.

Smoking and Pregnancy

Smoking and pregnancy is an important health concern. Smoking during pregnancy increases the risk of stillbirth, miscarriage, premature birth, and low–birth-weight infants (USDHHS, 1989, p. 19). There is evidence that heavy smoking (two or more packs per day) by pregnant women can cause birth defects such as mental retardation, facial anomalies, and heart defects (New pattern, 1985, A3). A study conducted by the University of Maryland School of Medicine showed that pregnant women who participated in antismoking intervention programs cut their smoking in half,

and on an average gave birth to infants who were heavier and larger than those who did not stop or cut back (APHA, 1984, Anti-smoking, p. 11). A self-help cessation program for pregnant women showed that this low-cost prenatal intervention can significantly affect smoking behavior (Ershoff, Mullen, and Quinn, 1989, p. 182). Unfortunately, many women are not aware of the risk factors smoking poses for pregnancy (USDHHS, 1989, p. 19), and their need for health education is great.

Passive Smoking and Smokeless Tobacco

Passive inhalation of smoke (passive smoking) and smokeless tobacco are public health issues related to smoking that have received increased attention in recent years. Studies have shown that nonsmokers are at increased health risks from passive inhalation and that smokeless tobacco use is related to certain cancers and conditions.

Nonsmokers are becoming increasingly concerned about their own health risks from passive smoking. Each year 46,000 nonsmokers die from exposure to cigarette smoke (Wells, 1989, p. 20), and an unknown number of people develop illnesses from such exposure. Many deaths from passive smoking involve exposure at the home and workplace. The Environmental Protection Agency has stated that nonsmokers in public buildings cannot avoid exposure to the ill effects of tobacco smoke unless smokers are quarantined and are provided with separate ventilation systems (Friend, 1989). Smoke persists in buildings long after smoking stops, and the most practical way to eliminate the exposure is to remove the source.

More than a dozen research studies have shown increased lung cancer risk among passive smokers (National Research Council, 1986) and several studies have pointed to increased heart disease risk in passive smokers (Sandler, Comstock, Helsing, and Shore, 1989, p. 163). There is some evidence that risk from passive inhalation of smoke increases with age. The health of children is adversely affected when parents smoke; they experience more episodes of bronchitis and pneumonia during the first years of life (Koop and Luoto, 1982, p. 323; Neuspiel, Rush, Butler,

Golding, Bijur, and Kurzon, 1989, p. 168; Byrd, Shapiro, and Schiedermayer, 1989, p. 209). Children in households that include adult smokers have more restricted activity and bed disability days than children living with nonsmokers (Byrd, Shapiro, and Schiedermayer, 1989, p. 209).

Smokeless tobaccos, such as snuff and chewing tobacco, are emerging as a health concern. It has been estimated that 12 million Americans, including 3 million under the age of 21, use snuff and chewing tobacco (National campaign, 1990, A10). Unfortunately, many states have not passed laws that prohibit the sale of smokeless tobacco to children. With the bans on smoking in public places increasing, it is thought that more Americans will turn to smokeless tobacco.

This threat to health was vividly described in *Sean Marsee's Smokeless Death* (Fincer, 1985), an article about a teenage athlete who died of oral cancer related to his use of smokeless tobacco. Such stories are appearing with increasing frequency. Annually there are 29,000 new cases of oral cancer and 9000 deaths from this cause, with 70 percent related to tobacco use. Research has linked snuff and oral cancer and former Surgeon General C. Everett Koop has declared that smokeless tobacco does pose a cancer threat.

In response to the threat, the Comprehensive Smokeless Tobacco Education Act of 1986 (Public Law 99-252) was passed. This law established a program of public education to inform people of the health dangers of smokeless tobacco products. It supports educational programs and public service announcements. The act supports research on the effects of smokeless tobacco on human health and regulates the labeling of smokeless tobacco products and advertising of them—provisions similar to those of the Cigarette Smoking Act of 1969.

The American Academy of Otolaryngology–Head and Neck Surgery, Inc., and the National Federation of State High School Associations sponsored a weeklong, nationwide educational campaign aimed at stopping the use of snuff and chewing tobacco among young people (National campaign, 1990, A10). The effort, "Through with Chew Week," was designed to educate teenagers

about the health risks of smokeless tobacco, including life-threatening cancers of the mouth and throat. As part of the campaign a 10-minute video that outlined the social and health risks of smokeless tobacco was made available for distribution to high schools.

THE COMMUNITY HEALTH NURSE'S ROLE IN MAINTAINING ADULT HEALTH

Health is a blend of developmental, physiologic, psychological, spiritual, and social factors. When one of these aspects of health breaks down, all are affected. When working to promote adult health, community health nurses must take into consideration all these factors and develop intervention strategies which comprehensively address clients' needs. The implementation of comprehensive intervention strategies frequently requires interdisciplinary team work.

Health is affected by human development, but only limited nursing research has focused on the adult from a developmental framework (Stevenson, 1984, p. 55). Stevenson (1984) states that a foundation of nursing research about adult development in relation to health promotion, illness, and crisis situations is needed on which to base nursing actions and activities. Without this knowledge, nursing must draw from the social and psychological sciences when incorporating individual and family development into health care.

Adults have a variety of health care needs but they are also busy people. They have responsibilities at home, at work, and in the community, and often spend so much time achieving and doing for others that their own health care needs are overlooked or neglected. It is not always an easy task to motivate adults to participate in health activities, especially if they consider themselves to be well. Well adults do not always recognize or act on health needs, and may ignore primary prevention activities.

Various approaches are often needed to plan nursing interventions that address the health needs of well adults. When working with adults, the community health nurse implements interventions on all levels of prevention—primary, secondary, and tertiary. Utilization of the referral process (refer to Chapter 9) is an integral part of promoting the health of the adult. Nurses can help adults become aware of the available resources that meet their health care needs and refer them to these resources when appropriate. However, many health care resources are organized to deal with acute health care episodes rather than with preventive health care measures.

Health Promotion through Preventive Intervention

As discussed in earlier chapters, health promotion begins with people who are basically healthy and encourages the development of lifestyles that maintain and support health and well-being (U.S. Department of Health, Education, and Welfare, 1979, p. 119). Although little is known about how individuals and families move toward more optimal health and about what assists them in the process (Chalmers and Farrell, 1983, p. 62), a great deal is known about many health promotion activities, such as nonsmoking, which enhance a healthy lifestyle.

Some examples of health promotion activities which help adult clients to improve or maintain their well-being are displayed in the box at right. The adult will have more control over some of these activities than others. Some areas of health promotion such as environmental health and occupational health and safety are as much matters of legislation and enforcement as individual decision making. Obtaining documented data about outcomes of health promotion and nursing interventions that facilitate improved health outcomes is critical while working toward influencing legislation and health policy. When encouraging health promotion activities, the nurse should remember that people bring their own beliefs, attitudes, and values to health care situations. Beliefs about individual and family susceptibility to illness, the severity of illness in terms of health and lifestyle disruption, the effectiveness of diagnostic and prevention measures, and barriers to care will affect the health promotion and prevention activities in which a person engages (Rosenstock, 1966).

Healthy Adults: Selected Activities and Decisions for Promoting Health
1. Cessation of smoking
2. Not drinking to excess
3. Adequate nutritional intake
4. Control of environmental hazards
5. Promotion of worksite health and safety
6. Prevention and control of hypertension
7. Pap smear at least every 3 years
8. Regular self-examination of the breasts and testicles
9. Knowledge of and action on cancer warning signs
10. Counseling to promote mental health
11. Regular dental care
12. Regular health care
13. Regular exercise

Adapted from USDHEW: Healthy people, The Surgeon General's report on health promotion and disease prevention, Washington, DC, 1979, US Government Printing Office, pp 152-154.

The community health nurse carries out many primary prevention activities when helping adults to act on personal health risks. She or he is particularly interested in helping the adult to learn about health problems that can be prevented and about health behaviors that can promote wellness. A major primary prevention activity with adults is health teaching and counseling about family and personal health risk factors, accident prevention and safety, nutrition, personal hygiene, health examinations, family planning, STDs, disease transmission, and immunizations. Such health teaching, with utilization of resources as appropriate, may help to prevent an illness or injury, dental caries, an unwanted pregnancy, marital disenchantment, a suicide attempt, a case of tetanus, a case of flu, an incident of child abuse, or an STD. Health teaching activities help the adult to look at health in relation to present as well as future functioning.

Primary prevention and health risk appraisal are major goals of health promotion, but are not always easily attainable. In recent years, there has been increased emphasis on primary prevention;

however, many preventive health care measures, such as yearly physical examinations, are not covered under many forms of health insurance and become out-of-pocket expenses for the client. Health screening programs can provide valuable health services to persons who otherwise would not obtain them.

The community health nurse can help clients to assess individual and family health risk factors on an informal basis and can encourage health actions which decrease these risks. Health risk appraisal can also be handled through an automated process in which an individual's health-related behaviors and personal characteristics are compared to mortality statistics and other epidemiological data. Relating individual and group data helps individuals to identify their risk of dying from a specific condition by a specified time and the amount of risk which could be eliminated by making appropriate behavioral changes in health practices (Wagner, Beery, Schoenbach, and Graham, 1982, p. 347). Although this automated approach is not readily accessible to the general public, it will be available in the near future. Health risk appraisal can have beneficial health consequences. However, the real challenge for health professionals is in assisting people to act on personal health risks.

Safety for the adult is a key factor to consider when developing health teaching and risk appraisal strategies. Accidents kill adults in astounding numbers and account for 45 percent of deaths in the 20 to 29 age group (refer to Table 15-4). Motor vehicle accidents make up a large portion of these deaths, but accidents also happen at home, at work, and in the community. The nurse should help the adult to assess for potential safety hazards and to identify ways to correct them. Suggestions on measures to promote safety such as having stairway handrails, conveniently located electrical outlets, indirect nonglare lighting, and safe water and sewage disposal; keeping equipment in proper working order; providing easy entry to and exit from bathtubs and showers; maintaining stairs and landings free from clutter; and making sure that rugs are not loose can help to prevent accidents in the home.

Health teaching of the young adult should focus on violence as well as accident prevention. Accidents, suicide, and homicide are the leading causes of death for persons 20 to 29 years of age. The suicide rate among young adults has increased dramatically (USDHHS, 1988, p. 19). It is important to try to determine the nature and timing of critical precedents that place individuals at high risk for committing violent acts against themselves or others and to identify significant persons or groups in contact with high-risk individuals who could save the individual's life. White males are most at risk for committing suicide (USDHHS, 1988).

In order to prevent certain conditions, nurses can assist adults in looking at their own personal health habits and risk factors. Smoking, excessive intake of alcoholic beverages, lack of sufficient rest, and an inadequate diet all have an impact on present and future health status.

When nurses function from a prevention perspective, they stress the importance of medical, dental, and ophthalmologic examinations for prevention, early diagnosis, and treatment of disease. Secondary preventive health measures for the adult include practicing self-examination of the breasts and testicles, yearly Pap smears, and adherence to prescribed medical and dental regimens. The adult should be assisted to see the value of monitoring and screening for conditions for which he or she has a familial or individual predisposition, such as cardiovascular accidents, diabetes, cancer, or hypertension. Appendix 15-1 summarizes adult screening procedures used with adult clients as well as the age at which they should be done. Information in this table provides parameters for discussion when the community health nurse is carrying out health counseling.

Tertiary prevention health activities that the nurse may utilize with the adult are related to rehabilitation activities which minimize the degree of disability of the condition. These activities are discussed in Chapter 17, where the nurse's role in rehabilitation of the handicapped adult is covered. They involve interdisciplinary functioning and focus on encouraging client compliance with prescribed medical and dental regimens, as well as exploring ways to promote coping behaviors.

When working with adults, the community health nurse carries out preventive activities in a variety of settings such as in the home, hospital, or place of work; at school; and in social, recreational, and clinic settings. Local health departments usually include clinics and other services for adults. However, many adults are not aware of the range of services provided by their local health department and the minimal fees charged for them.

Whatever the setting, the interventions selected must be based on detailed information about the client and what motivates him or her to change. It is important to incorporate the client into the decision-making process when establishing goals and interventions; lecturing usually does not facilitate change.

LEGISLATION AFFECTING ADULT HEALTH

Much of the legislation that influences the adult also makes an impact on other age groups. The Social Security Act of 1935 and its amendments provide many maternal-child health programs, which are discussed in Chapters 4 and 13. The Social Security Act also provides for Medicaid and Medicare, for which the medically indigent or terminally ill adult may qualify. The Public Health Service Act of 1944 and its amendments have helped to provide adult health care services. Health planning and environmental health legislation have also benefitted adult health (refer to Chapters 4 and 12).

A significant piece of legislation that specifically addresses the adult population is the Occupational Safety and Health Act of 1970, which is discussed in Chapter 16. It deals with maintaining the health of the adult in the workplace and focuses on maintaining wellness.

Senator Edward Kennedy has introduced an antismoking bill which would mandate a Center for Tobacco Products at the Centers for Disease Control; would create large scale, federal tobacco education programs; and would establish a new regulatory authority of tobacco products for the disclosure of additives and requirements of labeling (Kennedy introduces, 1990, p. 1). This would bring tobacco in line with the way other hazardous or dangerous products are regulated.

SOME CRISES OF ADULTHOOD AND NURSING INTERVENTION

Life comprises a series of *life change events* (refer to Table 6-6). The number, duration, and type of these events will vary with individuals. A life event that is major for one person may not be considered major for another.

Unlike young children, who have parents or others to support and guide them through the experience of life change events, the adult often does not have adequate support available during times of heightened stress or may not use the help that is available because dependency is feared. Our society emphasizes self-sufficiency during adulthood, and even a mature adult may experience feelings of insecurity when seeking assistance from others. Many adults must learn that *interdependency* is a mature state.

Examples of some life change events are leaving the parental home, obtaining job education and training, pursuing a career, marriage, childbearing, child rearing, child launching, providing for an aging parent, pursuing leisure-time activities, and experiencing the death of a parent. Life change events that are more or less expected usually evoke what could be termed *normative stress.* However, other life change events induce stress that goes beyond what could be considered normative, and may necessitate developing new interpersonal relationships, coping mechanisms, and resources. Examples of some of these life change events are divorce or separation, loss of a child, loss of a job, development of a chronic health condition, and career changes. If these events occur in rapid succession, the adult may have difficulty adapting and may experience crisis.

An example of what can happen when major life events occur in rapid succession is seen in the Stephen Johns case situation:

In a period of less than 14 years, Mr. Johns, now 32 years old, left home to enter college, completed a college education, entered a career, married, bought a house, had a child, changed jobs, moved to a new residence, became divorced, moved to another residence, changed jobs again, and experienced the death of a parent. These were all significant life events for Mr. Johns, and the rapid succession of their development left him in a confused and disorganized state. He was overwhelmed with his life and began to question whether it had meaning. Thus, he sought counseling through a local mental health clinic. Through work with a psychiatric nurse therapist, Mr. Johns was able to establish life goals and to take action to achieve these goals. This made him comfortable about himself as a person, and gave direction and meaning to his life. He began to recognize his own strengths and to work within and accept his limitations. He began to reach out to others and saw that interdependency can be therapeutic.

Mr. Johns is not atypical. Although major life events may not always be experienced this rapidly, or in this magnitude, many significant stresses do occur during adulthood. While experiencing these stresses, adults are also trying to achieve a balance between their responsibilities to family and society, to develop as individuals, and to maintain health. These tasks in themselves produce stress. Thus, when sudden or unexpected situational difficulties arise, such as divorce, death, or changes in job and residence, the individual is at risk for crisis.

It is important for the community health nurse to recognize that the crisis state may be experienced at any time throughout adult life. When mobilizing coping mechanisms during times of stress, the adult has many life experiences from which to draw. These experiences, however, do not necessarily prepare one to handle all the events that occur throughout adulthood. At each developmental stage there are new or different events requiring adaptation. The following quote from Knafl and Grace (1978, p. 265) vividly portrays the pressures one deals with during middlescence:

He (the middlescent) realizes that the choices of the past have limited his choices in the present. He can no longer dream of infinite possibilities. He is forced to acknowledge that he has worked up to or short of his capabilities. Goals may or may not have been reached; aspirations may have to be modified. The possibility for

advancement becomes more remote. He will have to go on with ever-brighter, ever-younger men and women crowding into competitive economic, political and social arenas. In the United States success is highly valued, and is measured by prestige, wealth or power. To be without these by middle age causes stress, and the likelihood of achieving them diminishes with age.

When working with the adult in crisis, it is important for the community health nurse to deal with the current realities of the situation. The individual should be helped to look at the circumstances that precipitated the crisis and modify them to reduce future occurrences. The nurse should be supportive of the client without leveling judgment, should help the client and family to assess the resources and support systems they have available, and make plans for the immediate future. As discussed in Chapter 7, the mastery of a crisis provides opportunities for personal growth and development.

A major goal of community health nursing practice in relation to crisis is prevention. In order to achieve this goal, the community health nurse must recognize early signs and symptoms of heightened stress (refer to Chapter 7) and must help individuals who are experiencing these symptoms to mobilize appropriate coping mechanisms.

The supports people utilize during crisis and time of need will vary. Emotional support, encouragement, assistance with problem solving, companionship, and tangible aid have been shown to be helpful to people who are dealing with a crisis. Individuals experiencing a crisis will look for care givers who provide these interventions (Figley and McCubbin, 1983, p. 11).

The following are some common crises of adulthood or situations that have gone beyond normative stress. Many of these crises can be resolved through supportive nursing intervention.

Depression

Depression is the most common, most treatable, and possibly the most painful of mental illnesses in the United States (Thompson, McFarland, Hirsch, Tucker, and Bowers, 1989, p. 1533). Depression in women is common between the ages of 25 and 44, and between 55 and 70 (National Mental Health Association [NMHA], 1988). Twenty-five percent of all women and 11.5 percent of all men will experience a depressive episode but only one third will seek treatment (NMHA, 1988). Research shows that depression is often recurrent.

Freud viewed depression as aggression turned inward. Depression has been described as chronic frustration stemming from environmental stresses in family, social, or work environments beyond the coping ability and resources of the client. Depression can result when stress is intensified. All persons experience times when they feel low or discouraged, but the depressed feelings are usually acute and self-limiting. Depression becomes a serious problem when it is chronic and affects the ability to cope with the events, roles, and responsibilities of daily living. Depression is often precipitated by a loss of some kind: a death or a separation or a loss of job, status, or health.

Some symptoms of depression include general sadness and despair, difficulty in making decisions, difficulty in carrying on a conversation, trouble concentrating, trouble sleeping, tiredness, listlessness, loss of appetite, eating binges, social regression, loss of or decreased libido, and decreased self-esteem. People who are depressed may be overly sensitive to what other people say or do, may be angry with others and not trust them, and may withdraw from others due to a fear of being among people.

Many causes have been linked to depression, but the etiology is often unknown. Genetic factors have been implicated in many studies, and the disorder has been found to be 1.5 to 3 times greater among first-degree biological relatives than in the general population (Thompson, McFarland, Hirsch, Tucker, and Bowers, 1989, p. 1533). Some studies indicate a biochemical imbalance, a factor over which the client has little control. Research has shown women are commonly at greater risk than men (Thompson, McFarland, Hirsch, Tucker, and Bowers, 1989, p. 1533). Other studies discuss psychosocial and maturational factors as determinants of depres-

sion. Chronic or severe medical conditions such as hypertension, multiple sclerosis, metabolic and chemical disorders, and systemic lupus erythematosus have been linked to depression. In fact, any chronic, painful, severe, or terminal condition has the potential to cause depression. Whatever the cause, depression is a painful experience for both clients and their families.

Depression has been directly associated with homicide, violent acts, and accidents. Suicide has been noted as a severe consequence of depression, and victims of depression account for 60 percent of all suicides (Depression, 1987, p. 48). The nurse must not overlook the fact that this is a possibility. Depression is associated with disruptions and stress in individual, family, and community life.

Persons who are depressed are often not aware that they are suffering from this condition. They know that they do not feel well and thus may seek medical help for minor physical problems. That is why it is so important for the community health nurse to systematically collect a complete health history (refer to Chapter 8) when working with adult clients. If data are collected only on the client's complaint about physical health, depression can be overlooked.

When working with clients who are depressed, the community health nurse should help to restructure their environment into one that is positive and hopeful. The depressed person should be given a chance to air complaints and grievances, and assistance which will help her or him to deal with problems. The nurse should remember that depressed persons may be angry at themselves or think that others have failed them. Attempts to help may be met with defensiveness, verbal abuse, and frustration. It may be difficult for them to develop a trusting relationship with another person. The client may need reassurance that he or she is cared about. The nurse should offer therapeutic support and understanding without fostering dependence. It is important to recognize that when a depressed client withdraws from the nurse-client interaction, it does not necessarily mean he or she does not want help. It probably means that the client is afraid to trust others or feels unworthy. People who are depressed find it hard to confide their innermost thoughts and feelings to another person and may need help and encouragement to talk things over.

Clients who are depressed are frequently unable to see any positive alternatives in their lives, and they dwell on their failures and weaknesses. It is critical that the nurse help the client to be objective and see alternatives to the current situation. Depressed clients can feel an intense sense of hopelessness. They feel immobilized, as if there were no solution to the situation. If persons can see that there are alternatives, the atmosphere of hopelessness is diluted.

When visiting depressed clients, the community health nurse needs to extend empathy without being sympathetic. Sympathy often serves to reinforce the person's depressed state. The nurse should encourage the client to be an active participant in the therapeutic process rather than a passive sufferer. The nurse must remember that the client may need support to be active, since it can be difficult for the person who is depressed to take action. Helping the client to recognize strengths and assets, instead of focusing on the negative aspects of the situation, frequently assists the client in assuming greater independence.

When working with depressed clients, maintaining a two-way communication between the client and nurse is essential. People who are depressed generally like feedback on what is going on, to know that someone has listened to them, and that someone is available for support and assistance. Unfortunately, all too often the depressed client is excluded from social contacts. Family, friends, and even professionals may isolate depressed clients in an attempt to protect the client from further hurt or stress. This social isolation serves to reinforce the client's feelings that no one cares.

Depressed individuals who are assessed to be potentially suicidal should be referred for psychotherapy. Some nurses are afraid to assess for suicide potential because they fear their questioning may precipitate a suicide attempt. Suicide is not prevented by avoiding conversation about it. Rather, it is prevented by helping clients get the assistance they need to deal with stresses in their daily lives.

Helping clients who are depressed can be discouraging because progress is often slow and the client may appear to resent assistance. The nurse may sometimes feel helpless, bewildered, and discouraged by the apparent lack of progress. The nurse needs to be aware of his or her feelings, and realize that these feelings are a normal response to the situation. The nurse will need to be a good and patient listener and help the client to see alternatives. When working with such clients, the nurse may find it helpful to talk with peers and supervisors about the feelings that he/she is experiencing and about alternatives for enhancing client action. Sometimes others who are not directly involved in the nurse-client interaction can be more objective about the situation and see alternatives.

Encountering clients who are depressed is common in community health nursing practice. At times, the client is able to resolve the depressed state by utilizing the supportive assistance of the community health nurse and significant others, such as family, friends, relatives, and lovers. At other times, additional mental health counseling is necessary. It should be remembered that depression will continue to exist until the individual is able to successfully mobilize coping mechanisms that enhance growth. Most chronic depressions are related to unresolved psychosocial difficulties. Crisis and normative stress are self-limiting; chronic depression is not.

Every six months, ten million Americans experience depression (NMHA, 1988). Unfortunately, only $10 per capita is spent on research for depressive disorders as compared with $161 for multiple sclerosis and $1000 for muscular dystrophy (NMHA, 1988). More research and research monies need to be invested in this important area of health.

The nurse can assist the client in community resource utilization such as community mental health centers and self-help groups. Other sources of information and referral for the client and family are groups such as the Foundation for Depressive Illness (1-800-248-4344), and the National

Mental Health Association (1-703-684-7722). On the federal level, the National Institute of Mental Health is charged with improving the understanding, treatment, and rehabilitation of the mentally ill; preventing mental illness and fostering the mental health of the people. NIMH is heavily involved in prevention activities. It sponsors Project D/ART (Depression/Awareness, Recognition and Treatment). Project D/ART is concerned with ameliorating the public health problem of depression and aims to improve the identification, assessment, treatment, and clinical management of depressive disorders through an educational program focused on the general public, primary care providers, and mental health specialists. Project D/ART is involved with many voluntary and professional organizations and provides information and materials for the general public as well as professional audiences. NIMH can be contacted at 1-301-443-4515.

Alcoholism

Alcoholism is the largest drug problem in the United States today; some 10 percent of the adult population has a chronic, heavy intake of alcoholic beverages (Williams, Stinson, Parker, Harford, and Noble, 1987, p. 81). Nearly 10.5 million adults show symptoms of alcoholism and 7.2 million are alcohol abusers. Seventy percent of 12- to 17-year-old youths have used alcohol (USDHHS, 1987, Prevention '86/'87, p. 40), and an estimated 4.6 million teenagers have serious alcohol problems (USDHHS, 1987, Prevention '86/'87, p. 61). The per capita consumption is above 2.65 gallons of alcohol for every resident above the age of 14 years—up from 2.25 gallons in 1945 (USDHHS, 1987, Prevention '86/'87, p. 41). Cirrhosis is the ninth leading cause of death among adults, and as many as 90 percent of cases are associated with excessive use of alcohol (USDHHS, 1987, Prevention '86/'87, p. 40). Nearly one half of all traffic deaths are alcohol related, fetal exposure to alcohol is the leading cause of mental retardation, and alcohol abuse and dependency cost the United States more than $136 billion in 1989 (Sperling, 1990, p. D1).

Besides contributing to cirrhosis of the liver, alcoholism contributes to such health problems as nutritional deficiencies, pancreatitis, and cancer. It is a factor in other leading causes of adult deaths including accidents, suicides, and homicides. Studies show that careless handling of smoking materials by intoxicated persons is dangerous and contributes to substantial numbers of burn injuries, death, and property damage.

The psychosocial consequences of alcoholism are immense. Such consequences include disruption of family life, loss of on-the-job productivity, and lowered self-esteem. The families of alcoholics are victims of alcoholism themselves.

The adverse effects of alcohol on fetal development has been a health concern for more than 250 years (Anderson and Grant, 1984, p. 3). The infants of mothers who consume large amounts of alcohol suffer from low birth weight, birth defects, and/or mental retardation (USDHHS, 1983, Health, p. 19). The terms *fetal alcohol syndrome* and *alcohol-related birth defects* are often seen in the literature. However, public awareness of these conditions is still limited (Anderson and Grant, 1984, p. 6). Unfortunately, the number of American women who drink heavily, especially in the childbearing years, is on the rise (McCarthy, 1983, p. 33). Women of childbearing years, and especially pregnant women, need to know the effects of drinking on their fetuses. The nurse's health history should include questions about drinking habits. However, adequate answers are not always provided when this question is asked. Thus, the nurse should observe for signs and symptoms of increased alcohol consumption during pregnancy. This, coupled with information on alcohol and pregnancy that should be shared with every expectant mother, may help to cut down on alcohol abuse during pregnancy. Alcohol abuse includes both chronic drinking and binge drinking: Studies have shown that binge drinking can have disastrous effects.

Passive intervention measures such as the use of flame retardant fabrics and smoke detectors, identification and reduction of stairway hazards, sanctions against the sale and use of alcohol, sanctions against drunk drivers, and greater alcohol intoxication screening in health care settings and at work can all help. Former Surgeon General C. Everett Koop recommended a massive increase of alcohol-related public service ads to match the number of beer, wine, and spirit ads; an increase in the federal excise tax on liquor as well as a state tax to be used for education programs; elimination of "happy hours" and drink discounts; an end to alcohol ads that use celebrities and ads that appear on college campuses; a halt to liquor makers sponsoring sports events, rock concerts, and other programs where the majority of the audience is under age 21; an immediate reduction in the legal blood-alcohol level for motorists to 0.08 percent and a further reduction to 0.04 percent by the year 2000 (Cox, 1989). These suggestions by the Surgeon General were considered drastic, did not meet with overwhelming support from the liquor industry, and have not been acted on to any degree. Although these measures would help to curb alcoholism in the United States, most of them are passive and do not involve the person who has an alcohol-related problem. Such measures, coupled with those in which the person is actively involved in treatment, are necessary.

Self-help groups such as Alcoholics Anonymous, Children of Alcoholics, and counseling services are available for alcoholics and their families. The National Council on Alcoholism (1-800-NCA-CALL) is a voluntary organization that offers information and referral services. Many places of work have alcoholism programs or work closely with community programs. The community health nurse can carry out health education activities, offer support, remain nonjudgmental, and encourage the client to use available resources.

The National Institute on Alcohol Abuse and Alcoholism (NIAAA) provides a national focus to increase knowledge and promote effective strategies to deal with the health and psychosocial problems associated with alcoholism. The NIAAA sponsors extensive research programs, much of which is targeted at prevention. NIAAA programs include youth awareness, fetal alcohol awareness, and national drunk driving awareness, among others. The National Clearinghouse on Alcohol and Drug Abuse (1-301-468-2600) offers information, educational materials, and referral resources.

Changing Jobs or Careers

The case situations on the worker role presented earlier in the chapter illustrate that making a decision to alter one's work role can result in crisis and indecision. During this time, a major reorganization is required in one's life and the stresses encountered should not be underestimated. This is particularly true if changing a job or a career was not a voluntary decision, such as when a person is fired or laid off from a job. However, even if the decision was a voluntary one, it still may not have consensus within the family.

The adult's and his or her family's perceptions of the situation should be ascertained. Does the individual see it as a new and challenging adventure or as a threat to personal and economic security? The community health nurse should be especially sensitive to the distresses that can occur when an individual is changing jobs or careers, since this is becoming a frequent occurrence in our society. Change is not always easy. It can result in a more satisfying life or it can result in dissatisfaction, depending on how the client views what is happening. Support or encouragement can facilitate individual growth and development and make the change more rewarding. Referral to outside counseling agencies, vocational rehabilitation, or employment service agencies may be necessary.

Unemployment

Unemployment is common in contemporary America; millions of people are out of work annually. It appears that no one is exempt from unemployment; the situation can create a devastating situation for a family.

Families experiencing unemployment may at first draw closer to work on common goals, but tension usually mounts as work responsibilities are redistributed, roles are altered, and family goals are modified (Kaforey, 1984). Role reversal between husband and wife may occur, and there is an increased frequency of marital disruption and role conflict (Moen, 1983). Unemployment can cause increased family violence, instability, and economic deprivation (Voyanoff, 1983).

Social stigma attaches to unemployment, because society does not sanction it. The unemployed family tends to become socially isolated; suffering from shock, shame, and altered self-esteem and lifestyle, the unemployed family tends to withdraw socially (Hill, 1978). Social isolation is not helpful and can produce more stress for the family; it should be minimized whenever possible.

The unemployed person and family are psychologically vulnerable. The unemployed worker may evidence lowered self-esteem, anxiety, apathy, decreased appetite, inertia, feelings of helplessness, and suffer from a variety of psychosomatic conditions (Swineburne, 1981; Krystal, Moran-Sackett, and Cantoni, 1983). Madonia (1983) found that approximately 80 percent of unemployed respondents stated that they were more frustrated then than when they were employed, and 70 percent stated that they were frequently agitated and experienced tension. Moreover, the children of the unemployed have shown symptoms of increased stress (Krystal, Moran-Sackett, and Cantoni, 1983). Such families need help working through these feelings. They have suffered a loss; they need to be able to recognize the validity of their loss and be able to grieve for it (Krystal, Stickney, and Thompson, 1983; Hill, 1978).

Unemployment generates stress that can cause health problems. People who are unemployed often do not feel well physically (Kasl, Gore, and Cobb, 1975; Madonia, 1983). The unemployed worker is likely to present with physical symptoms such as chest pains, shortness of breath, dizziness, dry mouth, eczema, weakness, and inability to sleep (Krystal, Moran-Sackett, and Cantoni, 1983). Children of the unemployed experience a higher rate of illness than other children (Margolis and Farran, 1981). People who are unemployed are often unable to afford health care services.

The community health nurse should recognize that unemployment is a major crisis physically, socially, emotionally, and financially. The nurse should help unemployed families to be aware of what is happening and encourage them to utilize appropriate community resources. Although unemployment necessitates family adjustment, change, and adaptation, the stress experienced can be minimized, and positive growth can occur.

Chronic Illness

Chronic illness is a major health problem in the American population (refer to Chapters 10 and 17). Illness for the individual or family is a normal part of the life cycle. We all expect at some point in time to have a case of the flu, a cold, or even minor surgery. Acute, nondisabling illness can often be handled by normal resources and coping mechanisms. It does not involve major lifestyle adaptation. If the illness becomes chronic, disabling, or terminal, however, the family situation can become quite stressful.

When the adult is afflicted with a chronic health condition, major life changes and hardships can occur. These hardships can include strained family relationships, modifications in family activities and goals, increased health care tasks and time constraints, increased financial stress, need for housing adaptation, social isolation, medical concerns, and grieving (Figley and McCubbin, 1983, pp. 25-26.) The individual and family may also demonstrate changes in work, school, and community experiences as a result of the illness.

The extent to which life-style changes occur during chronic illness varies, depending on the degree of disability encountered and the adult's perception of the event. Role reversal, changes in sexual behavior, and alterations in self-image are a few examples of the problems experienced by clients who have developed debilitating chronic illness during adulthood. The adult who is not progressing well along the developmental continuum may regress, become depressed, or become dependent when chronically ill. He or she may resist treatment and techniques to make recovery faster, or become self-absorbed, not relate to others well, and use the illness as an escape from responsibility.

Community health nurses must understand the difficulties encountered when one is chronically ill before they can effectively work with clients and families who are experiencing the effects of a chronic condition. The nurse should help the well-adjusted adult to resume as normal a level of independence and functioning as possible and provide the support and encouragement needed for the individual to do so. The nurse can assist the client and family by making them aware of the medical course of the client's condition, giving anticipatory guidance, and encouraging them to take an active role in health care decision making.

It is important for the community health nurse to maintain a therapeutic role with the chronically ill adult. It is easy for the nurse to fall into a pattern of encouraging clients to meet societal expectations of self-sufficiency, minimal dependency, and generativity. The nurse can help the chronically ill adult accept the interdependency needed to deal successfully with his or her condition. The nurse should not make unrealistic promises of recovery or an optimistic prognosis if this is not the case. There may be no guarantee that treatment will improve the level of disability. False hopes prevent the client from confronting and working through the crisis.

Use of both the educative and problem-solving approaches to nursing intervention is essential when one is working with families who are dealing with a chronic condition. These families frequently need increased knowledge to realistically evaluate the changes which are occurring and which may occur. These families also need to problem-solve in order to determine the most appropriate ways for them to adapt to changes, especially permanent ones. Chronic illness can be both emotionally and financially draining. Different coping mechanisms and resources must be mobilized to reduce tension and to maintain financial stability. The possibility of death may also be a matter for the nurse to work through with chronically ill adults and their families. Families should be encouraged to express their fears and, if the client's situation warrants it, to prepare for death. Reading materials written by Kübler-Ross (1974, 1975) can enhance a community health nurse's skill in working with clients who are dying.

The hospice care movement is gaining popu-larity in this country. Hospice care is designed to keep the chronically ill person who is terminal at home as long as possible. It is a cost-effective and humane method of health care. A family-centered, multidisciplinary approach is followed, with an emphasis placed on improving the quality of life for both the client and the client's family during the final stages of dying. Community health nurses are regular participants on this interdisciplinary team, and thus they must be prepared to deal with the concerns of dying clients and their families. It is becoming increasingly important for community health nurses to be skilled at caring for this group of people (refer to Chapter 19).

When working with any chronically ill adult, the community health nurse will more than likely utilize the referral process. There are a variety of community resources, such as the Lost Chord Club, the Multiple Sclerosis Association, the Cancer Society, Goodwill Industries, the division of vocational rehabilitation, and the department of social services, which will help clients and their families to adapt to chronic illness. It is critical, when working with clients who are chronically ill, for the community health nurse to know about resources that will help the client with his or her rehabilitation process.

Homelessness

Homelessness is a critical problem in America today, and one with which nurses are becoming increasingly involved. The days when a homeless person was an older, male alcoholic are gone. Entire families are now part of the homeless population. It is estimated that there are as many as 2 to 3 million homeless people in the United States (Lindsey, 1989, p. 78; Bowdler, 1989). Demographics on the homeless show that their average age is 35 to 40 years; at least one half are nonwhite; approximately one fourth are female; and approximately one third have a high school education (Bowdler and Barrell, 1987, p. 135). The homeless population is becoming ever younger, with more and more children being included in this group. Up to 90 percent of the homeless have a diagnosable mental illness (Bowdler, 1989).

New York City alone houses almost 10,000 individuals and 5000 families each night, with an annual budget of over $312 million (Lindsey, 1989, p. 78). Most homeless individuals have no regular source of health care, and the majority are without health insurance (Robertson and Cousineau, 1986, p. 561). There is a great need to enhance the mental health resources available to the homeless.

The health problems of the homeless are enormous. The transient nature of their lives makes it difficult for them to obtain regular health care and adequate treatment for health conditions. Even when they do find health care it is difficult for them to access it because of financial constraints. Giving a person who is homeless a prescription for medicine may not be helpful as the person may not have access to resources to fill it. It may be a better idea to give the person the necessary medication. Clinic facilities located in homeless shelters and areas with high rates of homelessness are often effective in helping to meet health care needs. Such a clinic could be a nurse-run clinic with appropriate referrals being made to community agencies.

People who are homeless have a high prevalence of physical problems, mental disorders, substance abuse, and infectious/parasitic diseases (Bowdler and Barrell, 1987, p. 135). They are nearly constantly exposed to the elements; experience overcrowding and unsanitary conditions; have high rates of alcoholism, hypertension, drug abuse, trauma, and mental illness; are more susceptible to communicable diseases and conditions such as tuberculosis, influenza, scabies, lice, and pneumonia; and suffer from a variety of nutritional deficiencies (With neither, 1989, pp. 21, 31). Homeless children may not receive the necessary immunizations, putting them at increased risk of serious communicable disease.

Peripheral vascular disease is common among homeless people who have been on the streets for long periods of time. This occurs because they stand for extended periods, which causes gravitational and mechanical obstruction to the deep venous system and increases venous pressure (With neither, 1989, p. 31).

The social implications of homelessness are enormous. Homeless people are often isolated from the mainstream of society. Children do not have regular schooling or friends. Families find themselves without the necessary support or resources to cope with even minor problems and difficulties.

Many groups and organizations have sponsored fund raising efforts and benefits to aid the plight of the homeless. Comic Relief has consistently raised funds. Not long ago a Notre Dame–Louisiana State basketball game raised money in excess of $100,000. Efforts like this are going on all over the country, yet voluntary efforts are not enough.

Knowing that something needed to be done on a national level, the Stewart B. McKinney Homeless Assistance Act (Public Law 100-77) was enacted to help meet the needs of the homeless population. The act provides urgently needed assistance to protect and improve the lives and safety of the homeless, with special emphasis on elderly, handicapped persons and families with children. It established the Interagency Council on the Homeless and numerous grant programs. The act authorized emergency food, emergency shelter, supportive housing, programs for primary health care, substance abuse services, community mental health care, adult education, education for children and youth, job training, and studies of homelessness.

Community health centers, federally supported by Section 330 of the Public Health Service Act, are emerging to assist disadvantaged populations. The purpose of these centers is to provide high quality, *managed* care for those people who are most likely to lack access to health services because of geographic isolation or financial barriers (National Association of Community Health Centers, Inc., 1986, p. 1). More than 600 such centers are active. They serve over 5 million people, of whom 60 percent are female, 64 percent are members of a minority group, 45 percent are children, and 60 percent have incomes under the poverty level (National Association of Community Health Centers, Inc., 1986, p. 1).

With the homeless evidencing increased physical health and mental health problems, the need for appropriate nursing service is critical. Nurses can help to decrease the incidence of communicable disease through immunizations, encouraging and promoting sanitary practices, helping clients to find regular sources of health care, and promoting the use of shelter-based, nurse-run clinics. Nurses can help to refer clients to appropriate resources in the community and can serve as client advocates. They can help to coordinate the many loose ends that seem to occur with health care for the homeless, and serve as a focal point for other health professionals involved with the client and family. There are no easy answers to the health care problems of the homeless. However, the nurse should be aware of their plight and respond to this contemporary health care issue.

Acquired Immune Deficiency Syndrome (AIDS): United States

AIDS has been classified as the number one priority of the U.S. Public Health Service. AIDS is a serious disease characterized by a defect in natural immunity which causes increased susceptibility to disease. There have been no cases of AIDS in which this lost natural immunity has been regained.

AIDS was first seen in this country in 1979, and the first cases were documented in 1981. All races and ethnic groups have been affected, and the age range is mainly 25 to 44 years. Approximately 2500 children have been diagnosed as having AIDS. Since it was first documented there have been more than 146,700 cases diagnosed in the United States (CDC, 1990, September, p. 5) and the number rises daily. An epidemiological summary of AIDS is presented in Table 15-8.

AIDS cases have been reported in all 50 states, the District of Columbia, and the four U.S. territories. California and New York have the highest incidence of AIDS; at this writing New York City alone has reported more than 22,665 cases. The distribution of AIDS in the United States is given in Figure 15-3. It is projected that 270,000 cases of AIDS cases will be diagnosed and reported to the CDC by the end of 1991, and that by the end of 1992 the number will be 365,000 (CDC, 1989, AIDS and human, p. 5). Of the 117,781 documented cases of AIDS there have been 70,313 deaths, yielding a case fatality rate of close to 60% (CDC, 1990, January, HIV/AIDS, p. 18). However, AIDS patients are now living longer; they have an average 12-month survival rate after being diagnosed. Drugs such as AZT (approved by the FDA for use in patients with AIDS in 1987) may prolong life; the long-term effect of new therapies on survival rates is not yet available.

The human immunodeficiency virus (HIV) responsible for AIDS was isolated in 1984. More recent information indicates that the virus is more complex than originally thought, and that the body's immune system becomes impaired soon after a person is infected (Hellinger, 1988, Forecasting, p. 309). AIDS cases are reported to the CDC based on a uniform case definition and case report form. The definition of AIDS was broadened in 1987 to incorporate a broader range of AIDS indicator diseases and conditions; the HIV diagnostic tests are used to improve the sensitivity and specificity of the diagnosis (CDC, 1989, HIV/AIDS, p. 15).

The time between infection with the AIDS virus and the onset of symptoms ranges from 6 months to 5 years or more. It appears that infection with the virus may not always lead to AIDS. About 78 percent of AIDS patients have one or both of two rare diseases: *pneumocystis carinii* pneumonia (PCP), a parasitic infection of the lungs; and a type of cancer known as Kaposi's sarcoma (KS) (USDHHS, 1987, Facts about AIDS, p. 4). Other opportunistic infections include unusually severe yeast infections, cytomegalovirus, herpesvirus, and parasitism. The early signs and symptoms of AIDS are similar to those of a cold or flu and include fever, shaking, night sweats, enlarged lymph nodes, unexplained weight loss, yeast infections, persistent cough, persistent diarrhea, fatigue, and loss of appetite.

Universal AIDS precautions were given in Appendix 10-1. Some precautions to prevent the spread of AIDS are the following:

TABLE 15-8 An epidemiological summary of AIDS

What is AIDS?	AIDS is a serious health condition characterized by a loss of, or defect in, a person's natural immunity against disease.
Scope	More than 146,700 cases in the United States since 1979 (approximately 2,500 cases are children).
	Almost a 60% case fatality rate to date among known cases.
Etiologic agent	A virus called human T-lymphotropic virus, type III (HTLV-III). Infection with this virus does not always lead to AIDS. Incubation period range: 6 mo. to 5 yrs.+
Symptoms	Often resemble the flu or a cold. A person may complain of tiredness, fever, loss of weight, loss of appetite, diarrhea, night sweats, and swollen glands. Many AIDS patients will develop one or both of two rare, opportunistic diseases: *Pneumocystis carinii* pneumonia (PCP) or Kaposi's sarcoma (KS).
Who has AIDS?*	90% of all AIDS patients are men, between 20 and 49 years old. AIDS patients fall into the following groups:
	1. Male homosexual and bisexual contacts with multiple sex partners (58%)
	2. IV drug users (18%)
	3. Persons with hemophilia or other coagulation disorders (1%)
	4. Heterosexual contacts of someone with AIDS or at risk for AIDS (5%)
	5. Persons who have had transfusions with blood or blood products (2%)
	6. Infants born to infected mothers (1%)
	7. Unknown etiology (3%)
	There has been no significant change over time in the distribution of AIDS by sex, age, or race (patients = 62% white, 25% black, and 14% Hispanic).
Diagnostic test	A blood test *has been* developed to test for antibodies to HTLV-III. Although a positive test does not indicate that the person has an active case of AIDS, the test provides a good screening mechanism. Antibody testing of donated blood and plasma is also done.
Transmission	AIDS appears to be transmitted by intimate sexual contact or by percutaneous inoculation of blood or blood products and by perinatal transmission. There has been no evidence of transmission by casual contact or airborne spread. Precautions for the general public and for health care personnel have been published by the Centers for Disease Control.
Treatment	Currently there are *no* antiviral drugs available that have been proven to cure AIDS. *No* treatment has been successful in restoring the immune system of an AIDS patient. There is no vaccine available.

*Percentages vary when adjusted for age; percentges are for AIDS cases with a single mode of exposure and thus do not equal 100 percent.

From US Department of Health and Human Services: Facts about AIDS, Washington, DC, 1987, US Government Printing Office; Centers for Disease Control: AIDS and human immunodeficiency virus infection in the United States: 1988 update, MMWR, 38(5-4):1-38, May 12, 1989; Centers for Disease Control: HIV/AIDS surveillance report, Atlanta, Ga, September 1990, The Centers, pp 1-18.

1. Do not have sexual contact with persons known or suspected to have AIDS.
2. Do not have sex with multiple partners or with persons who have had multiple partners.
3. If you are a health worker, use extreme caution when handling or disposing of hypodermic needles and when handling blood products.
4. Do not abuse IV drugs. If you use IV drugs do not share needles or syringes (boiling does not guarantee sterility).
5. Do not have sex with people who abuse IV drugs.
6. Practice "safe sex," in which no exchange of body fluids takes place and no contact is made with body fluids, especially contact with mucous membranes (i.e., use condoms, avoid oral-genital contact, avoid open mouth intimate kissing).

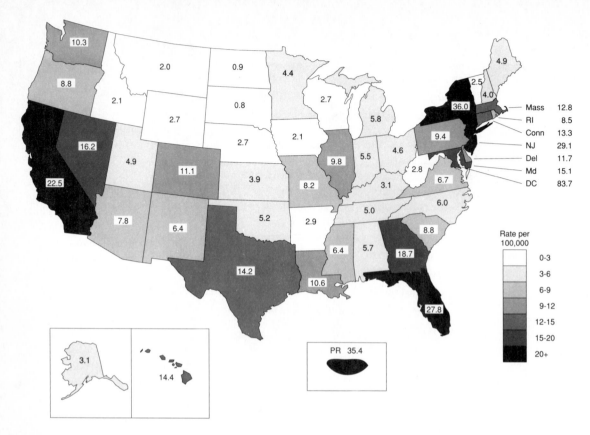

Figure 15-3 AIDS annual incidence rates per 100,000 population for cases reported November 1988 through October 1989, United States. (From Centers for Disease Control: HIV/AIDS surveillance. AIDS cases reported through October 1989, Atlanta, Ga, 1989, CDC, p 3.)

Based on estimates of a lifetime cost of treating an AIDS patient at $60,000, the cumulative lifetime medical care costs of treating all AIDS patients will be about $4.7 billion in 1990, $6 billion in 1991, and $7.5 billion in 1992 (Hellinger, 1988, National forecast, p. 469). This cost is less than had been projected in earlier years because health care professionals have learned how to treat patients more efficiently, and because numerous coordinated systems of care have been developed that depend less on hospital-based service and more on community-based service. It is difficult to predict whether technologic advances will decrease or increase future cost of lifetime treatment.

These lifetime costs do not take into consideration the social pain, grief, and suffering experienced by AIDS patients, their friends, and fami-

lies. AIDS victims are suffering from a serious disease, but they are also people with human needs. In working with AIDS victims, their families, and the community the nurse must draw from theory related to chronic illness, death, and stress. The nurse must realize that there is a fear of AIDS among the general public, a lack of public knowledge about AIDS, and a social stigma attached to it. AIDS victims will likely be in need of many health and social services, and at the same time may be unable to obtain them. It is important for these patients to know that the heatlh care system has not abandoned them and is responsive to their needs. Health education programs and community resources need to be developed for victims of AIDS, their families, and the community. People need to be educated about AIDS.

Education and information can play an important role not only in prevention, but also in helping people to understand the disease. A National Health Interview Survey was carried out in August 1987 to assess AIDS knowledge in the general population and again in August of 1988. The results showed an increase in knowledge among the public. For instance, over this period the percentage of adults who understood that AIDS was caused by a virus rose from 44 percent to 64 percent, the percentage stating that a pregnant woman can transmit HIV to her baby increased from 69 percent to 80 percent, and the percentage that knew there was no vaccine against AIDS increased from 65 percent to 76 percent (CDC, 1989, HIV epidemic, p. 354). At the same time, the percentage of adults stating they knew "a lot" about AIDS increased only from 20 percent to 22 percent. A substantial increase occurred in the percentage of adults who knew that the AIDS virus could not be transmitted through casual contacts. Figure 15-4 shows the percentage of adults who responded correctly to selected questions on the 1987 and 1988 National Health Interview Survey.

The community health nurse can be very helpful in educating people about AIDS. The National League for Nursing has developed the *Caring for Persons with AIDS Test* to assist nurses in learning more about AIDS. This test is intended for nurses working in hospitals, long-term care facilities, home health agencies, and schools of nursing to measure the nurse's knowledge and ability to apply basic principles in AIDS patient care (NLN, 1989, p. 563). For more information about this test the National League for Nursing can be contacted at 1-800-NOW-1-NLN, and in New York City at 1-212-989-9393.

The National Center for Nursing Research of the National Institutes of Health has awarded monies to promote research in nursing care of persons with AIDS (Research Reporter, 1989, p. 24). There are also resources at the federal level for AIDS education and information. The Centers for Disease Control oversees the National AIDS Information Hotline (1-800-342-AIDS), which offers information and answers questions; and the National AIDS Information Clearinghouse (1-800-458-5231), which provides many of

the same services as the Hotline but also is a direct source of free, government-approved educational materials such as brochures, posters, and displays. Orders for bulk quantities or single copies of publications can be placed through the Clearinghouse's toll-free number. The Centers for Disease Control can be called for AIDS statistics at 1-404-330-3020. There are often community support groups available for the AIDS client.

Marital Crises

It is not uncommon for the community health nurse to encounter families who are experiencing some form of marital crisis. The forms discussed here are disenchantment, separation and divorce, and family violence.

Disenchantment, Separation, and Divorce

The divorce rate has increased dramatically in the past three decades. Between 1965 and 1980, the rate more than doubled. Although the upsurge in divorce has occurred among adults of all ages, it has been greatest among those under 45 years of age (Glick and Lin, 1986). Whereas there is some evidence to suggest that this trend is slowing down, marital crisis is still a major life stress for the adult population group. Between 1980 and 1988, the number of one-parent situations increased by 2.4 million (U.S. Bureau of the Census, 1989). Reasons for this increase were divorce and separation, as well as a rise in the number of never-married parents.

Marital disenchantment, separation, and divorce occur throughout adulthood and should not be considered a problem of youth alone. During middlescence, for instance, spouses find that they have more time together, and if they are unable to reestablish intimacy or reinforce it, they may become disenchanted with their marital relationship. In addition, the sexual changes (menopause and climacteric) that occur during middlescence can also adversely affect the way in which spouses relate in the marital relationship.

Disenchantment, separation, and divorce have an impact on all family members. Adults as well as children need to make major changes. Experiencing feelings of uncertainty, betrayal, insecurity, failure, and loss is common during this time.

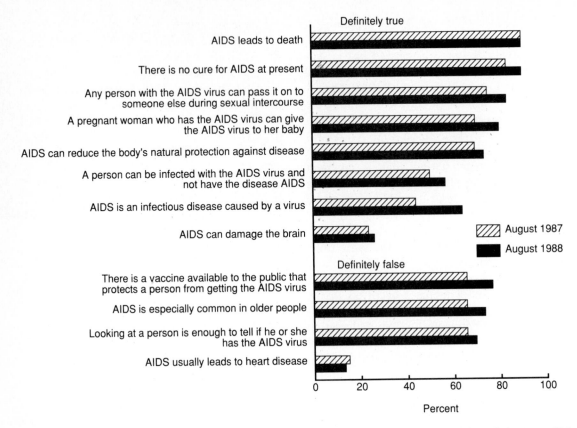

Figure 15-4 Provisional estimates of percentages of adults responding correctly to selected AIDS knowledge items, United States, August 1987 and August 1988. (From National Center for Health Statistics, Division of Health Interview Statistics: National Health Interview Survey, MMWR, 38(S-2), May 26, 356, 1989.)

As with all crises, the primary focus of the community health nurse with clients who are experiencing marital stress is on helping them to achieve homeostasis and growth. Adaptation could require divorce or separation, but it also may occur through renegotiation and alteration of family patterns which are dysfunctional. A therapeutic approach that encourages problem solving rather than blaming can best facilitate successful adaptation during this time of crisis.

Anticipatory guidance activities by the community health nurse may be instrumental in preventing marital crises. Preparing young adults to handle the stresses of parenthood or middlescent couples to deal with the conflicts during launch-

ing, for instance, may decrease the amount of distress experienced at these times.

Helping adults handle life crises such as those described above can be rewarding as well as challenging. Confusion, crisis, stress, and depression are all normal parts of life. If the adult has a supportive environment and assistance from others, he or she is better able to achieve health. Community health nurses are often in a favorable position to provide the extra assistance needed to adapt and grow during times of crisis and stress.

Domestic Violence

Domestic violence is not a normal situation, and it requires professional help. It involves battering as well as verbal/emotional abuse (National Coalition Against Domestic Violence [NCADV], 1989, What is; NCADV, 1989, On verbal/emotional). Battering often includes an attack by one spouse on another—pushing, slapping, punching, kicking, knifing, shooting, or throwing an object—with intent to do bodily harm. Both men and women are victims of domestic violence, but the more frequently and seriously injured are women.

Domestic violence has serious ramifications for the individual, family, and community. It can result in physical and emotional injury, death, temporary or permanent separation of families, and financial hardship. U.S. statistics about domestic violence reflect its overwhelming scope:

- Over 50 percent of all women will experience physical violence during the course of an intimate relationship, and in 24 to 30 percent of these women battering will occur regularly (NCADV, 1989, What is).
- Every 15 seconds the crime of battering occurs (NCADV, 1989, What is), and it is the single largest cause of injury to women in the United States (NCADV, 1988).
- In 50 percent or more marriages, there has been at least one incident of battering or assault on the woman (Drake, 1982, p. 40).
- A National Crime Survey found that, over a 12-month period, at least 2.1 million married, divorced, or separated women were victims of rape, robbery, aggravated or simple assault by their partners; and that 32 percent of these women were victimized more than once (NCADV, 1988). Estimates of battering range as high as 3 to 4 million women annually.
- In 1986, 30 percent of female homicide victims were killed by their husbands or boyfriends (NCADV, 1988).
- In 36 states, under many circumstances it is legal for a husband to rape his wife (NCADV, 1988).

Although assault and assault with intent to commit murder are crimes, police agencies hesitate to get involved in situations involving domestic violence. Frequently, police departments do not have uniform reporting procedures for domestic violence, and thus, cases of domestic violence are not reported to the police. Police may treat domestic violence as more of a social problem than a criminal one. Police follow-up of incidents of domestic violence account for a high percentage of deaths and injuries to police officers.

There are no stereotypes of battered wives; they come from all educational, social, and economic backgrounds. Some characteristics that have been observed with consistency include an early exposure to violence as a child, economic dependence on one's husband, lack of awareness of alternatives, poor self-image, and inadequate support systems. Oftentimes friends and relatives of the battered woman find it easier to ignore the situation or even sanction the abuse. The battered wife may be kept from contact with others who could provide help. She may be depressed and may frequently mention minor somatic complaints when seen by health care personnel, and may or may not show obvious signs of physical injury. She often believes that her husband will reform if she can just "wait it out."

The abusive spouse may be characterized as angry, resentful, suspicious, jealous, tense, insecure, moody, and a "loser" (National Mental Health Association, 1988). He often feels guilty and remorseful following an episode of abuse, and things may calm down for awhile. However, it does not take much to trigger a new episode of abuse. In fact, the abuse is very likely to occur again, and it may become more severe. A violent relationship can easily go on to become a violent system.

There are concrete linkages between battered wives and battered children (NCADV, 1988). Where one is occurring, community health nurses should look for the other. Children who have seen their parents use violence are more likely to use violence themselves as adults (Drake, 1982, p. 41). This supports the theory that abusive behavior is largely learned behavior. Female children who have been involved in domestic violence during their early years have a three times greater chance than other women of being abused or battered within their marital relationship (Drake, 1982, p. 41).

The dysfunctional patterns of the violent marriage impair the ability of the parents to meet the developmental and emotional needs of their children (Elbow, 1982, p. 465). Social and emotional development is delayed in as many as 70 percent of the children who come from families in whom domestic violence is occurring (Viken, 1982, p. 115).

When a family is involved in domestic violence, it is often difficult to be objective and not take sides in the matter. The family needs help to resolve the dysfunctional situation. Conjoint therapy between the abusive and abused spouse may be very helpful, if it is possible to get them to participate. During conjoint therapy, the couple can be encouraged to look at the management of stress and anger, positive ways to express anger, problem-solving techniques, the development of positive interactions and values, unrealistic expectations, and jealousy reactions (Taylor, 1984, p. 18). Taylor (1984) believes that the abuser role and the victim role grow in power and intensity over time, that stress and anger are closely interrelated within violent systems, that these stress and anger cycles can be interrupted, and that abusive systems create and are sustained by negative interactions and attitudes. Conjoint therapy facilitates working on these problem areas.

In situations of domestic violence, health care providers often seem to be more comfortable accepting spurious explanations or not getting involved than in probing for the truth (Drake, 1982, p. 40). The family needs help. The community health nurse is in a unique position to see the family at home, and may be the first to observe an abusive relationship. The nurse can help clients to look at the situation, and to see alternatives to their current lifestyle. This usually involves examining available community resources for both immediate and long-term assistance. Counseling services, shelters for battered women and their children, self-help programs, job training, and financial assistance are a few of the community services available to help domestic violence victims. Community health nurses provide supportive as-

sistance when the client is utilizing these community services. Community health nurses also facilitate comprehensive, ongoing care that is coordinated with other community groups and agencies, refer clients to safe houses, and serve as client advocates.

There are over 1400 shelters and safe homes for battered women servicing more than 375,000 women and children (NCADV, 1989, Statistics from). Increasingly, community health nurses are providing valuable services in shelters for battered women and their children. They complete health assessments, make appropriate referrals to community resources, provide health counseling, conduct group health education sessions, and provide consultation to the shelter staff relative to the health aspects of operating a group home. In this type of setting, community health nurses are active members of an interdisciplinary team and provide a unique perspective to the delivery of comprehensive health care. Their focus on preventive as well as curative services enhances the care provided to this population group. Because of the complex dynamics related to family violence, confidentiality in regard to the location of shelters for battered victims is maintained by health professionals throughout the community.

The nurse needs to be aware of these resources and refer families to them. Unfortunately, more than 40 percent of battered women and their children who need emergency housing are denied immediate shelter because of a lack of space (NCADV, 1989, Statistics from). Across the country domestic violence hotlines receive more than 2 million phone calls yearly, and the toll-free National Domestic Violence Hotline (1-800-333-SAFE) receives an average of 5000 calls every month (NCADV, 1989, Statistics from). The hotline is staffed 24 hours every day by people who respond to requests for information, discuss options, and provide shelter referrals. The National Coalition against Domestic Violence in Washington, D.C. (1-202-638-6388) is an excellent source of information and referral.

The Nursing Network on Violence against Women (NNVAW) was founded in 1985 during the first National Nursing Conference on Violence against Women, held at the University of Massachusetts at Amherst. The ultimate goal of NNVAW is to provide a nursing presence in the struggle to end violence in women's lives. NNVAW writes a quarterly column for *Response: To the Victimization of Women and Children,* a journal founded by and associated with the Center for Women's Policy Studies in Washington, DC. NNVAW can be contacted by writing NNVAW, Dr. Karen Landenburger, University of Washington, School of Nursing SC-74, Seattle, Washington 98195. A book written specifically for nurses on family violence is *Nursing Care of Victims of Family Violence* (1984) by Campbell and Humphreys. This book is an excellent resource for nurses.

SUMMARY

The adult is a significant member of our population and one who is often overlooked as having health needs. Adults who financially and emotionally support other age groups are vulnerable to some unique pressures and stresses. It is often hard for them to admit that they have health problems or are experiencing stress.

The role of the nurse in helping adults achieve their developmental tasks is an important one. Understanding human development and its impact on health is essential. It is easier for the adult to promote and to maintain health when he or she knows about health behaviors that enhance wellness and prevent stress. Major goals of the community health nurse when working with adults are to increase health promotion, prevention of illness, and self-care capabilities. Community health nurses play a vital role in enhancing the health of the adult population—a group of which the nurse is a part.

Screening Flow Chart for Health Promotion and Disease Prevention in Primary Care of Male and Female

I. *Screening tests found to be effective*	20	21	22	23	24	25	26	27	28	29	30	31	32	33	34	35	36	37	38	39	40
Hx Data base, initial (subsequently update only)	☐	☐	☐	☐			☐			☐			☐			☐			☐		
Alcohol use	☐						☐						☐						☐		
Smoking (nonsmokers)	☐						☐						☐						☐		
Rheumatic heart disease	☐																				
PE Complete physical examination																					
Weight	☐			☐			☐			☐			☐			☐			☐		
Blood pressure	☐			☐			☐			☐			☐			☐			☐		
Mouth, neck exam	☐			☐			☐			☐			☐			☐			☐		
Breast exam	☐			☐			☐			☐			☐			☐			☐		
Testicular exam	☐			☐			☐			☐			☐			☐			☐		
Prostatic exam	☐			☐			☐			☐			☐			☐			☐		
Pelvic exam	☐			☐			☐			☐			☐			☐			☐		
Lab Pap smear	☐	☐		☐			☐			☐			☐			☐			☐		
Stool guaiac																					
Mammography																☐					
Sigmoidoscopy																					
DT booster	☐									☐									☐		
Rubella titer	☐																				
PPD	☐									☐									☐		
VDRL	☐						☐						☐						☐		
II. *Screening tests possibly effective*																					
Serum cholesterol	☐																				
Tonometry																					
III. *Teach, counsel re:*																					
Exercise	☐			☐			☐			☐			☐			☐			☐		
Nutrition	☐			☐			☐			☐			☐			☐			☐		
Stress reduction, life change events	☐			☐			☐			☐			☐			☐			☐		
Seat belts	☐			☐			☐			☐			☐			☐			☐		
Report mouth sores	☐						☐						☐						☐		
BSE	☐						☐						☐						☐		
Neck, testicular palpation	☐						☐			☐			☐			☐					
Report postmenopausal bleeding																					
Obtain dental exam, dental prophylaxis	☐			☐			☐			☐			☐			☐			☐		

The Screening Flow Chart. Taking into account the findings of major studies and the recommendations of significant authorities, a flow chart has been developed. It is designed to facilitate a comprehensive, cost-effective lifetime preventive screening program for each patient.

It can best be used by inserting it into the patient chart cover, at the time the individual enters the NP's practice. The date should be plotted above the appropriate column, based on the patient's age. All screening tests recommended for the 20-year-old, as well as those indicated at the patient's current age, should be accomplished. Normal test results can be indicated by placing a ☐ in the appropriate box. An ☒ would signify an abnormal finding. Specific abnormal data could be recorded on an adjacent page. Subsequent visits could be planned for the asymptomatic, essentially healthy individual for the purpose of primary and secondary preventive screening at intervals, as indicated by the flow sheet.

41 42 43 44 45 46 47 48 49 50 51 52 53 54 55 56 57 58 59 60 61 62 63 64 65 66 67 68 69 70

This flow sheet should be regarded as a guideline, since ultimately each patient's prevention program should be tailored to individual needs, based on age, sex, risk factors, socioeconomic status, and mutual specific concerns of the patient and provider. It should be emphasized that these guidelines apply to asymptomatic persons. Patients with symptoms require a complete work up and persons at risk need a more intensive screening program.

From Lindberg SC: Periodic preventive health screening schedule for adult men and women: a guide for the primary care practitioner, Nurse Practitioner 5(5):9-13, 1980.

REFERENCES

American Cancer Society: Cancer facts and figures—1989, Atlanta, Ga, 1989, The Society.

American Heart Association (AHA): Fact sheet on heart attack, stroke, and risk factors, Dallas, 1988, The Association.

AHA: 1990 heart and stroke facts, Dallas, 1989, The Association.

AHA: 1990 research facts, Dallas, 1989, The Association.

AHA: Research. The heart of it all, Dallas, 1989, The Association.

American Public Health Association (APHA): Antismoking effort for pregnant women lowers rates of low weight babies, Nation's Health, March 1984, p 11.

Anderson SC, and Grant JF: Pregnant women and alcohol: implications for social work, Social Casework 65(1):3-10, 1984.

Antoine FS: Biological therapies: newest form of cancer treatment, Washington, DC, 1988, National Cancer Institute, Office of Cancer Communication.

Bowdler JE: Health problems of the homeless in America, Nurse Pract 14(7):44, 47, 50-51, 1989.

Bowdler JE and Barrell LM: Health needs of homeless persons, Public Health Nurs 4(3):135-140, 1987.

Byrd JC, Shapiro RS, and Schiedermayer DL: Passive smoking: a review of medical and legal issues, Am J Public Health 79(2):209-215, 1989.

Caldwell LR: Questions and answers about menopause, Am J Nurs 85(9):968-972, 1982.

Campbell JC and Humphreys JC: Nursing care of victims of family violence, Norwalk, Conn, 1984, Appleton/Lange.

Centers for Disease Control (CDC): Behavioral risk factor prevalence surveys—United States, second quarter 1982, MMWR 32:370-372, July 22, 1983.

CDC: AIDS and human immunodeficiency virus infection in the United States: 1988 update, MMWR 38(S-4):1-38, May 12, 1989.

CDC: HIV epidemic and AIDS: Trends in knowledge—United States, 1987 and 1988, MMWR 38(S-2):353-358, May 26, 1989.

CDC: HIV/AIDS surveillance. AIDS cases reported through October 1989, Atlanta, Ga, November 1989, The Centers.

CDC: HIV/AIDS surveillance report, Atlanta, Ga, September 1990, The Centers, pp 1-18.

Chalmers K and Farrell Pl: Nursing interventions for health promotion, Nurse Pract 8(11):62-64, 1983.

Cigarette advertising—United States, 1988, MMWR 39(16):261-265, April 27, 1990.

Cox J: Koop says up tax, cut liquor ads, USA Today, June 1, 1989, p A1.

Depression: Newsweek May 4, 1987, pp 48-52.

Division of Gerontology, The University of Michigan: Aging in the modern world, Ann Arbor, 1957, The University of Michigan.

Drake VK: Battered women: a health care problem in disguise, Image XIV(June):40-47, 1982.

Duvall EM: Family development, ed 2, New York, 1962, JB Lippincott.

Duvall EM and Miller BC: Marriage and family development, ed 6, New York, 1985, Harper & Row.

Elbow M: Children of violent marriages. The forgotten victims, Social Casework 63(8):465-471, 1982.

Erikson EH: Childhood and society, ed 2, New York, 1963, Norton.

Erikson EH: The life cycle completed: a review, New York, 1982, Norton.

Ershoff DH, Mullen PD, and Quinn V: A randomized trial of a serialized self-help smoking cessation program for pregnant women in an HMO, Am J Public Health 79(2):182-187, 1989.

Figley CR and McCubbin HI, eds: Stress and the family, vol 2, New York, 1983, Brunner/Mazel.

Fincer J: Sean Marsee's smokeless death, Reader's Digest, October 1985.

Frame PS and Carlson SJ: A critical review of periodic health screening using specific screening criteria. Part I: Selected diseases of respiratory, cardiovascular and central nervous systems, J Fam Pract 2(1):29-36, 1975.

Friend T: EPA: indoor smoking is big pollutant, USA Today, June 20, 1989, p 1A.

Friend T: High death rate among blacks hard to explain, USA Today, February 9, 1990, p 1D.

Glick PC and Lin SL: Recent changes in divorce and remarriage, Journal of Marriage and the Family, 48:737-748, 1986.

Havinghurst RJ: Developmental tasks and education, New York, 1972, David McKay.

Heart attacks, Newsweek, February 8, 1988, pp 50-54.

Hellinger FJ: Forecasting the personal medical care costs of AIDS from 1988 through 1991, Public Health Rep 103(3):309-319, 1988.

Hellinger FJ: National forecasts of the medical care costs of AIDS: 1988-1992, Inquiry 25(Winter):469-484, 1988.

Hill J: The psychological impact of unemployment, New Society 43:118-120, 1978.

Hypertension and strokes: a success story, Newsweek, February 8, 1988, p 60.

Kaforey EC: Crisis intervention and the new unemployed, AAOHN 32:154-157, 1984.

Kasl SV, Gore S, and Cobb S: The experience of losing a job: reported changes in health, symptoms, and behavior, Psychosom Med 37(2):106-122, 1975.

Kennedy introduces anti-smoking package, Nation's Health 1, January 1990.

Knafl KA and Grace HK: Families across the life cycle, Boston, 1978, Little, Brown.

Koop CE and Luoto J: The health consequences of smoking. Overview of a report to the Surgeon General, Public Health Rep 97(4):318-324, 1982.

Krystal E, Moran-Sackett M, and Cantoni L: Serving the unemployed, Social Casework 64(1):67-76, 1983.

Kubler-Ross E: Questions and answers on death and dying, New York, 1974, Collier Books.

Kubler-Ross E: Death: the final stage of growth, Englewood Cliffs, NJ, 1975, Prentice-Hall.

Langley R and Levy RC: Wife beating: the silent crisis, New York, 1977, Simon & Schuster.

Lindberg SC: Periodic preventive health screening schedule for adult men and women: a guide for the primary care practitioner, Nurse Pract 5(5):9-13, 1980.

Lindsey A: Health care for the homeless, Nurs Outlook 37(2):78-81, 1989.

Madonia JF: The trauma of unemployment and its consequences, Social Casework 64:482-488, 1983.

Margolis LH and Farran DC: Unemployment. The health consequences in children, NC Med J 66:268-269, 1981.

McCarthy PA: Fetal alcohol syndrome and other alcohol related birth defects, Nurse Pract 8:33-37, 1983.

Moen P: Preventing financial hardship: coping strategies of the unemployed. In McCubbin HI, Cauble AE, and Patterson JM, eds: Family stress, coping and social support, Springfield, Il, 1983, Charles C Thomas, pp 151-168.

Monmaney T: The fitness connection. Couch potatoes: off your duffs, Newsweek, February 8, 1988, p 60.

Monmaney T, Springen K, Hager M, and Shapiro D: The cholesterol connection, Newsweek, February 8, 1988, pp 56-58.

Murray R and Zentner J: Nursing assessment and health promotion through the life span, ed 6, Englewood Cliffs, NJ, 1989, Prentice-Hall.

National Association of Community Health Centers: Community health centers: a quality system for the changing health care market, McClean, Va, 1986, National Clearinghouse for Primary Care Information.

National campaign aims to snuff out smokeless tobacco use by young folks, Knoxville News-Sentinel, February 22, 1990, p A10.

National Cancer Institute (NCI): Taking time. Support for people with cancer and the people who care about them, (NIH Pub No 88-2059), Washington, DC, 1987, The Institute.

NCI: Questions and answers about PDQ the National Cancer Institute's Computerized Database for physicians, Washington, DC, 1989, The Institute.

National Center for Health Statistics, Division of Health Interview Statistics: National Health Interview Survey, MMWR May 25: 356, 1989.

National Coalition against Domestic Violence (NCADV): NCADV statistics. May 1988, Washington, DC, 1988, The Coalition.

NCADV: Statistics from 1987 NCADV domestic violence statistical survey, Washington, DC, 1989, The Coalition.

NCADV: What is battering? Washington, DC, 1989, The Coalition.

NCADV: On verbal/emotional abuse, Washington, DC, 1989, The Coalition.

National Institute for Disability and Rehabilitation Research: Stroke. Rehab brief, Washington, DC, 1989, US Government Printing Office.

National League for Nursing: Caring for persons with AIDS test, Nurs Health Care 10(10):563, 1989.

National Mental Health Association: Depression: what you should know about it, Alexandria, Va, 1988, The Association.

National Research Council: Environmental tobacco smoke—measuring exposures and assessing health effects, Washington, DC, 1986, National Academy Press.

National Safety Council: Accident facts, 1988 edition, Chicago, 1988, The Council.

Neuspiel DR, Rush D, Butler NR, Golding J, Bijur PE, and Kurzon M: Parental smoking and post-infancy wheezing in children: a prospective cohort study, Am J Public Health 79(2):168-171, 1989.

New pattern of birth defects linked to pregnant smokers, Knoxville Journal, October 12, 1985, p A3.

Newman RB and Newman PR: Development through life: a psychosocial approach, Homewood, Il, 1975, Dorsey Press.

Novotny TE, Warner KE, Kendrick JS, and Remington PL: Smoking by blacks and whites: socioeconomic and demographic differences, Am J Public Health 78(9):1187-1189, 1988.

Office of Minority Health-Resource Center (OMH-RC): Cancer hits some minorities hard. In Cancer and minorities: closing the gap, Washington, DC, 1989, Department of Health and Human Resources, p 1.

OMH-RC: In Cancer and minorities: closing the gap, Washington, DC, 1989, Department of Health and Human Resources, p 3.

OMH-RC: Cancer and minorities. In Cancer and minorities: closing the gap, Washington, DC, 1989, Department of Health and Human Resources, p 1.

Office on Smoking and Health (US Department of Health and Human Services): Office on Smoking and Health: the health consequences of smoking: Cancer. A report to the Surgeon General, Washington, DC, 1982, US Government Printing Office.

Research Reporter: Rush College of Nursing Awarded $500,000 AIDS grant, Nurs Res 38(1):24, 1989.

Robertson MJ and Cousineau MR: Health status and access to health services among the urban homeless, Am J Public Health 76(5):561-563, 1986.

Rosenstock I: Why people use health services, Milbank Q 44:94-127, 1966.

Sandler DP, Comstock GW, Helsing KJ, and Shore DL: Deaths from all causes in non-smokers who lived with smokers, Am J Public Health 79(2):163-167, 1989.

Sempos C, Fulwood R, Haines C, Carroll M, Anda R, Williamson DF, Remington P, and Cleeman J: The prevalence of high blood cholesterol levels among adults in the United States, JAMA 262(1):45-52, 1989.

Sheehy G: Passages: predictable crises of adult life, New York, 1976, Dutton.

Smoking also a cause of stroke, says 25th anniversary report, Nation's Health, February 1989, p 6.

Smoking ban in effect on 99% of flights, Knoxville News-Sentinel, February 25, 1990, p A5.

Sperling D: Alcohol is leading U.S. drug worry, USA Today, January 24, 1990, p D1.

Squitieri T: In tobacco country, fight is irritating, USA Today, February 21, 1990, p A1.

Stevenson JS: Adulthood. A promising focus for future research. In Werley HH and Fitzpatrick JJ, eds: Annual review of nursing research, vol 1, New York, 1984, Springer.

Stevenson JS: Issues and crises during middlescence, New York, 1977, Appleton-Century-Crofts.

Swineburne P: The psychological impact of unemployment on managers and professional staff, J Occup Psychol 54:47-64, 1981.

Taylor C, Lillis C, and LeMone P: Fundamental of nursing. The art and science of nursing care, Philadelphia, 1989, Lippincott.

Taylor JW: Structured conjoint therapy for spouse abuse cases, Social Casework 65:11-18, 1984.

Thompson JM, McFarland GK, Hirsch JE, Tucker SM, and Bowers AC: Mosby's manual of clinical nursing, ed 2, St Louis, 1989, CV Mosby.

US Bureau of the Census: Household and family characteristics: March 1988, Current population reports, Series P-20, No 437, Washington, DC, 1989, US Government Printing Office.

US Department of Health, Education, and Welfare (USDHEW): Smoking and health. Report of the advisory committee to the Surgeon General of the Public Health Service, Washington, DC, 1964, US Government Printing Office.

USDHEW: Healthy people. The Surgeon General's report on health promotion and disease prevention, Washington, DC, 1979, US Government Printing Office.

US Department of Health and Human Services: The 1990 health objectives for the nation: a midcourse review, Washington, DC, 1986, US Government Printing Office.

USDHHS: Prevention '86/'87: federal programs and progress, Washington, DC, 1987, US Government Printing Office.

USDHHS: Facts about AIDS, Washington, DC, 1987, US Government Printing Office.

USDHHS: Health United States: 1987, DHHS Pub No (PHS) 88-1232, Washington, DC, 1988, US Government Printing Office.

USDHHS: Promoting health/Preventing disease: Objectives for the nation, Washington, DC, 1980, US Government Printing Office.

USDHHS: Health United States, 1983, Washington, DC, 1983, US Government Printing Office.

USDHHS: The Surgeon General's 1989 report on reducing the health consequences of smoking: 25 years of progress, Washington, DC, 1989, USDHHS.

US Preventive Services Task Force: Guide to clinical preventive services: an assessment of the effectiveness of 169 interventions, Baltimore, Md, 1989, Williams & Wilkins.

Viken RM: Family violence. Aids to recognition, Postgrad Med 71:115-122, 1982.

Voyanoff P: Unemployment: family strategies for adaptation. In Figley CR and McCubbin HI, eds: Stress and the family, vol II, New York, 1983, Brunner/Mazel, pp 90-102.

Wagner EH, Beery WL, Schoenbach VJ, and Graham RM: An assessment of health hazard/health risk appraisal, Am J Public Health 72:347-352, 1982.

Warner KE: Smoking and health: a 25-year perspective, Am J Public Health 79(12):141-142, 1989.

Wells AJ: Deadly smoke, Occup Health Safety 58(10):20-22, 44, 60, 69, 1989.

Williams GD, Stinson FS, Parker DA, Harford TC, and Noble JN: Demographic trends, alcohol abuse and alcoholism 1985-1995, Alcohol Health Res World 11(3):80-83, 91, 1987.

With neither home nor health, Emerg Med 21(4):21-24, 27-28, 31-32, 35-36, 38, 43-44, 46, 1989.

SELECTED BIBLIOGRAPHY

Andrews B and Brown GW: Marital violence in the community. A biographical approach, J Psychiatry 153:305-312, 1988.

Campbell, JC and Sheridan DJ: Emergency nursing interventions with battered women, J Emerg Nurs 15(1):12-17, 1989.

Campbell JC and Sheridan DJ: Women's responses to sexual abuse in intimate relationships, Health Care Women Int 10:335-346, 1989.

Campbell JC and Sheridan DJ: The dark consequences of marital rape, Am J Nurs 89:946-949, 1989.

Campbell JC and Sheridan DJ: A test of two explanatory models of women's responses to battering, Nurs Res 38(1):18-24, 1989.

Duffy ME: Determinants of health promotion in midlife women, Nurs Res 37(6):358-362, 1988.

Flaskerud JH: Prevention of AIDS in blacks and hispanics. Nursing implications, J Community Health Nurs 5(1):49-58, 1988.

Silverman MM, Lalley TL, Rosenberg ML, Smith JC, Parron D, and Jacobs J: Control of stress and violent behavior: mid-course review of the 1990 health objectives, Public Health Rep 103(1):38-47, 1988.

Stuart EP and Campbell JC: Assessment of patterns of dangerousness with battered women, Issues Mental Health Nurs 10:245-260, 1989.

Talashek ML, Tichy AM, and Salmon ME: The AIDS pandemic: a nursing model, Public Health Nurs 6:182-188, 1989.

Tobacco and health: Am J Public Health, special issue, 79(2), 1989.

USDHHS: Surgeon General's workshop on violence and public health, Washington, DC, 1985, The Department.

Wynder EL: Tobacco and health. A review of the history and suggestions for public health policy, Public Health Rep 103(1):8-17, 1988.

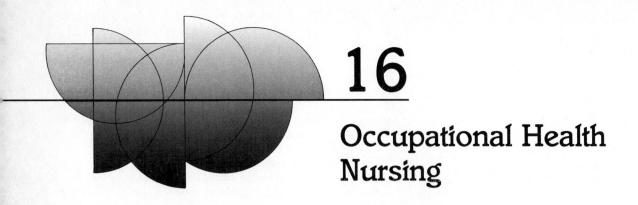

16

Occupational Health Nursing

Upon completion of this chapter, the reader will be able to:

*1. Discuss the national health objectives for
occupational health.*

*2. Summarize the purpose, intents, and mandates of
the Occupational Health and Safety Act of 1970.*

*3. Give an overview of the evolution of occupational
health nursing in the United States.*

*4. Describe recommended educational preparation and
opportunities for occupational health nurses.*

*5. Explain the functions of the occupational health
nurse.*

*6. Discuss the ten leading work-related diseases/
injuries in the United States.*

The first census in 1790 showed the United States to be an agricultural nation with limited industry. The Industrial Revolution, which began in the late 1800s, rapidly changed this situation. Between 1870 and 1910 the population rose 132 percent while the number of persons working in industry rose almost 400 percent (Morris, 1976, p. 109). There are now millions of workplaces and workers in the United States. The working population safeguards the economic security of our nation, and cuts across all socioeconomic levels, ethnic, religious, and cultural backgrounds, and levels of health.

The working population is basically a well population, and maintaining its health is extremely important. Occupational health professionals are actively involved in making the workplace a safe and healthy place to be, and emphasize primary prevention activities such as health protection and promotion. This chapter addresses the role of the occupational health nurse in promoting the health of workers and their families.

OCCUPATIONAL HEALTH IN THE UNITED STATES

Work is a major means of establishing individual, family, state, and national economic security. Historically, wages and not health issues were a major concern of workers. However, by the mid-1800s health concerns of workers began to emerge. Workers rallied for shorter work days, child labor laws, and health and safety measures. In 1850, at the urging of workers, Massachusetts became the first state to study occupational health and safety. Massachusetts was also the first state to require factory inspections and the reporting of industrial accidents.

In 1887, the Homestake Mining Company sponsored the first industrial medical department in the United States (U.S. Department of Labor [USDL], 1977, p. 15). In 1888 Betty Moulder, a nurse, was hired by a group of Pennsylvania coal mining companies to care for the miners and their families, but little is known of her duties or accomplishments (Parker-Conrad, 1988, p. 156; Pinkham, 1988, p. 20).

At the turn of the century, occupational medicine emerged. The federal government issued its first major report on occupational safety and health in 1903 (USDL, 1977, pp. 15-16). Physicians began to write about occupational disease, public awareness of occupational hazards increased, and occupational health legislation was beginning to be enacted. It was at this time that a pioneer in occupational medicine, Dr. Alice Hamilton, began her work. In 1910, Dr. Hamilton was named to chair the first Occupational Disease Commission in the United States, sponsored by the State of Illinois, and in 1911 she was asked to head a similar commission for the federal government. Dr. Hamilton researched many occupational diseases and conditions and carried out extensive studies on lead poisoning.

Dr. Hamilton achieved international recognition for her studies in industrial health, her staunch advocacy of the rights of workers, and for her prolific writings in the field. She is considered by many to be the founder of American occupational medicine. She died in 1970—the year that the first federal occupational safety and health act was passed—leaving a great legacy. Another leader in the field of occupational medicine, and a contemporary of Dr. Hamilton, was Dr. Carey McCord. Dr. McCord was also a prolific writer, and during his lifetime published more than 20 books and 3000 articles. He taught at the University of Michigan and many of his works are available at the University of Michigan School of Public Health historical library. He died in 1979 at the age of 93, leaving another great legacy in occupational health research.

During Dr. Hamilton's and Dr. McCord's time, the emergence of labor unions and the formation of the U.S. Department of Labor placed new emphasis on the rights of the worker. At this time, the health of the worker became a primary concern. Workers were concerned because if they were not healthy, their economic livelihood was threatened. The employer wanted a healthy worker because an unhealthy one threatened the economic stability of the workplace. Both the worker and the employer agreed on the value of maintaining worker health. A major point of difference between them, was what happened when an employee died or became ill, injured, or disabled due to work-related conditions. If the condition was job-related, the employees thought that the employer should compensate the worker. This view was not always shared by the employer. In fact, it had to be proved that *the employer was negligent* before the worker could receive financial compensation for medical care or lost wages. When compensation was granted to the workers, it was usually minimal.

Around the beginning of the century workers began to take a firm stand on the right to be compensated for job-related illness, injury, or disability. As a result, workers' compensation legislation was developed. The initial workers' compensation acts were met with much resistance from employers, and many were found to be unconstitutional. In 1911, New Jersey passed the first workers' compensation act to be upheld by the courts. Other states quickly followed, with nine more acts enacted in 1911; 11 in 1912; and 11 more in 1913

(USDL, 1977, p. 77). Organized industrial health services developed largely as a result of these acts (USDL, 1977, p. 77). It became more economical for the industry to keep workers healthy than to compensate them and their families for illness, injury, disability, and death.

By 1948, all 48 states and the territories of Alaska and Hawaii had enacted workers' compensation legislation. The primary function of this legislation was to compensate the worker for illness, injury, or disability related to the job. It places liability for workplace illness, injury, and disability on the *employer*. Workers' compensation is administered by the individual states; thus the benefits vary from state to state. Workers' compensation legislation, its cash benefits for loss of wages, and its health and disability components are discussed in detail in Chapter 4.

At about the same time that labor unions and the Department of Labor were emerging, health

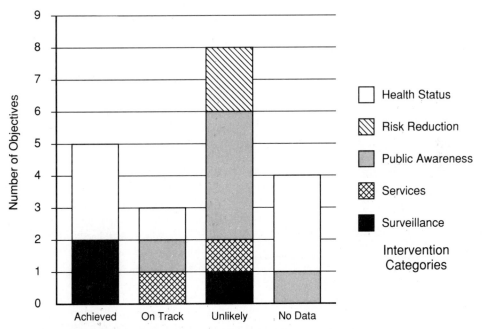

Note: Figure refers to the number of national occupational safety and health objectives in each intervention category that will or will not be achieved by the targeted 1990 date.

Figure 16-1 Status of occupational safety and health—1990 health objectives for the nation (20 objectives). (From US Department of Health and Human Services: The 1990 health objectives for the nation: a midcourse review, Washington, DC, 1986, US Government Printing Office, p 109.)

professionals began to appear in industry. Their numbers were scant, and they were usually employed at the discretion of the owner or operator of the workplace. Their primary function was to provide emergency care for on-the-job illness and injury.

Occupational Health and the 1990 Health Objectives for the Nation

The 20 objectives for occupational health that are included under the 1990 health objectives for the nation address the areas of improved health status (seven), reducing risk factors (two), increased public and professional awareness of occupational health (six), improved services/protection (two), and improved surveillance and evaluation (three). These objectives encourage health promotion activities at the workplace, reduction in death and disease from exposure to occupational hazards, design or alteration of the work environment to prevent exposures and injuries, studies for the surveillance of occupational health hazards, and epidemiological investigations (USDHHS, 1983, p. 255).

Many of the original 20 objectives remain unmet. Figure 16-1 shows the status of the 1990 occupational safety and health objectives. Gains in such areas as noise-induced hearing loss, occupational metal poisoning, health hazard plan implementation, and increased public awareness either are minimal or data are not available to evaluate them (USDHHS, 1986, pp. 116-126). The year 2000 health objectives will need to deal aggressively with occupational health and safety issues.

OCCUPATIONAL HEALTH LEGISLATION IN THE UNITED STATES

Appendix 16-1 presents an historical overview of some of the significant legislation and activities related to occupational health in the United States. Occupational health and safety legislation did not come early in our history. Many European nations were much more expeditious in developing such legislation. By 1884, Germany had already enacted a law which provided for a comprehensive system of occupational health, including compensation for occupational illness, injury, or disability irrespective of who was responsible for the condition occurring (McCall, 1977, p. 21).

For years, occupational health nurses, occupational physicians, and countless workers stressed the hazards involved in the workplace. In 1968, Dr. William Steward, Surgeon General at the time, told Congress that U.S. Public Health Service studies showed that 65 percent of industrial workers were exposed to toxic or harmful substances or conditions in their workplaces (Stellman and Daum, 1973, pp. xiii-xiv). The same year, an occupational health law was defeated by Congress. Many Americans thought that legislation in the workplace would endanger the free enterprise system. It was not until 1970 that the United States actually mandated a comprehensive, federal occupational safety and health program with the passage of the Occupational Safety and Health Act.

Occupational Safety and Health Act of 1970 (Public Law 91-596)

The landmark piece of occupational safety and health legislation in the United States is the Occupational Safety and Health Act of 1970. This act made the health of employees a public concern. It has been frequently amended and, in the last few years, has had many challenges to its authority.

Intents and Mandates of This Act

The intents of this act were to (1) prevent placing toxic substances in the workplace, (2) regulate exposure to toxic and dangerous substances already in the workplace, and (3) compensate workers for occupational illness and injury. To carry out these intents, the act had specific mandates:

1. Formation of the:
    a. *Occupational Safety and Health Administration (OSHA)*. Sets and enforces standards for occupational safety and health. Under the jurisdiction of the Department of Labor.
    b. *National Institute for Occupational Safety*

and Health (NIOSH). Researches and recommends occupational safety and health standards to OSHA and carries out training programs. Under the jurisdiction of the Department of Health and Human Services, Centers for Disease Control.

c. *Occupational Safety and Health Review Commission.* A quasijudicial agency that is charged with ruling on cases forwarded to it by the Department of Labor when disagreements arise over the results of safety and health inspections performed by the Department's Occupational Safety and Health Administration. Once a case is decided, a review of the decision can be obtained in the U.S. Court of Appeals.

d. *National Advisory Council on Occupational Safety and Health.* A consumer and professional council to make occupational safety and health recommendations to OSHA and NIOSH.

e. *National Commission on State Workers' Compensation Laws.* A temporary evaluative commission to study and make recommendations on the adequacy of state workers' compensation laws to the President. *Official termination date: October 30, 1972.* (The Office of Workers' Compensation under the Employment Standards Administration of the Department of Labor is still in existence.)

2. Establishment of federal occupational safety and health standards.

3. Imposition of fines and sentences for violation of federal occupational safety and health regulations.

The act also requires employers to keep records of work-related deaths, injuries, and illnesses for OSHA review. Under the act, states can develop their own occupational safety and health administrations as long as the state standards meet or exceed the federal standards.

Some Problems with the Act

A number of parts in the act have proven to be problematic. Consequently, the act has not been as effective as planned. Many of the problems center on the following areas.

Funding. Funding has been grossly inadequate since its inception and has greatly affected the ability of OSHA to carry out the intents and mandates of the act. According to the *Budget of the United States, Fiscal Year 1990, Appendix,* estimated funding is set at approximately $44,580,000 for NIOSH and $252,892,000 for OSHA. This amounts to slightly more than $1 per citizen per year. At the same time, the Black Lung Disability Trust Fund will spend approximately $640 million. This is twice the total NIOSH and OSHA budgets. It seems more logical, responsible, and humane to place money in programs attempting to minimize occupational illness, injury, and disability rather than to focus efforts on treating occupational conditions. The NIOSH budget has recently taken severe cuts.

Coordination of services. The services of OSHA and NIOSH have not been well coordinated in the past. These two agencies are under the jurisdiction of two different federal departments and the fact that one researches standards (NIOSH) while the other sets and enforces them (OSHA) has often complicated the issue. The two agencies have not always been in agreement on standards and regulations.

Fines and sentences. The fines and sentences set forth by the act are usually too low to serve as an incentive to employers to improve working conditions and sentences have usually not been imposed. Employers seem to be more concerned with the monetary amounts of employee lawsuits than with OSHA fines and sentences. However, fines have recently become stiffer.

Economic impact statements. Economic impact statements became policy in 1975. They are an occupational cost analysis study of a proposed OSHA standard or regulation. If the management can show that it would not be economically feasible to comply with a standard or regulation, they can appeal the proposed regulation. OSHA must then prove that the standard or regulation would not be detrimental to the economic stability of the workplace. The workplace often has better resources to finance such studies than does OSHA.

Scope of the problem. The scope of the problem is enormous: it has been estimated that there are more than 15,000 toxic agents in industry today. Standards exist for less than 500 (Plog, 1988, p. 806-809). It is estimated that every 20 minutes a new and potentially toxic chemical is introduced into workplaces (Serafini, 1976, p. 755), and revision of existing standards is far less than desirable. In its first 13 years, OSHA issued only 11 new or revised health standards concerning 24 chemical substances, one standard covering exposure to noise and 26 new or revised safety standards (Office of Technology Assessment, 1985, p. 22). This is beginning to change, and OSHA recently considered more than 400 industrial chemicals and substances during one regulatory proceeding (OSHA issues, 1989, p. 14).

Legal challenges. Through the legal system, various industries and groups are challenging the right of OSHA to set and enforce occupational safety and health standards. How these legal challenges are decided will be of great interest to the American worker.

Lack of trained personnel. There are severe shortages of occupational health professionals, which adversely affects our ability to enforce the mandates and intents of the act and promote worker health. NIOSH Educational Resource Centers (refer to Appendix 16-2) are making great efforts to train and educate professionals in the field. The American Public Health Association and the American Association of Occupational Health Nurses (AAOHN) are encouraging educational programs that prepare new health professionals to include knowledge and skills about occupational health needs.

What the Act Means to the Occupational Health Nurse

The Occupational Safety and Health Act of 1970 has many implications for the occupational health nurse. The nurse needs to be knowledgeable about the act and have a knowledge of occupational health and safety standards, regulations and prevention activities.

OSHA and NIOSH are the two best-known organizations under the act, and the ones that the occupational health nurse is likely to have contact with and utilize. The nurse often deals with OSHA regulations and enforcement, and must be prepared to assist in OSHA on-site visits. Frequently, it is the nurse who accompanies the OSHA investigators as they inspect and visit the workplace. OSHA tries to ensure that every worker has a safe and healthful workplace; its activities are oriented toward prevention and emphasize anticipation and abatement of potentially hazardous workplace conditions. The nurse can utilize OSHA consultation activities, legislative updates, and resource materials or may be involved in OSHA's agreements with state health authorities to monitor occupational health.

NIOSH is a prevention-oriented research and educational institute; the nurse often utilizes NIOSH educational and training programs and resource materials. The nurse may also be involved in NIOSH's "Comprehensive Plan for Surveillance of Occupational Illness and Injury in the United States," which serves to provide an improved, standardized nationwide system for identifying and monitoring occupationally related diseases, injuries, and hazards.

The demands placed on the nurse under this act and the many primary responsibilities that the nurse assumes in occupational health make it imperative that the nurse have adequate educational and experiential preparation for the job.

OCCUPATIONAL HEALTH NURSING IN THE UNITED STATES

The evolution of occupational health nursing in the United States closely followed other advances in the field of health care and occupational health. Occupational health nurses were originally called *industrial nurses.*

In 1895, the woman considered by many to be the first occupational health nurse in the United States, Ada Mayo Stewart, was hired by the Vermont Marble Company. Much has been written about Miss Stewart. Her sister Harriet, also a nurse, worked with her during the first year of her practice (Parker-Conrad, 1988, p. 156).

The Vermont Marble Company was ahead of

its time. It provided such worker benefits as housing, a library, profit-sharing, general accident insurance, and a company store (Felton, 1988; Pinkham, 1988, p. 20). When the company decided to offer nursing services Ada Mayo Stewart was an outstanding candidate for the job. She had studied the classics, history, mathematics, English, and Latin at Vermont Academy and had graduated from the Waltham Training School for Nurses where she had received training in "district nursing" (refer to Chapter 1) (Pinkham, 1988, p. 20).

Miss Stewart was employed as a visiting nurse who gave care in the home to company employees and family members who were sick, and went into the schools to teach health practices to the children of employees. She often traveled through town on bicycle, and "conversed" in sign language with many non–English speaking residents. As with other early community health nurses, the primary focus of her practice was on maternal-child health and control of communicable disease (Hannigan, 1984; American Association of Industrial Nurses, 1976). From those early days, the field has grown to number more than 20,000. Government studies have shown that thousands more are needed if worker health and safety are to be promoted and maintained.

In 1942, nearly 50 years after Miss Stewart began her work in occupational health nursing, the American Association of Industrial Nurses (AAIN) was founded. The first president of AAIN was Catherine Dempsey, and the new association published the journal *Industrial Nursing.* At its founding the AAIN had annual membership dues of 50 cents (Parker-Conrad, 1988, p. 158), and its membership numbered approximately 300 nurses from 16 states (Martin, 1977, p. 10). On January 1, 1977 the AAIN changed its name to the American Association of Occupational Health Nurses (AAOHN) and could boast membership in every state.

American Association of Occupational Health Nurses

The AAOHN is the professional association for registered nurses involved in occupational health,

and works in close cooperation with the American Nurses' Association (ANA). The mission of AAOHN is to promote occupational health nursing, maintain professional integrity, and enhance its professional status (AAOHN, 1989, A commitment). The association establishes standards of occupational health nursing practice, assists nurses in providing quality care, and serves as an advocate for occupational health (AAOHN, 1989, A commitment). The association has a membership of more than 12,000 nurses and is comprised of 180 local, state, and regional constituent groups. It publishes the *American Association of Occupational Health Nurses Journal* (AAOHN Journal). The AAOHN focuses on the program areas of professional affairs, governmental affairs, membership, and public affairs. The following descriptions of activities in these areas are adapted from these publications: *A commitment for excellence. American Association of Occupational Health Nurses* (1989) and *A year of progress . . . American Association of Occupational Health Nurses. 1988 Annual Report* (1989). For further information contact American Association of Occupational Health Nurses at 50 Lenox Pointe, Atlanta, Georgia 30324 (1-800-241-8104 or 1-404-262-1162).

Professional Affairs

The professional affairs activities of AAOHN are numerous. They involve many educational and research activities including continuing education (e.g., continuing education modules in the association's monthly professional journal, assisting constituent organizations with continuing education activities, and offering continuing education home study courses); promoting the inclusion of occupational health nursing courses in undergraduate and graduate nursing curricula; supporting and encouraging the certification program administered by the American Board for Occupational Health Nurses; encouraging and publishing professional research; publishing educational manuals and resource guides; setting and publishing standards of occupational health nursing practice; addressing questions related to ethics; sponsoring annual awards for outstanding achievement in occupational health nursing; and publishing position statements.

Governmental Affairs

The AAOHN has a strong governmental affairs program. AAOHN leaders have attended White House briefings, testified before Congress, and worked closely with the Occupational Safety and Health Administration (OSHA). The executive director of AAOHN has provided expert testimony to OSHA on such contemporary issues as workplace guidelines for AIDS. Other services offered by the governmental affairs arm include working with the Department of Health and Human Services (USDHHS) to set the Year 2000 Health Objectives; informing members of national legislation and issues; responding to legislative initiatives and regulations; maintaining regular contact with legislators and regulatory agencies; participating in coalitions with other occupational health organizations; and publishing the *Governmental Affairs Program Guide for Constituent Associations.*

Membership

As with all professional organizations, AAOHN is concerned with membership recruitment and retention and constituent association services. Along these lines the association has developed an aggressive 5-year plan whose goal is to increase membership by 10 percent. Membership activities and services include membership recruitment and retention (including advertising in professional journals); discounted professional liability insurance; constituent association manual; continuing education recordkeeping for members; annual membership awards and recognition; and statistical information and staff consultation as needed.

Public Affairs

The association makes numerous efforts to keep members informed of the latest developments in the field. To do this it carries out programs including publishing the *AAOHN News,* a monthly newsletter that discusses the activities of the association and includes an employment information service; publishing the *AAOHN Leadership Update,* a quarterly publication for association leaders; printing and distributing brochures and special publications about the association and significant issues in occupational health nursing; and compiling the Association's annual report to members.

Occupational Health Nursing Education

Occupational health nursing integrates public health and nursing theory, with an emphasis on community health nursing. In the United States, integration of occupational health nursing theory and concepts into nursing education has been very limited. Some of the early training was not offered through a school of nursing. For example, in 1917, Boston University College of Business Administration offered one of the first courses for occupational health nurses, consisting of 10 lectures per week for 16 weeks, a 2-week practicum, and assistance with job placement (Parker-Conrad, 1988, p. 159).

Discussions on integrating occupational health nursing content into baccalaureate curricula have been under way for over 45 years. In 1945, the National League for Nursing (NLN), the National Organization for Public Health Nursing, and the American Association of Industrial Nurses stated that specific courses in industrial nursing should not be a part of the undergraduate nursing program, and specialty education was encouraged at the graduate level (AAIN, 1976; Olson and Kochevar, 1989, p. 33). Faculty in undergraduate schools of nursing now recognize the importance of nursing students learning basic content on occupational health nursing (Rogers, 1986), and the NLN has adopted a position stating that graduates of baccalaureate programs should be prepared to practice in a variety of health care settings (Olson and Kochevar, 1989, p. 33). Occupational nursing should be a part of these various health care settings. The purpose of integrating occupational health content in baccalaureate programs is not to prepare occupational health nurses at the undergraduate level, but to prepare nurses to have an understanding of the relation of work and the work setting on health promotion, maintenance, and restoration (Olson and Kochevar, 1989, p. 38).

The fact that nursing faculty generally are not familiar with occupational nursing content and have not practiced in it is a major deterrent to content integration (Prestholdt and Holt, 1989, p. 465; Olson and Kochevar, 1989). Occupational health nursing content must become a part of baccalaureate as well as graduate nursing education. It is possible to integrate this content into existing curricula as well as to develop curricula specific to occupational health nursing. Research by Olson and Kochevar (1989) has indicated that occupational health content areas most often included in undergraduate curricula were health promotion and health education and that nursing faculty were actively interested in audiovisual materials and course materials on occupational health nursing. As a result of this research a 15-minute slide program entitled *Occupational Health Nursing: Meeting the Challenge* was developed by the Midwest Center for Occupational Health and Safety (640 Jackson Street, St. Paul, Minnesota 55101, 1-612-221-3992—Occupational Health Nursing) and is available for loan. A program designed to assist undergraduate nursing faculty in the integration of occupational safety and health content into nursing curricula was also proposed.

Talbot (1983) cited numerous instances in which experts in occupational health nursing stated that the largest portion of knowledge necessary for occupational health nursing is already in place in baccalaureate education today, because that knowledge is essential to all fields of nursing. What is lacking is the conceptual framework and clinical experience. A variety of techniques can be used to incorporate occupational health into nursing education including self-study modules, clinical preceptorships or extended experiences in occupational health settings, lectures on occupational health in community health nursing courses, electives in occupational health, using occupational health nurses as adjunct faculty, encouraging research or term papers on occupational health, and observational experiences.

Graduate Education

The National Institute for Occupational Safety and Health Educational Resource Centers (ERCs) offer graduate and continuing education in occupational health and safety for health professionals. They operate under federal grants, and student stipends are often available. The centers also offer courses on aerosols, asbestos recognition and removal, audiometric certification and training, hearing conservation, back injury prevention, computers, epidemiology, ergonomics, hazard communication/right-to-know, hazardous waste management, infectious disease, industrial hygiene, legal aspects of occupational health, occupational health management, noise control, occupational medicine, pulmonary function testing, radiation, radon testing, respiratory protection, risk assessment, occupational safety, toxicology, ventilation, and workers' compensation. These centers are located at major universities across the country and are often affiliated with schools of public health. They are listed in Appendix 16-2 and can be contacted directly or through the NIOSH Division of Training and Manpower Development, Robert A. Taft Laboratories, MS C-11, 4676 Columbia Parkway, Cincinnati, Ohio 45226-1998, 1-513-533-8225.

Qualifications of the Occupational Health Nurse

AAOHN supports the baccalaureate degree in nursing as basic preparation for entry into professional practice (AAOHN, 1986, Education preparation). In addition, it recommends coursework in occupational health nursing theory and practice, physical assessment, health care administration, epidemiology, toxicology, occupational health and safety practice and legislation, environmental health, health education, rehabilitation, business administration and management, ergonomics, human relations and psychology (Babbitz and Bodnar, 1989). Knowledge of individual and group skills is recommended.

AAOHN recommends a minimum of 2 years of professional nursing experience in a primary care setting, such as community health, ambulatory care, emergency, or critical care units before entering occupational health nursing practice.

Additional experience in areas such as mental health, rehabilitation, and medical-surgical nursing is desirable.

The AAOHN has offered certification in occupational health nursing since 1974. Certification is on a voluntary basis and is processed through the American Board for Occupational Health Nurses, Inc. It involves a combination of work experience, course work, and a written examination.

Standards of Practice

Standards of practice are a minimum baseline against which nursing actions can be measured. AAOHN (1988) has developed standards for guiding practice. These standards are frequently revised to reflect the changing scope and essence of the practice.

Objectives of Occupational Health Nursing

Primary objectives for the occupational health nurse are to

1. Protect the worker from occupational safety and health hazards
2. Promote a safe and healthful workplace
3. Facilitate efforts of workers and workers' families to meet their health and welfare needs
4. Promote education and research in the field

These objectives are carried out in a therapeutic milieu involving the worker, his or her family, the community, and the occupational health setting. Occupational health and safety is a team effort, and the nurse must work cooperatively with disciplines such as occupational safety, occupational health, management, occupational medicine, and toxicology. The nurse must also be aware of what community resources are available and be able to work with them. The nurse realizes that successful implementation of occupational safety and health objectives will help to result in high-level wellness, increased job productivity and a safer work environment. Ultimately a safer, healthier community is the result.

To accomplish these objectives, the occupational health nurse carries out specific nursing functions. These functions are broad and complex. They demand a number of nursing activities, responsibilities, and roles. Close to two thirds of occupational health nurses work alone, and often without direct medical supervision. Their high level of independence makes this type of nursing distinctly different from many other areas of nursing practice.

Functions of the Occupational Health Nurse

For the most part, workers are healthy people, and because of this the functions of the occupational health nurse are heavily oriented toward primary prevention—keeping the worker healthy. Occupational health nursing functions can be classified into the categories of *administration and management, environmental surveillance, direct nursing care, health education, counseling,* and *research*. These functions will have the nurse engaged in activities ranging from health promotion to rehabilitation.

The number of nurses required to handle occupational health nursing functions effectively is determined by the size of the company, the number of employees and their health status, the type of workplace, and actual as well as potential health and safety problems (AAOHN, 1989, Occupational health nursing). In general, to carry out nursing functions effectively, the ratio of nurses to workers should be one nurse for up to 300 employees in an industrial setting, and up to 750 in a nonindustrial setting; two or more nurses for up to 600 industrial employees; three or more nurses for up to 1000 employees in an industrial setting; and one nurse for each additional 1000 employees up to 5000 in either setting (AAOHN, 1989, Occupational health nursing; Lee, 1978). Larger or more hazardous work settings require additional nursing personnel, while smaller ones may be able to implement effective programs with only part-time nursing services.

Confidentiality and ethics play an important role in all occupational health nursing functions. The AAOHN (AAOHN code, 1986) has published a *Code of Ethics* for occupational health nurses to help guide them in this important area of nursing practice. In the past, ethical dilemmas have not received as much attention as other areas of nursing, but this is changing (Rogers, 1988, p. 100). Ethical issues confronting the occupational health nurse include, among others, risk of exposure to hazardous substances, informed consent, confidentiality of health care records, resource allocation, drug testing in the workplace, right-to-know issues, and numerous questions related to AIDS. The AAOHN code of ethics stresses the need to protect and promote the health and safety of the worker while at the same time safeguarding the worker's rights.

AAOHN (1988) has published a position statement titled *Confidentiality of Health Information.* The confidential treatment of health information and records and the worker's right to privacy are considered professional obligations of the occupational health nurse. AAOHN supports health information only being released if the employee has given written consent or if a law mandates release. This is not always an easy task in the occupational health setting. Management personnel may have access to health service records, and computerization of records may further jeopardize the ability to keep information confidential. To protect employees from unauthorized or indiscriminate access to health information, the AAOHN recommends that written policies and procedures be developed on record access; that educational activities be carried out to let employees, employers, and other health care providers know about policies in regard to record access, and that legal counsel be sought by the nurse in instances of unclear or questionable practice situations (AAOHN, 1988, Confidentiality).

The following describes the specific roles and responsibilities that occupational health nurses carry out. It should be noted that many of these roles and responsibilities overlap. The nurse's functions reflect emphasis on primary prevention.

Administration and Management

Administrative and management functions consume a significant part of the nurse's time. In carrying out these functions the nurse must be given the necessary authority, responsibility, and accountability for decision making and action (AAOHN, 1989, Occupational health nurse).

Administrative and management functions include planning, implementing, and evaluating the occupational health service; maintenance of occupational health records; development and maintenance of an occupational health nursing policy and procedure manual; training and supervising auxiliary health personnel; emergency procedures; cooperation with federal and state occupational health regulatory bodies; and participation in student educational placement programs. The nurse designs programs to meet the health needs of employees and employers, and develops alternatives to the traditional provider models (e.g., Employee Assistance Programs) (AAOHN, 1988, Delivery of). Although these functions are not all-inclusive, they are representative of the comprehensive and complex array of functions carried out by the nurse.

The operation of the occupational health service at the workplace is a major part of the nurse's administrative and management function. This service involves many responsibilities. AAOHN has published an excellent guide to assist the nurse in these various health service roles and responsibilities—*A Comprehensive Guide for Establishing an Occupational Health Service* (1987). This guide discusses health assessments, health planning, fields of knowledge fundamental to occupational health nursing practice, developing an occupational health service, staffing, environmental surveillance, employee assistance programs, immunization, health counseling, disaster planning, recordkeeping and reports, legislation, scope of practice, and accountability and evaluation. To assist the nurse in role description the AAOHN (1989) offers a publication called *Guidelines for Developing Job Descriptions in Occupational Health Nursing* which can be of great help to the nurse in establishing his or her role.

Record Keeping

The importance of maintaining occupational health records as part of the operation of an occupational health service cannot be overestimated! The nurse has legal and professional responsibility to keep accurate, comprehensive, up-to-date written records (Ossler, 1988, p. 8). Laws regulating medical documentation exist, and the nurse must adhere to them (Rabinow, 1988, p. 314).

Occupational health nursing records should conform to company policy, OSHA requirements, and nursing standards. The reason for each employee's visit to the occupational health service should be recorded. Records should note all employee contacts with the health service beginning with the preemployment physical and interview. They should include the results of screening tests, periodic health appraisals, health risk assessments, rehabilitation activities, community referrals, nursing plans of care, and educational programs in which the worker has participated. As usual in nursing, these records are confidential.

The occupational health nurse also keeps records of workplace observations and health statistics as they pertain to health and safety at the worksite. Interviews with workers and other health care personnel and the environmental surveillance done by the nurse can elicit this information. Such information can be utilized in health promotion activities.

Student Supervision

A major role of the occupational health nurse is that of educator (Randolph, 1988, p. 166). Part of the nurse's administrative and managerial responsibility involves participation in student educational programs. These students often are nursing students, but students of other disciplines, such as occupational health and safety, social work, vocational rehabilitation, toxicology, public health, and audiology also utilize the nurse as an educational resource. This educational supervision has included physicians involved in occupational medicine residency programs (Bertsche, Sanborn, and Jones, 1989). Occupational health nurses are in a unique position to further the education of students in occupational safety and health.

One area that occupational health nurses have not ventured into in any depth, but that has great potential, is that of educating school children in occupational health and safety. Comprehensive school health education curricula that incorporate concepts of occupational health was recom-

mended in *Promoting Health, Preventing Disease. Objectives for the Nation* (USDHHS, 1980, p. 42). Unfortunately, little progress has been made in this endeavor.

Occupational health education can start in elementary school. If occupational health nurses are not available to visit classrooms themselves, they could arrange with school nurses or administrators to have such content integrated. Health education modules could be developed for use with children.

Children can be encouraged to start thinking in terms of health and safety on the job and their future as workers. Guest speakers can be brought to health and science classes. Activities can involve, for instance, a demonstration of earplugs, masks, or helmets; the children might be invited to describe the jobs that would require these devices. Various work situations could be discussed. Older children might be asked to write a description of a job, then discuss its health component. Such life-span education can encourage workers to be informed about occupational health, and can serve as a recruitment tool by which young children become interested in occupational health nursing.

Community Resource Collaboration

Another administrative function involves developing collaborative and cooperative networks with community resources. The nurse works with community agencies and is knowledgeable about community resources. In this capacity, the nurse helps to promote ongoing, comprehensive health care for the worker in and away from the workplace. Networking also assists the nurse in handling the highly independent nursing role that is assumed in the occupational health setting. Resources of particular interest to the occupational health nurse include state and local health departments, vocational rehabilitation agencies, coalition groups whose aim is to improve environmental health and safety, counseling services for problems such as alcoholism, drug abuse, and domestic violence, and organizations such as the American Heart Association, American Lung Association, American Diabetic Association, and

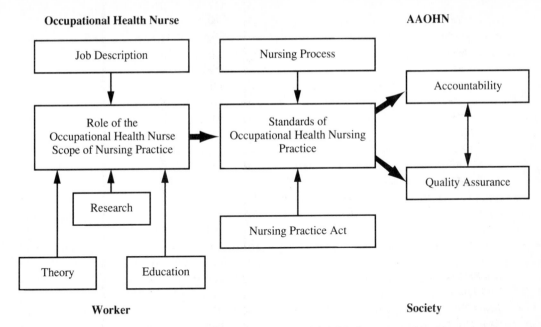

Occupational Health Nurse   **AAOHN**

Figure 16-2 Quality care in occupational health nursing. (From Randolph SA: Occupational health nursing. A commitment to excellence, AAOHN J 36:166, 1988.)

American Cancer Association (refer to Chapters 9 and 17 for additional information on community resources).

Quality Assurance and Accountability

These matters are extensively dealt with in the AAOHN publication *A Comprehensive Guide for Establishing an Occupational Health Service* (1987), mentioned previously (administration and management role). Workers expect, and should receive, quality occupational health nursing care (Randolph, 1988, p. 168). Phaneuf and Wandelt (1974) state that quality assurance was a method of accountability of health personnel for the quality of care they provide (Dirschel, 1986; Randolph, 1988, p. 168). Figure 16-2 presents interacting elements in accountability and quality care in occupational health nursing. It illustrates the importance of research, theory, and education working together with the nursing process, standards of practice, and the legal aspects of practice for quality assurance and accountability (Randolph, 1988, p. 167).

Evaluation of nursing care can be accom-plished through quality assurance activities such as peer review, self-evaluation, and audit. Evaluation is an essential administrative and managerial function of the occupational health nurse. Through evaluation, strengths and weaknesses can be assessed and appropriate measures taken to correct deficiencies. The recommendations coming from such evaluation measures are shared with other members of the occupational health team. As nurses evaluate services and detect service gaps, they will frequently find themselves in the position of advocating better and more comprehensive health care services for workers and their families. The occupational health nurse is continually involved in such activities. Chapter 22 discusses this function and the process for establishing and assuring a quality assurance program.

Environmental Surveillance

The nurse must continuously survey the work environment for health hazards and work toward establishing cause and effect relationships between health and illness or injury. The nurse has daily contact with workers in the workplace and is knowledgeable about the health problems of the workers and any potential or actual health hazards at the worksite. The nurse can be the first health professional in the workplace to recognize danger areas and risks to health.

These surveillance activities are carried out with other members of the occupational health care team: members of management, occupational safety personnel, industrial hygienists, and physicians. Surveillance activities may sometimes be carried out in conjunction with OSHA visits and inspections at the workplace.

Environmental surveillance involves evaluating which areas of the workplace have higher or lower-than-expected illness or injury rates, what kinds of illness or injuries occur, the timing of incidents (e.g., frequency and intervals), and the possible reasons why. Potential stressors, hazardous equipment, and known and suspected irritants should be routinely and regularly logged and monitored for their detrimental effects. It is through this careful kind of epidemiological study that hazards are pinpointed and minimized and the solutions found. The nurse needs to share these environmental observations and/or recommendations with management and seek solutions. An example of this process is illustrated in the following situation.

An occupational health nurse suspected that one area of the plant in which she worked had a higher-than-average noise area. After obtaining permission from the plant management to do periodic audiometric testing on the workers in this area in combination with testing on a control group, she began to collect data to confirm her hypothesis. Employees in both areas were tested every 6 months. Over a period of time, the nurse was able to show that the workers in this one area had increasingly abnormal audiograms and that the control group in another area had consistently normal ones. The workers themselves had not noticed any change in levels of hearing, but the audiograms told a different story. The results of the study were shared with management and the workers, and corrective measures were taken. In this example, the comparative screening tests, coupled with knowledge about protective measures, furthered the health of the workers in the plant.

Appendix 16-3 presents an assessment guide that assists occupational health nurses in completing an environmental survey in a systematic manner. An organized approach to environmental surveillance is essential for an accurate diagnosis of health and safety problems in the workplace. Occupational health nurses apply the principles of community assessment when carrying out surveillance activities at the worksite (refer to Chapter 11).

Direct Nursing Care

The direct nursing care given by the occupational health nurse ranges from assessment to rehabilitation. The nurse needs to be skilled in making physical assessment as well as in carrying out medical-surgical, rehabilitation, emergency care, and community health nursing practice.

Occupational health disorders can be very serious. Each year more than 10 million traumatic injuries occur on the job, 400,000 workers become ill from exposure to hazardous substances, and 100,000 workers die prematurely from exposure to occupational stressors (USDHHS, 1986, The 1990 health, p. 109). Studies have estimated that 240 people die every workday in the United States as a result of job-related accidents or illness, and 1.8 million Americans suffer crippling injuries on the job each year (Ubell, 1989, pp. 4-5). It is estimated that as many as 100,000 deaths occur each year as a direct result of occupational disease and illness (USDHHS, 1986, The 1990 health, p. 109), along with an incalculable number of diseases and illness. These figures help to give the reader an idea of the scope of the problem facing the occupational health nurse.

The nurse is in an excellent position to promote health in the workplace, and workers tend to relate well to occupational health nursing services. Workers often comply with nursing plans of care and view the nurse as someone who is concerned about them, cares about them, and wants to help them. The direct nursing care activities include, but are not limited to assessment and screening, rehabilitation, immunizations, emergency care, nonoccupational injuries and illnesses, and treatment of acute and chronic conditions. The nurse will utilize many health education strategies and community resources in these endeavors.

Physical assessment and screening procedures are done on a regular basis. The nurse needs to be skilled in physical assessment of the well adult, and often does employment and return-to-work physicals. The nurse carries out selected screening procedures on an ongoing basis during the employee's term of employment. These screening measures involve periodic blood pressure measurement, urinalysis, hematocrit, hemoglobin, vision testing, audiometrics, electrocardiograms, vision screening, and pulmonary function analysis. Such screening measures are very important, providing baseline and subsequent data for the study of occupational injury and illness and contributing to a comprehensive health history. Many workplaces offer special training to enable the occupational health nurse to carry out these screening activities (e.g., audiometrics and pulmonary function).

Rehabilitation services are another direct nursing care function. The nurse will often be involved in occupational, physical, and medical therapy rehabilitation plans. Many of these rehabilitation plans will have aspects that are to be carried out in the workplace on a regular basis for a given period of time.

Rehabilitation activities begin at the time of the initial referral. During this period, the focus is on prevention as well as on prompt, adequate treatment to minimize the consequences of the illness or injury. Once immediate care needs are met, the occupational health nurse maintains good communication and collaborative relationships with the client, his or her family, and other occupational health personnel, and utilizes community resources to facilitate care.

The occupational health nurse is aware that rehabilitation activities require immediate action. There is a direct correlation between the time the injury or illness occurred, the time of the rehabilitation referral, and the success of the rehabilitation program. The longer the time lapse between injury and referral, the greater the chance that rehabilitation efforts will not be effective (Donnelly,

1983, p. 40). A well-established referral mechanism which decreases this time lapse is critical. The occupational health nurse is usually responsible for setting up this mechanism.

The nurse may be involved in assessing the employee's ability to return to work following rehabilitation. The nurse serves as a facilitator for the client's return to work and health. The nurse realizes that rehabilitation is a family affair and can put stress on its members. The nurse will need to incorporate the family into the rehabilitation process, and refer the family to community agencies as necessary (refer to Chapter 9). Other components of the nurse's role in rehabilitation are discussed in Chapter 17.

Immunizations are another direct care function that may be provided by the occupational health nurse. It is estimated that as many as 80 percent of American adults are not fully immunized; the workplace can serve as a setting to maintain appropriate immunization schedules (Murphy, 1989). Permanent immunization records on employees should be kept and immunizations should be encouraged.

Statistics show that more than 15,000,000 work days are lost every year because of influenza alone; 25 to 300 cases of tetanus are reported every year; and at least 200,000 new cases of hepatitis B are reported every year (Murphy, 1989). These illnesses are preventable.

Emergency care is probably the most dramatic of the occupational health nurse's direct care functions. The nurse must be skilled in cardiopulmonary resuscitation, first aid, and emergency care techniques. The nurse is usually the first health professional in the workplace to have contact with the ill or injured worker, and often has to make a decision and take action immediately.

Nonoccupational illnesses and injuries are also part of the nurse's direct care function. Although these are incurred outside the workplace, they have an effect on work and the work setting. The occupational health nurse will treat these conditions initially and will often refer the client for further treatment to community agencies.

Among the nonoccupational conditions of which the nurse should be cognizant are alcoholism and drug abuse. If an employee comes to work intoxicated or under the influence of drugs and the employer allows the individual to remain, workers' compensation laws in many states would rule in favor of the worker in the event of occupational injury. For the safety of the worker and to protect the employer from liability, employees who are unfit to work should not be permitted to stay. In some cases, the worker's supervisor will make the decision regarding fitness for work, and in other cases the nurse or physician will. Unfortunately, most non-job-related conditions are not effectively managed in the workplace. The challenge exists for the occupational health nurse to influence management to initiate effective treatment programs dealing with all health problems of employees.

Acute and chronic conditions are treated on a day-to-day basis by the nurse. These conditions are evidenced in forms ranging from the common cold to the crippling effects of arthritis or a work-related injury. Providing services for these conditions takes up a large part of the nurse's time.

As our population ages, and the incidence of chronic conditions increases, the nurse will be increasingly involved in direct care activities to treat chronic conditions. Many community agencies (e.g., American Lung Association, American Heart Association, and American Diabetic Association) provide relevant services and information. Appendix 17-2 lists some agencies in the community that may be useful to the nurse in this effort.

The direct nursing care functions of the occupational health nurse are diverse and demand a high level of nursing skill, professional flexibility, and independence. To carry out these direct nursing care functions, the nurse must be able to assess both the worker and the workplace. An assessment guide for nursing in industry is included in this text (Appendix 16-3).

Health Education and Health Promotion

These activities focus on wellness, and there is unlimited opportunity to implement them in the workplace. Nurses and other health professionals are extremely interested in these programs for their ability to promote the workers' right to

health and improve the quality of life. Employers are often interested in such activities from the standpoint of cost containment and public relations (e.g., enhanced company image, reduced workers' compensation costs, fewer medical benefits used, less time lost from work, and increased productivity).

The cost of health care benefits is expected to rise to 50 percent of wages by the early 1990s (Whitmer, 1984; Selleck, Sirles, and Newman, 1989, p. 413), and employers need to look for ways to contain them. Health education and health promotion activities save money. The Johnson and Johnson Company has reported that it could save $1 million per year if its health promotion program was offered to all employees. Employee health promotion programs often exist because employers realize that it costs less to educate workers about many health risks than to pay the high cost of illness, injury, and disability (Selleck, Sirles, and Newman, 1989, p. 420). Occupational health nurses engaged in health education and health promotion activities are truly cost effective for industry.

Worksite health promotion programs are paying their way and occupational health nurses are well qualified to develop, implement, and evaluate these programs (Selleck, Sirles, and Newman, 1989, p. 412). The worksite has become a major setting for health education and promotion programs. *The National Survey of Workplace Health Promotion Activities* (USDHHS, 1987), carried out by the U.S. Department of Health and Human Services, showed that 66 percent of worksites having more than 50 employees sponsored at least one health promotion activity; the larger the worksite the more likely it was that such activities would be available; and many of these activities were carried out by worksite staff without the help of outside agencies. The most frequently cited programs were smoking control (35.6 percent), health risk assessment (29.5 percent), back care (28.6 percent), stress management (26.6 percent), and exercise/fitness (22.1 percent). Health risk assessments are becoming more popular at the worksite and nurses should include the health risk assessment method among their functions. (Sherman, 1990, p. 19). This method is an excellent way to promote wellness. Other components of worksite health education programs are blood pressure control, weight control, nutrition education, and lifestyle and behavioral change. It is often the occupational health nurse who carries out the program or is directly involved in it. Nurses provide quality, cost-effective care at the workplace and employers are quick to utilize them in such programs (Gillis, 1988). Nurses should target the activities toward three levels: awareness, lifestyle/behavioral change, and supportive environments (Selleck, Sirles, and Newman, 1989, p. 420).

When planning and implementing health education and promotion activities, the nurse needs to assess the competency level of the target group (including educational background); attitudes, values, and beliefs; cost effectiveness; and what teaching is necessary. The nurse should try to coordinate these activities with community activities. For example, if the community is celebrating health and fitness week, the nurse can build on this activity in the workplace.

Occupational health nurses frequently need to use creative approaches in reaching their targeted population. Some employers are not willing to grant work time for health education activities and employees are often not willing to use their personal time for such activities. In these situations, nurses plan health education programs that can be implemented during lunchtimes and breaks or they may bring in community programs normally used by employees on their own time. For example, many workers join Weight Watchers and appreciate having Weight Watchers' meetings at their employment site after work hours. Employees can also be reached through the distribution of educational materials. Distributing a health newsletter or flyer with paychecks is one way to inform all workers about current health issues.

Through health education and health promotion activities the nurse has the opportunity to have a great effect on the health of the worker. The opportunities are unlimited, and have great potential for cost containment as was mentioned earlier. They also have great potential for improving the health of our nation's workers.

Health education activities often include employee in-service programs on health and safety. In addition they involve health and safety counseling on a one-to-one or small-group basis. The Occupational Safety and Health Act of 1970 requires that workers be told of the hazards they are exposed to in the workplace (right-to-know), and making the worker aware of these hazards is often left to the occupational health nurse. Discussing with an employee how a given condition such as diabetes will affect the employee's job, job safety, and daily living is another aspect of this function.

An important aspect of health education and health promotion is the interpretation of health and welfare benefits to the employee. This means interpreting what is offered through the employer and also what is available through the community. The nurse can be instrumental in initiating a referral to counseling services or procuring services for family members of an employee. Clinical experience has demonstrated that when an occupational health nurse assists an employee in meeting family needs, there is less job-related injury and illness.

Another important task of health education and counseling is assisting the worker to see work as a developmental task. Using anticipatory guidance for meeting some of the possible crises and challenges that may arise in one's work career can assist workers to deal with their developmental tasks.

Counseling is an important occupational health nursing function. If the counseling required is beyond the scope of the nurse, a referral can be made to an appropriate community resource. When carrying out health education and promotion, nurses will need to make use of their knowledge of community resources and utilize them to facilitate worker, family, and community health, when the treatment is beyond the capability of the resources of the worksite.

Research

Research is an integral part of nursing practice and theory. The improvement of practice in any professional discipline is based on research activity and productivity designed to expand, advance, and refine the body of knowledge in the field

(Rogers, 1989). Until recently occupational health nurses were not extensively engaged in research activities. This has changed, largely because of the commitment to research by the AAOHN, the availability of research-oriented graduate education in the field, the research emphasis of the National Center for Nursing Research, the availability of grants by NIOSH, and research funding from private organizations (Rogers and Spencer, 1984; Rogers, 1989, p. 493).

In 1981 the AAOHN established a research committee for the purpose of promoting occupational health nursing research. At the 1982 annual American Occupational Health Nursing Conference, the first research session on occupational health nursing studies was held (Silberstein, 1983, p. 9). The *AAOHN Journal* includes a column on research and regularly publishes research articles. AAOHN offers research awards in occupational health nursing.

There is significant potential for research in this field, and the topics are limitless and exciting. In 1988, the research subcommittee and professional staff of AAOHN identified preliminary priority research areas to be surveyed among the general membership. A survey instrument was developed and sent to a random sample of AAOHN members, who were asked to rate the suggested research areas and to recommend others that were not included (Rogers, 1989). In a follow-up, Rogers (1989) conducted research that established 12 priorities for occupational health nursing. These priorities, listed in the box at right, were adopted by the AAOHN in 1990.

American Association of Occupational Health Nurses Research Priorities in Occupational Health Nursing

- Effectiveness of primary health care delivery at the worksite
- Effectiveness of health promotion nursing intervention strategies
- Methods for handling complex ethical issues related to occupational health (e.g., confidentiality of employee health records, truth telling)
- Strategies that minimize work related health outcomes (e.g., back injuries)
- Health effects resulting from chemical exposures in the workplace
- Occupational hazards of health care workers
- Factors that influence worker rehabilitation and return to work
- Mechanisms to assure quality and cost effectiveness of occupational health programs (e.g., effects of employee assistance programs or health surveillance programs on improving employee health)
- Effectiveness of occupational health nursing programs on employee productivity and morale
- Factors that contribute to behavioral changes among health care workers for self-protection from occupational hazards (e.g., HIV/AIDS)
- Factors that contribute to sustained risk reduction behavior related to lifestyle choices (e.g., smoking, substance abuse, nutrition)
- Effectiveness of ergonomic strategies to reduce worker injury and illness

From American Association of Occupational Health Nurses (AAOHN): Research priorities in occupational health nursing, Atlanta, Ga, February 1990, The Association. Used with permission of the author.

Work as a Developmental Task

Work is an activity carried out by people to provide economic security and by doing so helps to preserve and maintain life. Society expects that adults will work and be self-sufficient; in the past, being out of work often carried with it many negative societal connotations. Our nation sanctions work and promotes the work ethic.

Work is a point of social contact and of personal growth and expression. People identify closely with work, and their personal identity is focused around their work life (Thomas, McCabe, and Berry, 1980). Work has been described as a developmental task for the American adult (Duvall and Miller, 1985; Stevenson, 1977). The developmental tasks of work are carried out simultaneously with family and individual developmental tasks across the life cycle. Duvall and Miller (1985) see the young adult as facing the work-related task of selecting and training for an occupation, the adult and middlescent as carrying out a socially adequate worker role as well as balancing between work and leisure, and the aged adult as adjusting to retirement.

Stevenson (1977) describes the developmental tasks of the young adult as integrating personal values with career development and socioeconomic constraints, the early-middle-years adult as developing socioeconomic consolidation and assuming responsible positions in occupational activities; the late-middle-years adult as maintaining flexible views in occupational positions, preparing for another career when feasible, and preparing for retirement; and the adult in late adulthood as pursuing a second or third career and/or adjusting to retirement. If these work-related developmental tasks are left undone or are interrupted, sequential development can be affected and stress can occur. Looking at work from a developmental framework helps to sensitize one to changes that might affect the form and degree of linkages between the individual, family, and community, as a result of accomplishment or lack of accomplishment of work-related developmental tasks.

The occupational health nurse should be aware of the developmental tasks associated with work and help the worker to achieve task fulfillment. Illustrative of how occupational health nurses can do this is the opportunity to work with an employee who has been laid off due to an illness. For example, an employee with uncontrolled diabetes may not be able to return to the job until the diabetic condition is under control. The occupational health nurse can assist this worker to obtain needed medical treatment, discuss with the employee possible reasons for the uncontrolled condition, and help to see that the employee's job situation allows adequate care for meeting health requirements.

OCCUPATIONAL HEALTH STRESSORS AND THEIR RISKS TO WORKERS

Most occupational illnesses and injuries are preventable. It is unfortunate that they occur. The stressors in the workplace that cause occupational illness and injury are extensive and diverse. They can be categorized (with examples) as follows (Olishifski, 1979):

1. *Chemical:* liquids, gases, dusts, particles, fumes, mists, and vapors

2. *Physical:* electromagnetic and ionizing radiation, noise, pressure, vibration, heat, and cold
3. *Biologic:* insects, mold, fungi, and bacteria
4. *Ergonomic:* monotony, fatigue, boredom, stress; the effects of the environment on humankind

For diverse reasons, it is often difficult to formulate cause-and-effect relationships between occupational stressors and specific illnesses and conditions. A primary problem in formulating cause-and-effect relationships is that no immediate, observable effect of the stressor may be apparent. Long latency periods may exist between contact with the stressor and stressor effects. For example, occupational cancers usually do not become evident until 5 to 40 years after the initial exposure to the carcinogen (CDC, March 9, 1984, p. 127). In diseases and conditions with long latency periods, the worker may already have left the job where contact occurred, making it increasingly difficult to identify and trace the stressor.

The influence of multiple stressors is another factor which affects cause-and-effect relationships. Victims may have been occupationally, environmentally, and personally exposed to many stressors, the interactions between them may greatly increase the risk of contracting the condition, and their effects may not be easily separated (CDC, March 9, 1984, p. 126). It may also become difficult to ascertain which stressor caused the problem. How can the miner with emphysema prove that mine work rather than a heavy smoking habit was the primary factor in the causation of the disease?

The fact that valid, comprehensive occupational health statistics are often not readily available further complicates the situation (APHA, 1984, p. 283). Obtaining reliable data on occupational health is a prerequisite to research. The United States has not formulated national standards for reporting occupational disease and injury; a national occupational disease and industry registry is necessary.

Birth and death certificates are commonly used to obtain health statistics, but occupation and industry entries on these certificates are often missing or incomplete. The National Center for Health Statistics has published *Guidelines for Reporting Occupation and Industry on Death Certificates* to aid in this endeavor, but uniform reporting is lacking. Since 1980, NIOSH has sponsored a pilot program in six states to survey occupational disease, disability, and mortality as reflected in death certificates (Lalich and Schuster, 1987, p. 1310); since 1989 parental employment has been added to the standard *U.S. Fetal Death Certificate* (Lalich and Schuster, 1987, p. 1313).

Information gathered from death certificates can assist in helping others exposed to the reported occupational hazards. However, these data are of no use to the deceased worker. It has been suggested that workers' compensation data and hospital discharge data would provide a better basis for early diagnosis, treatment, and client follow-up (Schwartz and Landrigan, 1987, p. 1457; Lalich and Schuster, 1987, p. 1310).

Until additional occupational health data are routinely collected and analyzed, it will be difficult to formulate cause-and-effect relationships and to formulate effective plans for intervention (Whorton, 1983). It should be remembered by direct care practitioners that in gathering health information, occupational information must be routinely incorporated into their assessment.

In addition to their potential for causing serious illness and injury, stressors may also have a negative impact on the worker's psychological well-being. This fact has often been overlooked in studying stressors and their effects. Stressors can cause a worker to be anxious, depressed, irritable, and moody.

Occupational illness and injury are significant national concerns; the hardships experienced by individuals and their families are inestimable. From a financial standpoint, it is estimated that billions of dollars are lost annually due to job-related illness and injury, through wages, medical expenses, insurance claims, and production delays, and millions of workdays are lost each year to illness and absenteeism.

Reducing illness and injury on the job is a major task. One related problem is the difficulty in overcoming the attitudes and actions of the workers themselves. Unfortunately, many people who are exposed to occupational hazards deny the risks of working around them, and do not take steps to lessen their chances of developing health problems. This poses a problem for occupational health personnel.

Educating the worker to the hazards of the workplace and actions that can be taken to minimize them is a critical step in illness and injury reduction. Sometimes it is difficult to get the worker to realize that a stressor exists, because it is not visible to the human eye. If something cannot be seen, it is often difficult to conceptualize that a problem exists. People are less suspicious of, and tend to minimize, the hazards of those things they cannot visualize.

Table 16-1 shows the 10 leading work-related diseases, injuries, and conditions in the United States. It is readily seen that they are diverse and extensive and that they involve psychological as well as physical problems. NIOSH focuses research efforts on these areas.

Occupational Lung Diseases

Occupational lung disease heads the list of the 10 leading work-related diseases and injuries. The lung is both a target organ and a portal of entry for toxic substances. Annually more than 1.2 million workers are exposed to silica dust, and more than 500,000 workers are exposed to cotton dust (USDHHS, 1987, p. 73). The potential is high for workplace exposure to substances causing asbestos-related diseases, silicosis, coal workers' pneumoconiosis, byssinosis, emphysema, asthma, and chronic industrial bronchitis.

Asbestosis is expected to kill 10 to 18 percent of asbestos and shipyard workers exposed to it; byssinosis (brown lung) has disabled thousands of textile workers; silicosis will strike thousands of miners and foundry workers; pneumoconiosis continues to kill coal miners every year; and occupational asthma is rampant, affecting from 10 to 100 percent of workers in certain occupations; the list goes on and on (CDC, January 21, 1983).

TABLE 16-1 The 10 leading work-related diseases and injuries—United States

Diseases/conditions	Examples
1. Occupational lung diseases	Asbestosis, byssinosis, silicosis, coal workers' pneumoconiosis, lung cancer, occupational asthma
2. Musculoskeletal injuries	Disorders of the back, trunk, upper extremity, neck, lower extremity; traumatically induced Raynaud's phenomenon
3. Occupational cancers (other than lung)	Leukemia, mesothelioma; cancers of the bladder, nose, and liver
4. Traumatic injury and death	Amputations, fractures, eye loss, lacerations
5. Cardiovascular diseases	Hypertension, coronary artery disease, acute myocardial infarction
6. Disorders of reproduction	Infertility, spontaneous abortion, teratogenesis
7. Neurotoxic disorders	Peripheral neuropathy, toxic encephalitis, psychoses, extreme personality changes (exposure-related)
8. Loss of hearing	Noise-induced hearing loss
9. Dermatologic conditions	Dermatoses, burns (scaldings), chemical burns, contusions (abrasions)
10. Psychologic disorders	Neuroses, personality disorders, alcoholism, drug dependency

From Centers for Disease Control: Leading work-related diseases and injuries—United States (occupational lung diseases), MMWR, p 25, January 21, 1983.

A national health objective is that by 1990, among newly exposed workers, virtually no new cases of the four preventable occupational lung diseases will develop; asbestosis, byssinosis, silicosis, and coal miners' pneumoconiosis (USDHHS, 1986, The 1990 health, p. 115). At present there is no uniform method for reporting the diseases addressed in this objective, making it almost impossible to measure its success (USDHHS, 1986, The 1990 health, p. 116).

Musculoskeletal Injuries

Although musculoskeletal injuries result in few work-related deaths, they account for a great amount of human suffering and loss of productivity. Impairments to the musculoskeletal system are estimated to affect more than 12 million persons, and the workplace accounts for more than 20 percent of all back sprains and injuries reported to medical authorities (USDHHS, 1987, p. 73). Back injuries account for one of every five workplace injuries and are associated with improper handling of materials, repetitive motion, and vibration injuries. Improved equipment design, a minimum of biomechanical stress, rota-

tion of workers to jobs with different physical demands, safety training, and other worker education would all help to alleviate these injuries (CDC, April 15, 1983). Occupational health nurses play an active role in establishing and implementing these control measures. They focus on health risk appraisal and educational activities and emphasize ways to prevent musculoskeletal injuries.

Occupational Cancers

Estimates of the percentage of cancers related to the workplace are as high as 20 percent. Some cancers among occupational groups are so frequent that a causal relationship is obvious (e.g., cancer of the bone in radium dial painters and mesothelioma among asbestos workers) (USDHHS, 1987, p. 73). Occupationally induced cancers often appear decades after the exposure that initiated the cancer. Table 16-2 lists some occupational cancers and related agents by industry and occupation. Having an awareness of the data presented in Table 16-2 helps the occupational health team to design preventive strategies which will prevent unnecessary deaths due to cancer.

TABLE 16-2   Selected occupational cancers and related agents by industry/occupation

Condition	Industry/occupation	Agent
Hemangiosarcoma of the liver	Vinyl chloride polymerization	Vinyl chloride monomer
	Industry vintners	Arsenical pesticides
Malignant neoplasm of nasal cavities	Woodworkers, cabinet/furniture makers	Hardwood dusts
	Boot and shoe producers	Unknown
	Radium chemists, processors, dial painters	Radium
	Nickel smelting and refining	Nickel
Malignant neoplasm of larynx	Asbestos industries and utilizers	Asbestos
Mesothelioma (peritoneum) (pleura)	Asbestos industries and utilizers	Asbestos
Malignant neoplasm of bone	Radium chemists, processors, dial painters	Radium
Malignant neoplasm of scrotum	Automatic lathe operators, metalworkers	Mineral/cutting oils
	Coke oven workers, petroleum refiners, tar distillers	Soots and tars, tar distillates
Malignant neoplasm of bladder	Rubber and dye workers	Benzidine, alpha and beta naphthylamine, auramine, magenta, 4-aminobiphenyl, 4-nitrophenyl
Malignant neoplasm of kidney; other, and unspecified urinary organs	Coke oven workers	Coke oven emissions
Lymphoid leukemia, acute	Rubber industry	Unknown
	Radiologists	Ionizing radiation
Myeloid leukemia, acute	Occupations with exposure to benzene	Benzene
	Radiologists	Ionizing radiation
Erythroleukemia	Occupations with exposure to benzene	Benzene

From Centers for Disease Control: Leading work-related diseases and injuries—United States (occupational cancers other than lung), MMWR, p 126, March 9, 1984. Adapted from Rutstein DD, Mullan RJ, Frazier TM, Halperin WE, Melius JM, and Sestito JP: Sentinel health events (occupational): a basis for physician recognition and public health surveillance, Am J Public Health 73:1054-1062,1984.

Problems in documenting occupationally induced cancers can obscure important epidemiological associations and considerations (CDC, March 9, 1984). Some of these problems are described below (CDC, March 9, 1984).

1. Errors in diagnosis and classification of cancers can occur, and unusual neoplasms are often misdiagnosed.
2. There is a lack of meaningful occupational histories. In only a few states is information collected on the work histories of cancer victims; hence, crucial associations with occupational carcinogens are often missed.
3. Precise measurements of levels and duration of exposures have not been generally available, resulting in an inability to delineate dose-response relationships in a consistent manner.
4. The occupational etiology of a very rare cancer due to a specific agent, such as hemangiosarcoma of the liver to vinyl chloride, is much more readily documented than the occupational etiology of cancer caused by several factors.
5. Highly significant differences in the rates of cancer among small subgroups of a population may be overlooked because these rates affect the overall rate for cancer in the larger study population only slightly, if at all. This

creates what has been called the "dilution factor."

There are thousands of suspected carcinogens in the workplace that are not regulated. Exposure to carcinogens does not always cause cancer, and not everything is a carcinogen. *The dose and frequency of duration are often the key to the toxicity of a substance.* Many chemicals such as zinc, nickel, tin, and potassium are essential for health in small quantities, but are toxic in larger quantities.

Traumatic Injury and Death

NIOSH estimates that at least 10 million Americans suffer traumatic injuries on the job each year, of which some 30 percent are severe and 10,000 are fatal (USDHHS, 1987, p. 74). These traumatic injuries include amputations, fractures, severe lacerations, eye loss, acute poisonings, burns, and even death. Preventing these injuries rests largely with implementing engineering controls, use of protective equipment, worker education, putting barriers such as curtains and shields between the worker and the hazard, and monitoring the workplace for emergency hazards (CDC, April 27, 1984).

Cardiovascular Diseases

Cardiovascular diseases are the leading cause of death in the United States. The role of occupation in cardiovascular disease is not clear, and most researchers believe that personal risk factors play a much more important role than environmental ones. However, some occupational factors, such as cardiotoxins and stressors, are clearly associated with cardiovascular diseases (USDHHS, 1987, p. 74). Fortunately, the workplace is an excellent site for preventive programs in personal risk factors related to cardiovascular diseases such as smoking cessation, proper diet, blood pressure control, exercise, and stress reduction. Occupational health nurses assume a major role in developing and implementing these prevention programs. An increasing number of worksites have well-established health promotion programs designed to prevent premature deaths related to cardiovascular disease.

Reproductive Disorders

Research has shown that exposure to occupational stressors can cause disorders of reproduction. The data include information on male sterility in dibromochloropropane workers, impotence in workers exposed to specific neurotoxins, increased birth defects among children born to female pharmaceutical workers, and excessive spontaneous abortions among medical laboratory workers and hospital and dental personnel exposed to anesthetic gases (USDHHS, 1987, p. 74). NIOSH has developed a program to identify potential teratogens and mutagens that may exist in the workplace; to identify possible associations between parental employment and reproductive loss; and to target the epidemiological study of workers at high risk for reproductive disorders.

Neurotoxic Disorders

More than 850 chemicals in the American workplace have been identified as toxic to the central nervous system, and the number of workers exposed to these neurotoxic chemicals has been estimated at 8 million (USDHHS, 1987, p. 74). Peripheral neuropathy, characterized by numbness and tingling in the feet or hands, followed by clumsiness or incoordination, is one of the most common and serious. The worker may find his or her ability to work impaired on either a temporary or permanent basis. The nurse should monitor exposure to such chemicals and assess workers for symptomatology.

Psychological Disorders

Psychological stressors are present on any job and are often related to ergonomics. They can be brought on by such things as boredom, stress, monotony, and fatigue. At any one time, an estimated 8 to 10 percent of the work force is suffering from disabling emotional or psychological ill health (USDHHS, 1987, p. 75). Stress-related symptoms contribute to absenteeism, lost productivity, and company health care expenses at a cost of $50 to $75 billion annually (USDHHS, 1987, p. 75).

The occupational health nurse should be sensitive to the fact that family members are often the victims of the effects of work stress and psychological disturbance. Group sessions on stress awareness and management may be especially helpful for workers and their families. The nurse should refer workers to community mental health resources as appropriate.

One interesting work-related psychological phenomenon is epidemic psychogenic illness, sometimes called mass or contagious psychogenic illness. This phenomenon occurs when a number of workers simultaneously experience similar symptoms, seemingly contagious in nature, from a cause that appears to be work-related but for which no identifiable stressor except a psychological one can be found. NIOSH has done studies of mass psychogenic illness since 1974. They indicate that it occurs much more frequently in the workplace than the literature suggests (Colligan and Smith, 1978; Colligan and Murphy, 1979; Colligan, 1981; CDC, June 10, 1983).

The symptoms of mass psychogenic illness vary, but often include headaches, nausea, chills, blurred vision, muscular weakness, and difficulty breathing (Colligan and Stockton, 1978). The illness is frequently linked with worker's sense of smell and being overcome by strange odors (Colligan and Murphy, 1979). It has routinely been connected with stressful job situations. These jobs are often characterized by boredom, monotony, production pressures, hazardous physical stressors, poor labor-management relations, and lack of communication such as occurs in a noisy environment (Colligan and Murphy, 1979). A person who is unhappy or dissatisfied with work appears to be vulnerable to psychological work disorders, as does a person suffering bereavement, social isolation, abrupt social change and threat of uncertainty (Colligan, 1981). When outbreaks do occur, NIOSH recommends that symptomatic persons be removed to a quiet, out-of-the-way area and that the situation be handled as quietly as possible to contain the spread of pain and anxiety (CDC, June 10, 1983). According to Colligan (1981) there are some important questions about psychogenic illness: (1) by what mechanisms do psychological properties and processes become translated into physical symptoms; (2) are some individuals or work settings more susceptible to

such illnesses and outbreaks than others, and what are the precipitating conditions; and (3) to what extent do psychological stressors lower worker resistance to even mild irritants in the work environment, making the workers more susceptible? These questions afford excellent areas for further research.

There are numerous examples of mass psychogenic illness in industry. In one study cited by the CDC (June 10, 1983) 46 percent of the employees in one facility developed severe symptoms after diesel fumes accidentally entered the production area, and it was thought that the employees were being exposed to toxic chemicals. (Diesel fumes are noxious, but not toxic or disease producing.) That episode caused two separate plant closings, with six separate episodes of fume smelling.

In epidemic psychogenic illness, the nurse should be sensitive to the needs of the worker, while maintaining a focus on the reality of the situation. The symptoms are real to those who are experiencing them, and they should not be discounted. Talking openly with workers about this phenomenon will help to eliminate, minimize, and demystify the situation, and may be the most effective means of ending an epidemic. *One must be cautious, however, not to attribute everything to psychogenic illness. Each situation should be carefully evaluated, since there may actually be a hazardous occupational stressor present.*

Hearing Loss

Noise is a physical stressor that causes hearing loss. That workers in noisy environments lose their hearing has been known for at least the past 200 years. By the early twentieth century boilermakers' deafness, caused by boilermakers' riveting inside a metal boiler, was an occupational hazard of considerable magnitude (Lawrence, 1978, p. 22) Federal efforts to regulate occupational noise were begun in 1955. Noise-induced hearing loss is one of the most serious, common, and preventable occupational conditions.

Approximately 8 million workers in the United States are exposed to potentially harmful noise levels, 20 percent (1,600,000) may have impaired hearing, and some 5 percent (400,000) have compensable hearing loss (USDHHS, 1987, p. 74). Unfortunately, thousands of workers are exposed to noise levels in excess of the federal noise standard.

It has been determined that an industrial noise hearing loss is represented on audiograms by a notch at approximately 4000 Hz (Figure 16-3). This notch is often referred to as the industrial noise or industrial acoustic trauma notch. The person suffering from this loss may initially complain of tinnitus, which is a ringing in the ear. Many such persons are unaware of any hearing loss, and by the time a hearing loss is noticed, which may be years later, the person is experiencing difficulty communicating. Most workers are unaware of the continuing hearing damage until the damage is severe and permanent.

Nurses are active in hearing conservation in industry. A successful hearing conservation program in industry carries out the following activities (Garvey, 1983; Lacy, 1978, p. 18):

1. It provides noise surveys for analyzing the workers' environment for excess noise exposure.
2. It utilizes administrative and engineering controls for reducing noise levels.
3. It performs audiometric testing on each prospective employee and continues to measure an employee's hearing periodically.
4. It furnishes hearing protection for employees working in noisy areas.
5. It provides ongoing educational programs to encourage the employees' cooperation in hearing conservation.

The success or failure of an occupational hearing conservation program will depend largely on the occupational health nurse. It is the nurse who obtains the workers' medical and occupational history, carries out the audiometric testing, refers employees with ear complaints or poor audiograms to the physician, counsels the employees regarding industrial noise, and fits or supplies the employee with appropriate hearing protection devices. An industrial hearing conservation program reduces noise levels in the following three ways: (1) through primary prevention of the

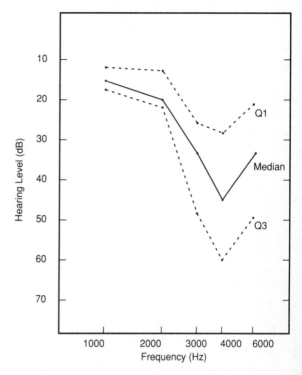

Figure 16-3 Noise-induced permanent threshold shift after 4 years on the job, based on 8 hours of exposure per day. (Adapted from American Industrial Hygiene Association: Industrial noise manual, ed 3, Akron, Oh, 1975, American Industrial Hygiene Association, p 35.)

noise; (2) through alteration of the noise source; and (3) through utilization of protective devices.

Dermatological Disorders

More than 40 percent of all reported occupational health diseases and conditions in the United States are disorders of the skin (USDHHS, 1987, p. 75), though their true incidence is estimated to be 10 to 50 times higher than what is reported (Moses, 1989, p. 118). Dermal absorption of chemicals may be more serious than absorption by inhalation, in the case of chemicals such as aniline, dimethylformamide, dibromochloropropane, and glycol ethers.

Workers in agriculture are at four times greater risk of contracting skin disease than workers in other industries (Moses, 1989, p. 118). This is largely due to their exposure to pesticides and chemicals. Personal protective clothing, the use of less toxic chemicals, and health education activities can all help to decrease the incidence of dermatitis. Dermatitis is usually an occupational illness that is amenable to early diagnosis and treatment.

AIDS IN THE WORKPLACE

The number of individuals diagnosed with AIDS increased from under 100 in 1981 to 146,746 by September 1990 (CDC, 1990, p. 5), and the number rises daily. This is more than a 1000 percent increase in less than 10 years. CDC estimates that by 1992 the total number of AIDS cases will exceed 365,000. It is estimated that nearly 2 million people in the United States are infected with the AIDS virus (Harris, 1990, p. 6). With no effective treatment or cure in sight the prospect that the situation will improve in the near future is dim.

The AIDS epidemic is being felt everywhere, including the workplace. To help meet the challenge, the AAOHN has published *Educational Resources on AIDS* (1988), a continuing education module for occupational health nurses; the comprehensive *AAOHN Resource Guide. HIV Infections/AIDS in the Workplace* (1988); and an abundance of articles in the *AAOHN Journal.* The resource guide is extremely helpful to the nurse: its three sections include (1) definitions, (2) HIV infection/AIDS information, and (3) resource information. It covers such topics as worker surveillance, counseling, policy development, research, ethics, confidentiality, and the right to work. The guide recommends that workers with AIDS be employed for as long as possible; confidentiality of HIV testing results and records be maintained; management take aggressive action to establish AIDS policy and education at the workplace; and discrimination against the HIV-positive employee be discouraged (AAOHN, 1989, A year). Occupational health nurses need to maintain up-to-date knowledge of HIV-related illnesses, and disseminate information to the workforce (AIDS taskforce, 1988, p. 286).

Close to 91 percent of all people diagnosed with AIDS are between the ages of 20 and 49 (USDHHS, 1986, Coping with; Harris, 1990, p.

6). It has been estimated that more than 8300 work years will be lost because of disability and premature death from AIDS, amounting to an economic loss in excess of 4.8 billion dollars and an incalculable amount of human pain and suffering (Newman, Sirles, and Williamson, 1988, p. 258). Most HIV-infected people are members of the workforce, and would prefer to continue to work as long as they are able.

The workplace has been slow to respond to the immense needs created by AIDS. While the number of companies employing HIV-infected workers has more than tripled since 1985, only 10 percent of all companies have adopted AIDS policies (Nyamathi and Flaskerud, 1989, p. 403). Additional companies are developing such policies, but the progress remains slow. It is as if many companies are not sure where to start or what direction to take.

Research by Hansen, Booth, Fawal, and Langer (1988) showed that most workers held some negative attitudes and myths about HIV-positive coworkers. There is a great need for information programs to educate workers and employers about AIDS. Education at the worksite must include factual information on disease transmission, personal risk behaviors, risk reduction activities, and data which dispel myths and misinformation (Williamson, Brown, and Packa, 1988, p. 265). The occupational health nurse has been, and likely will continue to be, the key figure in AIDS policy development and educational programming (Harris, 1990, p. 11). Research by Nyamathi and Flaskerud (1989) revealed statistically significant improvements in AIDS knowledge following an AIDS education program with employees. This education is one that occupational health nurses will be involved in far into the future, and they will be instrumental in shaping AIDS policies in the workplace.

OCCUPATIONAL HEALTH AND MINORITY WORKERS

The nurse needs to be aware that employment in hazardous occupations is much more common among minority workers (blacks, Hispanics, Asians, and Native Americans). This results in a disproportionate number of occupational illnesses, injuries, and deaths within these population groups. Because of socioeconomic factors, these minority workers are less likely to receive adequate health care, and are often not even properly diagnosed (Friedman-Jimenez, 1989, p. 70). Nurses need to consider this in their plans of care and when implementing health education and safety programs.

Unfortunately, this area of occupational health has not always received the attention, recognition, and research it deserves. In 1981 NIOSH held a national conference on occupational health and safety issues affecting minority workers, but the proceedings were never published (Alexander, 1989, p. 107).

Black and Hispanic workers tend to be particularly underrepresented in low-risk occupations, but highly overrepresented in dangerous high-risk ones (Morris, 1989, p. 53; Friedman-Jimenez, 1989, p. 65). Fifteen percent of the 7 million black workers are permanently disabled from work-related causes compared to 10 percent of white workers. Blacks have a 37 percent greater likelihood of suffering work-related illness or injury and a 20 percent greater likelihood of dying from a job-related condition than whites (Davis, 1980; Morris, 1989, p. 53). Hispanics are heavily represented in the hazardous occupations of farm work and manufacturing. Farm work is the most hazardous occupation in the United States, with more than 1600 deaths annually and 160,000 disabling injuries (Ubell, 1989, p. 5). Many of these deaths and injuries occur among seasonal, migrant farm workers of whom 75 percent are Hispanic and 20 percent are black (Morris, 1989, p. 53). It was for this reason that migrant farm work has been singled out for further discussion in this text. Many of the areas of concern discussed in the section below apply at least in part to other minority workers in other work settings.

Migrant Farm Workers

Migrant workers face many health hazards, and are not protected by many of the laws which govern the health and welfare of other workers. Farm workers are excluded completely or partially from federal laws including the National Labor Rela-

tions Act (which guarantees the right to join a union and bargain collectively), the Fair Labor Standards Act (which governs minimum wage and child labor), the Occupational Safety and Health Act (which governs standards of health and safety in the workplace), and state workers' compensation laws and unemployment insurance laws (Moses, 1989, p. 115). In general, family-owned farms are excluded from government safety supervision and inspection (Ubell, 1989, p. 5).

Some states have made provisions for the migrant worker, but these provisions are sparse, and the migrant worker has little legislative protection. Migrant farm workers face many problems including financial instability, child labor, poor housing, lack of education, and impaired access to health and social services

Financial Stability

Migrant farm workers represent a large, mobile supply of cheap labor. Their work is characterized by low wages, long hours, few benefits, and poor working conditions. They are the working poor, without many of the health and welfare benefits that other workers have. Many migrant farm workers earn less than $3500 a year (Goldfarb, 1981, pp. 15-17). This is well below the poverty level, and most migrant families live in chronic poverty.

Child Labor

Child labor has all but disappeared from U.S. industry, except in the agricultural sector. Many migrant children work, because it brings in additional family income. Growers continue to use child labor, because it is inexpensive and available. Migrant children who work are subject to the same job hazards and health risks as adults, including long hours and hazardous or faulty equipment and chemicals. They show increased incidence of accidental injury on the job. Working often keeps migrant children from school and other normal childhood activities.

Housing

It has been estimated that 42 percent of farm housing falls into the substandard category, compared to 14 percent of nonfarm housing (Goldfarb, 1981, p. 43). Housing is generally crowded and inadequate, and living conditions are not safe or sanitary. Migrant housing has been compared to slave quarters: horrible and dehumanizing, without adequate heat, light, or ventilation, and often without plumbing or refrigeration (Goldfarb, 1981, p. 42). These unsanitary and unsafe housing conditions are breeding grounds for diseases, disability, hopelessness, and death.

Migrant Education

Many migrant children never enter high school, and of those who do, few graduate. It is not that migrant families do not want an education for their children; they just have great difficulty obtaining it for them. Their mobility and the seasonal nature of farm work necessitate frequent school changes and absences. Local school officials hold attitudes toward migrants which range from indifference to hostility, and they are frequently lax in enforcing school attendance and other regulations for migrant children. The manner in which many of these children are handled within the school system can leave them scarred for life. They may be labeled slow, retarded, uncooperative, or uninterested, when actually the situation is more a social problem than a question of the children's educational ability or attitude.

The federal government authorizes funds for migrant education. A startling find is that often not all of this money is utilized. During three fiscal years, of $90 million that was given to the states for migrant education, $13 million was not spent (Goldfarb, 1981, p. 47).

The aspirations of migrant families that their children receive a good education go unfulfilled. As long as migrant children are poorly educated, it will be difficult for them to escape their present living conditions.

Access to Services

Although the migrant worker may qualify for federal aid programs, restrictive local and state policies often limit access to the health and welfare services within these boundaries. Migrant workers may be subject to rejection and hostility from the community in which they are working.

Many migrant workers are unfamiliar with local resources, personnel, and other individuals; they tend to stay together rather than mix in a community that does not welcome them or provide resources for them. Migrant workers generally have no voice in community planning and decision making and often do not feel any attachment, other than economic, to the community in which they work.

In 1969, a Supreme Court decision (*Shapiro v. Thompson*, 394 U.S. 618) ruled that a state could not exclude persons from welfare benefits because they were not residents of that state or had not resided in that state for a specific period of time. This was a great help to the migrant worker, because many of them became eligible for health and welfare services, such as food stamps.

The Department of Labor provides many benefits for migrant farm workers and their families. Programs such as child care, economic development, housing, subsidies, training, health services, legal aid, transportation, and others are provided for eligible migrant farm workers.

Health

Historically, the migrant farm worker has had minimal access to the health care system, even though federal funds are available for these services. The Health Revenue Sharing Act of 1975 (Public Law 94-63) authorized grants to public and other nonprofit agencies for cost sharing in the establishment and operation of migrant family health service clinics. These projects offer a comprehensive range of health services, such as diagnosis and treatment, dental services, preventive care, and health counseling. Services not available at these centers are often supplemented by referrals to other agencies and groups.

The transient nature of the migrant worker's employment makes it difficult to establish regular routes for health care. The pay base of the work does not allow sufficient funds for health care services, and many migrants are not covered under private health insurance plans. Migrant workers are often not aware of the health care services in the area where they reside. Migrant workers have limited access to health care services, yet often evidence significant health care needs. Research has shown they are at increased risk for developing malignant lymphoma, leukemia, multiple myeloma, testicular cancer, and cancer of the gastrointestinal tract (Moses, 1989, pp. 121-122). It is believed that this increased risk is related to the chemicals, especially pesticides, to which they are exposed during the course of the workday.

A major problem with estimating occupational illness and injury among migrant farm workers is that few reliable statistics are kept. Two occupational hazards for the farm worker which have been documented are (1) farm machinery and (2) pesticides and other chemicals.

At least 800,000 farm workers are injured from exposure to pesticides (Goldfarb, 1981, p. 35). Acute health effects from exposure to pesticides range from eye infections and upper respiratory tract irritability and contact dermatitis to systemic poisoning, which can cause death (Moses, 1989, p. 117). The primary route of exposure to pesticides, except for fumigants, is through the skin, and they may persist on the skin for many months (Moses, 1989, p. 116). Little is known about the chronic health problems related to pesticide exposure. Few studies have been done in this area, and record keeping on pesticide-related exposures and illnesses is lacking. The nurse should recognize the risks for such exposures and include this area in assessment.

With today's modern health technology, one could assume that migrant health would be making major strides forward, but it is not. Migrant workers still suffer from malnutrition and many turn-of-the-century communicable diseases not usually seen in the general population. Migrant children often are not properly immunized, and families frequently do not seek preventive medical care. One health survey showed that only 8 percent saw a physician during the year, compared to 70 percent of the general U.S. population; the survey also showed that 90 percent of the migrant population was not covered by any form of health insurance (Goldfarb, 1981).

The average life expectancy for the migrant worker is 49 years (Goldfarb, 1981, p. 34). This figure is statistically and *morally* significant considering that the life expectancy for the nation as a whole is 74 years.

Other health statistics also reflect the magnitude of the health problems facing migrant workers and their families. Ashford (1976, p. 522) stated that migrant farm workers experience (1) an infant mortality rate 125 percent higher than the national average, (2) death rates from influenza and pneumonia 200 percent higher than the national average, and (3) tuberculosis rates 250 percent higher than the national average. These statistics indicate the magnitude of the health problems facing the migrant worker and the family.

The stresses the worker must face are ones to which many of us have never been exposed. The poor working and living conditions, minimal health services, decreased educational opportunities for their children, and low wages all contribute to a poverty beyond what most Americans experience. The migrant farm worker is largely concerned with immediate, day-to-day survival, and plans for the future are almost a luxury.

The nurse working with migrant farm workers and their families can greatly facilitate their effort to obtain health care. The nurse needs firsthand knowledge of community resources, health care facilities, and occupational hazards. The nurse can assist the family in obtaining necessary services and is often in a position to be an advocate for their rights. The health of migrant workers is a vast and challenging field.

OCCUPATIONAL HEALTH NURSING AND THE FUTURE

The future of occupational health nursing is bright and exciting. The recent activities of OHN leaders who are conducting research, developing educational programs, and advocating legislative change has enhanced its professionalism and excellence. It is expected that these efforts will continue and offer many avenues for the new practitioner to pursue.

Research in occupational health nursing has been increasing by leaps and bounds. The AAOHN has made a commitment to research that will put the profession in the forefront of occupational health.

Educational opportunities have also been increasing. What is likely to be seen are major efforts to make nursing students aware of the field, integration of this content area into baccalaureate nursing education, and an expansion of coursework at the graduate level, all of which will produce a greater number of occupational health nurses holding masters or doctorate degrees. The education of school children and the general public about occupational health should also be on the nurse's agenda.

The political wisdom and expertise of the occupational health nurse will continue to grow. By monitoring the social, economic, and political forces affecting health, the nurse will be able to predict the effect of these forces on the role and scope of practice and on occupational health in general. The AAOHN has provided testimony to the U.S. Department of Health and Human Services in relation to the year 2000 occupational health objectives. Occupational health nurses undoubtedly will continue to play an active role in defining national and occupational health legislation and regulation (Cox, 1989, pp. 356-357).

Occupational health nurses already are largely autonomous, yet their role will undoubtedly expand in consulting, health care of the workforce with chronic conditions, and prevention and control of infectious diseases in the workplace. Nurses will have greater opportunity to take part in health promotion and primary prevention activities in the workplace, and will likely be called upon to develop, implement, and evaluate such programs. This prospect is exciting because it gives the nurse the opportunity to promote wellness instead of trying to treat and cure illness and disability.

Ethical issues will increase in scope, and the AAOHN and individual nurses will need to monitor them closely. Such issues as AIDS in the workplace, right-to-know, and cost containment that may be at the expense of worker health will remain at the forefront of ethical issues in occupational health.

The future for occupational health nursing is an exciting one. The hope is that many nursing students will look at occupational health nursing as a potential area of study and practice.

SUMMARY

Maintaining the health of the working population is an important task of all health care professionals. The health of well adults influences not only the status of the worker as an individual, but also the health of society as a whole.

Nursing plays a very significant role in promoting the health of the well-adult population. The occupational health nurse provides key services in an occupational health program. The nurse in the community setting must also be aware of, and act on, occupational health problems and concerns. Many workplace problems will be evidenced at home, and may first be noticed in the home setting. Routinely gathering pertinent occupational health histories should be a part of every nursing assessment.

Nurses also need to make other health care professionals aware of occupational health and safety issues. The nurse needs to take an active policy-making and legislative role in this field. It is through actions such as these that there will be more complete disclosure of harmful agents in the workplace, that adequate legislation and appropriations to control the effects of hazardous substances will be obtained, and that higher levels of worker and community health will be realized.

There have been more advances in the protection of workers from occupational health hazards in the United States in the last 25 years than in the entire history of the nation. Occupational health and safety is rapidly evolving and occupational health nursing is an expanding field. Occupational health nursing will gain the interest of many new graduates. Occupational health nursing is part of the nursing of the future; it is an exciting, challenging field with unlimited potential.

APPENDIX 16-1

Overview of Occupational Health in the United States—Significant Legislation and Activities

1836	First restrictive child labor law enacted in Massachusetts. At that time, two-fifths of all employees in New England factories were children from 7 to 16 years old.
1877	State legislation passed requiring factory safeguards (Massachusetts).
1879	State legislation passed requiring factory inspections (Massachusetts).
1886	State legislation passed requiring reporting of industrial accidents (Massachusetts).
1888	Betty Moulder, a nurse, is hired by a group of Pennsylvania mining companies.
1895	Ada Mayo Stewart, a nurse, is hired by the Vermont Marble Company.
1903	Federal government issues a report on occupational safety.
1904	National Child Labor Committee organized.
1905	State health inspection of occupational dangers established (Massachusetts).
1910	State legislation passed requiring formation of an Occupational Disease Commission (Illinois).
1911	Workmen's Compensation Act passed and not declared unconstitutional (New Jersey).
1911	Federal Occupational Disease Commission established.
1913	U.S. Department of Labor given cabinet status.
1917	First training course to educate occupational health nurses.
1919	Florence Wright publishes *Industrial Nursing.*
1935	Social Security Act passed establishing the state-federal unemployment insurance program.
1936	Federal legislation set occupational safety and health standards and minimum age limitations for workers employed in government contract work where the contract exceeded $10,000 (Walsh-Healy Act).
1938	Federal legislation set a minimum age for child labor: 16 years old for general work and 18 years for hazardous work, applicable to most industrial settings (Fair Labor Standards Act).
1942	American Association of Industrial Nurses (AAIN) founded.
1948	Finally, all states have workers' compensation acts.
1956	Mary Louise Brown writes *Occupational health nursing.*
1965	Federal legislation extended to include suppliers of government services the same protection as had been embodied in the Walsh-Healy Act of 1936 (McNamara-O'Hara Act).
1966	Federal legislation passed requiring mandatory inspections and health and safety standards in the mineral industry (Mine Safety Act).
1969	Federal legislation passed setting mandatory health and safety standards for underground mines (Coal Mine Health and Safety Act).
1970	*Occupational Safety and Health Act* of 1970 passed; the most important piece of occupational safety and health legislation in U.S. history.
1971	American Board for Certification of Occupational Health Nurses formed to establish certification standards and examinations, first examination given in 1974.
1973	The Rehabilitation Act of 1973 provided new vocational rehabilitation guidelines.
1976	The Toxic Substances Control Act (Public Law 94-469) enacted requiring testing, restriction, and control of certain chemical substances.
1977	Federal Mine Safety and Health Act passed consolidating all existing mine legislation into one act; intended to promote safety and health throughout the mining industry as well as to prevent recurring disasters.
	American Association of Industrial Nurses changed its name to American Association of Occupational Health Nurses (AAOHN) on January 1, 1977.
1981	AAOHN establishes a research committee.
1982	At the 1982 Annual AAOHN Conference, the first research session on occupational health nursing was held.
1989	AAOHN identifies priority research areas in occupational health nursing (refer to box on p. 634).

APPENDIX 16-2

NIOSH Educational Resource Centers (ERCs) and Other Graduate Education in Occupational Health Nursing

NIOSH EDUCATIONAL RESOURCE CENTERS

Alabama Educational Resource Center
Deep South Center for Occupational Health and Safety
University of Alabama at Birmingham
School of Public Health
Birmingham, Alabama 39294
1-205-934-7178

Northern California Educational Resource Center
University of California at San Francisco
Occupational Health Nursing Program
Community and Administrative Nursing
San Francisco, California 94143-0608
1-415-476-1504

Southern California Educational Resource Center
University of Southern California
Continuing Education Director
Institute of Safety and Systems Management—Professional Programs
3500 South Figueroa Street, Suite 202
Los Angeles, California 90007
1-213-743-6383 or 1-213-743-6523

University of Cincinnati Educational Resource Center
University of Cincinnati
College of Nursing and Health ML 38
Cincinnati, Ohio 45221-0038
1-513-558-5650

Harvard Educational Resource Center
Harvard University
Harvard School of Public Health
Office of Continuing Education
677 Huntington Avenue
Boston, Massachusetts 02115-9957
1-617-732-1171

Illinois Educational Resource Center
University of Illinois at Chicago
School of Public Health MC 922
Director of ERC Continuing Education
2121 West Taylor
Chicago, Illinois 60612
1-312-996-6620 or 1-312-996-7473

Johns Hopkins Educational Resource Center
The Johns Hopkins School of Hygiene and Public Health
Department of Environmental Health Sciences
Continuing Education Director
615 North Wolfe Street, Room 1003
Baltimore, Maryland 21205
1-301-955-2609

Michigan Educational Resource Center
University of Michigan
Center for Occupational Health and Safety Engineering
Director of Continuing Education or Training Coordinator
1205 Beal Avenue, 10E Building
The University of Michigan
Ann Arbor, Michigan 48109-2117
1-313-763-2243

Minnesota Educational Resource Center
Midwest Center for Occupational Health and Safety
Program Director
640 Jackson Street
St. Paul, Minnesota 55101
1-612-221-3992

New York/New Jersey Educational Resource Center
Department of Environmental and Community Medicine
Division of Consumer Health Education
UMDNJ—Robert Wood Johnson Medical School
Brookwood Plaza II, 45 Knightsbridge Road
Piscataway, New Jersey 08854
1-201-463-5062 or 1-201-463-4500

North Carolina Educational Resource Center
North Carolina Occupational Safety and Health Educational Resource Center
University of North Carolina
Occupational Health Nursing
109 Conner Drive, Suite 101
Chapel Hill, North Carolina 27514
1-919-962-2101

Texas Educational Resource Center
Southwest Center for Occupational Health and Safety
Texas A&M University

Continuing Education Director
P.O. Box 20186
Houston, Texas 77225
1-713-792-4604 or 1-713-792-4648

Utah Educational Resource Center
Rocky Mountain Center for Occupational and Environmental Health
University of Utah, Building 512
Continuing Education Program Director
Salt Lake City, Utah 84112
1-801-581-5710

Washington Educational Resource Center
Northwest Center for Occupational Health and Safety
University of Washington, SC-34
Department of Environmental Health
Seattle, Washington 98195
1-206-543-1069

APPENDIX 16-2

NIOSH Educational Resource Centers (ERCs) and Other Graduate Education in Occupational Health Nursing—cont'd

OTHER GRADUATE EDUCATION IN OCCUPATIONAL HEALTH NURSING

Emory University
Nell Hodgson Woodruff
School of Nursing
Atlanta, Georgia 30322

Hunter College
City University of New York
Bellevue School of Nursing
425 East 25th Street
New York, New York 10010

University of Pennsylvania
School of Nursing 420 Service Drive/S2
Philadelphia, Pennsylvania 19104

University of Pittsburgh
School of Nursing
426 Victoria Building
Pittsburgh, Pennsylvania 15261

Simmons College
Department of Nursing
300 The Fenway
Boston, Massachusetts 02215

Texas Women's University
College of Nursing
1130 M.D. Anderson Blvd.
Houston, Texas 77030

University of Wisconsin at Milwaukee
College of Nursing
P.O. Box 41
Milwaukee, Wisconsin 43201

APPENDIX 16-3

Assessment Guide for Nursing in Industry: A Model

1. Community in which industry is located

  a. Description of the community
    (1) Size in area and population

    (2) Climate, altitude, rainfall

    (3) Pollution (noise, radiation, etc.)

    (4) Housing

    (5) Transportation

    (6) Schools

    (7) Sanitation
    (8) Protection: fire, police, etc.
    (9) Trends

  b. Population

    (1) Age distribution

    (2) Sex distribution
    (3) Ethnic and religious composition

    (4) Socioeconomic characteristics

  c. Health information
    (1) Vital statistics

1. Just as industry affects the community, so the community affects industry.

  a. Use three or four key descriptive words.
    (1) How far do the employees travel to work and are the workers neighbors?
    (2) Are there times or seasons that are more hazardous than others?
    (3) Can the worker's dermatitis or hearing loss be attributed to the community or is it work related?
    (4) Is there adequate, safe housing in the area? Must the worker spend too great a percentage of his or her salary on housing?
    (5) Is there safe, adequate transportation to work as well as to a hospital or school?
    (6) Do children have to be bused to school or attend overcrowded classes?
    (7) Are roaches and rats common to the area?
    (8) Are the workers and the industry protected?
    (9) Is the area becoming more urban? Residential? Rundown? Deserted?

  b. How alike or different is the population of the industry from that of the community?
    (1) Are the families of child-rearing age or of retirement age?
    (2) Are there more men or more women?
    (3) Are there certain customs or languages that are predominant in the community?
    (4) What is the level of education of the community? What is the mean community income?

  c. Is it an ill or well community?
    (1) What is the infant mortality rate, birth rate, average life expectancy? Usually the local health department has this information.

Continued.

APPENDIX 16-3

Assessment Guide for Nursing in Industry: A Model—cont'd

(2) *Disease incidence and prevalence*

(3) *Health facilities available*

(4) Community resources

2. The company

a. Historical development

b. Organizational chart

c. *Policies*

(1) Length of the work week
(2) Length of work time

(3) *Sick leave*
(4) *Safety and fire provisions*

d. Support services (benefits)

(1) Insurance programs

(2) Retirement program
(3) Educational support

(4) Safety committee

(5) Recreation committee

e. Relations between worker and management

f. Projection for the future

3. The plant

a. General physical setting
(1) The construction

(2) Parking facilities and public transportation stops

(2) *What are the leading causes of morbidity and mortality?*

(3) *What physical facilities and professional services are available?*

(4) Are there day-care centers, drug rehabilitation facilities, Alcoholics Anonymous groups, etc.?

2. The official name and address of the company.

a. Get a perspective on how, why, and by whom the company was founded and compare it with the present situation.

b. What is the formal order of the system and to whom will the nurse be responsible?

c. *If there is a policy manual, try to obtain a copy. Are the workers aware of the manual?*
(1) How many days a week does the industry operate?
(2) Are there several shifts? Breaks? Is there paid vacation?
(3) Is there a clear policy, and do the workers know it?
(4) Is management aware of situations or substances in the plant which represent danger? Are there organized fire drills? *The Federal Register* is the source of information for federal standards and serves as a helpful guide.

d. What is the attitude of management concerning worker benefits?
(1) *Is there a system for health insurance and life insurance, and is it compulsory?* Does the company pay all or part? *Who fills out the necessary forms?*
(2) Are the benefits realistic?
(3) Can the worker further his or her education? Will the company help financially?
(4) The programmed Red Cross First Aid course is excellent. For information consult your Red Cross. *If there is no committee, do certain people routinely handle emergencies?*
(5) Do the workers have any communication with or interest in each other outside the work setting?

e. This is difficult information to get, but it is important to know how each perceives the other.

f. If the company is growing, workers may see themselves as having a secure future; if not, they may be worried about their job security. How will plant expansion affect the need for nursing services?

3. Draw a small map to scale, labeling the areas. When an accident occurs, place a pin in the exact location on your map. Different-color pinheads can be used for keeping statistics.

a. What is the gross appearance?
(1) What is the size and general condition of buildings and grounds?
(2) How far does the worker have to walk to get inside?

APPENDIX 16-3

Assessment Guide for Nursing in Industry: A Model—cont'd

---

(3) Entrances and exits

(4) Physical environment

(5) Communication facilities
(6) Housekeeping
(7) Interior decoration

b. The work areas

(1) Space
(2) Heights: workplace and supply areas

(3) Stimulation
(4) Safety signs and markings
(5) Standing and sitting facilities

(6) Safety equipment

c. Nonwork areas
(1) Lockers

(2) Hand-washing facilities

(3) Rest rooms

(4) Drinking water

(5) Recreation and rest facilities

(6) Telephones

(7) Ashtrays

4. The working population

a. General characteristics

(1) *Total number of employees*

(2) General appearances
(3) *Age and sex distribution*

(4) Race distribution

(5) Socioeconomic distribution

(3) How many people must use them? How accessible are they?
(4) Comment on heating, air conditioning, lighting glare, drafts, etc.
(5) Are there bulletin boards, newsletters?
(6) Is the physical setting maintained adequately?
(7) Are the surroundings conducive to work? Are they pleasing?

b. Get permission to examine them. Use *The Federal Register* as a guide.
(1) Are workers isolated or crowded?
(2) *Falls and falling objects are dangerous and costly to industry.*
(3) Is the worker too bored to pay attention?
(4) Is danger well marked?
(5) Are chairs safe and comfortable? Are there platforms to stand on, especially for wet processes?
(6) Do the workers make use of hard hats, safety glasses, face masks, radiation badges, etc.? Do they know the safety devices the OSHA regulations require?

c. Where are they located? Is there easy access?
(1) If the work is dirty, workers should be able to change clothes. Are they taking toxic substances home?
(2) If facilities and supplies are available, do workers know how and when to wash their hands?
(3) How accessible are they and what condition are they in?
(4) Can a worker leave the job long enough to get a drink of water when he or she wants to?
(5) Can a worker who is not feeling well lie down? Do workers feel free to use the facilities?
(6) Can a worker receive or make a call? Does a working mother have to stay home because she can't be reached at work?
(7) Are people allowed to smoke in designated areas? Is it safe?

4. Include worker and management, but separate data for comparison.

a. Be as accurate as possible, but estimate when necessary.
(1) Usually, if an industry has 500 or more employees, full-time nursing services are necessary.
(2) Heights, weights, cleanliness, etc.
(3) Certain screening programs are specific for young adults whereas others are more for the elderly. Some programs are more for women; others are more for men. Is there any difference between day and evening shift? Are the problems of the minority sex unattended?
(4) Does one race predominate? How does this compare with the general community?
(5) Great differences in worker salaries can sometimes cause problems.

Continued.

APPENDIX 16-3

Assessment Guide for Nursing in Industry: A Model—cont'd

(6) Religious distribution	(6) Does one religion predominate? Are religious holidays observed?
(7) Ethnic distribution	(7) Is there a language barrier?
(8) Marital status	(8) Widowed, single, divorced people often have different needs.
(9) *Educational backgrounds*	(9) *Can all teaching be done at approximately the same level?*
(10) Life-styles practiced	(10) Are certain life-styles frowned upon?
b. Type of employment offered	b. What percentage of the work force is blue-collar and what percentage is white-collar?
(1) Background necessary	(1) What educational level is required? Skilled vs. unskilled?
(2) Work demands on physical condition	(2) Strength needed: sedentary vs. active.
(3) Work status	(3) Part-time vs. full-time; overtime?
c. Absenteeism	c. Is there a record kept? By whom? Why?
(1) *Causes*	(1) *What are the five most common reasons for absence?*
(2) Length	(2) Absenteeism is costly to the employer. There is some difference between one 10-day absence and ten 1-day absences by the same person.
d. Physically handicapped	d. Does the company have a policy about hiring the handicapped?
(1) Number employed	(1) Where do they work? What do they do?
(2) *Extent of handicaps*	(2) Are they specially trained? Are they in a special program? Do they use prosthetic devices?
e. Personnel on medication	e. Know what medication and where the employee works.
f. Personnel with chronic illness	f. At what stage of illness is the employee? Where does the employee work? Will he or she be able to continue at this job?
5. The industrial process	5. What does the company produce and how?
a. Equipment used	a. Portable vs. fixed; light vs. heavy.
(1) General description of placement	(1) Mark each piece of large equipment on the scale map.
(2) Type of equipment	(2) Fans, blowers, fast moving, wet or dry.
b. Nature of the operation	b. Get a brief description of each state of the process so that you can compare the needs and abilities of the worker with the needs of the job.
(1) *Raw materials used*	(1) *What are they and how dangerous are they? Are they properly stored?* Check *The Federal Register* for guidelines on storage.
(2) Nature of the final product	(2) Can the workers take pride in the final product or do they make parts?
(3) Description of the jobs	(3) Who does what? Where? Label the map.
(4) Waste products produced	(4) What is the system for waste disposal? Are the pollution control devices in place and functioning?
c. *Exposure to toxic substances*	c. *Describe the toxins to which the worker is exposed and the extent of exposure.* Include physical and emotional hazards. Remember that chronic effects of industrial exposure are subtle; a person often gets used to having mild symptoms and won't report them. *The Federal Register* contains specifications for exposure to toxins and some states issue state standards.

APPENDIX 16-3

Assessment Guide for Nursing in Industry: A Model—cont'd

d. Faculties required throughout the industrial process

d. The need for speed, hearing, color vision, etc., can help determine the types of screening programs necessary.

6. The health program

6. Outline what is actually in existence as well as what employees perceive to be in existence.

a. Existing policies
   (1) Objectives of the program
   (2) *Preemployment physicals*

   (3) First-aid facilities
   (4) *Standard orders*

   (5) *Job descriptions for health personnel*

a. Are there informal, unwritten policies?
   (1) Are they clear?
   (2) Are they required? Are they paid for by the company? Is the information used to deselect?
   (3) What is available? What is not available?
   (4) Is there a company physician who is responsible for first aid or emergency policy? If so, work closely with him or her in planning nursing services.
   (5) If there are no guidelines to be followed, write some.

b. Existing facilities and resources

   (1) Trained personnel
   (2) Space

   (3) *Supplies*

   (4) *Records and reports*

b. Sometimes an industry that denies having a health program has more of a system than it realizes.
   (1) *Who responds in an emergency?*
   (2) Where is the sick worker taken? Where is the emergency equipment kept?
   (3) *Make a list and describe the condition* of each item.
   (4) What exists? The Occupational Safety and Health Act requires that employers keep three types of records: a log of occupational injuries and illnesses, a supplemental record of certain illnesses or injuries, and an annual summary (forms 100, 101, and 102 are provided under the act). Good records provide data for good planning.

c. *Services rendered in the past year*
   (1) Care needed
   (2) Screening done
   (3) Referrals made
   (4) Counseling done
   (5) Health education

c. Describe as specifically as possible.
   (1) Chronic or acute? Why?
   (2) Where? By whom? Why?
   (3) By whom? To whom? Why?
   (4) Often informal counseling goes unnoticed.
   (5) What individual or group education was offered by the company?

d. *Accidents in the past year*

d. Including those occurring after work hours, as some of these accidents may be directly or indirectly work-related.

e. *Reasons employees sought health care*

e. List the five major reasons.

From Serafini P: Nursing assessment in industry, Am J Public Health, 66:755-760, 1976. (Author's name is now P. Serafini Blanco.)

REFERENCES

AIDS taskforce resource guide approved. Recommendations issued for stopping spread of HIV/AIDS in the workplace, AAOHN J 36:286, 1988.

Alexander DL: Chronic lead exposure. A problem for minority workers, AAOHN J 37:105-108, 1989.

American Association of Industrial Nurses. The nurse in industry, New York, 1976, The Association.

American Association of Occupational Health Nurses (AAOHN): AAOHN code of ethics, Atlanta, Ga, 1986, The Association.

AAOHN: Education preparation for entry into professional practice (position statement), Atlanta, Ga, 1986, The Association.

AAOHN: A comprehensive guide for establishing an occupational health service, Atlanta, Ga, 1987, The Association.

AAOHN: Confidentiality of health information (position statement), Atlanta, Ga, 1988, The Association.

AAOHN: Continuing education (CE) module. AIDS in the workplace, AAOHN J 36:294-296, 1988.

AAOHN: Delivery of occupational health services (position statement), Atlanta, Ga, 1988, The Association.

AAOHN: Educational resources on AIDS, AAOHN J 36:284-285, 1988.

AAOHN: AAOHN resource guide. HIV infections/ AIDS in the workplace, AAOHN J 36:464-471, 1988.

AAOHN: Standards of practice, Atlanta, Ga, 1988, The Association.

AAOHN: A commitment for excellence, Atlanta, Ga, 1989, The Association.

AAOHN: A year of progress . . . American Association of Occupational Health Nurses 1988 Annual Report, AAOHN J 37(4), 1989.

AAOHN: Continuing education (CE) module. Achieving occupational health among minorities, AAOHN J 37:137-139, 1989.

AAOHN: Guidelines for developing job descriptions in occupational health nursing, Atlanta, Ga, 1989, The Association.

AAOHN: Occupational health nurse: a manager (position statement), Atlanta, Ga, 1989, The Association.

AAOHN: Occupational health nursing. The answer to health care cost containment, Atlanta, Ga, 1989, The Association.

AAOHN: AAOHN research priorities in occupational health nursing, Atlanta, Ga, 1990, The Association.

American Industrial Hygiene Association: Industrial noise manual, ed 3, Akron, Oh, 1975, The Association.

American Public Health Association (APHA): Policy statement No. 8129: occupational data on death certificates, Am J Public Health 72:206, 1982.

APHA: Policy statement No. 8313: the need for accurate job-related injury and illness data, Am J Public Health 74:283, 1984.

Ashford NA: Crisis in the workplace, Cambridge, Ma, 1976, MIT Press.

Babbitz MA and Bodnar EM: Promote wellness at the worksite: become an occupational health nurse, Atlanta, Ga, 1989, American Association of Occupational Health Nurses.

Bertsche PK, Sanborn JS, and Jones ER: Occupational medicine residency training programs. The role occupational health nurses play, AAOHN J 37:316-320, 1989.

Brockert JE: Occupation/industry of parents on birth certificates, Am J Public Health 74:623, 1984.

Budget of the United States government FY 1990: Washington, DC, 1989, US Government Printing Office.

Centers for Disease Control (CDC): Leading work-related diseases and injuries—U.S. (occupational lung diseases), MMWR, pp 24-27, January 21, 1983.

CDC: Leading work-related diseases and injuries—U.S. (musculoskeletal injuries), MMWR, pp 189-190, April 15, 1983.

CDC: Epidemic psychogenic illness in an industrial setting—Pennsylvania, MMWR, pp 287-289, June 10, 1983.

CDC: Leading work-related disease and injuries—U.S. (occupational cancers other than lung), MMWR, pp 125-128, March 9, 1984.

CDC: Leading work-related disease and injuries—U.S. (severe occupational traumatic injuries), MMWR, pp 213-215, April 27, 1984.

CDC: HIV/AIDS surveillance report, Atlanta, Ga, September 1990, The Centers.

Colligan MJ: Mass psychogenic illness: some clarification and perspectives, J Occup Med 23(9):635-638, 1981.

Colligan MJ and Murphy LA: Mass psychogenic illness in organizations: an overview, J Occup Psychol 52:77-90, 1979.

Colligan MJ and Smith MJ: A methodological approach for evaluating an outbreak of mass psychogenic illness in industry, J Occup Med 20:401-402, 1978.

Colligan MJ and Stockton W: The mystery of assembly-line hysteria, Psychology Today, June 1978, pp 93-99, 114-116.

Cox AR: Planning for the future of occupational health nursing. Part II: comprehensive membership survey, AAOHN J 37:356-360, 1989.

Davis M: The impact of workplace health and safety on black workers: assessment and prognosis, Labor Law J 31:274, 1980.

Dirschel KM: A mandate for standards of care, Nurs Health Care 7(1):27-29, 1986.

Donnelly DC: Rehabilitation and the occupational health nurse, Occup Health Nurs 31(8):39-42, 1983.

Duvall EM and Miller BC: Marriage and family development, ed 6, New York, 1985, Harper & Row.

Educational resources on AIDS, AAOHN J 36:284-285, 1988.

Felton JS: The genesis of American occupational health nursing. Part II, AAOHN J 34:31-35, 1988.

Friedman-Jimenez G: Occupational disease among minority workers. A common and preventable public health concern, AAOHN J 37:64-70, 1989.

Gafafer WM: Occupational diseases: a guide to their recognition, Washington, DC, 1964, US Government Printing Office.

Garvey J: At the workplace. The OHN and hearing conservation, Nurs Times 79:25-27, October 5, 1983.

Gillis DM: Employers ally with nursing in the war on health care costs, Nurs Health Care 9(4):173, 1988.

Goldfarb RL: A caste of despair, Ames, Ia, 1981, Iowa University Press.

Hannigan LJ: Occupational health nursing practice: state of the art, AAOHN J 32:17-20, 1984.

Hansen B, Booth W, Fawal HJ, and Langer RW: Workers with AIDS: attitudes of fellow employees, AAOHN J 36:279-283, 1988.

Harris J: AIDS policy and education in the workplace, AAOHN J 38:6-11, 1990.

Lacy SE: Dow nurses make hearing conservation a reality, Occup Health Safety 47(1):18-20, 1978.

Lalich NR and Schuster LL: An application of the sentinel health event (occupational) concept to death certificates, Am J Public Health 77:1310-1314, 1987.

Lawrence M: Researchers seek to pinpoint physiological mechanisms of noise-induced hearing loss, Occup Health Safety 47(1):22-24, 1978.

Lee JA: The new nurse in industry (NIOSH Pub), Washington, DC, 1978, US Government Printing Office.

Levine C: AIDS: an ethical challenge for our time, 12(8):273-277, 1986.

Martin G: New roles for the occupational health nurse, Job Safety Health 5(4):9-15, 1977.

McCall B: How West Germany protects its workers, Job Safety Health 5(7):21-25, 1977.

Midwest Center for Occupational Health and Safety: National Institute for Occupational Safety and Health (NIOSH) Educational Resource Centers, St Paul, Mn, 1989, The Center.

Miller MA: Social, economic, and political forces affecting the future of occupational health nursing, AAOHN J 37:361-366, 1989.

Morris LD: Minorities, jobs, and health, AAOHN J 37:53-55, 1989.

Morris R: The American worker, Washington, DC, 1976, US Government Printing Office.

Morris R and Alexander DL: Minority workers: educational models for workers, health providers, and planners, AAOHN J 37:101-104, 1989.

Moses M: Pesticide-related health problems and farmworkers, AAOHN J 37:115-130, 1989.

Murphy DC: The primary care role in occupational health nursing, AAOHN J 37:470-474, 1989.

National Center for Health Statistics: Guidelines for reporting occupation and industry on death certificates, Hyattsville, Md, 1983, The Center.

National Institute of Occupational Safety and Health (NIOSH): NIOSH recommendations for occupational health standards, MMWR (suppl):1S, October 7, 1983.

Newman KD, Sirles A, and Williamson KM: Nurse management of the HIV-infected employee, AAOHN J 36:258-261, 1988.

Nyamathi A and Flaskerud JH: Effectiveness of an AIDS education program on knowledge, attitudes and practices of state employees, AAOHN J 37:397-403, 1989.

Office of Technology Assessment: Preventing illness and injury in the workplace (OTA Pub No OTA-H-257), Washington, DC, 1985, US Government Printing Office.

Olson DK: Framework for tomorrow. The future of occupational health nursing, AAOHN J 35:501-504, 1987.

Olishifski JB, ed: National safety council handbook of occupational safety and health, Chicago, Il, 1979, National Safety Council.

Olson DK and Kochevar L: Occupational health and safety content in baccalaureate nursing programs, AAOHN J 37:33-38, 1989.

OSHA issues huge rule revamping exposure rules, Nation's Health, 19(2):14, February 1989.

Ossler CC: Record keeping, AAOHN J 36:8-14, 1988.

Parker-Conrad J: A century of practice. Occupational health nursing, AAOHN J 36:156-161, 1988.

Phaneuf MC and Wandelt MA: Quality assurance in nursing, Nurs Forum 13(4):328-345, 1974.

Pinkham J: 100 years of industrial nursing has vastly improved workplace safety, Occup Safety Health 57(4):20-23, 1988.

Plog BA, ed: Fundamentals of industrial hygiene, ed 3, Chicago, Il, 1988, National Safety Council.

Prestholdt C and Holt BA: Balancing baccalaureate student nursing education, AAOHN J 37:465-469, 1989.

Rabinow J: Occupational health records. Documentation and confidentiality, AAOHN J 36:314-317, 1988.

Randolph SA: Occupational health nursing. A commitment to excellence, AAOHN J 36:166-169, 1988.

Rogers B: Environmental and occupational health content in undergraduate nursing education programs, Nurs Environ Health Watch 7(1):4, 1986.

Rogers B: Ethical dilemmas in occupational health nursing, AAOHN J 36:100-104, 1988.

Rogers B: Establishing research priorities in occupational health nursing, AAOHN J 37:493-500, 1989.

Rogers B and Spencer GA: Nursing research in occupational health, AAOHN J 32:552-553, 1984.

Rutstein DD, Mullan RJ, Frazier TM, Halperin WE, Melius JM, and Sestito JP: Sentinel health events (occupational): a basis for physician recognition and public health surveillance, Am J Public Health 73:1054-1062, 1984.

Schmutz JF: An industrial response to chronic health hazards. In Sax N, ed: Dangerous properties of industrial materials, ed 5, New York, 1979, Van Nostrand Reinhold, pp 303-307.

Schwartz E and Landrigan P: Use of court records for supplementing occupational disease surveillance, Am J Public Health 77:1457-1458, 1987.

Selleck CS, Sirles AT, and Newman KD: Health promotion at the workplace, AAOHN J 37:412-422, 1989.

Serafini P: Nursing assessment in industry, Am J Public Health 66(8):755-760, 1976.

Sherman A: Health risk appraisal at the worksite, AAOHN J 38:18-24, 1990.

Silberstein C: Nursing research in occupational health, AAOHN J 31:9, 1983.

Stellman JM and Daum DM: Work is dangerous to your health, New York, 1973, Vintage Books.

Stevenson JS: Issues and crisis during middlescence, New York, 1977, Appleton-Century-Crofts.

Talbot DM: An educational model to prepare the baccalaureate nurse for occupational health nursing, AAOHN J 30(5):20-25, 1983.

Thomas LE, McCabe E, and Berry JE: Unemployment and family stress: a reassessment, Family Relations 29:511-516, 1980.

Thompson H: The occupational health nurse's role in rehabilitation, AAOHN J 30(1):25-28, 1982.

Ubell E: How dangerous is your job? Parade, January 8, 1989, pp 4-7.

US Department of Health, Education, and Welfare (USDHEW): A guide to the work-relatedness of disease, Washington, DC, 1976, US Government Printing Office.

US Department of Health and Human Services (USDHHS): Promoting health. Preventing disease. Objectives for the nation, Washington, DC, 1980, US Government Printing Office.

USDHHS: Health United States, 1983, Washington, DC, 1983, US Government Printing Office.

USDHHS: The 1990 health objectives for the nation: a midcourse review, Washington, DC, 1986, US Government Printing Office.

USDHHS: Coping with AIDS: psychological and social considerations in helping people with HTLV-III infection, Pub No ADM 85-1432, Washington, DC, 1986, US Government Printing Office.

USDHHS: The National Survey of Workplace Health Promotion Activities, Washington, DC, 1987, US Government Printing Office.

USDHHS: Prevention 86/87, Washington, DC, 1987, US Government Printing Office.

US Department of Labor: Important events in American labor history, 1778-1975, Washington, DC, 1976, US Government Printing Office.

US Department of Labor: Labor firsts in America, Washington, DC, 1977, US Government Printing Office.

Whitmer RW: Healthy employees mean healthy profits, Sunbelt Exec 40:63-64, 1984.

Whorton MD: Accurate occupational and injury data in the US: can this enigmatic problem ever be solved? Am J Public Health 73(9):1031-1032, 1983.

Williamson KM, Brown KL, and Packa J: AIDS education at the worksite, AAOHN J 36:262-265, 1988.

SELECTED BIBLIOGRAPHY

Brodeur P: Expendable Americans, New York, 1974, Viking.

Brown ML: Occupational health nursing, New York, 1981, Springer.

Felton JS: Teaching occupational health at the secondary level, J Occup Med 23:27-29, 1981.

Finn P: Occupational safety and health education in the

public schools. Rationale, goals, and implementation, Preventive Med 7(3):245-259, 1978.

Goldstein DH: The occupational safety and health act of 1970, Am J Nurs 71:1535-1538, 1971.

Hamilton A: Industrial poisons in the United States, New York, 1925, Macmillan.

Moses M: Cancer in humans and potential occupational and environmental exposure to pesticides. Selected epidemiological studies and case reports, AAOHN J 37:131-136, 1989.

Murphy DC: The primary care role in occupational health nursing, AAOHN J 37:470-474, 1989.

Nelson LN and Hellman SL: Counseling employees at risk for HIV, AAOHN J 37:404-411, 1989.

Page JA and O'Brien MW: Bitter wages, New York, 1973, Grossman.

Robinson JC: Trends in racial inequality and exposure to work-related hazards, 1968-1986, AAOHN J 37:56-63, 1989.

Scott R: Muscle and blood, New York, 1974, Dutton.

Turner JG, Gauthier DK, Ellison KJ, and Greiner DS: Nursing and AIDS. Knowledge and attitudes, AAOHN J 36:274-278, 1989.

Yorker BC: AIDS testing. A legal perspective on testing in the workplace, AAOHN J 36:231-232, 1988.

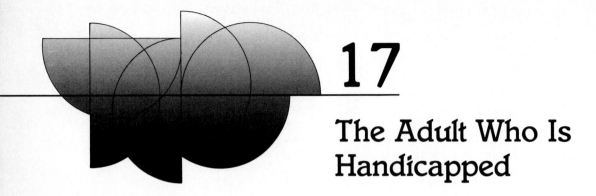

17

The Adult Who Is Handicapped

When one is working with people who are handicapped, it must be remembered that first they are people and, secondary to that, they have a handicapping condition.

Upon completion of this chapter, the reader will be able to:

1. *Distinguish between the terms chronic condition, disability, and handicap.*
2. *Discuss the concepts of normalization and mainstreaming.*
3. *Explain individual, family, and societal variables that influence adaptation to a handicap.*
4. *Describe areas of major concern for people with a handicap.*
5. *Discuss the health promotion role of community health nurses when working with adults who are handicapped.*
6. *Summarize major resources which assist adults who are handicapped.*
7. *Identify legislation which provides health care resources for adults who are handicapped or which promotes awareness of the needs of this population group.*

From early in recorded time people have noted the handicapping conditions among them. Handicapping conditions were recorded as early as 384 B.C. by Aristotle (Buscaglia, 1983, p. 162). Later Hippocrates, Galen, and others studied such conditions and sought answers to why they existed. Answers were not often found, and myths and misinformation prevailed. In early times, few people who were handicapped lived to adulthood, and many died in childhood.

Throughout history societies have dealt in various ways with members who were handicapped. Attitudes toward the handicapped have ranged from acceptance to rejection and from understanding to fear. The Elizabethan Poor Law of 1601 equated handicapping conditions with crime, and under this law, people who were handicapped were often disenfranchised, publicly punished, and imprisoned (Sussman, 1966, p. 3). The classic story of the *Hunchback of Notre Dame* clearly illustrates society's reaction to disfigurement during the eighteenth century.

Although being handicapped is no longer considered criminal, people who are handicapped often arouse anxiety and discomfort in others and are socially stigmatized (Fine and Asch, 1988, p. 8).

It is estimated that there are more than 37 million disabled citizens in the United States (National Council on the Handicapped, 1988, On the threshold of independence, p. 9; Meyerson, 1988, p. 180). Approximately 14 percent of Americans are limited in activity because of a chronic, disabling health condition (What is disability?, 1988, p. 2; Kraus and Stoddard, 1989, p. 2). Disabilities cannot be ignored if we are to maximize the potential of the individual, the family, and society. Individuals with disabilities make up one of the largest minority groups in the United States. Like other minority groups, the disabled population group has been subjected to various forms of exploitation, prejudice, and oppression (Hahn, 1988, Politics, p. 41). However, in recent years, the more than 20 million disabled adults of voting age have been learning how to voice their needs and issues, and are beginning to exert political and social influence (Calkins, 1988, p. 11).

CHRONIC AND HANDICAPPING CONDITIONS: RELATED BUT DISTINCT PHENOMENA

As the U.S. population ages, and technology advances to combat the limitations of chronic conditions, the number of people with such conditions continues to grow. It is important to remember that not all people who have chronic conditions are handicapped. Chronic and handicapping conditions are related yet distinct phenomena.

Chronic Conditions

Chronic conditions exist long term and often have an uncertain outcome. They were defined in Chapter 10 as impairments or deviations from normal that have at least one of the following characteristics: permanency, residual disability, irreversible pathological causation and alteration, need for special rehabilitation and training, and need for a period of long-term supervision and care (Commission on Chronic Illness, 1957, p. 4). Chronic conditions include but are not limited to cancer, heart disease, diabetes, cerebral palsy, deafness, drug addiction, alcoholism, epilepsy, spinal cord injury, mental or emotional illness, mental retardation, multiple sclerosis, muscular dystrophy, orthopedic impairment, speech or visual impairment, and perceptual handicaps such as dyslexia, minimal brain dysfunction, and developmental aphasia. Chronic conditions affect millions of Americans. Some 12.8 million people (7.1 percent of the population) have trouble reading standard newspaper print, even when wearing glasses or contact lenses, and approximately 1.7 million cannot read it at all; about 7.7 million people have trouble hearing a normal conversation and 500,000 are unable to hear such a conversation; and 2.5 million Americans have a speech impairment severe enough that others have difficulty understanding them (National Council on the Handicapped, 1988, On the threshold of independence, p. 9).

Chronic conditions can adversely affect an individual's ability to carry out one or more major life activities such as communication, ambulation, self-care, socialization, education, vocational training, transportation, housing and employment. Chronic conditions may become handicapping conditions, according to the following schema of disease (WHO, 1981, p. 8):

Disease/condition → impairment → disability → handicap

A chronic condition becomes a handicap based on the *level of disability* it imposes on an individual.

What Is Disability?

Traditionally in the United States disabilities have been medically defined, but definitions are now broadening to incorporate psychosocial aspects. The World Health Organization (1981, p. 8) has defined a disability as any restriction or lack of ability to perform an activity in the manner, or within the range, considered to be normal for a human being. Several national surveys have defined disability as a limitation, related to a chronic health condition or set of conditions, in the type or amount of activities that a person would oth-

TABLE 17-1   Conditions with highest risk of disability, by type of disability, all ages: United States, 1983-1986

Chronic condition	Number of conditions (1,000s)	Percent causing activity limitation	Rank	Percent causing major activity limitation	Rank	Percent causing need for help in basic life activities	Rank
Mental retardation	1,202	84.1	1	80.0	1	19.9	9
Absence of leg(s)	289	83.3	2	73.1	2	39.0	2
Lung or bronchial cancer	200	74.8	3	63.5	3	34.5	4
Multiple sclerosis	171	70.6	4	63.3	4	40.7	1
Cerebral palsy	274	69.7	5	62.2	5	22.8	8
Blind in both eyes	396	64.5	6	58.8	6	38.1	3
Partial paralysis in extremity	578	59.6	7	47.2	7	27.5	5
Other orthopedic impairments (not in back or extremities)	316	58.7	8	46.2	8	14.3*	12
Complete paralysis in extremity	617	52.7	9	45.5	9	26.1	6
Rheumatoid arthritis	1,223	51.0	10	39.4	12	14.9	11
Intervertebral disk disorders	3,987	48.7	11	38.2	14	5.3	—
Paralysis in other sites (complete/partial)	247	47.8	12	43.7	10	14.1*	13
Other heart disease/disorders†	4,708	46.9	13	35.1	15	13.6	14
Cancer of digestive sites	228	45.3	14	40.3	11	15.9*	10
Emphysema	2,074	43.6	15	29.8	—	9.6	15
Absence of arm(s)/hand(s)	84	43.1	—	39.0	13	4.1*	—
Cerebrovascular disease	2,599	38.2	—	33.3	—	22.9	7

*Figure has low statistical reliability or precision (relative standard error exceeds 30 percent).

†Heart failure (9.8%), valve disorders (15.3%), congenital disorders (15.0%), all other and ill-defined heart conditions (59.9%).

Note: Data are estimates (annual averages) based on household interviews of the civilian noninstitutionalized population.

From National Health Interview Survey, 1983-1986. As cited in Disability risks of chronic illnesses and impairments, Disability Stat Bull 2(Fall):2, 1989.

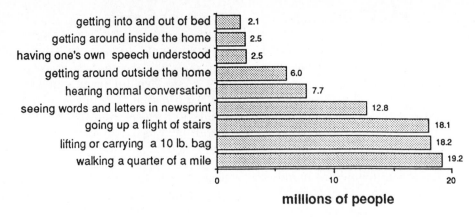

Figure 17-1   Functional limitations of adults with disabilities. (From Kraus LE and Stoddard S: Chartbook on disability in the United States, an InfoUse Report, Washington, DC, 1989, National Institute on Disability and Rehabilitation Research, p 3.)

erwise be expected to be able to perform (What is disability?, 1988, p. 2). Regardless of existing definitions, what constitutes a disability is often determined by public opinion and policy, and disability tends to become whatever the law says it is (Scotch, 1988, p. 168). As evidenced in Table 17-1, there are a number of chronic conditions that cause activity limitation.

Based on the WHO definition, more than 20 percent of all noninstitutionalized persons in the United States above the age of 15 years have a functional limitation; in approximately 40 percent, the disability is severe enough that they need assistance to perform the function (Kraus and Stoddard, 1989, pp. 3-4). Figure 17-1 illustrates functional limitations of adults with disabilities.

The level of disability is determined by combining the results of multiple assessment, including clinical evaluation, utilization of standardized performance tests and scales, assessment of client and family perceptions and knowledge, and measurement of ability to carry out activities of daily living (ADL). While definitions for levels of disability vary among disciplines, the majority of these definitions include activities of daily living (ADL) and employment abilities. Below are four general levels of disability, taking into consideration ADL and employment abilities:

Level 1: Partial disability characterized by slight limitation in one or more of the major life activities; able to take part in school, competitive employment, and self-care

Level II: Partial disability characterized by moderate limitation in one or more of the major life activities; generally able to attend school, work regularly or part-time (but the employment may need to be modified); may need assistance with self-care

Level III: Partial disability characterized by severe limitation in one or more of the major life activities; usually unable to attend school or work regularly (considered occupationally disabled); often requires assistance with self-care

Level IV: Total disability characterized by complete, or almost complete dependency on others for activities of daily living, self-care and economic support; usually unable to work or attend regular school

When a chronic condition becomes severely disabling (Levels III and IV), it substantially limits an individual's ability to carry out normal life functions, and becomes a handicapping condition.

Handicapping Conditions

A *handicap* is a condition that *substantially* limits one or more of an individual's major life activities and fulfillment of normal roles (President's Committee on Employment of the Handicapped,

1978, Affirmative Action; WHO, 1981). A handicap is not desirable, and in most cases, it will cause at least some physical pain, discomfort, embarrassment, and expenditure of a great deal of time and money (Buscaglia, 1983, p. 14). The possibility of developing a handicap increases with age, but handicapping conditions occur across the life-span.

Many handicapping conditions are not preventable and, once they occur, full restoration or cure is impossible. People with handicapping conditions are often caught in the double bind of not qualifying for the special privileges society accords the acutely ill while not having the status of the able-bodied (University of Michigan, 1981).

Handicapping conditions may be congenital or acquired, and can encompass the entire range of disability. For example, individuals with cerebral palsy may evidence functional abilities ranging from independence to complete dependence. The level of disability caused by a handicapping condition is used to determine client needs, intervention strategies, and effectiveness of care. However, individuals with handicapping conditions usually need to redefine family roles, relationships, and division of labor; deal with social, emotional, physical, educational and financial problems; and utilize a complex array of community resources.

Normalization and Mainstreaming

In recent years people with handicaps have risen to a higher level of social visibility and responsiveness than in the past. Acknowledgment of their right to equal opportunity and quality of life is increasing (Meyerson, 1988, p. 181). In line with this, people who are handicapped have been assisted in assuming as normal a life as possible (normalization) and have been increasingly brought into the mainstream of society (mainstreaming).

Mainstreaming refers to integrating the person who is handicapped into the everyday life of the community. The person functions in the "mainstream" of the community and is not separated from it. Many people who are handicapped blend easily and readily into the community; they are difficult to discern from the community's non-

handicapped members. For those who do not blend readily, special efforts must be taken for the integration to occur.

Normalization refers to assisting persons who are handicapped to live as normal a life as possible, in a manner analogous to the rest of society. They are aided and encouraged to participate in the same activities as other members of the community, such as adhering to laws, working, housekeeping, using public transportation, going to school, and shopping.

Normalization and mainstreaming reflect a humanistic approach to working with people who are handicapped, and focus on maximizing their strengths. Successful implementation requires careful planning, supportive community attitudes, adequate resources, and recognition that people who are handicapped are entitled to the same rights, privileges, and respect as other members of society. Normalization and mainstreaming necessitate practicing the philosophy that people who are handicapped are people first, and that secondarily they have a handicapping condition.

ADAPTATION TO THE HANDICAP

Adaptation to a handicap is a complex process and is influenced by individual, family, community, and societal variables. It is the combination of these variables that determines how well a person adapts to a handicap.

Societal Attitudes toward People Who Are Handicapped

Society creates handicaps (Scotch, 1988, p. 168; Buscaglia, 1983). Societal attitudes toward people who are handicapped play a major role in individual and family adaptation to the handicapping condition. They are a crucial component of the surroundings with which people who are handicapped must contend (Hahn, 1988, Politics, p. 40). In fact, the debilitating aspects of a handicap often result not so much from the disability as from the manner in which others define and respond to it (Hahn, 1988, Can disability).

Unfortunately, many societal attitudes toward people who are handicapped are negative. Prejudice, stereotyping, and discrimination, in relation to physical and mental handicaps, are common in the United States (Bogdan and Taylor, 1988). These attitudes are frequently due to a lack of knowledge among the general public about the etiology, treatment, and prognosis of handicapping conditions. Societal attitudes have been referred to as "the invisible barriers" (Kendrick, 1983, p. 17). The impact of these barriers is seen in the quote from Deborah Kendrick, a mother who is blind:

The difficulty is neither in being blind nor in being a mother. It is in the attitudes of others, the *invisible barriers* which can separate me from other mothers and my children from their children. (Kendrick, 1983, p. 18)

People with disabilities are often characterized as being helpless, permanently suffering, dependent, and emotionally unstable; they are often held at least partially responsible for their disability (Seifert, 1981).

In our society, ambivalent feelings about handicapping conditions are prevalent and continue to inhibit achievement among persons who are experiencing a disability. This is not true in all cultures. Donald Sims (Figure 17-2), a young man who has impaired functioning of his lower extremities because of a motorcycle accident, found that when he visited the Choco Indians in Panama, his strengths were respected and his differences accepted: the attitudes of the Choco Indians helped him to realize his potential and to accept his differences:

An unbelievable experience! They treated me as though I was no different—I was accepted as a person—a people, a culture with no concept of handicapped. I did what I could, they did their thing, and we all worked and played together. No one shied away from the chair. The Choco Indians made my Panama trip the most wonderful experience since my accident. They helped reinstate my faith in people, in life itself, and a positive attitude toward all things.

Societal attitudes toward the handicapped are influenced by multiple variables, some of which

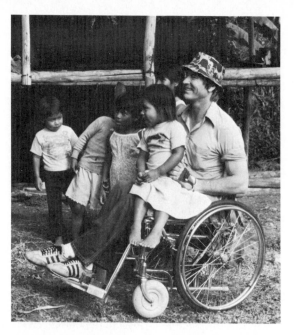

Figure 17-2 Societal attitudes influence how individuals, families, and groups perceive differences among individuals in a society and can either facilitate or inhibit individual growth and development. (Courtesy of Donald Sims and photographer H. Morgan Smith, Explorations, Brigade Quartermasters. Morgan Smith has more than 30 years membership in the Explorers Club, is an honorary member of the Choco Indian tribe, and is an anthropologist and naturalist who has conducted numerous archeological excavations.)

are discussed below (Safilios-Rothschild, 1982, p. 4):

1. *Beliefs regarding the value of physical and mental integrity.* The values held in regard to physical and mental integrity will greatly affect the acceptance of handicapping conditions and the services rendered to people who are handicapped. The values placed on physical and mental integrity are usually high, and the higher the value placed, the more likely there is to be prejudice and discriminatory action against those who are physically and mentally handicapped.

2. *Beliefs in relation to illness.* There is often a difference between the role given someone who is acutely ill and one who is chronically

impaired. If a chronic condition is of long term and severely limiting, there is a tendency to separate the person from the mainstream of society through institutional, nursing home, or long-term placement. If the condition is only mildly to moderately limiting, the person is often expected to perform "normally," even when this normal behavior is difficult. Once a condition has become chronic and has existed for a long time people often believe it is more bearable. This is not always the case.

3. *Beliefs regarding condition occurrence.* If it is believed that the individual had a high degree of responsibility in the occurrence of the handicapping condition, less aid is generally accorded that person. Obesity, alcoholism, mental illness, AIDS, and drug abuse are examples of this.

4. *The role of the government in alleviating social problems.* If a society does not believe that the government should assume an active role in alleviating social problems and subsidizing those who cannot support themselves, there may be little public assistance or empathy for people who are handicapped.

5. *Beliefs regarding the origins of poverty.* Many people who are handicapped frequently fall below the poverty level. If a society believes that poverty is generally a matter of self-will, there may be less willingness to assist the handicapped.

6. *The rate of employment and economic development.* When unemployment is high, preferential hiring practices are often accorded the nonhandicapped individual. If an economy is unstable, there is less inclination to financially subsidize those who are handicapped.

Studies of societal attitudes toward people who are handicapped reflect that persons who are handicapped have many negative attitudes to overcome when they are working toward full potential. Buscaglia (1983) described a study involving nonhandicapped people viewing nonhandicapped people (1) in a wheelchair, giving one the

impression of being handicapped, and (2) out of a wheelchair and nonhandicapped. Seen in the wheelchair, the nonhandicapped individual was described as helpless, hopeless, and of decreased value; however, the same person, out of the wheelchair, was described positively. The same sort of responses occurred with a nonhandicapped person viewed (1) with leg braces and (2) without leg braces. Other studies have shown that even people with handicapping conditions showed negative attitudes toward people with handicapping conditions (Dixon, 1977, p. 308). Handicapping conditions can pose a threat to one's self-image.

Nearly everyone is poor at communicating with people who are handicapped, not because they do not wish to communicate, but because they are uncomfortable with the communication and are not sure how to communicate. (Penrose, 1983; University of Michigan, 1981). This inability to communicate about handicapping conditions, and with people who are handicapped, compounds a very significant problem: it increases their social isolation. It is this social isolation that has traditionally prevented the person who is handicapped from achieving maximum productivity and fulfillment (University of Michigan, 1981; Strauss, Corbin, Fagerhaugh, Glaser, Maines, Suczek and Wiener, 1984, p. 16).

It is not uncommon to find that there are inadequate residential, educational, occupational, medical, or social programs to meet the needs of the person who is handicapped in the community. When services do exist, they are often fragmented, of questionable quality, and poorly monitored. Many services are geared to an acute care orientation rather than a chronic, long-term orientation.

The community health nurse can help to eliminate societal prejudices that exist toward the handicapped, and can be instrumental in the passage of health legislation which will reflect a humanistic philosophy toward individuals who need special services to maximize their potential. Too often, people look at individuals who are disabled in terms of their limitations, not their strengths. Through health education activities, the nurse can facilitate clients and others in gaining a realistic understanding of the nature of handicapping conditions. Health education can also help others to gain an appreciation of the strengths as well as needs of individuals who have handicaps.

Health education activities in the school setting are especially beneficial in changing attitudes toward individuals who have handicaps. It is not uncommon for children in elementary classrooms to encounter peers who deviate from what is defined as normal. A sensitive teacher and school nurse can help these children to accept peers who are different, understand why these differences have occurred, and promote normalization and mainstreaming.

Individual and Family Variables Influencing Adaptation to a Handicap

In addition to societal variables, individual and family variables also affect adaptation to a handicap. Because these variables interact, it is difficult to separate the effects of one from another.

The Family with a Handicapped Member

Many families include members who are handicapped. Each family will adapt and cope with caring for a handicapped family member differently and, as indicated in Chapter 7, some families are more vulnerable to the stresses involved than others (Brillhart, 1988, p. 316). Handicapping conditions can produce stress for the entire family. Research has found that families of persons who are handicapped may be treated as if they were different from other families or somehow to blame for the handicap (Buzinski, 1980). This creates even more stress, and makes it more difficult for families to adjust.

A handicapping condition requires that a family make many difficult decisions regarding such things as family priorities, time allocation, allocation of financial resources, and provision of care. Families are often forced to reorganize economic, social, and emotional priorities around the needs of the impaired member. The financial demands of the handicapping condition may place many hardships on the family.

Family roles, goals, and division of labor may need to be redefined. For example, parents of handicapped children may not go through launching when the child reaches adulthood, and may need to reexamine the goals they had for themselves and their children.

In addition to caring for a handicapped family member, families are expected to carry out other life activities and responsibilities such as school, work, and household maintenance. Despite all this, families remain the primary caregivers for their handicapped members (Bubolz and Whiren, 1984). Family care givers frequently experience considerable stress, and supportive intervention is needed to prevent family burnout.

Studies have shown that families are more likely to place handicapped members outside the home when the following variables exist: the person is severely disabled; the family structure is incapable of providing adequate time, care, and resources; there is a high level of family conflict and discord, such as marital dissatisfaction; and community supports and resources are insufficient or not utilized (Sherman and Cocozza, 1984; Giele, 1984). Having an awareness of these variables helps community health nurses to identify families who need their services as well as community resources to care for a handicapped member at home. Every attempt should be made to minimize the stresses that lead to institutionalization. An especially important factor which influences individual and family adjustment to a handicap is the availability of social supports and resources (McCubbin and Patterson, 1983; Walkover, 1988).

In recent years greater emphasis has been placed on identifying strategies to promote family stability and growth after a handicapping condition has been diagnosed. The Beach Center on Families and Disabilities is sponsored by the National Institute on Disabilities and Rehabilitation Research (NIDRR). Its research focuses on individualizing services to families; determining positive contributions by family members; enhancing family capacities; increasing the quality of life for families with handicapped members; providing advocacy services; and strengthening parent-to-parent networks (Research and training focuses, 1989, p. 13). For further information contact Beach Center on Families and Disabilities, University of Kansas, Bureau of Child Research, 2045

Haworth Hall, Lawrence, Kansas 66045 (1-913-864-4295).

Variables Affecting Adaptation Growth

The impact of a handicapping condition on the individual and family as a whole is often greatly influenced by a combination of the following variables:

1. The stage the individual has reached in the grief and mourning process associated with the handicap
2. Age at which the handicapping condition occurred
3. Age appropriateness of the handicap
4. Rapidity of onset of the handicap
5. Level of disability caused by the handicap
6. Visibility of the handicap
7. Value of the handicapped area
8. Attitudes regarding self
9. Attitudes of significant others
10. Community resources available and utilized
11. Coping mechanisms utilized
12. Prognosis and/or expected duration of the handicap

The first variable, dealing with grief and mourning, poses some unique aspects, because there are few data on grief and mourning in relation to chronic illness and handicapping conditions (Lewis, 1983). The person and family experiencing chronic illness have definitely suffered a loss. This loss may take many forms, such as loss of health, independence, control over life, privacy, body image, personal relationships and roles, social status, financial stability, material possessions, and self-fulfillment (Lewis, 1983). It can be compounded by the fact that there may be no immediate end in sight, and the individual is often grieving personally while experiencing the effects of significant others grieving also (Werner-Beland, 1980). Stages of grief and mourning are experienced by the individual and family in relation to a handicap (Bower, 1977; Vargo, 1978; Lewis, 1983). These stages closely resemble the stages discussed by Kübler-Ross (1969) when looking at death and dying. The following describes the grief and mourning process that a person and family go through when adapting to a handicapping condition:

Denial: The individual/family is not prepared to accept the reality and ramifications of the handicap and deny that it is occurring.

Awareness: The individual/family realizes that the handicap is real, the loss becomes real, and feelings of hostility, bitterness, and anger can arise in response to it.

Mourning: The individual/family actively grieves for the loss that has occurred.

Depression: The individual/family realizes the permanency, long-term nature or other ramifications of the condition and experiences feelings of rejection, helplessness, altered self-esteem, and despair. This is often a very encompassing and time-consuming stage.

Adaptation: The individual/family becomes capable of coping with the handicap, gradually having realized that one cannot function in a constant state of depression, even though periods of depression may occur periodically. The goals of this stage are equilibrium and rehabilitation.

Until grieving has been successfully carried out, rehabilitation, and ultimately adaptation and growth, cannot be fully successful. Unresolved grief can seriously alter and affect interpersonal relationships and family functioning.

Community health nurses play a major role in helping families to experience a healthy grieving process, because they are frequently responsible for coordinating health care services for these families. Being able to accept that grief is normal when adapting to a handicapping condition, helps the community nurse to better assist families to work through the grieving process in a constructive manner. Writings by Kübler-Ross (1969) help professionals as well as clients to deal with grief.

The age at which a handicapping condition occurs and the age appropriateness of the condition are also critical to adaptation. Handicapping conditions that occur after the development of a self-image are frequently more difficult to handle than others. A child born without an arm will have a different adjustment process than the child who loses an arm at age 5 or the adult who loses an arm at 50. The internalized body image of the adult makes it difficult to accept, much less incorporate, drastic alterations of body structure (Safilios-Rothschild, 1982, p. 80). An age-appropriate handicap is more easily accepted than one not commonly found among individuals of a particular age group. For example, an elderly person with a hearing impairment or arthritis is often more readily accepted than is a preschooler with the same conditions.

The rapidity of a condition's onset is also critical to adjustment (Payne, 1988, p. 191). If a condition develops gradually, as does rheumatoid arthritis, the adjustment time is lengthened and there is an opportunity to develop skills, resources, support systems, and coping mechanisms. If the occurrence is sudden, as with traumatic injury, there is little or no adjustment time. Any person needs time to adapt to a condition, and rehabilitation techniques may need to be delayed until adaptation can take place. Sudden change is often difficult to incorporate into one's body image (Safilios-Rothschild, 1982, p. 88). Similarly, a sudden alteration in the image of oneself held by others is difficult to absorb.

The level of disability associated with a condition will have a great deal to do with the adjustment the individual/family is able to make. Generally, the higher the level of disability, the more difficult it is to adjust. An individual with a paralyzed hand will likely have less difficulty in adjustment than a paraplegic or a person who is severely mentally retarded. The level of disability will be a major determinant of the functional capacity the individual is able to attain.

The level of disability has an impact on the person's ability to accomplish the age-specific developmental tasks discussed throughout this text. They include such things as establishing an occupation and a companionship lifestyle, utilizing leisure time, and taking part in civic activities. The person who is handicapped is often impeded in accomplishing developmental tasks.

The visibility of the condition affects the adjustment made to it. People generally 'have stronger reactions to visible than to invisible signs and symptoms. Any visible condition will gener-

ally elicit more discriminating individual and societal responses than a nonvisible or slightly visible condition.

The value of the handicapped part is of major importance. A person becomes more upset when something happens to a part of the body that is highly valued. The value placed on body parts will vary from individual to individual; however, some parts seem to have a higher value than others. Facial disfigurement illustrates well the value placed on certain body parts. Although facial disfigurement causes few physical limitations, it is one of the most difficult handicapping conditions to adjust to because of the high value placed on facial characteristics (Safilios-Rothschild, 1982, p. 126). Conditions that create sexual handicaps are also difficult for most people to accept. The social value placed on body parts or functions significantly affects the type and degree of stigma attached to the handicap.

The attitudes held about oneself and the attitudes about oneself held by significant others are critical to the outcome of a handicapping condition. If such attitudes are negative, their impact can be detrimental to the outcome of the condition. Community health nurses, and others in therapeutic roles, should build upon the positive attitudes found and help the client and significant others to analyze why negative attitudes exist. Since attitudes have an important effect on an individual's social and psychological adjustment to his or her handicap, it is crucial for the community health nurse to identify attitudes that may hamper successful adaptation.

Rehabilitation services play a key role in handicap outcome. Handicap adjustment is impeded if rehabilitation services are not available, appropriate, or accessible. Rehabilitation is an extremely important concept and will be discussed in a separate section of this chapter.

SOME AREAS OF MAJOR CONCERN FOR PEOPLE WHO ARE HANDICAPPED, THEIR FAMILIES, AND HEALTH PROFESSIONALS

People who are handicapped are at a disadvantage in contemporary society. As they try to keep up with the rapid pace, social, educational, and occupational demands and a number of other concerns emerge. Not all people who are handicapped will evidence the special needs and concerns mentioned here. Many people who are handicapped function well in the mainstream of society and are difficult to separate from their nonhandicapped counterparts. However, a large proportion of people who are handicapped evidence these concerns, and thus the health care professional needs to be aware of them.

Education

People who are handicapped have often been put at an educational disadvantage. This lack of education makes it difficult for the adult who is handicapped to find a job. Lack of education stems not from a lack of interest among the handicapped in seeking education, but from a lack of provision of such education by the public. It was not until the 1970s that states began enacting mandatory education laws for people who were handicapped. Prior to this time, if a person did not "fit" the existing school district programs, and most individuals who were handicapped did not, the school district was not responsible for the education of this person. As mandatory education programs for the handicapped evolved, they often applied to children, and the adult who was handicapped was frequently excluded. The Federal Education for All Handicapped Children Act of 1975 (Public Law 94-142) instituted educational services for children who were handicapped from ages 3 to 18 as of September 1, 1978, and provided incentive monies for services to people from 3 to 21 as of September 1, 1980. After age 21 the federal law does not mandate educational programs for the adult who is handicapped. Some states have enacted education laws for the handicapped that are more comprehensive than the federal law. For example, in some states, people who are handicapped have a right to a free public education from birth through age 25.

What happens to a person's educational training program after he or she reaches the age at which the mandatory education laws no longer apply is a contemporary educational dilemma. Nevertheless, the provisions of the Developmental Disabilities Assistance and Bill of Rights Act (Public Law 95-602) are encouraging. This act provides grants for federally assisted state programs designed to (1) assist in the provision of comprehensive services not already covered under the Education for All Handicapped Children Act, the Rehabilitation Act of 1973 and other legislation, (2) assist the states in educational planning activities, and (3) train professional staff (Michigan State Planning Council for Developmental Disabilities, 1983, pp. 7-8).

By law, the handicapped adult who applies for college entrance, job training, or adult basic education must be considered on academic records and cannot be discriminated against because of the handicap. Also, such programs cannot limit the number of handicapped students admitted. Colleges are not required to lower academic standards or alter degree requirements for people who are handicapped. However, if the college is receiving a federal subsidy, it may be required to modify teaching methods and provide teaching aids as necessary to accommodate the student who is handicapped.

Students with disabilities need to be exposed to career options and employment potentials (What should, 1989, p. 25); vocational education is an important component of the student's educational program and of the rehabilitation programs discussed later in this chapter.

Homebound Instruction

A number of people who are handicapped utilize homebound instruction to learn a skill or train for a number of careers. The U.S. Department of Education recognizes the National Home Study Council (1601 Eighteenth Street, N.W., Washington, D.C. 20009 phone: (202) 234-5100) and its handbook *Directory of Accredited Home Study Schools* as a valid resource for locating quality schools of home study.

Some companies offer educational assistance to people who are handicapped that could readily be adapted to the home. Apple Computer, Inc., has established an Office of Special Education to help make their computers more accessible to people with disabilities. Apple's Office of Special Education maintains a database called Special Education Solutions that describes thousands of adaptive devices, software programs, disability-related organizations, publications, and networks; and it publishes a computer resource guide called *Connections* that lists books, learning and assessment programs, resources for communication aids, and disability-based organizations and publications (Apple finds a place, 1988, p. 4). To receive more information on Apple services contact Apple Computer, Inc., Office of Special Education and Rehabilitation, 20525 Mariani Avenue, Cupertino, CA 95014 (1-408-996-1010).

IBM also offers educational assistance to people with disabilities through the IBM National Support Center for Persons with Disabilities. This support center helps individuals learn how health technology and computers can improve the quality of life for the person with a disability at school, home, and work (IBM center offers, 1988, p. 5; Seaver, 1989, p. 513). To receive more information contact IBM National Support Center for Persons with Disabilities, P.O. Box 2150, Atlanta, GA (1-800-IBM-2133).

Financial Stability

An adult who is handicapped is financially responsible for himself or herself. Almost 25 percent of families with a chronically ill family member report having major financial problems as a result of the illness, and this figure rises to 40 percent for those families at or below poverty levels (The Robert Wood Johnson Foundation, 1984, p. 17). Financial stability is a major concern for adults and families of those who are handicapped. Many adults who are handicapped are financially independent; however, some are unable to achieve this independence and must rely on assistance programs for financial support. One third of the people who are disabled receive public assistance income (Watson, 1988, p. 139).

Most of the financial assistance available to the adult who is handicapped comes from either the state department of human or social services (DHS or DSS) or the federal Society Security Administration (SSA). Under DHS/DSS the adult is eligible for all forms of categorical aid such as General Assistance and Aid to Families of Dependent Children (AFDC). Under the Social Security

Administration the person who is handicapped may be eligible for Social Security Disability Insurance or Supplemental Security Income (SSI). These programs and their payment rates have been discussed in Chapter 4. Many adults who are handicapped rely on Social Security Administration programs for income maintenance.

To qualify for SSI under aid-to-the-disabled a person must have a medically determinable physical or mental impairment expected to result in death or one that is expected to last for an unbroken period of at least 12 months. SSI may be applied for through the local SSA office. Generally, individuals are not eligible for SSI if they have resources of about $2500 ($3000 for a couple), and have income greater than $4416/year. Certain resources are excluded, most commonly a home, an automobile whose current market value is $4500 or less, household goods and personal effects of reasonable value, and life insurance with a face value of $1500 or less. In 1989 approximately 2.5 million people who were disabled received SSI payments (Loeff, Bretz, and Kerns, 1989, p. 63).

It is not mandatory that the adult who is handicapped apply for financial assistance. Many times the family totally or partially supports the person. This may be sufficient for an indefinite period of time, but there is great likelihood that it will eventually prove inadequate or unacceptable. The community health nurse should encourage the adult who is handicapped, and his or her family, to explore the different employment and funding possibilities available. Local DHS and SSA offices can be contacted for specific information regarding available programs and opportunities.

Employment

Employment is of great concern to persons with disabilities (National Council on the Handicapped, 1988, On the threshold of independence, p. 45). The President's Committee on Employment of the Handicapped was established by President Harry S Truman in 1947 to facilitate employment of people who were handicapped. The name has been changed to President's Committee on Employment of People with Disabilities. The committee strives to eliminate environmental and attitudinal barriers impeding handicapped persons. It sponsors an ongoing public information campaign, publishes *Worklife,* a quarterly periodical dealing with employment and people with disabilities, and sponsors a speakers bureau. It is involved in National Disability Employment Awareness Month (October) and National Employ the Handicapped Week (the first full week of October each year), and addresses such issues as advocacy and affirmative action, vocational education, sheltered workshops, independent living access to employment, public attitudes, employment rights, training and legislation. The National Symposium on Employment of Americans with Disabilities (President's Committee, 1988) has recommended that the federal government provide responsible leadership with the aim of developing a national disability employment policy to enhance the work opportunities for people who are disabled.

Employment offers the possibility of dramatically improving an individual's lifestyle, and it is a prerequisite to economic self-sufficiency and quality of life. The number of noninstitutionalized people with a work-related disability is esti-

mated to be at least 13.3 million (18.6 percent of the working population), of whom 7.25 million have a severe disability that often results in unemployment (Kraus and Stoddard, 1989, pp. 36, 40). Close to 16 percent of people with a work-related disability are unemployed—approximately three times that of the nondisabled population. The median annual income of persons with work disabilities is $6434, whereas for the nonhandicapped population it is $13,403 (Kraus and Stoddard, 1989, p. 45). The condition most frequently reported to cause work limitation is heart disease. Figure 17-3 lists the five leading chronic conditions causing work limitation.

America's work ethic makes employment a central part of life. It is a societal expectation that people will work and be self-sufficient. Work has a great deal to do with how people identify themselves, as well as how they are identified by others. The personal identity and assessed self-worth of a person is often focused around work life. Work situations for the adult who is handicapped are limited and largely dependent on the presenting handicap.

Adults who are handicapped are found in com-

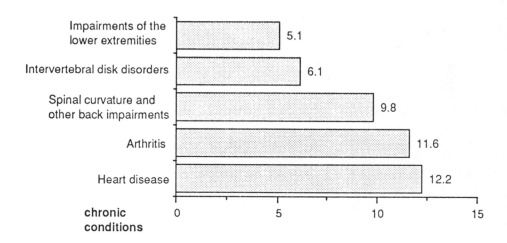

percent of all conditions causing work limitation

Figure 17-3   The five leading chronic conditions causing work limitation. (From Kraus LE and Stoddard S: Chartbook on disability in the United States, an InfoUse Report, Washington, DC, 1989, National Institute on Disability and Rehabilitation Research, p 42.)

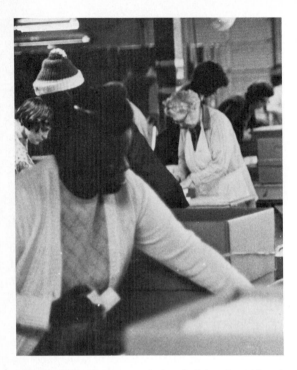

FIGURE 17-4　The great majority of adults who are hand-icapped can achieve skills that permit them to be gainfully employed. Sheltered workshops provide job training and placement services which enhance their abilities to function in competitive as well as noncompetitive work environments. (Courtesy of Sunshine Workshop, a nonprofit voluntary agency, sponsored by the Association of Retarded Citizens/Knox County, Tennessee and the photographer, Mary Louise Peacock.)

petitive, modified, and sheltered employment. *Competitive employment* is work with nonhandi-capped members of the work force on an equal basis, such as a job on the assembly line at an automotive factory. *Modified employment* is work done with nonhandicapped members of the work force in a work environment that has been modified to meet the needs of the handicapped worker. *Sheltered employment* (refer to Figure 17-4) is work that is open only to the handicapped and is done under direct supervision and guidance. The Association for Retarded Citizens and Goodwill Industries frequently sponsor sheltered workshops. The Wagner-O'Day Act of 1938, and its amendments of 1971, provide for special pref-

erence in bidding on government contracts to sheltered workshops for the severely handicapped.

A critical factor in the placement of the hand-icapped is the attitude of employers (Knight, 1988, p. 14; Kennedy, 1989, p. 8B). The placement process is facilitated when the employer is willing to accept the person with a handicap as an individual and to see him or her as a valuable worker. People with disabilities make very good employees and are highly rated by employers on overall job performance, willingness to work, reliability in attendance and productivity (O'Bryant, 1988, p. 8). In general, employers find people who are handicapped to be trustworthy, loyal, dependable, and dedicated employees (Kennedy, 1989, 8B). Handicapped workers do not increase employer insurance costs (O'Bryant, 1988, p. 10).

A study done by deBalcazar, Bradford and Fawcett (1988) showed that people who were handicapped thought that their job opportunities were very limited. They also thought that many employers did not provide reasonable accommodations for handicapped workers, that work disincentives still exist within the Social Security system, that people with disabilities are discriminated against because of their disability in the workplace, and that people with disabilities often do not know where to go for job training or placement.

The Washington Business Group on Health/ Institute for Rehabilitation and Disability Management (IRDM) has shown that employers, employees, and the general public were often misinformed about what handicapped workers can do, and that this misinformation is a serious deterrent to employment of the handicapped (O'Bryant, 1988, p. 9). The IRDM is presently involved in the Community Partnership Initiative with the Dole Foundation to build strong relationships between local employers, foundations, and disability service providers. This initiative is designed to enhance understanding about and employment of people with disabilities and to coordinate disability services (Dole foundation's, 1988, p. 13). The Initiative will give communities across the nation the means to develop or expand local programs to improve employment opportunities for people with disabilities.

A recent national publication, *Careers and the Handicapped,* is helping to serve the needs of people with disabilities. It was given the 1988 Media Award from the President's Committee on Employment of People with Disabilities, and it has the distinction of having published the first job recruitment ad in the world in Braille (Schneider, 1988, p. 15). It is published by Equal Opportunity Publications (44 Broadway, Greenlawn, New York 11740) and is available through them. Its sister publication, *Independent Living and Health Care Today,* assists people who are handicapped with independent living and health care options. These publications may be of interest to the person who is handicapped as well as the health care professional.

Although there are few incentives for employers to hire the handicapped worker, some do exist. The Internal Revenue Service allows tax incentives for businesses employing people who are handicapped (Coyle, 1989, p. 29). Tax credits are available to offset the cost of worksite accommodations for the handicapped. The Paralyzed Veterans of America publishes a guide to such accommodations entitled *Design Guidelines Qualifying for the Tax Advantages of Section 190,* and the President's Committee on Employment of People with Disabilities sponsors the Job Accommodation Network, a free national referral service to employers who are interested in accommodating disabled workers (1-800-526-7234).

In many cases self-employment for the person who is handicapped may be a viable option. The Small Business Administration makes loans to people who are handicapped to establish, acquire, or operate a business when other loans are not available on reasonable terms. Being self-employed provides individuals with the ability to have more control over their work environment and address their own employment needs (Handicapper small business, 1989, p. 18).

The Rehabilitation Act of 1973 mandates that federal agencies and federally contracted agencies take action to hire and promote handicapped persons. According to this law, no employer receiving federal assistance can discriminate against the handicapped employee in recruitment, hiring, promotion, demotion, transfer, layoff, firing, or rehiring. Further, an employer receiving federal assistance is required to take reasonable steps to accommodate the handicapped worker.

A handicapped job applicant or employee has the same rights and privileges as nonhandicapped applicants and employees. A person's handicap must not be considered in employment unless it keeps him or her from performing adequately.

If a person with a handicap believes that he or she has been discriminated against in relation to a federal job, the person should file a complaint with a federal job information center. Employers who discriminate against the handicapped face legal action and penalties. For further information about employment and the person who is handicapped contact:

President's Committee on Employment of
   People with Disabilities
1111 Twentieth Street N.W.
Washington, D.C. 20036-3470
Phone: (202) 653-2087

Transportation

A major barrier to employment and other life activities for the handicapped person is transportation. Accessible transportation is a critical component of self-reliance and self-sufficiency (National Council on the Handicapped, 1988, On the theshold of independence, p. 5).

Many people who are handicapped are either unable to drive or cannot afford a car. Public transportation such as buses, trains, trolleys, and subways is often lacking, and when it is available, it is often not readily accessible to the handicapped (Dietl, 1983). Although some communities in the United States have made provisions on public transportation for persons with a handicap, other countries have made much greater strides with the transportation needs of handicapped persons than has the United States. In Sweden, all public vehicles are accessible to the handicapped, France has a rail system that has specially equipped cars for the disabled, Japan has a totally accessible rail system, and Great Britain requires that all taxis be accessible (Dietl, 1983).

In the United States, many people who are handicapped must rely on friends, relatives, Dial-a-Rides, taxis, and voluntary transportation services, such as FISH. This shortage of available, consistent, and reliable transportation prevents persons who are handicapped from taking part in many activities. Federal legislation has mandated that no person be denied the use of public transportation because of a handicap. However, this goal is far from being realized.

Health Care

People with handicapping conditions utilize and require more health care services than the general population. Although people who are handicapped account for approximately 15 percent of the U.S. population, they account for 30 percent of all U.S. hospital days (Verville, 1981, p. 43).

Many people who are handicapped are eligible for the state and federally funded programs of Medicaid and Medicare. However, these programs often do not adequately provide for assistive devices and other necessary health care. Private health insurance is difficult for handicapped persons to obtain either because the condition precedes their insurance application or because they are considered high risk. The CIGNA corporation has offered a plan to provide major medical coverage to people who are mentally retarded, but such plans are scarce (Major medical plan, 1989, p. 2). Many people who are handicapped do not have health insurance that adequately covers their needs.

People who are handicapped often have difficulty accessing health care. They report that an increasing number of doctors are refusing to take Medicaid or Medicare; they cannot afford regular medical care; transportation to medical providers is often difficult; medical professionals are often insensitive and unaware of the special medical or physical assistance needs imposed by a disability; the general public is unaware existing programs do not provide adequate medical care for people with disabilities; and assistive devices (e.g., wheelchairs) are often too expensive or simply not available (deBalcazar, Bradford, and Fawcett, 1988, pp. 30, 32, 34).

Preventive health care services are often underutilized by the disabled because of a lack of accessible facilities and because of the negative attitudes of health care professionals (deBalcazar, Bradford and Fawcett, 1988). For the mobility-impaired client, certain equipment and procedures present almost insurmountable barriers to health care resources, unless health care personnel are responsive and innovative enough to adapt the situation to the client's needs. During health care procedures, factors such as positioning, privacy, and comfort must not be overlooked for the person who is handicapped.

Many health care professionals prefer not to work with people who are severely handicapped, especially those who are mentally handicapped. Even when funding is adequate the handicapped may be unable to find a private health care provider and it is difficult for them to obtain other medical or dental care. The community health nurse can be instrumental in procuring these health services. Transportation to medical and dental appointments is sometimes facilitated if the person has Medicaid, since Medicaid may provide funds for transportation to medical appointments.

The cost of medical care for the person who is totally disabled can be at least three times that for the nonhandicapped population (Social Security Administration, 1977). Many of these costs are not covered by insurance since handicapped people are less likely to have comprehensive insurance coverage.

Social and Recreational Opportunities

Few social and recreational programs are specifically designed for people who are handicapped. Recreation is one of their most neglected needs (Spiegel and Podair, 1981, p. 305), and many handicapped adults suffer from social isolation (Strauss, Corbin, Fagerhaugh, Glaser, Maines, Suczek, and Wiener, 1984, p. 16). Community support of social and recreational activities will play a major role in their availability. Community health nurses can help secure such support.

Some adults who are handicapped, especially those who are mentally retarded, often find great enjoyment in participating in social and recreational activities planned especially for them. Others, such as the severely diabetic, often mix freely in social and recreational activities that nonhandicapped adults enjoy. Whatever the level of disability, these people are social beings and should have social programs and activities available to them. Unfortunately, many buildings and areas where social and recreational programs are offered are physically inaccessible to them.

Access to social and recreational activities is important (Weiss, 1988, p. 8). Robert Zywicki, an internationally recognized expert on travel and recreation for handicapped people, is editor of *The Itinerary,* a magazine for travelers with disabilities, and is president of Whole Person Tours, Inc., which specializes in accessible vacations. Mr. Zywicki is himself confined to a wheelchair. Some of the accessible vacations he recommends are Disney World in Florida, the national parks, the Smithsonian Institute in Washington, D.C., and the Island of Oahu in Hawaii (Weiss, 1988, p. 8).

Guides to the national parks for people who are handicapped are becoming available. *Access America: an atlas and guide to the National Parks for visitors with disabilities* and *Access Yosemite National Park: an atlas and guide for visitors with disabilities* are available (New accessibility, 1988, pp. 1, 15). These publications were prepared with the cooperation of the National Park Service and health professionals. For ordering information contact Northern Cartographic, P.O. Box 133, Burlington, Vermont 05402 (1-802-655-4321).

Sexuality

Being disabled does not change a person's need for intimacy, even though it may alter the experience of sexual fulfillment (Cole and Cole, 1981, p. 279). Many myths and misconceptions surround sexuality and people who are disabled: the disabled are often treated as if they were asexual or as if sex were inappropriate for them (Haring and Meyerson, 1981; Peters, 1982). Adults who are handicapped often find that the sexual aspects of their disability are ignored or viewed as unim-

portant. Preconceptions about what is sexually appropriate for the person who is handicapped often deny, limit, or inhibit the person from expressing sexuality.

Like the rest of the population, people with disabilities may have sexual problems at some time or another. Medical evaluation of their problems and counseling is helpful. It is only recently that sexuality has been an acceptable part of rehabilitation counseling (Cole and Cole, 1981, p. 279), and many counselors still do not feel comfortable handling this type of counseling with individuals who are handicapped. The lack of counseling resources and the reluctance of professionals to deal with the topic can leave the disabled client with minimal support in working out sexual problems and concerns.

The person who is disabled needs the same knowledge about love and caring, sexual functioning, intimacy, and sexual responsibility that other people need. It cannot be expected that individuals will make informed, appropriate decisions if they do not have the information needed to make such decisions. Like other persons, individuals who are handicapped should be made aware of community resources, such as family planning clinics and Planned Parenthood, which can help them to deal with their sexual needs.

Depending on the handicap, the person may or may not have any sexual dysfunction. If dysfunction exists, the person should be helped to find avenues of expression and fulfillment of sexual needs. Achievement of intimacy with a partner often leads to increased self-esteem and provides encouragement for achievement in other areas.

Nurses have recognized and written about sexuality concerns and needs of people who have chronic and handicapping conditions (Hahn, 1989; Burgener, 1989). The Sex Information and Education Council United States (SIECUS) regularly publishes annotated bibliographies on sexuality and disability (Sexuality, 1988, p. 29). In general, health care professionals need to look closely at their own feelings and attitudes about sexuality and the person who is handicapped. Professionals must be aware that sometimes even an unconscious facial gesture can convey negative meaning to handicapped persons and affect how they feel about themselves and about the service they are utilizing. If a professional does not feel capable or comfortable with sexuality counseling, the client should be assisted in finding another resource.

Guardianship

Many people who are handicapped do not need guardians. They are able to go through their entire life making and acting on their own decisions. This is especially true of people who are physically handicapped. Guardianship is usually considered for individuals who are severely disabled, especially those who are severely mentally ill or mentally retarded.

Once the age of majority is reached, a person is legally responsible for himself or herself unless a legal guardian has been appointed by probate court. The court decides if a guardian should be appointed, and whether the guardian should be plenary (complete) or partial. Partial guardianship is not allowed in every state. Partial guardianship implies that the person is able to carry out some functions alone but needs assistance in carrying out other functions. If no guardian is appointed the person is responsible for making his or her own decisions. Until guardianship is applied for, none generally is appointed by the court. Guardians are frequently appointed for people who are mentally handicapped, but may be appointed for other adults who need assistance in carrying out the activities of everyday life.

Parents are "natural" guardians of their own minor children and can make legal decisions for them. Parents are *not* natural guardians of their adult offspring who are handicapped and cannot make their legal decisions without having guardianship. Many parents are unaware of this fact, which can present a problem when their adult offspring needs medical care or other social services. If the adult who is handicapped is unable to make a rational decision, medical care or services may be denied until a legal guardian is appointed. Anticipatory guidance with parents or significant others can prevent this from happening.

Handling guardianship issues is difficult for many families. Families who have handicapped adult offspring frequently experience a crisis when they realize that their offspring are not able to make rational decisions at the age of maturity. Parents at this point can no longer avoid the reality that their offspring may never develop the skills to function independently. Feelings of sadness and hopelessness at this time are not uncommon. It is crucial for the community health nurse and other health care professionals to recognize the distress these parents are experiencing and to provide support during this critical transition period. Helping families to identify the strengths their adult offspring have, as well as the potential for benefitting from experiences that are developmentally within their reach, can reduce their anxiety and increase their ability to plan for the future.

When helping a family to deal with guardianship issues, it is crucial for the community health nurse to focus on the entire family system. Siblings are often asked at this time to make a commitment to assume responsibility for the care of an adult sibling who is handicapped after the parents are no longer able to do so. This can stimulate feelings of fear, shame, guilt, or hostility, especially if the siblings do not want to make such a commitment. Families may need assistance in analyzing what is best for all family members.

At times, community health nurses have found that some families assume that adults who are handicapped are unable to care for themselves just because they are handicapped. It is important to remember that not all adults who are handicapped need guardians. In fact, most of them do not.

Community Residential Opportunities

It is the right of persons who are handicapped to live their lives as normally as possible in the mainstream of the community. All people belong in the community regardless of their degree of disability, and community integration involves participation in community life—not just being there.

Many people who are handicapped do not require any specialized form of housing and live independently. For some people who are handicapped, especially those with mobility limitations or those who are wheelchair-bound, adaptations must be made to make housing facilities accessible. Housing problems are related to discrimination, affordability, and accessibility. The number of federally subsidized housing units has dropped sharply in recent years, making affordable housing harder to obtain. There is a shortage of accessible, affordable housing for people with disabilities.

Builders and contractors are often unaware of laws, access codes, and modifications necessary for handicap accessibility, and may not comply with existing laws, including those that require a certain percentage of handicap-accessible units in public housing (deBalcazar, Bradford, and Fawcett, 1988, p. 33). People who are handicapped often end up making the necessary housing modifications themselves.

Accessible housing is essential if people with handicaps are to be able to live independently in the community (Carling, 1989, p. 6). The Center for Accessible Housing, the nation's first research and training center focusing on making housing accessible to people with handicaps, is funded by the National Institute for Disability and Rehabilitation Research (NIDRR). The center has a dual mission: to improve the quality of housing environments for people with disabilities and to increase the availability of such housing (Research and training, 1989, p. 4). The center plans to offer training sessions for people with disabilities, their families, and the construction industry. For further information about center programs, publications, and activities contact Center for Accessible Housing, Box 7701, North Carolina State University, Raleigh, North Carolina, 27695-7701 (1-919-737-7714).

Community living arrangements should be geared to the level of disability being experienced by the person. These placements can encompass independent living, living in the household of a relative, foster care, group homes, nursing homes, public medical care facilities, and state residential facilities. The recruitment, funding, placement, and monitoring aspects of residential placements vary from state to state, and even county to county. People looking for specific placements should check with local departments of social or human services, departments of mental health, or specialty agencies dealing with the conditions involved. Some examples of such agencies are the local association for retarded citizens, the National Association for Multiple Sclerosis, and various associations for blind persons. These agencies are often aware of available community placements and can refer people to appropriate agencies.

In selecting residential placement, one should carefully evaluate the facility and establish placement objectives for the individual. If placement objectives, such as extent of personal freedom and educational goals, are not being met, contact promptly the agencies responsible for licensing and monitoring the facility and report the deficiencies. These agencies vary from state to state.

In many areas restrictive zoning regulations do not allow group homes for people who are handicapped. Zoning laws have changed in some states to become more liberal in regard to community placement of people who are handicapped (McGuire and Guernsey, 1978). Restrictive zoning policies in the past led to clustering of community residential facilities in areas where zoning policies were not restrictive. These areas were often the less desirable residential areas. Examine the geographic clustering of facilities when considering a residential facility. If handicapped people are to be integrated into the mainstream of the community, they should not be clustered together in settings apart from the mainstream. There is often much community education that needs to be done to assist the person who is handicapped in adjusting to community life.

In recent years there has been a marked return to the community of people who resided in institutional settings, particularly those who are mentally handicapped. For example, the number of psychiatric mental hospital residents has decreased from 560,000 in 1955 to 125,000 (Shadish, Lurigio, and Lewis, 1989, p. 2). People who are leaving institutional settings need to be prepared to return to the community, and the community also needs to be prepared for their return. If this preparation is not done many problems can arise. If not adequately prepared the individual will have difficulty adapting to this new setting; if the community is not prepared it will not facilitate the individual's adjustment. Many communities have gone to court to prevent, remove, or restrict residences for the handicapped, who often are mentally handicapped.

The community health nurse can do much to help educate the community and its leaders regarding the needs of a person who is handicapped. Actively participating on community advisory boards established to facilitate community placement programs provides many opportunities to influence community leaders and to educate the public.

Families, like the handicapped adult and the community, need assistance in dealing with the deinstitutionalization process. Frequently they need help to reestablish their relationship with their adult offspring, especially if this individual has been institutionalized for several years and they have had limited contact with him or her. Often families must reevaluate all the decisions that were made in relation to the future of an adult who is handicapped. If the handicapped member returns home, the family may again have to decide how to ensure adequate care, as well as deal with increased physical, mental, social, and economic responsibilities. If he or she returns home or to another setting in the community, such as an adult foster care home, the family may have to deal with feelings of guilt and inadequacy in regard to the original placement, concern regarding financial and parental responsibility, and uncertainty as to the appropriateness of the placement. An example of the dilemma that this transition from institution to community can pose with a family is seen with Mrs. Bartel.

Mrs. Bartel, a 75-year-old widow receiving social security, was being seen by the community health nurse for hypertension. Mrs. Bartel's blood pressure was unusually high on this home visit and she seemed openly troubled. When the nurse asked her if something was upsetting her, she began crying and stated that her 52-year-old son, who was moderately retarded and had been in a local institution for 35 years, was now being considered for community placement in an adult foster care home. She had received a letter inviting her to a case conference to discuss this placement, but she had no way to get there. Mrs. Bartel was worried that her son was not being appropriately placed and that she would be expected to pay for the community placement. With Mrs. Bartel's permission, the nurse contacted the case conference coordinator and shared her concerns. It was established that the nurse on the community placement team would visit with Mrs. Bartel and the community health nurse to discuss the situation.

The nurse visited and explained the process of community placement to Mrs. Bartel. She arranged for her to visit John's tentative foster home so that she could meet the people who would be responsible for John's care. She assured Mrs. Bartel that John's needs would be met and that there would be no charge to her for the placement. The nurse assured Mrs. Bartel that she would be able to visit John, that his placement would be regularly monitored, and that a change in placement would be made if necessary. After visiting the adult foster home, Mrs. Bartel said, "I wish I had had this choice 35 years ago. I would never have placed John in the institution. I know I cannot take care of him, but here it is more like a home. He will have a more normal life and I am happy for him. I will be able to die in peace."

The community health nurse, by utilizing available resources, was able to help ease this transition for Mrs. Bartel and aid in her adjustment to her son's deinstitutionalization. Concerns like Mrs. Bartel's are not uncommon.

Attendant Services

The person who is handicapped may not be able to carry out all the activities of daily living. When this happens the person can benefit from attendant services. The attendant assists the person in such activities as maintaining personal appearance and hygiene (e.g., feeding, dressing, grooming), mobility, household maintenance, safety, and interactions within the community through communication assistance (Attendant services, 1989, p. 2). It is estimated that more than 850,000 Americans currently use some form of community-based attendant services (Litvak, Zukas, and Heumann, 1987; Consumer management, 1988), and that at least 7.7 million noninstitutionalized Americans age 15 and above have personal care limitations and need personal assistance to carry out activities of daily living (Kraus and Stoddard, 1989, p. 5). This means that four out of five Americans who need attendant services are not receiving them. Personal care limitations are assessed using one of two scales: activities of daily living (ADLs) and instrumental activities of daily living (IADLs). ADLs include bathing, dressing, eating, walking, and other personal activities, whereas IADLs encompass preparing meals, shopping, using the phone and communicating, doing laundry and other measures of being able to live independently (Kraus and Stoddard, 1989, p. 5).

For many people who are handicapped the availability of attendant services is a major determinant to their ability to live independently and to obtain employment (Opie and Miller, 1989, p. 196). Unfortunately, there is a lack of adequate attendant services in the United States; no comprehensive, uniform system for providing such services exists; and services vary greatly from state to state. These services are sometimes obtainable through Medicaid, Department of Human Services (Social Services Block Grant Title XX), Older Americans Act provisions, Veterans Administration, and various state and locally funded programs. The community health nurse can be instrumental in helping clients to obtain such services.

Respite Care

It is unfair to expect the caretakers of persons who are handicapped to provide 24-hour-a-day care and to assume all the burden for this care. However, this frequently happens and, increasingly, caretakers are experiencing burnout.

Respite care is one solution to the problem of caretaker overload. It provides short-term, 24-hour-a-day placement, including, but not limited to, the following settings: nursing homes, clients' homes, private homes, foster care, group homes, hospitals, and institutions. Respite care provides relief for the caretaker and may avoid institutionalization. It is also successful in decreasing stress and increasing coping ability, attitudes, and

adaptability (Sherman and Cocozza, 1984). A caretaker may request respite care for personal reasons such as illness, vacation, or mental health. Whatever the reason, it is legitimate for the caretaker to request time away from his or her charge.

Most people are unfamiliar with the concept of respite care, and in the United States it is difficult to obtain. Where it exists privately, the costs are often prohibitive. Some families and organizations have developed respite co-op groups where they exchange periods of time in caring for their respective handicapped family members. The Omnibus Budget Reconciliation Act of 1981 allowed Medicaid waivers for reimbursement of respite care if the cost is the same or less than institutional care (Hildebrandt, 1983). More bills related to respite care are being introduced into Congress.

When assisting a client in looking for respite care, agencies that deal with the specific condition(s) involved should be contacted, along with the local department of social or human services. The community health nurse can be instrumental in advocating respite care services for clients and in making this very important need known to the community. If only from a cost-effectiveness standpoint, the community should be interested, because it is more economical to finance respite care services than it is to provide institutional care or long-term care. The humane reasons for providing such care cannot be measured.

LEGISLATION

An overview of federal legislation and voluntary efforts is presented in Appendix 17-1. Major pieces of legislation have provided the mechanisms for meeting many of the needs of people who are handicapped. Some of these pieces of legislation include the following:

Developmental Disabilities Act (1971)
Rehabilitation Act of 1973
Developmental Disabilities and Bill of Rights Act (1975, 1984)
Education for All Handicapped Children Act (1975)
Mental Health Systems Act (1980)

Civil Rights of Institutionalized Persons Act (1980)

Protection and Advocacy for Mentally Ill Individuals Act of 1986 (1986, 1988)

Americans with Disabilities Act (1990)

Newer legislation has promoted awareness of the needs of people who are handicapped. Legislation in the 1980s has focused on providing access so the person can participate in society; provision of increased financial benefits; and increased service provision (Watson, 1988, p. 137). The most recent piece of legislation addressing the needs of people who are handicapped, the Americans with Disabilities Act, is designed to provide a clear and comprehensive mandate to end discrimination against individuals with disabilities. It deals with such issues as housing, employment, public transportation, and communication services (Americans, 1989, p. 22; Moses, 1989, p. 9) The act is meant to ensure the civil rights of persons who are handicapped, and extend to them the protection given in other federal civil rights legislation (Americans, 1989, p. 22; Moses, 1989). It is considered to be the most significant piece of legislation of the past decade for people who are disabled. At this writing, governmental officials are examining how to implement the mandates of this act.

The United Nations General Assembly has proclaimed the years of 1983 through 1992 as the International Decade of Disabled Persons; former President Reagan issued a proclamation naming the same time period as the United States National Decade of Disabled Persons.

Despite the recent national and international interest generated by legislative proclamations, disability-related programs continue to be underfunded. One needs to stay knowledgeable about the legal issues facing people who are disabled in order to advocate for reform effectively. Some good sources of legal information on disability are *Mental and Physical Disability Law Reporter* (bimonthly); *Handicapped Requirements Handbook,* updated monthly; and *Education of the Handicapped Law Report* (Goldman, 1984). Legislative advocacy which promotes reform will be needed in order to ensure forward movement in the Decade of Disabled Persons.

REHABILITATION

Rehabilitation is the process of restoring an individual to the fullest physical, mental, social, vocational, and economic usefulness possible. A major goal of rehabilitation is to integrate the individual into society. A key component of many rehabilitation programs is vocational rehabilitation. Here, a chief goal is to place a client in a job with a stable employer and good benefits (Handicapper small business, 1989, p. 18). Vocational rehabilitation efforts frequently involve assessment of the client's work potential, vocational education and training, purchase of the assistive devices necessary for employment, vocational counseling and employment placement, evaluation, and follow-up. Many vocational rehabilitation services are provided for under the Rehabilitation Act of 1973 through its state-federal vocational rehabilitation programs. In order to qualify for these programs a person must be at least 16 years old, have a physical or mental disability that constitutes an employment handicap, and be able to become employable as a result of the education, training, and rehabilitation. To apply for rehabilitation services the person should contact the local office of the state Department of Education, Division of Vocational Services. Other rehabilitation programs are offered through hospitals, long-term care facilities, and outpatient settings.

Rehabilitation is important since cures do not exist for many chronic and handicapping conditions. Comprehensive programs are multidisciplinary and combine medical treatment with physical and occupational therapy, as well as sociological, psychological, and economic counseling and services. Rehabilitation is a comprehensive, long-term process and demands a high level of commitment.

Federal Government Rehabilitation Resources

The U.S. Department of Education offers many services to people who are handicapped. The Rehabilitation Services Administration (RSA) administers vocational and rehabilitation programs. Its state-federal vocational rehabilitation program provides important employment/vocational services. RSA works for the removal of architectural barriers for the handicapped, and is actively involved in education, training, and advocacy. It publishes the quarterly periodical *American Rehabilitation.* RSA can be contacted at Rehabilitation Services Administration, Department of Education, Mary E. Switzer Building, Room 3024, 330 C. Street SW, Washington, D.C. 20202 (1-202-732-1296).

The department's National Rehabilitation Information Center (NARIC) (1-800-34-NARIC) was established in 1977 to supply information and publications on disability and rehabilitation. NARIC publishes the *NARIC Quarterly, NARIC Guide to Disability and Rehabilitation Periodicals,* and *Resource Guides* on selected topics. These guides include topic description; a listing of national and international organization involvement, periodicals, and information resources; Rehabilitation Research and Training Centers; REHABDATA descriptors; and a brief annotated bibliography of major NARIC holdings (NARIC prepares, 1989). NARIC's online computerized databases REHABDATA (1-800-34-NARIC) includes bibliographic information and abstracts; and ABLEDATA (1-800-344-5405) provides information about commercial rehabilitation products. NARIC is a service of the department's National Institute on Disability and Rehabilitation Research (NIDRR). NIDRR gathers disability data that can be accessed by calling InfoUse at 1-415-644-9904. It sponsors the publications *Disability Statistics Bulletin* (a free, semiannual publication), *Disability Statistics Abstracts,* and *Disability Statistics Reports.* All are available from the Institute for Health and Aging, University of California, 201 Filbert Street, Suite 500, San Francisco, California 94133-3203 (1-415-362-3620).

The Department of Education also houses the Clearinghouse on Disability Information (Department of Education, Mary E. Switzer Building, Room 3132, 330 C. Street SW, Washington, D.C.

20202; [1-202-732-1244]). This Clearinghouse was established in 1975 to respond to inquiries from handicapped people and serves as a resource to organizations and professionals who supply information to people who are handicapped. The Clearinghouse library is open to the public.

The Rehabilitation Process

Rehabilitation programs involve casefinding, multidisciplinary assessment, planning, intervention, and evaluation; restorative services; vocational counseling and placement, and retraining. Family involvement is extremely important. The rehabilitation process follows the same steps as the systematic nursing process (refer to Chapter 8). It involves data gathering, formation of diagnosis and rehabilitation prognosis, goals, plans, follow-up, and ongoing evaluation. Records are kept and discharge planning is done as the process proceeds (refer to Chapter 9).

The plan of care is done in conjunction with the client, family, and significant others, and has both rehabilitation facility and home care foci. The family is of central importance in the rehabilitation process. When a crisis such as illness or disability strikes one member of a family, all family members are affected in some way, and family variables such as coping patterns, knowledge of the disability, expectations, and economic status will greatly affect the family's ability and willingness to adapt and help (Watson, 1989, p. 318). Individual and family adaptation to the handicap is crucial to active and successful client participation in the rehabilitation process. Factors related to this adaptation have been discussed previously in this chapter.

Unfortunately, rehabilitation is too often more under the control of professionals rather than the client and family (Walkover, 1988). This practice fosters client and family dependence and can inhibit the rehabilitation process. There is a need to shift the responsibility for achieving rehabilitation goals to the client and family and to focus on self-management (Sawyer and Crimando, 1984). Professionals must realize that the client and family will need to handle their situation long after health care professionals are no longer involved and must have self-care skills to make appropriate health care decisions.

Self-management techniques are directed toward developing the capacity in clients to regulate and make decisions about their own behavior (Sawyer and Crimando, 1984). Self-management has also shown to increase an individual's motivation toward achievement of rehabilitation goals, which is critical to the successful outcome of the rehabilitation process (Sawyer and Crimando, 1984).

Motivation is increased if the client believes that the rehabilitation program is realistic and will result in increased independence. It is important for the nurse to discover and utilize methods that promote belief in the rehabilitation activities.

The client must also be willing to participate in the demanding process of rehabilitation and realize many major life changes may need to occur. The client must make the effort necessary to improve his or her condition, endure the therapeutic procedures and adjust to assistive devices.

The problems do not end with rehabilitation. In fact, rehabilitation may often accentuate some of them because it will restore the person to a level where it will be necessary to deal with the non-handicapped population on his or her own. The person often needs help in seeing the value of becoming part of the mainstream. This may be a difficult task, especially if society is not willing to accept the person who is handicapped, either socially or emotionally, even after successful rehabilitation.

THE COMMUNITY HEALTH NURSE'S ROLE WITH THE HANDICAPPED ADULT

Community health nurses carry out many roles with adults who are handicapped. These include roles as resource coordinator, counselor, case finder, advocate, health educator, direct care provider, and health planner. When implementing these roles, community health nurses use the nursing process and are involved in primary, secondary, and tertiary preventive activities. A deterrent to primary prevention is that the etiology of many chronic and handicapping conditions is unknown. Due to the long-term nature of handicap-

ping conditions, the client is likely to be involved in rehabilitation activities for extended periods of time.

When working with the adult who is handicapped, the community health nurse must include the caretakers in establishing, implementing, and evaluating the plan of care. Caretakers should be helped to use anticipatory guidance, plan for the long-term implications associated with the condition, set realistic expectations, and use self-management techniques. Health care professionals can provide support, guidance, knowledge, and assistance, but only the client and his family can evoke change.

Allowing for meaningful expression of feelings that may range from despair and hopelessness to unrealistic optimism is one of the most significant functions of a community health nurse when working with individuals who are handicapped (Safilios-Rothschild, 1982, p. 90). The nurse must be equipped to deal with this range of feelings.

Nurses have a variety of personal feelings which can inhibit or enhance their ability to function effectively. When working with clients who are handicapped, professionals must be careful not to temper their empathy for clients with patronizing and dependency (Peters, 1982, p. 36). Because of the complexities of providing therapeutic services to people who are disabled, community health nurses have found it beneficial to have peer collaboration in which they have the opportunity to examine their feelings in relation to clients' needs and nursing interventions.

Community Resource Utilization

Crucial to the successful control of chronic and handicapping conditions is the utilization of community resources (Bubolz and Whiren, 1984; Nelson, 1984; Sargent, 1983; McCubbin and Patterson, 1983; and Watson, 1989). The knowledgeable community health nurse refers clients to community resources as appropriate (refer to Chapter 9), because clients often are not aware of the resources available to them or how to work with these resources.

Some excellent resources were noted previously under federal government rehabilitation resources. Many resources are available, but often it is difficult for the client to locate them. The nurse can help the client and family be aware that they need to be persistent when exploring resources, and not become discouraged and give up too easily. Searching out available resources can be a trying experience even for the experienced health care professional. Oftentimes word-of-mouth or other people with the same condition can make the client aware of resources. Self-help groups can provide clients with valuable information about community resources.

The search for resources can be harrowing. The nurse may want to make telephone or direct contacts on behalf of the client, because this can both help to avoid client discouragement and can make the nurse more aware of community resources. Resources we take for granted such as appropriate clothing and household furnishings, tools, and appliances can be difficult to obtain for the person who is handicapped.

One significant national resource to which the nurse can direct clients is the Clearinghouse on Disability Information (1-202-743-1244) mentioned earlier. The clearinghouse can help the client to obtain needed resources and can provide valuable information. The *Directory of National Information Sources on Handicapping Conditions and Related Services* was originally published by the clearinghouse, and is now published privately under the title *Handicapping Conditions and Services Directory*. It is available through Harold Russell Associates, 8 Winchester Place, Suite 304, Winchester, Massachusetts 01890 (1-617-245-7099), at a reasonable cost.

Another helpful publication is *Health Information Resources in the Federal Government*. This publication is available from the Office of Disease Prevention and Health Promotion (Contact: National Health Information Center, U.S. Department of Health and Human Services Public Health Service, P.O. Box 1133, Washington, D.C. 20013-1133; 1-800-336-4797 or 1-202-429-9091). The magazine *Exceptional Parent* publishes an annual directory of organizations that provide services to people who have handicaps. It is available at a minimal cost from Exceptional Parent Magazine, 1170 Commonwealth Avenue, Boston, MA, 02134 (1-617-730-5800). The Na-

tional Spinal Cord Injury Association (1-800-962-9629) publishes *National Resource Directory,* which provides resource information and is available through them for a reasonable cost or as a benefit of membership.

The local telephone book is a valuable source of information. Some books include specific sections on human and community services. Many agencies are located under the governmental phone listings, or under specific headings in the yellow pages such as hospitals, hospital equipment, rehabilitation, and mental health. Local health departments and departments of human services, federal Social Security Administration offices, state Developmental Disability Councils, United Way, and public libraries are all valuable sources of information. A list of resources is given in Appendix 17-2. Many have local affiliates.

The nurse can also refer clients to such travel and recreational services as the American Automobile Association (AAA) and the Society for the Advancement of Travel for the Handicapped (SATH). AAA publishes *The Handicapped Driver's Mobility Guide* that lists hundreds of services for the handicapped driver including hand-control devices. This publication is available through local AAA offices. SATH offers travel tips and has listings of travel agents who are experienced in dealing with handicapped people. It can be reached at 26 Court Street, Brooklyn, New York 11242 (1-718-858-5483).

Another comprehensive resource guide for people who are handicapped is: *Resource. A Free Guide to Needed Information, Equipment, Clothing and Supplies for Persons with Disabilities,* published by the Castelwood Corporation. (This guide has been in Sears, Roebuck and Company Home Health Care catalogs). Other guides are often obtained from the local library, and local telephone books carry comprehensive agency telephone listings.

Nurse's Responsibility in Rehabilitation

The community health nurse is in a key position to help the client and family accept and implement the rehabilitation program. A resource that the nurse may find helpful in providing such services is the Association of Rehabilitation Nurses.

Preadmission information

How did you find out about the rehabilitation unit? (Check one)

☐ Doctor

☐ Nurse

☐ Other health person

☐ Friend

☐ Other (please name) _____

Did the nurse or doctor talk to you before you came?　☐ Yes　☐ No

If yes, did you get your questions answered?　☐ Yes　☐ No

If yes, did you understand what the unit was like?　☐ Yes　☐ No

What should patients know about the rehabilitation unit before coming to the unit?

About your care	Always	Often	Sometimes	Rarely	Never	NA
I was included in planning my care.	☐	☐	☐	☐	☐	☐
The staff listened to my problems.	☐	☐	☐	☐	☐	☐
Questions about sex were answered.	☐	☐	☐	☐	☐	☐
My call light was answered quickly.	☐	☐	☐	☐	☐	☐
I learned about my medications.	☐	☐	☐	☐	☐	☐
Nurses explained things to be done to me.	☐	☐	☐	☐	☐	☐
Therapists explained things to be done to me.	☐	☐	☐	☐	☐	☐
Family						
My family was included in planning my care.	☐	☐	☐	☐	☐	☐
My family was taught how to care for me.	☐	☐	☐	☐	☐	☐
My family had their questions answered.	☐	☐	☐	☐	☐	☐
My family went to family support group.	☐	☐	☐	☐	☐	☐
My family rate this group as helpful.	☐	☐	☐	☐	☐	☐
If you had speech problems, please answer the following:						
Therapist helped me learn to talk.	☐	☐	☐	☐	☐	☐
My speech improved.	☐	☐	☐	☐	☐	☐
Staff understood my speech problem.	☐	☐	☐	☐	☐	☐
I learned to talk with the staff.	☐	☐	☐	☐	☐	☐
Family was taught to understand my speech.	☐	☐	☐	☐	☐	☐

Results and evaluation

Did you have special things to learn before you came?　☐ Yes　☐ No

Did you learn what you wanted to learn?　☐ Yes, definitely.　☐ Yes, I think so.　☐ No, I don't think so.　☐ No, definitely not.

If needed, would you return to the unit?　☐ Yes　☐ Probably　☐ No

Would you tell others to come to the unit?　☐ Yes　☐ Probably　☐ No

What I liked most about the rehabilitation center:

_____

_____

_____

What I liked least about the rehabilitation center:

_____

_____

_____

_____

Figure 17-5　Sample items on a patient satisfaction survey. (From Courts NF: A patient satisfaction survey for a rehab unit, Rehab Nurs 13(2):80, 1988. Reprinted from Rehabilitation Nursing, Volume 13, Issue 2, with permission of the Association of Rehabilitation Nurses, 5700 Old Orchard Road, First floor, Skokie, Il. 60077-1024. Copyright © 1988 Association of Rehabilitation Nurses.)

This association deals specifically with the application of rehabilitation concepts to nursing practice and can be contacted for information at ARN, 5700 Old Orchard Road, Skokie, Illinois, 60077 (1-708-966-3433).

The community health nurse frequently encounters rehabilitation clients in the home, outpatient, long-term care, and clinic environments. The nurse collaborates with other members of the rehabilitation team and promotes a multidisciplinary approach to treatment. The nurse has the objectives of helping the client and family to adjust to the changes imposed by the handicap, and helping the client's family and significant others to become partners in the rehabilitation process (Power, 1989, p. 73). Community health nurses work closely with clients and families to enhance their abilities to cope and adapt. They are actively engaged in coordinating community resources, providing support and encouragement, helping to minimize discouragement, and facilitate program evaluation.

Evaluating the client's rehabilitation regimen is an important role that is often left up to the nurse. A client satisfaction survey can be an effective tool in rehabilitation evaluation. It provides data that can serve as a basis for decision making about patient care, enhances public relations because it conveys to clients and their families that their opinions are valued, and enhances client care (Courts, 1988, p. 79). Sample items for such a survey are given in Figure 17-5.

The nurse's role in rehabilitation is varied and comprehensive. The nurse will need to be flexible and adaptable in implementing rehabilitation care and sensitive to the needs of the client and family. The nurse needs to work in close collaboration with other members of the rehabilitation team.

The Nurse, Affirmative Action, and Advocacy for the Person Who Is Handicapped

The nurse is the health professional most familiar with the health care system in its totality, including its gaps and inequities. Sometimes the gaps and inequities in the system can be managed, but sometimes they need to be challenged.

The person who is handicapped is at risk in the system, and often finds it difficult to advocate for herself or himself. It is frequently someone other than that person who is in the best position to advocate change.

Client advocacy among health professionals is a recent phenomenon. Many health professionals hesitate to put themselves in client advocacy positions for the following reasons:

1. *Advocacy is an unfamiliar role.* Professionals have generally not been trained to be advocates and are not used to undertaking such a role. The person assuming an advocacy role is not conforming to the established system and may be pressured to conform. The advocate may find advocacy difficult, awkward, and uncomfortable.
2. *Fear of reprisal.* There are many ways that an individual can be punished for advocacy actions. Often the greater the impact of the advocacy action, the greater the risk of reprisal. The advocate must be aware of the possibility of reprisal and must decide the possible outcomes of his or her behavior.
3. *Role conflict.* It can be difficult for the professional to remain separate from the professional role and place himself or herself in the role of advocate, especially if the advocate role is in conflict with the professional one. It is difficult to take stands contrary to the stand of other professionals in the field or contrary to the organization for which one works.
4. *Apathy.* Some will choose to be apathetic and not be involved. If one is not personally or directly affected, this role may be assumed.
5. *Lack of support.* If one finds oneself standing alone, or almost alone, it is often difficult to take a firm stand on any position. If one lacks the support of significant others, the stand also becomes difficult.
6. *Change implications.* Professionals realize the implications of changing a situation. To encourage change, to take a stand, is often to encourage stress. Are we willing to give up a system, possibly a stable one, to invoke an unstable one?

Health professionals and the organizations they represent have many frequently used excuses for not advocating on behalf of the client in addition to the ones listed. Excuses such as not enough time, not enough money, no one to help, not wanting to get involved on an emotional level, and the system not being ready for such a change all enter in. It is easy to feel empathy with these excuses as most of us have probably used them at one time or another. Taking or not taking an advocacy stand often boils down to one common denominator—one's philosophy in life. If one believes that all people are equal, and as such deserve equal rights and treatment, the question of advocating or not advocating becomes almost secondary whenever one sees an individual's rights being violated or ignored.

The impact that a nurse can have on the system as an advocate should not be underestimated. An example of this is the case of a nurse working with a local association of parents of retarded children.

The parents in a local association for retarded citizens were increasingly aware of instances of suspected abuse to their children in the institutional setting in which they resided. The parents had talked with the institution administration and felt they were not receiving adequate information; some of the parents felt intimidated. The parents were concerned about the implications of their actions on their institutionalized children. If they continued to press for information, they were worried about reprisals. If they did not press for information, they were worried that the situation would get worse. A nurse who was a member of the association was able to take action because she did not fear reprisal and she had the support of the parent group.

The nurse met with the parents and the institution administration. After assessing that there was a problem and that the administration was resistant to change, the nurse examined the laws of the state regarding child abuse. One section of the law clearly stated that an institution must be independently investigated when there were suspected cases of child abuse or neglect. The nurse knew that state institutions were not adhering to that section of the law. By obtaining legal counsel, and working with the established grievance procedure for state mental health clients, the community health nurse was able to help effect change in the system. The state

now has impartial investigations of all cases of child abuse in state institutions, and parents or guardians have access to the results.

The advocacy efforts of this community health nurse had many positive effects. Reporting procedures for institutional cases of suspected abuse and neglect have been clearly written and implemented in that state. The state legislature has appropriated a large sum of money to be used in further protection and advocacy services for people who are developmentally disabled. In addition, the general public has become increasingly aware of the needs of people who are mentally handicapped.

Nurses are in a position to correct public misconceptions about people who are handicapped. They can work to gain greater acceptance of individuals who are handicapped in whatever setting they reside. The nurse can be instrumental in promoting a positive attitude toward the handicapped by the general public.

SUMMARY

The number of individuals in society who are accurately characterized as disabled can be expected to increase. Demand for services to these individuals will increase concomitantly as they assert their needs to society and demand services.

Adults who are handicapped are confronted with adapting to their handicaps amidst societal, family, and individual variables, which influence adaptation and growth-promoting activities. Many handicapping conditions are long term and require ongoing utilization of a number of community resources. The need for better communication, coordination, and cooperation among these resources is great, as well as for greater accessibility to services and greater availability of attendants for handicapped people.

Community health nurses are in a unique position to assist clients who are handicapped to obtain services that will enhance adaptation in a way which will promote client growth. They assist clients with rehabilitation, and work cooperatively with the clients and their families to establish plans of care. A sensitivity to the needs of this population group and an awareness that there are individual differences among clients who are handicapped are both essential for the community health nurse to function effectively with clients who have special needs.

Increasingly, health care professionals are becoming actively involved in advocacy for this population group. Advocacy has been critical in the procurement of many essential services for these clients. While legislation in the last decade has reflected a more positive attitude toward people who are handicapped, there remain numerous unmet needs. Professionals must continue to facilitate public awareness about handicapping conditions and the needs of people who are experiencing them. Adults who are handicapped are at risk and deserve their share of our country's health resources.

APPENDIX 17-1

An Overview of Legislation and Voluntary Efforts for the Handicapped in the United States

1798 U.S. Congress established a marine hospital to provide for disabled seamen (England had established such a facility in 1588).

1902 Goodwill Industries was originated by a minister, Dr. Edgar Helms. Provided employment opportunities for people who were handicapped.

1918 Federal Board of Vocational Rehabilitation was established. Provided vocational rehabilitation services to the disabled veterans of World War I.

Massachusetts became the first state to establish public provisions to aid in the vocational rehabilitation of disabled citizens.

1920 The first Vocational Rehabilitation Act (Public Law 565) was passed. Services under the act were primarily for physically disabled military personnel. This act was administered by the Vocational Rehabilitation Administration.

1935 Social Security Act was passed. It resulted in increased federal appropriations to states for vocational rehabilitation with direct relief provided for the disabled. Amendments to this act have provided for SSI, Disability Insurance, Medicare, and Medicaid.

1943 Amendments to the Vocational Rehabilitation Act of 1920 broadened vocational rehabilitation services to include facilitating a disabled person to engage in competitive employment and included such services as diagnosis, medical and surgical treatment, prescriptions, hospitalization, books, tools, and occupational equipment.

Baruch Committee on Physical Medicine was established by the son of Dr. Simon Baruch, a confederate army surgeon and pioneer in the field of physical medicine. The committee supported research and scholarship in physical medicine.

1944 The Public Health Act of 1944 (Public Law 78-410) has provided for professional education, training, and research on many handicapping conditions.

1945 Joseph Bulova School of Watchmaking established a training program in watchmaking for people who were handicapped. Forerunner of many companies offering employment and training opportunities to the handicapped.

1946 National Mental Health Act (Public Law 79-487) authorized extensive federal support for mental health research, diagnosis, prevention, and treatment, established the National Institute of Mental Health and state grant-in-aid programs for mental health under the U.S. Public Health Service.

1947 The Department of Rehabilitation and Physical Medi-

cine was started at New York University College of Medicine at Bellevue Hospital under the direction of Dr. Howard Rusk. The first comprehensive program in rehabilitation at Bellevue was made possible by a grant from the Baruch committee. This department served as a model for the development of rehabilitation centers all over the world.

1953 Establishment of the Department of Health, Education, and Welfare with the Office of Vocational Rehabilitation as a part.

1954 Federal provisions made to support training and education programs for professional rehabilitation personnel in the form of scholarships, stipends, research, and construction grants.

1956 Amendments to the Social Security Act gave benefits to workers and their families during periods of extended disability.

The Mental Health Study Act (Public Law 84-812) authorized grants to facilitate a program of research into resources and methods of care for the mentally ill. The act authorized grants for participation in a national study and reevaluation of the human and economic problems of mental illness.

1963 Mental Retardation Facilities and Community Mental Health Centers Construction Act of 1963 (Public Law 88-164) provided assistance in combating mental retardation through grants for construction of research centers and facilities for people who were mentally retarded. It provided assistance in improving mental health services through construction of community mental health centers.

1965 Amendments to the Vocational Rehabilitation Act of 1920 provided for increased flexibility in financing and administrating state rehabilitation programs and for assisting in the expansion and improvement of rehabilitation services financed by a state-federal payment sharing plan. The word *handicapped* was substituted for *physical disability.* The Federal Board of Vocational Education was established.

Medicaid and Medicare established by federal law. Both programs provide essential health and health related services for individuals who are handicapped (refer to Chapter 4).

The Mental Retardation Facilities and Community Mental Health Centers Construction Act Amendments of 1965 (Public Law 89-105) authorized assistance in meeting the initial cost of professional and technical personnel for comprehensive community mental health centers.

1968 Architectural Barriers Act (Public Law 90-480) passed.

*NOTE: Laws that have had, or have the potential for having, major impact on the person who is handicapped are indicated by an asterisk.

APPENDIX 17-1

An Overview of Legislation and Voluntary Efforts for the Handicapped in the United States—cont'd

The act mandated that almost any public building, constructed or leased by federal funds must be accessible to the physically handicapped, and that all construction after 1968 using federal funds ensure building accessibility to handicapped persons with no exceptions allowed. The act affected many educational settings and was enforced by the Architectural Barriers Compliance Board. However, the mandates of this law were ignored, and in 1978 Congress created a compliance board to enforce the law (Goldman, 1984).

1971 Developmental Disabilities Act* (Public Law 91-517) passed. The act stated that each state would receive federal funds to establish and maintain services which are required by developmentally disabled children and adults. These services include diagnosis, evaluation, treatment, personal care, special living arrangements, training, education, sheltered employment, recreation, counseling, protective and sociolegal services, information services, transportation services, and follow-up services.

Urban Mass Transportation Act (Public Law 91-453) passed. The act stated that special efforts would be made in federally funded mass transportation to include utilization by persons who are handicapped.

1973 Rehabilitation Act of 1973* (Public Law 91-453) was a landmark piece of legislation that replaced the 1920 act. It authorized vocational rehabilitation services; emphasized services to those with severe handicaps, expanded the federal role in service and training programs, defined services necessary for rehabilitative programs, established the National Architectural and Transportation Barriers Board, and began affirmative action programs to facilitate employment of the handicapped. This act is the basis for rehabilitation services and programs.

Social Security Act of 1935 amendments eliminated previous categories of Aid to the Blind, Aid to the Aged (Old Age Assistance), and Aid to the Disabled under which direct financial assistance was given to people who were handicapped. Supplemental Security Income was established as of January 1, 1974, under which the aged, blind, and disabled could qualify.

1974 Rehabilitation Act Amendments of 1974 (Public Law 93-576) authorized the White House Conference on the Disabled.

Numerous transportation legislation including the following:

1. Amtrak Improvement Act (Public Law 93-140) stated that the Amtrak corporation must ensure that the handicapped would not be denied transportation because of the handicap. Provisions did not apply to commuter and short-haul service.

2. Federal Aid Highway Act (Public Law 93-87) stated that funding could not be approved for any state or federal highway not granting reasonable access for the movement of the physically handicapped across curbs.

3. National Mass Transportation Act (Public Law 93-503) stated that mass transit funds could not be approved unless the rates charged persons who are handicapped were reduced rates from regular fare.

4. Federal Bus Act (Public Law 93-37) stated that all federally funded projects to improve bus transportation must include plans to facilitate usage by people who are handicapped.

1975 Developmental Disabilities Assistance and Bill of Rights Act* (Public Law 94-103) created a system of advocacy on the state level to pursue legal and other actions necessary to eliminate the problems facing citizens with mental retardation, epilepsy, autism, and cerebral palsy and also expanded the national effort to protect the rights of the developmentally disabled.

Education for All Handicapped Children Act (Public Law 94-142) passed. Enabled by September 1, 1980, a free, appropriate public education to all persons aged 3 to 21 years old regardless of handicapping condition involved. Recently, the federal government has tried to deregulate the act, but proposed changes created such a furor among the disabled, their families, and advocates that the changes were withdrawn.

1977 Reorganization of the Department of Health, Education, and Welfare with creation of the Office of Human Development. The Administration for Handicapped Individuals (AHI) is under the Office of Human Development and oversees (1) Rehabilitation Services Administration, (2) President's Committee on Mental Retardation, (3) Architectural and Transportation Barriers Compliance Board, (4) White House Conference on Handicapped Individuals, (5) Developmental Disabilities Office, and (6) Office of Handicapped Individuals.

Federal Aviation Act of 1958 amended (Public Law 95-163) to provide special rates (reduced) on a space-available basis to persons with severe visual or hearing impairments and other physically or mentally handicapped people as defined by the Civil Aeronautics Board, as well as any attendant required by such persons.

1978 Rehabilitation Act Amendments established the Council on the Handicapped to function as a steering committee to make recommendations to the President concerning the needs of disabled individuals, and established the National Center for Rehabilitation Research.

1980 Mental Health Systems Act* (Public Law 96-398) gave the states more authority to plan community mental health centers, to increase the quality of mental health

Continued

APPENDIX 17-1

An Overview of Legislation and Voluntary Efforts for the Handicapped in the United States—cont'd

services, and to reach more people. Included advocacy provisions and a Bill of Rights of Mental Health.

Civil Rights of Institutionalized Persons Act* (Public Law 96-247) authorized actions for redress in cases involving deprivations of rights of institutionalized persons that were secured or protected by the Constitution of the United States. The act stated that when an action has been commenced in any court of the United States seeking relief from conditions which deprive persons residing in such institutions of any rights, privileges, or immunities secured or protected by the Constitution or laws of the United States that causes them to suffer grievous harm, the Attorney General of the United States may intervene.

1982 Telecommunications for the Disabled Act (Public Law 97-140) amended the Communication Act of 1934 to provide that persons with impaired hearing are insured reasonable access to telephone service by requiring that all coin-operated telephones, telephones frequently used by hearing-impaired persons, and emergency telephones provide an internal means of coupling with hearing aids. Retrofitting could be required on coin-operated and emergency telephones.

The Surface Transportation Assistance Act (Public Law 97-424) encouraged removal of architectural barriers.

1984 Rehabilitation Amendments (Public Law 98-221) modified the definition of severely disabled and placed the age limit for disability benefits at 16 years. Made the National Council on the Handicapped an agency independent from the Department of Education.

Developmental Disabilities Assistance and Bill of Rights Act (Public Law 98-527) formally established a Bill of Rights for the developmentally disabled.

1986 Protection and Advocacy for Mentally Ill Individuals Act of 1986* (Public Law 99-319) established protection and advocacy services for individuals who are mentally ill. Restated the Bill of Rights for mental health patients. Promoted the establishment of family support groups for the families of people with Alzheimer's disease.

Education of the Deaf Act (Public Law 99-371) consolidated several free-standing statutes relating to federally supported educational institutions for the deaf into one effective piece of legislation.

Rehabilitation Amendments (Public Law 99-506) emphasized the rehabilitation needs of disabled native Americans, provided funding for disability technology, and expanded the influence of the National Council on the Handicapped.

Employment Opportunities for Disabled Americans Act (Public Law 99-643) amended the Social Security Act to improve employment opportunities for disabled Americans.

Air Carrier Access Act of 1986 greatly improved access to air transportation for people who are handicapped.

1988 Numerous pieces of technology-related legislation including

1. Hearing Aid Compatibility Act of 1988 (Public Law 100-394) required telephones manufactured or imported into the United States after August 16, 1989 be hearing-aid compatible

2. Technology-Related Assistance for Individuals with Disabilities Act of 1988 (Public Law 100-407) established a competitive grant program to enable participating states to develop and implement programs to promote technology-related assistance to individuals with disabilities.

3. Telecommunications Accessibility Act (Public Law 100-542) assured that the federal telecommunication system is fully accessible to hearing-impaired persons who use telecommunications.

Protection and Advocacy for Mentally Ill Individuals Amendments Act of 1988 (Public Law 100-509) amended the 1986 act to reauthorize the act and to establish a governing authority for protection and advocacy in each state.

1990 The Americans with Disabilities Act* (Public Law 101-336) was passed. A landmark piece of legislation designed to provide a clear and comprehensive mandate to end discrimination against individuals with disabilities. It addresses such issues as housing, employment, public transportation, and communication services.

APPENDIX 17-2

Community Resources for the Person Who Is Handicapped*

Privately Funded/Voluntary Organizations:

Alcoholics Anonymous (1-212-686-1100)
American Cancer Society (1-800-227-2345)
American Civil Liberties Union (1-202-457-0800)
American Council of the Blind (1-800-232-5463)
American Diabetes Association (1-800-ADA-DISC)
American Heart Association (1-214-373-3600)
American Kidney Fund (1-800-638-8299)
American Liver Foundation (1-800-223-0179)
American Lung Association (1-212-315-8700)
American Mental Health Fund (1-800-433-5059)
American Paralysis Association (1-800-225-0292)
American Red Cross (1-202-737-8300)
Anorexia Bulimia Treatment and Education Center (1-800-33-ABTEC)
Arthritis Foundation (1-800-283-7800)
Association for Retarded Citizens (1-202-636-2950)
Asthma Information Line (1-800-822-ASMA)
Cooley's Anemia Foundation (1-800-221-3571)
Cystic Fibrosis Foundation (1-800-634-5895)
Disabled But Able to Vote (1-703-525-3268)
Dyslexia Society (1-800-ABCD-123)
Epilepsy Foundation of America (1-800-EFA-1000)
Human Services Research Institute (1-617-876-0426)
Huntington's Disease Society of America (1-800-345-4372)
Independent Living Research Utilization Program (1-713-960-9961)
Juvenile Diabetes Foundation International (1-800-223-1138)
Lupus Foundation of America (1-800-558-0121)
Muscular Dystrophy Association (1-212-586-0808)
National Association for Sickle Cell Disease (1-800-421-8453)
National Council on Alcoholism (1-800-NCA-CALL)
National Council on the Handicapped (1-202-267-3846)
National Foundation for Depressive Illness (1-800-248-4344)
National Headache Foundation (1-800-843-2256)
National Kidney Foundation (1-800-622-9010)
National Multiple Sclerosis Society (1-800-624-8236)
National Neurofibromatosis Foundation (1-800-323-7938)
National Organization for Rare Disorders (1-800-447-NORD)
National Parkinson Foundation (1-800-327-4545)
National Spinal Cord Injury Association (1-800-962-9629)
Parkinson's Education Programs (1-800-344-7872)
Scleroderma Foundation (1-800-722-HOPE)
Spina Bifida Information and Referral (1-800-621-3141)
United Cerebral Palsy Associations, Inc. (1-202-371-0622)
United Way (1-703-549-4447)

Publicly Funded Organizations:

ABLEDATA—information on rehabilitation products (1-800-344-5405)

AIDS Information Hotline (1-800-342-AIDS)
Cancer Information Service (1-800-4-CANCER)
Clearinghouse on Disability Information (1-202-742-1244)
Disability Statistics Program—InfoUse (1-415-644-9904, 9901)
Institute for Rehabilitation and Disability Management (1-202-877-1946)
Job Accommodation Network (1-800-526-7234)
Local Department of Human Services
Local Health Department
Local School District
National AIDS Information Clearinghouse (1-800-458-5231)
National Arthritis and Musculoskeletal and Skin Diseases Information Clearinghouse (1-301-468-4235)
National Clearinghouse for Alcohol and Drug Information (1-301-468-2600)
National Diabetes Information Clearinghouse (1-301-468-2162)
National Digestive Disease Information Clearinghouse (1-301-468-2162)
National Information Center for Handicapped Children and Youth (1-703-522-3332)
National Institute on Disability and Rehabilitation Research (1-202-732-1134)
National Institute on Drug Abuse Helpline (1-800-622-HELP)
National Rehabilitation Information Center (1-800-34-NARIC)
National Technical Institute for the Deaf (1-716-475-6283)
President's Committee on Employment of People with Disabilities (1-202-653-2087)
State Department of Education
State Department of Human Services
State Developmental Disabilities Council
State Health Department
State Protection and Advocacy Services for People Who Are Developmentally Disabled
U.S. Alcohol, Drug Abuse, and Mental Health Administration (1-301-443-3783)
U.S. Department of Education (1-202-732-3366)
U.S. Department of Education—Rehabilitation Services Administration (1-202-472-3814)
U.S. Department of Education Resource Center (1-202-732-3366)
U.S. Department of Health and Human Services (1-202-245-6296)
U.S. Social Security Administration—Office of Public Inquiries (1-301-965-7700)
World Institute on Disability (1-415-486-8314)

---

*The numbers given are national listings. *Consult your phone book or operator for local listings.* The 800 numbers have varying hours of service; some are open 24 hours a day and others only during work hours. For state 800 numbers please consult information at 1-800-555-1212. The government section in the phone book lists many local, state, and federal government agencies. Local health departments (nursing division) and United Way agencies often have extensive community resource listings and can be helpful in resource location. *Remember that telephone numbers, especially the government listings, frequently change. If one of the above numbers is no longer in service contact telephone information for the new listing. Making contact with agencies is not always easy. Don't get discouraged—keep trying.*

REFERENCES

Americans with Disabilities Act: What does it mean for the nation and the nation's businesses? Worklife 2(3):22-23, 1989.

Anderson EA, and Lynch MM: A family impact analysis: the deinstitutionalization of the mentally ill, Family Relations 33(1):41-46, 1984.

Apple finds a place in special education: NARIC Q 1(3):4-5, 1988.

Attendant services: Rehab Briefs 11(4):1-4, 1989.

Bogdan R and Taylor T: Toward a sociology of acceptance: The other side of the study of deviance, Social Policy 18(2):34-39, 1988.

Bower FL, ed: Distortions in body image in illness and disability, New York, 1977, Wiley.

Brillhart B: Family support for the disabled, Rehab Nurs 13(6):316-319, 1988.

Bubolz MM and Whiren AP: The family of the handicapped: an ecological model for policy and practice, Family Relations 33(1):5-12, 1984.

Bureau of the Census: Statistical abstract of the United States, 1984, ed 104, Washington, DC, 1983, US Department of Commerce.

Burgener S: Sexuality concerns of the post-stroke patient, Rehab Nurs 14(4):178-181, 1989.

Buscaglia LF, ed: The disabled and their parents: a counseling challenge, ed 2, Thorofare, NJ, 1983, Slack.

Buzinski P: Groups for brothers and sisters of developmentally disabled children: one component of a family-centered approach, Issues Compr Pediat Nurs 4(1):45-50, 1980.

Calkins P: The disability vote in 1988. Learning to make a difference, Worklife 1(3):11-12, 1988.

Carling PJ: Access to housing: cornerstone of the American dream, J Rehab 55(3):6-8, 1989.

Cole TM and Cole SS: Sexual adjustment to chronic disease and disability. In Stolov WC and Clowers MR, eds: Handbook on severe disability, Washington, DC, 1981, US Government Printing Office, pp 279-288.

Commission on Chronic Illness: Chronic illness in the United States, vol I: Prevention of chronic illness, Cambridge, Ma, 1957, Harvard University Press.

Consumer management of attendant services: benefits and obstacles, NARIC Q 1(2):1, 6-14, 1988.

Courts NF: A patient satisfaction survey for a rehab unit, Rehab Nurs 13(2):79-81, 1988.

Coyle JJ: Employment of people with disabilities, Worklife 2(4):29, 1989.

deBalcazar YS, Bradford B, and Fawcett SB: Common concerns of disabled Americans: issues and options, Social Policy 19(2):29-35, 1988.

Dietl D: The phoenix: from the ashes and looking to the ultimate barrier: our own attitude, J Rehab 49(3):12-17, 1983.

Disability risks of chronic illnesses and impairments: Disability Stat Bull 2(Fall):1-2, 4, 1989.

Dixon JK: Coping with prejudice: attitudes of handicapped persons toward the handicapped, J Chron Dis 30:307-321, 1977.

Dole foundation's innovative community partnerships: Worklife, 1(4):13, 1988.

Fine M and Asch A: Disability beyond stigma: social interaction, discrimination, and activism, J Soc Issues 44(1):3-21, 1988.

Giele JZ: A delicate balance: the family's role in the care of the handicapped, Family Relations 33(1):85-94, 1984.

Goldman CE: Advocacy in the 80's, Disabled USA 1:21-23, 1984.

Gordon S: Sexual rights for the people who happen to be handicapped, Syracuse, NY, 1974, Syracuse University.

Hahn H: Can disability be beautiful? Social Policy 18(3):26-32, 1988.

Hahn H: The politics of physical differences: disability and discrimination, J Social Issues 44(1):39-47, 1988.

Hahn K: Sexuality and COPD, Rehab Nurs, 14(4):191-195, 1989.

Handicapper small business association provides assistance, J Rehab 55(2):18, 1989.

Haring M and Meyerson L: Attitudes of college students toward sexual behavior of disabled persons. In Spiegel AD and Podair S, eds: Rehabilitating people with disabilities into the mainstream of the population, Park Ridge, NJ, 1981, Noyes Medical, pp 29-35.

Hildebrandt ED: Respite care in the home, Am J Nurs 83:1428-1431, 1983.

IBM center offers technological advice, NARIC Q 1(3):5, 1988.

Kanger FH: Self-management methods. In Kanger F and Goldstein A, eds: Helping people change: a textbook of methods, New York, 1980, Permagon, pp 334-389.

Katz AH and Martin K: A handbook of services for the handicapped, Westport, Ct, 1982, Greenwood.

Kendrick D: Invisible barriers. How you can make parenting easier, Disabled USA 1:17-19, 1983.

Kennedy M: More companies hire the retarded. Worker's dedication impresses firms, USA Today, p 8B, January 9, 1989.

Knight J: The employer's expectations from the job applicant, Worklife 1(3):13-14, 1988.

Kraus LE: Disability by the numbers, Worklife 2(2):10-11, 1989.

Kraus LE and Stoddard S: Chartbook on disability in the United States, an InfoUse report, Washington, DC, 1989, National Institute on Disability and Rehabilitation Research.

Krusen FH: Concepts in rehabilitation of the handicapped, Philadelphia, 1964, Saunders.

Kubler-Ross E: On death and dying, New York, 1969, Macmillan.

Langer E and Rodin J: The effects of choice and enhanced personal responsibility: a field experiment in an institutional setting, J Personality Social Psychol 34(2):191-198, 1976.

Lewis KS: Grief in chronic illness and disability, J Rehab 49(3):8-11, 1983.

Litvak S, Zukas H, and Heumann J: Attending to America: assistance for independent living, Berkeley, Ca, 1987, World Institute on Disability.

Loeff J, Bretz J, and Kerns W: Social security programs in the U.S.—income support programs, Social Sec Bull 52(7):62-77, 1989.

Major medical plan for people who are mentally retarded: Helping Hand (Newsletter of Knox County Association for Retarded Citizens), p 2, October 1989.

Maraldo P: Nursing as a political force—making our own destiny. Paper presented at the First Annual Alumni Reunion, University of Tennessee, Knoxville—College of Nursing, June 16, 1984.

Mastin P: Final report of the joint legislative committee to study community placement in Michigan, Lansing, Mi, 1976, State of Michigan.

McCubbin HI and Patterson J: Family transitions: adaptation to stress. In Figley CR and McCubbin HI, eds: Stress and the family, vol 1, New York, 1983, Brunner/Mazel, pp 5-25.

McGuire SL and Guernsey C: Residential placement opportunities in Michigan for people who are mentally retarded, Lansing, Mi, 1978, Michigan Association for Retarded Citizens.

Meyerson L: The social psychology of physical disability: 1948 and 1988, J Social Issues 44(1):173-188, 1988.

Michigan State Planning Council for Developmental Disabilities: Developmental disabilities three year state plan: FY 1984-1986, State of Michigan, Lansing, Mi, 1983, Michigan Department of Mental Health.

Moses H: Extending civil rights protection, NARIC Q 2(2):2, 9-13, 1989.

NARIC prepares resource guides: NARIC Q 2(2):5, 1989.

National Council on the Handicapped: On the threshold of legislative changes, NARIC Q 1(2):5, 1988.

National Council on the Handicapped: On the threshold of independence: progress on legislative recommendations from Toward Independence. A report to the President and the Congress of the United States, Washington, DC, 1988, The Council.

Nelson D: Nurse-managed rehabilitation, Nurs Management 15(3):30-39, 1984.

New accessibility atlas opens national parks, NARIC Q 1(2):1, 15, 1988.

O'Bryant T: Facts about hiring people with disabilities, Worklife 1(3):8-10, 1988.

Opie ND and Miller ET: Attribution for successful relationships between severely disabled adults and personal care attendants, Rehab Nurs 14(4):196-199, 1989.

Park L: The law says . . . , Disabled USA 1(4):11-13, 1977.

Patterson JA and McCubbin HI: The impact of family life events and changes on the health care of a chronically ill child, Family Relations 32:255-264, 1983.

Payne MB: Utilizing role theory to assist the family with sudden disability, Rehab Nurs 13(4):191-194, 1988.

Penrose J: Double handicap. Does he take sugar? Nurs Times 79:52-54, 1983.

Peters L: Women's health care. Approaches in delivery to physically disabled women, Nurse Pract 7:34-37, 48, 1982.

Power DW: Working with families: an intervention model for rehabilitation nurses, Rehab Nurs 14(2):73-76, 1989.

President's Committee on Employment of the Handicapped: Affirmative action to employ handicapped people, Washington, DC, 1978, US Government Printing Office.

President's Committee on Employment of People with Disabilities: National symposium on employment of Americans with disabilities: utilizing a national resource, Conference proceedings, Stanford, Ca, Stanford University, December 15-16, 1988.

Research and training center for accessible housing opens, NARIC Q 2(4):4, 1989.

Research and training focuses on families and disability, NARIC Q 2(2):13, 1989.

Robert Wood Johnson Foundation: Annual Report 1983, New York, 1984, Robert Wood Johnson Foundation.

Roessler R and Bolton B: Psychosocial adjustment to disability, Baltimore, Md, 1978, University Park Press.

Ruesch JH and Bradsky C: The concept of social disability, Arch Gen Psychiatry 19:394-403, 1968.

Safilios-Rothschild C: The sociology and social psychology of disability rehabilitation, New York, 1982, University Press of America.

Sargent JV: An easier way, Ames, Ia, 1982, Iowa State University.

Sargent JV: Something good from Ames, Iowa, Disabled USA 2:17-20, 1983.

Sawyer HW and Crimando W: Self-management strategies in rehabilitation, J Rehab 50(1):27-30, 1984.

Sawyer HW and Morgan BG: Innovative trends in adjustment services, Vocat Evaluat Work Adjust Bull 14:20-27, 1981.

Schneider J: Careers and the handicapped, Worklife 1(4):15-16, 1988.

Schrader B and Brown D: The rehabilitation process, Disabled USA 1:16, 1983.

Schwartz HD: Further thoughts on a "sociology of acceptance" for disabled people, Social Policy 19(2):36-39, 1988.

Scotch RK: Disability as the basis for a social movement: advocacy and the politics of definition, J Social Issues 44(1):159-172, 1988.

Seaver ME: Employing persons with disabilities, Am Assoc Occupat Health Nurses J, 37:513-517, 1989.

Seifert KH: The attitudes of working people toward disabled persons, especially in regard to vocational rehabilitation. In Spiegel AD and Podair S, eds: Rehabilitating people with disabilities into the mainstream of society, Park Ridge, NJ, 1981, Noyes Medical.

Sexuality and the developmentally disabled: SIECUS Reports: 29, November/December, 1988.

Shadish WR, Lurigio AJ, and Lewis DA: After deinstitutionalization: the present and future of mental health long-term care policy, J Social Issues 45(3):1-15, 1989.

Sherman BR and Cocozza JJ: Stress in families of the developmentally disabled: a literature review of factors affecting the decision to seek out-of-home placements, Family Relations 33(1):95-103, 1984.

Social Security Administration: Work disability in the United States, Washington, DC, 1977, US Government Printing Office.

Spiegel AD and Podair S: Rehabilitating people with disabilities into the mainstream of society, Park Ridge, NJ, 1981, Noyes Medical.

Stolov WC and Clowers MR, eds: Handbook of severe disability, Washington, DC, 1981, US Government Printing Office.

Strauss A, Corbin J, Fagerhaugh S, Glaser B, Maines D, Suczek B, and Wiener CL: Chronic illness and the quality of life, ed 2, St. Louis, 1984, CV Mosby Co.

Sussman MB, ed: Sociology and rehabilitation, Washington, DC, 1966, American Sociological Association.

University of Michigan: Toward a barrier-free society: breaking the isolation of handicap, Research News: 22, November-December, 1981.

US Department of Health and Human Services: Health characteristics of persons with chronic activity limitation: United States, 1979, Washington, DC, 1981, US Government Printing Office.

Vargo JW: Some psychological effects of physical disability, Am J Occupat Ther 32(1):31-34, 1978.

Verville RE: The disabled, rehabilitation and current public policy. In Spiegel AD and Podair S, eds: Rehabilitating people with disabilities into the mainstream of society, Park Ridge, NJ, 1981, Noyes Medical, pp 41-50.

Walkover M: Social policies: understanding their impact on families with impaired members. In Chilman CS, Nunnally EW, and Cox F, eds: Chronic illness and disability, Newbury Park, Ca, 1988, Sage, pp 220-247.

Watson PG: Rehabilitation legislation of the 1980s: implications for nurses as healthcare providers, Rehab Nurs 13(3):136-141, 1988.

Watson PG: Indicators of family capacity for participating in the rehabilitation process: report on a preliminary investigation, Rehab Nurs 14(6):318-322, 1989.

Weiss dV: Accessible vacations, J Rehab 54(3):8-9, 1988.

Werner-Beland JA: Grief responses to long-term illness and disability, Reston, Va, 1980, Reston.

What is disability? Disability Stat Bull 1 (Spring):2, 1988.

What should our priorities be? A report on the Stanford Symposium, Worklife 2(1):24-25, 1989.

World Health Organization Expert Committee on Disability Prevention and Rehabilitation: Disability prevention and rehabilitation, Technical Report Series 668, Geneva, 1981, The Organization.

SELECTED BIBLIOGRAPHY

Ayrault EW: Sex, love, and the physically handicapped, New York, 1981, Continuum.

Burish GG and Bradley LA: Coping with chronic disease: definitions and issues. In Burish GG and Bradley LA, eds: Coping with chronic disease, New York, 1983, Academic, pp 3-12.

Cornelius DA: Who cares? A handbook on sex education and counseling service for disabled people, ed 2, Baltimore, Md, 1982, University Park Press.

DeJong G and Lifchez R: Physical disability and public policy, Sci Am 248(6):40-49, 1983.

Disability in the working ages: Disability Stat Bull 1(Spring):2, 1988.

Gordon S: Sexuality and the disabled, Aust J Sex Marriage Family 2(4):157-164, 1981.

Gordon S and Snyder C: Family life education for the handicapped, School Health 50(5):272-274, 1980.

Haber LD: Identifying the disabled: concepts and methods in the measurement of disability, Social Sec Bull 51(5):11-28, 1988.

Hahn H: Civil rights for disabled Americans. In Gartner A and Joe T, eds: Images of the disabled, disabling images, New York, 1987, Praeger, pp 181-203.

Makas E: Positive attitudes toward disabled people: disabled and nondisabled persons' perspectives, J Social Issues 44(1):49-61, 1988.

Norback J and Weitz P: Sourcebook of aid for the mentally and physically handicapped, New York, 1983, Van Nostrand Reinhold.

Peterson Y: The impact of physical disability on marital adjustment: a literature review, Family Coordinator 28(1):47-51, 1979.

Topolnicki DM: The gulag of guardianship, Money 18(3):149-152, 1989.

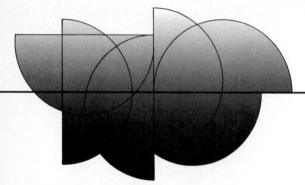

18

The Well Elderly: Needs and Services

There's no shame in growing old—We're all doing it. Age is, after all, the one thing we all share.

MAGGIE KUHN

———————————————— OBJECTIVES ————————————————

Upon completion of this chapter, the reader will be able to:

1. Construct a personal philosophy about aging.
2. Differentiate between the health problems of the young-old, the middle-old, and the oldest-old.
3. Rank and discuss the major causes of mortality and morbidity for the aging population.
4. Discuss principles of primary, secondary, and tertiary prevention used by community health nurses with aging people.
5. Identify significant legislation that provides funding for services for the aging.
6. Summarize major resources that assist aging persons.
7. Describe barriers to health care for the aging.
8. Discuss significant health promotion activities for the aging and the community health nurse's role in promoting health among the aging.

Meet 91-year-old Hattie Harris: From her upstairs apartment in Rochester, New York, she is known as the "elder statesman of the Republican Party" and the "Mayor of Strathallan Park." In these positions, she advises candidates and political leaders of the major parties, seeks financial backing from business leaders, sets up candidates' meetings with senior citizens' groups and rallies neighborhood organizations.

She may not have a diploma, but one drawer in her apartment is stuffed with awards and tributes: an honorary deputy sheriff's badge awarded to her in a public ceremony last July, the 1982 Jefferson Award for public service, an award from the city of Rochester declaring April 24, 1975, "Hattie Harris Day," the South East Area Coalition award, the Rochester Federation of Women Club's 1973 Susan B. Anthony award, an award from Rochester's Bureau of Parks for her work for Goodwin Park, the Mayor's Rehabilitation Award.

But ask Hattie which of her many accomplishments she is proudest of and she'll say defiantly, "That in my 86th year I was strong enough mentally to take off 40 pounds." And that she has built for herself a secure, self-sufficient life. ("I'm still saving for my old age—like my mother. When she died at 97 she was saving for her old age.") And that she has friends who will remember her "for my conviviality, and that I was honorable, trustworthy" (Jacobson, 1983, p. 1C).

The description of Mrs. Harris's attitude toward life and its approaching end are in direct contrast to the concept of acute loneliness and unproductiveness in old age held by many people of all ages. One cannot help but wonder why some people are old and weary at 65 and others, like Mrs. Harris, are vigorous and productive long after that age. Examining certain concepts of aging sheds light on this question and helps us to better prepare ourselves for this part of our own life cycle as well as to better care for aging clients.

AGING DEFINED

The aging process is a series of complex changes that occur in all living organisms. It is a process that continues over a lifetime at different rates among people. The rate varies among populations and among individuals of the same population. The terms *aged, old,* and *elderly* are used to describe persons who have achieved a certain chronological age. The reasons for using age 65 to designate the beginning of old age in the United States are basically legislative and social. In some underdeveloped nations, a person 40 years old is often considered aged.

Older people vary, like persons in any other age group, and caution must be used when they are discussed as a group. Myths and stereotypes result from the habit of expecting people to act in certain ways simply because they have reached a specific chronological age. It should be remembered that aging is an individual process.

SOME PERSPECTIVES ON AGING

There is a tendency to focus on the pathologic and negative aspects of aging. However, there are positive, healthy, active roles for older people that also need to be recognized. Productiveness like that of Mrs. Harris should become the usual rather than the unusual. Changes in physical, mental, and psychological capabilities associated with aging occur very gradually (NCOA, 1986, p. 40).

American Attitudes toward Age and Aging

America is an ageist society. Robert Butler, a renowned gerontologist, coined the term *ageism* in 1968 and defined it as a process of systematic stereotyping of, and discrimination against, people because they are old (Sheppard, 1990, p. 4). The Gray Panthers (Figure 18-1), an organization which staunchly advocates the rights of older people, defines ageism as the use of age to define capability and role. The National Institute on Aging defines ageism as prejudice against people because they are old. Whatever the definition, the costs of ageism are great: as with other forms of prejudice it is dehumanizing, inhibits people from maximizing their potential, and limits the forms people's lives may take.

As a society, Americans do not value the elderly, and have a fear of growing old (McGuire, 1986, p. 322). In our youth-oriented culture peo-

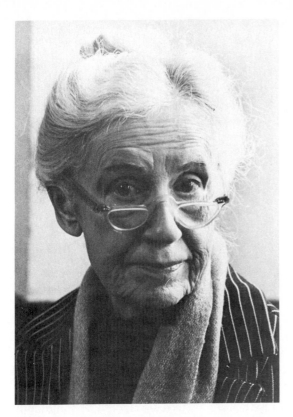

Figure 18-1 Maggie Kuhn, founder of the Gray Panthers, thrives because she has accepted aging. (Photographer: Julie Jensen.)

ple often disengage socially and emotionally from aging and view aging negatively. The advantages of youth are constantly emphasized in our society, and Americans invest much time, money, and energy in staying young. Vigorous! Active! Attractive! Independent! are words often used to describe a person of 20, 30, or 40, but rarely one of 60, 70, or 80. The American view of aging has not encouraged positive attitudes or expectations toward life's later years. Even young children have negative feelings about growing old and about older people (McGuire, 1986, p. 322). The negative attitudes about aging often become self-fulfilling prophecies. Such attitudes inhibit healthy development and the quality of life in later years.

Older people have a wealth of knowledge and experience to offer. They are, and have been, America's leaders, and helped to make America a great nation. It is older people who have knowl-edge of the trades and crafts that have been all but lost to later generations. Older people are the gatekeepers of our nation's history, values, culture, and traditions. It cannot be denied that with aging come many changes; but with aging also comes continued human growth and development and new life experiences.

Unfortunately, there is a lack of knowledge and understanding about aging in our society. In general, Americans are not educationally, socially, or emotionally prepared for old age (McGuire, 1987, p. 174). As the elderly population increases Americans will be forced to reevaluate their attitudes about growing old and to become knowledgeable about the aging process.

Ultimately, our professional nursing care, our social interactions, our personal decisions, and our decisions as citizens are affected by society's ageist attitudes. Today's Americans will most likely spend a significant part of their lives as older people. In order to maximize these later years, people need to develop realistic, positive attitudes toward aging. Nurses work with people who are elderly in many community settings. They have unique opportunities to facilitate adaptation to aging, educate people about this process, promote healthy development in later years, and to shape more positive attitudes about aging. Nurses need to help people differentiate between the actual limits of aging and the limits society has placed.

Other Cultures' View of Aging

History, anthropology, and art imply that aging has not always been equated with deterioration. The negative focus on aging is relatively recent. Throughout history, aging persons have been portrayed in the literature and through art as wise individuals, strong in character, and leaders of their people.

The Chinese philosopher Confucius, speaking to his followers about aging, said, "At fifteen, my mind was bent on learning. At thirty, I stood firm. At forty, I was free from delusions. At fifty, I understood the laws of Providence. At sixty, my ears were attentive to the truth. At seventy, I could follow the promptings of my heart without overstepping the moon."

Other cultures have said that aging leads to deterioration or growth, depending upon a person's inner resources, dedication, strengths, attitudes towards aging, and some luck. This period of life can give a person insight, knowledge, and freedom if it is seen as a manageable process with developmental tasks that need to be accomplished (Figure 18-2). In some cultures elderly people are given elevated status and treated with great respect. Unfortunately, individuals from such cultures (e.g., Asian) may lose the advantageous position of older people seen in their society when their families immigrate to a Western culture (Chae, 1987).

Valuing different cultural views relative to the aging process, life, health, and health care can assist community health nurses in providing quality nursing care to various older client groups. Cultural sensitivity helps professionals to elicit from clients cultural beliefs, values and practices which affect how they respond during times of stress and illness. The cultural assessment guide found in Appendix 6-1 aids the community health nurse in obtaining appropriate cultural data during the assessment phase of the nursing process.

Developmental Tasks of Aging

Duvall and Miller (1985, p. 318) identified eight developmental tasks for aging persons:

1. Making satisfying living arrangements as aging progresses
2. Adjusting to retirement income
3. Establishing comfortable routines
4. Safeguarding physical and mental health
5. Maintaining love, sex, and marital relations
6. Remaining in touch with family members
7. Keeping active and involved
8. Finding meaning in life
9. Remaining active in community activities when it is physically and financially possible
10. Feeling a sense of worth as a person, of which independence is a valuable part

Aging persons who achieve these tasks progress along the developmental continuum with a sense of dignity.

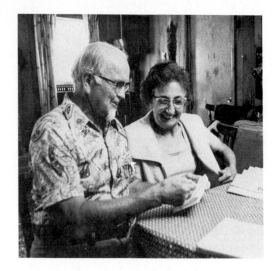

Figure 18-2   A happy healthy aging couple.

Concepts Basic to a Positive Philosophy of Aging

Manney (1975) has presented three concepts about aging that are important to understand if caregivers are to develop a positive philosophy about aging.

1. Aging has no chronological rules. The notion of "older" people is a demographic one because no matter how we look at it, aging varies in its onset and course.
2. The processes of aging are interrelated. Society's attitudes toward older people and the roles it assigns them affect intellectual performance, motivation, and interest in learning. Mandatory retirement typically cuts an individual's income in half. This affects the person's ability to obtain health care, to eat well, and to visit friends and family, as well as to maintain adequate housing.
3. Aging is a developmental process. Old age cannot be studied apart from middle age, adulthood, adolescence, childhood, and infancy. At each stage there are losses and gains. The gains and losses of old age do not arise immediately at age 65 and they do not stay the same until death. Aging is a part of the life cycle, which is constantly changing.

People need to view aging as a natural and life-long process, see the similarities between young and old, recognize that older people are valuable and contributing members of society, realize that different generations learn from each other, and that they must plan for old age (McGuire, 1987, p. 176). People have much control over the older person that they become.

DEMOGRAPHY OF AGING PERSONS

Statistical information is helpful in planning for the health needs of the aging population. The United States is definitely aging! Never before have there been so many older people; never before have people lived so long. The following statistics reveal a demographic overview of this population (American Association of Retired Persons, 1988; Aging America, 1987):

- People age 65 have an average life expectancy of an additional 16.9 years.

- A child born in 1987 can expect to live 74.9 years (28 years longer than a child born in 1900).
- The older population accounts for more than 12 percent of the U.S. population, or 30 million people. (In 1900 older people accounted for 4 percent of the population or approximately 3 million people.) This percentage is expected to climb to 21.8 percent by the year 2030, accounting for more than 65 million people.
- The older population grew more than twice as fast as the rest of the population during the past two decades.
- The "old-old," 85+ population group, is the most rapidly growing segment in our population today and is expected to be seven times as large by 2050 as it was in 1980.
- Elderly women outnumber elderly men three to two.
- More than half of the elderly live in the eight states of California, New York, Florida, Penn-

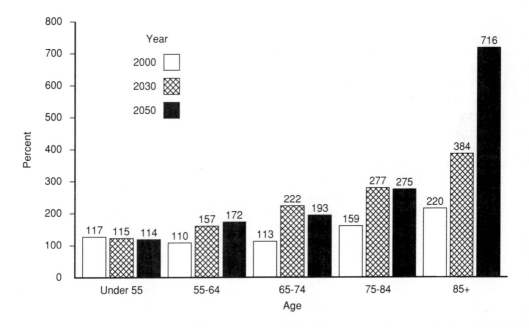

Note: 1980 = 100%. Bars represent projected population as a percent of 1980 population.

Figure 18-3 Projected growth in population by age group, 1980-2050. (From Spencer G: U.S. Bureau of the Census. Projections of the population of the United States by age, sex and race 1983 to 2080, Current Population Reports Series P-25, No. 952, Washington, DC, May 1984, US Government Printing Office.)

sylvania, Texas, Illinois, Ohio, and Michigan.
• Five percent of American elderly reside in institutional settings (1 percent of those age 65 to 74, 6 percent of those age 75 to 84, and 22 percent of those age 85+).

Of particular importance is the expanding age group of people above 85 years of age. Figure 18-3 displays the growth of this age group in comparison to other age groups. The number of people over 85 is expected to quadruple between 1980 and 2030. In this over-85 group are an increasing number of centenarians, people who are 100 years old or older. There are an estimated 25,000 centenarians in the United States today, and the Census Bureau predicts there will be 1 million by 2080; if mortality is less than projected, there could be as many as 5 million centenarians by year 2080 (U.S. Bureau of the Census, 1987, p. 1). From a health care aspect, it needs to be remembered that these old-old Americans are more vulnerable to physical, emotional, and social problems. They will require an increasing number of services from the health care system.

Close to 29 million people over age 65 live in the community; approximately one third of this group, or 8.5 million people, live alone (Commonwealth Fund Commission on Elderly People Living Alone, 1988, p. 13). Poverty rates are nearly five times higher for elderly people who live alone than for elderly couples, and 43 percent of those who live alone are either poor or near-poor (Commonwealth Fund Commission on Elderly People Living Alone, 1988, p. 16). Most often, the aged living alone are women above the age of 75. For the millions of elderly who live alone, the threats of loneliness and isolation are very real. Many of them have serious health or economic problems that are not being met.

The *Commonwealth Fund Commission on Elderly People Living Alone* was created in 1985 in response to this growing population group and their immense needs. The Commission has issued the reports: *Old, Alone and Poor, Medicare's Poor,* and *Aging Alone.* It has advocated for resources and services for elderly people living

alone. Copies of commission reports can be obtained by calling the commission at (301) 955-3775 or by writing to the commission at 624 North Broadway, Baltimore, Maryland 21205.

HEALTH CARE AND AGING

Although the 65+ age group represents 12 percent of the U.S. population, it accounts for more than 30 percent of total personal health care expenditures (American Association of Retired Persons [AARP], 1988, p. 14). In 1988, health care for the elderly cost more than $175 billion dollars (including $70 billion Medicare expenditures and $21 billion Medicaid expenditures), or approximately $5749 for each senior citizen—three times the amount spent by people under age 65 (House Select Committee on Aging, 1989, p. 10). Of this amount, $2394 was out-of-pocket expense paid by the individual (amounting to 18 percent of the median income of an older American) (House Select Committee on Aging, 1989, p. 10).

The number of days in which usual activities are restricted because of illness or injury increases with age. In 1987 older people accounted for 31 percent of all hospital stays and 42 percent of all days of care in hospitals. The average length of stay for the older person was 8.6 days as compared to 5.4 days for people under age 65 (AARP, 1988, p. 14). Hospital care costs accounted for 41 percent of the cost of health care for the elderly; and nursing homes, for 21 percent of the cost (House Select Committee on Aging, 1989, p. 10).

The quality and coordination of health care for the elderly are often in question. No single health profession has yet claimed service to the elderly as its unique task—an opportunity nursing must not allow to slip past (Strumpf, 1987, p. 447). In a position paper, the World Health Organization recommended that nurses be the primary workers responsible for providing comprehensive health care to the elderly (World Health Organization, 1980; Strumpf, 1987, p. 446). Nursing has been described as the last and best hope of the aged for decent health care (Yarling, 1977; Strumpf, 1987, p. 447). Less than 10 percent of practicing registered nurses work with elderly persons (Strumpf,

1987, p. 448), and many nursing programs have little content in gerontology.

HEALTH RISKS AND AGING

Older people generally view their health positively. According to the results of the 1986 Health Interview Survey, conducted by the National Center for Health Statistics, 70 percent of older people living in the community describe their health as excellent, very good, or good (AARP, 1988, p. 12). There was little difference between the sexes on this measure, though older blacks were more likely to rate their health as fair or poor (45 percent) than older whites (29 percent) (AARP, 1988, p. 12).

The incidence of chronic illness increases with age; 80 percent of people age 65 or over have one or more chronic conditions (Abbott, 1986, p. 7). These can significantly affect physical functioning and often cause activity limitations (refer to Figures 18-4 and 18-5). More than half (58.5 percent) of elderly persons are functionally limited and about 40 percent are limited in activities, whereas fewer than 10 percent of those under 45 report activity limitation. Figure 18-5 illustrates that physical functional limitations increase dramatically among persons 75 years of age and older (Kraus and Stoddard, 1989, p. 28). Elderly persons most affected by health limitations are women, the poor, and minorities. Native Americans and blacks report the greatest activity limitation (Kraus and Stoddard, 1989). Nevertheless, income has a greater effect than race on activity lim-

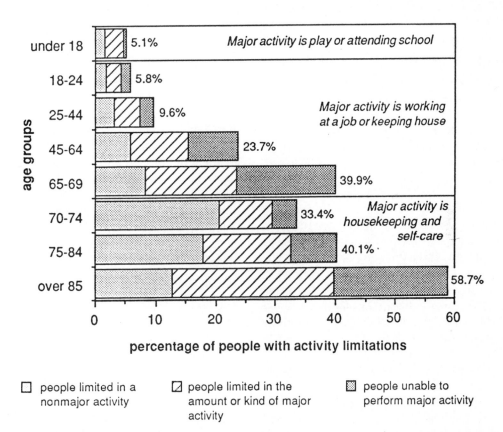

Figure 18-4 Activity limitations of all degrees by age groups. (From Kraus LE and Stoddard S: Chartbook on disability in the United States, an InfoUse Report, Washington, DC, March 1989, US National Institute on Disability and Rehabilitation Research, p 10.)

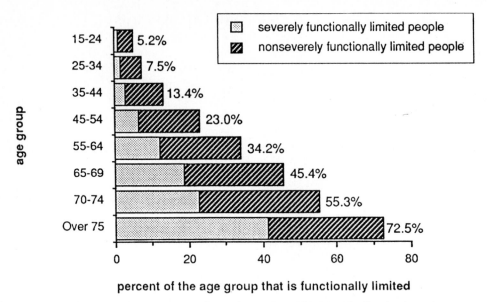

Figure 18-5 Functional limitations by age groups. (From Kraus LE and Stoddard S: Chartbook on disability in the United States, an InfoUse Report, Washington, DC, March 1989, US National Institute on Disability and Rehabilitation Research, p 11.)

itation. Both white and minority individuals with annual incomes below $10,000 suffer the greatest activity limitation, and those with incomes $35,000 and above, the least (USDHHS, Public Health Services, 1986, p. 46). A variety of conditions cause activity limitation in older years.

Major Causes of Mortality and Morbidity

An understanding of mortality and morbidity trends helps nurses to be more effective in planning and implementing care for aging clients. The past 20 years have seen great improvement in life expectancy as a result of the significant declines in death rates for the older age groups. Heart disease, cancer, and stroke (cerebrovascular disease) account for three out of four fatalities among elderly people. The death rate from cancer continues to rise in the elderly, as in all other segments of the population (refer to Figure 18-6). Other significant causes of death among the elderly are chronic obstructive pulmonary disease, diabetes mellitus, pneumonia, and accidents. Although atherosclerosis is not a major cause of death for persons 65 to 74 years of age, it is significant among those 75 years of age and older (National Safety Council, 1988).

The nature of illness and disease in older people has changed throughout the century. In the early 1900s, communicable diseases such as pneumonia and acute health conditions were predominant. Today, communicable diseases have been greatly reduced, and chronic conditions are prevalent. The chief chronic conditions affecting the elderly are heart disease, arthritis, hypertensive disease, hearing impairment, and orthopedic impairment (refer to Figure 18-7). In addition, the aging population experiences significant mental and psychosocial health problems.

Mental Health

The United States has failed to ensure older persons access to community mental health services, and many older people's mental health needs go unmet. It is estimated that the older population uses mental health services at only about half the rate of the general population (NCOA, 1986, p. 20). Yet, research by the National Institute of Mental Health estimates that as many as 25 percent of the aged in the community have some degree of mental health impairment and could benefit from mental health services (NCOA, 1986, p. 20). Dementia (discussed in Chapter 19) and de-

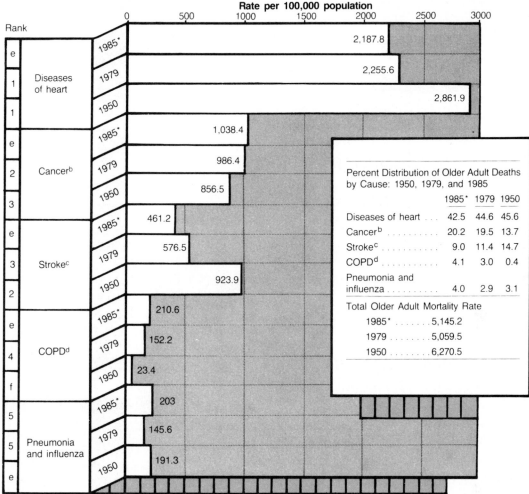

Figure 18-6   Leading causes of older adult deaths: 1950, 1979, and 1985. (From USDHHS: Prevention '86/'87: federal programs and progress, Washington, DC, 1987, US Government Printing Office, p 45.)

pression are considered to be significant problems; 30 percent to 50 percent of those above the age of 65 will experience an episode of depression severe enough to interfere with activity of daily living. It is the main cause of psychiatric institutionalization among the elderly (Harper, 1989).

Signs and symptoms of depression in the el-

derly often do not follow the patterns seen in younger individuals (Salamon, 1989). Aging persons frequently complain of physical rather than emotional illness. Thus, depression can be easily misdiagnosed. Depression is treatable, but left untreated or misdiagnosed it can lead to serious problems. This is evidenced in the high rate of sui-

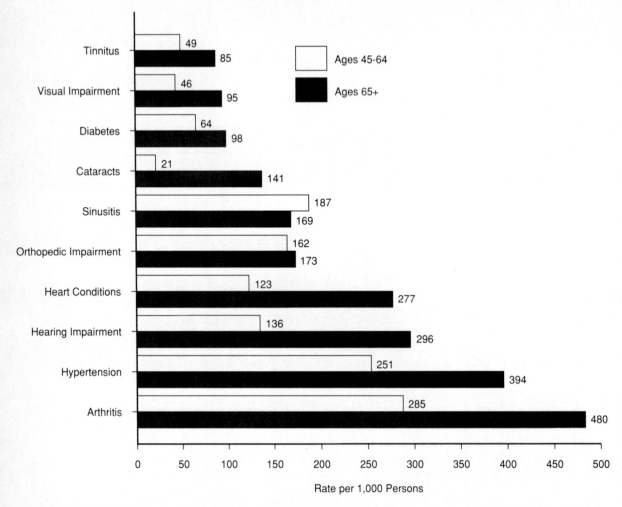

Figure 18-7 Morbidity from top 10 leading chronic conditions: 1986. (From National Center for Health Statistics: Current estimates from the National Health Interview Survey, United States, 1986, Vital and Health Statistics, Series 10, No. 164, Washington, DC, October 1987, U.S. Government Printing Office.)

cide among the elderly as compared to the general population.

Suicide

Suicide is a large mental health concern and a major cause of death among the elderly. The American Association of Retired Persons (AARP, 1989) has published *Elder Suicide: A National Survey of Prevention and Intervention Programs,* to increase understanding among the general public about this problem. Among Americans above age 65, the suicide rate is *50 percent higher* than that of the general population. Important high-risk indicators for suicide include social isolation and loneliness; pain and illness; status changes in employment, income, and independence; a sense of hopelessness; and previous suicide attempts. The AARP survey found that there are few suicide prevention and intervention programs which specifically target older persons and few professionals who are trained in elder suicide prevention and counseling. The nurse needs to assess clients regarding risk factors, counsel and support those under stress, and refer to community resources as appropriate.

Elder Abuse and Neglect

It has been estimated that more than 1,000,000 older Americans are mistreated annually. Elders living alone, with their families, and those in institutional settings are the victims. The abuse may be physical, psychological, or financial. Neglect may be passive or active. Passive neglect is the *unintentional* failure to fulfill a caretaking obligation. It frequently results when significant others assume responsibility for the care of a dependent older person even though they are not capable of meeting the needs of that person. Active neglect is the *intentional* failure to fulfill a caretaking obligation. Examples of neglect are nonprovision of food or health-related services, deprivation of dentures or eyeglasses, and abandonment (Douglass, 1988). Most states have legislation in place, similar to child abuse legislation, to protect the elderly.

Murray and Zentner (1989, p. 503) state that signs and symptoms of elder abuse include bruises, fractures, malnutrition; undue confusion not attributable to the physiological consequences of aging; conflicting explanations about the senior's condition; unusual fears exhibited by the senior; a report of the daily routine that contains many gaps; apparent impaired functioning or abnormal behavior by the caregiver; and indifference or hostility displayed by the caregiver in response to questions. Avoidance of questions and vague responses may also indicate risk of neglect or abuse. A knowledge of these signs and symptoms helps professionals to recognize the signs of mistreatment and to prevent further abuse and neglect. Hamilton (1989) has developed and validated an instrument for nurses to use in evaluating the risk of elder abuse in the home. This tool provides a systematic framework for identifying factors related to elder abuse. Elder abuse is a serious problem and one on which the nurse must be ready to assess and act.

Prevention is the key to resolving this problem. Educating the public about how to protect themselves against maltreatment in later years is a primary prevention activity being implemented by community health professionals. Individuals are being encouraged to plan for future care needs while they are healthy and capable of making these arrangements for themselves. From a secondary prevention perspective, efforts are focused on early case-finding and treatment. Interventions might include, but are not limited to, crisis intervention with the elderly and their families, respite for caregivers, and provision of skilled nursing and maintenance services.

CONSIDERATIONS IN HEALTH PROMOTION IN THE AGED

The 1990 health objectives for the nation had specific objectives aimed at improving the health of older Americans. In line with these objectives, the Office of Disease Prevention and Promotion for the Public Health service sponsors a national public education program called *Healthy Older People* that focuses on improving the quality of life of aging Americans. The program is designed to encourage older Americans to adopt healthy habits such as exercising regularly, eating nutritiously, using medicines safely, stopping smoking, preventing accidents and injuries, and adapting to the changes of aging (Gilbert, 1986, p. 11).

Normal Changes of Aging

We begin aging at the moment of birth. Aging brings about physical, social, and emotional changes. The medical model has often been used to study aging. This model defines health as the absence of disease and seeks to improve health by preventing and eliminating disease. It looks at the physical aspects of normal aging, but often does not integrate the social and emotional changes that accompany the aging process.

Aging is a natural and lifelong process. It brings with it normal body changes. Listed in Table 18-1 are major physical changes that occur with aging along with their implications. Elderly people as well as nurses caring for the elderly must take these changes into account if the client's health potential is to be maximized and changes

TABLE 18-1   Physical changes with age

Change	Implications
Skeletal system	
1. Calcification of vertebral ligaments	1. Postural change
2. Fibrocartilaginous atrophy; muscle atrophy	2. Loss of muscle power; contractures; paralysis; decreased respiration efficiency
3. Osteoporotic bone change	3. Diminished weight bearing; spontaneous fractures
4. Ossification of joint cartilage	4. Joint stiffness; ankylosis
Gastrointestinal system	
1. Atrophy of mucosal linings; diminished production of hydrochloric acid (achlorhydria)	1. Delayed gastric emptying; decreased secretion of enzymes; impaired absorption; diminished food appeal
2. Smooth muscle weakness; muscle atrophy	2. Decreased excretory efficiency; incontinence; constipation; diminished peristalsis
Respiratory system	
1. Increase in residual lung volume	1. Distressed breathing; fear, anxiety; CO_2 retention; limited mobility
2. Muscle atrophy	2. Impaired ventilation, reduced ability to cough or deep breathe
3. Thickened membranes, alveoli, and capillaries	3. Impaired diffusion of O_2; diminished lung resiliency; impaired circulation
Nervous system	
1. Atrophy of brain surface and brain cells	1. Behavioral changes: diminished emotions; disrupted self-image; less adaptability; confusion; disorientation; narrowing of interests
2. Atrophy of tendon reflexes	2. Stimuli-response change
3. Spinal cord synapse degeneration	3. Diminished overall coordination of neuromuscular, circulatory, glandular systems; increased susceptibility to shock
Genitourinary system	
1. Muscle weakness; muscle atrophy	1. Retention; guilt or embarrassment; incontinence
2. Kidney; reduced filtration; reduced blood flow; atrophy of glomeruli, tubules, nephrons; interstitial fibrosis	2. Urine retention; infection; pain, fear, anxiety; urinary stones; polyuria; nocturia; diminished excretion of toxic substances; diminished bladder capacity
3. Increased bladder-urethra infection	3. Urinary stasis
4. In females, atrophy of ovarian, uterine, vaginal tissues; thinning of vaginal walls	4. Decreased lubrication; loss of fertility; need for increase in stimulation time
5. In males, diminished spermatogenesis; decreased number of sperm; atrophy of testes; enlargement of prostate	5. Increased time for erection; reduced intensity of sensation; reduced volume and viscosity of seminal fluid; reduced force of ejaculation
Nutrition and metabolism	
1. Vitamin deficiencies: lack of vitamin B, inflammation of mucous membranes of the mouth; lack of vitamins C and K, capillary fragility	1. Discomfort; decreased food appeal; multiple bruises; disturbed self-image; fear, anxiety
2. Metabolic rate decrease—estimated at 1 percent per year after 25	2. Changes in nutrition, drug reaction, hypothermia

TABLE 18-1 Physical changes with age—cont'd

Change	*Implications*
3. Depletion of water	3. Increased stress in excretion; constipation
4. Increased proportion of body fat	4. Less muscle mass, weakness; storage of nutrients in body fat
5. Mineral intake deficiency	5. Malnutrition; bone demineralization
6. Teeth: diseased, lost, ill-fitting dentures	6. Dehydration, malnutrition
7. Decreased digestive enzymes gastric acidity, saliva	7. Impaired digestion; swallowing stress; cracking of mucous membranes of the mouth
Cardiovascular system	
1. Protein degeneration; lipofuscin accumulation	1. Diminished cardiac output—decreased blood flow to brain, heart, kidneys, liver
2. Fibrosis of blood vessel lumen; calcification of arteries; elongation of arteries	2. Increased systolic blood pressure; vasal sluggishness
3. Thickening of vessel membranes	3. Impaired tissue nourishment; impaired removal of waste; edema
4. Increased perivascular fibrosis tissue	4. Increased peripheral resistance to blood flow; edema
Skin and cutaneous tissue	
1. Atrophy of sweat glands, hair follicles, subcutaneous tissue	1. Decreased perspiration; balding; increased susceptibility to trauma, abrasions, bed sores; inability to regulate body temperature
2. Deposits of melanin	2. "Age spots"
3. Thickening of connective tissue	3. Finger- and toenail thickening and hardening

NOTE: Listed in the left-hand column are major physical changes associated with normal aging; among these are changes often compounded by chronic disease. In the right-hand column are listed implications of these changes. It is often helpful to take these implications into account in day-to-day dealings with older persons.

From Linda David, Institute of Gerontology, as Consultant to Relocation Preparation Program, Pennsylvania Department of Public Welfare. References utilized: Rossman I: Human aging changes. In Burnside IM ed., Nursing and the aged, New York, 1976, McGraw-Hill; Kimmel DC, Biological and intellectual aspects of aging. In Kimmel DC, ed: Adulthood and aging, New York, 1974, Wiley, chap 8, pp 369-376; Jennings M, Nordstorm M, and Schumake N. Physiologic functioning in the elderly, Nurs Clin North Am 7:237-246, June 1972; Cameron M, Views of aging: a teacher's guide, Ann Arbor, 1967, Institute of Gerontology, University of Michigan-Wayne State University, pp 146-148.

of aging are to be accommodated. For instance, smooth muscle weakness and muscle atrophy causing constipation are inherent in aging. However, diet can be changed to overcome this problem and the client may not need to take laxatives or other treatments. Another change that comes with aging is thinning of the vaginal walls in women and atrophy of the testes in men. As a result, sexual experiences are different from those of earlier years. However, sexual needs continue throughout life! Sexuality is often overlooked in care of the aging client. Community health nurses

should be aware of these sexual changes and needs and help older clients to obtain the information, counseling, and encouragement they need to fulfill their sexuality.

Postponement or avoidance of chronic diseases and conditions can be facilitated by eliminating risk factors such as lack of exercise, cigarette smoking, passive inhalation of smoke, excessive alcohol intake, obesity, high cholesterol diets, environmental toxins, and injuries. Unfortunately, the prevalence of chronic conditions and limitation of activity among the oldest-old (people 85 and above) often leave the younger generation with the impression that elderly people are all in poor health.

The end of the aging process is death, and nurses, the aged, and their families must come to terms with this. The nurse may be involved in death education and in helping the client and family work through this final stage of growth. Kubler-Ross's (1969) five stages of grief are well known and provide a structure with which the nurse can educate and guide clients and families. We tend to ignore death as a topic of education, thus nurses need to evaluate their own feelings and preparation for death in order to enhance client care.

Community health nurses should familiarize themselves with the numerous books written for the lay person that serve as excellent resources for elderly people who wish to remain well and enjoy old age. The noted psychologist B.F. Skinner has written (with M.E. Vaughn) *Enjoy Old Age: A Program of Self Management* (1983) out of his own life experience. A practical guide is Uris's *Over Fifty: The Definitive Guide to Retirement* (1981). Maggie Kuhn has written *Maggie Kuhn on Aging* (1977) and Alex Comfort has written *A Good Age* (1978). A common theme in all of these books is that aging is individual, can be modified, and can be enjoyable.

The changes of aging listed in Table 18-1 cannot be modified. However, aging can be enjoyed, the quality of life can be improved, and aging can be a time of great personal and family growth and development. Americans are fortunate to live in a country where they are able to grow old. They need to take advantage of, and look forward to, these added years of life.

Health Promotion and Wellness

Health promotion has the potential to maintain health and minimize the effects of chronic conditions. The community health nurse takes into consideration multiple variables when planning health promotion activities for the aged. The nurse utilizes the principles of primary, secondary, and tertiary prevention and knowledge of the natural life history of diseases/conditions when identifying nursing services that will maximize the older person's potential for growth and development (refer to Chapter 10).

Primary prevention activities that the community health nurse may implement when working with the aged are numerous. They include counseling and education measures to prevent accidental injuries, promote good nutrition, decrease risk of communicable diseases, maintain immunization levels, and prepare the individual and family for significant life changes such as retirement and loss of family and friends through death.

Although primary prevention is the focus of community health nursing practice, the needs of clients frequently reflect situations that require secondary and tertiary prevention activities. Secondary prevention activities often involve early diagnosis and treatment. This includes encouraging and facilitating regular medical and dental care, obtaining periodic screening for conditions to which the person is predisposed (e.g., hypertension and diabetes), encouraging adherence to medical treatment regimens, carrying out of self-monitoring activities such as self-examination of the breasts and testicles, and assessing for the danger signs of cancer.

Tertiary prevention involves rehabilitative and restorative activities. The community health nurse is often involved in helping elderly persons to carry out a physical or speech therapy program and to adjust activities of daily living to their changing physical, mental, social, and emotional level of functioning.

Health promotion activities need to start early in life. People, beginning when they are young, must realize that they have a responsibility for their health throughout life. Research has consistently shown that lifestyle, health practices, and environmental factors are integrally related to disease and condition occurrence. If health is to be improved in the elderly, these variables will often need to be changed. Predisposition to conditions such as coronary heart disease can be altered with a program of exercise, proper diet, avoidance of smoking, and protection from stress. Community health nurses, working with well adults in occupational, clinical, and home settings, are in a key position to help them see the value of taking responsibility for maintaining their health and preparing for life's later years. They can help people to recognize the long-term detrimental consequences of such practices as smoking, and can assist them in establishing a preventive health maintenance program that will decrease their risks for later health problems.

The National Council on Aging (NCOA) includes a National Center for Health Promotion and Aging. This center works in cooperation with the U.S. Office of Disease Prevention and Health Promotion to promote health maintenance awareness among older Americans and stimulate the development of health promotion programs. The center offers publications about peer group health education for seniors, health promotion materials, and resource kits such as "Stepping Out" for establishing walking programs. Information can be obtained about the center's health promotion activities by calling NCOA at 1-202-479-1200.

Wellness and health promotion activities are integrally linked, and wellness activities help the elderly to maintain physical functioning. Wellness is a major theme in the health care of today. Maintaining functional independence for as long as possible is a reasonable and obtainable goal for senior wellness programs (Abbott, 1986, p. 7). Wellness programs incorporate such topics as exercise and safety education, blood pressure control, diet, stress control, and smoking cessation. Senior wellness programs are beginning to emerge countrywide. These programs are often offered through local senior centers, churches, and fitness organizations.

According to Abbott (1986), the benefits of such programs include reduced risk of illness and disability; more effective management of chronic conditions; more appropriate use of the health care system and reduced medical expenditures; increased sense of control and independence; increased sense of strength and well-being; and increased sense of value as a participant in community life. The NCOA offers a wellness year-round planning calendar for senior citizens that suggests monthly topics and learning activities, provides factual wellness information, and identifies wellness resources.

Exercise

Regular exercise helps optimize physical and mental health throughout life (National Voluntary Organizations for Independent Living for the Aging [NVOILA], 1986, The importance). Exercise is important for everyone, and gradual, sensible exercise is not a danger to health. There is growing evidence that older people can obtain significant benefits, both physical and mental, from exercise and that seniors who participate regularly in properly designed exercise programs may improve their cardiovascular fitness, flexibility, strength, and general well-being (National Health Information Center, 1987). Certain exercises can help to prevent or alleviate low back pain and reduce the pain of arthritis. However, research shows that only 27 percent of people age 65 and older exercise regularly (Gilbert, 1986, p. 11).

Many older people report that they are unsure of what types of exercise they should be doing and the duration of such exercise. As with everyone else, older people with existing disease conditions should consult a physician before engaging in an exercise program. Many communities have YMCAs, YWCAs, and other fitness centers that offer senior exercise programs. The National Association for Human Development (1620 Eye Street NW, Washington, D.C., 20006; 1-202-331-1737) provides inexpensive exercise guides for seniors that range from basic warmup, stretching, and muscle-toning through more demanding aerobic exercises. Two free publications—*Pep up Your Life: A Fitness Book for Seniors* (American Association of Retired Persons, 1909 K Street NW, Washington, D.C. 20049; 1-202-872-4700) and *Staying with It: A Guide to Lifetime Adherence to a Physical Fitness Program* (President's Council on Physical Fitness and Sports, 405 Fifth Street NW, Room 7103, Washington, D.C. 20002; 1-202-272-3430)—may be helpful to seniors who want to exercise and keep fit. There are many publications on exercise targeted for seniors, and each person will want to assess what best meets his or her needs.

Safety

Accidents are among the leading causes of death among elderly people. Among persons 65 to 74 years of age, motor-vehicle accidents are the leading cause of accidental death, followed by falls, surgical or medical complications, ingestion of food, and fires. Falls are the leading cause of accidental death among individuals 75 years and over (National Safety Council, 1988). Even if a person is not injured during a fall, a fall can undermine confidence and increase the likelihood of future falls.

Accident rates are higher among those who are limited in their activities. Also, most accidents occur at home. Experts estimate that nearly 90 percent of accidents could be prevented if people followed simple safety rules and eliminated hazards in their environment (NVOILA, 1986, Preventing accidents). The contributing factors to accidents are physiological as well as environmental. Slowed reaction time, uncertain gait, and changes in hearing and vision are examples of physiological factors. To aid in accident prevention, older adults should have their hearing evaluated at 1- or 2-year intervals and obtain the necessary corrective aids.

The nurse should assist the client in learning about and taking safety precautions. Since most falls occur in or around the home, the home should be made as safe as possible. Stairs are the most hazardous location for falls. They need to be adequately lighted, free of clutter, and be equipped with handrails and nonskid surfaces whenever possible. It may be helpful to outline the edge of each step with a luminescent or contrast tape or color and to paint top and bottom steps so that they are easily noticed.

Other safety precautions around the home include having light switches within easy reach; using a light if it is necessary to get up at night; using nonskid soles on shoes; eliminating throw rugs, casters on chairs, linoleum, and extension cords; avoiding sedation; placing distinct labels on medications; having a telephone at the bedside; and placing emergency numbers in a handy location. Smoking in bed should be eliminated.

For their own safety and the safety of others, older persons should have frequent reevaluation of their ability to drive motor vehicles. In trying to prevent motor vehicle accidents, it may be

helpful for the older person to minimize or avoid night driving, and avoid congested areas and rush-hour traffic. As with all other drivers, the older driver should not drink and drive and should always use a seat belt. To avoid pedestrian accidents, the older person should be encouraged to use designated crosswalks, ask for help if signals are hard to see, avoid congested areas, wear white or reflective clothing, and walk with a companion if possible.

The nurse can be of great assistance in making seniors aware of the health risks of accidents and in helping to prevent them. The nurse can help older adults see that safety is an area over which they have an immense amount of control, and that safety precautions can help to promote health and maintain quality of life. Older adults owe it to themselves to "play it safe."

Nutrition

As with all other age groups, nutrition is an important part of health. There is good reason for concern about the diets of older Americans; research has estimated that 20 percent of those above age 65 are malnourished (NCOA, 1986, p. 53).

Maintaining good nutrition is not always easy. Problems such as ill-fitting dentures, loss of teeth, periodontal disease, decreased senses of taste and smell, diminished efficiency of the digestive and excretory systems, reduced income, and loneliness all have the potential to affect nutritional status. Older people are well aware of what should be avoided in their diets, such as salt, cholesterol, and sweets; but they are often unable to describe the elements of a balanced diet and are somewhat confused about nutrition in general (Gilbert, 1986, p. 12).

Deficiencies in intake of protein, calcium, iron, and vitamins C and A are present often as a result of limited income and resources. Foods such as cheeses, yogurt, and buttermilk may help to meet this need and are good sources of protein. Older people often want foods that can be prepared and chewed easily.

Fluid intake of at least seven 8 ounce glassfuls of water is essential. Fluid intake is often less because the aging process reduces the thirst sensation, and the person limits fluid intake to ease problems with incontinence; and if fewer meals are eaten the desire for fluids is less apparent (Murray and Zentner, 1989, p. 509). Yet fluids maintain kidney function, aid in the absorption of medications and high fiber foods, decrease side effects of some medications, aid in expectoration, help to soften stools, and prevent dehydration.

The nurse plays an important role in senior nutrition counseling, realizing that the older person's physical, emotional, and economic status must all be considered in nutrition education and counseling. Older people living alone are especially vulnerable to problems of inadequate nutrition, and often lose interest in meal planning and preparation. The frail elderly often lack manual dexterity, have declining energy or functional limitations, and are frequently unable to feed themselves. They can pose a unique nutritional challenge for professionals and family caregivers (Hogstel and Robinson, 1989).

During assessment of nutritional status, a 3-day diet recall can be an excellent tool. The nurse can evaluate this information for nutritional adequacies and deficiencies, as well as overnutrition. Such a recall can also lead to discussions of food preparation and preferences, buying habits, and eating problems and can be an excellent teaching/learning tool. The nurse needs to remember that nutrition habits are not easy to change. Older persons have developed a lifetime of food practices, and may find food one of the few pleasures in life. They may not be willing to implement diet restrictions even when this could improve their health. Cultural, ethnic, and religious beliefs may also strongly influence nutritional practices.

Much is written about inadequate nutrition among older people, but overnutrition, with the possibility of resulting atherosclerosis, obesity, and diabetes is frequently overlooked. A diet rich in carbohydrates, fats, sweets, and alcohol can quickly lead to overnutrition. Unfortunately, many of these foods may be tempting to the older client. The nurse should assess the client's diet for sources of overnutrition.

The nurse can also assist in low-cost food buying and preparation. "Spending down" for food is difficult when food prices keep increasing and senior income remains relatively static. Ingenuity in using dried legumes, beans, whole cereal grains, poultry, fish, dried fortified milk, and organ meats is often helpful. Although not always inexpensive, foods such as low-fat cheeses and yogurts are good sources of protein and keep well when refrigerated. Making seniors aware of the various meal programs and supplements in the community can help to stretch the food budget. Programs such as Meals on Wheels and meals at senior centers may be useful. Alternating meal preparation and sharing with a friend can help to curb food costs as well as provide companionship and offer variety in meals. Special food-preparation techniques such as cooking larger quantities and freezing foods in freezer dinner trays may also be useful. Many local restaurants offer senior discounts, and local churches frequently sponsor low-cost meals that are open to the general public.

Foods served in an attractive, pleasant manner often enhance appetite. Good oral hygiene should be encouraged and helps to promote appetite. Fixing meals in such a way that they are simple to prepare and easy to eat can be helpful. Foods with different textures and aromas should be served at each meal; eating each food separately, rather than mixing foods, helps to increase the ability to taste the food (Murray and Zentner, 1989, p. 509).

Physical barriers to proper nutrition need to be considered. Lack of transportation to well-stocked stores where clients can use food stamps or get their money's worth can be a problem. Physical disabilities such as foot problems or vision and hearing problems, can inhibit the ability to shop. Individuals with these problems may need assistance with shopping. This assistance may be available through local homemaker services, senior centers, or friends and family.

When the nutrition problems are beyond the scope of the nurse a dietitian or physician should be contacted. Most health departments include dietitians on the staff, and dietitians are also available through local hospitals and county extension services.

Physical Examinations

Annual physical examinations, dental examinations, and hearing and vision checks need to continue into the aging period. Unfortunately, they are not currently part of Medicare coverage.

These actions cannot slow aging, but they can help to detect disease early, minimize the effects of existing problems, and prevent further complications. Health habits regarding sleep, exercise, alcohol, and cigarette consumption need to be examined and discussed with clients so that they understand the relationship of these habits to health. Health risk screening (discussed in Chapter 8) at the time when a physical examination is completed assists the professional in focusing preventive counseling activities.

Medications

The elderly account for 25 percent of all drug use (Gilbert, 1986, p. 11). The physiological changes that come with aging make older adults particularly susceptible to adverse drug effects, and alter responsiveness to drugs. Among this group of people, changes in behavior and mental status are often attributed to age, senility, and depression, and a drug reaction may go unrecognized.

The elderly not only respond in a modified way to drugs, they also respond in a much more variable way than do younger adults. Their response is caused by a number of factors. The effects of primary aging are foremost. As people age, many of the organ systems lose some of their efficiency. The kidney, liver, and heart are the most important systems as far as the capacity to handle drugs is concerned. Quite simply, the elderly do not distribute, metabolize, and excrete drugs as easily and as efficiently as do younger people. Therefore, drugs may have a tendency to accumulate, leading to toxic side effects (Lamy, 1982, p. 39).

Older people frequently have chronic disease conditions that require long-term multiple-drug therapy. Errors of omission and commission in self-administration of drugs are not at all uncommon. Health care professionals are not always careful enough in explaining medications to older people. One national survey showed that less than 25 percent of people 55 and over felt informed about the prescription drugs they were taking (Gilbert, 1986, p. 12).

The community health nurse is in an excellent position to help clients avoid medication errors. During home visits, a 24-hour medication history is essential. "Let's take yesterday, starting with when you woke in the morning. What was the first medicine you took?" "How much?" "How many times a day?" "What are you taking the medicine for?" Checking a client's medication and assessing changes needs to be done on each visit. An alert student nurse made a visit to an 84-year-old woman and discovered an error in the client's dose of digitalis. The very independent client was somewhat deaf and during a phone call to the doctor described symptoms which the doctor felt necessitated cutting the digitalis dose in half. The client tripled the dose. During a 24-hour medication check, the student realized the mistake just as the client was beginning to experience symptoms of drug toxicity.

Appendix 18-1 provides a guide to use when doing a medication assessment with elderly persons. A medication assessment should be completed on a regular basis, because factors which bear on drug use can change dramatically in a very short time period.

Employment and Retirement

About 3.1 million (11 percent) older Americans, or 2.6 percent of the labor force, are working (AARP, 1988, pp. 11-12). Approximately half of these workers are employed part time (AARP, 1988, p. 12). The NCOA has offered the *Senior Community Service Employment Program* (SCSEP) for the past 20 years. This program has demonstrated that low- and moderate-income older workers, given training and encouragement, can help themselves and their communities (Changing the, 1989, p. 17). NCOA's *Prime Time Productivity Program* (PTPP) works with employers in helping them to see the advantages of hiring older workers and in keeping older workers in the workplace. Occupational health concerns have been discussed in Chapter 16. Although millions of senior citizens are working, many more have retired from the workplace.

Retirement is a contemporary phenomenon. Before the passage of the Social Security Act of 1935, few Americans retired or could afford to retire, and retirement was a privilege of the well-to-do. People who retired usually did so only after they were too ill or disabled to work, and not really capable of enjoying their retirement years. With the advent of retirement benefits, people were able to retire from work, and a new developmental task had begun. The Age Discrimination in Employment Act of 1967 protects workers from forced retirement.

Today, most people are able to retire from work while they are still in good health, and have the potential for enjoying retirement. Some people retire early, many retire between the ages of 60 and 70, and some never retire. Retirement is a personal matter. The span of one's life that is spent in retirement has grown from 3 percent in 1900 to 20 percent in 1980 (Growing old, 1985).

A strong correlation exists between successful retirement and retirement planning. NCOA and AARP have a great deal of information available that helps in planning for this life activity. Many businesses have retirement planning programs, or work with groups such as the NCOA to implement on-site training programs for future retirees.

Planning for retirement is essential, and must begin well before it occurs. It requires more than merely planning for the financial aspects of retirement; it involves planning for the psychosocial and emotional aspects as well. Retirement is looked forward to by some and dreaded by others. It is a time of role restructuring and redefinition. It can be a time of major decisions and issues such as deciding to move or stay where one lives; deciding on a new career or educational pursuits; reestablishing links with friends and family; deciding what to do with leisure time; and reassessing finances.

In a national survey of people 55 and older, conducted by AARP, 74 percent of those still working said they would prefer to continue working in some capacity after retirement even if it was not an economic necessity (Growing old, 1985). Many older people continue to work after retirement in a variety of positions. One in four older

Americans perform volunteer services, and the dollar value of such services amounts to more than $12 billion annually (NCOA, 1986, p. 53). Many retired persons volunteer their time to various organizations and activities that interest them—in line with AARP's philosophy "To serve, not to be served." Elder volunteers are a valuable resource. The Service Corps of Retired Executives (SCORE) is a well-known volunteer effort of retired people that is sponsored by the Small Business Administration. SCORE matches retired executives with businesses that can use their services. The business benefits from the expertise of the retired worker, and the retired worker makes a productive contribution to society.

Leisure time pursuits are an integral part of retirement and should be considered during retirement planning. Participation in fulfilling leisure time activities can greatly assist retirement adjustment. For many, retirement is the first period when one has significant amounts of time for leisure pursuits.

The nurse can be instrumental in helping people recognize the need for retirement planning. The nurse can assist persons in seeing the many options open to them, make them aware of the community resources available, and offer support and encouragement during this stage of transition and growth.

Housing

Housing is a primary health concern for the elderly. The majority of older Americans live in their own homes (NCOA, 1986, p. 33). However, housing for the elderly is generally older and less adequate than for all other population groups; some 45 percent of homes owned by older persons were built before 1950 (AARP, 1988, p. 11). Many of them need expensive repairs. They need to be carefully assessed for safety hazards. Many area agencies on aging offer chore services which can help older people with home maintenance and minor repairs at a nominal cost.

More than 40 percent of public housing units and rental assistance units are occupied by the elderly (NCOA, 1986, p. 33). Unfortunately, funding for these federally subsidized housing units has been on the decline in recent years. Problems in the Department of Housing and Urban Development have complicated this matter.

Lack of federally subsidized low- to moderate-income housing has made it difficult for many older people to find housing that they can afford and that is suitable to their needs. There is now interest in innovative housing ideas for the elderly such as home sharing, home equity conversion, group homes, "Granny flats" and rehabilitation to suit the home to the individual's changing needs (NCOA, 1986, p. 35). Whether to live in their own homes or apartments, live with relatives, or live in a long-term care facility are just some of the many issues that confront the elderly. The NCOA's Institute of Senior Housing is in the forefront of advocating adequate senior housing.

Rural Elderly

One of every three older Americans dwells in a rural setting, and yet there is no central body, inside or outside the federal government that monitors and takes action to meet their needs (NCOA, 1986, p. 57). There needs to be a rural network through which regional delegates can link the needs of rural elderly within and between states (NCOA—Direct, 1989, p. 7). The health promotion needs of the rural elderly are extensive. They are often isolated from the services provided the elderly living in cities. Many rural hospitals have closed, or are threatened with closing, with the advent of prospective payment. Rural elderly generally lack access to public transportation and may not have transportation available to health care services. The NCOA's National Center on Rural Aging (NCRA) advocates the rights of the rural elderly. The Office of Rural Health Policy within the Health Resources and Services Administration of the U.S. Department of Health and Human Services has the potential for addressing problems of this elderly subgroup. The National Institute on Aging has proposed a Center on Studies of Aging Rural Populations that could help meet the needs of this population group (NCOA—direct, 1989, p. 7). Community nurses need to help link the rural elderly to the services that are available and advocate further services.

TABLE 18-2   A life-cycle view of older people's needs

50-65	65-75	75-85	85-death
Departure of children from home, career stabilization, nagging health problems	Retirement, income problems, widowhood, chronic health problems, death of friends	Further loss of health, friends, strength; threat to independence	Serious loss of health, critical income need, dependency

Role reorientation _____
  Social intervention _____
    Personal intervention _____
      Personal maintenance _____

From Manney JD: Aging in American society: an examination of concepts and issues, Ann Arbor, 1975, Institute of Gerontology, University of Michigan—Wayne State University, p 14.

Life-Cycle View of People's Needs

Manney has constructed a life-cycle view of older people's needs which is accompanied by the system of services that responds to these needs (Table 18-2). This chart appears to show a continuum of loss in the lives of aging persons. The lines on the chart indicate that services continue throughout the life-span but that priorities for services change. Services can be arranged so that people can compensate for their losses and live the fullest lives possible.

Role reorientation, needed during the 50- to 65-year-old period, includes services such as recreation, education, and employment; opportunities for volunteer work; and preventive health care.

Social intervention, beginning during the 65- to 75-year-old period, includes income maintenance programs such as social security, Medicare, Medicaid, and housing and transportation assistance.

Personal intervention, beginning with age 65 to 85, maximizes the individual's personal independence. Dresen (1978) has elaborated on the need for autonomy in an aging person's life and has discussed ways in which this can be accomplished, such as using the family network, homemakers, home health aides, friendly visitors, Meals-on-Wheels, and intergenerational living.

Finally, at the end of life the aged person may become almost completely dependent on others and require either institutional care or complete care by the family.

SIGNIFICANT LEGISLATION

Politicians have begun to grasp the value of supporting programs to benefit the elderly. This has happened in part because of the voting power that the elderly population now represents. The legislation discussed below has previously been addressed in Chapter 4. It is briefly summarized here, specifically in relation to the older population.

Older Americans Act

Congress passed the Older Americans Act (OAA) in 1965. It has since been amended several times. The act provides funds for service, research, and training and is carried out by the Administration on Aging of the Department of Health and Human Services.

The OAA provides funding to states to establish state agencies on aging, and in turn, to help states to establish local area agencies on aging. The OAA provides grant money for research and demonstration projects that have regional or national value, grant money for the specialized training of persons who want to work with the aged, transportation and health education services for the elderly, senior nutrition programs, in-home health care services for the frail elderly, and preventive health services. For more information on the OAA, refer to Chapter 4, Appendix 4-3.

Social Security Act of 1935

The Social Security Act of 1935 mandates many programs that serve elderly people. The main parts are the income support programs of Social Security and Supplemental Security Income, and the health components of Medicare and Medicaid. Medicare and Medicaid are used extensively by the elderly.

Medicare

Medicare, a legislative program passed in 1965, is administered by the Social Security Administra-

tion, Department of Health and Human Services. It is a health insurance program that is available to almost every person over 65. There are two parts to Medicare:

1. Part A provides hospital insurance that helps to pay for care when an aging person is in the hospital. It also pays for some health-related services after the person leaves the hospital. There is no monthly premium for part A, though clients do have to pay a small part of the total cost of their hospital stay.
2. Part B provides supplementary medical insurance that costs the elderly person a small monthly premium. It covers doctors' services, outpatient hospital services, skilled home health services, medical services, physical therapy, and speech pathology services. The exclusions in part B are numerous and significant. Routine physical examinations, eye refractions, immunizations, hearing examinations, prescription drugs, false teeth, and eyeglasses are among those items not covered by Medicare.

Medicare is discussed further in Chapters 4 and 19.

Health Maintenance Organizations and Medicare

Comprehensive health plans for people who have Medicare are developing around the country. Such plans combine Medicare coverage and HMO Benefits (described in Chapter 4) into one program. The benefits of such a program include convenience because no claim forms have to be filled out by clients and *all* health care is provided in one center. Moreover, the program boasts a *preventive* approach to health care. In Table 18-3, one HMO lists its benefits for such a plan and compares them with traditional Medicare coverage.

Medicaid

Medicaid is a medical assistance program that helps pay the medical bills for low-income people. Each state administers its own Medicaid program and thus eligibility requirements and benefits differ. Generally, an elderly person may receive Medicaid if he or she receives public assistance

TABLE 18-3   A comparison of health services covered by Medicare Parts A and B and Group Health, Blue Cross and Blue Shield in the Rochester, New York area.

Medicare benefits	SeniorCare benefits[1]
Summary of Part A and Part B Medicare Benefits.	For persons with Medicare Part A and Part B
(For definitive explanation of Medicare benefits and exclusions, call the local Social Security office.)	(Except in certain emergency situations, you are not entitled to the following benefits and services unless they are provided, arranged or approved by the medical group. There is (one) $5.00 registration fee per calendar day for all benefits and services received in a health center. There is (one) $10.00 registration fee per calendar day for all benefits and services received outside a health center[4].)

In the hospital:

- Semiprivate room with meals
- Radiation therapy
- Drugs, casts, dressing and appliances
- Blood after first three pints
- Physical, speech and occupational therapy
- Intensive care
- Coronary care
- Laboratory services
- X-ray services

Unlimited number of days of acute care after yearly deductible. Yearly deductible amount is revised periodically by Medicare.

There is no limit on the number of acute days of medical care, board, semiprivate room and hospital services in a Hospital for which Group Health will pay, except with respect to psychiatric care as set forth below.

Mental health services: inpatient

Unlimited number of days of acute care after yearly deductible. Yearly deductible amount is revised periodically by Medicare.

No charge for unlimited days of acute care in an acute general hospital.

Psychiatric hospital

190 days lifetime limit.

Outpatient

There is no charge for 190 lifetime (non-renewable) days of care.

Outpatient psychiatric care is covered under a special payment rule. Medicare pays a maximum amount per year (revised periodically) after the beneficiary pays the yearly deductible.

20 visits per calendar year for diagnosis, evaluation, and treatment of mental disorders, but in no case will the benefit coverage be less than the maximum Medicare benefit per calendar year.

(One) $5.00 registration fee for all in-center services, OR (One) $10.00 registration fee for all out-of-center services per calendar day.

Skilled nursing facility (SNF):

Care in a skilled nursing facility is paid by Medicare for up to 150 days per calendar year. Daily coinsurance of 20% for days one through eight. 142 days at no charge.[3]

There is no charge for 150 days of skilled care per calendar year.[2]

Home health care:

Medicare covers home health care services not including meals, housekeeping, or personal comfort items when provided by a participating Medicare home health agency.

Home Health Care services are paid in full except for meals, housekeeping or personal comfort items.[2]

Hospital emergency room:

Medicare pays 80%[3] of "reasonable charges" after the yearly deductible has been met.

No charge when authorized by the medical group for a medical emergency whether in or outside the service area.

TABLE 18-3   A comparison of health services covered by Medicare Parts A and B and Group Health, Blue Cross and Blue Shield in the Rochester, New York area—cont'd

Medicare benefits	*SeniorCare benefits[1]*

Out of Area

Medical emergency and urgent problems (non-life-threatening medical care resulting from an unforeseen illness or injury).

Medicare pays 80%[3] of "reasonable charges" after the yearly deductible has been met.

There is no charge.

Additional medical services:

- Podiatrist.
  Podiatry services are covered except for routine foot care, which may be covered if the person has a medical condition affecting the lower limbs (such as severe diabetes) which requires that such care be performed by a podiatrist.

Benefits are the same as Medicare except covered services are paid in full, subject to (one) $5.00 registration fee for all in-center services, OR (one) $10.00 registration fee for all out-of-center services per calendar day.

- Chiropractor.
  Medicare only pays for the manual manipulation of the spine to correct subluxation that can be demonstrated by x-ray. Other diagnostic or therapeutic services, including x-rays, are not covered.

Benefits are the same as Medicare except covered services are paid in full, subject to (one) $5.00 registration fee for all in-center services, OR (one) $10.00 registration fee for all out-of-center services per calendar day.

- Speech pathology
- Outpatient physical therapy
- Mammogram (annually or biannually depending on age)

(One) $5.00 registration fee for all in-center services, OR (One) $10.00 registration fee for all out-of-center services per calendar day.[5]

- Ambulance Services

Services are covered in full when medically necessary.

- Durable medical equipment, such as orthopedic appliances, wheelchairs, oxygen equipment and prostheses (artificial limbs and eyes)

Medicare services referred to at the left are paid in full.

Medicare pays 80%[4] of "reasonable charges" after the yearly deductible has been met.

Medical and surgical services:

Medical and surgical services performed by physicians for the treatment of illness or injury including hospital (in- and out-patient services), office, house calls and skilled nursing facility care will be covered by Medicare at 80%[4] of "reasonable charges" after the yearly deductible has been met.

Medical and surgical services in the hospital are paid in full.

Physician house calls are subject to a $5.00 fee. House calls will only be made in the service area.

(One) $5.00 registration fee for all in-center services, OR (One) $10.00 registration fee for all out-of-center services per calendar day.[5]

Medicare Exclusions

Routine health care including:
- Physical examination
- Physician office visits for health screening
- Routine eye exams
- Hearing testing
- Nutrition Counseling
- Laboratory and x-ray procedures
- Immunizations (except pneumococcal and hepatitis B vaccine)

Routine health care (listed at the left as excluded under Medicare) is provided in full in the health centers or arranged or approved by the medical group for services provided out-of-center.

(One) $5.00 registration fee for all in-center services, OR (One) $10.00 registration fee for all out-of-center services per calendar day.

Continued.

TABLE 18-3 A comparison of health services covered by Medicare Parts A and B and Group Health, Blue Cross and Blue Shield in the Rochester, New York area—cont'd

Medicare benefits	SeniorCare benefits[1]
• Eyeglasses Coverage at 80% of "reasonable charge" for cataract glasses or lenses after yearly deductible.[4]	One pair of eyeglasses, purchased at a Group Health optical shop, will be provided at 50% of charge per calendar year. Cataract glasses or lenses are covered at 80% at a Group Health optical shop.
• Prescription Drugs	Prescription drugs provided at 50% of normal and customary charge when prescribed by the medical group and filled at a Group Health pharmacy. Prescription drugs qualifying for this discount are limited to those drugs normally stocked at Group Health pharmacies.
• Hearing Aids	One hearing aid is covered at 80% every 36 months.
• Personal comfort items • Routine dental care • Private Duty Nursing • Custodial Care[2] • Cosmetic Surgery[3]	Same exclusions as Medicare.

NOTES:

[1]**Contract does** provide supplement insurance as defined by the New York State Insurance Department.

[2]**Custodial Care**—You are not entitled to benefits for custodial care. Custodial care means any care (institutional, outpatient or professional) which is not rendered for purposes of diagnosis or treatment; is not restorative in nature; and/or, will not foreseeably result in an improvement in your condition.

[3]**Cosmetic Surgery**—Group Health will pay for services if needed because of accidental injury or to improve functioning of a malformed part of the body.

[4]This percentage is subject to change depending on legislation regulating Medicare payment.

[5]Visits for radiation therapy, chemotherapy, renal dialysis, PUVA treatments and physical therapy outside of a health center will have a $200 maximum copayment per calendar year per type of treatment or therapy.

payment. Medicare and Medicaid may be received concurrently.

All state Medicaid programs pay for at least the following services to people who are 65 and older: inpatient hospital care, outpatient hospital services, lab and x-ray services, skilled nursing home services, physicians' services, and home health services.

SELECTED RESOURCES ON AGING

Many resources for older people exist in both the public and private sectors. Public sector resources are supported by tax dollars and exist on the federal, state, and local levels.

Governmental Resources

The Department of Health and Human Services (DHHS) is the major federal agency involved in providing services to older people. Found within this department is the Administration on Aging (1-202-245-0641), as well as the National Institute on Aging (1-301-496-5345). The Administration on Aging (AOA) is the principal agency charged with carrying out the many provisions of the Older Americans Act. The Administration on Aging publishes *Aging Magazine.* Each year, AOA sponsors Older American's Month in May. The National Institute on Aging (NIA) (1-301-496-1752) was established in 1974 to conduct and support biomedical and behavioral research and training related to the aging process for the purpose of increasing knowledge about this process and the associated physical, psychological, and social factors resulting from advanced age. It includes the Gerontology Research Center in Baltimore, Maryland. The department's Social Security Administration is in charge of the Social Security Act programs of Medicare, Medicaid, Social Security, and Supplemental Security Income that are utilized extensively by senior citizens. Social Security district offices are located throughout the country to assist in filing for Social Security benefits. These offices can be identified in the local telephone directory under Federal Government listings. Chapter 5 gives more information on resources provided by the DHHS.

Numerous other federal agencies provide assistance to the elderly. The Department of Agriculture offers many food and nutrition programs. The Department of Housing and Urban Development subsidizes low-cost public housing. The Department of the Treasury offers assistance relating to tax problems through the Internal Revenue Service. The Department of Labor enforces the Age Discrimination in Employment Act. The Department of the Interior issues Golden Age (free) and Golden Eagle Passports (low cost) to senior citizens allowing them to enjoy the federal park system. The Department of Transportation underwrites funding to assist in providing mass transportation facilities and services. The Department of Defense offers programs for retired veterans, and Veteran's Administration hospitals offer many services to retired veterans.

The Small Business Administration (1-202-653-6554) sponsors the SCORE program discussed earlier in this chapter. ACTION is another independent federal agency. It is the principal federal agency that administers volunteer programs. Its purpose is to mobilize Americans for voluntary service throughout the United States through programs that help meet basic human needs and support self-help efforts of low-income families and communities. Under its older American volunteer programs it offers Foster Grandparents (1-202-634-9349), Retired Senior Volunteers (RSVP) (1-202-634-9353), and Senior Companions (1-202-634-9349). Many older Americans volunteer time through these programs.

As previously discussed, the Older Americans Act provides funding to states to establish state agencies on aging and, in turn, to establish local area agencies on aging. There are 664 such local area agencies on aging across the United States (NCOA, 1986, p. 37). State and local area agencies on aging plan and coordinate programs for aging persons. The local area agency on aging can be identified by calling the Federal Information Center, located in most telephone directories under United States Government, or can be located by checking the local telephone listing under county or city government listings under Area Agency on Aging.

Unfortunately, the old adage, "What is everyone's business is no one's business" very often applies to the elderly. Services for the aging are spread so thinly over the entire government that many individuals "fall through the cracks."

Private, Voluntary Resources

Private resources are numerous and vary from community to community. On a national level, two groups which work very actively with and for the elderly are NCOA and AARP. These two groups, along with the activist Gray Panthers, have lobbied on state and national levels for more favorable legislation and services for older people.

National Council on Aging (NCOA)

Established in 1950, the NCOA is a private, nonprofit organization with a membership consisting of individuals, voluntary agencies, associations, businesses, labor unions, and others united by a common commitment to improve the lives of older Americans. NCOA's membership units include National Association of Older Worker Employment Services (NAOWES), National Center on Rural Aging, National Institute of Senior Centers (NISC), National Institute of Senior Housing (NISH), National Institute on Adult Daycare (NIAD), National Institute on Community-Based Long-Term Care (NICLC), and National Voluntary Organizations for Independent Living for the Aging.

NCOA serves as a national source of information, training, technical assistance, advocacy, and research on every aspect of aging. NCOA forms cooperative relationships with governmental, business, private foundations, and other funding sources to educate the public and professionals about the aged and their needs and to anticipate and signal challenges and opportunities of the future for the aged.

NCOA sponsors the country's only gallery devoted exclusively to the creative accomplishments of older artists. It has been a part of NCOA headquarters since 1981 and is called the NCOA Gallery Patina. Patina is defined as a surface appearance of something grown beautiful, especially with age or use. The gallery is an extension of NCOA's Center on Arts and Aging.

In 1987, NCOA was cofounder with the Child Welfare League of America of *Generations United.* This is a coalition of more than 100 national organizations around the country dedicated to linking the needs and resources of generations. Generations United provides positive themes about intergenerational opportunities for cooperation and programs that bring young and old together (Another kind, 1989, p. 11). It works closely with such groups as the Center for Understanding Aging, in Framingham, Massachusetts (1-508-626-4979); the Center for Intergenerational Learning, housed at Temple University; Institute on Aging in Philadelphia (1-215-787-6970); New Age, Inc. of Ann Arbor, Michigan (1-313-663-9891); and Generations Together at the University of Pittsburgh (1-412-638-7155), to promote intergenerational activities and aging education (Programs that, 1989, pp. 12-16). These affiliations have been successful in developing many programs which benefit both the young and the old. One program is the Senior Center/Latchkey program in which older volunteers spend time with youngsters after school; a manual on this program is available from NCOA. NCOA is headquartered in Washington, D.C., and can be contacted at 600 Maryland Avenue, SW, West Wing 1090, Washington, D.C. 20024.

American Association of Retired Persons (AARP)

The AARP was established in 1958 by Dr. Ethel Percy Andrus, founder of the National Retired Teachers Association. It represents millions of older people across America. AARP has over 30 million members and is the largest nonprofit and nonpartisan membership organization in the world (AARP, 1989, All about, p. 1).

The purposes of AARP are to enhance the quality of life for older persons; promote independence, dignity, and purpose for older persons; lead in determining the role and place of older persons in society; and improve the image of aging (AARP, 1989, All about, p. 1). Membership in the group is limited to those age 50 years and older and costs $5 annually. It has local affiliates across the country.

AARP publishes a bimonthly magazine, *Modern Maturity,* that offers retirement advice, travel ideas, and health tips, and also publishes the monthly *AARP News Bulletin.* It is a strong voice in speaking up on legislative issues for older people. It offers savings on health aids and prescriptions from AARP's nonprofit order-by-mail pharmacy. It also offers travel, health, home, auto, and road insurance; investment opportunities; and other benefits including discounts across the country at many participating businesses. It sponsors a tax assistance program to help older low- and moderate-income taxpayers. It publishes an excellent intergenerational publication, *Growing Together: An Intergenerational Sourcebook,* that outlines intergenerational programs and resources across the country and is available at no cost. AARP can be contacted at 1909 K Street NW, Washington, D.C. 20049 (1-202-872-4700).

Other community resources include senior centers, adult day care programs, home care agencies, family services agencies, geriatric counselors and health care professionals, churches, community service groups, and caregiver support groups. Listings for many such agencies can be found in the local telephone directory or can be obtained through local health departments or United Community Service agencies. The nurse needs to be aware of resources and services for the elderly in the community and refer clients to them when appropriate. The nurse can advocate services when none exist.

BARRIERS TO HEALTH CARE

The mindset of caregivers, of aging people, and of our culture toward aging is a barrier to health care. Until we all see aging as a natural and even beautiful part of the life cycle, we will not "age gracefully." People do have at least some control over their own health and they may need assistance in recognizing this. Developing healthy ways of living and planning for the years after retirement when we are young means that life after 65 or 70 can be both healthy and enjoyable. We have to believe that this is the case, however, and believe that people can still be productive and valuable as they age.

There are two outstanding barriers to achieving health care in this age group, aside from the attitude that "to be old is to be sick, lonely, and tired." These are transportation and income.

Transportation

Research has consistently shown that transportation problems present a considerable barrier for aging persons (Biegel, Petchers, Snyder, and Beisgen, 1989; Burnside, 1988). Getting to health care facilities, service agencies, or grocery stores may be impossible without a car or public transportation. The inability to drive or physically to get around due to mobility limitations contributes to the problem. In some communities, Dial-a-Ride and the Red Cross have provided some transportation to solve this problem.

There is little public transportation in this country. Rising costs and proposals to reduce funding are endangering the progress that has been made in meeting the transportation needs of older persons (NCOA, 1986, p. 54). Close to 10 percent of Older Americans Act funds are used to provide transportation services (NCOA, 1986, p. 54).

Seniors living in rural settings are especially affected by the problems of transportation and access to resources and services. For the first time in recent history, more seniors are living in the suburbs (10.1 million) than in central cities (8.1 million) (NCOA, 1986, p. 54), and their transportation needs are becoming acute.

Income

Financial stability is a very real concern for the elderly. Limited income is a major barrier for many elderly Americans seeking health care. AARP (1988, pp. 8-11) reports that:

- The median income of older persons in 1987

was $11,854 for males and $6734 for females.
- Families headed by persons age 65 and older reported a median income in 1987 of $20,813 ($21,474 for whites, $14,107 for blacks, and $14,377 for Hispanics).
- Elderly persons living alone or with nonrelatives were likely to have low incomes in 1987, with 41 percent reporting incomes of $7000 or less.
- The major source of income for older families and individuals is Social Security, followed by asset income and earnings (24 percent each), public and private pensions (15 percent), and payments such as Supplemental Security Income, unemployment, and veteran's payments (2 percent).

The prices of food, medicine, doctors' visits, and gas continually rise, yet many older people live on a fixed income. Older people often cannot afford services that they need. They should be encouraged to utilize programs that can be of direct financial assistance to them, such as Social Security, Supplemental Security Income, Food Stamps, and senior discounts at many stores and businesses, as well as programs which provide services to reduce financial expenditures, such as Meals-on-Wheels and congregate meals. The many services that are available in the community can help to stretch the dollars available in later life and assist the older person in enjoying retirement and having sufficient income to eat nutritiously, seek health care, pursue hobbies, visit family and friends, and travel.

ROLE OF THE COMMUNITY HEALTH NURSE

Care of aging persons holds unique challenges for community health nurses, such as helping elderly people who lack a feeling of self-worth to find it, helping them to maintain independence, and assisting them to be contributing citizens, as well. Some of these challenges are the result of the special economic, biological, and psychological characteristics of people who have lived a long life.

The main role of community health nurses has been that of working in the area of health maintenance and prevention of disease and disability.

TABLE 18-4 Ranking of services according to need for provision of additional resources by public health nurses and individuals 65 or over

Service	Rank assigned by public health nurses	Rank assigned by the elderly
Ambulance service	21	23
Hospital service	17	20
Access to physicians	23	21
Nursing and custodial homes	16	14
Services of a public health or visiting nurse	14	9*
Homemaker-health aide services	9*	8*
Meal and nutrition services, such as group meals, home-delivered meals	10*	5*
Availability of large print (books, records, tapes, etc.)	19	13
Services to deliver books, tapes, and records to shut-ins	20	18
Social and recreational center for, or including, older people	3*	16
Church relationships with older people	5*	15
Education or training in subjects of special interest to older people	8*	19
Employment service for older people in the community who wish to work	6*	12
Handyman service	12	7*
Help for older people in finding housing	11	6*
Information and referral service	13	10*
Legal help for those who cannot afford to pay	2*	2*
Preretirement training programs	15	22
Program of reassurance by regularly scheduled telephone calls to the elderly	7*	4*
Senior citizens club	18	11
Transportation services	1*	1*
Visiting program to older people in their homes, hospitals, nursing homes, retirement homes	4*	3*
Agency or organization that offers older people opportunities to volunteer their services	22	17

*Services ranked in the top 10 in terms of priority for provision of additional resources.

From Keith PM: A preliminary investigation of the role of the public health nurse in evaluation of services of the aged, Am J Public Health, 66:379, 1976.

An example of this role is health teaching and counseling about the use of medications.

Underlying this role are many others that the nurse must participate in if comprehensive care is to be given. Some of these are discussed below.

Evaluating Available Services for the Aging

Four community health nurses in a city of 30,000 people were asked to assess the needs for further services to the elderly in their community. Because of their knowledge of currently available services as well as their contacts with clients, the nurses were in an excellent position to be able to evaluate services for this population group.

Table 18-4 lists the services that elderly people of the community, as well as the community health nurses, felt were needed. It then compares the way in which these two groups rank the needs with each other. The table demonstrates that aging people desire services that will help them to remain independent in the community. Nurses want aging people to have recreational centers and church relationships. The elderly desire the services of the community health nurse or visiting nurse as well as home-delivered meals. In summary, the expansion of programs to include more prevention and maintenance activities by nurses receives *more* support from clients than from nurses. Perhaps we have underestimated the importance of our role with aging persons! As with other age groups, the community health nurse needs to ascertain the services that clients need, in addition to those they are already receiving. The survey discussed here is one way of accomplishing this.

Political Involvement

Good nursing care must involve a knowledge of the political system and how to work within it. Many of the services that aging clients need, such as an adequate income and transportation, can be obtained only when caring people work to obtain them on the local, state, and federal levels. Nurses need to know their legislators, inform them of the needs in the community, and help to organize aging people into power groups. Only with this kind of action will major changes take place. Chapter 23 describes the forms that legislative and political involvement can take for community health nurses.

Home Visiting

Home is an extremely significant place to most older people. It is a place where things are familiar and where one is able to remain independent and have a sense of autonomy. A home visit is a useful way of making an individualized assessment of the needs and strengths of older people. The needs can be met by making necessary referrals to available services and by working out solutions with clients. The physical environment, interpersonal relationships, and the client's physical and psychological capabilities need to be assessed. Rauckhorst, Stokes, and Mezey (1980) have constructed tools to assess these different areas.

Support Services

Mental health intake, screening, and evaluation

Mental health care

Physicians' services

Nursing services

Homemaker-home health aides

Physical therapy

Occupational therapy

Speech therapy

Inhalation therapy

Dental care

Nutrition service (Meals-on-Wheels, group dining, food distribution programs)

Health education

Laundry services

Social services:

   Information and referral

   Financial support

   Legal services

   Personal needs (transportation, telephone, reassurance, grooming, shopping, companions, friendly visitors, pets)

   Family "respite" services

   Night sitters (for short-term illnesses)

   Home safety

   Chore services (handyman) or home maintenance repairs

   Recreation (community center, senior center)

   Employment and volunteer work (VISTA, Senior Aides, SCORE, Peace Corps, Foster Grandparent, Green Thumb, etc.)

   Education (home library service, academic courses)

Religious support (clerical or pastoral counseling, "practical" ecumenism)

Police assistance

Outpatient care in clinics, community mental health centers, day hospitals, day-care centers

Multipurpose senior centers

Protective services

Screening before hospital admission

From Butler RN and Lewis MI: Aging and mental health: Positive psychosocial approaches, ed 2, St Louis, 1977, CV Mosby Co, p 215.

Maintaining the Elderly in the Home

The home assessment may show that the aging person needs help to remain at home. Most people prefer home care to institutionalization, which separates them from familiar patterns.

There are many support services that the nurse can mobilize. A summary of some of these support services is given in the box on page 725. Few communities will have all of these services.

If the home assessment indicates that care outside the home is needed, the community health nurse can be a resource person for help in this decision. The nurse has the opportunity to help the family work through this difficult, often guilt-producing situation as well as to help in choosing a good institution. This is not an easy situation, because the community health nurse is helping to make radical changes in the lives of clients and families. Chapter 19 provides the nurse with information that facilitates the placement process.

SUMMARY

Aging persons have unique characteristics. The views of our culture about aging have to change if aging people are to experience healthy aging and receive quality care. Some of the common health problems of this group stem from the negative view held by young people and by older persons themselves. Old age may be a positive part of life if it is planned for and if good health habits are begun early in life. One of the health promotion needs is that of preparation for retirement. Significant legislation, including the Older Americans Act, Medicare, and Medicaid, are of great help to aging people, but many people "fall between the cracks" and are not helped by them. Four major barriers to achieving health among the aging are attitudes about the elderly, inadequate services, lack of transportation and limited income. Community health nurses can play a significant role in meeting the health needs of this group. This begins with the nurses' understanding of how they themselves view aging. Involvement in the political process is essential if the system of health care of the aging is to be improved.

The expected growth of the population over 65 ensures the continued existence of subgroups within this population group that will require assistance to maintain their independence. These subgroups are the very ones that are expected to grow the most rapidly in the coming years: minorities, women, and those over 85. Planning and implementing policy for these subgroups at risk is a significant challenge for community health nurses.

APPENDIX 18-1
Kent County Health Department: Seniors Substance Abuse Project

ASSESSMENT FORM

Name _____ ID# _____

Occupation _____

Language in the home _____

Current living arrangements _____

_____

Number of children _____

Significant others _____

_____

RELEASE OF INFORMATION

I, _____ , agree to participate in a Seniors Substance Abuse Project conducted by the Kent County Health Department. I authorize Donna Spruit, R.N., from the Kent County Health Department to release information regarding my medication and health status to _____
(doctor or agency).
I also authorize _____ (doctor or agency) to give information regarding my medication and health status to Donna Spruit, R.N.
Recipients of substance abuse services have rights protected by State and Federal Law and promulgated rules. For information, contact Seniors Project Supervisor, Kent County Health Dept., 700 Fuller, N.E., GR, MI., 49503, 774-3040 or the Office of Substance Abuse Services, Recipient Rights Coordinator, P.O. Box 30035, 3500 North Logan, Lansing, MI 48909.
   Client's signature _____
   Date _____
   Witness _____
   Relationship to Client _____

Interviewer's name _____ Date _____

Site of interview _____

Continued.

page 2

Seniors Project Questionnaire

ID # _____

Date _____

KNOWLEDGE OF MEDICATIONS

List each medication (including over-the-counter and home remedies) the client is taking in the left-hand column. In the right-hand column, write down what the client says is the reason [for] taking this drug. Include how much and how often he [or she] claims to take each. Use the client's words if possible. It is important that the *client's perceptions* be recorded, not the interviewer's.

Name of drug	*Reason for taking*	*Amount of frequency (with meals/ without meals)*

KENT COUNTY HEALTH DEPARTMENT SENIOR SUBSTANCE ABUSE QUESTIONNAIRE
MEDICATION USE/MISUSE

Risk Factor Analysis: Date _____ ID # _____
Evaluate the status of each risk factor and circle the number on the left which best describes the client's risk. 0 for not-at-all to 5
for very much a problem. On the right of each risk factor write in any comments which may help clarify the specific situation,
e.g., "diet implications"—*special weight reduction 1500 cal. diet, lo Na lo chol.;* "side effects"—*C/O dry mouth, excessive
tiredness;* "sensory deprivation"—*poor vision, cataracts both eyes.*

0 1 2 3 4 5   Cost _____
0 1 2 3 4 5   Confusion _____
0 1 2 3 4 5   Diet implications _____
0 1 2 3 4 5   Difficulty opening safety closures _____
0 1 2 3 4 5   Depression _____
0 1 2 3 4 5   Drug intolerance _____
0 1 2 3 4 5   Forgets to take medication _____
0 1 2 3 4 5   Fear of taking medication _____
0 1 2 3 4 5   Inappropriate storage:
               _____ temperature, humidity_____
               _____ removal from original container_____
               _____ medication stored at bedside_____
0 1 2 3 4 5   Language barrier _____
0 1 2 3 4 5   Lack of knowledge regarding meds _____
0 1 2 3 4 5   Living alone _____
0 1 2 3 4 5   Multiple prescriptions _____
0 1 2 3 4 5   Multiple pharmacies _____
0 1 2 3 4 5   Multiple physicians _____
0 1 2 3 4 5   Physician hopping _____
0 1 2 3 4 5   Outdated medications _____
0 1 2 3 4 5   Over-the-counter use _____
0 1 2 3 4 5   Reading disability _____
0 1 2 3 4 5   Sensory deprivation _____
0 1 2 3 4 5   Side effects _____
0 1 2 3 4 5   Stopping medication _____
0 1 2 3 4 5   Stretching medication _____
0 1 2 3 4 5   Sharing medication _____
0 1 2 3 4 5   Not following prescribed regimen _____
0 1 2 3 4 5   Transportation difficulty _____
0 1 2 3 4 5   Use of household remedies (i.e., baking soda) _____
0 1 2 3 4 5   Mood-altering drugs _____
0 1 2 3 4 5   Use of alcohol _____
0 1 2 3 4 5   Other (list):

0 1 2 3 4 5   _____
0 1 2 3 4 5   _____
0 1 2 3 4 5   _____

Total Risk Factor Score_____

_____
Interviewer's Signature

Continued.

KENT COUNTY HEALTH DEPARTMENT
Seniors Substance Abuse Questionnaire Guide
Risk Factor Analysis

Review each risk factor with client and determine applicability. Rate the risk factor from 0 (not applicable, no risk) to 5 (high risk), and circle the appropriate number. This analysis requires your professional judgment and is based upon your assessment of the client and his personal situation.

Cost

The client may consider some of his medications to be very costly. If his income level is low and/or fixed, he may not be able to afford these medications. Determine his priority for expenses—medications may not be high priority, and therefore, the risk of omission is increased.

Confusion

Rate this according to how well oriented the client seems to be. Does he relate appropriately to time and place, etc.?

Diet Implications

Is the client on a special diet such as low sodium, low cholesterol, weight reduction, diabetic? Some medications contain sodium, i.e., Milanta, Maalox. Some medications are to be taken on an empty stomach, while others are to be taken with meals. Milk is to be avoided with certain drugs. It is important to determine whether the client adheres to these recommendations.

Difficulty Opening Safety Closures

Patients with arthritis may have increased difficulty opening safety caps. They may omit a dose just because of the hassle or worse yet, they may transfer drugs to an unmarked container. (See inappropriate storage.) Determine how likely this risk is. Client may be unaware that easy-open caps are available from the pharmacy.

Depression

Is the client now depressed or does he have a history of depression? Because of the many losses suffered by the elderly, some degree of depression is fairly common. Depression may influence adherence to a medical regimen. Likewise, depression may be a side effect of some drugs.

Drug Intolerance or Allergy

History of intolerance or allergy would have implications for current drug use. It would be important that this information be readily available in case of emergency. Rate this risk according to the severity and likelihood of recurrence.

Forgets to Take Medication

Does the client state that he sometimes forgets to take medication? Determine how likely this is. This risk may go hand-in-hand with confusion, or it may stand alone. Not all persons who forget to take medication are confused. They may be overwhelmed by the number of medications they are to take or they may be distracted by other activities. Listen for key phrases like, "Don't know if I remembered." Client may be threatened or embarrassed to admit forgetfulness. Good, non-threatening interviewing will be helpful here.

Fear of Taking Medication

Some clients are reluctant to take drugs, even those that are prescribed. Determine if the client has any such reluctance. Some clients may be very open and verbal about this fear. Rate this risk according to how likely it is that the client would not take needed medication.

Inappropriate Storage

Temperature, Humidity: Medications are subject to deterioration in certain temperature extremes and high humidity. Storage in the bathroom is undesirable. Storage in the refrigerator is required for certain drugs and contraindicated for others. Check labels or check with pharmacist if necessary.

Removal from Original Containers: Many clients are tempted to put all pills together in one container, especially when they travel. This is a very unsafe practice. All medications should remain in the original containers until needed. It is considered safe to place medications in special dispensers. These are best when divided by time of day they are to be taken. This helps the problem of forgetfulness. However, a list of what each drug is should be available nearby for emergency information, especially if traveling.

KENT COUNTY HEALTH DEPARTMENT
Seniors Substance Abuse Questionnaire Guide
Risk Factor Analysis

Medication Stored at Bedside: Although this may seem like a very convenient storage site, it runs the risk of error if the client should happen to take medications when not fully awake. Also, too easy access may make over-using certain medications more likely, such as pain medication or mood-altering drugs. Having to go to the storage site allows a more purposeful effort and hopefully a more accurate dosage.

Language Barrier
Labels and directions written in a language not understood by a client could lead to misuse. Also, if the client does not understand verbal instructions given by the doctor or pharmacist, there is increased potential for misuse.

Lack of Knowledge Regarding Medications
See first part of Questionnaire, "Knowledge of Medications." How well does the client understand what the medications he/she is taking are for, how to take them, how much to take, and how often?

Living Alone
This may or may not be a risk factor, depending on how well the client has adapted to living alone. Living alone can be a problem if there is no support system to encourage the client to take good care of himself. Motivation to comply with a medical regimen will be affected in some cases.

Multiple Prescriptions
The more medications the clients are taking, the more likely they are to have a problem with adverse drug interactions, side effects, confusion about dosage and schedule, etc.

Multiple Pharmacies
Going to more than one pharmacy to have prescriptions filled is undesirable. The pharmacist may be unaware of other drugs being taken by the client and he/she will be hampered in his/her ability to do a drug profile and advise the client on possible incompatibility of certain drugs.

Multiple Physicians
Since the elderly tend to have a number of chronic illnesses, they frequently find themselves being treated by a number of specialists, i.e., internist, rheumatologist, cardiac specialist, gastroenterologist. This is sometimes unavoidable, and it is important that each physician be aware of what drugs the other has prescribed. The client has responsibility for conveying that information.

Physician Hopping
This is different from "multiple physicians." Here clients go from one doctor to another within a short span of time because they are not satisfied with their care. This can be a dangerous and fruitless practice and frequently results in multiple prescriptions for similar drugs, i.e., mood-altering drugs, antibiotics, pain medication. The client rarely informs the new doctor of his recent previous visits to other doctors. There are clients who have gotten three prescriptions for the same drug from three different doctors and ended up taking all three, and therefore, three times the desired dosage.

Outdated Medication
All drugs should be discarded once they are outdated. *Saving drugs* is a potentially dangerous practice because they can change in composition and may be harmful if used. Also, their presence in the medicine chest could result in someone accidentally taking the old drug instead of the desired one. This risk factor can be most accurately evaluated by a home visit where the medicine chest can be viewed or by asking the client to bring all drugs to the next visit.

Over-the-Counter Use
Clients who regularly use over-the-counter drugs run the risk of drug interactions, especially if they are taking other prescription medication. Sometimes clients do not count over-the-counter drugs as "real" drugs. They do not realize that these drugs also have side effects and contraindications. The more over-the-counter drugs used by the client and the greater the frequency, the higher the risk rating they would receive for this risk factor.

Reading Disability (Comprehension)
This is not to be confused with the "language barrier" problem. What is considered here are perceptual difficulties that could be the result of a stroke (aphasia) or possibly a life-long condition. If a client is unable to read and understand the information on the label, it would signal a risk of misuse.

Continued.

KENT COUNTY HEALTH DEPARTMENT
Seniors Substance Abuse Questionnaire Guide
Risk Factor Analysis

Sensory Deprivation
Visual, auditory, or other sensory-related problems that may influence the client's ability to follow directions or correctly self-administer medications, i.e., reduced vision or blindness, loss of feeling in fingertips, deafness.

Side Effects
Undesirable effects caused by the drug may influence a client to avoid taking a needed drug, i.e., disagreeable taste, dry mouth, dizziness, nausea, drowsiness, lingering bad taste in mouth, impotence.

Stopping Medication
When the client stops taking a prescribed drug before the desired therapeutic results are obtained, this is a medication misuse. This risk factor could occur as a result of unpleasant side effects, cost, emotional reasons, denial of illness, symptoms reduction (blood pressure medication, antibiotics), embarrassment.

Stretching Medication
The client tries to make the medication last longer by skipping doses or taking less than the prescribed dose. This is usually done for financial reasons or because the client desires to minimize the amount of drugs he is taking.

Sharing Medication
Usually a misplaced friendship gesture. The friend tells the client that this drug worked for him, "why doesn't he take one." A very dangerous practice.

Not Following Prescribed Regimen
This may or may not be a *deliberate* act on the part of the client. It could be the result of "confusion," "forgetfulness," or "stretching medication." Adjusting dosage schedules ad lib can be potentially hazardous depending upon the drug and its intended action.

Transportation Difficulty
This may not be a problem unless it results in not getting a prescription filled or related effect such as not making a follow-up visit to the doctor, which might be a necessary component in monitoring a drug's effectiveness.

Use of Household Remedies
The use of such items as baking soda for upset stomach could be a problem if the client were on a low sodium diet and/or hypertensive, since baking soda is high in sodium. The household remedy would need to be evaluated as to the contents, amount taken, and frequency.

Mood-Altering Drugs
This category of drug runs a risk of its own because of the nature of the drug and the condition it is intended to alleviate. These drugs may be habit forming. A depressed client may overdose himself.

Use of Alcohol
Some drugs interact or are increased by the use of alcohol. It would be important to determine how much and how often the client utilized alcohol. A history of alcohol abuse would be significant.

Asking the following questions developed by John A. Ewing, Director for the Center for Alcohol Studies at the University of North Carolina may be helpful:
1. Have you felt the need to cut down your drinking?
2. Have you ever felt annoyed by criticism of your drinking?
3. Have you had guilty feelings about drinking?
4. Do you ever take a morning eye-opener?
If two or three questions receive a positive response, the likelihood that the person is an alcoholic is high.

Add up the total risk factor score and place in the designated space. By looking over the form, you can determine which risk factors you can help eliminate or reduce through intervention. Write up a plan with the client. After six to eight weeks, readminister the tool and determine if the total risk factor score has been lowered.

Reproduced by permission of the Nursing Division, Kent County Health Department, Grand Rapids, Mi; Wanda Bierman, RN, MS, Family Health Services Supervisor and Donna Spruit, RN, Geriatric Services, Principal Developers.

REFERENCES

Abbott SD: Wellness programs for older adults, Perspect Aging 15(3):7-8, 1986.

Aging America. Trends and projections (1987-88 edition): Washington, DC, 1987, US Special Committee on Aging.

American Association of Retired Persons (AARP): Growing together: an intergenerational sourcebook, Washington, DC, 1986, The Association.

AARP: A profile of older Americans, Washington, DC, 1988, The Association.

AARP: Elder suicide: a national survey of prevention and intervention programs, Washington, DC, 1989, The Association.

AARP: All about AARP. In Modern Maturity 32(4):insert, 1989.

Another kind of network—generations united, Perspect Aging 18(3):11, 1989.

Biegel DE, Petchers MK, Snyder A, and Beisgen B: Unmet needs and barriers to service delivery for the blind and visually impaired elderly, Gerontologist 29(1):86-92, 1989.

Burnside IM: Nursing and the aged: a self-care approach, ed 3, New York, 1988, McGraw-Hill.

Butler RN, and Lewis MI: Aging and mental health. Positive psychosocial approaches, ed 2, St Louis, 1977, CV Mosby Co.

Cameron M: Views of aging: a teacher's guide, Ann Arbor, 1967, Institute of Gerontology, University of Michigan—Wayne State University.

Chae M: Older Asians, J Gerontol Nurs 13(11):18–25, 1987.

Changing the world of work: Perspect Aging 18(3):17-19, 1989.

Comfort A: A good age, New York, 1978, Simon and Schuster.

Commonwealth Fund Commission on Elderly People Living Alone: Aging alone. Profiles and projections, Baltimore, Md, 1988, The Commission.

Douglass RL: Domestic mistreatment of the elderly—towards prevention, Washington, DC, 1988, American Association of Retired Persons.

Dresen SE: Autonomy: a continued developmental task, Am J Nurs 78(8):1344-1346, 1978.

Duvall EM and Miller BC: Marriage and family development, ed 6, New York, 1985, Harper & Row.

Fact vs. myth, Perspect Aging 15(3):22-23, 1986.

Gilbert S: Health older people: a national public education campaign, Perspect Aging 15(3):11-13, 1986.

Growing old in America: An ABC News closeup, TV Doc Viewers Guide, December 28, 1985.

Hamilton GP: Prevent elder abuse: using a family systems approach, J Gerontol Nurs 15(3):21-26, 1989.

Harper MS: Depression, suicide significant risks in elderly, Mental Health, Suppl Rep to AAHA Provider News, Washington, DC, February 24, 1989, American Association of Homes for the Aging.

Hogstel MO and Robinson NB: Feeding the frail elderly, J Gerontol Nurs 15(3):16-20, 1989.

House Select Committee on Aging: Per capita health care costs for persons age 65 and over—1988, Public Policy Aging Rep 3(2):10, 1989.

Jacobson S: Hattie Harris, Times-Union, pp 1C-3C, November 8, 1983.

Jennings M, Nordstorm M, and Schumake N: Physiologic functioning in the elderly, Nurs Clin North Am 7(6):237-246, 1972.

Keith PM: A preliminary investigation of the role of the public health nurse in evaluation of services of the aged, Am J Public Health 66(4):379, 1976.

Kimmel DC: Biological and intellectual aspects of aging. In Kimmel DC, ed: Adulthood and aging, New York, 1974, Wiley, Chap 8.

Kraus LE and Stoddard S: Chartbook on disability in the United States, an InfoUse Report, Washington, DC, March 1989, US National Institute on Disability and Rehabilitation Research.

Kubler-Ross E: On death and dying, New York, 1969, Macmillan.

Kuhn ME: Maggie Kuhn on aging, Philadelphia, 1977, Westminister.

Lamy P: Drugs and the elderly: a new look, Family Community Health 5(2):34-44, 1982.

Manney JD: Aging in American society. An examination of concepts and issues, Ann Arbor, 1975, Institute of Gerontology, University of Michigan—Wayne State University.

McGuire SL: Promoting positive attitudes toward aging among children, J School Health 56(8):322-324, 1986.

McGuire SL: Aging education in schools, J School Health 57(5):174-176, 1987.

Murray RB and Zentner JP: Nursing assessment and health promotion strategies through the life span, ed 4, Norwalk, Ct, 1989, Appleton & Lange.

National Center for Health Statistics: Current estimates from the National Health Interview Survey, United

States 1986, Vital and Health Statistics, Series 10, No 164, Washington, DC, October 1987, US Government Printing Office.

National Center for Health Statistics: Health United States 1987, DHHS Pub No (PHS) 88-1232, Washington, DC, March 1988, US Government Printing Office.

National Council on Aging (NCOA): Public policy agenda 1986-1987, Perspect Aging 15(2):1-64, 1986.

NCOA—direct lines to action networks, Perspect Aging 18(3):6-10, 1989.

National Health Information, Center Office of Disease Prevention and Health Promotion, US Public Health Service: Exercise for older Americans, Washington, DC, 1987, The Center.

National Safety Council: Accident facts, 1988 edition, Chicago, 1988, The Council.

National Voluntary Organizations for Independent Living for the Aging (NVOILA): Preventing accidents, Perspect Aging 15(4):insert, 1986.

NVOILA: Preventing accidents, Perspect Aging 15(4):insert, 1986.

NVOILA: The importance of exercise, Perspect Aging 15(5):insert, 1986.

Programs that bring people together: Perspect Aging 18(1):12-16, 1989.

Rauckhorst LM, Stokes S, and Mezey M: Community and home assessment, J Gerontol Nurs 6(6):319-326, 1980.

Rossman I: Human aging changes. In Burnside IM, ed: Nursing and the aged, New York, 1976, McGraw-Hill.

Rossman I and Burnside IM: The United States of America. In Brocklehurst JC, ed: Geriatric care in advanced societies, Baltimore, 1975, University Park Press.

Salamon MJ: Wide variety of treatable mental disorders seen among elderly, Mental Health, Suppl Rep to AAHA Provider News, Washington, DC, February 24, 1989, American Association of Homes for the Aging.

Sheppard HL: Damaging stereotypes about aging are taking hold: how to counter them? Perspect Aging 19(1):4-8, 1990.

Skinner BF and Vaughn ME: Enjoy old age. A program of self-management, New York, 1983, Norton.

Spencer G: U.S. Bureau of the Census, Projections of the population of the United States by age, sex, and race: 1983 to 2080, Current Pop Rep Series P-25, No 952, Washington, DC, May 1984, US Government Printing Office.

Strumpf NE: A new age for elderly care, Nurs Health Care 8(8):444-448, 1987.

Subcommittee on Aging of the Committee on Labor and Public Welfare: Legislative history of the older Americans comprehensive services amendments of 1972, Washington, DC, 1972, US Government Printing Office.

Travis J: Wellness workbook: a guide to high level wellness, Mill Valley, Ca, 1977, Wellness Resource Center.

US Bureau of the Census: America's Centenarians, Current Pop Rep, Series P-23, No 153, Washington, DC, 1987, US Government Printing Office.

USDHHS: Prevention '86/'87: federal programs and progress, Washington, DC, 1987, US Government Printing Office.

USDHHS, Public Health Service: Health status of the disadvantaged chartbook 1986, DHHS Pub No (HRSA) HRS-P-DU86-2, Washington, DC, 1986, US Government Printing Office.

Uris A: Over fifty: the definitive guide to retirement, New York, 1981, Bantam.

World Health Organization: Draft position paper on health care of the elderly, Geneva, October 1980, The Organization.

Yarling R: The sick aged, the nursing profession, and the larger society, J Gerontol Nurs 3:42-51, 1977.

SELECTED BIBLIOGRAPHY

Brower HT and Crist MA: Research priorities in gerontologic nursing for long-term care, Image 17(1):22-27, 1985.

Editorial: An aging nation presents new challenges to the health care system, Public Health Rep 103(1):1-2, 1988.

Hankes D: Self-care: assessing the aged client's need for independence, J Gerontol Nurs 10(5):27-31, 1984.

Lank NH and Vickery CE: Nutrition education for the elderly: concerns, needs and approaches, J Applied Gerontol 6(3):259-267, 1987.

Richardson JL: Perspective in compliance with drug regimens among the elderly, J Compliance Health Care 1(1):33-45, 1986.

Shaw B and Cristol J: Bridges: intergenerational approaches to health promotion for the well elderly, Public Health Rep 104(1):91-93, 1989.

USDHHS: Staying healthy. A bibliography of health promotion materials, Washington, DC, 1987, US Government Printing Office.

Weissert W, Credy CM, and Pawelak JE: The past and future of community-based long-term care, Milbank Q 66(2):1988.

Weiter PG, Chi I, and Lubben JE: A statewide preventive health care program for the aged, Public Health Rep 104(3):215-221, 1989.

Wilson HS: Family caregiving for a relative with Alzheimer's dementia: coping with negative choices, Nurs Res 38(2):94-98, 1989.

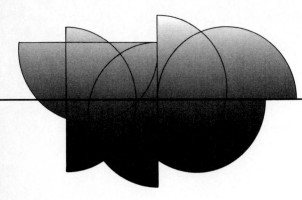

19

Clients with Long-Term Care Needs: A Growing At-Risk Population

Like good cheese
She sits idly waiting to be
*   selected or needed*
But the ugly mold of age
Repels life's amateurs
And turns them away
Ignorant of the quality inside

RUTH NAYLOR

OBJECTIVES

Upon completion of this chapter, the reader will be able to:

1. Describe the factors influencing the growing need for long-term care.

2. Discuss population groups at risk for needing long-term care services.

3. Identify the settings where long-term care services are provided.

4. Discuss the concept of home care and the range of home care services available in the community.

5. Summarize governmental financing for long-term care.

6. Explain legislation influencing long-term care service delivery.

7. Discuss barriers to the provision of community-based long-term care and methods for improving long-term care service delivery.

8. Analyze the role of the community health nurse in long-term care.

This text stresses the importance of working with populations at risk in the community in order to prevent major community health problems. Of all the groups discussed, none is growing more rapidly or has more primary, secondary, or tertiary prevention needs than the population which requires long-term care: the elderly, the chronically ill, and the disabled across the life-span. Members of these groups are often ignored by society because their qualities are not recognized.

Multiple institutional and community settings provide long-term care services for individuals across the life-span. While this chapter focuses on the role of the community health nurse in providing services at home for people who have long-term care needs, community health nurses must be critically aware of the role institutional settings play in long-term care. Institutional settings provide the most extensive, formal long-term care services and consume a major portion of the long-term health care dollar.

An inevitable result of the current financing of health care for many Americans is to be made powerless by sickness and poverty (Getzen, 1988). This occurs because often dependent individuals must deplete their life savings to pay for extended institutional long-term care. A significant amount of the funds for long-term care comes from consumers: of the estimated $45 billion spent on long-term care in 1985, private funds, primarily out-of-pocket payments, accounted for 48 percent (Polich, 1989).

Long-term care is a significant women's issue. Older women are twice as likely as older men to be institutionalized. The person most likely to enter a nursing home is the oldest-old female; one in four women 85 years of age or above resides in a nursing home, compared to one in seven men in this age group (Hing, 1987). Although they use institutional services more frequently, women often do not have the financial resources to pay for them. Women constitute 72.4 percent of the elderly poor (Ross, Danzinger and Smolensky, 1987). A significant number of older women who reside in nursing homes are impoverished either upon entering the institution or sometime during the nursing home stay (Sekscenski, 1987). Fur-

ther, since women are the traditional caregivers in our society, they experience social, emotional, and physical burdens related to long-term care as well as financial ones. Stone, Cafferata, and Sangl (1987) found, in a national sample of informal caregivers who were assisting frail elderly persons, that the majority of these caregivers (71.5 percent) were female. Caregiving responsibilities can place an individual at risk of social isolation and physical or emotional health problems (Deimling and Bass, 1986; Pruchno and Resch, 1989).

Since there is a growing demand for long-term care, the focus in this chapter is on examining the role of the community health nurse in this area of practice. Emphasis is placed on identifying current long-term care resources, gaps in the present system, and future needs of this rapidly growing population.

DEFINING LONG-TERM CARE

Approaches and attitudes to caring for the aging and for the chronically ill in the United States are changing rapidly. Long-term care today implies a continuum of health and social services and includes both institutionalized and noninstitutionalized care. Broadly defined, long-term care services

are those typically needed by persons in declining health or by those suffering from chronic or terminal illnesses. These services include homemaker, chore, and social services; nutrition and health education; personal care aid; occupational, physical and speech therapy; and skilled nursing. Individual requirements may vary from minor personal care or homemaker services in normal housing to a full range of nursing, rehabilitative, and personal services that can be provided only in an institutional setting. The distinction between long-term care and acute care lies in whether the primary reason for the service is to diagnose or treat an illness or to assist an individual whose capacity for functioning has been impaired by illness or age. (Congressional Budget Office, Technical Analysis Paper, 1977, p. 1).

The General Accounting Office has defined long-term care as:

one or more services provided on a sustained basis to enable individuals whose functional capacities are chronically impaired to be maintained at their maximum levels of psychological, physical, and social well-being. The recipients of services can reside anywhere along a continuum from their own homes to any type of institutional facility (GAO, 1983, p. 1).

Although long-term care entails a variety of institutional and community-based services, public programs disproportionately support institutional care. In 1987, 66 percent of Medicare funds were used to purchase hospital care; 72 percent of Medicaid funds were used for institutional services (evenly split, 36 percent, between hospital and nursing home care) that same year (Letsch, Levit, and Waldo, 1988). A very small portion of public funds are spent on home-based services. Medicare expenditures for home health care services account for about 3 percent of total Medicare outlays (Rivlin and Wiener, 1988): Medicare primarily covers acute care and is not intended to provide coverage for the long-term care needs of the dependent elderly (GAO, November, 1988). Although Medicaid funds about 50 percent of nursing home care, it funds only approximately 12 percent of home-based services (GAO, November, 1988).

A crisis exists in the long-term care system because financing for services has not kept pace with the growing need for services (Getzen, 1988). The present system requires significant out-of-pocket spending for nursing home care and other long-term care services, which had not been anticipated by its users. Consequently, incomes are strained, life savings are used up and an increasing number of individuals are becoming dependent on welfare funding for services. Being dependent on welfare assistance is degrading for many elderly persons (Rivlin and Wiener, 1988). Consumer inability to pay for extended care has created a two-class system of long-term care, one for the poor and one for the wealthy. This has, in turn, stimulated quality of care concerns, especially in relation to the delivery of nursing home services. Nursing homes which accept only private-pay patients generally provide higher-quality

care than those dependent on Medicaid patients (Rivlin and Wiener, 1988).

FACTORS INFLUENCING THE GROWING NEED FOR LONG-TERM CARE

Sanger (1983) has described three explanations for the increased need for organized long-term care services: epidemiological, industrial, and sociodemographic. These explanations have worked independently as well as synergistically to increase the use of long-term care services.

Epidemiologic Factors

Americans are living longer, the causes of death are changing, chronic illness is increasing, and the gap between male and female longevity is widening. It is crucial to the subject of long-term care to recognize that the rise in numbers and percentages of people in this country is among the very groups who need long-term care services the most. As medical technology and public health practice have advanced, an increasing number of vulnerable infants and disabled children and adults have been saved and life expectancy has risen dramatically, causing a significant expansion in the numbers of people 65 years of age and older. Persons in these population groups often have multiple chronic conditions and frequently require institutional or community-based long-term care services. Home health and other long-term care services are primarily delivered to the aging and the chronically ill (Berk and Bernstein, 1985, p. 22).

Not all elderly are at risk for long-term care. As studies of functional dependency and chronic illness consistently indicate, those most vulnerable are among the subgroup 85 years of age and older. Although only a small number (5 percent) of the elderly are in institutional settings, over 22 percent of the oldest-old (persons aged 85 and over) reside in nursing homes (Aging America, 1987). This segment of the elderly population is the fastest growing. This trend was identified in Figure 18-3 and is further illustrated in Figure 19-1. Between 1960 and 1987, the oldest old increased from 5.6 percent to 9.6 percent of the elderly. By

Total (65 and over)

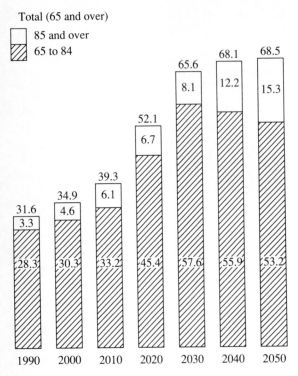

Figure 19-1 Projections of the elderly population by age: 1990 to 2050 (middle series projections in millions). (From US Bureau of the Census: Population profile of the United States: 1989, Current Population Reports, Series P-23, No. 159, Washington, DC, 1989, US Government Printing Office, p 40.)

year 2050, the number of persons aged 85 and over is projected to be 15.3 million, or 23.8 percent of the elderly population (U.S. Bureau of the Census, 1989, p. 40).

Although several factors (age, poverty, health status, sex, and living arrangements) have been associated with the use of long-term care services, data suggest that the key variables are poverty, age, and health status. Data from the National Medical Care Expenditure Survey (NMCES) related to the use of home health care, showed that the poor and near-poor were about twice as likely as the nonpoor to receive these services. These data also reflected that persons with activity limitations and those who consider themselves as having a poor health status were much more likely to use home health care services than the

nonlimited and individuals who consider themselves having a good health status. However, the elderly with activity limitations and poor health status were more likely to use home health services than either the younger limited population (6.7 percent versus 3.3 percent) or the nonelderly with poor health status (6.9 percent versus 1.5 percent). The elderly were also found in this study to use home health care much more intensively than younger home health care users. Although elderly women were more likely than elderly men to use home health services, women less than 65 years of age did not use more home health services than nonelderly men. Individuals living alone used more health services than persons living with their spouses (2.4 percent versus 1.5 percent) or children or other relatives (2.4 percent versus 0.7 percent) (Berk and Bernstein, 1985). Among the elderly, women are more likely than men to live alone: in this country 80 percent of the 8.8 million elderly persons who live alone are women. Elderly persons living alone are almost five times as likely to be poor as elderly couples and are twice as likely as other aging persons to have no children. Children are a major source of care and assistance for the elderly person (Commonwealth Fund Commission on Elderly People Living Alone, 1987, April).

People are living longer because they are dying of different diseases than was the case 80 years ago. Infectious diseases are no longer the leading cause of death as was the case in the early 1900s (refer to Chapter 1). Cancer, heart disease, and stroke are now the chief killers, and they are often degenerative and chronic. As previously mentioned, individuals affected by these conditions usually require long-term care services. It is clear that epidemiological factors and demographic changes will make significant demands upon the long-term care delivery system in the near future. It is estimated that the number of older persons in nursing homes will nearly double, to about 2.2 million residents by the year 2000 (Burke, 1988, December).

Industrial Factors

The availability of informal supports is one of the prime keys to disabled people living in the community. Over 4 percent, or 7.7 million persons of the age 15 and above, among the noninstitutionalized population, need assistance with daily activities. Of these, more than 5 million need help with instrumental activities of daily living (IADLs) (e.g., meal preparation, shopping, and doing laundry)—and 2.5 million need assistance with activities of daily living (ADLs) (e.g., bathing, dressing, eating, and toileting) (Kraus and Stoddard, 1989, p. 5). Many individuals with IADL and ADL dependencies could not reside in the community without assistance from informal supports.

The family is the primary source of care for the disabled and the frail elderly (Doty, 1986; OTA, 1987; Kraus and Stoddard, 1989). Close to 80 percent of the 13.3 million persons of working age who have a work disability live with their families (Kraus and Stoddard, 1989). About 75 percent of the disabled, older persons residing in the community rely solely on family and friends and most of the remainder depend upon a combination of family care and paid help (Soldo, 1983; Liu, Manton, and Liu, 1986). In 1982, about 2.2 million informal caregivers were providing unpaid assistance to 1.2 million noninstitutionalized, functionally impaired, elderly persons who reported problems with at least one ADL. A significant number of informal caregivers also provide assistance to elderly persons who have problems with IADLs but who are not ADL dependent. Informal caregivers for the elderly are predominantly female with adult daughters providing about one third of the long-term care (Stone, Cafferata, and Sangl, 1987, pp. 10-11).

Sanger (1983) states that four consequences of industrialization—geographic mobility, rising incomes, urbanization, and careers for women—have all changed the ability of families to provide informal support.

Rising incomes allow people to live apart and to negate the dependence families have for one another. Small urban homes are not designed for intergenerational families. Industrialization has made it both possible and necessary for women to take on a career outside the home. During recent decades, females have increasingly joined the paid labor force. This will make it more difficult for

them to provide informal care for elderly relatives (Scanlon, 1988, December). It is anticipated that work obligations may conflict with caregiving responsibilities to a greater extent in the future than they do now (Stone, Cafferata, and Sangl, 1987).

Sociodemographic Factors

There are three sociodemographic factors that have increased the need for people to use formal long-term care services. Sanger (1983) lists these as the decline in the number of children a family chooses to have, the aging of the providers of care, and the increasing rates of divorce and remarriage. Simply summarized, there are fewer children to care for parents who are living longer lives. These children are also older when they are required to care for their parents. Data from the 1982 National Long-Term Care Survey showed that the average age of the caregivers assisting the disabled and/or frail elderly was 57.3 years (Stone, Cafferata, and Sangl, 1987). Further, divorce may change the bonds of affection and obligation, and children and stepchildren may face extremely difficult decisions about those for whom they should care. Aging persons themselves may be alone as the result of divorce or death.

PROFILE OF THE LONG-TERM CARE POPULATION

Certain population groups may be presumed to be at risk for needing long-term care services, and in the minds of many people the category of people at greatest risk is the elderly. There is no question that the elderly population experiences more chronic illness (refer to Figure 18-7), physical functional limitations (refer to Figure 18-5), and activity limitation (refer to Figure 18-4) than younger age groups. However, not all elderly are disabled and the aged alone are not the only individuals needing long-term care services: more than 660,000 persons aged 25 to 44 years need assistance in IADL and another 250,000 individuals in this age category need help in ADL. The number of persons 45 to 64 years of age needing assistance in IADL is close to 1.4 million and 540,000 more need help with ADL. The percentage of people in any age group needing assistance with

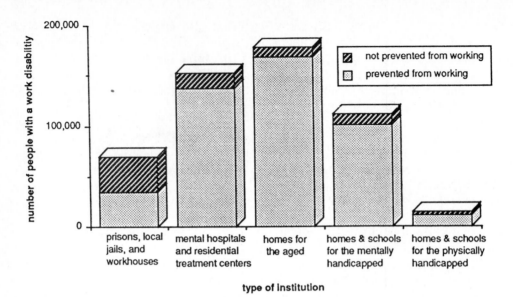

Figure 19-2 Number of persons of working age with work-related disabilities, in institutions. (From Kraus LE and Stoddard S: Chartbook on disability in the United States, an InfoUse Report, Washington, DC, 1989, National Institute on Disability and Rehabilitation Research, p 47.)

ADL and IADL is relatively small (under 10 percent) until advanced age (Kraus and Stoddard, 1989, p. 29).

Several groups of nonaged people who use long-term care services are easily identified: the physically and mentally disabled and the mentally ill. In recent years, the deinstitutionalization of clients with chronic conditions such as mental illness, mental retardation, and immobilizing physical problems has resulted in a significant increase in the number of individuals of all ages who need long-term care resources in their local communities.

The Physically and Mentally Disabled

Approximately 13.6 million noninstitutionalized people in the United States above the age of 15 report severe functional limitations. An estimated 13.3 million noninstitutionalized persons, accounting for 8.6 percent of the working age population (16 to 64 years old) have a work disability. Of those with work disability, it is estimated that 7.25 million have a disability that severely limits work ability. Work disabilities for institutional-

ized people (2.5 million persons) are more pervasive and usually are severe enough to prevent them from working (Figure 19-2). A high percentage of people with work disabilities is found among persons of working age receiving care in mental hospitals and residential treatment centers (81.8 percent), in homes for the aged (93.8 percent), homes and schools for the mentally handicapped (94.5 percent), and homes for the physically handicapped (91.1 percent) (Kraus and Stoddard, 1989).

Although many elderly are included in the figures for functional limitations, a significant number of Americans age 64 and under are functionally limited or mentally disabled. About 9 percent of families care for a chronically ill family member at home, and close to one third of these individuals are adults (Figure 19-3) in the prime of life (Robert Wood Johnson Foundation, 1984, p. 16).

The chronically ill experience a variety of health problems which can cause activity limitations. Chronic health conditions which most often cause activity limitations of any kind include multiple sclerosis, paralysis of extremities,

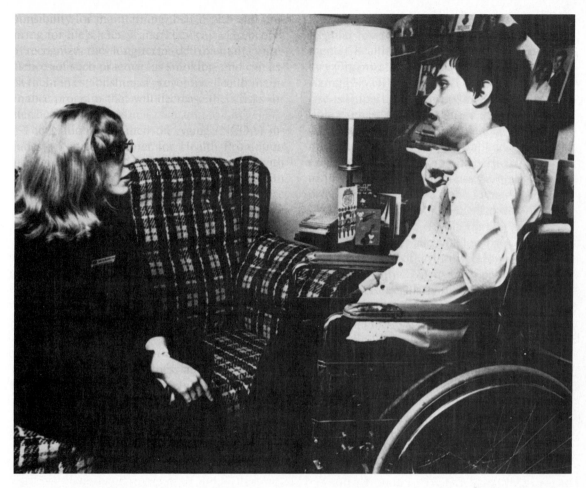

Figure 19-3 Young physically disabled adults frequently have extensive health care needs that cannot be neglected in planning of long-term care services. Often these young people can become productive members of society if they have social and community supports to help them handle their disabling conditions. (From Genesee Region Home Care Association, Rochester, NY.)

emphysema, intervertebral disk disorders, and epilepsy (Kraus and Stoddard, 1989, p. 24). These conditions mandate changes in lifestyle and careers, and alter family functioning (Pitzele, 1986).

Children as well as adults have activity limitations and disability. Over 3.2 million children under the age of 17 have limitations in activity and about 2 million children under the age of 18 have a physical, mental, or emotional disability. Among this population, males, blacks, and the poor are more highly represented (Kraus and Stoddard, 1989, p. 31). The types of chronic

handicapping conditions causing disability in childhood were presented in Table 14-3.

Children who have functional disabilities often need a complex array of long-term care services. Appendix 9-1 presents a case history of one such child and vividly illustrates that younger as well as aging Americans are highly dependent on our long-term health care system.

The profile of the mentally disabled or retarded population is not clear, because estimates of their percentage range from 0.67 percent (1.6 million people) to 3 percent (6.5 million people). Of these individuals, approximately 89 percent are mildly retarded; 6.0 percent are moderately retarded; 3.5 percent are severely retarded; and 1.5 percent are profoundly retarded (Kraus and Stoddard, 1989, p. 6). Individuals moderately to profoundly retarded (176,000 to 715,000 people) usually need ongoing long-term care. The long-term care services needed by the mentally retarded were discussed in Chapter 17. An estimated 23 million American adults currently suffer from a major mental or behavioral disorder other than substance abuse and about twice that number experience mental illness sometime throughout their lives (USDHHS Public Health Service, 1989). Mental illnesses cost the public billions of dollars annually; yet a significant number of individuals in need of mental health services are not receiving them. Those at risk are the disadvantaged, women, aged, and handicapped (Belk, 1987; NCOA, 1986; President's Commission on Mental Health, 1978; Weissman, 1987).

Among the mentally ill, the most neglected and most needy are the chronic mentally ill. It is estimated that about 2.8 million adults in the United States have severe and persistent mental disorders; of these, 2 million suffer schizophrenia. Whereas anxiety and depression are the most common of the major mental disorders, schizophrenia is the one most likely to result in functional disabilities (USDHHS Public Health Service, 1989). The majority of individuals with chronic mental illness reside in the community, as a result of the deinstitutionalization trend of the early 1970s.

The Mentally Ill

A comprehensive and accessible array of biopsychosocial and supportive long-term services is needed to address the needs of the chronic mentally ill. Individuals among this population group frequently have multiple and complex physical and mental difficulties and a broad range of functional problems such as impaired capacity to work in competitive employment, problems with basic tasks of daily living, difficulty coping with stress and minor everyday issues, and inability to seek out sustained assistance.

A significant number of people who receive and need mental health assistance require long-term care services. Chapter 17 discusses in greater detail the service needs of people who are physically and mentally disabled. When working with the chronic mentally ill in the community, it is important not to overlook their physical health problems, because often these problems greatly limit their functional abilities.

The Aging and the Availability of Long-Term Care

The only universal feature of the older population is age. Most aging people are leading healthy, independent lives. "The great majority of elderly Americans are the wealthiest, best fed, best housed, healthiest, most self-reliant older population in our history" (Fowles, 1983, p. 6). However, a large number of individuals in this population group have difficulty functioning independently due to poor health and to lack of money, transportation, employment, and social interaction. The elderly from minority groups, aging individuals over 85, and aging women are affected to a greater degree by these problems than other elderly groups.

It has consistently been identified that the needs of older people increase with age. The young old, or individuals 65 to 74 years of age, are generally able to remain functionally independent. Those above 75 want to be independent but often need much more help to do so. The aged above 85 represent, however, the greatest concern: the proportion of the aged dependent in 1984 ranged from 18 to 48 per 1000 for persons 65 to 74 years of age, from 37 to 97 per 1000 for persons 75 to 84 years of age, and from 90 to 286 per 1000 for persons 85 years of age and older. These data reflect that the proportion dependent among persons 85 years of age and over is from double to triple the proportion dependent among persons 75 to 84 years of age (Fulton, Katz, Jack, and Hendershot, 1989, March, p. 10).

Approximately 7 million elderly people need some type of long-term care assistance, ranging from need for help with ordinary household tasks to need for total assistance in every activity of

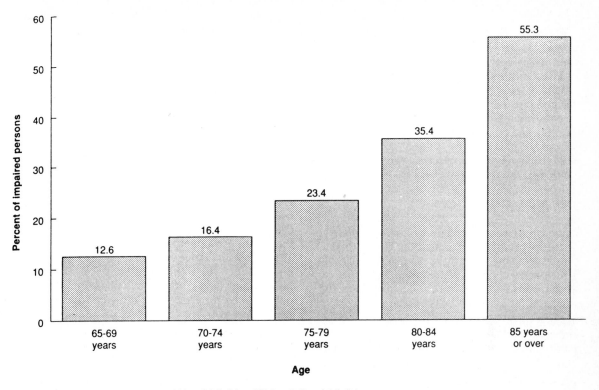

NOTE: IADL is instrumental activities of daily living; ADL is activities of daily living.

Figure 19-4   Effect of age on the probability of risk of IADL or ADL impairment, 1984-85. (From Scanlon WJ: A perspective on long-term care for the elderly, Health Care Financ Rev, 1988 Annual Suppl. p 9.)

daily living. Approximately 30 percent or 2 million older persons needing long-term care assistance have only limited long-term care dependencies. However, a significant number (20 percent or 1.4 million elderly) of aging persons needing long-term help are almost totally dependent (Scanlon, 1988, December, p. 7). The need for assistance with ADLs and IADLs increases markedly in the old-old or fragile-elderly age group (Figure 19-4). Among the young-old population, only about 13 percent need help with long-term care, but among the oldest-old, 55 percent require assistance (Scanlon, 1988, December, p. 7).

Dementia

The notion that dementia among the elderly is inevitable and affects the majority of older people is not supported by statistical data. The prevalence of severe dementia among elderly subgroups

ranges from 1 percent (ages 65 to 74), to 7 percent (ages 75 to 84), to 25 percent (above age 85): an estimated 1.5 million Americans suffer from severe dementia and require constant care. Between 1 million and 5 million others have mild or moderate dementia. Dementia places a person at risk of requiring institutionalization. It is estimated that at least half of nursing home residents in the United States have dementia (OTA, 1987).

Although a relatively small percentage of the elderly suffer from dementia, interest in this condition as a significant health problem is growing for a number of reasons. A large reason is the anticipated increase in the number of persons with dementia. It is estimated that by the year 2040, 7.4 million Americans will be demented, which is five times as many persons as today. Concern about dementing illnesses is also rising because financial costs as well as personal stresses related to

DISORDERS CAUSING DEMENTIA

Degenerative Diseases
Alzheimer's disease
Pick's disease
Huntington's disease
Progressive supranuclear palsy
Parkinson's disease (not all cases)
Cerebellar degenerations
Amyotrophic lateral sclerosis (ALS) (not all cases)
Parkinson-ALS-dementia complex of Guam and other
  island areas
Rare genetic and metabolic diseases (Hallervorden-
  Spatz, Kufs', Wilson's, late-onset metachromatic
  leukodystrophy, adrenoleukodystrophy)

Vascular Dementia
Multi-infarct dementia
Cortical micro-infarcts
Lacunar dementia (larger infarcts)
Binswanger disease
Cerebral embolic disease (fat, air, thrombus
  fragments)

Anoxic Dementia
Cardiac arrest
Cardiac failure (severe)
Carbon monoxide

Traumatic Dementia
Dementia pugilistica (boxer's dementia)
Head injuries (open or closed)

Infectious Dementia
Acquired immune deficiency syndrome (AIDS)
  AIDS dementia
  Opportunistic infections
Creutzfeldt-Jakob disease (subacute spongiforn
  encephalopathy)
Progressive multifocal leukoencephalopathy
Post-encephalitic dementia
Behcet's syndrome
Herpes encephalitis
Fungal meningitis or encephalitis
Bacterial meningitis or encephalitis
Parasitic encephalitis
Brain abscess
Neurosyphilis (general paresis)

Normal Pressure Hydrocephalus (communicating
  hydrocephalus of adults)

Space-Occupying Lesions
Chronic or acute subdural hematoma
Primary brain tumor
Metastatic tumors (carcinoma, leukemia, lymphoma,
  sarcoma)

Multiple Sclerosis (some cases)

Auto-Immune Disorders
Disseminated lupus erythematosus
Vasculitis

Toxic Dementia
Alcoholic dementia
Metallic dementia (e.g., lead, mercury, arsenic,
  manganese)
Organic poisons (e.g., solvents, some insecticides)

Other Disorders
Epilepsy (some cases)
Post-traumatic stress disorder (concentration camp
  syndrome—some cases)
Whipple disease (some cases)
Heat stroke

DISORDERS THAT CAN SIMULATE DEMENTIA

Psychiatric Disorders
Depression
Anxiety
Psychosis
Sensory deprivation

Drugs
Sedatives
Hypnotics
Antianxiety agents
Antidepressants
Antiarrhythmics
Antihypertensives
Anticonvulsants
Antipsychotics
Digitalis and derivatives
Drugs with anti-cholinergic side effects
Others (mechanism unknown)

Nutritional Disorders
Pellagra (B-6 deficiency)
Thiamine deficiency (Wernicke-Korsakoff syndrome)
Cobalamin deficiency (B-12) or pernicious anemia
Folate deficiency
Marchiafava-Bignami disease

Metabolic Disorders (usually cause delirium, but can
  be difficult to differentiate from dementia)
Hyper- and hypothyroidism (thyroid hormones)
Hypercalcemia (calcium)
Hyper- and hyponatremia (sodium)
Hypoglycemia (glucose)
Hyperlipidemia (lipids)
Hypercapnia (carbon dioxide)
Kidney failure
Liver failure
Cushing syndrome
Addison's disease
Hypopituitarism
Remote effect of carcinoma

Adapted from Katzman R, Lasker B, and Bernstein N: Accuracy of diagnosis and consequences of misdiagnosis of disorders causing dementia. Contract report prepared for the Office of Technology Assessment, US Congress. In Office of Technology Assessment: Losing a million minds: confronting the tragedy of Alzheimer's disease and other dementias, Washington, DC, 1987, US Government Printing Office, 1987, pp 13-14.

these conditions are great. From a financial perspective, it costs billions of dollars each year to care for these individuals (OTA, 1987, p. 5). The fact that caregivers of persons with dementia experience burdens and stresses related to their caregiving obligations is well documented (Eagles, Beattie, Blackwood, Restall, and Ashcroft, 1987; Fitting, Rabins, Lucas, and Eastham, 1986; George & Gwyther, 1986; OTA, 1987; Zarit, Todd, and Zarit, 1986). It has also been demonstrated that caregiving places individuals at risk for developing health problems (George and Gwyther, 1986; Haley, Levine, Brown, Berry, and Hughes, 1987; OTA, 1987).

Dementia designates a group of illnesses characterized by a progressive and usually irreversible loss of mental function (Prochazka, Henschke, Skinner, and Last, 1983, p. 1). Some 70 conditions can cause dementia (see box on p. 746). The diseases classified as degenerative are those whose progression cannot be arrested. Alzheimer's disease is the most common degenerative dementing illness, found in 66 percent of all cases (OTA, 1987, p. 12).

Alzheimer's Disease

Alzheimer's disease was named for Alois Alzheimer, a German doctor who in 1907 accurately described the typical brain alterations related to morphologic, neurochemical, and physiological dysfunction. These alterations are irreversible. The cause is unknown; nevertheless, distinctive alterations in and loss of nerve cells are detectable in the brain tissue of affected persons. It is believed that Alzheimer's disease is actually a group of related disorders distinguished by their symptoms, rate of progression, inheritance patterns, and age of onset. Researchers are exploring genetic and environmental causes as well as defects in the immune system as explanations for the disease. Until the cause is known, treatment can be only symptomatic (Burns and Buckwalter, 1988; OTA, 1987).

Affected people manifest various stages as the disease progresses, from forgetfulness with long-term and short-term memory, to confusion, and finally to dementia. These stages differ in length and intensity from one person to another. The symptoms include a decline in mental status involving changes in memory, language, praxis, mood, concentration, cooperation, thought process, perception, with progressive deterioration. Mood changes occur until finally the person becomes completely passive. During the end stages, help is needed with the simplest activities of daily living, and the person commonly assumes the fetal position (Buckwalter, Abraham, and Neuendorger, 1988).

The onset of symptoms is usually noticed first by the affected person, family, friends, or peers at work, rather than by health care professionals. The person usually hides early symptoms such as memory loss and decreased mental ability, for as long as years. Progression is insidious, with a diagnosis frequently made more than 4 years after the onset of symptoms. The average duration of Alzheimer's disease is 8.1 years, but duration is unpredictable: in some people it has remained as long as 25 years. The individuals usually die from other illness such as pneumonia, heart disease, or kidney failure (OTA, 1987).

Alzheimer's disease causes mental anguish for the affected person as well as for the significant others. Caring for the individual places a constant burden on families and taxes their resources. Community health nurses play a major role in helping afflicted persons and their families to obtain appropriate care. A mental health model which focuses on adapting to the individual's behavior appears to benefit them more than a medical model focused on correcting a disability. A specific pattern of care that emphasizes medical evaluation and drug management, combined with mental health care in nursing homes and day care centers that coordinate their services with social and aging services, is emerging (OTA, 1987, p. 43).

A variety of social and aging services are frequently available in the community to assist demented persons and their families to enhance the quality of their lives (see box on p. 748). Community health nurses are often in a unique position to help families to obtain needed services. The Alzheimer's Disease and Related Disorders

Care Services for Individuals with Dementia		
Adult day care	Information and referral to services	Physician services
Case management	Legal services	Protective services
Chore services	Mental health services	Recreational services
Congregate meals	Occupational therapy	Respite care
Dental services	Paid companion/sitter	Skilled nursing
Home delivered meals	Patient assessment	Speech therapy
Home health aide services	Personal care	Supervision
Homemaker services	Personal emergency response systems	Telephone reassurance
Hospice services	Physical therapy	Transportation

From Office of Technology Assessment (OTA): Losing a million minds: confronting the tragedy of Alzheimer's disease and other dementias, Washington, DC, 1987, US Government Printing Office, p 36.

Association (ADRDA) is an extremely valuable resource for both health care professionals and clients. This association provides resource materials that help families to establish an effective management program at home, offers group support services for families experiencing the related stresses, and assists families in identifying community resources skilled in working with affected persons. However, many health care services do not address the needs of individuals with dementia. Persons especially likely to be unable to obtain adequate services are those without families, individuals from minority and ethnic groups, individuals experiencing disease onset in middle age, individuals residing in rural areas, veterans, and the poor (OTA, 1987, p. 45).

Support for informal caregivers is essential. The problems faced by families dealing with dementia are complex and very stressful and place them at high risk for experiencing financial difficulties as well as health problems. "The primary needs of informal caregivers are respite care, information on the diseases and care methods, information about services, and a broadened range of services" (OTA, 1987, p. 63). The range of services for persons with dementia and their families is very limited in many communities.

There is no question that the long-term care resources must be expanded. Statistical data show that the number of persons needing long-term ser-

vices will increase dramatically in the next several decades. Defining at-risk aggregates in the community, and subgroups within these aggregates who need these services, and pinpointing exactly at what intensity they need the services will be the future challenge of health care providers.

ANALYSIS OF LONG-TERM CARE SETTINGS

Contrary to popular belief, long-term care services are provided by diverse institutional and community-based settings rather than only by large state hospitals and county facilities. In fact, focus has been placed on developing a wide variety of alternative community-based services for all at-risk aggregates who need long-term care resources.

Institutional Settings

Figure 19-5 displays the types of institutions which provide long-term care services. By far, the largest number of institutionalized residents who require long-term care are served by various types of nursing homes: skilled nursing facilities, intermediate care facilities, and personal care facilities. The majority of residents in nursing homes (90.4 percent), mental hospitals (79.1 percent), and residential facilities (73.1 percent) are elderly. However, in facilities for mentally retarded persons, al-

Of the more than 2 million people served in institutions many are over the age of 65.

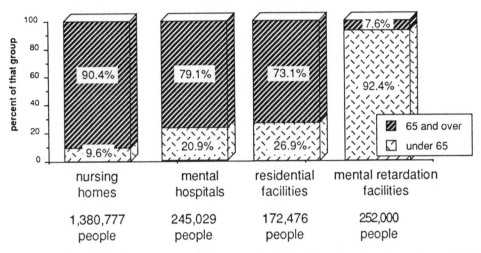

Figure 19-5   Numbers of residents in long-term care institutions and percentage of residents in each type of facility, by age. (From Kraus LE and Stoddard S: Chartbook on disability in the United States, an InfoUse Report, Washington, DC, 1989, National Institute on Disability and Rehabilitation Research, p 21.)

most all (92.4 percent) are under the age of 65; 76 percent are between 22 and 64 years of age (Kraus and Stoddard, 1989, p. 21).

As a result of the projected aging of the U.S. population and societal trends which bear on the availability of informal caregivers, there is a growing concern about access to long-term care services. It is anticipated that the elderly long-term care population will increase from an estimated 6.2 to 6.5 million in 1985 to about 14.3 million in 2020. During this same time period, the nursing home population is expected to increase to about 4.2 million because the most rapidly growing segment of the disabled elderly is the extremely dependent—those with five or more ADL limitations (GAO, 1988). ADL dependency dramatically increases a person's risk of being institutionalized: 5 percent of dependent elderly with only IADL limitations and approximately 12 percent of those with only one or two ADL dependencies reside in nursing homes; however, 50 percent of the aged with five or six ADL limitations reside in nursing homes (Scanlon, 1988, p. 7). Severely dependent elderly have difficulty obtaining

nursing home care (GAO, 1988). It is unlikely that this situation will improve, because the increase in nursing home beds has not kept pace with the aging of the American population. This has occurred because states have vigorously attempted to control Medicaid costs by limiting the supply of nursing home beds (Scanlon, 1988, December, p. 9).

During the 1970s and early 1980s, focus was placed on determining whether dependent elderly could be cared for in the community at a lower cost than in nursing homes. Medicare and Medicaid waiver programs and demonstration projects were established which allowed a percentage of the funds (less than the cost of nursing home care) that would normally have been used for nursing home care to be utilized for community-based services (Kemper, Applebaum, and Harrigan, 1987). Under those programs, case management mechanisms were established to ensure that individuals who could receive appropriate care at less cost in their own home or other settings could obtain the assistance needed to do so. However, because of the difficulty in identifying at-risk individuals who were likely to enter a nursing home, few of these projects demonstrated that this process and expanded community services decreased overall health care expenditures (Hughes, 1985; Kane, 1988; Weissert, Cready, and Pawelak, 1988). In spite of this finding, the case management model for delivering services to long-term care populations continues to be advocated, because some projects have demonstrated cost effectiveness and many persons with long-term care needs prefer to remain in their homes as long as possible (Capitman, 1988; GAO, 1988; Zawadski and Eng, 1988).

Defining who does and who does not need nursing home care is difficult, because nursing home need is a product of complex interactions among individual, medical, social, and economic circumstances. For example, individuals whose medical problems limit their functional abilities but who have available support systems are less likely to enter a nursing home than individuals with the same type of medical problems and functional difficulties who have no support systems to provide ongoing assistance.

Estimates of the number of persons likely to use nursing home care are based on characteristics of people who have used nursing homes in the past. On the basis of a study which merged data files estimating these characteristics for both the institutionalized and noninstitutionalized populations, the major predictors of nursing home use among the elderly are (General Accounting Office, 1983, p. 38):

- Whether they are dependent in the basic activities of daily living for eating, toileting, bathing, and dressing
- Whether they are mentally ill or have received a diagnosis of injury, cancer, or digestive, metabolic, blood, or genitourinary disorders
- How old they are (young-old or old-old)
- Whether, with these characteristics, they live alone or have help from spouse, family, or friends

Recent studies reflect similar characteristics among nursing home residents (GAO, 1988; Scanlon, 1988, December).

The importance of informal support networks in preventing institutionalization cannot be overestimated. As previously discussed, about 75 percent of the dependent elderly are cared for in their homes. Most families want to care for their disabled family members and keep them at home as long as possible. Often in doing so, these families experience extreme financial costs and stress and place themselves at risk for experiencing health problems (OTA, 1987). Families usually opt for institutional care as a solution for dealing with their stress only after their personal resources for coping have become exhausted (Johnson and Johnson, 1983; Pallett, 1990; Zarit and Zarit, 1982).

When visiting in the home environment, community health nurses should assess characteristics which place people at risk of requiring nursing home placement and should work with the client and family to explore other long-term care options. Adult day-care programs, respite care, alternative family care homes, residential care facilities, and domiciliary care facilities are a few examples of such options.

Community health nurses play a crucial role in assessing the level of care needed by clients who require long-term care services. Reducing inappropriate use of nursing home beds by people who are capable of living at home—a "gatekeeping mechanism"—can save costly and scarce health care resources and can better meet clients' physical and emotional needs.

Community-Based Settings

Community-based and home care settings are becoming increasingly important sites for the provision of long-term and acute-care services. Escalating health care expenditures in the early 1980s provided the impetus for refocusing health care delivery patterns; outpatient ambulatory care and office settings now provide many services once performed only in the inpatient setting, and home health care is increasingly being used to reduce the length of hospital stays. As a result of these trends, a new subindustry—the walk-in clinic—for providing acute care has arisen, home health care is increasing at an estimated average annual rate of 20 to 25 percent, and new methods for financing and delivering long-term care have emerged (GAO, 1988; Waldo, Levit, and Lazenby, 1986).

There are a variety of formal community settings that provide long-term care services including, but not limited to, board and care facilities, continuing care retirement communities, social/ health maintenance organizations, adult day care, community mental health and senior centers, outpatient facilities and clinics, sheltered workshops, and numerous voluntary organizations such as the Alzheimer's Disease and Related Disorders Association. However, the majority of the dependent disabled are cared for in their homes by informal caregivers (GAO, 1988; OTA, 1987). Formal community-based and home care services are usually used only when the informal care system breaks down, or informal supports are not available (OTA, 1987), and to supplement the care of informal providers.

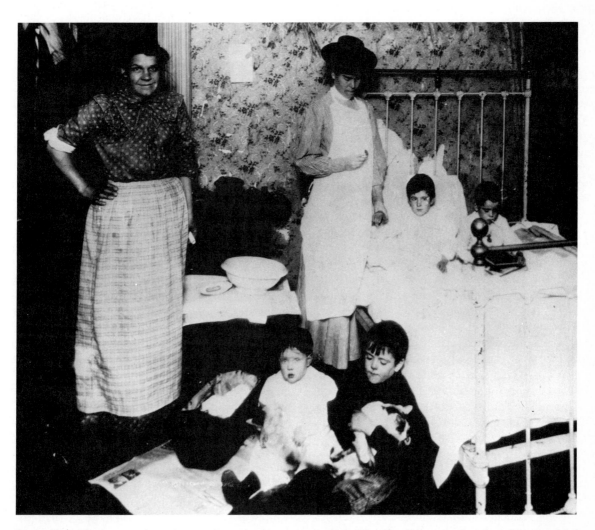

Figure 19-6   The increased emphasis on home health care is not new. Home health care services have been provided by public health nurses since the late 1800s. Individuals across the life-span benefit from these services. (Courtesy of Metropolitan Life Insurance.)

Formal Home Care Services

Home care is not a new long-term care concept. In fact, modern community health nursing practice originated from the organized provision of home nursing services to the sick poor (refer to Figure 19-6). In the early 1900s care of the ill and disabled in their home environments was the traditional form of health care for most people (Spiegel, 1987). Over the years, this type of care has been reaffirmed as an essential community service from a public health perspective (Administration of home health, 1945; Bedside nursing care, 1945; Haupt, 1953; Olson, 1986).

Home care includes a broad range of home-based health and social services such as home management assistance, personal care, consumer education, and financial counseling services. Social home care services are covered under Title XX of the Social Security Act, for clients who qualify for Title XX assistance (Title XX is discussed later in this chapter). These services are provided by diverse community agencies such as local departments of social service, family service organizations, and councils on agencies.

During the past 10 years, demonstration projects have experimented with different approaches for delivering home care. One approach has been to mix formal (professionally directed) services with informal supports (family and friends). Others extend the informal system with homemaker services and Meals on Wheels. Another approach has been to place nursing home candidates in foster homes; the paid caregiver in the foster home provides a private room, meals, laundry, assistance with ADLs, and 24-hour assistance. A community health nurse provides nursing care, education of the caregiver, and ongoing assessment. The life satisfaction scores of people in foster home settings such as these have been high (Oktay and Volland, 1987).

A very important component of home care is home *health* care. Based on materials prepared by multiple professionals organizations (such as the National Association of Home Health Agencies, the ANA, and the NLN), the Department of Health, Education and Welfare (now the Department of Health and Human Services) defined home health care as (Warhola, 1980, p. 9)

that component of a continuum of comprehensive health care whereby health services are provided to individuals and families in their places of residence for the purpose of promoting, maintaining or restoring health, or of maximizing the level of independence, while minimizing the effects of disability and illness, including terminal illness. Services appropriate to the needs of the individual patient and family are planned, coordinated, and made available by providers organized for the delivery of home health care through the use of employed staff, contractual arrangements, or a combination of the two patterns.

Home health services are made available based upon patient care needs as determined by an objective patient assessment administered by a multidisciplinary team or a single health professional. Centralized professional coordination and case management are included. These services are provided under a plan of care that includes, but is not limited to appropriate service components such as medical, dental, nursing, social work, pharmacy, laboratory, physical therapy, speech therapy, occupational therapy, nutrition, homemaker–home health aide service, transportation, chore services, and provision of medical equipment and supplies.

Multiple types of agencies (refer to Table 19-1) provide home health care services. Both the governmental and private sectors of our health care delivery system are active in delivering home health services. The number and types of home health care agencies have proliferated in the past two decades, mainly due to the passage of the Medicare health insurance program for the elderly and the Medicaid health program for the poor in 1965. Both programs established mechanisms for reimbursing home health services and provided an impetus for the expansion of these services across the country. Proprietary and institutional affiliated agencies (hospital and skilled nursing facility) are growing the most rapidly.

The proliferation of home health care agencies provided an impetus for the development in 1986 of *Standards of Home Health Nursing Practice* by the American Nurses' Association. These standards guide agencies and nurses in providing care of the highest quality for home health care clients and read as follows (ANA, 1986, pp. 5-19)*:

---

*Reprinted with permission from Standards of Community Health Nursing Practice. © 1986, American Nurses' Association, Kansas City, Mo.

TABLE 19-1   Types of home health care agencies in the United States*

Type of agency	Description of agency
Official	A governmental or public agency, usually a local health department, which is supported by state and local taxes. Official agencies are mandated by law to provide certain specific services, such as communicable disease follow-up. They provide health promotion and disease prevention services as well as home health care.
Voluntary	A private, nonprofit agency whose operating funds come largely from individual contributions, fees-for-service, united community funds, contracts for service, grants, and other nonofficial sources of funding. Voluntary agencies are governed by a board of directors. These agencies are not required by law to provide specific types of services; they primarily, but not exclusively, provide home health care services. The visiting nurse associations traditionally have been the major voluntary organizations which provide home health care services in a local community.
Combination	A combined governmental (a local health department) and voluntary agency (a VNA), whose operating funds came from both official and nonofficial sources. This organizational structure was promoted for the purposes of preventing duplication of services, decreasing continuity of care difficulties and reducing the cost of delivering local health care services. A combination agency provides both health promotion/disease prevention and home health care services.
Private, nonprofit	A privately owned agency which is tax exempt because of its nonprofit status. Unlike voluntary agencies, these agencies are governed by the owner(s) of the organization. Their major source of revenue is fee-for-service. Private nonprofit agencies are usually established to provide home health care services only.
Proprietary	A private agency established to make a profit. These agencies are not eligible for tax exemption. They are governed by their owner(s), who are increasingly large corporations. Their major source of revenue is a fee for service. Like the private, nonprofit agencies, proprietary agencies are usually established to provide home health care services only.
Hospital-based	A home health care agency run and governed by a hospital. Sources of revenue and tax status vary depending on the type of hospital (governmental, voluntary, private, nonprofit, or proprietary) which has established the home health care agency. It is predicted that the numbers of hospital-based home health care agencies will increase dramatically in the next decade.

*Refer to Chapter 5 for further discussion of official and voluntary agencies.

From Health Care Financing Administration: Medicare program; home health agencies: conditions of participation and reduction in recordkeeping requirements, 42 CFR, Part 484, Sections 484.1 through 484.52. Washington, DC, October 1989, US Department of Health and Human Services; Hirsh L, Klein M, and Marlowe G: Combining public health nursing agencies: a case study in Philadelphia, New York, 1967, Department of PHN, NLN, p 3.

STANDARD I. Organization of Home Health Services

All home health services are planned, organized, and directed by a master's-prepared professional nurse with experience in community health and administration.

STANDARD II. Theory

The nurse applies theoretical concepts as a basis for decisions in practice.

STANDARD III. Data Collection

The nurse continuously collects and records data that are comprehensive, accurate, and systematic.

STANDARD IV. Diagnosis

The nurse uses health assessment data to determine nursing diagnoses.

STANDARD V. Planning

The nurse develops care plans that establish goals.

The care plan is based on nursing diagnoses and incorporates therapeutic, preventive, and rehabilitative nursing actions.

STANDARD VI. Intervention.

The nurse, guided by the care plan, intervenes to provide comfort, to restore, improve, and promote health, to prevent complications and sequelae of illness, and to effect rehabilitation.

STANDARD VII. Evaluation

The nurse continually evaluates the client's and family's responses to interventions in order to determine progress toward goal attainment and to revise the data base, nursing diagnoses, and plan of care.

STANDARD VIII. Continuity of Care

The nurse is responsible for the client's appropriate and uninterrupted care along the health care continuum, and therefore uses discharge planning, case management, and coordination of community resources.

STANDARD IX. Interdisciplinary Collaboration

The nurse initiates and maintains a liaison relationship with all appropriate health care providers to assure that all efforts effectively complement one another.

STANDARD X. Professional Development

The nurse assumes responsibility for professional development and contributes to the professional growth of others.

STANDARD XI. Research

The nurse participates in research activities that contribute to the profession's continuing development of knowledge of home health care.

STANDARD XII. Ethics

The nurse uses the code for nurses established by the American Nurses' Association as a guide for ethical decision making in practice.

Presented on pp. 754-755 are four case histo-

ries which represent the type of care offered by voluntary home health agencies across the country. The Visiting Nurse Service of the Toledo District Nurse Association, the agency which published these case histories, has been caring for elderly and disabled persons for more than 83 years. Throughout these years, this organization has provided millions of home visits to needy persons (Visiting Nurse Service, 1984, p. 57.)

These case histories clearly illustrate that individuals across the life-span need community-based home care services. They also reflect the increasing complexity of client care demands and the need for coordinated, multidisciplinary home health services. Most importantly, they show that skilled home-based nursing services can make a difference: they help families to strengthen their coping abilities and they assist disabled persons to improve their functional capabilities and avoid unnecessary institutionalization.

VNS Caring in Toledo, Ohio: Four Case Examples*

CASE EXAMPLE ONE

Sixteen-year-old boy run over by train which inflicted massive trauma resulting in amputation of left hindquarter, amputation of arm, multiple pelvic fractures, fracture of transverse process, avulsion of urethra-prostate-testes and L-sileium exposing peritoneal sac, laceration L. ureter and L. iliac arteries, resulted in colostomy, supra-pubic cystotomy, hemi-pelvectomy, bilateral orchiectomy, skin grafts to hip sockets, etc.

After only five weeks in the hospital, client was allowed to go home (on Coordinated Home Care, saving over 30 hospital days) with a 24″ × 24″ graft in L pelvic area with open draining area. The VNS Home Care Coordinator managed this complex referral, coordinated arrangements for special dressing supplies and equipment and facilitated care throughout the period of need. The case nurse said, "The coordinator made it all come together and work." Clearly, the value of the coordinator having home care experience and familiarity with agency operations was evident.

Nursing visits were daily for two weeks, then reduced to three times a week as the family became more confident in care. Nursing activities included aseptic wound care, supervision of colostomy care, suprapubic catheter care, observation for complications with prompt intervention, instruction of family in all aspects of care and encouraging this adolescent to become independent in ADL's. To promote usual family activities, the nurse supported their decision to go on a weekend

camping trip within the first two weeks and arranged to make visits at the local campsite.

Physical and occupational therapy services were provided for ADL's, gait training, transfers, strengthening and stump wrapping. Since this boy was left-dominant, he had to relearn all activities one-handed with the nondominant side. When a left arm prosthesis was secured, the OT (who, herself has an upper extremity prosthesis) resumed visits to aid in learning its use.

A total of 129 home health visits were provided over a nine-month period to aid in his excellent recovery, and he has now returned to school.

Although several intervening hospitalizations were required for re-evaluations and surgical revisions, none were necessary for complications, e.g., infection.

This example of teamwork included various surgery specialists, numerous VNS staff, and, of course, the family.

CASE EXAMPLE TWO

A 70-year-old patient who had transhepatic biliary disease, probably cancer of head of pancreas and a history of cancer of gallbladder was admitted to service after insertion of a transhepatic ring catheter which allows bile to drain from the common duct to the duodenum.

GOVERNMENTAL LONG-TERM CARE FINANCING

The Health Care Financing Administration (HCFA) is the primary source of funding for long-term services. The major portion of public expenditures for long-term care services goes to institutional care, with the Medicaid program being the principal payor for this type of care. The Medicaid program pays for over half of all nursing home expenditures. It supports long-term institutional care in a variety of facilities, including skilled nursing facilities (SNFs), intermediate care facilities (ICFs), intermediate care facilities for the mentally retarded (ICFs/MR), and mental hospitals. The Medicare program pays for skilled and complementing skilled (home health aide services) home health care services, and care in

---

Four Case Examples—cont'd

The patient and family were quite anxious re: involved procedures. The visiting nurse instructed the family in home care including such things as withdrawing of bile, irrigating ring catheter technique, dressing changes using aseptic technique, changing catheter plug, and teaching of signs of complications, in addition to monitoring hypertension status, nutrition/hydration, reactions to x-ray treatment, medications and pain control.

After verbal and demonstrative teaching, the family was able to provide the necessary care and patient was discharged in stabilized condition.

CASE EXAMPLE THREE

A 5-month-old infant who had been normal at birth developed pneumococcal meningitis with resulting hydrocephalus, severe neurologic deficits and seizure disorders. The mother, who was single and 16 years old, wanted to care for the child at home as long as possible so a referral was made to VNS.

At the time of hospital discharge, the child was totally unresponsive and had no purposeful movements, was on continuous gastric tube feedings with a Kangaroo pump, and required a suction machine and vaporizer. Nursing care consisted of providing and teaching re: dressing changes around the G-tube, tube irrigation, frequent repositioning, ROM, skin care and hygiene, relaxation and stimulation techniques, and use of Kangaroo pump. Additionally, the home care nurse assessed neurological and respiratory status and provided frequent intervention related to medication regimen, irritability, and seizure control. A home health aide assisted the mother with care, bathing and stimulation techniques. A total of 54 home health visits were provided over a five-month period.

The Maternal Child Health nurse supported this young mother in her difficult decision to place the child in an extended care unit for the developmentally disabled at one year of age (where she visits frequently and takes her home every other weekend) so she could return to school.

At the time of discharge from VNS, this young child could take water orally, respond to the mother and had some purposeful movement.

CASE EXAMPLE FOUR

A 76-year-old client had a long history of Crohn's disease and malabsorption syndrome, and after multiple admissions for weight loss, malnutrition and dehydration, a permanent subclavian line was inserted in early summer of 1981 for total parenteral nutrition. It became apparent that adequate nutrition could only be attained through TPN and she would need regular infusions of amino acids, electrolytes, minerals and, eventually, fatty acids through this subclavian line. VNS nurses worked closely with physicians, hospital nurses, nutritionists, pharmacists, social workers, and patient's family in planning for adequate predischarge teaching and adequate home support for this patient. Through a joint effort between VNS and the community hospital, the patient's elderly brother has been successfully managing her four-times-a-week home TPN infusion, and once-a-week lipid infusion. This patient has the original subclavian line in place (for over two years) and it has remained free of any signs and symptoms of infection for over two years. In addition to care for the subclavian line and TPN infusions, VNS has helped the brother learn to care for the patient's permanent colostomy and chronic abdominal fistula.

Patient's condition has deteriorated gradually over the last two years; she now has an indwelling foley catheter and is essentially bed bound, requiring the services of a home health aide. Patient appears to have suffered at least one CVA and has been hospitalized for erratic blood sugars, and abnormal blood values which reflects the necessary and frequent nursing intervention. Nutritionally she has remained stable, demonstrating a weight gain of sixteen pounds over two years (originally weight was 88 pounds and now is 104 pounds).

Through the joint efforts of VNS, the community hospital, and the family, this patient has been able to go home and remain at home, without serious nutritional compromise, over the last two years.

---

*From Visiting Nurse Service (VNS) of Toledo—Eighty-three years of caring. Caring, 3:61, 1984. Case examples were written by Janet Blaufuss, RN, former Executive Director of the Visiting Nurse Service of the Toledo District Nurse Association, Toledo, Ohio, 1984.

skilled nursing facilities during acute phases of illness. This program does not support long-term care in nursing homes and other facilities providing unskilled or custodial services (GAO, 1988).

Noninstitutional long-term care or home care is currently funded by four federal programs—title XVIII (Medicare), title XIX (Medicaid), title XX (block grants to states for social services) of the Social Security Act, and title III of the Older Americans Act (O'Shaughnessy, Price, and Griffith, 1985, October 17, pp. XI-XII). The basic characteristics of each of these programs were discussed in Chapter 4. The type of home care services financially supported by each program is presented below.

Medicare (Title XVIII)

The largest governmental expenditures for home health care services are made by Medicare. Medicare expenditures for home health care are increasing dramatically: Between 1968 and 1985, Medicare spending for home health care had an annual growth rate of 24 percent. Medicare expenditures for home health care in 1968 were $60 million and in 1985 were $2.3 billion. It is anticipated that Medicare outlays for home health care will increase significantly because of the aging of the population (Waldo, Levit, and Lazenby, 1986, p. 11). It has been estimated that individuals 65 years of age and above receive 85 to 90 percent of the home health services provided in the United States (Cassak, 1984; Ginzberg, Balinsky, and Ostow, 1984).

Both Part A (hospital insurance) and Part B (supplemental medical insurance) of Medicare include provisions for home health care. Medicare reimburses a home health care agency for the following services (HCFA, 1989, October):

- Part-time or *intermittent* skilled nursing services provided by or under the supervision of a registered nurse
- *Intermittent* physical, occupational, or speech therapy provided by or under the supervision of a qualified therapist
- *Intermittent* medical social services provided by or under the supervision of a qualified social worker

- *Intermittent* home health services provided by a home health aide who has completed a competency evaluation program supervised by a registered nurse who possesses a minimum of 2 years of nursing experience, at least 1 year of which must be in the provision of home health care, and who has supervised home health aide services for at least 6 months
- Medical supplies (other than drugs and medications) and the use of medical appliances
- Hospice services including short-term inpatient care, nursing care, therapy services, medical social services, home health aide services, physician services, and counseling.

Provisions of the Omnibus Budget Reconciliation Act of 1980 (Public Law 96-499) expanded the home health benefits offered by Medicare so that beneficiaries are permitted unlimited home health visits without the requirement for a prior hospital stay or payment of a deductible amount. To qualify for those benefits, Medicare beneficiaries must be *homebound;* the services must be prescribed and periodically reviewed by a physician (at least once every 60 days); and the client must need part-time or *intermittent, skilled* nursing care and/or therapy services (physical, occupational, or speech therapy). When home health aide services are needed, the registered nurse, or appropriate professional staff member if only therapy services are provided, must make a supervisory visit to the client's residence at least every 2 weeks (HCFA, 1989, October).

Landmark changes in the Medicare program have occurred as a result of a lawsuit brought against Medicare by the National Association for Homecare (NAHC) in the late 1980s. The suit contained two essential claims: (1) the challenge to the part time or intermittent policy for length of care allowed clients, and (2) how "medical necessity" is interpreted to qualify a client for care. The successful conclusion to the lawsuit did not change Medicare regulations but did change HCFA's interpretation of them, so that more services could be provided. Several of these changes are noteworthy (Staggers' Lawsuit, 1988, pp. 1-3):

1. Clients are considered homebound if they

attend adult day care centers, renal dialysis clinics, or outpatient radiation or chemotherapy facilities when the purpose is to receive medical care. Regarding adult day care patients, it is the agency's responsibility to demonstrate that attendance at the day center is for the purpose of receiving medical care.

2. A new skilled service is described—skilled nursing management and evaluation of a patient care plan—which allows coverage for nurses who need to manage certain complex unskilled care cases.

3. Specific coverage standards are set out for venipuncture in stable and unstable patients. For example, a client receiving prothrombin whose blood test results indicate stability within the therapeutic range will qualify for a skilled nursing visit once a month to continue appropriate monitoring.

4. A client cannot be denied solely on the basis of having a chronic disease or terminal illness.

5. An order for "personal care" of a home health aide is allowed, with the boundaries of that personal care to be determined by the nurse following a care plan, rather than by a physician.

6. Coverage of family counseling is specifically recognized as part of the function of a medical social services visit, in which family counseling is incidental to beneficiary counseling and designed to remove an impediment to the delivery of safe and effective care.

The *Medicare Home Health Agency Manual,* known as HIM 11 (HCFA, 1989), has been rewritten to address these changes. It contains many case examples clarifying coverage criteria and is useful on a daily basis for the staff nurse.

With its statutory emphases on part-time acute and postacute treatment of illness, the Medicare program does not adequately address the long-term care needs of the aging population (GAO, 1988). The homebound and the part-time or intermittent skilled nursing criteria for eligibility make it impossible for many chronically ill or disabled aging persons to qualify for Medicare home health care benefits. With public expenditures on health care rising dramatically, it is unlikely that the Medicare program will be expanded to cover additional long-term care services for the aged. Finding new approaches for meeting the long-term care needs of the elderly is a growing challenge for health care providers.

Managed health care systems are emerging as a way of financing home health care. Managed care controls, monitors, reviews, and directs health care in the most efficient manner and recommends the most appropriate treatment in the most efficient environment. Client's symptoms are usually controlled by the payor in a way that does not overutilize the delivery system.

Managed systems include health maintenance organizations (HMOs) and preferred provider organizations (PPOs). Home health agencies have developed relationships with HMOs because the federal government has encouraged Medicare beneficiaries to join HMOs. Under a managed care system, community health nurses have greater control placed on the delivery of home care services so that the care plan is well organized. Usually an assessment visit is authorized; following the nursing assessment, the plan of care is discussed with the system reviewer, who then gives authorization for care, usually 1 week at a time. The goal is cost containment and systematic allocation of resources (Daniels, 1988; McNiff, 1988; St. Armand, 1988). Finding new approaches for meeting the long-term care needs of the elderly is a growing challenge for health care providers.

Medicaid (Title XIX)

Current Medicaid statute provides states with the authority to include a variety of home and community-based services in their Medicaid programs. Medicaid programs can cover case management, personal care services, day care, private duty nursing, and home health services (GAO, 1988). Unlike the requirements of the Medicare program, home health under Medicaid includes *skilled* and *unskilled* services. To qualify for home care benefits under Medicaid, clients must meet income eligibility requirements, have the services ordered by a physician, and have the plan of care reviewed by a physician every 60 days. Clients do not need to be homebound to receive Medicaid benefits.

Since Medicaid is a state-administered program, the range of home care benefits offered varies from state to state. However, in order to be federally subsidized under Medicaid, a state must provide at least home health services. Personal care services are not mandated by the federal government (Federal Register, 1985, March). States also have the freedom to determine eligibility requirements and the amount of service they will reimburse under Medicaid. Some states extend home care benefits to the "medically needy," those persons who do not qualify for regular Medicaid benefits but who have inadequate financial resources to meet health care costs.

Section 2176 of the Omnibus Budget Reconciliation Act of 1981 (Public Law 97-35) expanded the range of long-term services which can be offered by the Medicaid program; this act established the Medicaid Waiver Authority to implement 2176 Waiver programs of home- and community-based care. "Under these programs, states can provide a comprehensive array of medical and social services including case management, homemaker and home health aides, personal care, adult day care, habilitation care and respite care to avoid more costly institutional care" (United States Senate, Committee on Finance, 1984, p. 78). These programs serve individuals in the community who would require the level of care provided in a skilled nursing facility or intermediate care facility if they did not receive 2176 Waiver services. The costs of the community-based waiver services cannot exceed the cost of institutional care.

Although the major portion of public expenditures for long-term care for poor people is provided under the Medicaid program, many low-income persons still have unmet long-term care service needs. In some states, home health agencies are finding it increasingly difficult to serve Medicaid clients, because they are often reimbursed for their services at a cost less than the true cost of providing the service. In other states, eligibility requirements are restrictive, and the range of services offered by the Medicaid program is inadequate. Discrepancies such as these can prevent a large number of people from receiving needed long-term care.

Social Services Block Grants to States (Title XX)

The Title XX program was established by the 1975 Amendments to Social Security Act. The Omnibus Budget Reconciliation Act of 1981 (Public Law 97-35) altered Title XX, reformulating it as a federally funded Social Services Block Grant (Blancato, 1986). The Social Services Block Grant, like other block grants, provides the states freedom in determining the populations to be served and the types of services to be offered. The Social Services Block Grant program provides funding for a comprehensive array of social services directed toward the following goals (GAO, 1986, May):

- Achieving or maintaining economic self-support to prevent, reduce, or eliminate financial dependency
- Achieving or maintaining self-sufficiency, including reduction or prevention of dependency for daily care
- Preventing or remedying neglect, abuse, or exploitation of children and adults unable to protect their own interests; or preserving, rehabilitating, or reuniting families
- Preventing or reducing inappropriate institutional care by providing for community-based care, home-based care, or other forms of less intensive care
- Securing referral or admission for institutional care when other forms of care are not appropriate, or providing services to individuals in institutions

A broad range of home-based services can be provided by the states under Title XX including homemaker, home health aide, home management, personal care, consumer education, and financial counseling services. As with Medicaid, the benefits offered under this program vary from state to state. In order to qualify for Title XX services, clients must meet income eligibility requirements.

In order for states to participate in the Title XX program, they must establish a Comprehensive Annual Service Program plan that outlines the services they will provide, to whom, and by what methods. Federal spending under Title XX is capped, and funds are allocated among states on the basis of their populations. Social Services Block Grant funds aid states in meeting local needs not met by other social service agencies in the community (GAO, 1986, May). However, the limited funding for this program does not allow states to expand home care services significantly.

Title III under the Older Americans Act of 1965

The Older Americans Act of 1965 established the Administration on Aging in the Department of Health, Education, and Welfare and authorized a variety of health and social services projects for aging citizens (refer to Chapter 4). In 1978, amendments to the Older Americans Act consolidated several existing titles (Titles III, V, and VII) of the original act and revised and expanded Title III. Title III is now designed to encourage and help state and local agencies to concentrate resources on developing a comprehensive and coordinated system to serve elderly citizens age 60 and over (House Select Committee on Aging, 1985).

TABLE 19-2   Comparison of essential characteristics of four governmental programs funding in-home services

	Social Security Act			Older Americans Act
	Title XVIII	Title XIX	Title XX	Title III
Services authorized				
Nursing	Yes	Yes	No	Yes
Therapy	Yes	Yes	No	Yes
Home health aide	Yes	Yes	Yes	Yes
Homemaker	No	No	Yes	Yes
Chore	No	No	Yes	Yes
Medical supplies and appliances	No	No	Yes	Yes
Program eligibility				
Client must meet age requirement	Yes	No	No	Yes
Client must meet income requirement	No	Yes	Yes	No
Client must need part-time or intermittent skilled nursing care	Yes	No	No	No
Client must be homebound	Yes	No	No	No
Services to client must be authorized by a physician in accordance with a plan of care	Yes	Yes	No	No
Services must be included in state plan	*	Yes	Yes	Yes
Administration	Federal	State	State	State
Funding	Open ended	Open ended	Capped	Capped

*Federally administered program—no state plan required.

From General Accounting Office (GAO): Improved knowledge base would be helpful in reaching policy decisions on providing long-term, in-home services for the elderly, HRD-82-4, Washington, DC, October 26, 1981, US Government Printing Office, p 26.

Title III mandates a broad range of social services for the elderly, including but not limited to home health, home health aide, homemaker, and nutritional services. The only client eligibility requirement for participation in the Title III program is age 60 and over. Unlike Medicare, clients do not need to be homebound and do not need skilled nursing care in order to qualify for home health benefits.

Title III is a state-administered program, carried out under the direction of the Department of Health and Human Services. Federal expenditures under Title III are capped. In fiscal 1985, appropriations for Title III totaled $785 million. Of these funds, $265 million were allocated for supportive services and $68 million for home-delivered nutrition services. A significant amount ($336 million) of these monies was also appropriated for congregate nutrition services. Recently, emphasis has been placed on using OAA monies for home care and supportive services because of the increasing number of the oldest-old. These fragile elderly frequently find it difficult to use community-based services. Legislation allows states to transfer a percentage of their OAA allocation among funding categories and increasingly states are doing so in order to expand homecare services (Senate Special Committee on Aging, 1985, February). The 1987 Admendments to this act authorized nonmedical in-home services (e.g., in-home respite, telephone and visiting reassurance, and chore maintenance) for the *dependent* elderly (GAO, 1988, p. 287).

Displayed in Table 19-2 is a comparison of the essential characteristics of the four governmental funding programs just described.

Increasingly, federal and state governments are focusing attention on in-home services under all of their programs in order to reduce inappropriate, costly institutional care. As this shift occurs, emphasis is being placed on evaluating the cost effectiveness of community-based services. There is a concern that increasing the numbers of people eligible for home care and liberalizing coverage of services, would increase the overall national health bill (Rivlin and Wiener, 1988). The cost effectiveness of community alternatives to institu-

tionalization has not yet been conclusively proved (U.S. Senate Committee on Finance, 1984, p. 80).

LEGISLATION INFLUENCING LONG-TERM CARE SERVICE DELIVERY

In addition to the legislation which authorizes funding for long-term home care services, several other pieces of federal legislation influence long-term care service delivery. Some of this legislation is discussed below.

Omnibus Budget Reconciliation Act (OBRA) of 1980

In December 1980, President Jimmy Carter signed into law the Omnibus Budget Reconciliation Act of 1980. Included in this law are provisions relating to home care benefits under Title XVIII (Medicare). The emphasis of the act was to encourage the use of noninstitutional services such as home health care to fight escalating health care costs.

The amendments relating to home health care were as follows:

1. Unlimited home health visits would be available under parts A and B of the Medicare program.
2. The existing 3-day prior hospitalization requirement for home health benefits under part A would be eliminated.
3. The $60 deductible, which home health benefits under part B are subject to, would be eliminated.
4. The need for occupational therapy would be added to the list of qualifying criteria for home health benefits.
5. The elimination of the requirement that proprietary (for-profit) home health agencies have state licenses to participate in the Medicare home health program.

OBRA legislation since 1980 has in some years contained amendments that expand or restrict long-term care services. For example, as discussed previously in this chapter, this legislation in 1981 created a Social Services Block Grant and 2176 Medicaid Waivers. The latest OBRA Act (OBRA-

89) increased Medicare and Medicaid payments for hospice care but froze fees for durable medical equipment (DME) (NAHC, 1989, December). Omnibus Budget Reconciliation legislation needs to be monitored carefully by health professionals because amendments significantly influence the type of long-term care/services funded by the federal government.

Channeling: A National Long-Term Care Demonstration

In 1980, Congress appropriated $20 million for a long-term care demonstration program, with focus on the concept of channeling. The responsibility for managing this money was placed in the Office of the Assistant Secretary for Planning and Evaluation, which is funded by the Health Care Financing Administration and the Administration on Aging. Channeling entailed creating new agencies with three interrelated functions: to "channel" all or part of the long-term care population—that is, to match those in need with appropriate long-term care service settings; to plan for the long-term care service system to ensure that sufficient suppliers of needed services and settings would be available; and to coordinate directly or indirectly the provision of long-term care services (Baxter, Applebaum, Callahan, Christianson, and Day, 1983).

The National Long-Term Care Demonstration was based on the assumption that channeling—a managed system of community-based long-term care for the disabled elderly—could be established, operated, and produce results more favorable than the present arrangements for long-term care. Channeling was not designed to address all the problems of long-term care, nor was it necessarily seen as the only alternative for improving the match of needs with services. It was not, for example, designed as a source of extensive funding to be used to establish new or expand existing service programs on a communitywide basis. Nor was it intended to intervene directly in the professional practice of doctors, nurses, and other individual practitioners. It was intended to address a specific set of deficiencies in the current system and to achieve the following objectives (Baxter,

Applebaum, Callahan, Christianson, and Day, 1983):

- *Improved targeting* of service resources to those in greatest need
- *Improved matching* of client needs and services (both formal and informal)
- *Outreach* to identify and attract the target population
- *Screening* to determine whether an applicant is part of that target population
- *Comprehensive needs assessment* to determine individual problems, resources, and service needs
- *Care planning* to specify the types and amounts of care to be provided to meet the identified needs of individuals
- *Service arrangement* to implement the care plan through both formal and informal providers
- *Monitoring* to ensure that services are provided as planned and modified as necessary
- *Reassessment* to adjust care plans to changing needs

These core channeling functions were designed to identify the population most appropriate for community care, to provide information about individual needs and services, and to arrange for and coordinate services that most appropriately and efficiently meet those needs. Although the channeling demonstration projects were not successful in reducing overall aggregate health care costs, they were moderately successful in improving quality of life (GAO, 1988, pp. 36-37).

Diagnostic-Related Groups

Another piece of legislation has significantly challenged the long-term care system. On April 20, 1983, President Reagan signed Public Law 98-12, which includes the establishment of a prospective payment system (PPS), based on the 467 diagnostic related groups (DRGs), that allow pretreatment diagnosis billing categories for almost all hospitals reimbursed by Medicare. "Culminating a series of hospital billing and reimbursement reforms that were initiated decades ago, these changes will permanently alter the nature of health care delivery as we have known it" (Shaffer, 1983, p. 388).

The importance of prospective payment for hospital discharges is that health care providers are paid at rates that are set in advance and are fixed for certain periods. Thus, if a hospital treats a client for less than the amount fixed under the DRG, it can keep the profit; if it charges more, it must absorb the loss. Greater efficiency in client care became imperative; under the traditional system, the more a hospital spent, the more it was paid by Medicare.

DRGs have influenced hospital care in two ways: patients are experiencing much shorter hospital stays, and they are being discharged sicker than before the advent of DRGs ("quicker and sicker"). These changes have influenced the complexity and quantity of community health nursing services: there are more requests for service and the requests are technically more complicated (Kornblatt and Fisher, 1985). Further, community health nurses are spending more time teaching the family to care for the ill members, families are learning to work with complex equipment such as morphine pumps, hyperalimentation lines, and Hickman catheters. Nurses with critical care and "high tech" skills are moving from the hospital setting to the home. Community-based nurses are updating their technical expertise, and are learning to administer total parenteral nutrition, intravenous antibiotic therapy, intravenous chemotherapy, oxygen, and feeding tubes. Testing of blood levels for cholesterol, glucose, and clotting factors is also routine, as are blood pressure monitoring, apnea monitoring, cardiac pacing, rate and rhythm, and fetal monitoring.

One development that vividly demonstrates the growth of high technology in home care is pediatric home care, which is the fastest-growing segment of the home care field (Laxton, 1989). This is occurring because of a recent phenomenon in childbirth—infants born with the human immunodeficiency virus infection or anomalies requiring complex care. Another reason for growth is that home care is less costly than institutional care. Neonatology has made tremendous advances in the past few years, and babies who would have died are now living. Nationally there are about 2000 children whose respiratory function depends daily on the assistance of mechanical ventilators. Thousands more depend on parenteral nutrition, intravenous drugs, and other advanced devices. Helping parents deal with these issues on a daily basis has made unprecedented demands on both professionals and the lay public (Lidke 1989, Fall). Many children would remain in the hospital if pediatric home care services were not available. Thus, pediatric home care is becoming a subspecialty in the home care field.

Balanced Budget and Emergency Deficit Control Act of 1985 (Gramm-Rudman-Hollings Act)

Signed into law on December 12, 1985, this act mandated that the federal budget be balanced ($0 deficit) by 1991. To accomplish this, stipulations were established to reduce the federal deficit by a specified amount each year for a 6-year period, beginning in 1986. The General Accounting Office (GAO) had the responsibility of analyzing federal spending to determine whether the deficit reduction targets could be met. If they could not be met, across-the-board reduction sufficient to bring the deficit in line with the targeted goal of the Gramm-Rudman-Hollings Act was to be made in domestic spending programs. Selected antipoverty programs (e.g., Medicaid and AFDC) were exempt from cuts, and health programs such as Medicare and Migrant Health Centers could be reduced by no more than 2 percent per year.

Although the U.S. Supreme Court declared the Gramm-Rudman-Hollings Act unconstitutional on July 7, 1986, members of Congress indicated at that time their intention to rectify the constitutional shortcomings of this act to achieve a balanced federal budget (Spiegel, 1987, p. 404). Gramm-Rudman-Hollings reduction is now addressed in the OBRA legislation. The 1989 OBRA contained reduction stipulations for Part A and Part B Medicare payments (NAHC, 1989, December). Achieving a balanced federal budget is necessary and long overdue. The federal deficit is creating a crisis. However, legislation that mandates across-the-board cuts, regardless of worth, is not a sound way to address this crisis.

BARRIERS TO ADEQUATE COMMUNITY-BASED LONG-TERM CARE

Various problems in the community and in the health care delivery system make it difficult for clients who have long-term care needs to avoid unnecessary institutionalization. These problems can be summarized under four categories: (1) lack of community resources, (2) acute-focused reimbursement mechanisms, (3) fragmentation and lack of coordination, and (4) family burnout.

Lack of Community Resources

A significant factor preventing many of the chronically disabled to obtain adequate long-term care is the scarcity of formal alternatives to institutionalization (GAO, 1988; NCOA, 1986; OTA, 1987). After it is ascertained by care givers and families that an individual cannot live at home without support or health care, staying in the community depends upon social supports, adequate financial resources, and the availability of health and social services.

Many older people, and especially those above 75, have characteristics that place them at risk for being institutionalized. Unfortunately the very dependent elderly often find it difficult to obtain needed services in the home. Data from the 1982 National Long-Term Care Survey showed that 5 percent (168,000 aging persons) of the dependent elderly needed more help with ADLs and 34 percent (1.1 million persons) were not receiving the help they needed with IADLs (GAO, 1986, December, p. 50).

The lack of adequate housing (and especially supportive congregate or domiciliary housing for people who live alone) for the frail elderly and disabled is a major barrier to community long-term care services. One problem with current housing arrangements is affordability: fuel prices, interest rates, and construction costs have all made housing costs difficult to manage on a limited income. Another problem is that households are becoming smaller; while rents are increasing, the number of people paying rent is decreasing as a result of increasing divorce rates and increasing numbers of aged and deinstitutionalized people living alone.

In large cities, single room occupancy (SRO) hotels, formerly a source of housing for many, are being converted into condominiums.

In some communities, innovative housing programs, sponsored by the Department of Housing and Urban Development, have provided suitable alternatives to institutionalization. The National Housing Act, Section 202, provides a direct loan program based on the current securities marketed by the Treasury Department. The level of these interest rates makes housing projects attractive to builders; they are financially sound as well. Section 8 of the same act provides for direct subsidies to individuals who occupy Section 8 housing. The sponsors of such housing, usually nonprofit organizations, receive full market rent. However, the federal government pays a portion of the rent.

Acute-Focused Reimbursement Mechanisms

Another barrier to effective long-term care is inadequate financial coverage for needed long-term care services. The Medicare program was specifically designed to provide protection for acute-care needs (Rivlin and Wiener, 1988). Once a client's condition becomes stable or once skilled services such as nursing, speech, or physical therapy are no longer needed, Medicare coverage for home health care ceases. Medicare specifically prohibits payment for custodial care. According to the Official *Medicare Manual* "Care is considered custodial when it is for the purpose of meeting personal needs and could be provided by persons without professional skill or training; for example, help in walking, getting in and out of bed, bathing, eating, dressing, and taking medicine" (HCFA, 1989, October). These are precisely the functions needed by many clients with long-term care needs.

Other problems with Medicare home health benefits are that housekeeping and food services arrangements are not covered. One of the most serious problems is that services must be *intermittent* to be covered. For example, home health aides, in conjunction with other services and for a finite period of time, may work only a few hours a day, several days a week, and their hours may not exceed 32 per week. This type of care is often inadequate when a client needs help with activities of daily living on a constant basis.

Private insurance plans offer little or no coverage for long-term care. Most major medical insurance plans exclude nursing home or home health care, or they cover only private duty nursing in the home. In 1985, private insurance paid for only 1.0 percent of all nursing home costs and even a smaller fraction of home care (Waldo, Levit, and Lazenby, 1986).

Medicaid, the assistance program for the very poor, does cover long-term care, but clients must deplete their own resources to qualify as "medically needy" in order to receive these funds. However, for persons who meet the eligibility requirements, the Medicaid program more effectively meets the long-term care needs of clients than does Medicare. Services do not have to be skilled (a client may have custodial needs met), and the services may be delivered by a person who has received some training for personal care services.

Medicaid expenditures for home care remain small (Rivlin and Wiener, 1988). Because Medicaid is a state-administered program, services vary considerably from state to state. In some states participation is limited in home and community-based services because these states view the services as (1) potentially costly and difficult to manage and (2) not permitting targeting of services to address the specific long-term care needs of the elderly (Justice, 1988, April, p. 121). States are unable to target specific population groups because Medicaid requirements mandate that all eligible recipients in the state must have access to available services developed with Medicaid financing (GAO, 1988, November, p. 27).

Fragmentation and Lack of Coordination

It has consistently been documented that fragmentation and lack of coordination in the long-term care system make it extremely difficult for clients to obtain needed long-term care services (OTA, 1987; Rivlin and Wiener, 1988). Consequently, a significant number of the noninstitutionalized population need but do not receive long-term care.

Existing formal long-term care services are provided by an array of state and local agencies which have differing eligibility requirements and finance mechanisms. Clients who have multifaceted needs frequently find it difficult, if not impossible, to identify the appropriate service provider. In most communities, there is no central organization or professional which assists the chronically impaired client in locating and coordinating needed long-term care services (Rivlin and Wiener, 1988).

Obtaining needed long-term care services often places unnecessary hardships on the client. It is not unusual for clients to have to make separate trips to several agencies in order to arrange a comprehensive package of services. An aged client, for example, may have to apply separately for Medicaid, Meals-on-Wheels, transportation services, Title XX homemaker services, and home nursing services.

Fragmentation and lack of coordination have left many gaps in the long-term care delivery systems. Thus, we continue to have unnecessary institutionalization among high-risk groups and the costs for long-term care services are rising dramatically. Efforts to develop comprehensive, coordinated systems for delivering community-based services must be expanded.

Family Burnout

It has been estimated that between 60 and 85 percent of all disabled or impaired people are helped by the family in a significant way. It has been demonstrated over the years that the family is the primary source of care for the frail elderly in the community (Callahan, Diamond, Giele and Morris, 1980; Doty, 1986; Stone, Cafferata, and Sangl, 1987). Family caretakers play a pivotal role in helping chronically disabled family members to avoid institutionalization. Caring for impaired family members, however, can place a heavy and expensive burden on the family, especially when care is required for an extended period of time. Many chronically impaired persons have been placed in nursing homes because their families are unable to bear the emotional, physical, and financial strain of providing home care in the absence of support from community programs (Kane and Kane, 1987).

Currently, only a few community resources provide temporary relief for family caregivers. Where community resources do exist, eligible families often lack adequate knowledge of long-term care options. In a caregiver survey conducted for the U.S. Congress, Office of Technology Assessment (OTA), the majority of the respondents who listed respite care as "essential" either knew these services were not available or did not know whether they were available (OTA, 1987, p. 63).

In order for long-term care programs to be effective, the needs of family caregivers as well as dependent family members must be addressed. As discussed previously, caregivers of the dependent disabled need respite care, information about services, a broad array of community- and home-based health and social services, and knowledge about health conditions and care methods (OTA, 1987).

METHODS FOR IMPROVING
THE LONG-TERM CARE SYSTEM

With population estimates that project dramatic increases in the over-75-year age group and with health care costs expanding, it is obvious that the present system is not meeting and will not meet the need for long-term care services in the future. A number of methods for improving the system have been suggested:

1. Expansion of noninstitutional forms of long-term care while developing disincentives to constructing more institutional capacity
2. Emphasis on appropriate discharge planning
3. Effective gatekeeping and initial placement of clients assessed as appropriate for institutionalization
4. Targeting home care services to the people who need them the most

Discharge planning has been discussed in Chapter 9 and thus will not be expanded on here. It is im-

portant to remember, however, that chronically ill and disabled clients often need extensive discharge planning services.

Expansion of Noninstitutional Alternatives

A number of demonstration projects have been funded at the state and federal level to evaluate the appropriateness of expanding noninstitutional alternatives and decreasing capacity levels in institutional settings. In New York state, for example, the Nursing Home without Walls program was initiated in 1978 to encourage noninstitutional alternatives as an appropriate cost-effective policy for long-term care of the elderly (Lombardi, 1987). Four components of the program include (1) intervention in the actual process of nursing home placement so that clients are exposed to home care before a nursing home placement decision is made, (2) cost containment with a limit set on the per capita cost of services, (3) case management of services so that social and medical services are integrated into the system, and (4) waivered services so that services not included in the Medicaid law such as respiratory therapy and home improvement can be offered to those needing them.

Another demonstration of the expansion of noninstitutional forms of long-term care is Enriched Housing (Nursing home without walls, 1982, p. 107). Enriched Housing serves that portion of the population who is able to live independently but needs some help with personal care, meal preparation, housekeeping, shopping, laundry, heavy cleaning, transportation, and 24-hour emergency coverage. The typical person entering this program does not have an informal support network to help him or her to live independently. The program differs from the Nursing Home without Walls program, because the client must also need housing. In this program, the person enters the housing secured by the program, usually a portion of a rent-subsidized building. Payment is generally through SSI.

Adult foster care is another mandated service in many states for people over 18 who are socially, mentally, or physically handicapped. Its purpose is to provide the opportunity for normal family and community life as well as help with problems. A foster home for adults is usually operated by individuals in their own homes and provides room, board, housekeeping, personal care, and supervision to four or fewer adults on a 24-hour basis. Those eligible for the program include people who receive AFDC (Aid to Families with Dependent Children) or SSI. Talmadge and Murphy (1983) found that both patients and their families can benefit from well-planned foster home placements.

Economical shared or sheltered housing for the elderly and disabled deserves greater effort. Improved federal funding of long-term care services should accompany efforts to utilize volunteer efforts on behalf of this population. One mutual aid scheme involving the exchange and banking of time in long-term care could be centered on congregate housing developments or similar concentrations of older citizens. These would ordinarily be built without adequate service supports. Residents could be admitted initially across a range of ages and disabilities. When able, they could be encouraged to help care for one another in a variety of ways. Those on waiting lists for apartments could be encouraged to help as well. In exchange, subsequently, residents would receive aid from new and more able helpers. These exchanges are in existence today and can probably be increased in number and intensity by a mild effort to back them publicly. People who help others would be guaranteed help in return. If no one volunteered to provide that subsequent help, it would be financed publicly and delivered by paid workers. Time devoted to helping others would be backed hour for hour by the full faith and credit of the United States—probably the best form of currency since the silver certificate. In this way, we could build faith in a currency of altruism (Sanger, 1983, p. 104).

Developing Effective Gatekeeping Mechanisms

Developing models, such as local-area management organizations (LAMOs) and social–health maintenance organizations (S/HMOs), is another solution for dealing with the problems in the long-

term care system (Ruchlin, Morris, and Eggert, 1982). Both are methods of financing and organizing health care for the elderly and are variations of the Health Maintenance Organizations (HMOs) described in Chapter 4. Funding for LAMOs and S/HMOs comes from all public monies currently designated for short-term and long-term medical care, rehabilitation, and custodial services. The LAMO enrolls all people with functional deficits and provides the services necessary to help them at home, utilizing informal supports whenever possible. The S/HMO enrolls all elderly people, anticipating that low use of services by the relatively well elderly compensates for extensive use by the vulnerable and severely ill. Both models function as gatekeepers into the long-term care system; case managers function as brokers for the services needed by the population served, and they also certify the level of care needed. ACCESS in New York is a LAMO that has been successful in saving millions of dollars,

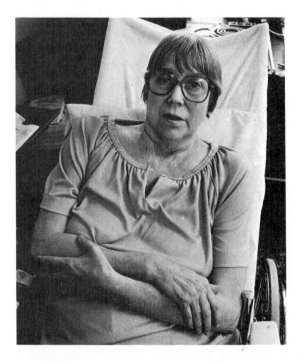

Figure 19-7 Jane Richards, who lost both legs to gangrene, lives at home rather than in a nursing home. (Anne Lennox/Times-Union.)

———————————————— **A Woman Is Rescued from a Nursing Home** ————————————————

Henrietta homemaker Jane Richards lost a leg to gangrene in June 1978.

But Mrs. Richards, then a 63-year-old widow, convinced herself that life would go on, that she would learn to get around again through physical therapy.

By the time she had mastered solo trips to the bathroom, her circulation problem flared again. Four months after her first operation, she lost her other leg.

She recalls being devastated. Where would she go? How would she take care of herself? To whom could she turn? There seemed no good answers for a woman who was still relatively young, still lively, still involved in the world around her and yet trapped in a helpless, immobile body.

After she spent 10 months in the extended care facility of Genesee Hospital, a social worker suggested a possible answer: round-the-clock skilled nursing care at home, arranged by ACCESS, a federal demonstration project, run by Monroe County Long-Term Care Inc., an independent non-profit corporation.

ACCESS is testing the assumption that encouraging long-term care at home and in nursing homes will cut medical costs, relieve the backup of patients waiting to leave hospitals, and also provide more comfortable, humane medical care for the elderly, Executive Director, Gerald M. Eggert said.

Its goal is to help people who need long-term health care receive it in the least costly setting appropriate to their needs, he said.

Mrs. Richards believes ACCESS liberated her. After undergoing a battery of medical, financial and social evaluations arranged through the program, a caseworker found her an apartment accessible to a wheelchair-bound tenant, and supplied equipment, such as a hospital bed, trapeze and a specially designed wheelchair.

Bills were paid primarily through Medicaid, the government's health program for the poor.

Finally, in October 1979, after 1½ years in various medical institutions, Mrs. Richards went home. At first, she depended on help from around-the-clock aides. Two years later, that care was reduced to eight hours a day, four hours in the morning and four in the evening, where it remains today.

"I've been very pleased with what they've done for me," she said, chatting in her sun-drenched living room. "I'd recommend it to anybody. I'd have nothing left, no spirit if they put me in a nursing home. I would figure they had stuck me in a nursing home to die."

Until a few years ago, programs aimed at keeping the elderly and chronically disabled out of nursing homes were rare. If Mrs. Richards lost her legs a decade ago, chances are she would have spent the rest of her life in a nursing home.

Today, however, she is among hundreds of Monroe County residents who, despite serious disabilities and handicaps, live at home rather than in hospitals or nursing homes, and who stress the personal and economic advantages of that decision.

Since its 1977 start, ACCESS has received 19,558 referrals from families, physicians, community health nurses and agencies and hospital discharge staff members in Monroe County, said Belinda S. Brodows, deputy director.

ACCESS works like a broker, assessing patients' needs, arranging home health aides, social workers and other services through existing private agencies and conducting periodic follow-ups.

But its key feature is the authority to approve Medicaid and Medicare payments for long-term care services. Since November, the program has been authorized to approve Medicare benefits for 100 days of home health care and nursing home care without the usual requisite three-day hospital stay.

In the past, Eggert said, a major obstacle to encouraging long-term health care was the tilt in government health insurance programs toward acute-care coverage, which encouraged people to go to hospitals or nursing homes.

As a result of ACCESS, increasing numbers of chronically ill or disabled people in Monroe County are getting medical care and living at home: Between 1978 and 1982, the percentage of hospital patients referred to ACCESS—patients who were assessed as needing skilled nursing level care and who returned home—increased to 61 percent from 19 percent.

The percentages are higher for patients referred from the community: In 1978, 81 percent of the patients assessed at home stayed at home; the percentage rose to 96 percent in 1982.

At a time when rising health care costs and the burgeoning population of elderly are threatening Medicare's solvency, many doctors, geriatric specialists, and policy-makers believe programs like ACCESS may be the wave of the future.

From Eisenberg C: A woman is rescued from a nursing home, Times-Union, Rochester, NY, p 8, May 3, 1988.

primarily through the reduction of acute hospitalizations (Eggert and Brodows, 1982).

The story of ACCESS client Jane Richards (refer to Figure 19-7 and box above) made newspaper headlines when the public heard what the agency had to offer (Eisenberg, 1983).

When they examine various ways for expanding noninstitutional long-term care alternatives, community health nurses must understand that although the demand for home care services is likely to grow, home health care does not necessarily ensure cost reduction. A study carried out by the Government Accounting Office (GAO, 1982) showed that when expanded home health care services were made available to those in need of long-term care services, client satisfaction improved. However, those services did not reduce nursing home, hospital, or total service costs. The study concluded that the focus of research should be on how to provide services most effectively and efficiently in various health care settings. Researchers in the study agreed that *targeting* services to people in the community in the most cost-effective manner was crucial. Simply expanding home health care to all those in need of long-term care was neither efficient nor cost-effective (Capitman, 1988).

Targeting Services

When they think of targeting long-term care services, community health nurses must know that a relatively small group of elderly are extremely high users of medical care. In Colorado, 0.5 percent of Medicare beneficiaries who were enrolled continuously for 4 years accounted for 57 percent of the acute hospital use, and 18 percent accounted for 88 percent of overall Medicare use (McCall and Wai, 1983). This pattern is part of a larger phenomenon known as Pareto's law that has been recognized in the business world for many years:

The fact that a small number of people account for a disproportionate share of activities is common knowledge among management experts. There is a basic phenomenon that is encountered in many human activities. It is couched in these general terms. In a given activity, only a few of the actors contribute to (account for) a major and disproportionate share of the action. This distribution is variously called the Pareto Law (after the noted Italian economist who recognized the universality of the phenomenon); the Lorenz curve (after an economist who applied it to distributions of family incomes); the A-B-C curve where the "A" items are the small number accounting for the major share of the activity while the "C" items, large in number, account for a small percentage of the activity, whereas the "B" items are intermediate; the 80-20 curve since 20% of the items accounting for 80% of the activity is a common distribution (Gavett, 1983).

Targeting needed services to the 20 percent of the long-term care population who utilize 80 percent of the resources is the key to effective and efficient use of services. The choice should not be between institutional and noninstitutional care but between acceptable and unacceptable care. Hospice programs, for example, focus on helping families to care for ill family members by providing services that are most appropriate for each individual family.

Hospice is a humanistic approach to the care of the dying. One of the three main diagnoses of home care clients is cancer. This disease is a chronic one that requires services much more important than medical care. For the elderly, cancer often progresses slowly and thus, leads to a longer period of home care than other diseases. Hospice presents a solution to many of the needs of this population group as well as to clients across the life-span who are dealing with the difficulties associated with cancer.

The hospice concept is an approach to providing care for terminally ill clients and their families: it is a way of dying rather than a place where dying people receive care. It focuses on helping people to die with dignity and on assisting families with the grieving process. It emphasizes relieving psychological as well as physical distress.

The hospice movement developed from the work of Cicely Saunders, a physician from England. She founded St. Christopher's Hospice in 1960, which became a model for similar programs in the United States. In the early 1970s, the first American hospice was organized in New Haven, Connecticut.

The development of the hospice movement in the United States is relatively recent, beginning only 20 years ago. However, the growing number of aging people as already discussed, the tremendous growth in medical technology that extends life, the growing awareness and fear of cancer, and the involvement of educated consumers who desire a voice in treatment have led to rapid growth in this movement in recent years. Further, cost containment has been another important issue since caring for the terminally ill in the cure-focused setting of a high-technology hospital is more expensive and less comfortable than the home setting. Since the inception of the movement, more than 1500 hospices have been opened in the United States (Paradis, 1985, p. 8).

Hospice is a movement that emphasizes (Coping with Cancer, 1980, p. 180):

- Help in dealing with emotional, spiritual, and medical problems
- Support for the entire family
- Keeping the patient in his or her home for as long as appropriate and making his or her remaining life as comfortable and as meaningful as possible
- Professional services from a health care team supplemented by volunteer services, as appropriate to individual circumstances
- Relief of pain and other symptoms

Organizations providing hospice services vary, ranging from small homes run by church groups to hospitals or home health agencies. There are five models: the free-standing hospice, the hospital-affiliated free-standing hospice, the hospital-based hospice that includes either a centralized team or a specialized hospice team, a hospice within an extended care facility, and finally, home care programs that are hospital, community, or nursing based (Paradis, 1985). Figure 19-8 depicts the inpatient hospice unit of Genesee Region Home Care. It complements the home hospice program of this agency and provides terminally ill patients help with pain control, gives their families respite for short periods, and teaches families how to deal with the signs of terminal illness in the home setting.

Hospice programs which meet the standards of care developed by the National Hospice Organization are medically directed by a qualified physician and provide both inpatient and home-based care as needed. Care is provided by an interdisciplinary team 24 hours a day, 7 days a week. Volunteers are an integral part of this team. The patient and his or her family are the central figures on the team as well as the unit of service and, as such, are actively involved in developing the management plan. Plans of care address pain and symptom management, psychosocial and spiritual difficulties, coping with dying, and bereavement. Support services for staff are an essential component of a Hospice, as staff members must be able to deal with the grieving process first in order to assist the families (Paradis, 1985).

THE ROLE OF THE COMMUNITY HEALTH NURSE IN LONG-TERM CARE

If current demographic trends continue, we will clearly be faced with increased numbers of people at advanced ages. The unknown variable will be the health of this group. If the health of this group in the future is not considerably different from the health of the present cohort, a huge proportion of the population will be suffering from chronic diseases. Today, health-care resources are stretched to the point at which federal entitlement programs for the health care of the elderly have become a major political issue. Increased pressures on the limited resources of our society will require difficult decisions in terms of the quantity and quality of health care for older Americans. The only approach that can forestall these consequences of increased life expectancy is for substantial inroads to be made in the prevention, treatment, or management of the common chronic diseases of aging (Schneider and Brody, 1983, p. 855).

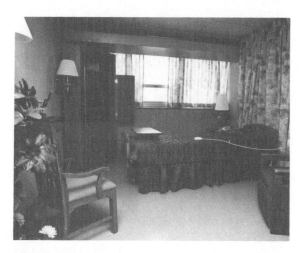

Figure 19-8   The homelike atmosphere of the inpatient hospice unit of Genesee Region Home Care complements the Home Hospice program. (Used with permission of Genesee Region Home Care, Rochester, NY.)

Nurses are increasing their involvement with this growing at-risk long-term care population and are becoming leaders in caring for people who have long-term needs. In fact, long-term care is very likely to become a key growth area for professional nursing (Reif and Estes, 1983, p. 149). Nurses already represent the largest number and percent of professional workers involved in long-term care; however, estimates suggest that there is a growing shortage of nurses in the areas of long-term care and gerontology.

There are seven areas upon which community health nurses should focus to provide more adequate long-term care. These are: prevention at all three levels among people across the life-span, functional independence for clients rather than a cure, families coping abilities, case management, interdisciplinary functioning, evaluation of services, and responsible public policy making.

Utilizing Levels of Prevention

Throughout this text, the concepts of disease prevention and health promotion have been stressed. The importance of these concepts cannot be overemphasized, especially when one examines the problems encountered by long-term care population groups. In order to decrease the number of people needing long-term care, it is essential to concentrate our efforts on the primary prevention of chronic problems.

Since the prepathogenesis period of disease (refer to Chapter 10) begins early in life, primary prevention and health promotion activities which address many problems encountered by chronically disabled persons and the aged must be introduced when working with young people. Health education programs which address such matters as lifestyle modification, stress management, and retirement planning, and counseling services which help individuals to develop a risk profile are examples of such activities. Other examples are integrated throughout Chapters 13 through 18.

Community health nurses are uniquely able to apply the concepts of prevention as they work with clients who need long-term care. Primary, secondary, and tertiary preventive activities are commonly implemented by nurses who provide home health care services. Examples of primary prevention activities include accident prevention education and teaching about control of infection. Helping a client who has diabetes to learn how to self-administer insulin injections and to handle postsurgical wound care are examples of secondary prevention activities.

Tertiary prevention, continuing care and rehabilitation, is frequently carried out with people who need long-term care. These people often need help with physical, occupational, and/or speech therapy to return to or maintain their optimal level of functioning. The challenge facing the community health nurse at the tertiary level of prevention is how to maintain an ongoing working relationship with clients so that the care plan can be adjusted in response to the client's and family's changing circumstances and conditions. Strategies that community health nurses can utilize to help clients manage chronic diseases include medical record coauthoring, self-monitoring, educational support groups, family involvement, and telephone or postcard contact with clients. Excellent literature is available that describes how to use these strategies (American Hospital Association, 1982).

Helping Families to Cope

The family is the primary support system for the elderly person residing in the community (Norris, Sherwood, and Gutkin, 1981). The family is also the primary resource in maintaining the aged in the community when chronic illness and functional decline begin to appear.

Approaches to develop long-term care services should first seek ways to buttress the family and its competence and capacity to cope with the increasing demands and strains, then augment the family resources with community services that permit the family to maintain its supportive involvement (Koff, 1982, p. 16).

Most aging people have some informal support systems which provide assistance with activities of daily living when necessary (Stone, Cafferata, and Sangl, 1987). Community health nurses should not, however, expect families and other informal supports to do the impossible—to provide care with no relief over long periods of time. Helping families to cope and not burn out is crucial. One way for informal supports to be strengthened is to provide for respite care, or time off, from caring for a chronically disabled family member. *Respite care* is a pioneering field in the United States, and unfortunately relatively few programs are available which clients can afford (Hildebrandt, 1983; Lawton, Brody, and Saperstein, 1989).

There is no one model for respite care, some bring care givers to clients, paying for aide service in the home. Others bring clients to hospitals and other facilities.

Respite care is a wise financial investment. There is evidence which shows that this type of care can delay nursing home admission, keep families together, and keep public expenditures at a minimum (Ellis and Wilson, 1983).

Helping families to find an affordable respite program, and helping a community to initiate a home or institutional respite program, are very significant community health nursing functions. The Omnibus Budget Reconciliation Act of 1981 allows Medicaid waivers for reimbursement of respite care if the cost is the same as or less than institutional care. Also, the Tax Equity and Fiscal Responsibility Act of 1982 includes a hospice benefit provision that allows money to be used for respite care if the client is terminally ill. OBRA legislation has been increasing these benefits since 1982.

Family members and other informal supports need to be nurtured. Supportive counseling helps families to deal with feelings of guilt and frustration that arise when caring for an ill family member. When they provide care for a chronically disabled person, community health nurses must focus attention on the needs of the family as well as the client. Ignoring the family may result in the client not getting the assistance that he or she needs.

Focus on Functional Independence

Clients with long-term care needs often have conditions that cannot be cured. The goal for their care is to help them to maintain quality in their lives and to continue to function at the highest possible level. With the cure orientation that pervades our health care system, this can be a difficult orientation for a community health nurse to develop and maintain. This orientation becomes easier to handle as one sees through practice that clients can live satisfying lives even when they have not been cured. The story of Jane Richards, discussed previously in this chapter, is an example of a client who was not cured but yet is able to function independently and peacefully in the community. Community health nurses play a significant role in assisting clients to achieve greater functional independence.

Case Management

Historically, case management has been an integral part of community health nursing practice. Renewed focus on this process has developed because dramatic changes in the health care delivery system have increased the complexity of client care issues and the need for increased community resources to address client needs. Case management is being advocated as a means to improve client access to health care resources and the effective and efficient use of these resources. As discussed earlier in this chapter, case management projects have emerged to address the needs of special population groups such as the frail elderly and the mentally ill. Case management should be integrated into every nurse's practice. Most clients using long-term care services need assistance in dealing with the multiple resources required to meet their needs.

Case management is an essential component of comprehensive health care in all client settings. It is a problem-solving process which involves the assessment of the client's and family's total health care needs; coordination of resources and the delivery of health care services; and the continual monitoring of client and family progress (ANA, 1986). A major component of case management involves making decisions about which health care professional or community resource can best meet current client needs and what plan of care is the most appropriate to address these needs. Use of the nursing process (discussed in Chapter 8) and the referral process (discussed in Chapter 9)

TABLE 19-3   Role descriptions for select members of the long-term health care team*

Discipline	Role description
Community health nurse†	*An essential professional member of the health care team*—The professional nurse utilizes the nursing process to determine client needs, to establish a plan of care in conjunction with the client, to provide skilled nursing services, and to evaluate care delivered by the nursing team. Traditionally, the professional nurse has assumed a case management role on the health care team. As a case manager, the community health nurse focuses on determining the comprehensive needs of the client and the client's family, makes referrals to appropriate community resources as needed, and coordinates care among the multiple agencies providing services to a family.
Homemaker-health aide	*A paraprofessional who is trained to assist clients with personal care and light household tasks*—According to the Medicare conditions of participation for home health agencies, a home health aide's "duties include the performance of simple procedures as an extension of therapy services, personal care, ambulation and exercise, household services essential to health care at home, assistance with medications that are ordinarily self-administered, reporting changes in the patient's condition and needs, and completing appropriate records" (HCFA, 1989, October). Home health aides must be supervised by professional nurses, who must make supervisory visits to the client's home at least every *2 weeks.*
Nutritionist	*A professional team member who assists clients in meeting their basic nutritional needs*—The nutritionist assesses a client's nutritional status, helps the client to plan an adequate and appropriate dietary intake, suggests ways to plan economical nutritious meals, helps clients to learn about therapeutic diets, and teaches about food purchasing and preparation. These professionals are often used as resource persons by other members of the health care team.
Physician	*A professional team member who is either a doctor of medicine or osteopathy*—The Medicare conditions of participation for home health agencies specify that the physician must establish and authorize the client's plan of treatment in writing and must review this treatment plan at least once *every 60 days* to determine if care is appropriate and necessary (HCFA, 1989, October). In addition to establishing a plan of treatment, the physician evaluates the client's medical status and provides medical care as needed. A physician also serves on a home health agency's professional advisory committee.
Social worker, medical	*A professional member of the home health care team who works with clients who are experiencing significant psychosocial, financial, or environmental difficulties*—Medical social workers apply the principles of social case work to help clients to enhance their emotional and social adjustment and to adapt to change. The primary purpose of their intervention is to reduce psychosocial, financial, and environmental barriers which are adversely affecting a client's health status or response to health care. Medical social workers provide direct counseling services, refer clients to community resources, assist clients in attaining needed social and health care services, and help plan for institutional community placements such as nursing home or extended-care facility placements. They also serve as resource persons for other members of the health care team who are dealing with difficult psychosocial, financial, or environmental problems.
Therapists, occupational	*Professional members of the team who work with clients that have difficulty carrying out activities of daily living*—After determining the self-care activities most important to the client, the occupational therapist assesses the environment to identify safety hazards and barriers to self-care, recommends environmental modifications which would help the client to increase independence and to prevent accidents, and assists the client in learning techniques, such as the use of simple eating and dressing devices which promote effective and efficient client functioning. The occupational therapist focuses on helping the client to improve motor coordination and muscle strength so that the client can reach his or her maximum level of functioning.
Therapists, physical	*Professional members of the team who work with clients who have functional impairments related to neuromuscular problems*—After assessing the client's functional abilities, physical therapists help clients to preserve, restore, and improve neuromuscular functioning and to increase their self-care capabilities. Physical therapists carry out a broad range of activities to help clients reach their maximum level of functioning. Performing needed range-of-motion, strengthening, and coordination exercises; recommending the use of appropriate orthopedic and prosthetic devices; and teaching clients ambulation techniques and how to use assistive appliances are a few examples of the activities performed by physical therapists.

TABLE 19-3   Role descriptions for select members of the long-term health care team*—cont'd

Discipline	Role description
Therapists, speech	*Professional members of the team who work with clients who have communication problems—* After assessing the client's speech, language, and hearing abilities, speech therapists concentrate on helping clients to increase their functional communication skills. Based on client needs, the speech therapist may initiate exercises to increase functional speaking skills, teach esophageal speech, recommend the use of communication appliances such as intraoral devices or hearing aids, identify barriers in the environment which inhibit effective communication, and teach significant others in the environment how to communicate with the client.

*The central figures on any long-term health care team must be the client and his or her family.

†In order to be certified for Medicare and Medicaid funding, a home health agency must provide nursing services.

From Health Care Financing Administration (HCFA): Medicare program; home health agencies: conditions of participation and reduction in recordkeeping requirements, 42 CFR, Part 484, Sections 484.1 through 484.52, Washington, DC, 1989, US Department of Health and Human Services.

aids the community health nurse in making these decisions.

Utilize All Members of the Health Care Team

No *one* discipline can address the array of needs experienced by long-term care clients. The problems involved with long-term care demand that all members and levels of health care providers be involved. The community health nurse must be attuned to drawing on the health care team's sources whenever possible. Jane Richards' care plan, for example, utilized a physical therapist, an occupational therapist who carried out an assessment of the environment, a vendor of medical supplies and equipment who ordered materials including a wheelchair specifically prepared for her, a rehabilitation home economist who taught her to be self-sufficient in her kitchen, and a social worker who helped her to think through long-range plans and to find housing. In addition, she received daily ongoing personal care from a home health aide. Many of these people continue to be involved at intervals.

The community health nurse often functions as the coordinator of the health care team, an extremely important role which must not be neglected. The client can easily feel that care is fragmented if no one person has overall responsibility for complete care. Understanding the roles of each team member (refer to Table 19-3) can facilitate planning and coordination. The role defi-

nitions presented in Table 19-3 should be regarded only as a starting point for developing effective team relationships. When entering any new service agency, spend time with each member of the team to determine how they function.

The central figures on any long-term health care team must be the client and his or her family. In order to achieve the highest level of functioning possible for the client, the client must be actively involved in establishing a plan of care appropriate to his or her needs. Engaging families in the therapeutic process is essential, because often they have needs of their own that must be addressed. In addition, families are frequently participants in the rehabilitation process and provide continuing support for disabled family members after health care providers leave the home environment.

Evaluate Services

An integral part of working in any health care setting is evaluation. The evaluation process helps health care professionals to determine whether they are providing appropriate and quality services in an effective and efficient way. In this era of decreasing resources, it is essential for community health professionals to monitor carefully how they use available resources. The needs of at-risk aggregates, such as those comprising the long-term care population, can only be met if resources are allocated and used in a responsible manner.

Community health nurses at all levels must assume responsibility for evaluating the way in which nursing services are delivered. While nursing administrators have the overall task of seeing that evaluation is done, staff-level professionals must be accountable for assessing their own practice. They must also supervise the care they have delegated to others, such as home health aides and homemakers. When community health nurses delegate or assign tasks to others, they are responsible for seeing that these tasks are performed in an acceptable way.

A variety of direct and indirect measures are currently used by community health nurses to evaluate the delivery of nursing services, such as direct observation of care, case management conferences, annual performance evaluations, and record reviews. The Standards of Home Health Nursing Practice (ANA, 1986) referred to earlier in this chapter should guide the development of an evaluation plan that includes criteria for measuring quality and methods for assuring that care is consistent with professional standards (refer to Chapter 22). Requirements of reimbursement sources must also guide the development of evaluation measures. Community health nurses in home health agencies must, for example, fulfill the following evaluation requirements in order to receive Medicare reimbursement for health services provided by their agency (Health Care Financing Administration, 1989):

- Conduct an overall evaluation of the agency's total program at least once a year to examine to what extent the agency's program is *appropriate, adequate, effective,* and *efficient*
- Establish a professional *advisory* group which includes at least one physician, one registered nurse, one member who is neither an owner nor an employee of the agency, and appropriate representatives of other professional disciplines, such as social work, physical therapy, and speech therapy, who are providing service for the agency; the group must meet frequently to advise agency staff on professional issues and to participate in overall agency evaluation
- Review with the patient's physician the ap-

propriateness of the plan of treatment, as often as the severity of the patient's condition requires, but at *least once every 60 days*
- Have the registered nurse, or appropriate professional staff member, if other services are provided, make a supervisory home health aide visit *at least every 2 weeks*
- Conduct a clinical record review on active and closed records *at least quarterly* to ensure that established policies are followed in providing services
- The agency must employ only home health aides who have completed a competency evaluation program

Two types of record reviews are conducted in the home health setting: quality care audit and utilization review. During the *quality care audit* process, health care providers focus on appraising the quality of care received by clients, using predetermined standards of care, as evidenced by documentation in the client's record (refer to Chapter 22). During a *utilization review,* the client's records are assessed for the purposes of evaluating the appropriateness of the client's admissions and discharges; the appropriate and adequate use of personnel; and over- and underutilization of services (NLN, 1980, p. 48).

Staff-level community health nurses can play a very important role in all evaluation review procedures. Staff involvement in evaluation processes helps administrators to obtain a clearer picture about service delivery issues. As case managers, staff-level nurses are in a unique position to identify gaps in service and deficiencies of care.

Work toward Responsible Public Policy

Thus far in this chapter, ample evidence has been presented to demonstrate that public policy for long-term care in this country is inadequate. Carolyn Williams, a leader in community health nursing, writes:

It is important that nurses—particularly those who consider themselves community health nursing specialists—assign a high priority to participation in the formation of health policy and broader public policy (1983, p. 225) . . . primarily because this is a crucial modality for influencing the health of defined populations (p. 228).

Involvement in forming public policy can be at any one of a number of levels. These levels range from apathy and no participation, to voting, to holding public office. All levels require knowledge of the issues; community health nurses in long-term care possess this as an outcome of their experience.

Involvement in the political arena is both fun and professionally rewarding. Working with professional organizations, such as the National Association for Home Care and the American Public Health Association, is a good way to get started in the political arena. These organizations are making a concerted effort to analyze key health care issues and to promote strategies which may resolve some of the current health care delivery problems.

SUMMARY

Increasing numbers of people across the life-span have long-term care needs that must be addressed by local communities throughout our nation. Elderly persons, who constitute the most rapidly growing population group in America, are particularly at risk for needing long-term care services. Although most elderly people experience good health, certain chronic, disabling illnesses do increase with aging.

The fastest-growing component of the United States health care delivery system is long-term care. Diverse and multiple social, health-related, and health care organizations deliver a variety of long-term care services to people in need. Despite the dramatic growth in the long-term care industry, there are still many chronically disabled persons who do not receive the services they need. Developing strategies to eliminate barriers to adequate community-based, long-term care must receive greater attention by health care providers in this decade. There is no question that the aging of the American population will increase the need for long-term care services in the future.

Long-term care presents challenges and opportunities for the community health nurse. Developing solutions to overcome the deficiencies and to fill the gaps in the long-term care system will require major policy changes at all three levels of government. However, community health nurses at all levels of practice can be instrumental in effecting change in the health care delivery system. Innovative projects which more adequately address the needs of at-risk long-term care populations are beginning to emerge across the country.

REFERENCES

Administration of home health nursing: care of the sick by health departments, Public Health Nurs 37:339-342, 1945.

Aging America. Trends and projections: 1987-88 ed, Washington, DC, 1987, US Special Committee on Aging.

American Hospital Association: Strategies to promote self-management of chronic disease, Chicago, 1982, The Association.

American Nurses' Association: Standards of home health nursing practice, Kansas City, Mo, 1986, The Association.

Baxter R, Applebaum R, Callahan J, Christianson J, and Day S: The planning and implementation of channeling: early experiences of the national long-term care demonstration, Princeton, NJ, 1983, Mathematica Policy Research.

Bedside nursing care by official agencies, Public Health Nurs 37:333-334, 1945.

Belk J: Federal policy and disabled people, Caring 6(8):6-9, 52-54, 1987.

Berk ML, and Bernstein A: Use of home health services: some findings from the National Medical Care Expenditure Survey, Home Health Care Serv Q 6(1):13-23, 1985.

Bishop CE: Living arrangement choices of elderly singles: effects of income and disability, Health Care Financ Rev 7:65-73, 1986.

Blancato R: The Older American Act as a vehicle, Pride Institute J Special Issue, 29-32, 1986.

Buckwalter KC, Abraham IL, and Neuendorger MM: Alzheimer's disease. Involving nursing in the development and implementation of health care for patients and families, Nurs Clin North Am 23(1):1-9, 1988.

Burke TR: Long-term care: the public role and private initiatives, Health Care Financ Rev, 1988 Annual Suppl, pp 1-5, December 1988.

Burns EM and Buckwalter KC: Pathophysiology and etiology of Alzheimer's disease, Nurs Clin North Am 23(1):11-29, 1988.

Callahan JJ, Diamond LD, Giele JZ, and Morris R: Responsibilities of families for their severely disabled elders, Health Care Financ Rev 1:29-49, 1980.

Capitman JA: Case management for long-term and acute medical care, Health Care Financ Rev, 1988 Annual Suppl, pp 53-56, 1988.

Cassak D: Hospitals in home health care: an industry in transition, Health Industry Today 47(7):16-28, 1984.

Commonwealth Fund Commission on Elderly People Living Alone: Old, alone and poor: a plan for reducing poverty among elderly people living alone, Baltimore, Md, 1987, The Commission.

Congressional Budget Office, Budget Issue Paper: Long-term care for the elderly and disabled, Washington, DC, February, 1977, US Congress.

Congressional Budget Office, Technical Analysis Paper: Long-term care actuarial cost-estimates, Washington, DC, 1977, US Congress.

Coping with cancer. A resource for health professionals, NIH Pub No 80-2080, Bethesda, Md, 1980, National Cancer Institute.

Daniels K: Will nurses control care at home? Home Healthcare Nurse 6(2):18-23, 1988.

Doty P: Family care of the elderly: the role of public policy, Milbank Q, 64:34-75, 1986.

Deimling GT and Bass DM: Symptoms of mental impairment among elderly adults and their effects on family caregivers, J Gerontol 41:779-784, 1986.

Eagles JM, Beattie JAG, Blackwood GW, Restall DB, and Ashcroft GW: The mental health of elderly couples. 1. The effects of a cognitively impaired spouse, Brit J Psychiat 180:299-303, 1987.

Eggert G and Brodows B: The access process: assuring quality in long-term care, Quality Rev Bull 8(2):10-15, 1982.

Eisenberg C: A woman is rescued from a nursing home, Times-Union, Rochester, NY, p 8, May 3, 1983.

Ellis V and Wilson D: Respite care in the nursing home unit of a veteran's hospital, Am J Nurs 83(10):1433-1434, 1983.

Federal Register: Medicaid program: home and community-based services, Final Rule 50(49):10013-10028, March 1985.

Fitting M, Rabins P, Lucas MJ, and Eastham J: Caregivers for dementia patients: a comparison of husband and wives, Gerontologist 26:248-252, 1986.

Fowles D: The changing older population, Aging 339:6-11, 1983.

Fulton JP, Katz S, Jack SS, and Hendershot GE: Physical functioning of the aged, 1984, Series 10: Data from the National Health Survey, No 167, DHHS Pub No (PHS) 89-1595, Hyattsville, Md, USDHHS March 1989.

Gavett J: Hospital experimental program high cost patient study, Rochester, NY, 1983, University of Rochester School of Management, unpublished study.

General Accounting Office (GAO): Improved knowledge base would be helpful in reaching policy decisions on providing long-term, in-home services for the elderly, HRD-82-4, Washington, DC, October 1981, US Government Printing Office.

GAO: The elderly should benefit from expanded home health care but increasing these services will not insure cost reductions, Washington, DC, December 1982, US Government Printing Office.

GAO: Medicaid and nursing home care: cost increases and the need for services are creating problems for the states and the elderly (GAO IPE-84-1), Washington, DC, October 1983, US Government Printing Office.

GAO: Community services: block grant helps address local social service needs, Pub No HRD 86-91, Washington, DC, May 1986, US Government Printing Office.

GAO: Medicare: need to strengthen home health care payment controls and address unmet needs, Pub No HRD-87-9, Washington, DC, December 1986, US Government Printing Office.

GAO: Long-term care for the elderly: issues of need, access, and cost, Washington, DC, November 1988, US Government Printing Office.

George LK, and Gwyther LP: Caregiver well-being: a multidimensional examination of family caregivers of demented adults, Gerontologist 26:253-259, 1986.

Getzen TE: Longlife insurance: a prototype for funding long-term care, Health Care Financ Rev, 10(2):47-55, 1988.

Ginzberg E, Balinsky W, and Ostow M: Home health care: its role in the changing health services market, Totowa, NJ, 1984, Rowman and Allanheld.

Haley WE, Levine EG, Brown SL, Berry JM, and Hughes GH: Psychological, social, and health consequences of caring for a relative with senile dementia, J Am Geriat Soc 35:405-411, 1987.

Haupt AC: Forty years of teamwork in public health nursing, Am J Nurs 1:53, 1953.

Health Care Financing Administration: Medicare

home health agency manual, Pub 11, Washington, DC, 1989, USDHHS.

Health Care Financing Administration: Medicare program; home health agencies: conditions of participation and reduction in recordkeeping requirements, 42 CFR, Part 484, Sections 484.1 through 484.52, Washington, DC, October 1989, USDHHS.

Hildebrandt ED: Respite care in the home, Am J Nurs 83(10):1428-1430, 1983.

Hing E: Use of nursing home by the elderly: preliminary data from the 1985 National Nursing Home Survey, Advance Data from Vital and Health Statistics, No. 142, USDHHS Pub No (PHS) 87-1250, Hyattsville, Md, 1987, Public Health Service.

Hirsh L, Klein M, and Marlowe G: Combining public health nursing agencies: a case study in Philadelphia, New York, 1967, Department of PHN, NLN.

Holghan JF and Cohen JW: Medicaid: the trade-off between cost containment and access to care, Washington, DC, 1986, Urban Institute.

House Select Committee on Aging: Building a long-term policy: home care data and implications, Pub. No. 98-484, Washington, DC, 1985, US Government Printing Office.

Hughes SL: Apples and oranges? A review of evaluations of community-based long-term care, Health Serv Res 20:460-488, 1985.

Johnson CL and Johnson FA: A micro-analysis of "senility": the response of the family and the health professionals, Culture Medicine Psychiat 7:77-96, 1983.

Justice D: State long-term care reform: development of community care systems in six states, Washington, DC, April 1988, National Governors Association.

Kane RA: The noblest experiment of them all: learning from the national channeling evaluation, Health Serv Res 23:189-198, 1988.

Kane R and Kane R: Long-term care: principles, programs, and policies, New York, 1987, Springer.

Kemper P, Applebaum R, and Harrigan M: Community care demonstrations: what have we learned? Health Care Financ Rev 8:87-100, 1987.

Koff T: Long-term care. An approach to serving the frail elderly, Boston, 1982, Little, Brown.

Kornblatt E and Fisher M: The impact of DRGs on home health nursing, Quality Rev Bull 11(10):290-294, 1985.

Kraus LE and Stoddard S: Chartbook on disability in the United States, an InfoUse report, Washington, DC, 1989, National Institute on Disability and Rehabilitation Research.

Lawton MP, Brody EM, and Saperstein AR: A controlled study of respite service for caregivers of Alzheimer's patients, Gerontologist 29(1):8-16, 1989.

Laxton CE: Editorial introduction, Caring 8(5):2, 1989.

Letsch SW, Levit KR, and Waldo DR: National health expenditures, 1987, Health Care Financ Rev 10(2):109-122, 1988.

Leutz W: Long-term care for the elderly: public dreams and private realities, Inquiry 23:134-140, 1986.

Lidke K: Technology-dependent children: addressing problems that arise from success, Advance, Ann Arbor, Fall 1989, University of Michigan Medical Center, pp 2-15.

Liu K, Manton K, and Liu BM: Home care expenses for noninstitutionalized elderly with ADL and IADL limitations, Health Care Financ Rev 7(2):52, 1986.

Lombardi T: Nursing home without walls, Caring 6(5):4-9, 1987.

McCall N and Wai H: An analysis of the use of medical services by the continuously enrolled aged, Med Care 21(6):1983.

McNiff ML: Impact of managed care systems on home health agencies, Home Health Nurs 6(2):10-13, 1988.

National Association for Home Care: Home care and hospice provisions contained in the Omnibus Budget Reconciliation Act of 1989, HR3299 Special Rep No 341a, Washington, DC, December 1989, The Association, pp 1-3.

National Council on Aging (NCOA): Public policy agenda 1986-1987, Perspect Aging 15(2):1-64, The Council, 1986.

National League for Nursing: Criteria and standards manual for NLN/APHA accreditation of home health agencies and community nursing services, New York, 1980, The League.

Naylor R: Christian living, March-April 1983, p. 21.

Norris J, Sherwood S, and Gutkin C: Meeting the needs of the impaired elderly: the power and resiliency of the informal support system, Boston, 1981, Hebrew Rehabilitation Center for Aged.

Nursing home without walls. Its progress and future: summary of proceedings of meeting, Albany, NY, June 22-23, 1982, New York State Senate Health Committee.

Office of Technology Assessment (OTA): Losing a million minds: confronting the tragedy of Alzheimer's disease and other dementias, Washington, DC, 1987, US Government Printing Office.

Oktay J, and Palley H: Home health and in-home service programs for the chronically limited elderly: some equity and adequacy limitations, Home Health Care Serv Q 2(4):5-28, 1981.

Oktay JS and Volland PJ: Foster home care for the frail elderly as an alternative to nursing home care: an experimental evaluation, Am J Public Health 77(12):1505-1510, 1987.

Olson HH: Home health nursing, Caring 5(8):53-61, 1986.

O'Shaughnessy C, Price R, and Griffith J: Financing and delivery of long-term services for the elderly, Pub No 85-1033, Washington, DC, October 17, 1985, Congressional Research Service, Library of Congress.

Pallett PJ: A conceptual framework for studying family caregiver burden in Alzheimer's type dementia, Image: J Nurs Schol 22(1):52-58, 1990.

Paradis LF: Hospice handbook guide for managers and planners, Rockville, Md, 1985, Aspen.

Phillips EK and Cloonon PA: DRG ripple effects on community health nursing, Public Health Nurs 4(2):84-87, 1987.

Pitzele SK: We are not alone: learning to live with chronic illness, New York, 1986, Workman.

Polich CL: Financing long-term care: the role of the federal government, Caring 7(4):16-19; 22-23, 1989.

President's Commission on Mental Health: Task panel reports submitted to the President's Commission on Mental Health, vol III, Washington, DC, 1978, US Government Printing Office.

PROs for nurses, Nurs Health Care 4(9):405, 1983.

Prochazka Z, Henschke P, Skinner E, and Last P: Memory loss and confusion: dementia, a guide for caring people, Adelaide, Aust, 1983, Health Promotion Services, South Australian Health Commission.

Pruchno RA and Resch NL: Husbands and wives as caregivers: antecedents of depression and burden, Gerontologist 29:159-165, 1989.

Reif L and Estes C: Long-term care: new opportunities for professional nursing. In Aiken, L, ed: Nursing in the 1980s: crises, opportunities and challenges, Philadelphia, 1983, Lippincott.

Rivlin AM and Wiener JM: Caring for the disabled elderly, Washington, DC, 1988, Brookings Institution.

Robert Wood Johnson Foundation: Annual report 1983, New York, 1984, Robert Wood Johnson Foundation.

Ross C, Danzinger S, and Smolensky E: The level and trend in poverty in the United States, 1939-1979, Demography 24, 1987.

Ruchlin H, Morris J, and Eggert G: Management and financing of long-term care services, New Engl J Med 306:101-106, 1982.

Sanger AD: Planning home care with the elderly—patient, family, and professional views of an alternative to institutionalization, Cambridge, Ma, 1983, Ballinger.

Scanlon WJ: A perspective on long-term care for the elderly, Health Care Financ Rev, 1988 Annual Suppl, pp 7-15, December 1988.

Schneider EL and Brody JA: Sounding board. Aging, natural death, and the compression of morbidity: another view, New Engl J Med 309:854-856, 1983.

Sekscenski ES: Discharged from nursing homes: preliminary data from the 1985 National Nursing Home Survey, Advance Data from Vital and Health Statistics, No 142, USDHHS Pub No (PHS) 87-1250, Hyattsville, Md, 1987, Public Health Service.

Senate Special Committee on Aging: Developments in aging: 1984, vol 1, Report 99-5, Washington, DC, February 1985, US Government Printing Office.

Shaffer FA: DRGs: history and overview, Nurs Health Care 4:388-396, 1983.

Slow, steady and heartbreaking Time, p 56, July 11, 1983.

Soldo B: The elderly home care population: national prevalence rates, selected characteristics, and alternative sources of assistance, Working Paper 1466-29, Washington, DC, 1983, Urban Institute.

Spiegel AD: Home health care, ed 2, Owings Mills, Md, 1987, Rynd Communications.

St. Armand L: Managed care: fitting pieces of the puzzle together, Home Health Nurse 6(2):14-17, 1988.

Staggers' Lawsuit: Part II, NAHC Report, No 275, Washington, DC, August 12, 1988, National Association for Home Care, pp 1-3.

Stone R, Cafferata GL, and Sangl J: Caregivers of the frail elderly: a national profile, Washington, DC, 1987, US Government Printing Office.

Stone RI: The feminization of poverty among the elderly, Women's Stud Q 17(1&2):20-34, 1989.

Talmadge H and Murphy D: Innovative home care program offers appropriate alternative for elderly, Hosp Progr 50-51, 72, 1983.

US Bureau of the Census: Population profile of the United States: 1989, Current Population Rep, Series P-23, No 159, Washington, DC, 1989, US Government Printing Office.

USDHHS, Public Health Service: Promoting health/preventing disease: year 2000 objectives for the nation, Draft for public review and comment, Washington, DC, September 1989, US Government Printing Office.

United States Senate, Committee on Finance: Long-term health care: hearing before the subcommitttee on health of the committee on finance, United States Senate, ninety-eighth Congress, Washington, DC, 1984, US Government Printing Office.

Upstate Health System, Inc: Data book for the chronically ill and aged task force, Rochester, NY, January 1983, Upstate Health Systems, Inc.

Visiting Nurse Service of Toledo—eighty-three years of caring, Caring 3:57-61, 1984.

Waldo DR, Levit KR, and Lazenby H: National health expenditures, 1985, Health Care Financ Rev 8(1):1-22, 1986.

Warhola C: Planning for home health services: a resource handbook, Department of Health and Human Services, DHHS Pub No HRA 80-14017, Washington, DC, 1980, US Government Printing Office.

Weissert WG, Cready CM, and Pawelak JE: The past and future of home- and community-based long-term care, Milbank Q 66:309-390, 1988.

Weissman MM: Advances in psychiatric epidemiology: rates and risks for major depression, Am J Public Health 77(4):445-451, 1987.

Williams CA: Making things happen: community health nursing and the policy arena, Nurs Outlook 31:225-228, 1983.

Zarit SH, Todd PA, and Zarit JM: Subjective burden of husbands and wives as caregivers: a longitudinal study, Gerontologist 26:260-266, 1986.

Zarit SH and Zarit JM: Families under stress: interventions for caregivers of senile dementia patients, Psychother Theory Res Practice 19:461-471, 1982.

Zawadski RJ and Eng C: Case management in capitated long-term care, Health Care Financ, 1988 Annual Suppl, pp 75-82, 1988.

SELECTED BIBLIOGRAPHY

Brechling BG and Kuhn D: A specialized hospice for dementia patients and their families, Am J Hospice Care 6(3):27-30, 1989.

Dush D: Trends in hospice research and psychosocial palliative care, Hospice J 3(4):13-28, 1988.

Hollingsworth C: Clinical procedure manual for home health care, ed 2, Baltimore, Md, 1990, Williams & Wilkins.

Home health and hospice manual: regulations and guidelines, Owings Mills, Md, 1988, National Health Publishing.

Jones ML: Home care for the chronically ill child, New York, 1985, Springer.

Kalnins I: Home health agency preferences for staff nurse qualifications, and practices in hiring and orientation, Public Health Nurs 6(2):55-61, 1988.

Keating SB and Kelman GB: Home health care nursing concepts and practice, Philadelphia, 1988, Lippincott.

Pasquale DK: Characteristics of Medicare-eligible home care clients, Public Health Nurs 5(3):129-134, 1988.

Pawling-Kaplan M and O'Connor P: Hospice care for minorities: an analysis of a hospital-based inner city palliative care service, Am J Hospice Care 6(4):13-21, 1989.

Ryan MA: Education and service collaboration in hospice, Am J Hospice Care 6(6):23, 1989.

Shamansky SL, ed: Home health care, Nurs Clin North Am 23(2):1988.

Stiller SB: Success and difficulty in high tech home care, Public Health Nurs 5(2):68-75, 1988.

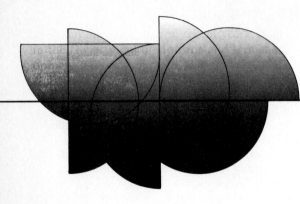

20

Methods for Meeting the Health Care Needs of People: Group Work and Clinic Services

Upon completion of this chapter, the reader will be able to:

1. *Discuss the advantages and disadvantages of using the group approach to promote the health of population groups.*
2. *Describe six ways that groups can meet health needs of clients.*
3. *Discuss how a group is formed and the functions of the community health nurse as a group leader.*
4. *Summarize the phases in the life of a group.*
5. *Discuss how developments in society have contributed to the development of clinic and ambulatory care services.*
6. *Explain how community health nurses establish and maintain clinic services.*
7. *Describe the role of the community health nurse in the clinic setting.*

"There are many ways to skin a cat" is one way of saying that a goal can be reached by numerous routes. This axiom applies to meeting the health care needs of people in community health nursing. The nurse who visits people in their homes is taking one route. As discussed in Chapters 13 and 18, nurses visit parents of newborns to help them with the unique tasks that accompany parenthood and they visit aging people to help them with changing developmental tasks. Other routes, explained in Chapters 14 and 16, are the school nursing role and the occupational health nursing role.

In this chapter, two more methods of meeting people's health care needs are presented: group work and clinic services. Both methods can be used by nurses to provide primary, secondary, and tertiary preventive services to population groups so that they achieve their maximum level of functioning. Both methods focus on groups of people rather than on the nurse-to-family approach utilized in home visits. Clients come to the nurse rather than the nurse serving the family members in their own personal environment.

GROUP WORK IN COMMUNITY HEALTH NURSING

Community health nurses have long worked with groups of people to meet health care needs effectively. In this context *group* is defined as a gathering of people who are together for a specific reason. An example of the use of group work in community health nursing practice is a parent effectiveness training class. Parents in this situation come together to discuss ways to rear children effectively. A gathering of people at a bus stop is not defined as a group.

Community health nursing agencies frequently utilize the group intervention strategy. Community health nurses focus on delivering services to populations in census tracts and on caseloads rather than on individual clients only. Thus, needs common to an area are more readily apparent, particularly if caseload analyses and a community assessment are done. One community health nurse realized that she continually re-

ceived numerous referrals from the intermediate school district to visit families with children who had developmental delays, and that many of these families were clustered close together. To help meet the needs of these families, the nurse formed a parent support group to serve the many primary and secondary health needs of this population.

The History of the Group Approach to Health Care Needs

Kurt Lewin is generally considered to be the founder of modern group process. His research during World War II was aimed at increasing work production as well as changing food consumption patterns. Lewin found that group discussion and group decision helped people to change their ideas much more effectively than lectures or even individual instruction (Lewin, 1947). Giving people information only did not motivate them to change personal attitudes and behavior. Rather, discussion in groups helped persons to become involved, conceptualize ideas, and take health action. Group participants learned something about their own behavior in group settings, and the information gained was relevant to their personal lives.

Another development in the group approach to health was *group psychotherapy.* It became a part of the treatment plan of psychologists and psychiatrists in the 1920s and 1930s, but it was not until the 1960s that group process and group psychotherapy came together (Loomis, 1979, p. 5). During the decade of the 1960s, the *encounter group* movement proliferated and the differences between sensitivity groups and psychotherapy groups blurred. It was realized that everyone, not just "sick" people, could benefit from group process.

The terms *group process, group dynamics,* and *group interaction* all refer to the way groups work and give us ways to assess and observe group functioning. Groups are formed for a variety of psychological, social, and educational purposes such as losing weight, controlling drug usage and smoking, and giving support during divorce and death. Nurses are part of a group on the health team and in professional associations, in choirs, parent-teacher organizations, League of Women Voters, and synagogues. Clearly, group work is an integral part of life in the United States today.

Advantages and Disadvantages of the Group Approach

The definition of community health nursing states that promoting and preserving the health of populations is its goal. Thus, nurses are constantly viewing ways of helping people to look critically at their own health behavior.

Telling people about healthy behavior is not enough—the low immunization levels of preschool children discussed in Chapter 13 is verification of that statement. There must be a way of helping people to value preventive health practices so that they will change their health behavior. Lewin's work, among that of many others, gives evidence that groups can help to accomplish this. A major reason for using the group approach is that different kinds of people with similar concerns can work on these concerns together. Feelings of isolation and aloneness that are so often a part of crisis can be worked through. "I'm not the only one who feels this way, and that's a relief" becomes a frequent comment.

It must be emphasized that the group approach will not meet all clients' health needs. Some people will never feel secure enough to leave their own familiar surroundings, to find transportation, to have the needed energy and skill, or even want to become part of a group. There are people who lack the social expertise, experience, and motivation required to become involved in a group. This behavior can be learned, but it requires patience and skill on the part of the nurse to teach it. An overwhelmed 17-year-old single mother with two children under 2 years of age who has exhibited poor bonding behaviors with her newborn probably needs an intense one-to-one relationship with a nurse before she can profit from a group discussion about parenting.

Nurses gain valuable information about a family when they see individual family members interacting in their own surroundings. A data base on the family system as discussed in Chapter 6 is very difficult to collect when the client is a member of a larger group. Situations that warrant a family-centered nursing approach are best handled in the home environment.

Some people like to function in groups; others do not. These differences need to be respected because an individual's attitude and beliefs regarding the group experience will have an effect on group learning and outcomes.

Luft (1970, p. 30), in his writings on group process, summarized the advantages of group versus individual productivity and problem-solving:

1. There are definite advantages and disadvantages to group versus individual problem-solving and productivity.
2. When a problem demands a single overall insight or an original set of decisions, an individual approach may be superior to a group effort.
3. Problems calling for a wide variety of skills and information or the cross checking of facts and ideas seem to call for a group approach. Feedback and free exchange of thinking may stimulate ideas that would not have emerged by solo effort.
4. If goals are shared, then there is greater likelihood for cooperative effort; when the group goal is not shared by members, morale and productivity may suffer. Consequently, when the goal is decided upon by group discussion and participation, there is greater likelihood of full member involvement.
5. The greater the group members' desire for individual prominence and distinction, the lower will be their friendly sharing or group morale.
6. When members decide on the need for group effort, the smaller size of the group the better it will function, provided that the necessary diversity of skills and group maintenance resources are present.
7. A group may be a source of strong interpersonal stimulation; a group will also generate its own conformity pressures. In order to decide between group and individual work, these two sets of forces (stimulating and binding) should be kept in mind.

8. A society which places highest value on the worth and freedom of the individual also encourages the strongest independent thought, independent work, and independent responsibility. An inherent goal of a sound group in such a society is the reaffirmation of true independence while meeting group needs concerning tasks and morale.

How Community Health Nurses Utilize the Group Approach

Loomis (1979, pp. 3-11) has discussed six ways that groups can be used to meet the biopsychosocial health needs of clients: support, task accomplishment, socialization, learning—behavior change, human relations training, and psychotherapy—insight and behavior change.

Support. This text focuses on the developmental needs of clients throughout the life cycle. Many people are healthy, but during periods of rapid development and change, they need help to manage the maturational and situational crises that can occur. La Leche League groups, classes of expectant parents, and widow-to-widow programs come under this category. Primary prevention of problems is the thrust of support groups because they help those participating to develop healthy methods of dealing with potentially difficult situations.

Because of limited resources, a recognition of the value of support group interaction, and the complex nature of current health problems, community health nurses are increasingly initiating support groups for at-risk clients and/or their families. Support groups are established in a variety of settings including schools, clinics, industries, neighborhood centers, and other community facilities. They are developed for multiple purposes, such as to promote self-esteem among elderly clients (Janosik and Miller, 1982); to help role-reversal couples to adjust to changes in their lifestyles (Moch, 1988); to assist families in dealing with the burden of caregiving (Schmitt, 1982; Watson, 1987); and to help families deal with grief (Demi, 1984). The support group intervention strategy can be a cost-effective and efficient way to meet the needs of at-risk groups. Com-

munity health nurses who guide these types of group experiences find them to be rewarding and meaningful.

Task accomplishment. Large complex tasks need more than one person to carry them out. The interdisciplinary team of a health department which includes nurses, physicians, environmentalists, nutritionists, and physical therapists is one example of how meeting the health care needs of people is accomplished by a group.

Clients in a group can help each other to accomplish goals as well. One large senior citizen's center uses retired volunteer physicians, nurses, and lay people to carry out monthly health screening. The workers *are* needed and *feel* needed, and the clients screened feel that they are helped "by people who understand them."

On a larger scale, community action groups or coalitions have been developed to address major health problems in society. One significant example of this type of group is the national Healthy Mothers, Healthy Babies Coalition, which has affiliated coalitions in the majority of the states. This coalition is a cooperative venture of 80 national voluntary, health professional, and governmental organizations established to accomplish the specific task or goal of improving maternal and infant health through education (Arkin, 1986). Public health leaders believe that coalition building is essential in order to deal with the public health needs evident in our nation (Institute of Medicine, 1988). Community action groups are being developed on national, state, and local levels and are becoming powerful in influencing health care delivery issues. These groups are involved in areas such as fund raising for innovation health planning activities, informing the public about major health problems, and influencing public policy by developing relationships with legislators and other public officials. All of these are important activities for community health nurses, and enhance the effectiveness of clinical practice.

Socialization. Situational and maturational crises such as death, divorce, and retirement can produce pain and isolation. Parents Without Partners, Welcome Wagon Clubs, and senior citizens' activity clubs provide fellowship for those experiencing common needs. As with support groups, clients can learn to develop new ways of dealing with crises through socialization.

Learning–behavior change. Having a new colostomy and coping with a new diagnosis of diabetes or leukemia are situational crises common to the community health nurse. Clients must learn completely new methods of functioning and living with irrigations, diet, and approaching death. Groups composed of clients with common problems provide support as well as teach new methods of coping. Ostomy clubs, Weight Watchers, and Parents Anonymous are examples of learning–behavior change groups.

Group learning/behavior change sessions should be carefully planned and related to the purpose of the group experience. The community health nurse may focus on providing information unknown to group participants, for example, when the nurse is working with a group of expectant parents who want to learn about labor and delivery processes. At other times, the community health nurse focuses on the facilitator role, especially when group members are learning how to cope with changes in their lifestyle.

When establishing a learning/behavior change group, it is essential for the nurse to obtain baseline data about what is already known by the group, as well as the interests and needs of individual group members. This data base can help the nurse to select appropriate content, educational materials, and educational strategies.

Major functions of community health nurses are health education and problem solving with groups as well as with individuals. Current practice trends emphasize group intervention when appropriate, to reach the greatest number, while containing costs. Community health nurses make significant contributions to public health through group work. Research has demonstrated that group health educational experiences can effect changes in health-related knowledge, practices, and attitudes (Centers for Disease Control, 1986).

Human relations training. The National Training Laboratory (now the NTL Institute for Applied Behavior Science) was established in Maine in 1947 to look at informal experimental methods of teaching group process (Luft, 1970, p. 4). It was designed as a 3-week workshop for professional people who wanted to deal more effectively with coworkers. T-groups or skills-training groups grew from the NTL. The subsequent encounter group movement was another later outgrowth. The purpose of these human relations groups is education. Such groups usually meet for a specific number of hours with the purpose of learning cognitively and affectively about human relations. Assertiveness training, body workshops, emotive therapy, and sexuality workshops are all kinds of human relations training groups. They have grown rapidly and their effectiveness depends greatly upon the skills of the leader. Before community health nurses refer clients to them or attend them, they should investigate the quality and preparations of the leader.

Psychotherapy—insight and behavior change. Therapy groups are conducted to treat clients. Usually these clients are people who are discontented and want to change something about their lives. Such groups are usually led by people with graduate degrees in nursing, medicine, or psychology. This group classification is different from the other five because it focuses on the goal-directed alteration of how the client relates to himself and others in an overall way. Psychotherapy may include altering specific behaviors or learning new ways of relating to other people, but it also includes specific assistance with how one feels about oneself (Loomis, 1979, p. 11). Staff-level community health nurses usually do not conduct these types of groups. If clients need psychotherapy, they are referred by the community health nurse to a mental health specialist.

Developing a Group

Before nurses think about using the group approach to meeting health needs, they must be familiar with the policies of their employing agency. Some agencies will not permit nurses to form groups under their auspices. Others will actively support group efforts if they are compatible with agency philosophy and resources. The nurse must also know whether or not her or his workload can support the added responsibility of group work.

This can be ascertained by discussion with the nurse supervisor. Chapter 21 deals more fully with this aspect of the nurse's role, that is, dealing with caseload management issues.

Since community health nurses work with populations such as a county, a city, or a township, common needs that can be met by a group may be expressed by clients, staff nurses, or others (for example, school officials). If the client and the nurse are so inclined, almost any health need can be met by the group process except those for which clients need one-to-one relationships (Loomis, 1979, p. 19). The very young single mother referred to earlier is a client whose needs may not be met by the group process. Frequently it can be useful to combine group and individual intervention strategies. For example, one nurse, had a family in her caseload which included a child with spina bifida and resultant paraplegia. The nurse visited the home to assess family functioning and the environment, as well as to help the mother with the child's daily routine. The nurse also referred the parents to a parent group at the intermediate school, where they received support from families with similar problems.

Once a need that is common to a number of people has been established, the potential group members need to be contacted. The nurse should discuss with them the objectives of what can be accomplished in a group. The important principle involved is that the nurse must have objectives in mind for the group, that the client must have needs in mind, and that the two should be congruent. This principle is also valid when the nurse is considering a referral to an already established group; it must meet the needs of the client. For example, a support group for new parents would probably not be helpful for a client with severe postpartum depression.

To facilitate this principle, contracting is suggested when working with groups. A contract is a written statement of the mutual expectations of both client and nurse for each other. Chapter 8 discusses contracting with families, and the same principles can be applied to groups. Contracts provide a basis for evaluation of the progress that takes place; the key question to consider is have

we or have we not met the objectives we set out to achieve?

The setting plays a crucial role in groups. Several questions, such as those below, should be asked in order to determine whether a particular setting is appropriate.

- Is the group meeting in a place that is easily accessible, that can be reached by public transportation or personal cars easily?
- Is the meeting place near the population being served?
- Is the location of the meeting place safe after dark?
- Does the meeting room provide privacy and warmth?
- Do seating arrangements facilitate group interaction?
- Will the facility be consistently available?

Besides the setting, there are many other factors to consider when developing a group. The size of the group is a major consideration. Though there are no clear rules, five to 15 people usually facilitate good communication. When the group should meet is another important variable. If it is composed of unemployed persons, mornings may be fine. Wage earners, on the other hand, are likely to be free only in the evenings. The frequency and length of meetings and child care arrangements are other issues that need to be decided by nurse and clients. If small children are to be brought along with clients, there needs to be a place with equipment and a caretaker provided. None of these details have "right" and "wrong" answers, but it is essential that clients know them and help to plan them.

Many nurses are hesitant to use the group approach to nursing care because they lack experience with this intervention strategy. Careful planning, staff development activities which facilitate the understanding of group dynamics, and guidance from professionals comfortable with this process will reduce fear.

The Life of a Group

It is helpful for nurses who lead groups to understand that a group goes through phases which include the initiation phase, the working phase, and the termination phase (Knopke and Diekelmann, 1978, p. 135). During the initiation phase, the group is oriented to its goals and purposes. Included in this information are the time limitations and behavior expected of group members. The working phase encourages problem solving through discussion. The final phase, termination, encourages expressions of warmth, anger, and depression as distancing devices for the final separation that will occur as part of the group process.

The Functions of the Community Health Nurse as Group Leader

Effective leadership is fundamental to a positive group experience; there are four functions that are appropriate for nurse group leaders (Marram, 1978, pp. 124-127):

1. The leader facilitates benefits of group membership. People join groups for the reasons discussed earlier and the leader can help the group to meet expected objectives by outlining a direction for the group and interpreting group objectives.
2. The leader maintains a viable group atmosphere by keeping relationships within the group pleasant or relatively secure. Group members need to feel free to be present and to be able to discuss their concerns. Being able to experience new behaviors is also important to growth.
3. The leader oversees group growth by keeping members attuned to the objectives and by clarifying issues in terms of how they relate to the objectives. The leader also needs to periodically help the group evaluate the progress made toward their objectives.
4. The leader regulates individual members' growth within the group setting. People will move toward objectives at different rates of speed and some members may need more specific objectives than others. The leader is concerned not only with the progress of the group toward objectives but also with the growth of individuals within the group.

To succeed in implementing leadership responsibilities in a group, a nurse must have an awareness of how people interact with each other. Community health nurses must utilize basic interviewing and communication skills in all settings, and group work is no exception. People want to be able to communicate and this can be facilitated by asking open-ended questions, asking direct questions, and using other techniques such as reflection and role playing. Games and audio-visual aids are different methods that can be used to stimulate interaction between group members.

Table 20-1 is a summary of the interventions that community health nurses use when they are group leaders. The table presents the types of interventions utilized along with end goals of each intervention. Having an awareness of group intervention strategies and why they are used helps one to effectively guide the group process and to develop criteria for evaluating group dynamics.

Nurses who are interested in working with groups but who have never done so should ask for supervision and a preceptor to help them with the process. Effective communication with group members and agency personnel, careful scheduling, and attention to small details of organizing the group can help this to be a successful experience. Review of the literature is also helpful when community health nurses consider developing groups in the clinical setting. Zander (1982) has written a readable practical book for neophytes who are concerned about creating a group and practicing group process skills.

Using Clinic Services in Community Health Nursing

Another route community health nurses use to meet the health care needs of population groups is through clinic services.

Clinics, often called *ambulatory health services,* are centers that examine and treat ambulatory clients on an outpatient basis. They are frequently operated under the auspices of a larger institution such as a hospital, medical school, group practice, HMO, health department, church, or community organization. Defining their services is difficult because they vary from one institution to the next.

TABLE 20-1 A summary of leader interventions

Type of intervention	Goals of intervention
Support	Provides supportive climate for expressing ideas and opinions, including unpopular or unusual points of view.
	Facilitates members continuing with their ongoing behavior.
	Helps reinforce positive forms of behavior.
	Creates a climate in which silent members may feel secure enough to participate.
Confrontation	Aids in growth and development; helps unfreeze members from being stuck in one mode of functioning.
	Helps reduce some forms of disruptive behavior.
	Helps members deal more openly and directly with each other.
Advice and suggestions	Shares expertise, offers new perspectives.
	Helps focus group on its task and goals.
Summarizing	Helps keep group on its task by reviewing past actions and by setting agenda for future sessions.
	Brings to focus still unresolved issues.
	Organizes past in ways that help clarify; brings into focus themes and patterns of interaction.
Clarifying	Helps reduce distortion in communication.
	Facilitates focus on substantive issues rather than allowing members to be sidetracked into misunderstandings.
Probing and questioning	Helps expand a point that may have been left incomplete.
	Gets at more extensive and wider range of information.
	Invites members to explore their ideas in greater detail.
Repeating, paraphrasing, and highlighting	Helps members continue with their ongoing behavior; invites further exploration and examination of what is being said.
	Clarifies and helps focus on the specific, important, or key aspect of a communication.
	Sharpens members' understanding of what is being said or done.
Reflecting: Feelings	Orients members to the feelings that may lie behind what is being said or done.
	Helps members deal with issues they might otherwise avoid or miss.
Reflecting: Behavior	Gives members the opportunity to see how their behavior appears to others and to see and evaluate its consequences.
	Helps members to understand others' perceptions and responses to them.
Interpretation and analysis	Renders behavior meaningful by locating it in a larger context in which a causal explanation is provided.
	Helps members understand both the likely bases of their behavior and its meaning.
	Summarizes a pattern of behavior and provides a useful way of examining it and working to modify it through the insights gained.
Listening	Provides an attentive and responsive audience for those who participate.
	Models a helpful way for members to relate to one another; gives a feeling of sharing and mutual concern.
	Helps members sharpen their own ideas and thinking as they realize that indeed others are listening and concerned about what they are saying.

From Sampson E and Marthas M: Group process for the health professions, New York, 1981, Wiley, pp 258-260. Reprinted by permission of John Wiley and Sons, Inc.

The clinic setting offers a wide range of preventive health services. Clinics may provide only primary intervention; this is usually the main focus in immunization clinics. Or clinics may provide screening, diagnosis, and treatment services, such as those provided by clinics treating sexually transmitted diseases which identify the disease, administer appropriate treatments, and locate contacts of the infected client for screening.

Clinics may serve only specific populations. Well-baby clinics usually provide assessment services for children from birth to 5 years of age, and family planning clinics usually serve females of childbearing age. Other clinics may serve anyone who comes, any time, with any problem, as do walk-in clinics of large teaching hospitals and neighborhood health care centers. Emergency rooms function as ambulatory clinics in many towns where there are no other resources.

The majority of official local health agencies provide preventive clinic services on a continuing basis for selected population groups. It is common to find Well Child, EPDST, WIC, immunization and communicable disease (e.g., sexually transmitted diseases and tuberculosis) clinic services provided on a regular basis in most health departments. Many also provide family planning, prenatal, dental health, primary care, and multiphasic diagnostic clinic services on an ongoing basis. The high pregnancy rate among adolescents provided an impetus for initiating comprehensive health services to youth through school-based health clinics (Dryfoos, 1985; Hirsch, Zabin, Streett, and Hardy, 1987). The St. Paul Maternal and Child Health Program, one of the oldest school-based clinic projects, offers a wide range of services to students during school hours, such as immunizations, mental health counseling, prenatal care, family planning, and support groups (Maternal and Child Health Program, undated). Other significant health problems have also provided the stimulus for the development of clinic services by private and official community health agencies. For example, an increasing number of official health departments are providing primary health care services for the homeless and other medically indigent groups.

As discussed in Chapter 15, community health centers (CHCs) are also emerging across the country to assist medically underserved aggregates. These centers, federally supported under Section 330 of the Public Health Service Act, are located in every territory and state except Wyoming. They are located in both urban and rural settings and serve persons with special needs, such as coalminers with respiratory and pulmonary impairments, the elderly, people who are confined to their homes, and migrant and seasonal farmworkers. Most migrant health centers are operated together with CHCs. Data reveal that these centers have significantly influenced the health status of the population groups they are serving. Clients served by a CHC have a lower incidence of hospitalization than clients cared for in other health care settings. Studies have also shown a dramatic reduction in infant mortality in specific regions of the country after the establishment of a CHC: in the rural south, infant mortality decreased by 50 percent, and in Denver's CHC program it decreased by 25 percent (National Association of Community Health Centers, Inc., 1986).

The type of care provided through clinics may be episodic, in which only the immediate needs of the clients are handled, or comprehensive, providing four levels of preventive services: primary preventive, diagnostic, therapeutic, and rehabilitative services. Primary preventive and diagnostic services (e.g., screening for communicable diseases or health risks such as high blood cholesterol) are frequently the focus in clinics sponsored by official health agencies.

The Evolution of Clinic Services over Time

Community health nurses have long worked in clinics. Beginning with the era of Lillian Wald, they have had to assume a considerable amount of responsibility, make independent judgments, and use skill in teaching clients. These competencies especially fitted them to work in the relatively independent clinic setting.

Early efforts at the beginning of the century to improve maternal child health and to control communicable disease frequently resulted in the development of clinic services for underserved aggregates. For example, between 1900 and 1930, many milk dispensaries evolved into preventive health centers. The Kentucky Frontier Nursing Service also hired nurses to provide care through home visiting and health centers for all residents in the region. Additionally, large-scale health demonstration projects were sponsored by the Metropolitan Life Insurance Company to combat tuberculosis and other communicable diseases, and included programs of mass screening and health assessment, as well as community education activities (Kalisch and Kalisch, 1986).

By the 1930s, child health conferences and maternity conferences or clinics were well established. Books on public health nursing practice written at this time addressed the role of the nurse in the clinic and stressed the need for conferences to achieve a well-balanced child welfare program (Gardner, 1928; National Organization for Public Health Nursing, 1939).

Clinic services were developed in the beginning of the century because a significant number of families could not afford other types of care. They were also established to reach a large number of individuals very quickly during epidemics of communicable diseases. These services have been maintained over the century because early efforts dramatically demonstrated their effectiveness in improving maternal/child health and in combating communicable diseases.

The nurse practitioner movement of the 1960s and 1970s significantly altered the role of nurses in community-based clinics. This movement evolved because the needs of disadvantaged aggregates across the life-span were neglected. It was believed that well-trained nurses with expanded skills could help to eradicate the problem of inaccessible and fragmented health-care services, especially in underserved areas. Increasingly, local health departments and other community health clinics are utilizing nurse practitioners to provide comprehensive services for at-risk aggregates (Lawler and Valand, 1988, pp. 187-188).

During the decade of the 1980s, there has been tremendous growth in ambulatory care or clinic services, particularly because of the introduction of the prospective payment system for Medicare-sponsored hospital stays. As the length of hospital stays has decreased, patient acuity at discharge has increased. This has resulted in the need for increased continuing care after discharge and has shifted the responsibility for patients' care to their families and community-based providers. Further, to increase cost-efficient care, insurers have encouraged people to have preadmission testing done on an outpatient basis, and have moved many surgeries such as lens implantation to an outpatient basis. As a result, the number of days being spent in community hospitals is decreasing significantly while the number of outpatient visits is rising dramatically. In fact, ambulatory care is one of the fastest growing specialities in nursing.

Establishing and Maintaining Clinic Services

Community health nurses frequently assume a major role in planning, implementing, and evaluating clinic services for populations with unmet needs. When establishing any new health care service, the nurse utilizes the health planning process described in Chapter 12; some specific factors to consider when setting up clinic services follow.

Determining the need for clinics is the first responsibility of a health care professional interested in developing such services. Factors to consider during this process are the health status, lifestyle patterns, and demographic characteristics of the population being studied; community resources available to the population under consideration; health care utilization patterns; and health care accessibility variables such as location of resources and client referral processes. Chapter 11 describes how and where community health nurses obtain these data. When analyzing these data, it is important to examine trends over time and to identify strengths as well as limitations in the health care delivery system. The goal is to determine if services are lacking or if services are adequate but not utilized because of unique characteristics of the population being served or service delivery problems. For example, community health nurses may find that clients do not use clinic services because their location makes them inaccessible, or clients are unaware they exist. If a need is verified, careful planning should take place before starting a clinic.

Several preclinic organizational activities need

to be accomplished in order to ensure effective and efficient service delivery. Establishing specific objectives for a clinic before development begins helps the nurse to determine what types of services to offer and what resources are needed to provide them. For example, the resources needed to staff a comprehensive child health conference would be significantly greater than those needed to staff an immunization clinic. Prospective clients should be part of the planning team to help ensure that clients' needs can be met through the proposed clinic.

Other preclinic organizational activities include determining the location for the clinic; securing necessary clinic equipment and supplies; organizing clinic facilities to ensure client privacy and effective and efficient service delivery; establishing clinic procedures such as follow-up policies that promote quality care; obtaining adequate professional staff with the skills needed to manage client health needs; securing and training of volunteers; and developing marketing strategies. All of these activities require careful thought and planning, and include several components. For example, securing necessary clinic equipment and supplies involves such things as identifying what is needed, determining where to purchase it, and establishing appropriate storage procedures for vaccines and other medications.

Determining a site for a clinic requires special attention because location of a clinic influences the way it will be utilized. Some clients are affected more than others by the location, namely, the poor and the aged. Difficulty and expense of access are important, so a knowledge of the possible transportation alternatives is important. Accessibility also involves appointment delay time, waiting time, clinic hours, services offered, health care given, and client/professional relationships.

During the preclinic organizational phase, evaluation procedures should be established. If this activity is neglected during the initial development phase, procedures will not be established to ensure collection of data needed to complete an evaluation once the clinic has been in operation. An overall evaluation of clinic operations should occur at least once a year, but evaluation is an ongoing process that needs attention throughout the

year. Procedures need to be established to evaluate overall clinic operations and utilization patterns. Questions for planners to consider when evaluating clinic services are shared in a later section of this chapter.

The importance of adequate planning when establishing and maintaining a clinic cannot be overstressed. Neglecting significant details during the planning phase can result in poor use of services. For example, one health department decided to open a well-baby clinic because it was determined that a rural portion of a large county was underserved. The first decision made was to send a staff nurse to school for preparation as a pediatric nurse practitioner. However, steps of the planning process were not logically followed after preparing this staff nurse for new role responsibilities. Thus, even though there were no other facilities for well-child care in the area, the clinic closed because of lack of clients. It was isolated with no public transportation available, so clients could not use the service.

The Role of the Community Health Nurse in the Clinic

The community health nurse can function in various ways to meet the health needs of populations in the clinic setting. As previously discussed, the expanded role of the nurse has aided community health nurses in more adequately meeting the health care needs of people in clinics. The client population being served in many clinics has become more complex and acute. Nurses no longer serve as schedulers and receptionists. Their roles have enlarged to include management of clients with both acute and long-term care needs, handling of complex treatments and procedures, client counseling and health education. In addition, nurses are often the primary providers for many clients and their families. Verran (1986), when studying the nursing care requirements of ambulatory clients attending a hospital-based ambulatory care center, developed a taxonomy which clearly illustrates the extensive range of activities assumed by nurses in clinic settings (refer to box on p. 792). Verran's taxonomy identifies six major responsibility areas that are assumed by ambulatory care nurses as well as activities to ful-

Taxonomy of Ambulatory Care Nursing Activities

PATIENT COUNSELING

Client advocacy
Terminal/chronic illness
General support
Clinic procedures

HEALTH CARE MAINTENANCE

General assessment
Preventive care instruction
Provide information
Follow-up assessment

PRIMARY CARE

Referral
Physical
Triage
History
Protocol care

PATIENT EDUCATION

General instruction
Standardized instruction
Plan of care
Illness/condition program
Individual instruction
Health care maintenance program

THERAPEUTIC CARE

Surgical preparation
Applications
Appliances
Noninvasive IV medications
Irrigations
Specimens
Recovery
Dressings
Blood therapy
Respiratory treatments
Measurement
Invasive medications
IV therapy

NORMATIVE CARE

Directing
Chaperoning
Documents coordination
Transporting
Assisting
System
Communication
Preparation
Comfort

From Verran JA: Testing a classification instrument for the ambulatory care setting, Research Nurs Health 9:280, 1986.

fill these responsibilities. Verran's taxonomy has been widely used and referenced in the development and application of tools for primary care (Schroeder, 1987; Smyth, 1987).

The range of activities implemented by a nurse in a clinic setting will vary based on the objectives of the clinic and the needs of clients. Common roles assumed by the nurse in most community health settings are discussed below.

Manager

The role of manager was the main nursing function in clinics for many years. Nurses attended to the many details necessary in order for clinics to run smoothly: distributing client caseload, following up on clients with problems, bringing needed reports to physicians, preparing clients physically for examinations, performing procedures, supervising aides and practical nurses, and carrying out clerical work. Although all this is necessary, the nurse should perform *nursing* activities, that is, helping clients when they are unable to help themselves. The nurse should supervise other members of the health team as described in Chapter 21 so that they can carry out the functions which do not require the professional skills of a registered nurse. This means that the nurse will understand the different levels of functioning of team members and utilize them appropriately. Clerks and aides as well as volunteers can be valuable assets in the clinic. They can weigh and measure babies, file and pull records, label and carry specimens to the laboratory, act as receptionists, and take temperatures. Smooth flow of clients from waiting to examining rooms is important and can be done by aides. As a manager, the community health nurse must understand that she or he is responsible for the care that these team members give. The nurse's supervision of team members is fundamental to the care given clients in the clinic setting.

Group Leader and Teacher

Many clinics have as one of their most important functions group sessions in which information is discussed that is designed to promote health. One example is an ostomy information clinic which disseminates information and helps clients to cope with problems related to their ostomies (Yahle, 1975, p. 457). Another example is a prenatal education program in a hospital setting in which the community health nurse meets with clients before appointments to share information about pregnancy, childbirth, childcare, and role transition concerns. The concepts presented earlier in this chapter on developing and leading a group are applicable to the nurse's role in clinics as group leader and teacher.

Practitioner

The expanded role of the nurse has provided nurses with physical assessment and client management skills. Practitioners are able to identify the current health status of clients, including emotional and physical components, and to plan interventions which meet clients' needs. Practitioners carry out a variety of functions in both adult and child health clinics. Providing physical, mental, social, and emotional support, educating clients about their health conditions, and referring clients to needed community resources are examples of functions implemented by the practitioner. Practitioners often work with an interdisciplinary team and actively participate in client care conferences. They provide a continuum of nursing services, especially for clients who have chronic health conditions or preventive health needs.

Evaluator

An integral part of working in the clinic setting is evaluation. This process was discussed in-depth in Chapter 12. Some specific questions one should ask when evaluating clinic services include the following: Are the objectives of the clinic being met? If this is the immunization clinic in Smith County, for example, are children upon school entrance at age 6 completely immunized? Are the numbers of clients being served increasing or decreasing? If the number of clients being served is changing, is it because the health service area population is changing or because clients feel that they are not being served adequately? The way clients feel about the care they receive determines whether or not they will use the health facility. Some method of client contact on a regular basis, either questionnaire or interview, provides data concerning this factor. Knowing who is served also means that a record system will be in operation so that numbers of visits and kinds of visits can be tabulated easily. A good record system will also provide for continuity of care from one visit to the next and yet not be overly time consuming.

Promoting the Community Health Nurse Philosophy in the Clinic

Increasingly, community health nurses are working in nontraditional public health clinic settings, such as hospital-based outpatient departments, or with ambulatory care health providers who do not share the same orientation to practice as theirs. This is occurring because health care delivery trends emphasize the provision of ambulatory care services, while funding sources do not reimburse primary prevention efforts. Thus, focus is on developing a comprehensive package of services, including preventive and curative services, which will be reimbursed by third-party payors. To achieve this focus, a team of health providers, with various backgrounds and skills, is often involved in many clinic settings. A large role for community health nurses on these teams is to promote the philosophy of community health practice: orientation to wellness rather than illness; family-centered versus individual-centered practice; continuity rather than episodic intervention; and population-based or community health planning. Regardless of where community health nurses function, these concepts should be central to their practice. As was discussed in Chapter 2, it is the nature of the practice—not the setting— which distinguishes community health nursing from other specialty nursing areas. The concepts of community health nursing greatly enrich service delivery and nursing care in any clinic setting.

Community health professionals are developing creative approaches for providing and obtaining funding for essential clinic services. The state of Missouri, for example, is demonstrating that it is possible to coordinate primary care that focuses on the population as a whole as well as on the

TABLE 20-2 Collaboration of community health nurse and nurse practitioner in prenatal care

Community health nurse	Advanced practice nurse
Client and family history	Review data
Current health status	
Screenings	
Weight, blood pressure	Risk assessment
Laboratory work	Physical examination
Urinalysis, blood	Pap smear and pelvic examination
Diet review	Fetal heart tones
Danger signs	Fundal height
Education	Education
Case management	Referral

From Riner MB: Expanding services: the role of the community health nurse and the advanced nurse practitioner, J Community Health Nurs 6:227, 1989.

health of individuals within the community (Riner, 1989, pp. 224-228). This state utilizes three levels of community health nurses: (1) the *generalist nurse* whose role responsibilities include clinical nursing, general in nature, epidemiological follow-up, case management, community resource coordination, and home health care; (2) the *mastery nurse* who has had special training for performing a complete physical examination, which increases early diagnosis and treatment through casefinding; and (3) the *advanced practice nurse* which includes certified nurse practitioners, nurse midwives, and clinical nurse specialists. These nurses collaborate to promote a continuum of nursing services. Table 20-2 delineates the different role responsibilities of a CHN generalist and the advanced practice nurse when providing prenatal clinical nursing service in the Missouri system. In this system, the services provided by all three levels of nursing are reimbursed by third-party payors. The case management activities of the generalist are reimbursed through Medicaid. Medicaid also funds services provided by the mastery nurse because of the difficulty in recruiting physicians for underserved areas. Payment for nurse practitioners comes

from a variety of sources such as federal block grant monies, special state grants, and Medicaid.

Developing new ways of providing services for at-risk populations is essential in this era of cost containment. In order to handle the demands in the health care delivery system and the changing nature of current health problems, coordinated, community-wide approaches must be emphasized. Community health nurses have unique skills and knowledge to deal with these challenges.

A FINAL COMMENT ON GROUP WORK AND CLINIC SERVICES

As adequate finances for health care delivery become a scarcer commodity, health care agencies are moving in the direction of using clinics and groups to meet the needs of people. One large health department in the midwest uses clinics almost exclusively; home visits to families are a rare occurrence. At a time when each home visit is costing taxpayers up to $100, it is not difficult to see why alternatives to home visiting are being considered.

It is important to remember that no one method will meet everyone's health needs and that nurses need "in every enterprise to consider where you would come out." Families generate as well as help to solve health problems, and this important aspect can be lost in group and clinic work. However, clinics and groups do have a place in health care, and each will increase in number. Remember, though, to start with the needs of clients to decide what route to use to assist them. This kind of choice contributes to the challenge, excitement, and creativity of community health nursing.

SUMMARY

Nurses can use many routes to meet the health care needs of clients. Group work and clinic services are two possible routes. Advantages and disadvantages of the group approach are many and nurses need to be familiar with them. Understanding the methodology followed to develop a group, the phases of a group, and the functions of the nurse as a group leader is essential if the nurse is going to function effectively in a group setting.

Clinics have long been a place where community health nurses have served varied populations. The location aspect of clinic facilities plays an important part in how well they are utilized. Clinic services need to be well planned if they are to be effective. Thus, it is crucial for the community health nurse to be familiar with the planning process.

The community health nurse carries out multiple roles and functions in the clinic setting—manager, group leader and teacher, practitioner, and evaluator. The nurse's major function is to assist clients to help themselves. The nurse must learn to appropriately delegate tasks to other members of the health care team, so that she or he has sufficient time to work with clients.

Increasingly, health care agencies are using clinics and groups to meet the needs of populations in the community. It is known, however, that a more effective and efficient health care delivery system must be established if the needs of all are to be met. Nurses must become involved in planning for the future so that a viable role for nursing is maintained in the evolving health care system.

REFERENCES

Arkin EB: The Healthy Mothers, Healthy Babies Coalition: four years of progress, Public Health Rep 101:147-156, 1986.

Centers for Disease Control: The effectiveness of school health education, MMWR 35(38):593-595, September 26, 1986.

Demi AS: Hospice bereavement program: trends and issues. In Schraff SH, ed: Hospice: the nursing perspective, New York, 1984, National League for Nursing.

Dryfoos J: School-based health clinics: a new approach to preventing adolescent pregnancy? Family Planning Perspect 17(2):70-75, 1985.

Gardner MS: Public health nursing, ed 2, New York, 1928, Macmillan.

Hirsch MB, Zabin LS, Streett RF, and Hardy JB: Users of reproductive health clinic services in a school pregnancy prevention program, Public Health Rep 102:307-316, 1987.

Institute of Medicine: The future of public health, Washington, DC, 1988, National Academy Press.

Janosik EH and Miller JR: Group work with the elderly. In Janosik EH and Phipps LB, eds: Life cycle group work in nursing, Monterey, Ca, 1982, Wadsworth, pp 248-265.

Kalisch PA and Kalisch BJ: The advance of American nursing, ed 2, Boston, 1986, Little, Brown.

Knopke HJ and Diekelmann NL: Approaches to teaching in the health sciences, Reading, Ma, 1978, Addison-Wesley.

Lawler TG and Valand MC: Patterns of practice of nurse practitioners in an underserved rural region, J Community Health Nurs 5:187-194, 1988.

Lewin K: Group decision and social change. In Newcomb TM and Hartley EL, eds: Readings in social psychology, New York, 1947, Holt.

Loomis ME: Group process for nurses, St Louis, 1979, CV Mosby Co.

Luft J: Group process. An introduction to group dynamics, ed 2, Palo Alto, Ca, 1970, Mayfield.

Marram GP: The group approach in nursing practice, St Louis, ed 2, 1978, CV Mosby Co.

Maternal and Child Health Program: St. Paul Adolescent Health Services Project, St Paul, Mn, undated, St Paul-Ramsey Medical Center.

Moch SD: Promoting health with role-reversal couples, J Community Health Nurs 5:195-202, 1988.

National Association of Community Health Centers, Inc: Community health centers: a quality system for the changing health care market, McLean, Va, 1986, National Clearinghouse for Primary Care Information.

National Organization for Public Health Nursing: Manual of public health nursing, ed 3, New York, 1939, Macmillan.

Riner MB: Expanding services: the role of the community health nurse and the advanced nurse practitioner, J Community Health Nurs 6:223-230, 1989.

Sampson E and Marthas M: Group process for the health professions, New York, 1981, Wiley.

Schmitt MH: Groups for the chronically ill. In Janosik EH and Phipps LB, eds: Life cycle group work in nursing, Monterey, Ca, 1982, Wadsworth, pp 266-290.

Schroeder MA: Computers in nursing: applications for ambulatory care, Nurs Econ 5(1): 27-31, 1987.

Smyth K: Justice and cooperation: moving ambulatory care practice into the 21st century, J Ambulatory Care Manage 10(3):76-81, 1987.

Verran JA: Testing a classification instrument for the ambulatory care setting, Research Nurs Health 9:279-287, 1986.

Watson WL: Intervening with aging families and Alzheimer's disease. In Wright LM and Leahey M, eds: Families and chronic illness, Springhouse, Pa, 1987, Springhouse, pp 381-404.

Yahle ME: An ostomy information clinic, Nurs Clin North Am 14:457-467.

Zander A: Making groups effective, San Francisco, 1982, Jossey-Bass.

SELECTED BIBLIOGRAPHY

Chamberlin RW: Beyond individual risk assessment: community wide approaches to promoting the health and development of families and children, Washington, DC, 1988, National Center for Education in Maternal and Child Health.

Grimes R: Developing neighborhood nurse offices, Nurs Health Care 4(3):138-139, 1983.

Hazard M and Kemp R: Keeping the well-elderly well, Am J Nurs 83(4):567-569, 1983.

Henshaw SK, Kenney AM, Somberg D, and Van Vort J: Teenage pregnancy in the United States: the scope of the problem and state responses, New York, 1989, Alan Guttmacher Institute.

Lewis S: Teaching patient groups, Nurs Manage 15(5):49-56, 1984.

O'Brien M: Reaching the migrant worker, Am J Nurs 83(6):895-897, 1983.

Oda DS and Boyd P: The outcome of public health nursing service in a preventive child health program: phase 1, health assessment, Public Health Nurs 5:209-213, 1988.

Selby ML, Riportella-Muller R, Sorenson JR, and Walters CR: Improving EPSDT use: development and application of a practice-based model for public health nursing research, Public Health Nurs 6:174-181, 1989.

Select Committee on Children, Youth, and Families: Opportunities for success: cost-effective programs for children, Washington, DC, 1985, US Government Printing Office.

Stimson DH, Charles G, and Rogerson CL: Ambulatory care classification systems, Health Serv Research 20(6):683-703, 1986.

Thibodeau JA and Hawkins J: Evolution of a nursing center, J Ambulatory Care Manage 10(3):30-39, 1987.

Thornton J: Developing a rural nursing clinic, Nurse Educator 7(2):24-29, 1983.

Wyka-Fitzgerald C: Long term evaluation of group education for high blood pressure control, Cardiovasc Nurs 20(3):13-18, 1984.

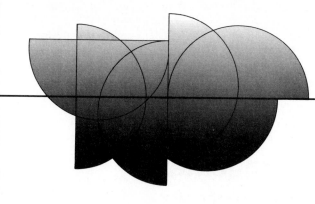

UNIT SIX

Management of Professional Commitments

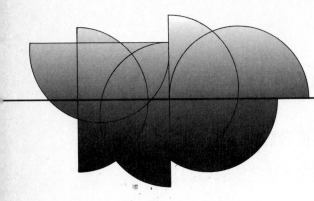

21

Utilizing Management Concepts in Community Health Nursing

This is my work; my blessing, not my
   doom;
Of all who live, I am the one by whom
This work can best be done in the right way.

HENRY VAN DYKE

Upon completion of this chapter, the reader will be able to:

1. Explain how a staff-level community health nurse
utilizes management skills in the practice setting.
2. Distinguish between the informal and formal
structure of an organization.
3. Describe the five management functions used by
community health nurses.
4. Discuss the elements involved in analyzing a
caseload and a client care situation.
5. Differentiate between the terms team nursing,
primary nursing, and case management.

6. Describe factors to consider when scheduling
community health nursing activities.
7. Explain factors which affect priority determination
and intensity of community health nursing service in
caseload management.
8. Describe the use of delegation in community health
nursing practice.

The community is an exciting setting which provides challenging opportunities for community health nurses. An outstanding characteristic of community health nursing is the independence of its practitioners. In any one day, a community health nurse may decide what families to visit and in what order they will be visited. During that day, the nurse may make a nursing diagnosis and carry out nursing interventions without nursing supervision, without a doctor's order, or without even talking to another nurse. That day, he or she may also receive new referrals and make decisions on their priority. Furthermore, the nurse may be carrying out nursing care indirectly through delegation to registered nurses, licensed practical nurses, or home health aides. When these health personnel are caring for clients under the nurse's supervision, the nurse is responsible for the care given by them.

This independence and delegation in community health nursing practice must be accompanied by knowledge of management concepts. Knowledge of management concepts helps the community health nurse to provide care, directly and indirectly, to families and population groups as well as to evaluate the quality of health services that the client receives. Available resources, such as finances and personnel, need to be managed so that maximum productivity, efficiency, and quality of care are achieved.

Managing the extensive amounts of data which community health nurses must collect and utilize is increasingly complex. Computerized management information systems are crucial for today's community health nurse manager: these systems are being used by CHN agencies across the country to facilitate effective and efficient resource management.

Whatever role a nurse assumes in the community setting, be it staff nurse, supervisor, or administrator, the nurse will participate in leadership and management functions to some degree. Community health nursing, like the management process, is a logical activity that helps clients, families, and groups to make goal-directed changes. The nurse facilitates these changes through the work of others. Thus, a conscious application of the management process to nursing care at any

level can make the nurse more effective in arranging his or her own personal workload as well as in functioning in a larger system.

This chapter briefly analyzes concepts of management and then examines how community health nurses can utilize them. A limited discussion of the historical development of management thought is also shared. Knowledge of the evolution of management concepts provides the information an individual needs to formulate a personal philosophy of management.

THE HISTORICAL DEVELOPMENT OF MANAGEMENT CONCEPTS

There are numerous leaders in the field of management who contributed to its development. To list them all here would be an almost impossible task. When reviewing the development of management thought, however, one can see that modern concepts of management have evolved over time. Historically, emphasis was placed on analyzing the functions and processes of management tasks, without taking into consideration the needs of the worker (see Chapter 16). Today, there is a trend for managers to apply systems concepts (see Chapter 6) in the work environment in order to determine how to maintain employee satisfaction and to increase productivity and efficiency.

Frederick Taylor is the founder of the scientific management movement. His belief was that the planning of tasks needed to be separated from their performance. In relation to this thought, he felt that managers should be responsible for the planning and controlling of tasks and that employees should assume responsibility for production. He conducted time and motion studies to determine the best way to accomplish tasks, to develop work standards, and to identify how to divide the work between managers and employees. Taylor's book, *The Principles of Scientific Management,* was published in 1911.

Henri Fayol expanded on Taylor's thoughts by identifying a composite of well-defined functions and tasks for managers. In 1916 he published his ideas about management, which were that managers had five basic functions: plan, organize, command, coordinate, and control (Koontz,

O'Donnell, and Weihrich, 1986, p. 11). With some minor changes in this list, these functions are still used by most authorities on management.

Significant criticism of management occurred during the first half of the twentieth century, because managers emphasized task performance without looking at worker satisfaction. As a result of this criticism, modern management trends which stressed the importance of examining employee needs emerged. The classic Hawthorne experiment conducted by Elton Mayo clearly demonstrated to management the value of looking at employees as people.

The Hawthorne studies of the Western Electric Company during the 1920s and 1930s applied the principles of psychology, social psychology, and sociology to the understanding of organizational behavior. The researchers of this study began by investigating the relationship between physical conditions of work and employee productivity; however, they found that social variables were much more important to productivity. The outgrowth of the Hawthorne study was the development of the concept of human relations, or the study of human behavior for the purposes of attaining higher production levels and personal satisfaction (Koontz, O'Donnell, and Weihrich, 1986, p. 13). The human relations concept has expanded into the behavioral science approach to management. A trend toward emphasizing employee satisfaction to increase production on the job can still be seen. Employee motivation, the workplace as a social system, leadership within the organization, communication within the system, and personal and professional employee development are five major areas of concern to managers who use behavioral science methods and principles. Writings by Chris Argyris, Chester Barnard, Douglas McGregor, Kurt Lewin, Rensis Likert, Robert Tannenbaum, and others give a more in-depth perspective on the behavioral science movement.

The systems approach to management was another development among management concepts. With the systems approach, both the structure and the processes of an organization are analyzed. Emphasis is placed on examining how all the parts of an organization interact and interrelate to achieve the goals of the organization. Systems managers recognize that a change in one part of the organizational system affects all the other parts, just as practitioners using a systems approach recognize that a change (illness) in the family unit affects all other members of the family system (see Chapter 6).

Today, community health nurses work in complex systems. To function effectively in these modern health care systems, the community health nurse must know not only nursing theory but management theory as well. Traditionally, management concepts were not emphasized during a nurse's academic study, even though nurses were expected to carry out management responsibilities in practice. Now it is recognized that the task of organizing health care delivery can be made easier and more powerful with knowledge of management concepts. That is why principles of management are covered during a nurse's basic educational preparation.

THE ORGANIZATIONAL STRUCTURE OF HEALTH CARE DELIVERY

The number of health care delivery systems in which community health nurses may work is increasing. They work in diverse health and health-related organizations, each of which may have a differing organizational structure and way of delivering nursing services.

Nurses must know the organizational structure of their employing agencies so that they can determine how to utilize agency resources and to identify appropriate ways to effect change within the organization. Organizational structure encompasses the formal and informal patterns of behavior and relationships in an organization. This includes both formal and informal position allocations, as well as the chain of command and the channels of communication.

The Informal Organizational Structure

The informal organizational structure refers to the personal and social relationships of people who work together. Informal relationships have no formal power. However, they can have a major impact on the organization and its management.

The way in which a manager is viewed by the staff does influence the manner and effectiveness of her or his management.

The Formal Organizational Structure

Formal organizational structure defines which people will do which tasks so that the objectives of the organization can be accomplished. It is the power structure of the organization. The rules, policies, procedures, control mechanisms, and financial arrangements of the organization are all part of the formal structure. The schematic organization is part of this formal structure and can be seen in an organizational chart.

Organizational Chart

An organizational chart diagrams the relationship among members of the organization and indicates the structure of authority, formal lines of communication, and levels of management and delegation. These all interrelate to accomplish the goals of the organization. An example of an organizational chart is presented in Figure 21-1.

An organizational manual supplements an organizational chart by supplying information about the requirements of the various job positions represented on the chart. Organizational charts and manuals are useful tools which describe the formal relationships in a particular organization. They do not show the informal relationships that exist.

Usually there are two types of positions in an organization: *staff* and *line.* Figure 21-1 shows how staff and line positions are depicted on an organizational chart. The line structure is the basic framework of an organizational structure. The staff nurse is in a direct line position and is accountable to the person directly above him or her on the organizational chart. The term *staff nurse* should not be confused with *staff personnel.* The staff personnel supplement the line personnel in an advisory capacity. They are extensions of the administrator but usually have no authority to direct the actions of persons in the line position. Authority can, however, be delegated in several directions from both staff and line positions.

The line organization is characterized by a di-

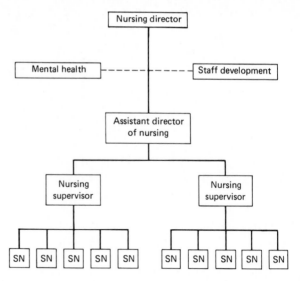

Figure 21-1   An organizational chart showing staff and line positions.

rect flow of authority from top to bottom. Each position has general authority over the one directly below it. Authority is inherent in line positions. For example, the assistant director of nursing has authority over the nursing supervisor who in turn has authority over the staff nurse. Persons in staff positions, on the other hand, are delegated authority by top-level administrators (nursing director) to carry out specific tasks and responsibilities. Authority is not inherent in staff positions.

A manager must have a basic understanding of organizational power relationships in order to manage effectively. Four types of power relationships evolve in any organization:

1. Authority: the power to direct the actions of others
2. Responsibility: the obligation to carry out or perform tasks in an acceptable way
3. Accountability: the obligation to answer for one's actions
4. Delegation: assigning and empowering one person to act for another with the responsibility for the act remaining with the person who assigned it

Organizational structure and resulting power relationships in a health care agency assist personnel in all positions to carry out effectively the functions of management. It would be impossible to manage if such a structure did not exist. Effective and efficient management can occur only when personnel understand what they are responsible for and to whom they are accountable. Ignoring the power relationships in an organization can create real difficulties. Illustrative of this are the actions taken by the community health nurse in the following situation.

A community health nurse identified a need for a family planning program in two of the census tracts she served. Knowing that the county health department did not include these services, she independently arranged a group meeting in the clubhouse at a local park to discuss the need for these services with the people of the community. This was done without discussing the action with her supervisor.

Twenty community members attended the meeting. They quickly became emotionally involved in the issue and wanted immediate action taken by the health department to initiate such a service. The nurse became uncomfortable because she recognized that she did not have the power to make a definite commitment regarding the establishment of a new program. The community members became frustrated with the nurse's lack of action.

Had proper channels within the agency power structure been utilized, this situation would probably have been handled differently.

When looking at this situation, one can quickly ask the following questions: Did the nurse have the authority to organize this meeting, and was she acting in a responsible and an accountable manner? What were her objectives for the meeting and did she clarify them for herself and the group?

When one is planning a meeting with a group such as the one above, it is crucial to seek the advice of individuals within the organization who have the authority to make decisions. When this is not done, it can result in stress and frustration for all parties involved. If the nurse had gone to her supervisor prior to the meeting, she would have been aware of the types of commitments she could make during the meeting. If, for instance, the health department did not have adequate re-sources to staff a family planning clinic, the group goal might be to look at alternative ways to obtain funding for family planning services in the community, rather than only to discuss how the health department might provide these services.

Organizational Policies

Another component of the formal organization structure which maximizes functioning is organizational policies. Policies define the limits of acceptable activities and provide structure and guidelines for employee decision making. They are generally developed to handle situations that occur consistently in daily practice. Policies that address how to handle referrals (see Chapter 9), when and how to conduct nursing audits (see Chapter 22), and benefits staff will have, such as travel allowance, are a few examples of policies commonly found in a community health agency. These types of policies provide direction for decision making.

When policies are absolute, with no flexibility, they are considered *rules.* Rules are usually established in order to ensure client and staff safety and quality of care. The following are examples of rules:

- "No home visits are to be made at night in census tract 3 without an escort."
- "No immunizations are to be given until an allergy history has been taken."
- "Every fifth record closed to service must be audited."

When nurses accept employment within a health setting, it is assumed that they accept responsibility for following, enforcing, and informing others about agency policies. This means that the conditions of employment should be clearly understood before the nurse accepts a position within an organization. Otherwise, the nurse may be in a situation where it is necessary to follow certain policies that are inconsistent with her or his philosophy of practice.

Nursing personnel at all levels may be involved in writing policies. Policy statements should include the following items:

1. Reason for establishing the policy (philosophy behind the policy)
2. Actual policy statement
3. Guidelines for implementing the policy

If used effectively, policies can increase the efficiency and ease with which individuals carry out their functions within an organization. Difficulties with implementing a policy will occur, however, if employees do not understand the reason for the policy, if employee input is not obtained when the policy is being formulated, if the policy is not clearly written, or if policies become numerous and prevent necessary flexibility for nursing practice.

DEFINING MANAGEMENT LANGUAGE

Management is the planning, organizing, directing, coordinating, and controlling of activities in a system so that the objectives of that system are met. For community health nurses, that system may be represented by any number of settings in which the nurse practices, such as a public health agency, ambulatory care setting, a school, or an industrial plant.

Administration is a term that is often mistakenly used interchangeably with *management.* The principles of management and administration are the same, but the scope of functioning for managers and administrators varies. For instance, both administrators and managers set goals, but the administrator sets goals for a department, whereas a staff nurse sets personal goals when managing her or his workload responsibilities.

Leadership is influencing others to reach desired goals. In any organization, there are both formal (appointed) leaders and informal (those chosen by the group) leaders. "A leader is able to command trust, commitment, and loyalty of followers. Most work is done by people who do not have a formal leadership position. Many of these people are leaders who take responsibility for reaching group goals. A leader is the person who communicates ideas to others and influences their behavior to reach an objective" (Douglass, 1988, p. 3). Thus, effective nurses at any organizational level use leadership and management skills: they positively influence those about them to promote the common good and they apply management principles to their practice.

THE MANAGEMENT FUNCTIONS OF THE COMMUNITY HEALTH NURSE

The five management functions carried out by the community health nurse are planning, organizing, directing, coordinating, and controlling. These management functions help to link the entire organizational system together and assist the nurse in effectively managing workload responsibilities. Managing is done on many levels by nurses, depending upon their place in the organizational structure as well as their interest, skills, and educational background.

The director of nursing in an agency will probably spend more time in managing than the staff nurse, and at a level which affects all staff members. Staff nurses must, however, utilize management functions to deliver nursing services. They can also influence how a director of nurses carries out management functions.

Management is a process which has both interpersonal and technical aspects and which utilizes human, physical, and technological resources to achieve well-defined goals (Koontz, O'Donnell, Weihrich, 1986). Figure 21-2 depicts all the variables that influence how the manager implements the five functions of management. It also illustrates the cyclical nature of the management process (planning, organizing, directing, coordinating, and controlling); the functions overlap and do not always follow a sequential pattern.

Planning

Planning means deciding in advance what must be done and what the organization wants to achieve. Without planning, no set goals will be accomplished.

Planning gives purpose and direction to the decision-making process. It is the management function most often neglected because of the emphasis placed upon carrying out day-to-day activities, the attitude that planning takes too much

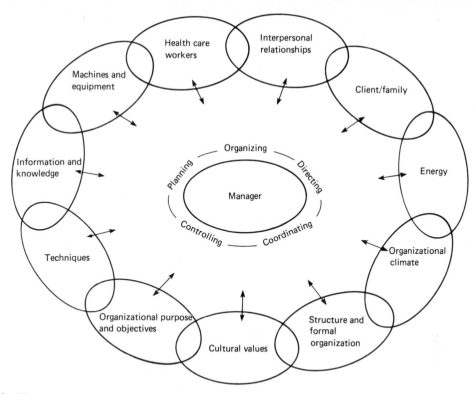

Figure 21-2 The manager links together subsystems of the organization. (From Clark CC and Shea CA: Management in nursing. A vital link in the health care systems, New York, 1979, McGraw-Hill, p 9.)

time, and the tendency for an individual to resist change. Planning is an important activity because it helps the organization to remain dynamic, to identify standards, and to determine what or who requires organization or direction. It increases the likelihood that activities will be orderly, predictable, and less costly. Most important, planning improves the quality and effectiveness of nursing care. Although planning does not guarantee the quality of outcomes, the evaluation aspects of this process help a manager to identify strengths and needs within the organization.

Health care planning should include both the provider and the consumer. Emergencies may necessitate individual decision making and planning. In these situations, it is important for the decision maker to explain to others involved in the process the circumstances and reasons for the emergency decision.

Planning uses past, present, and future information to project what services should be provided. Currently, the impact of political, social, economic, and technical forces is directly influencing the types of services provided by community health agencies and the type of personnel needed to implement these services. For instance, in health departments that provide bedside care, money allocated from taxes is increasingly scarce and third-party payments for home health care are an increasingly larger part of the health department budget. This budget change comes about because of demographic changes in the population as well as social and political policy about the appropriateness of tax money for tertiary health care. Some of the results of these changes include a greater emphasis on delivering home health care, greater use of ancillary personnel such as home health aides, and a greater focus on older people who need "hands-on" care rather than on clients who need health teaching and anticipatory guidance.

Careful planning is needed to successfully implement nursing services when the focus of these services has changed. Activities such as in-service education for staff, planning for increased time for the supervision of home health aides, and the added paperwork involved in carrying out a home health care program are a few examples of factors that should be considered when one is planning for increased home health services.

An example of a staff nurse putting the planning process into action would be when working with the nursing supervisor to establish a well-child conference in the staff nurse's area. Together they would develop a written plan which might include the following:

1. Specific, measurable objectives related to establishment of the conference
2. Time schedule for achieving objectives
3. Process for carrying out the objectives, including necessary resources
4. Evaluation methods to measure the success of the plan in relation to completion of objectives
5. Timetable for periodic evaluation

A staff community health nurse also implements the planning function when structuring the workday and when carrying out caseload management activities. The data gathering, diagnosis, and goal-setting phases of the nursing process are used for activities such as those described above.

During planning, many needs and goals may be identified and priorities for them must be set. The following points should be considered when priorities are being set.

Economic impact. Considering the results if something is or is not done is crucial. Although an immunization campaign against rubella may be costly, it is much less expensive socially and economically than paying for the care of children who have congenital deformities resulting from in utero rubella. The cost-benefit aspect must also be considered. In one community, for instance, the health department discontinued a screening clinic

for the geriatric population because it was not cost effective. It cost the health department $40 per client to do the screening, and 90 percent of those screened had recently received the same screening from their private physicians and planned to do so again in the future. This was duplication of services at a high cost to the health department. Methods other than a screening clinic could be utilized to reach the 10 percent of the population not receiving the screening privately.

Practicality. Is the program necessary? What is being done currently? Will enough people benefit from it to make it worthwhile? Are there sufficient resources available, such as work force and money, to accomplish the stated goals? Is there enough organizational and community support to carry out the program? Does it meet the needs of the community? All of these are questions to be answered in relation to the practicality of the program.

Feasibility. Does the program fit the organization's policies and priorities? Are the resources available to carry out the program?

Legal mandates. The organization must follow its legal mandates. The official health department, for example, has a legal mandate to control communicable disease.

Urgency of the situation. An emergency situation is usually given top priority. In one urban community, for instance, a large Mexican restaurant used home-canned chili peppers that were improperly prepared. Many of the restaurant's patrons developed botulism. This produced an emergency health situation which required urgent action to pinpoint the source of the poisoning and all patrons affected by the botulism agent. The county health department launched an immediate epidemiological investigation to pinpoint the cause. Many other health department activities were stopped or modified so that this serious problem could be given top priority. Once priorities are established, a manager must organize activities so priority goals can be implemented.

Organizing

Organizing determines how a manager implements planning to achieve stated goals. The organizational structure, as previously discussed, facilitates decision making and assigning of tasks. There are three principal components of any organizational structure: people, work, and relationships. The interrelationship of these three variables is analyzed during the organizing phase to determine the best way to organize activities. A manager's major concerns when organizing are fourfold:

1. *Analysis of the system:* identifying strengths and needs of the present system in order to make it more effective and efficient in the future. Comparing present staff capabilities to the needs evidenced by clients being served is one example of how a system is analyzed.
2. *Analysis of functions:* defining all the tasks that are involved in a particular job and determining the relationships between various jobs. A nurse and supervisor analyzing a staff nurse's responsibilities when she or he has a caseload of eight bedside-care clients, 40 families needing health supervision, and work in six schools and two clinics weekly is an example of this principle.
3. *Assigning job responsibilities:* grouping tasks to minimize duplication of effort and assigning responsibilities to individuals who have the knowledge and competence to carry out the job. Responsibility and authority limits should be clearly defined. Again, work with clients who need bedside care illustrates this principle. The home health aide should be assigned only basic physical care and the community health nurse should assess and supervise the care given by the home health aide.
4. *Implementation:* developing an atmosphere which allows for successful completion of the work to be done by identifying the structure of authority and support mechanisms in the system. Team meetings that provide support, case consultation, and identification of needs illustrate this concept.

Organizing requires a cooperative effort by a health care team working together to achieve the goals of the organization. This managerial function is familiar to community health nurses because they must organize the care of a family around the family's expressed needs and the resources of the health team working with them.

Directing

The purpose of directing is to convey to workers what has occurred during the planning and organizing phases of management. The activities of directing include order giving, direction, leadership, motivating, and communicating.

Order giving involves helping an employee to identify what needs to be done in a way that fosters understanding and acceptance. A community health nurse who clearly and completely tells an aide the details of the physical care needed by a client with a cerebrovascular accident and also allows the aide to ask questions and provide input illustrates how effective order giving can be accomplished.

Direction refers to the effort made in an organization to ensure that all the work is done. Personal and professional guidance for people is basic to the concept of direction. In the community health setting, work activities are focused on the provision of services both to families and to the community. Thus, the focus of direction should include guidance which helps staff to effectively intervene both with families and with the community. This helps staff to provide the services and the agency to achieve stated goals.

Employees are more likely to carry out directions if they understand the justification for them and if there is no doubt regarding what is expected to be done. If directions are clearly given, there should not be a need for constant supervision or follow-up.

Leadership is the ability to influence and inspire others to reach the objectives of the organization. Success in leadership is the result of interaction between a leader and those for whom the leader is responsible in a work situation. No single type of leadership is always successful. Rather, a successful leader chooses a method that works for her or him in a particular situation. Leadership is critical to the climate of the organization. Leaders can command people to do things, but the most effective style is to lead so that people want to reach organizational objectives. A successful leader develops a style that fits him or her and the situation. A nursing leader, for instance, may be directive (authoritative or dictatorial) with new nursing staff members because they need more structure in an unfamiliar work environment and democratic with more experienced staff members because they need less direction. Both of these styles can be appropriate. The leader must decide what to use and when. Each person in a leadership position should analyze her or his own assumptions and develop a style that is comfortable, meets the needs of the situation, and provides motivation for staff. This is defined as leadership and management by situation.

Motivating focuses on analyzing the needs of individual workers. Maslow's hierarchy of needs can provide a theoretical framework for examining worker needs. Maslow has developed a priority schema based on a continuum of needs beginning with those that are physiological and ending with self-actualization. He believes that a worker must satisfy lower-level needs (physiological) before the higher-level ones (self-actualization) become significant (Maslow, 1954). When working with other employees or when analyzing one's own behavior in the job setting, it may be found that work is not satisfying because lower-level needs are not being met. If this is the case, an effective manager would attempt to build into the management system rewards that would help the employee to meet these basic human needs.

McGregor (1960) has done considerable research into the effect of management attitudes upon employee motivation. His studies have provided the X and Y theories of motivation. Theory X illustrates a negative attitude in its assumptions about human nature, and theory Y reflects positive attitudes about human nature (McGregor, 1960, pp. 33-35, 45, 49).

Theory X makes the following assumptions:

1. The average human being has an inherent dislike of work and will avoid it if at all possible.
2. Most people must be coerced, controlled, directed, or threatened with punishment to get them to put forth adequate effort toward achievement of organizational objectives.
3. The average human being prefers to be directed, wishes to avoid responsibility, has relatively little ambition, and wants security above all.

Theory Y makes the following assumptions:

1. The expenditure of physical and mental effort is as natural as play or rest.
2. A person will exercise self-direction and self-control in the service of objectives to which that person is committed.
3. Commitment to objectives is a function of the rewards associated with their achievement.
4. The average human being learns, under proper conditions, not only to accept but to seek responsibility.
5. The capacity to exercise a relatively high degree of imagination, ingenuity, and creativity in the solution of organizational problems is widely, not narrowly, distributed in the population.
6. Under the conditions of modern industrial life, the intellectual potential of the average human being is only partially utilized.

McGregor promoted theory Y for the development of a directing style that would motivate employees. It is a more positive approach to working with people. McGregor's theories, like Maslow's framework, can be used as guidelines for managers.

Theory Z was published in 1981 (Ouchi, 1981). It expanded Theory Y and the democratic approach to leadership and focused on developing better ways to motivate and satisfy workers with the goal of increasing productivity. Based upon successful Japanese organizations, Theory Z is a participative mode of decision-making that involves everyone who is affected by a decision.

When using any set of guidelines to develop a management style, it is necessary to remember that work is more satisfying when workers are able to meet their own needs in the work situation. The nurse gives care to, and cares about, clients daily, and this is emotionally taxing. The needs of the nurse must also be met in the work setting.

Communicating with workers is crucial. The manager must be able to convey what is to be done, how it is to be done, who is to do it, and why it is to be done and to provide feedback on the activity. This feedback should emphasize the strengths, as well as the weaknesses, inherent in the employee's activity. The interviewing skills that are a primary tool of community health nurses should be used in communicating with health care workers. These skills will help the manager to direct, coordinate, and control activities within the organization.

Coordinating

Coordination links people on the health care team together to function in such a way that objectives are achieved. A problem arises when health care workers look at objectives in different ways. One nurse may consider nursing in the school setting as a low priority. The supervisor may think it a high priority. Thus, coordinating can mean managing conflict. Conflict can promote growth but it can also reduce productivity. Effective coordination reduces and prevents growth-restricting conflict.

Controlling

Controlling is a process that measures and corrects the activities of people and establishes standards so that objectives are reached. The controlling function has three steps: establishing standards, measuring performance criteria, and correcting deviations from normal. The nursing audit, described in Chapter 22, is an example of a controlling function, as is a supervisory or evaluation conference between a staff nurse and a supervisor.

The following are the six characteristics of effective control:

1. *Adjustability:* a control mechanism must be flexible enough to respond to changing situations.

2. *Purposefulness:* a control measure should focus on a specific problem area, not an entire system.
3. *Practicality:* a control measure should not be instituted until it can be implemented reasonably.
4. *Meaningfulness:* a control measure must give direction to other controls and activities, not work against them.
5. *Enforceability:* a control measure should not be instituted until it is possible to put it into effect and to carry out the mandates of the control.
6. *Congruence:* the control measure should be consistent with other control measures and allow the manager to perform other responsibilities and activities.

The staff nurse who delegates care to a home health aide can utilize these characteristics of control so that quality care is given consistently. The nurse and aide must be flexible in their expectations of each other; an aide who has an ill child at home may not work as well on that day as on another. If the nurse is concerned about a particular client care problem, such as the aide's lack of understanding about maintaining skin integrity, she or he can utilize conference time to discuss that problem but should not bring all other concerns to the conference. The nurse needs the supervisor's support when working with the home health aide so that the solutions to the nurse's concerns are enforceable and not opposed by the supervisor.

The controlling function can provide direction for growth and thus should be considered a positive function. It is important to examine *strengths* of workers as well as areas of concern when one is implementing the controlling function of management.

MANAGEMENT INFORMATION SYSTEMS (MIS)

Processing data and utilizing information efficiently and effectively is vital in any health care organization. Appropriate data and information management can facilitate decision making and increase productivity. With the current emphasis on cost containment, and the highly competitive nature of today's health care market, there is no question that methods must be identified to improve productivity, to enhance decision-making processes, and to use resources more effectively. One such method, the use of computerized information systems, is being advocated across the country. Community health agencies using computer-based processing systems are finding that these systems can be invaluable. The San Bernardino County Public Health Department found, for example, that a computerized format of the nursing process decreased charting time by 50 percent (Buelow, 1983, p. 1). A copy of one of this agency's computerized records is found in Appendix 21-1.

Computerized management information systems are being developed to support the management functions of planning, organizing, controlling, and evaluating. These systems enhance long-range planning processes and assist in resource allocation, personnel management, policy making, and client care documentation. Another primary function of such systems is to provide information needed to ensure efficient personnel performance (Parks, 1982, p. 6).

Management information systems provide systematic, comprehensive information which supports day-to-day activities and future planning. Information is more than raw data or facts that describe places, things, or events. Information is "data that has been processed into a form that is meaningful to the recipient and is of real or perceived value in current or prospective decisions" (Davis, 1974, p. 33). Computer software packages convert data into information.

Management information systems are currently being used by numerous community health care agencies. In 1983, the National Association for Home Care sent a computer services survey to all its members. Of those agencies responding, 72.9 percent were presently using computer services (NAHC, 1983, p. 14). One of the best-known management information systems for community and home health care is the one de-

veloped by the Visiting Nurse Association of Omaha, Nebraska. This system uses a classification scheme for client problems in community health nursing, which adapts easily to a computerized system of record keeping (Simmons, Martin, Crews, and Scheet, 1986). As was previously discussed in Chapter 8, this scheme provides a very useful framework when developing nursing diagnoses for community-based practice.

Nationally, there is a movement which supports the development of computerized nursing information systems (NIS). In 1982, a group of health care leaders met in Cleveland, Ohio, to dis-

TABLE 21-1　1982 Study group on nursing information systems: functions for which nursing information is needed

Nursing functions	Activities under each function
Patient care	Making nursing diagnoses
	Setting nursing care goals
	Choosing nursing actions
	Monitoring the quality of care
	Supporting patient education
Resource allocation	Nurse staffing
	Nurse scheduling
	Nursing care demand
Personnel management	Individual nurse-employee data on date of hire, work availability, performance capability, benefits received, experience, education, length of service, salary, etc.
Education	Patients
	Employees
	Students
Planning and policy making	Reports on care provided, resources used and outcomes achieved
	Nursing care cost (patient charges and revenue production)
	Institutional financial management
Investigations	Clinical evaluation
	Nursing research

From Study Group on Nursing Information Systems: Computerized nursing information systems: an urgent need, Res Nurs Health 6:104, 1983.

TABLE 21-2 Information needs of community health nurses: areas of computerized data collection, Contra Costa County Health Department

Information needs	*Purposes for obtaining information*
Knowledge of health needs of those served	
Identity	Provides a baseline for program development or deletion.
Place of residence	Provides a sampling for the correlation of services in any one group.
Family size	Provides a comparative sampling of services needed in a given area.
Age groups	Assists in the evaluation of the validity of ongoing programs.
Socioeconomic levels	
Cultural background	
Kinds of services given	
Nursing personnel statistical requirements	
Actual nurse work hours available for service	If we commit our division to deliver skilled nursing to meet the nursing commitments of a great variety of medical programs, community developments, and research and study projects, we need to be sure we have access to funding and recruitment of the required skills, so that we can adequately meet our commitment.
Variety of referrals and problems handled by nurse	
Distribution of services per nurse	Data provide information about the resources and skills presently available as well as baseline information with which to project skills, time and materials that will be needed in the future to meet new or changing programs and/or changing priorities for unchanging programs.
Correlation of use of nurse work hours with known priority needs	
Variety of work load by nurse, by area	
Ratio of population to nurse coverage	
Ratio of supervision to nurses	
Review for nurse staff evaluation	
Departmental needs from nursing statistics	
Profile of persons receiving nursing service	Provide appropriating bodies with a meaningful description of nurse activity and levels of operation.
Profile of services given family, clinic and community	Provide agency personnel with a better understanding of community needs.
Profile of community itself	Provide mandatory statistical reports for state and federal agencies, (e.g., such as funded medical programs and home health agency reports.)
Supplemental reporting of personal observations, and knowledge of person giving the specific service	
Adequacy of service and pertinency of service in relation to agency expectations	

From Keyes G: Why we need nursing statistics. In Management information systems for public health/community health agencies, NLN Pub No 21-1506, New York, 1974, National League for Nursing, pp. 56-57.

cuss issues related to the development of an NIS. It was believed by this group that an NIS could advance nursing knowledge, develop nursing practice, and improve patient care. The NIS study group stressed that in order for an NIS to be valuable to the nursing profession, it must provide nursing practice information as well as management data. The study group identified several functions for which nursing practice information is needed. These functions are presented in Table 21-1 (Study Group on Nursing Information Systems, 1983, pp. 101 and 104).

Developing an MIS which meets the information needs of nurses takes careful planning and input from nurses. Computer experts can provide technical knowledge, skill, and advice about appropriate computer packages. However, in order for computer experts to select computer equipment, nurses must be able to identify the information they need for decision making, as well as the nursing activities that must be supported by specific information sets. Information frequently needed by nurses in community health agencies and why the information is important is presented in Table 21-2.

When developing an MIS, nurses must take into consideration nursing ethics. They must en-sure that the rights of both client and staff are protected when information is computerized. Nurses must carefully monitor access to client and personnel data; usually these types of data have limited access requirements placed on them when entered into an MIS.

The development of an MIS can create stress within an organization, especially when staff members have not previously worked with computers. When experiencing this stress, it helps to focus on what can be achieved long range through the use of an MIS. Initially, it takes additional time out of one's schedule to become knowledgeable about the functioning of this type of system. However, a new system can, if used effectively, help an agency to improve the delivery of client care services and can reduce indirect service time.

APPLYING MANAGEMENT CONCEPTS IN COMMUNITY HEALTH NURSING

In the community health nursing setting, nurses have multiple responsibilities. They may have a large number of families in their caseload as well as a number of other nursing services to be performed. In addition, community health nurses need to develop collaborative relationships with

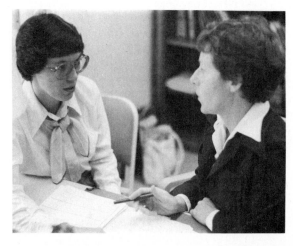

Figure 21-3 A staff nurse and supervisor in conference. Nurse/supervisor conferences are a common occurrence in community health nursing practice. Community health nurses find it helpful to meet with their supervisors on a regular basis to discuss caseload management and staff development issues.

other disciplines in order to coordinate family care and to establish priorities for home visits and other activities, such as school and clinic services. Community health nurses must also learn how to effectively delegate tasks to other nursing personnel.

Organizing and scheduling community health nursing activities is not an easy task for an experienced practitioner and, therefore, it is often overwhelming to a new staff member. These activities are easier to handle, however, if a new staff member applies management concepts while carrying out daily responsibilities.

Using Planning Functions of Management as a Staff Nurse

The nurse can more readily carry out responsibilities if the following planning activities of management are utilized.

Scheduling Regular Conferences with the Nursing Supervisor

This can assist in analyzing the nurse's caseload responsibilities and in establishing priorities for service (Figure 21-3). With the supervisor's help, the nurse should do both a case analysis of each family that is being seen and a caseload analysis of all the work that is being done.

Case analysis: The nurse should learn to "diagnose" each case by answering questions such as the following:

1. What are the health problems of this family as viewed by the family and the nurse?
2. What resources does the family have for meeting these problems?
3. What movement does the family wish to make?
4. What resources are there in the community for meeting these needs?
5. What nursing activities are needed to contribute to the solution of the problems and to bring family and community resources into proper relationship with family needs?
6. Are there some parts of the problems or needs which cannot be met at present with the resources available?

7. What has the family done to work toward solving the problem?
8. How effective have nursing interventions and family actions been in resolving current health problems?

This case analysis should be done on a periodic basis, at least every 6 months, so that families who do not wish to make progress can be closed to service until such time as they wish to again work on an area of need. In addition, case analysis helps nurses to look at their approach to families and alter it so that they can be more effective. A written summary, as well as supervisory conferences, facilitates case analyses. A written summary of work with a family, after a given number of visits in a specified time frame, helps nurses to organize their care and their work. In general, nurses find it valuable to summarize a family record after 10 visits have been made or after they have seen the family for 6 months. The controlling function of management is in effect when case analysis is done because work with clients is being measured and corrected.

Caseload analysis. Study of the caseload will also improve the planning ability of the nurse and will reveal gaps in service. A caseload analysis differs from a case analysis in that it focuses more on examining the quantity of work the nurse is responsible for and the multiple activities assigned than on the needs of individual families. Caseload analysis is done to determine whether a nurse has sufficient time to implement all assigned responsibilities, to ascertain whether time is being used effectively and efficiently, and to identify whether the needs present in a caseload of families reflect the needs of the population being served. Analysis of the caseload may be in relation to many aspects of service—the types and numbers of cases carried, the complexity of problems in the cases visited, the age groups served, the proportion of new referrals received, and the number of emergency or crisis situations, such as individuals with positive sputums for tuberculosis. In addition, it examines all the other activities a nurse engages in, such as school visits, clinic services, group work, committee meetings, coordination with other community agencies, and recording and planning time. When the caseload is studied, it is wise to graph or tabulate the findings so that they may be readily used and compared with caseloads in other areas or with the same area over time.

Simultaneous caseload study by several nurses may be encouraged occasionally to give a general picture of the services provided by the health agency and to allow for comparisons between nurses. When this was done in one health department, it was found that two of 15 census tracts had a disproportionate number of referrals. The result was that workload assignments were reallocated so that work was more evenly divided. The strength of such a procedure is its usefulness for the individual nurse to identify the uniqueness of cases in her or his own area and to examine if there is adequate time to handle the demands of the workload. Freeman (1949, p. 358), in her writings on public health nursing supervision, stressed that nurses should not try to develop an "average" in the caseloads they carry but should develop a caseload pattern which will provide optimum community service. This is a key principle to follow today, because of the diverse health problems in society and the dramatic changes in the population structure of the United States. When making comparisons, nurses must keep in mind that caseloads should reflect community needs and population characteristics (see Chapter 11 for how one determines these needs and characteristics). One nurse may have a higher geriatric clientele than another nurse because of the uniqueness of the census tract she or he serves.

Use a Tickler System

A tickler system is a card file wherein each family in the nurse's caseload has an identification card displaying data such as name, address, telephone number, and service classification. It assists in scheduling family visits, determining what families need service and when, as well as the type of service needed. When a nurse makes a home visit, the date of this visit and the month and day for the next visit are indicated on the card. The card is then placed under the appropriate month in an index file box. If a tickler system is used effec-

tively, a new nurse can quickly identify priorities for home visiting by noting how frequently the previous nurse visited a family and when the nurse planned the next visit. When a staff nurse has a caseload of families, an organized method such as a tickler file for determining when to see whom is essential.

Set Priorities

This allows the nurse to put activities in their order of importance or caseload priority. The following should be considered when one is establishing priorities:

Nursing knowledge. The nurse has a strong theoretical background on which to base priorities for nursing service. This knowledge helps the nurse to analyze the nursing service needs of families who have particular types of problems and direct interventions as well. The developmental framework discussed in Chapters 12 through 18 of this book, along with the nurse's knowledge of crisis theory, for instance, helps a nurse to identify problems across the life-span that present stress, and in some cases, crisis. For example, a single, pregnant adolescent may receive higher priority than a 25-year-old pregnant married person. The first client is dealing with the developmental tasks of two age periods—the adolescent and the young adult—and thus is more likely to experience a crisis than the 25-year-old, who is dealing with developmental tasks of only one age period.

Third-party payors. To be reimbursed by third-party payors for nursing services, the community health nurse must follow established guidelines. For instance, Medicare requires that nursing care be given to clients who need skilled care and are homebound. If these conditions are not met and substantiated by documentation in the client record, Medicare will not pay for nursing services. Nurses do need to consider the financial constraints of their organization so that they meet the requirements established by funders. An organization cannot run without adequate funding.

Community needs. Statistical data, input from consumers, and reports from other professionals can often alert the community health nurse to critical community problems or lack of health services in certain areas. For example, if the herd immunity for measles is 10 percent in a certain section of a county, the community health nurse needs to spend time planning for the provision of immunization service to the total population in this section of the county. This may leave the nurse less time for home visiting. In the long run, however, an immunization campaign could reduce the time the nurse needs for home visits. It takes far more time to individually contact families who need to up-date their immunization status than to conduct a mass campaign which alerts the total community to the need for immunization protection.

Agency policies and priorities. A community health nurse is responsible for following agency policy. Some agency policies read: "Premature infants should be seen weekly for 6 weeks" or "All newborns in the community are to be visited once." If the nurse finds, after analyzing the caseload, that it is impossible to implement an agency policy, she or he should not ignore the policy, but rather should take concrete action to see that it is changed. Many agencies, for instance, have recently found that it is impossible to visit all newborns because of the multiple needs present in the community. Unfortunately, sometimes it is found that an old policy is not changed because staff do not take the initiative to have it changed. This can create frustration, especially if staff members are trying to implement an unrealistic policy.

Nursing services should also reflect agency priorities and, hopefully, these priorities will coincide with communities' needs. If a community has a high geriatric population, a health department may place priority on delivering service, such as home health care to the elderly. If an agency places a high priority on home health services, the staff nurse will have to schedule other health supervision visits (maternal-child health, school health, mental health) around home health services. If, on the other hand, community statistics reflect high infant and maternal mortality rates, maternal-child health cases at risk may receive top priority for follow-up. Priorities may vary from one census tract to another, depending on the needs evidenced in each census tract.

Legal mandates. Communicable disease follow-up is mandated to the official health department by law and as such must receive priority when caseload needs are analyzed. Communicable disease follow-up is also a high priority because of its potential threat to the community.

Agency resources

1. *Staffing:* The availability of health personnel influences the type of services that can be provided. Where limited personnel and other resources exist, only clinic and crisis intervention services may be provided. If only limited resources are available, the community health nurse will have to examine carefully what nursing services are essential and how the most people can be reached in the time available. Some agencies have increased clinic services and group work and decreased home visits because of personnel shortages. If changes such as these do not meet the needs of the population being served, careful documentation may help the agency to obtain additional resources. Too often, however, nurses and other health professionals accept their current state and fail to document the need for increased resources.

2. *Funding:* Financing can affect the type and amount of staffing available within a health agency and also the type of services provided by a particular department. When nursing divisions in a health agency contract for special services, such as school health, family planning, and home health services, they often can expand their nursing staff, but there usually are conditions for the type of services which need to be provided, as well as a time frame designating when these services should be delivered. Health departments, for example, are sometimes paid for school health services by the board of education. Nurses in these instances may be required to visit the schools at least once a week from September through June.

Use Data from Time and Cost Studies

This is useful in determining the average time needed to accomplish certain nursing activities and costs related to these activities. Time studies help a new nurse to be more realistic about the

A.M.	Monday	Tuesday		Wednesday	Thursday	Friday
8:30	Prepare for conferences with personnel regarding assigned cases			Office Preparation Conferences with team TCs Recording		Prepare for shared home visits
9:00	TC Lerner, Mayor, and Vinant families re: time for home visit	School			Mary Jones, 16-year-old AP	Shared visit with LPN to Johnson family—diabetic
10:00	Hartsford family, cleft lip and palate, new parents	Gilbert child, recheck vision, TC to parents if indicated		Hartsford family follow-up visit		
11:00				Vinant family, premie, in hospital	Spartan, first baby	Shared visit with HHA—White family
12:00	Lunch					
P.M.						
1:00	Mayor family, threatened abortion	Mayor family, follow-up visit		Well-child conference set up by RN in A.M.	Endicott family, new in area, multiple sclerosis	Bond family, follow-up visit
2:00	Bond family, new TB	Lerner family, new parents		Conference		Make necessary TCs in relation to referrals or family needs
3:00				Follow-up on referrals from the well-child conference	Staff meeting	Complete recording
4:00	Recording and referrals if any; TCs to MDs or sources of referral	Ring family, rheumatic fever child		Hastings family, TB contacts encourage to go to clinic for exam		Plan for next week's work
5:00						

Figure 21-4   A sample weekly calendar of a staff community health nurse in a county health department which provides both home health care and health supervision services.

quantity of service that can be provided and the cost of the service being delivered. Time studies are not designed to evaluate the performance of an individual staff nurse. They are done to analyze the average time it takes for all staff members to accomplish certain activities. Even though they are time consuming and taxing, time studies are extremely valuable because they help a staff nurse and the nursing division to gain a better perspective on the cost-effectiveness of nursing service. In addition, time studies can provide the documentation needed to request additional funding for increased personnel and resources. They also provide guidelines that help a nurse to schedule nursing activities more efficiently.

Factors to Consider When Scheduling Community Health Nursing Activities

The community health nurse has a work schedule that frequently changes. As was discussed, there are guidelines that help the nurse to give priority to work. Establishing priorities helps the nurse to schedule activities more effectively. There are several other factors that need to be considered as the nurse schedules work. Ideally, at the beginning of each month, the nurse will develop a calendar that identifies her or his scheduled activities for the month and allows the nurse to see how much time is available for other requests such as new referrals. If new demands for service exceed the time available, the nurse will then have an organized calendar to share with the nursing supervisor which documents the excess demand and which helps to rearrange priorities as necessary. Figure 21-4 presents a portion of a monthly calendar to illustrate how a community health nurse uses it to schedule activities. As can be seen, the nurse's workload for this week is heavy. If too many new referrals are received, the nurse should seek assistance from the supervisor. Often it is found that staff nurses use the time set aside for office work to handle excess workload. It is not wise to do so consistently, because office time is essential for appropriate planning, adequate follow-up, and high-quality recording.

The community health nurse should consider the following parameters when scheduling community nursing activities for the coming month:

I. Schedule every case and activity requiring service during the month.

II. Schedule new visits around scheduled commitments.

III. Make daily visits at the same time each day, if possible.

IV. Establish priorities for visits according to need and timing of visits, as illustrated by the following examples:

   A. Families with new babies—around feeding or bath time, to assess how these activities are handled by the family

   B. Crisis cases as soon as possible

   C. Infectious diseases last in the day, if possible, to decrease potential for exposure to other families

V. Provide for follow-up of families with long-term and chronic diseases.

   A. Handicapped or ill individuals

   B. Chronic problems

VI. Set time aside for shared home visits, when care is delegated to:

   A. Home health aides

   B. Licensed practical nurses

VII. Plan time for:

   A. Office activities

     1. Planning of visits for the week; planning activities for next week

     2. Assignment of cases

     3. Supervisory conferences

       a. Ancillary personnel

       b. Supervisor

     4. Recording and reporting

     5. Follow-up

       a. Referrals

       b. Phone calls to agencies, physicians, families

     6. Team meetings

   B. Clinic activities

     1. Setting up

     2. Time in clinic

     3. Follow-up and evaluation

   C. School activities

   D. Agency or community committee activities

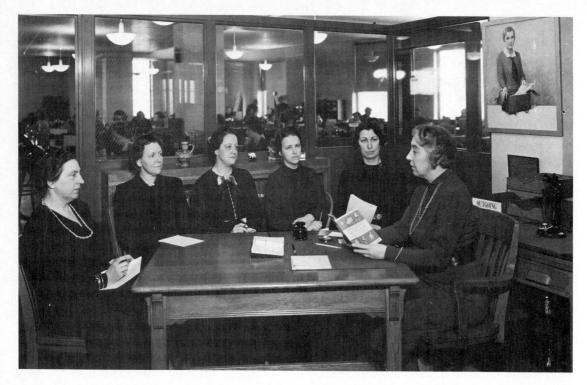

Figure 21-5   The value of team conferences to deal with caseload management concerns, community needs, and agency issues has long been recognized in the field of community nursing. Depicted above is a staff conference being conducted by Alma Haupt (first right in picture), the Director of Metropolitan's nursing service. This nursing service was founded in 1909 and significantly influenced the development of management practices in the field of public health nursing. Currently, with the trend toward decreasing the amount of time community health nurses spend in the office, there is a renewed interest in having regular staff meetings in community health agencies. Community health nurses at all levels find it essential to maintain supportive communication with their colleagues. This communication helps them to deal with workload demands, to maintain an objective perspective about practice issues, and to achieve cohesiveness among agency personnel. (Courtesy of Metropolitan Life Insurance Company.)

*Organizational Staffing Patterns
for Community Health Nurses*

Another area of concern to nurses who are managing the care of families and groups is the staffing pattern used in a health care organization. Some agencies utilize a system of primary nursing whereas others use a team nursing system or a case management model. The method of staffing selected by an agency will determine how the nurse schedules and implements monthly activities.

Primary nursing. If this pattern of organization is used, the community health nurse is assigned a geographical area and is responsible for all open cases, new referrals, and schools in that district. The advantages of this method of assignment are several. First, the same nurse follows all clients over time, which results in better continuity of care. Second, this method allows for independent planning and decision making, which is often less time-consuming and, therefore, less expensive than group decisions. Last, one person serves a geographic area, which requires less travel time than if the same person would have to travel in several different geographic areas.

The greatest disadvantage for primary nursing

is the lack of flexibility of work assignment. If an individual nurse becomes very busy with referrals or if the nurse becomes ill, coverage for the workload is difficult.

The primary nursing organizational pattern does not, or should not, eliminate peer and supervisory guidance with case analysis. Weekly team conferences (refer to Figure 21-5) can be very important to the successful implementation of the primary nursing concept. The nurse can use weekly conferences to increase knowledge in specific areas, such as available community resources, or to analyze the needs of complex families, such as failure-to-thrive families.

Team nursing. Other agencies use a team nursing method to deliver nursing services to clients in the community. This involves assigning a personnel team consisting of one or more community health nurses, RNs, LPNs, and HHAs to serve a larger geographical area or larger caseload than that in a primary nursing assignment. Each member of the team covers the same geographic area. Team nursing offers the advantage of lending more flexibility to work assignments because there are several team members to share new referrals or care of clients. Perhaps its greatest advantage is that quality of service can improve as a result of the shared planning and problem solving which occurs in regularly planned *team conferences.* Disadvantages are that more time is needed for planning because of the number of people involved and travel expenses are often increased.

Case management. Case management aims, by case type, to achieve quality care at low cost. This is accomplished by standardizing resources with a very clear direction toward specific client interventions for like problems, and with specific expected caregiver and system outcomes. Case managers promote collaboration among all disciplines to provide ongoing care from preadmission to postdischarge while involving the family in the process. Though this sounds like typical community health nursing, emphasis in case management models used by many community agencies is on *case types.* Illustrative of this concept is the case management focus on high-risk children at the Gloucester County Health Department in

New Jersey. This health department uses the case management model to promote early identification, evaluation, diagnosis, and treatment of children with special needs and potentially handicapping conditions. The case manager, a nurse who has a caseload of 300 families, is responsible for a team that counsels families, assesses the need for services, promotes and facilitates communication among the team providing services, and monitors the services received (ANA, 1988). With this model, nursing personnel are used efficiently, expected client outcomes are well delineated, timely discharge is facilitated, material resources are used appropriately, and collaborative practice is promoted. (Refer to Chapter 19 for further discussion of case management from a generalized perspective.) The disadvantage is that this model is case specific rather than general in scope.

Team, primary nursing, and case management can work. Some advantages and disadvantages of each were shared so that nurses will recognize the importance of analyzing strengths and limitations of different organizational patterns. Examining both strengths and limitations helps nurses to identify mechanisms which would minimize limitations when an agency selects a particular organizational pattern.

Determining Priorities in Community Health Nursing Practice

When setting up a calendar for the month, the staff nurse may find that there is not enough time to carry out all the responsibilities that she or he would like to be able to do. Community health nurses cannot meet all the health needs that are evidenced in the community setting. Money, time, and personnel are not limitless, and all three, in fact, are becoming scarcer commodities. As was indicated in Chapters 2, 10, and 11, our responsibilities to groups in need are based on their vulnerability and their degree of risk. Thus, one way of determining whom community health nurses will service is to set priorities for service. Several factors to consider when one is establishing priorities have already been discussed in the section which addresses how the community health nurse uses the planning function of management in the work setting. In addition to the variables mentioned in that section, such as funding, legal mandates, community needs, and agency priorities, determining priorities based on client needs is useful. Ruth Rives, in 1953, wrote a classic work for public health nurses on the establishment of priorities according to client needs; it was updated in 1958. An update of Rives's article which provides a basis for determining priorities for nursing services is provided in Appendix 21-2. Many priorities defined by Rives are still entirely appropriate. Others have been added and some have been deleted.

UTILIZATION OF VARIOUS LEVELS OF HEALTH PERSONNEL*

A variety of staffing patterns in agencies deliver community health nursing services. In nearly any community health setting staff members are involved in offering nursing services who are prepared at various levels. In some agencies, RNs (BSN-, AD-, and diploma-prepared), LPNs, and home health aides (HHAs) are hired. In others, only RNs and HHAs are available. In yet others, only BSN-prepared RNs are used. Knowledge of the educational preparation of these persons and the agency job descriptions are most helpful tools when nurses need to decide how to utilize personnel appropriately and determine what type of orientation and staff development is needed.

Home health aides are often prepared with noncredit courses that last from 8 weeks to 1 year. Course work usually includes classroom activities and in-hospital clinical preparation. In the community setting, HHAs can give personal care and assist with housekeeping, marketing, and preparation of meals. Home health aides can give the kinds of personal care that can be taught easily to a family member if there is someone to teach.

The licensed practical nurse is prepared to give physical care, to make observations about physi-

cal conditions, to carry out special rehabilitative measures after being instructed by the community health nurse, to continue teaching of clients begun by the registered nurse, and to contribute to the nursing care plan of a client. There is a significant difference in the level of care given by LPNs and HHAs. The licensed practical nurse has knowledge and skill that helps in making limited patient assessments and contributing to the development of nursing interventions. Home health aides have knowledge and skill to provide *unskilled* patient care. Both the LPN and HHA, however, were prepared to function under the supervision of a registered nurse. They both make valuable contributions on the health care team.

The registered nurse prepared at the AD or diploma level has been prepared mostly in acute care institutions, where there is a patient-centered approach to care. The RN is usually highly skilled in the care of home health service clients who are ill and who need expert care and observations in the home. Because the RN often has developed expertise in technical procedures, she or he can teach these techniques to other staff and family members. The RN has skill and knowledge to assist in the development of the nursing care plan, especially with clients who have disease conditions. Because the registered nurse's preparation has been primarily patient-centered, she or he should receive orientation in relation to family-centered nursing practice, concepts related to analyzing the needs of populations, and principles relative to the coordination of care and prevention, if she or he is expected to implement all the services provided by community health nurses in a health department. This orientation is a necessity. It is unfair to expect the registered nurse, prepared at the AD or diploma level, to provide comprehensive community health nursing services. She or he has not been prepared to do so. If circumstances exist where only these registered nurses are available, an agency has the responsibility to provide them with orientation and staff development opportunities which adequately prepare them to carry out the demands of the job.

The community health nurse has been prepared at the baccalaureate level in community

*The authors are indebted to Ruth Carey, former Vice President of Clinical Services, Michigan Home Health Care, Traverse City, Michigan for the use of this material.

health, with an emphasis in the educational program on wellness and prevention as well as experience in the community health setting. She or he is expected to have a family-centered focus and to function in a comprehensive fashion. This entails identifying client strengths and needs and all variables that affect health and illness (physical, social, and emotional), facilitating identification of family health goals and assisting families to reach their goals. The community health nurse initiates, plans, and evaluates care. In addition, she or he participates in planning for the health needs of the community and works in schools, clinics, and community groups, giving service as well as functioning as a planning participant to see that needed services are provided.

The agency job description is a helpful tool for nurses who are in positions where they have to delegate care to various levels of personnel. A job description defines what tasks or functions are appropriate for each level of personnel, based on their educational preparation. Identifying tasks and functions that different levels of staff are capable of handling facilitates the utilization of all personnel and also the delegation process. The following illustrates how this is so: In the well-child, immunization, or clinic for sexually transmitted diseases, many tasks need to be done, including taking histories, weighing and measuring children, teaching clients, giving immunizations or injections of medication, and drawing blood samples. Some of these are best done by the community health nurse, but others can be done effectively by the LPN or HHA. Knowledge of the educational preparation of personnel and agency job descriptions can help the nurse to decide what may be delegated or assigned. For instance, in one large health department, there were five kinds of personnel working in the well-child clinic because there were activities to be accomplished which could be handled by nurses prepared at various levels: the HHA weighed and measured children and set up the equipment needed to run the clinic; the LPNs and RNs gave immunizations; the RNs and community health nurses took immunization histories (determining with parents what their child had had and what was to be given that

day); the community health nurse took health and illness histories and counseled and provided education for parents. The pediatric nurse practitioner on the staff carried her own caseload of clients, doing physical examinations and teaching and counseling with parents. Assignments in this situation were based on the complexity of the tasks involved and the preparation each staff member had. Pediatric nurse practitioners, for example, usually have more in-depth preparation to handle complete physicals than does the generalized community health nurse.

Another example of how various levels of personnel can be used to implement nursing services in the community setting is the follow-up of vision and hearing failures from schools. Health departments often have hearing and vision technicians who screen school children, retest the failures, and then refer the retest failures to the community health nurse for follow-up and referral. It is then the community health nurse's responsibility to see that the follow-up is done. However, lesser-prepared personnel, such as an LPN or clerk, may be taught how to appropriately do the initial contacting of parents by phone to ascertain whether or not medical care has been obtained, and if so, what the results were. Using lesser prepared personnel to handle the above activities provides more time for the community health nurse to follow up with families who are having difficulty obtaining medical care. In addition to clinic and school activities, home health activities are commonly implemented by differing levels of personnel.

Many home health service clients need to be visited two or three times a week. After the nurse has established a plan of care, visits can often be shared with other personnel such as the LPN or HHA. Remember, though, that when care is delegated to other personnel, responsibility for care of that client or family remains with the community health nurse. The community health nurse must plan adequate time in her or his schedule to supervise the care delegated to other personnel. Some third-party payors, such as Medicare, require that supervisory visits be made by an RN in a specified time period.

Using Delegation as a Management Function in Community Health Nursing

In order to carry out the diverse responsibilities of the position, the community health nurse frequently needs to delegate tasks to other health care personnel. When planning responsibilities for others, the community health nurse should:

1. Analyze the nature of the task to be delegated, considering the complexity as well as the time involved to complete it
2. Determine the capability of the individual staff member to handle the assigned responsibility, especially noting the staff member's educational and experience background and other workload responsibilities
3. Identify the willingness of the staff member to accept responsibility for the assigned activity
4. Determine how much time will be needed to supervise if tasks are delegated to others

Delegation is the process of designating tasks and bestowing on others the authority needed to accomplish these assigned tasks. Delegation does not mean, however, that the community health nurse negates personal responsibility for providing quality care to the families she or he serves. Care given by home health aides or LPNs should never be increased so rapidly that it is impossible for the community health nurse to adequately supervise the care delegated to them. The community health nurse must have sufficient time available to apply the principles of the five management functions when carrying out the following supervisory activities with HHAs and LPNs:

1. Shared home visits with the LPN or HHA on the initial visit to a family (planning, organizing)
2. Development of nursing care plans on each family in the caseload, based on assessment data and input from the LPN or HHA (planning, organizing)
3. Regular conferences with the LPN or HHA to determine guidance and assistance needed in specific situations (directing, organizing, coordinating)
4. Periodic shared visits with the LPN or HHA for supervision and reevaluation of the status of the family (directing, coordinating, controlling)
5. Periodic review of family records to evaluate the status of the family and the level of nursing service (controlling)
6. In-service education related to the needs of the staff and the families in the nurse's caseload (directing)

In community health nursing, management functions are utilized daily by nurses at every level. The five functions of management—planning, organizing, directing, coordinating, and controlling—are useful tools to nurses as they work with peers, ancillary personnel, supervisors, and the community in providing nursing care.

SUMMARY

Community health nurses have multiple and diverse responsibilities to handle in the practice setting. They have found that by applying the principles of management they are more effective in dealing with the multiple and diverse demands in the work environment. Knowledge of the five functions of management is especially helpful. These are planning, organizing, directing, coordinating, and controlling. The use of a management information system supports these management functions by utilizing data effectively and efficiently.

The development of management thought has changed over time. Reviewing the historical evolution of management helps nurses to understand why it is useful to implement the five functions of management in the work setting. Analysis of this evolution is also beneficial because it provides a basis for defining a personal philosophy of management.

The utilization of management concepts in the community health nursing setting is essential. Management principles help the community health nurse to organize and schedule activities, to establish priorities for nursing service, to effectively and efficiently utilize time, and to appropriately delegate responsibilities. All these tasks must be accomplished if the community health nurse is going to deliver quality care to clients in the community.

APPENDIX 21-1

High-Risk Infant and Well Child, Birth to 12 Months

County of San Bernardino

Department of Public Health

163 HRI Program |_|
164 CHS Program |_|

1 Name _____

2 Address _____ 3 Census Tract_____

4 Birthdate _____ 5 Gest. Age_____

6 Referring Hospital_____

7 Initial Assessment |_| 10 Date Planned
                           For Next HV_____

8 Follow Up Assessment |_| 11 Flowsheet Closed |_|

9 PHN _____   12 Date_____

A = Assessment
  ✓ = WNL
  P = Problem
  + = Optimal Problem
      Management

I = Intervention and
    Anticipatory Guidance
  T = Teach   S = Supervise
  D = Demonstrate C = Contract
  L = Literature   P = Physical Care
  R = Refer

I = Outcome
  1=Goal Met
  2=Goal Not Met At This
    Time
  3=Lost to Follow Up
  4=Refused
  5=Client Failed to
    Follow Thru
  6=Referred to Another
    Dist. or Co.
  7=Continue on Appro-
    priate Flow Sheet

I. PHYSICAL ASSESSMENT   A

13 General____ |_|
14 Hygiene____ |_|
15 Alert____ |_|
16 Lusty Cry____ |_|
Skin
17 Condition____ |_|
18 Color____ |_|
19 Temp.____ |_|
20 Turgor____ |_|
21 Birth Marks____ |_|
Head
22 Shape____ |_|
23 Fontanels____ |_|
24 Scalp____ |_|
Eyes
25 Pupillary
   Response____ |_|
26 Clear____ |_|
Ears
27 Responds to
   Voice____ |_|
28 Nose____ |_|
29 Mouth____ |_|
30 Throat____ |_|
31 Neck Supple____ |_|
43 Heart Rate____ |_|
Abdomen
33 Shape____ |_|

34 Cord____ |_|
35 B.Sounds____ |_|
Chest
36 Symmetrical
   Movement____ |_|
Lungs
37 Clear____ |_|
Back
38 Spinal Cord____ |_|
Genitalia
39 Penis/Scrotum
   Testes____ |_|
40 Vulva____ |_|
Extremities
41 Symmetrical
   Movements____ |_|
42 Muscle Tone____ |_|
43 ROM____ |_|
44 Gluteal folds____ |_|
Neuro Reflex
45 Palmar Grasp
   (0-4 mos.)____ |_|
46 Rooting
   (0-4 mos.)____ |_|
47 Fencing
   (0-7 mos.)____ |_|
48 Moro
   (1-4 MOs.)____ |_|

Anticipatory Guidance   1
49 Fever Management____
50 Colic Management____
51 Thermom. Use____
52 URI____
53 Ear Infect____

Goal   0
54 P.A. will be WNL____ |_|
55 Optimal Management
   of Problems____ |_|

Interventions
56 Identify
   Abnormalities____ 1 |_|
57 Physical Care
   Required____ |_|
58 PMD Coordination____ |_|

II. GROWTH
         Birth Today % A
59 Ht | | | | |
60 Wt | | | | |
61 HC | | | | |
Goal
62 Growth Components   0
   Within 5-95% |_|
63 Demonstrate growth____ |_|
Interventions   1
64 Normal Growth Curve____ |_|
65 PMD Coordination____ |_|
66 Nutrition____ |_|

III. NUTRITION
                   Data A
67 Breast-min | | |
68   Freq. | | |
69 Formula type | | |
70   Amt. | | |
71   Freq. | | |
72 NCAST | | |
Anticipatory Guidance
                           I
73_____ | |
74_____ | |
75_____ | |
76_____ | |
77_____ | |
78_____ | |
Goal
79 Age Appropriate   0
   Diet____ |_|
Intervention
80 Nec. Nutrition   1
   Components____ |_|
81 Feeding Tech.____ |_|
82 Equip/BreastCare____
83 Feeding Sched____

IV. ELIMINATION   A
84 Stool____ |_|
85 Urine____ |_|
Anticipatory Guidance   1
86 Diaper Care____ |_|
87 Constipation
   Management____
88 Diarrhea Manage.____ |_|
Goal
89 Elimination Pattern   0
   WNL____ |_|
90 Optimal Management
   of problems____
Interventions
91 Normal Elimination   1
   Patterns____ |_|
92 Diet & Fluids____
93 PMD Coordination____ |_|

V. DEVELOPMENT   A
94 DDST-ADj____ |_|
95 DDST-Chrono____
96 Phn Assess.____ |_|
Anticipatory Guidance   1
97 Emotional Exp.____
98 Social Exp.____
99 Physical Exp.____
100 Sleeping/Crying____
101_____
102_____ | |
103_____ | |
104_____ | |
105_____ | |
106_____ | |
107_____ | |
108_____ | |
Goal
109 Overall Development   0
    WNL____ |_|
Intervention   1
110 Normal Development____ |_|
111 Stimulation____
112 PMD Coordination____ |_|

VI. BONDING   A
113 Harrison____ |_|
114 Phn Assess____ |_|
115 NCAST____ |_|
Goal
116 Bonding will be   0
    WNL____ |_|
Intervention   1
117 Parenting Skills____ |_|
118 Caregiver Needs____ |_|

VII. CAN POTENTIAL   A
119 CAN Scale____ |_|
120 Phn Assess____ |_|
Goal
162 CAN Absent   0
121 Low Risk for CAN____ |_|
Intervention   1
122 CAN Flow Sheet____ |_|
123 Agency Coord.____ |_|
124 Mandated Report____ |_|

VIII. SAFETY   A
125 Phn Assess____ |_|
Anticipatory Guidance   1
126_____
127_____
128_____
129_____
Goal
130 Physically Safe   0
    Environment____ |_|
Interventions   1
131 Basic Corrections____ |_|
132 Agency Coord.____

IX. HEALTH CARE SYS.
                       Data A
133 Source | | |
134 ER Source | | |
135 FIND | | |
Goal   0
136 Reg. Health Care |_|
Intervention   1
137 Correction of
    Barriers____ |_|
138 PMD/Agency Coord.|_|

IMMUNIZATIONS (Date Received)
139 DPT _____   144 HGb _____
140 _____   145 _____
141 _____   146 _____
142 Polio _____ 147 PPD _____
143 _____

REFERRALS

Prob. No.	Ref. Agency	Appt. Date	Appt. Kept	Consult
148				
149				
150				
151				

MEDICAL HISTORY

Severe Illness   152 1_____
                 153 2_____
Hospitalizations 154
165 Preventable |_| 155 1_____
166 Nonprevent |_| 156 2_____
Meds-Dose   157 3_____

Prob. No.	Pathology/Deviation	Clinical Notes/Plan	Anticipated Date of Goal Completion
158			
159			
160			
161			

**SAN BERNARDINO COUNTY DEPARTMENT OF PUBLIC HEALTH
DIVISION OF COMMUNITY HEALTH SERVICES**

Definition of Legend — High Risk Infant and Well Child Flow Sheet

Assessment

Problem = deviation from definition of WNL
+ = deviation from definition of WNL, except problem is being managed
   by caregiver following health care provider guidelines and expectations.

Outcome

1 - Goal met: Achievement of WNL and/or optimum problem management of
    appropriate assessment areas.

2 - Goal not met at this time: Goal not met at this time, caregiver and
    PHN have initiated interventions to achieve goal.

3 - Lost to follow-up: All resources to locate client have been
    exhausted.

4 - Refused: Client/caregiver unwilling to plan interventions for goal
    achievement.

5 - Client failed to follow thru: Client/caregiver appears willing to
    follow thru with plans but no action is evident.

6 - Referred to another district or county: Client/caregiver has moved
    and a referral has been initiated.

7 - Continue on appropriate flow sheet: Problem area indicates need for
    more intensive assessments and interventions than can be documented
    on this flow sheet.

**SAN BERNARDINO COUNTY DEPARTMENT OF PUBLIC HEALTH
DIVISION OF COMMUNITY HEALTH SERVICES**

Anticipatory Guidance Categories - High Risk Infant and Well Child Flow Sheet

Age	Safety	Nutrition	Development
0-3 months	S-0-1 Bathing	N-0-1 Bottle care	D-0-1 Bonding
	S-0-2 Bedding	N-0-2 Bottle carries	D-0-2 Eye tracking
	S-0-3 Car and infant seat	N-0-3 Bottle propping	D-0-3 Infant swing
	S-0-4 Prevent falls	N-0-4 Breast/formula	D-0-4 Mobile
		N-0-5 Burping	D-0-5 Muscle exercise
		N-0-6 Vol. Exp.	D-0-6 Sibling jealousy
			D-0-7 Smile response
			D-0-8 Tactile stimulation
3-6 months	S-3-1 Baby proofing	N-3-1 Intro of solids	D-3-1 Cradle gym
	S-3-2 Choking	N-3-2 Review formula or	D-3-2 Hand toys
	S-3-3 Prevent falls	Breast feeding	D-3-3 Imitates sounds
	S-3-4 Toy selection	N-3-3 Spoon vs bottle	D-3-4 Roll over
		N-3-4 Teething	D-3-5 Sitting Exp.
			D-3-6 Stranger distrust
6-9 months	S-6-1 Baby proofing	N-6-1 Cup drinking	D-6-1 Babbling
	S-6-2 Food aspiration	N-6-2 Finger foods	D-6-2 Busy Box
	S-6-3 Toy selection	N-6-3 Food selection	D-6-3 Crawling
	S-6-4 Walker risks	N-6-4 3 meals/day	D-6-4 Exploration
			D-6-5 Object permanence
			D-6-6 Pincer grasping
			D-6-7 Separation anxiety
9-12 months	S-9-1 Climbing	N-9-1 Dental Hygiene	D-9-1 Body parts
	S-9-2 Poison prevention	N-9-2 Finger feeding	D-9-2 Consistent limits
	S-9-3 Streets	N-9-3 Table foods	D-9-3 Discipline
	S-9-4 Wall/floor heater	N-9-4 Weaning	D-9-4 Midline activities
		N-9-5 16-24 oz. formula	D-9-5 Nesting toys
			D-9-6 Nursery rhymes
			D-9-7 Push and pull

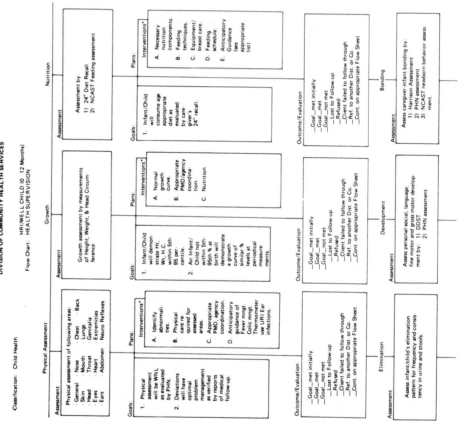

SAN BERNARDINO COUNTY DEPARTMENT OF PUBLIC HEALTH

DIVISION OF COMMUNITY HEALTH SERVICES

Classification: Child Health

Flow Chart: HRI/WELL CHILD (0 - 12 Months)
HEALTH SUPERVISION

Physical Assessment

Assessment

Physical assessment of following areas:

- General · Nose · Back
- Skin · Mouth · Lungs·
- Head · Throat · Genitalia
- Eyes · Heart · Extremities
- Ears · Abdomen · Neuro Reflexes

Goals:

Plans: Interventions*

1. Physical assessment will be WNL as evaluated by PHN.
2. Deviations will have optimal problem management as verified by reports of medical follow-up.

A. Identify abnormalities.
B. Physical care required for assessed areas.
C. Appropriate PMD, agency coordination.
D. Anticipatory guidance of Fever mngt. Colic mngt. Thermometer use URI Ear infections.

Outcome/Evaluation

__Goal__met initially
__Goal__met
__Goal__not met
__Lost to Follow-up
__Refused
__Client failed to follow through
__Ref. to another Dist. or Co.
__Cont. on appropriate Flow Sheet

Growth

Assessment

Growth assessment by measurements of Height, Weight, & Head Circumference

Goals:

Plans: Interventions*

1. Infant/Child will demonstrate Ht, Wt, H.C. within 5th-95th per-centile.
2. An Infant/Child not within 5th-95th % at birth will demonstrate a growth curve of similar % levels at periodical measurements.

A. Normal growth curve.
B. Appropriate PMD/agency coordination.
C. Nutrition

Outcome/Evaluation

__Goal__met initially
__Goal__met
__Goal__not met
__Lost to Follow-up
__Refused
__Client failed to follow through
__Ref. to another Dist. or Co.
__Cont. on appropriate Flow Sheet

Development

Assessment

Assess personal-social, language, fine motor and gross motor development by: 1) DDST 2) PHN assessment

Nutrition

Assessment

Assessment by
1) 24° Diet Recall
2) NCAST Feeding assessment

Goals:

Plans: Interventions*

1. Infant/Child will consume age appropriate diet as evaluated by care-giver's 24° recall.

A. Necessary nutrition components.
B. Feeding techniques.
C. Equipment/ breast care.
D. Feeding schedule.
E. Anticipatory Guidance (see appropriate list)

Outcome/Evaluation

__Goal__met initially
__Goal__met
__Goal__not met
__Lost to Follow-up
__Refused
__Client failed to follow through
__Ref. to another Dist. or Co.
__Cont. on appropriate Flow Sheet

Bonding

Assessment

Assess caregiver infant bonding by:
1) Harrison Assessment
2) PHN assessment
3) NCAST newborn behavior assessment.

Elimination

Assessment

Assess infant/child's elimination pattern for frequency and consistency in urine and stools.

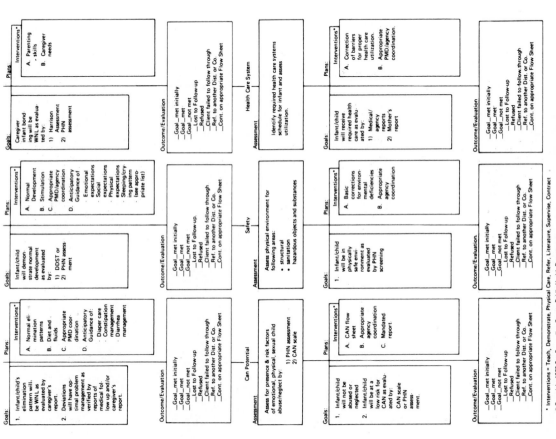

Goals:

1. Infant/child's elimination pattern will be WNL as evaluated by caregiver's report.
2. Deviations will have optimal problem management as verified by reports of medical follow up and/or caregiver's report.

Plans: Interventions*

A. Normal elimination patterns
B. Diet and fluids
C. Appropriate PMD coordination
D. Anticipatory Guidance of:
- Diaper care
- Constipation management
- Diarrhea management

Outcome/Evaluation

__Goal__met initially
__Goal__met
__Goal__not met
__Lost to Follow-up
__Refused
__Client failed to follow through
__Ref. to another Dist. or Co.
__Cont. on appropriate Flow Sheet

Can Potential

Assessment

Assess for presence & risk factors of emotional, physical, sexual child abuse/neglect by:
1) PHN assessment
2) CAN scale

Goals:

1. Infant/child will not be abused or neglected
2. Infant/child will be at a low risk for CAN as evaluated by: CAN scale or PHN assessment.

Plans: Interventions*

A. CAN flow sheet
B. Appropriate agency coordination
C. Mandated report.

Outcome/Evaluation

__Goal__met initially
__Goal__met
__Goal__not met
__Lost to Follow-up
__Refused
__Client failed to follow through
__Ref. to another Dist. or Co.
__Cont. on appropriate Flow Sheet

Goals:

Infant/child will demonstrate normal development as evaluated by:
1) DDST or
2) PHN assessment

Plans: Interventions*

A. Normal Development
B. Stimulation
C. Appropriate PMD/agency coordination
D. Anticipatory Guidance of:
- Emotional expectations
- Social expectations
- Physical expectations
- Sleeping/crying pattern (see appropriate list)

Outcome/Evaluation

__Goal__met initially
__Goal__met
__Goal__not met
__Lost to Follow-up
__Refused
__Client failed to follow through
__Ref. to another Dist. or Co.
__Cont. on appropriate Flow Sheet

Safety

Assessment

Assess physical environment for following areas:
• structural
• sanitation
• hazardous objects and substances

Goals:

1. Infant/child will be in physically safe environment as evaluated by PHN screening

Plans: Interventions*

A. Basic corrections for environmental deficiencies
B. Appropriate agency coordination

Outcome/Evaluation

__Goal__met initially
__Goal__met
__Goal__not met
__Lost to Follow-up
__Refused
__Client failed to follow through
__Ref. to another Dist. or Co.
__Cont. on appropriate Flow Sheet

Goals:

Caregiver infant bonding will be WNL as evaluated by:
1) Harrison Assessment
2) PHN assessment

Plans: Interventions*

A. Parenting skills
B. Caregiver needs

Outcome/Evaluation

__Goal__met initially
__Goal__met
__Goal__not met
__Lost to Follow-up
__Refused
__Client failed to follow through
__Ref. to another Dist. or Co.
__Cont. on appropriate Flow Sheet

Health Care System

Assessment

Identify required health care systems schedule for infant and assess utilization.

Goals:

Infant/child will receive required health care as evaluated by:
1) Medical/agency reports
2) Mother's report

Plans: Interventions*

A. Correction of barriers for proper health care utilization.
B. Appropriate PMD/agency coordination.

Outcome/Evaluation

__Goal__met initially
__Goal__met
__Goal__not met
__Lost to Follow-up
__Refused
__Client failed to follow through
__Ref. to another Dist. or Co.
__Cont. on appropriate Flow Sheet

---

* Interventions = Teach, Demonstrate, Physical Care, Refer, Literature, Supervise, Contract

© Copyright 1983 San Bernardino County Public Health Department

APPENDIX 21-2

Priorities in Community Health Nursing

PURPOSES

1. To identify target population groups requiring community health nursing service

2. To identify realistic spacing of nurse service contacts according to identified target population group

3. To utilize levels of prevention and health promotion in planning nursing service to a community

CODE

- *Classification I: intensive visiting* is defined as visits spaced daily to 3 times a week
- *Classification II: periodic visiting* is defined as visits spaced every 1 to 2 weeks
- *Classification III: widely spaced visiting* is defined as visits spaced every 2 to 3 months

---

	I. Intensive visiting	*II. Periodic visiting*	*III. Widely spaced visiting*
Communicable disease			
A. Tuberculosis (by law a priority)	To families who 1. Have young adults and unexamined contacts living in crowded home conditions with a patient who has positive sputum 2. Have a recently diagnosed patient with positive sputum 3. Have a recently diagnosed patient without positive sputum 4. Have a diagnosed patient with positive sputum, who is recalcitrant 5. Have a patient receiving chemotherapy	To families who 1. Have the patient with positive sputum hospitalized; have no young adults in the family; have good living standards but have some unexamined contacts 2. Need preparation for the hospital admission of the patient 3. Need preparation for the discharge of the patient	To families who 1. Have an arrested patient returned to good home conditions 2. Have had all contacts examined and the patient hospitalized, under adequate medical supervision. 3. Are under adequate medical supervision, with the source of infection located
B. Acute reportable dangerous communicable diseases	To families who 1. Have been contacts to reportable dangerous communicable disease 2. Have a diagnosed patient needing home care 3. Have food handlers as a case/contact to *Salmonella*	To families who 1. Are unimmunized 2. Have a patient under medical care but complications develop 3. Need follow-up for defects after recovery from acute stage	To families who 1. Are known to have immunization against communicable disease 2. Are receiving adequate medical care 3. Have a typhoid carrier in the home
C. Sexually transmissible diseases	To clients who 1. Need treatments and education on the prevention and spread of disease 2. Have known contacts they will name	To clients who 1. Need follow-up clinical examinations (for example, spinal taps)	

	I. Intensive visiting	*II. Periodic visiting*	*III. Widely spaced visiting*
	3. Need examination, advice on treatment, and education on how to arrest and prevent the transfer of infection		
	4. Need posttreatment observation		
	5. Need to be convinced of the necessity of the treatment ordered by the doctor		
	6. Need to be taught how to prevent further manifestations of the disease		
	7. Have babies born of mothers with active STD at time of delivery		
	8. To families who need instruction and assistance to care for a person with AIDS		
Home care of the sick			
A. Cardiovascular disease	To clients who	To clients who	To clients who
	1. Have cardiac failure or have had an acute cardiac episode from any cause	1. Have a congenital heart disease: nonoperable, postoperative	1. Have a history of rheumatic fever, but no clinical heart disease
	2. Have a chronic cardiac disability requiring active treatment: medical, nursing, dietetic	2. Have a murmur of undetermined origin with a history of rheumatic fever	2. Are under medical care, stabilized for cardiovascular diagnoses
	3. Have had a CVA and require active treatment: medical, nursing, occupational, and physical therapy	3. Have congenital heart disease (to be followed until a thorough medical evaluation is completed)	
	4. Have cardiac surgery	4. Have diagnosed hypertension	
B. Diabetes	To clients who	To clients who	To clients who
	1. Are newly diagnosed, not stabilized by diet or insulin	1. Are newly diagnosed, administering own insulin but still needing supervision	1. Are under medical care, stabilized as to diet or insulin, or both
	2. Cannot take own insulin (blind, aged, low mentality, and so forth)	2. Are suspected of having diabetes	
	3. Have difficulty understanding diet or administering their own insulin		

Continued.

Priorities in Community Health Nursing—cont'd

	I. Intensive visiting	II. Periodic visiting	III. Widely spaced visiting
	4. Have uncontrolled diabetes 5. Have diabetes with gangrene 6. Have diabetes complicated by an infection		
C. Kidney disease	To clients who 1. Are on dialysis 2. Need help with medications and diet and understanding disease	To clients who 1. Understand medications and diet but are not stabilized	To clients who 1. Are under medical care and are stabilized
D. Cancer	To clients who 1. Are discharged from a hospital and need active nursing care, instruction for themselves, and interpretation of their physical and emotional needs to the family 2. Have symptoms suspicious of cancer; need medical supervision, completion of all tests and examinations, and, if required, treatment on the earliest possible date 3. Are diagnosed but who, without consulting the physician, have interrupted their treatment or discontinued having medical checkups 4. Are under observation for malignancy but delinquent from regular medical supervision (the urgency of a patient's problem can be determined only by the attending physician) 5. Have hospice/terminal care needs 6. Need complex, high technology interventions such as TPN intravenous feedings	To clients who 1. Have precancerous lesions and are delinquent for periodic checkups (cervical erosions, leukoplakias, keratoses, mastitis, and others) 2. Have cancer apparently treated successfully but are not reporting for medical reexamination (cancer of the skin with no apparent recurrence) 3. Have advanced disease and need care (some of these patients may need to be in classification I) 4. Have families that have been taught to carry out medical orders but need support in continuing medical supervision	To clients about whom 1. Information is needed for statistical purposes (cured, deceased, or other)

Priorities in Community Health Nursing—cont'd

	I. Intensive visiting	II. Periodic visiting	III. Widely spaced visiting
E. Other noncommunicable diseases, acute or chronic	To clients who 1. Are acutely ill and need nursing care 2. Are helpless or bedridden and need nursing service 3. Are senile and do not receive adequate home care 4. Are acutely ill or helpless but have families who can be taught how to give the necessary care 5. Are receiving terminal care	To clients who 1. Are acutely ill or helpless but whose families can provide care under nursing supervision 2. Need encouragement to continue medical care 3. Need emotional support to carry out health instructions	To clients who 1. Are under adequate medical supervision and are given good home care (by the family, a registered nurse, or a practical nurse)
Health teaching and supervision			
A. Maternity-antepartum	To women who 1. Are primiparas 2. Are under 17 or over 40 years of age 3. Are single parents 4. Are of low socioeconomic status 5. Are hypertensive 6. Have poor nutrition 7. Are not under medical care 8. Have had six or more pregnancies 9. Have had conditions associated with pregnancy resulting in infant deaths 10. Have had complications in past pregnancies or have signs of complications in the present pregnancy, including psychosomatic disturbances 11. Have a chronic disease, such as tuberculosis, diabetes, syphilis, anemia, nephritis, cardiac disease, or rheumatic fever 12. Have previously had premature deliveries 13. Are HIV + and/or drug abusers	To women who 1. Have adequate medical supervision for apparently normal pregnancies 2. Are in good physical and mental condition 3. Are able to follow advice 4. Have questions and desire help	(No antepartum patients in this category)

Continued.

	I. Intensive visiting	*II. Periodic visiting*	*III. Widely spaced visiting*
B. Maternity-postpartum	To women who 1. Have nursing problems or breast complications, such as engorgement or abscess 2. Are not receiving adequate medical supervision or competent nursing care 3. Had complications or accidents of labor: stillbirths, abortions, or other difficulties resulting in a mishap to the mother or baby 4. Delivered prematurely 5. Had multiple births 6. Delivered a baby with a congenital defect 7. Had a baby that died during the first month of life 8. Evidence poor maternal-infant bonding 9. Have no or few support systems 10. Are single 11. Are economically stressed (low socioeconomic status)	To women who 1. Had problems but are making normal progress 7 days after delivery 2. Have adequate medical supervision 3. Are coping but need guidance and support related to care of the baby, the family's adjustment, and socioeconomic variables	To women who 1. Are receiving good care and supervision 2. Stabilizing in parenting skills and family adjustment
C. Infancy (higher priority is given to infants, regardless of whether they are first-born, when they live in low economic districts where the mortality rate is highest)	To infants who 1. Are premature 2. Are newborn, especially if firstborn 3. Have difficulty in breast-feeding 4. Have consistently lost weight 5. Are being weaned 6. Have inadequate medical care 7. Have a reportable dangerous communicable disease	To infants who 1. Are past the first month and are gaining slowly 2. Are not being fed properly 3. Have questionable physical and emotional delays 4. Need immunizations	To infants who 1. Are receiving adequate medical supervision 2. Are receiving good home care

	I. Intensive visiting	II. Periodic visiting	III. Widely spaced visiting
	8. Have a physical handicap resulting from a birth injury or a congenital defect—"high tech" babies such as those on respirators and who have been hospitalized at length		
	9. Need immunization		
	10. Are from substandard poorly managed homes, or homes where there are problems of inadequate parenting		
	11. Are considered difficult babies by parents		
	12. Are born to drug abusers		
	13. Are born to HIV risk mothers		
	14. Fail to thrive		
D. Preschool period	To children who	To children who	To children who
	1. Have a reportable dangerous communicable disease	1. Are insecure	1. Have adequate medical supervision
	2. Have a physical defect	2. Have lost weight	2. Have good home care
	3. Need immunization	3. Lack medical supervision	
	4. Need dental care	4. Have poor health habits	
	5. Have nutritional deficiencies	5. Deviate from normal physical and emotional behavior	
	6. Are inconsistently disciplined		
	7. Are from homes where there is inadequate parenting		
	8. Are reported for suspected child abuse and neglect		
E. School health	To children who	To children who	To children who
	1. Have acute health problems	1. Need follow-up of allergies: hives, eczema, asthma	1. Have a chronic health condition that is stabilized and under medical care
	a. Communicable diseases: immunization reactions or complications developing from acute communicable diseases	2. Have inadequate medical care	2. Have a congenital defect which does not require remedial work at the time
		3. Have not had diagnosed defects corrected within a reasonable period of time	

Continued.

APPENDIX 21-2

Priorities in Community Health Nursing—cont'd

	I. Intensive visiting	II. Periodic visiting	III. Widely spaced visiting
	b. Skin conditions: scabies, impetigo, ringworm, pediculosis c. Other: pregnancy, unexpected loss or gain of weight, abuse, neglect, diabetes, epilepsy 2. Have had an accident in school requiring hospitalization 3. Need immediate attention for defects discovered on physical examination: vision, hearing, cardiac, kidney, scoliosis, or other serious defects 4. Need follow-up of incidents indicating intense or serious emotional disturbance 5. Need follow-up as a contact of a diagnosed dangerous communicable disease 6. Have growth and other developmental delays	4. Are on medication for a duration of more than 3 weeks during the school year 5. Need to be observed in relation to their growth pattern (those with structural scoliosis, those wearing braces, and so forth) 6. Need follow-up of minor defects: poor eating and health habits, poor dental and personal hygiene, foot and posture problems	
F. Adult health	To clients who 1. Are in situational or maturational crisis 2. Are disorganized as a family and at risk for abuse and neglect of children or spouse 3. Have suspected dangerous communicable or chronic disease symptoms 4. Have no medical supervision for diagnosed physical, emotional, psychosocial problems 5. Are needing help adapting to chronic illness: heart disease, arthritis, multiple sclerosis, depression	To clients who 1. Are in crisis but have support systems 2. Recognize their disorganization and are working on ordering their lives 3. Have diagnosed disease and are receiving medical treatment; need help with referral to resources 4. Are needing help dealing with developmental tasks of parenting: sexuality and death education tasks of their children	To clients who 1. Have needed nursing care, are currently coping well, but are at risk for physical, emotional, and psychosocial problems

APPENDIX 21-2

Priorities in Community Health Nursing—cont'd

	I. Intensive visiting	*II. Periodic visiting*	*III. Widely spaced visiting*
G. Health of aging people	To clients who 1. Have no medical supervision 2. Have symptoms of a dangerous communicable, nutritional, or chronic disease 3. Have a diagnosed disease and need help following the treatment plan 4. Have no support systems 5. Have evidence of situational or maturational crisis especially in relation to: loss of income, loss of spouse, loss of friends 6. Have evidence of intentional or unintentional alcohol or drug abuse 7. Are unable to maintain an environmentally safe housing situation	To clients who 1. Have a diagnosed medical problem 2. Have a complex treatment regimen and are following it 3. Are able to live independently but need referral sources and support	To clients who 1. Are under medical supervision 2. Have readily available support systems

Adapted from Rives R: Priorities according to needs, Nursing Outlook, 6:404-408, 1958. Copyright American Journal of Nursing Company. Updated by F. Armignacco, Director of Patient Services and Community Nursing, Monroe Co. Department of Health, Rochester, NY

REFERENCES

American Nurses' Association: Nursing case management, Kansas City, Mo, 1988, The Association.

Buelow J: A computerized format of the nursing process in community health, unpublished paper presented to the American Public Health Association, Dallas, Tx, November 1983.

Clark CC and Shea CA: Management in nursing: a vital link in the health care systems, New York, 1979, McGraw-Hill.

Davis GD: Management information systems: conceptual foundations, structure and development, New York, 1974, McGraw-Hill.

Douglass LM: The effective nurse: leader and manager, ed 3, St Louis, 1988, CV Mosby Co.

Freeman RB: Techniques of supervision in public health nursing, ed 2, Philadelphia, 1949, Saunders.

Keyes G: Why we need nursing statistics. In Management information systems for public health/community health agencies, NLN Pub No 21-1506, New York, 1974, National League for Nursing, pp 56-57.

Koontz H, O'Donnell C, and Weihrich H: Essentials of management, ed 4, New York, 1986, McGraw-Hill.

Maslow AH: Motivation and personality, New York, 1954, Harper & Row.

McGregor D: The human side of enterprise, New York, 1960, McGraw-Hill.

National Association for Home Care: NAHC reports results of a computer services survey, Caring 2:14-15, 1983.

Ouchi WG: Theory Z: how American business can meet the Japanese challenge, Reading, Ma, 1981, Addison-Wesley.

Parks SJ: Introduction to health care facility: food service administration, University Park, Pa, 1982, Pennsylvania State University.

Rives R: Priorities according to needs. In Stewart DM and Vincent PA, eds: Public health nursing, Dubuque, Ia, 1958, Wm C Brown. Copyright 1958, American Journal of Nursing Company. Reproduced with permission from Nurs Outlook 6:404-408, July 1958.

Simmons DA, Martin KS, Crews CC, and Scheet NJ: Client management information system for community health nursing agencies, NTIS Accession No HRP-0907023, Springfield, Va, 1986, National Technical Information Service.

Study group on nursing information systems: Computerized nursing information systems: an urgent need, Research Nurs Health 6:101-106, 1983.

SELECTED BIBLIOGRAPHY

Bly JL: Measuring productivity for home health nurses, Home Health Care Serv Q 2:23-39, 1981.

Churness VH, Kleffel D, Onodera ML, and Jacobson J: Reliability and validity testing of a home health patient classification system, Public Health Nurs 5:135-139, 1988.

Corriveau, CL and Rowney RH: What is a day's work? Nurs Outlook 31:335-339, 1983.

Gleeson S: Helping nurses through the management threshold, Nurs Administration Q 7(2):11-16, 1983.

Halloran E and Kiley M: Case mix management, Nurs Manage 15(2):39-45, 1984.

Knollmueller RN: Community health nursing supervisor: a handbook for community/homecare managers, New York, 1986, National League for Nursing.

Marriner-Tomey A: Guide to nursing management, ed 3, St Louis, 1988, CV Mosby Co.

Peters DA: Development of a community health intensity rating scale, Nurs Research 37:202-207, 1988.

Saba VK and McCormick KA: Essentials of computers for nurses, Philadelphia, 1986, Lippincott.

Stanfill P: Participative management becomes shared management, Nurs Manage 18(6):69-70, 1987.

Tappen RM: Nursing leadership and management: concepts and practice, ed 2, Philadelphia, 1989, Davis.

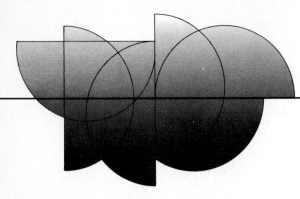

22

Quality Assurance in Community Health Nursing Practice

One characteristic of a profession is the presence of a professional association that is cohesive, self-governing, and a source of professional self-discipline, standards, and ethics.

JEROME P. LYSAUGHT, 1970, p. 41

Upon completion of this chapter, the reader will be able to:

1. *Identify reasons why quality assurance is increasingly important in health care systems.*
2. *Define the term quality assurance.*
3. *Describe the common elements in all quality assurance models.*
4. *Explain how values held by health care professionals influence quality assurance.*
5. *Discuss the terms structure, process, and outcome as they relate to quality assurance.*
6. *Identify several types of measurement tools and procedures used to evaluate quality of care.*
7. *Explain the concepts of risk management and utilization review and how they relate to quality assurance.*
8. *Identify the community health staff nurse's role in a quality assurance program.*

Health care professionals have entered an era of quality assurance. Increasingly they are being challenged by legislative action, third-party payors, and consumers to assume accountability for the services delivered by members of their profession. Legislative emphasis on quality assurance began in the 1970s. The professional standard review organizations (PSROs) established by the 1972 amendments to the Social Security Act were developed to ensure that federal monies spent for Medicaid, Medicare, and other federal health care programs would be used effectively, efficiently, and economically. The PSRO law (Public Law 92-603) mandated review of health care delivered by physicians and nonphysician health practitioners when such care was paid for by federal funds (Public Law 92-603, 1972). This has created the necessity of developing standards for practice, because the review examines current practice to see how it compares with established norms for quality care.

The passage of the National Health Planning and Resources Development Act of 1974 (refer to Chapter 12), like the PSRO legislation, also provided an impetus for the development of quality assurance programs. This law mandated that health care professionals promote activities that improve the quality of health care services to all segments of the population. It set forth as a national priority "equal access to quality health care at a reasonable cost" (Papers on The National Health Guidelines, 1977, January, p. 1). It called for the development of national health planning goals and standards.

Quality assurance became a major focus among legislators in the 1980s and a resulting avalanche of new requirements to protect the quality of client services emerged. Illustrative of this are the competency evaluation stipulations for home health aides and the patient rights requirements mandated by the Omnibus Budget Reconciliation Act of 1987 (refer to Chapters 4, 8, and 19). Federal involvement in the assessment and monitoring of quality care also increased in the 1980s. In 1986, results of a quality assurance investigation by the House Select Committee on Aging and the American Bar Association's Com-

mission on Legal Problems of the Elderly were presented to the House of Representatives. The document summarizing the findings of this investigation, and known as the "Black Box" report on home care quality, raised questions about the quality of care provided to vulnerable groups in our society (Sabatino, 1986). This has resulted in increased governmental involvement in the monitoring of quality in the health care delivery system. For example, the establishment of a home health toll-free hotline and investigative unit, which clients may call if they have complaints about local home health agencies, was mandated in the Omnibus Budget Reconciliation Act of 1986. The Medicare Conditions of Participation require home health agencies to inform their patients how they can reach this hotline (HCFA, 1989).

In addition to federal influences, private nonprofit third-party payors (refer to Chapter 4) have encouraged professionals to monitor both the cost and the quality of health services. They have established criteria for the type of care they will reimburse, and they require as well that health services be audited by professional audit committees.

Consumers are also motivating health care professionals to evaluate the care they provide. Consumers are becoming more sophisticated about the health care they desire and are demanding that current practice keep up with societal changes and needs. In addition, through legislative action, they are becoming more actively involved in reviewing services delivered by health care professionals. Influential organizations, such as the American Association of Retired Persons (AARP), are spearheading this involvement.

Nursing shares with all health care professionals the need to examine carefully the delivery of their services in light of changing societal demands. To validate itself as a profession and to maintain the right to govern nursing practice, nursing must take the responsibility to control the activities of its members. There is no question that if nursing does not assume accountability for its actions, others will control nurses' actions for them in this era of quality assurance. The challenge for the 1990s will be to ensure quality while containing health care costs.

QUALITY ASSURANCE DEFINED

Quality assurance is a dynamic process through which nurses assume accountability for the quality of care they provide. It involves both the evaluation of care and the implementation of measures to improve care, based on data obtained from evaluation efforts. It is a commitment to excellence with an emphasis on ensuring that all nurses provide safe nursing care and that all clients receive quality care. Quality assurance is a guarantee to society that services provided by nurses are being regulated by members of the profession. It is a series of actions aimed at governing nursing practice so that all clients receive nursing services that are *equal or* are *better than* the standard of care designated appropriate for clients who have like characteristics. Quality assurance is also a systematic, ongoing evaluation of care delivered by nurses for the purpose of determining what type of care is provided and the outcome of this care.

Selected definitions of quality assurance are presented in Table 22-1. Schmadl proposed an additional definition after analyzing what nurses should be assuring, for whom nurses are assuring quality, and what measures identify quality nursing care. His definition is given below because it is clearly stated, comprehensive, and provides direction for the development of a quality assurance program.

Quality assurance involves assuring the consumer of a specified degree of excellence through continuous measurement and evaluation of structural components, goal-directed nursing process, and/or consumer outcome, using pre-established criteria and standards and available norms, and followed by appropriate alteration with the purpose of improvement (Schmadl, 1979, p. 465).

Since its origin, the American Nurses' Association (ANA) has emphasized the importance of quality assurance in nursing practice. The first objectives for the Nurses' Associated Alumnae of the United States and Canada, established in 1897 and known as the ANA since 1911, focused on lack of standardization in nurses' training, as well as the need for licensure laws to protect the public from inadequately trained nurses. By 1912, there were 33 nurses' associations that had secured nurse practice acts (Christy, 1971, pp. 1778-1779).

Since 1966, the American Nurses' Association has diligently pursued the development of a quality assurance program for nurses. At that time the divisions on practice, including community health nursing, geriatric nursing, maternal and child health nursing, medical-surgical nursing, and psychiatric and mental health nursing, were established with a mandate to consider the development of standards for nursing practice as their major priority. After 6 years of concentrated efforts, all divisions on practice presented standards of care for their division based on their beliefs about nursing practice at the 1972 biennial ANA convention in Detroit (American Nurses' Association, 1975, p. 1). In 1973 the community health nursing standards were made available for distribution to all members of the community health nursing division. The most recent standards for community health nursing practice are delineated below. They address the responsibility of the nurse for assuring quality of nursing practice (American Nurses' Association, 1986, Standards of Community Health, pp. 5-15).

STANDARD I. Theory
The nurse applies theoretical concepts as a basis for decisions in practice.
STANDARD II. Data Collection
The nurse systematically collects data that are comprehensive and accurate.
STANDARD III. Diagnosis
The nurse analyzes data collected about the community, family, and individual to determine diagnoses.
STANDARD IV. Planning
At each level of prevention, the nurse develops plans that specify nursing actions unique to client needs.
STANDARD V. Intervention
The nurse, guided by the plan, intervenes to promote, maintain, or restore health, to prevent illness, and to effect rehabilitation.

TABLE 22-1 Selected definitions of quality assurance

Author	Definitions
American Nurses' Association	Estimation of the degree of excellence in (1) the alteration of the health status of consumers attained through providers' performances of (2) diagnostic, therapeutic, prognostic, and other health care activities.[1,2]
	Quality assurance is a relatively new term conveying the broad idea that superiority or excellence in care is made secure or certain.[3]
	A program executed to make secure or certain the excellence of health care; the term is applied to programs as limited as that of an administrative unit of a health care agency or as broad as that of a community, a region, a state, or a nation. The program must have two major components:
	1. The securing of measurements and ascertaining of the degree to which stated standards are met;
	2. The introduction of changes based on information supplied by the measurements, with the view to improvement of the total effort and product of the unit or agency.[4]
	Quality assurance is an ongoing program in the nursing profession, constructed and executed to secure and implement the excellence of health care.[5]
Brown	Quality assurance, when used in reference to health care, refers to the accountability of health personnel for the quality of care they provide.[6]
Davidson	Quality assurance is a process for attainment of the highest degree of excellence in the delivery of patient or client care.[7]
	A commitment to excellence of care; an estimation of the health status of consumers attained through nursing performance.[8]
Lang	Activities done to determine the extent to which a phenomenon fulfills certain values and activities done to assure changes in practice which will fulfill the highest levels of values.[9]
Mayers	Quality assurance has as its central goal making certain that care practices will produce good patient outcomes.[10]
Nichols	The term quality assurance is used to describe a process in which standards are set and action is taken to ensure achievement of the standards.[11] It involves the description of the level of quality desired and feasible, and a system for ensuring its achievement.[12]
Zimmer	Quality assurance is estimation of the degree of excellence in patient health outcomes and in activity and other resource cost outcomes.[13]

REFERENCES:
1. American Nurses' Association (ANA): Guidelines for Review of Nursing Care at the Local Level, Publ. NP-54, Kansas City, Mo, 1976, The Association, p A-2.
2. American Nurses' Association: Standards of Home Health Nursing Practice, Kansas City, Mo, 1986, The Association.
3. ANA: A Plan for Implementation of the Standards of Nursing Practice, Publ. NP-51, Kansas City, Mo, 1975, The Association, p 5.
4. Ibid, p 30.
5. Ibid, p 6.
6. Brown B: Quality assurance (editorial), Nurs Admin Q 1:v, Spring 1977.
7. Davidson SVS: PSRO: Utilization and audit in patient care, St Louis, 1976, CV Mosby Co, p 5.
8. Davidson SVS: Nursing care evaluation: concurrent and retrospective review criteria, St Louis, 1977, CV Mosby Co, p 408.
9. Lang N: A model for quality assurance in nursing, Milwaukee, 1974, Marquette University, p 11 (unpublished doctoral dissertation).
10. Mayers MG: Quality assurance for patient care: nursing perspectives, New York, 1977, Appleton-Century-Crofts, p 3.
11. Nichols ME and Wessells VG, eds: Nursing Standards and Nursing Process, Wakefield, Ma, 1977, Contemporary Publishers, pp 1–2.
12. Ibid, p 37.
13. Zimmer MJ: Quality assurance in the provision of hospital care: a model for evaluation nursing care, Hospitals, 48:91, 131, March 1, 1979.
From Schmadl JC: Quality assurance: Examination of the concept, Nursing Outlook, 27:462-465. Copyright 1979, American Journal of Nursing Company. Reproduced with permission from Nursing Outlook.

STANDARD VI. Evaluation
The nurse evaluates responses of the community, family, and individual to interventions in order to determine progress toward goal achievement and to revise the data base, diagnoses, and plan.
STANDARD VII. Quality Assurance and Professional Development
The nurse participates in peer review and other means of evaluation to assure quality of nursing practice. The nurse assumes responsibility for professional development and contributes to the professional growth of others.
STANDARD VIII. Interdisciplinary Collaboration
The nurse collaborates with other health care providers, professionals, and community representatives in assessing, planning, implementing, and evaluating programs for community health.
STANDARD IX. Research
The nurse contributes to theory and practice in community health nursing through research.*

The ANA's standards of home health nursing practice are listed in Chapter 19. Quality assurance is emphasized in these standards under the concepts of evaluation and the organization of home health services. The ANA believes that managers must assume responsibility for creating an environment which promotes quality assurance and for establishing a quality assurance program which measures both the clinical and administrative aspects of the organization (American Nurses' Association, 1986, Standards of Home Health, pp. 5-6). The ANA standard documents provide a valuable framework for developing a quality assurance program.

Beliefs and standards for nursing practice should never be static. As societal changes, expansion of knowledge, and technological advances occur, beliefs and standards should be reevaluated to determine whether they reflect the values of the profession and society. The ANA Standards for Practice of 1973 were presented only as a working document to be continually evaluated and revised. This has been done twice since they were initially developed.

*Reprinted with permission of the American Nurses' Association.

MODEL FOR QUALITY ASSURANCE

The development of standards for practice is only one component of quality assurance. Donabedian (1966) stressed that quality assurance efforts should be focused on evaluating the structure, process, and outcome aspects of health care delivery, as well as on the implementation of measures to improve care when warranted. Actions to improve care in the community health setting include such elements as securing more nursing staff, hiring better-prepared personnel, providing additional nursing supervision, increasing the frequency of home visits to given families, and planning health programs for specified at-risk population groups. All aspects of community health nursing practice, including services to individuals, families, and the community as a whole, must be evaluated when one is implementing a quality assurance program.

Like the nursing process described in Chapter 8, quality assurance involves a series of circular, dynamic actions which are client centered. Shared responsibility between nurses and consumers is essential if clients are to be protected from incompetent practitioners. The circular nature and the shared partnership aspects of quality assurance are illustrated in the quality assurance model (Figure 22-1) developed by participants at an ANA leadership workshop (Model shows, 1976, p. 23). When graphically depicted, the monitoring of quality assurance appears simple. In reality, it is a complex process requiring time, effort, and commitment to the value of professional accountability.

COMPONENTS OF A QUALITY ASSURANCE PROGRAM

Quality assurance is a broad and encompassing concept which presents many challenges for the health care professional. Use of a conceptual framework or model for organizing quality assurance activities facilitates the development and implementation of a meaningful quality assurance plan in the practice setting. Such a model is presented in Figure 22-1. This model identifies the

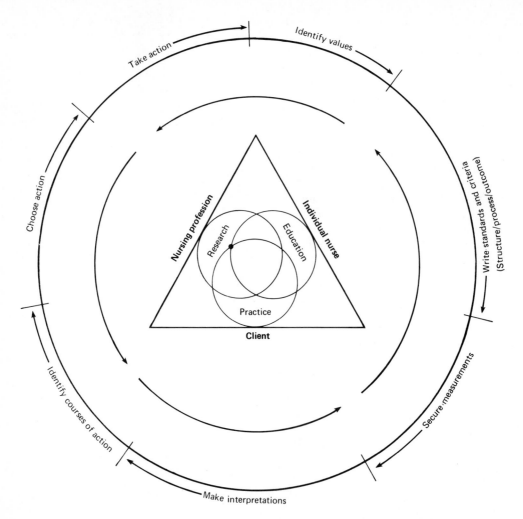

Figure 22-1 A quality assurance model. (From Model shows dynamic concept of quality assurance, Am Nurse, February 28, 1976, p 23. Adapted from the ANA Quality Assurance Model, a plan for implementation of the standards of nursing practice, Kansas City, Mo, 1975, The Association, p 15.)

basic components of quality assurance. These are listed below and will be discussed in detail later.

- Identify values
- Write standards and criteria (structure, process, and outcome)
- Secure measurements
- Make interpretations
- Identify courses of action
- Choose action
- Take action

Because of external and internal environmental pressures, quality assurance programs in many organizations and agencies are developing rapidly. Some programs are being implemented so quickly that nursing staff do not have adequate time to assimilate the changes that are occurring. Nursing personnel may need to conduct nursing audits or establish standards and criteria for care without fully understanding the concept of quality assurance. It is crucial that careful attention be given to *how* each aspect of a quality assurance program is initiated, because many of the changes being proposed may be foreign to staff nurses. Change to the unknown produces anxiety, especially when those involved do not understand why change is necessary, how the change may affect them, or how to accomplish the specific tasks required of them.

Continuing education is often the essential first step in developing a quality assurance program. Many staff nurses and their supervisors have not been prepared in the academic setting to develop standards of care, because emphasis has only recently been placed on identifying standards for practice. In addition, technological advances, changes in the health care delivery system, and current views on the rights and responsibilities of clients have altered the nature of community health nursing practice. As a result of these changes, nurses have found it necessary to seek opportunities for advanced education in order to work effectively with clients in the practice setting.

When a quality assurance program is implemented, the continuing education needs of all staff should be ascertained. *Quality is not assured if only a small committee evaluates care* and understands the quality assurance program. All personnel need the opportunity to provide input and to have administrative support that affords time and encouragement for learning. Research since the late 1970s supports the view that both staff nurses (Keller, 1978; Bappert and Blom, 1983) and management personnel (Knollmueller, 1987; Duffy and Fairchild, 1989) perceive a lack of knowledge to address some of the clinical and/or administrative changes in community health nursing service delivery. A sound quality assurance program measures both clinical and administrative aspects of the organization (ANA, 1986, Standards of Home Health, p. 5). For this to occur, adequacy of knowledge related to role responsibilities is essential.

As was previously mentioned, there are several components of quality assurance. Factors to consider when implementing each of these components will be shared in the following section of this chapter. By using the model presented in Figure 22-1 and the information presented below, the reader should be able to evaluate the progress made in implementing a quality assurance program in specific practice settings.

Identify Values

Attitudes, beliefs, and values influence how we think, how we act, and how we evaluate. In terms of quality assurance, they affect one's commitment to the concept and how quality is defined based upon one's beliefs about health, humanity, and the nature of nursing practice. Identifying values in relation to quality, however, is a difficult task because many factors influence how nursing services are delivered. Available resources, consumer needs and wants, and professional philosophies all determine the scope of practice in a particular community. It is unrealistic, for instance, to assume that an agency can plan nursing services without taking into consideration the restrictions of limited resources. Providing fragmented services for all is not assuring quality.

Establishing a philosophy of nursing practice is fundamental to the identification of quality in nursing care. A philosophy provides direction for the nature and scope of services provided by both an agency and an individual practitioner. Based on available resources, it identifies clients' needs, why activities are being carried out, and the population to be served. A philosophy also describes the type of relationship the practitioner and client will have.

When a philosophy for nursing practice is being defined, discussion related to key general concepts should occur. Often concepts are accepted as truths, but their meaning to each practitioner varies. Concepts such as "clients' right of self-determination," "active client participation," "individualization of client care plans," and a "family-centered preventive approach" to the delivery of health care are difficult to internalize. Practitioners need time to analyze how these concepts can be applied in the practice setting. They need to understand what it means to their practice when they subscribe to a broad concept such as "the right of self-determination." When dealing with this concept, for example, nurses need time

Statement of Philosophy: Visiting Nurse Association of Hartford, Incorporated

In 1969 a committee composed of Board members, supervisors and administrators was formed to develop the following Statement of Philosophy of the Visiting Nurse Association of Hartford, Inc. This was approved by all staff members and the Board of Directors.

The VNA of Hartford exists to provide services to people. It draws its authority from a 1923 Constitution in which the purpose ". . . to furnish . . . skilled services of a Visiting Nurse . . . including instruction in prevention of disease and preservation of health" is stated.

More specifically, the nature of the service is:

1. To provide, with a family centered approach, skilled nursing and other therapeutic services on a part-time basis in the home or other appropriate place.

2. To promote health and prevent illness—both mental and physical.

3. To help individuals get other necessary community services appropriate to their needs.

4. To recognize and bring to the attention of appropriate people unmet needs of the community and to participate in planning to meet these needs.

We believe:

1. The agency has a responsibility to honor all requests for services and to do an assessment of the situation involving the patient and the family and other appropriate professions or agencies, e.g., doctors, social workers, etc.

2. All planning and goal setting is done with the individual being served, his family and others involved in implementing care.

3. Planning and goal setting is a continuing process between nurse, patient and family, one of the goals being maximum independence of patient and family in taking care of their health needs.

4. Plans for the termination of VNA services should be made with the individual, family and all others involved when family needs exceed the capabilities of the nursing agency and the family.

5. All planning includes the giving of consideration to the coordination of services, the appropriate use of manpower and the avoidance of duplication of effort.

6. We believe the above can be best achieved through the practice of primary nursing.

A. The designation of the primary nurse for each patient/family will be based on geography, nurses' skill and nurses' availability.

B. The primary nurse will interpret her role to the patient/family. The primary nurse is responsible and accountable for the nursing care delivered on a 24 hour basis until the patient is discharged. Her responsibility for directing and evaluating the care of other nurses mandates holding other nurses accountable and responsible for the care they give.

C. The responsibilities of the primary nurse include:
(1) Assessment of patient's/family's condition.
(2) Identification of patient's/family's problems on the problem list.
(3) Development of the nursing care plan to meet the identified needs.
(4) Maintenance of the current problem list and plans, based on continuing assessment of the patient's/family's status.
(5) Implementation of the plan of care to the extent possible.
(6) Collaboration with nursing staff, physicians and other health workers in the care of the patient/family.
(7) Evaluation of the effectiveness of nursing intervention.

to share feelings about client situations where their value systems differ from their clients' value orientations.

It was said in Chapter 2 that a community health nurse's "dominant responsibility is to the population as a whole" (American Nurses' Association, 1986, Standards of Community Health). This concept, like the above concepts, is difficult to grasp and to apply. An agency that has limited resources and subscribes to this belief must identify ways in which it can implement this concept. It is impossible for any agency to provide direct service to all individuals within a community. However, a community health agency can identify nursing service needs it can provide and then apply the principles of health planning to see that gaps in services are met by other community agencies.

Agencies must determine what is realistic for them to accomplish in view of the resources available or potentially available to them. If this is not done, they will never be able to determine when quality has been achieved. Being "all things to all people" is an impossible goal, but defining what one can do is not impossible. For instance, in the accompanying statement of philosophy (see box on p. 846), the Visiting Nurse Association of Hartford, Inc., clearly spelled out that they would provide *skilled* nursing services, including instruction in prevention of disease and preservation of health and other therapeutic services, on a part-time basis. They meet the needs of the population as a whole by referring individuals to other community agencies and by participating in health planning activities when unmet needs were recognized. Although developed in the late 1960s, this agency philosophy statement remains a good model to follow when examining what is realistic for an agency to achieve.

It should not be assumed that all community health nurses have a clear understanding of or an appreciation for their agency's philosophy and beliefs. Even when an agency has had a written philosophy statement, discourse should occur among staff members periodically so that a common framework for practice becomes explicit to all. A philosophy document given to new employees may receive little attention. This frequently happens because new employees are naturally more interested in finding out what they have to do to achieve success in their new job situation than in the philosophy behind what they are doing. Thus, agency philosophy and beliefs about nursing practice must be reinforced by supervisors as new employees become comfortable with their job responsibilities. These beliefs must also be reexamined by staff who have been employed for a length of time. When the demands of the workload become heavy it is easy to lose sight of the beliefs and goals of the agency.

Write Standards and Criteria: Structure, Process, and Outcome

A philosophy of practice states the values and beliefs of an agency and guides the activities of all agency staff. It does not provide measurable elements by which a practitioner can judge the quality of care given by nurses. Standards and criteria must be developed so that the measurement of quality is possible. *Standards* are a "model or example established by authority, custom, or general consent" (Ramey, 1973, p. 18). They are rules that help the practitioner to establish a consistent data base in an organized manner so that consistencies and deficiencies of care are easily identified. They are specific statements that reflect the outcomes or goals toward which an agency is working. For example, in the ANA community health standards, one identified goal is "to promote, maintain, or restore health, to prevent illness, and to effect rehabilitation" (Standard V).

Criteria are predetermined measurable elements which reflect the intent of a standard (American Nurses' Association, 1975, p. 16). They identify expected levels of performance by practitioners (process criteria) or clients (outcome criteria) or organization (structure criteria). One process criterion for measuring ANA community health nursing standard V might be "community health nurse provides instruction in the prevention of disease and the preservation of health when client situation warrants such activities."

The development of standards and criteria for evaluation of nursing care should occur from three perspectives: structure, process, and outcome. According to Donabedian (1966, pp. 169-170), *structure* standards appraise the environment in which health care is provided. Such things as the organizational framework, the availability of resources, the qualifications of staff, and the adherence to legal mandates are examined with structural standards. Both the American Nurses' Association and the National League for Nursing have been actively engaged in the development of structural standards. Licensure, certification, and accreditation standards provide guidelines for agencies by which to evaluate their structural characteristics. One such standard requires that agencies have adequate resources to achieve their stated goals. Criteria in relation to such things as numbers of staff and amount of funding are used to measure this standard.

Process standards and criteria describe how care should be delivered (Donabedian, 1969, p. 1833). They focus on reviewing the activities carried out by nurses in order to help clients meet their specific health care needs. They are designed *to evaluate the use of the nursing process* to determine if it was appropriately applied with individual clients. Process standards and criteria help nurses to examine their behavior and skills in relation to client-nurse interactions, the formulation of nursing diagnoses and client goals, the implementation of various intervention strategies, the process of evaluation, and the coordination of care with other health professionals. Process standards and criteria determine if nursing services were appropriate to the needs of the family or a specified at-risk group. They also identify where nursing intervention was needed but not implemented. The ANA community health standards listed earlier are process standards. "Community health nurse documents a biopsychosocial health history on the client service record" could be one process criterion used to determine whether the ANA Standard II, in relation to data collection, has been achieved.

Outcome standards and criteria focus attention on the end results of care (Donabedian, 1969, p. 1833). They measure the behavioral change within the client rather than the process nurses used to effect client change. They evaluate what a client has learned, not what or how a nurse has taught. For example, an outcome standard might read, "Caregiver demonstrates knowledge of parenting skills." Some outcome criteria to measure achievement of this standard could be (1) care giver appropriately discusses three safety needs of infants; (2) caregiver verbalizes four basic physical care needs of infants; (3) caregiver appropriately discusses the recommended preventive health care schedule for infants.

There are limitations in all three approaches—structure, process, and outcome—to the evaluation of nursing care. Structural standards and criteria define essential system characteristics necessary for successful implementation of nursing care in a particular setting. They do not ensure that system resources are used effectively or efficiently in the delivery of care. Having sufficient staff, for instance, does not guarantee that quality care will be provided. Process standards and criteria appraise only how nurses carry out their functions to effect change. They do not evaluate if change has occurred as a result of nursing activities. Outcome standards and criteria are difficult to articulate because client health outcomes are influenced by multiple, interrelated factors. The biopsychosocial characteristics of a client, the environmental conditions of the client's setting, and the contributions of various disciplines all affect the health outcome status of a client. Outcome criteria do not specify which contributing factor was most relevant (Donabedian, 1966, pp. 167-169). It takes considerable skill to isolate elements which measure client outcomes that have occurred as a result of nursing actions alone.

There is a trend toward emphasizing the use of outcome standards and criteria. These types of measurements are extremely important, but they should not be the only type of measurement used to evaluate quality. They do not eliminae the need to evaluate process and structural aspects of health care delivery.

It is apparent that all three approaches to the evaluation of care are essential if quality is to be ensured. When using any of these approaches, it is important to be realistic about what one can accomplish. The realities of an agency's situation should be analyzed carefully to determine what is possible to operationalize. *Standards and criteria that are all-inclusive can seldom be reached and tend to cause frustration and anxiety among staff.* In the community health setting it is often stated, for instance, that comprehensive health care services will be provided to clients in the home, school, and clinic settings. Resources, however, are frequently not sufficient to achieve this goal. When this is the case, services to all clients are diluted, because the available work force is not adequate to meet all the health care needs in each of these settings. It would be more realistic to identify selected services, such as consultation to teachers and follow-up on children with chronic health problems, that will be provided in any one setting.

Developing standards and criteria presents special challenges to the nurse in the community health setting. A goal of community health nursing practice is to help groups (families, populations, and communities) to obtain their maximum level of functioning. Groups in all stages of the life-span are the recipients of community health nursing services. Health supervision activities versus curative treatment are the major orientation when community health nurses are working with these groups. Measurement of health supervision activities with groups, however, is not a well-defined art. In general, most community health agencies have not focused attention on evaluating systematically the quality of health supervision services. Morbidity care provided by home health agencies is more frequently evaluated systematically, because third-party payors mandate that it be done.

Quantitative counts such as numbers of home, school, and clinic visits, changes in mortality and morbidity statistics, and figures obtained from cost-benefit studies have traditionally been used to determine the effectiveness of nursing services in community health. *None of these measurements evaluates quality.* These measurements do not take into consideration the types of services required based on client needs, how well services are provided, and the results of nursing interventions.

Measuring health supervision activities is not an easy task, because often psychosocial variables have a greater impact on health outcomes than do biological variables. There are few absolutes when it comes to defining healthy psychosocial functioning. This is becoming increasingly true as societal values change, allowing for and accepting various lifestyles. In addition, there is little research aimed at validating the effectiveness of health supervision activities carried out by nurses.

Although it is not easy to develop health supervision standards, it is not impossible. They are being established. The ANA community health standards are designed to evaluate *process* with all types of nursing activities, including health promotion ones. An audit tool (refer to Figure 22-3) discussed later in this chapter illustrates how one agency has used process standards, based on the nursing process framework, to evaluate health supervision visits in its agency. The Ervin Quality Assessment Measurement Instrument (Ervin, Chen, and Upshaw, 1989) is another example of a process-oriented quality assurance tool appropriate for evaluating community health nursing service delivery.

Outcome standards for health supervision visits are also being developed by some agencies. These have been written in a variety of ways: according to development age categories such as infant, preschool, school, adolescent, adult, and aging; according to like conditions or health-related phenomena such as pregnancy, parenthood, mental retardation, or child abuse; or according to disease categories such as cancer, arthritis, or heart problems (Buck, 1988; Lalonde, 1988; Minnesota Department of Health, 1979; More and Masterson, 1987; Rinke and Wilson, 1988, Outcome measures, and 1988, Client oriented project objectives).

There is no "right" way to develop health promotion standards. Regardless of the format selected, however, a conceptual framework should be used to provide a consistent frame of reference for all. Maslow's hierarchy of needs, the developmental task approach, Roy's adaptation model, and the systems theory approach are a few examples of frames of reference that can be used. These frameworks assist the community health nurse in examining all parameters of functioning. They are especially appropriate for use in the community health setting because they have a health rather than an illness orientation. For example, Libey and Storfjell (1978) selected Maslow's hierarchy of needs as a conceptual framework and combined this with the developmental task approach when they developed the accompanying standards of care for community health nurses who are working with aging clients (refer to Figure 22-2). These two frameworks were selected because they provide parameters for assessing current and potential health needs and help to focus on health promotion and primary preventive activities as well as on curative services.

Libey and Storfjell's standards for the aging

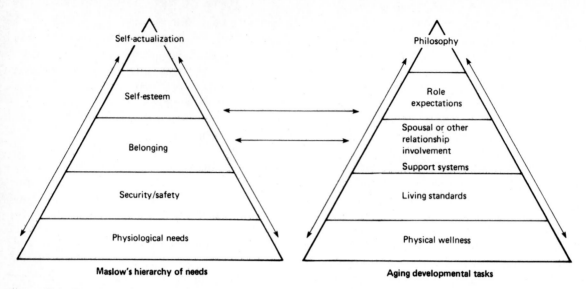

Figure 22-2 Standards of care for the aging, based on Maslow's hierarchy of needs and the developmental tasks of aging. (From Libey T and Storfjell J: Standards of care for the aging, 1978, p 6. A course paper submitted in partial fulfillment of course requirements for N515, Advanced Study of the Nursing Process, University of Michigan, Community Health Nursing Graduate Program, Ann Arbor, Mi.)

have been used, with favorable results, by undergraduate baccalaureate nursing students and staff in a home care agency. Their standards help these nurses to better organize their use of the nursing process and to focus on health promotion and preventive activities, because under each standard of care, Libey and Storfjell have identified categories to assess, key considerations to note when collecting data, and optimal client-family outcomes. Under standard I they examine family history, past health history, and general health status including hygiene, sleep, nutrition, health habits, activities of daily living, psychosocial status, and a review of functioning in relation to each body system. An example of how they have organized this material is shared in Table 22-2.

If community health nurses choose to organize standards of care according to disease categories, it is extremely important to guard against focusing attention on the disease process. How the client is *coping* with the disease condition, as well as the client's current health status, should be the

TABLE 22-2 Standard I: Maintain optimal physical and emotional wellness

Assessment	Considerations	Optimal client or family outcomes
Family history	Relatives with history of: cardiovascular or hypertensive, ocular, degenerative, lung, endocrine, or renal disease(s); cancer (breast, colorectal, prostate, lung, other); arthritis; psychosocial disorders; tuberculosis	Awareness of possible familial predisposition to disease and recognition of the importance of follow-up, referral, and care

From Libey T and Storfjell S: Standards of care for the aging, A course paper submitted in partial fulfillment of course requirements for N515, Advanced Study of the Nursing Process, University of Michigan, Community Health Nursing Graduate Program, Ann Arbor, 1978.

major emphasis in these types of standards. The role of the community health nurse is to provide information, to help the client problem-solve, and to improve the client's self-care capabilities in a way that will facilitate adaptation to stresses being experienced.

Developmental and family health supervision standards are needed in the community health setting, even when condition or disease standards are available. This is necessary since a major role of the community health nurse is to encourage health-promotion activities, even if disease is not present, among individuals, families, and groups across the life-span. In order to implement this role, community health nurses need a framework for assessing family structure, functions, and processes and for analyzing strengths and needs of family functioning. They also need a framework that will assist them to identify strengths and needs of individuals across the life spectrum and that will help them to modify intervention strategies according to the individual needs of a developmental age group.

Health supervision standards must be sufficiently broad so that cultural differences are not discounted. They must be flexible enough to allow for professional judgment and client participation in the formulation of specific outcomes. They should be individualized by providers in each health care setting, based on the needs of the community and the resources of the particular organization. Use of conceptual frameworks such as those previously discussed will more likely ensure that the above provisions will be included in standard formulation. Maslow's hierarchy of needs, for instance, postulates that people must meet their physical needs before they will achieve self-esteem or self-actualization. Based on this belief, a family health supervision standard which states "that the family provides for the basic needs of its members" could be developed and used with families from all cultures. Such a standard does not provide specific directives for how a family should accomplish this goal. This is important because cultures vary as to how food, shelter, and clothing are provided, as well as how health care is obtained. One criterion for evaluation of this stan-

dard could be "family members have an adequate intake of iron, which is demonstrated by all family members having a normal hemoglobin value." This criterion does not specify that a particular type of food must be eaten, and thus takes into consideration cultural variations in relation to eating patterns. There are several other criteria which could be used to measure whether this standard has been achieved. For any standard there will likely be many criterion measurements used to evaluate how well the standard has been met.

A strong knowledge base about specific cultural values and religious beliefs is essential in order for the community health nurse to use standards of care appropriately. Factors such as dietary patterns, traditional ways of dealing with child rearing, allocation of family roles, methods for obtaining health care and treating illness, and rituals during periods of joy or sadness must be known. Only when a community health nurse has this information can she or he make accurate professional judgments about a family's pattern of functioning. Judaism, for example, has a complex set of rituals during mourning which allows for various levels of grief and which encourages the release of emotional tension. A memorial prayer, the *kaddish,* is recited by many Jewish families at daily services for 11 months after the death of a loved one (Kensky, 1977, p. 199). This is *normal, traditional* behavior. A community health nurse who is not aware of these rituals may erroneously label this behavior "a prolonged grief reaction."

The importance of having an appreciation for the inherent worth of different cultural values and religious beliefs cannot be overemphasized. A community health nurse's ability to work effectively with families from different cultural groups is dependent upon the ability to understand them in terms of their background as they view it. Cultural values and religious beliefs dictate behavior and must be respected.

Secure Measurements

After standards and criteria are specified, tools and methods for evaluating and measuring quality must be selected. Nursing audits, utilization review procedures (see Chapter 19), interviews, observation of clients, peer review procedures, observation of staff performance, supervisory evaluation, and staff self-reviews are some of the most commonly used methods for evaluating the quality of nursing care. In addition, evaluative research studies are being conducted more frequently than in the past. Universities and agencies are combining their resources for the purpose of developing methodologies that assess the effectiveness and deficiencies in the delivery of nursing services.

Three evaluation tools—the Quality Patient Care Scale (Qualpacs) (Wandelt and Ager, 1974), the Slater Nursing Competencies Rating Scale (Wandelt and Stewart, 1974), and the Phaneuf Audit (Phaneuf, 1976)—were developed in the 1970s to assist practitioners in evaluating client care or staff performance and are still utilized. The Qualpacs instrument was designed to evaluate care as it is being given. The Slater scale was developed to evaluate individual nurse performance. The Phaneuf Audit was constructed to appraise the quality of nurse care retrospectively (Phaneuf, 1976, p. 33). Of these three tools, the audit is used most often in the community health nursing setting. It usually is modified to address the unique processes involved in community-based practice.

Nursing Audit

Phaneuf (1976, p. 32) defines the nursing audit as "a method for evaluating quality of care through appraisal of the nursing process as it is reflected in the patient care records for discharged patients." How well each aspect of the nursing process was carried out is examined when a client record is audited.

The nursing audit encompasses a systematic review of a specified number of service records, in a given period of time, and the development and implementation of corrective measures when deficiencies in quality are identified. It emphasizes the importance of accurately documenting nursing services, because judgments about quality are made solely on the basis of what has been recorded in the client service record.

The nursing audit is a *process* evaluation

method structured so that it ensures consistency of interpretation by all reviewers. This structure is obtained through the use of a nursing audit tool that has a *set of care standards, criterion measurements* for each care standard, and a *quality rating scale.* Criteria are predetermined, measurable characteristics of a variable (care standard) which are used to make judgments about the quality of care provided. One criterion used to determine how well a nurse makes assessments might read, "community health nurse collects and records data in relation to a client's family history."

The categories of care standards on a nursing audit tool should be selected so that they reflect the essential functions of nursing, not the functions of other disciplines. Phaneuf (1976, pp. 2-3) devised seven care standards from the seven nursing functions described by Lesnik and Anderson (1955). As can be seen from the list below, Phaneuf's care standards are components of the nursing process. She selected a nursing process framework, because she felt that the nursing process was a constant variable in practice, which was not likely to change over time.

Phaneuf's seven care standards
1. Application and execution of physician's legal orders
2. Observation of symptoms and reactions
3. Supervision of the patient
4. Supervision of those participating in care
5. Reporting and recording
6. Application of nursing procedures and techniques
7. Promotion of health by direction and teaching

Phaneuf's care elements have been valuable in providing a framework for the nursing audit process. Some community health agencies, however, have found that making terminology changes in Phaneuf's list has made the nursing audit tool more practical when the agency is evaluating the delivery of health supervision services. One health department, the Oakland County Health Department, Pontiac, Michigan, redefined their categories of care standards after consultation with Maria Phaneuf. This agency's care standards are as follows:

The Oakland County Health Department's care standards

1. Observation of situation
2. Evaluate total situation and draw up plans for nursing action
3. Implementation of nursing plans
4. Coordination of other services—intra- and inter-agency
5. Recording format

Upon examining Phaneuf's categories of care standards and the Oakland County categories of care standards, it is apparent that both use the nursing process as a framework for identifying nursing functions. The changes in terminology are due to variations in nursing approaches, roles, and responsibilities in the community setting as opposed to those in the hospital setting. A major role of the nurse in the community health setting, for instance, is to coordinate services with other community agencies. Thus, the Oakland County Health Department believed that this responsibility should be identified as a major care standard.

The complete audit tool, including care standards, criterion measurements, and a quality rating scale, developed by the Oakland County Health Department is presented in Figure 22-3. Definitions that assist their nurses in applying the criterion measurements and in using their rating scale are included in Appendix 22-1. This material is included so that the reader can gain an understanding of how one agency has chosen to look at the care delivered by community health nurses in their setting. Using these tools for several years has demonstrated to the Oakland County nursing staff that they do have consistency between reviewers.

A nursing audit tool does not eliminate the need for professional judgment. Members of the audit committee at Oakland County Health Department, for example, must use their nursing knowledge to determine if public health nurses collect sufficient data to evaluate the needs of all family members. No audit tool can list all the information needed in every family situation, because needs of families vary depending on their circumstances and resources.

Donabedian (1969, p. 1835) has found that "the validity of assessments of care rests largely on agreed-upon professional judgment." He believes that "reliable judgments can be obtained through the audit of medical records." However, in order to achieve valid, reliable reviews of quality, orientation of new audit committee members is essential. They must learn how the criterion measurements are interpreted, as well as how to analyze the results of a nursing audit.

Many community health agencies have found that it is necessary to change their recording format in order to achieve valid, reliable audit reviews. Traditionally, a narrative style of recording had been used in the community health setting. This type of recording is difficult to audit, especially if a nursing process framework has not been used to organize the narrative notes. Use of the problem-oriented medical record (POMR) developed by Weed (1970) has facilitated the auditing process in some community agencies. Nursing classification schemes are being developed to standardize and computerize the identification of client problems in the POMR. Two of these were presented in Chapter 8 (Gordon, 1989; Simmons, Martin, Crews, and Scheet, 1986). These two classification schemes fit easily into a nursing process framework and can be adapted readily to a computerized system of record keeping.

Computerized recording is beginning to occur in community health nursing and will continue into the future (refer to Figure 22-4). As previously discussed, Appendix 21-1 presents a copy of one of the San Bernadino County Public Health Department's computerized records. This record provides an excellent model to use when developing a *nursing* recording system, because it focuses on the use of the nursing process. It is revised regularly to reflect current practice in the community setting.

The new recording systems being developed can facilitate the auditing of nursing records. However, no one particular recording format can ensure quality. Nurses must understand how to *apply the nursing process* before they can implement quality nursing care or before they can effectively use any recording style.

I. Observations of situation	Yes (8)	No (0)	Partial (4)	
A. Physical environment	_____	_____	_____	_____ A
B. Social environment	_____	_____	_____	_____ B
C. Economic environment	_____	_____	_____	_____ C
D. Educational environment	_____	_____	_____	_____ D
E. Emotional environment	_____	_____	_____	_____ E
F. Problems and needs as seen by family	_____	_____	_____	_____ F
G. Problems and needs as seen by PHN	_____	_____	_____	_____ G
H. Resources	_____	_____	_____	_____ H
II. Evaluate total situation and draw up plans for nursing action	Yes (8)	No (0)	Partial (4)	
A. Available information is reviewed	_____	_____	_____	_____ A
B. Assessment of needs	_____	_____	_____	_____ B
C. Family and patient coping abilities	_____	_____	_____	_____ C
D. Acceptability of nursing service	_____	_____	_____	_____ D
E. Barriers to action	_____	_____	_____	_____ E
F. Nursing diagnosis	_____	_____	_____	_____ F
G. Written expected outcomes	_____	_____	_____	_____ G
H. Written nursing plans	_____	_____	_____	_____ H
III. Implementation of nursing plans	Yes (6)	No (0)	Partial (3)	
A. Evidence of planning with family	_____	_____	_____	_____ A
B. Evidence of PHN action	_____	_____	_____	_____ B
C. Evidence of follow-up	_____	_____	_____	_____ C
D. Evidence of flexibility	_____	_____	_____	_____ D
E. Assessment of expected outcomes	_____	_____	_____	_____ E
F. Legal practice	_____	_____	_____	_____ F
IV. Coordination of other services—intra- and inter-agency	Yes (4)	No (0)	Partial (2)	
A. Referral to other services	_____	_____	_____	_____ A
B. Follow-up of referrals made by PHN	_____	_____	_____	_____ B
C. Feedback to source of referral	_____	_____	_____	_____ C
D. Clarification of agency roles	_____	_____	_____	_____ D
E. Conferences on behalf of the family	_____	_____	_____	_____ E
V. Recording format	Yes (2)	No (0)	Partial (1)	
A. Family record forms complete	_____	_____	_____	_____ A
B. Agency dictation guide used	_____	_____	_____	_____ B
C. Summaries—periodic, transfer, closing	_____	_____	_____	_____ C
D. Family record in sequential order	_____	_____	_____	_____ D
E. Evidence of supervisor review	_____	_____	_____	_____ E
F. Evidence of PHN review	_____	_____	_____	_____ F

Comments: Please complete on back of this page.

Figure 22-3 Oakland County Division of Health, Public Health Nurse Family Record Audit: audit tool. (Reproduced by permission of the Nursing Division, Oakland County Division of Health, Pontiac, Mi.)

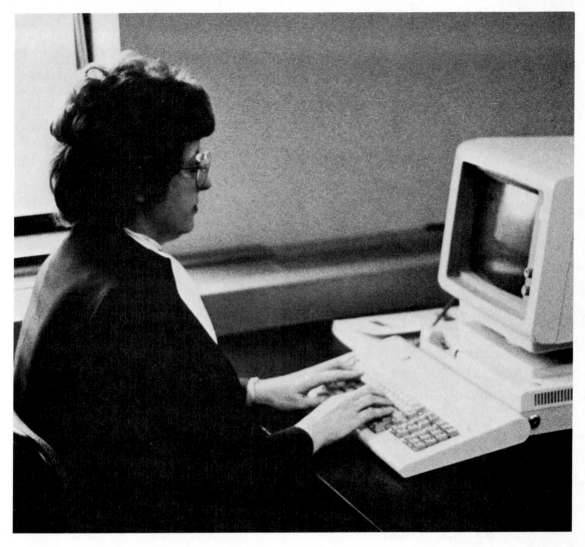

Figure 22-4 Community health nurses across the country are using computers to facilitate recording, quality assurance, and other documentation processes. Computerized information systems help nurses to effectively and efficiently document client data and nursing services and to obtain easy access to planning data. This, in turn, provides nursing administrators with information needed to support current or projected staffing patterns and relevant nursing programs. (Courtesy of photographer, Henry Parks.)

The nursing audit should not be used to evaluate individual staff performance. An agency is more likely to obtain an accurate assessment of the care provided by nurses in that agency if the audit tool is not used to identify weaknesses of individual staff. Rather, peer and supervisory conferences, observation of nursing care, staff self-evaluations, and supervisory evaluations should be used to determine the strengths and needs of individual community health nurses.

Individual Staff Evaluation

All nurses have the professional responsibility to evaluate the quality of care they are providing. Indirectly, the audit approach aids the individual nurse in examining her or his practice in relation

TABLE 22-3   Milwaukee Visiting Nurse Association's job and personnel specifications for a public nurse II

Section A—job description and specifications

Job Summary: Under supervision, has responsibility for case management of patients and families with a wide variety of complex health and social problems, including multiproblem families. Is expected to be able to function independently in most situations. Identifies need for consultation or supervisory help. May be assigned additional responsibilities which require leadership ability.

Duties and responsibilities	**Basic requirements**
1. Functions independently in case management of complex situations, using supervision appropriately	Interviewing skills. Physical assessment skills.
2. Admits patients and family members and gives service utilizing the nursing process.	Knowledge of health problems and illnesses.
a. Assessment—collects physiological, psycho-social, and financial data. Can identify the need for further data and pursues sources of data independently.	Knowledge of normal growth and development. Ability to make nursing judgments based on scientific nursing principles.
b. Assesses family members' health status and coping ability. Able to evaluate the family as a unit.	Knowledge of data sources within the community.
c. Identifies covert and overt nursing health and social problems of patients and families based on data collection.	Knowledge of family dynamics. Ability to see and interpret relationships in data and to arrive at a nursing care plan.
d. Implements nursing care plan as outlined. Adapts nursing procedures to the home setting.	Ability to identify objective parameters for evaluation of nursing care plan.
e. Evaluates results of care plan in terms of expected outcomes and takes appropriate action.	
3. Recognizes and interprets behavior patterns as influenced by basic physical and emotional needs, cultural and socioeconomic differences. Sensitive and accepting of these needs and differences and adapts plan of care accordingly.	Knowledge of cultural and socioeconomic factors. Knowledge of behavioral principles. Knowledge of self. Sensitivity and ability to listen. Knowledge of dependent and independent nursing functions.
4. Contacts physician to report alterations in patient's health status, to secure and share information, or to obtain medical orders.	Ability to collaborate with other disciplines regarding health care.
5. Independently identifies need for consultation and initiates referral.	Knowledge of consultants available and their role in the agency.
6. Independently refers patients and families to other VNA or community services.	
7. Communicates with other disciplines and services inter-agency and intra-agency to promote continuity and coordination of services.	Knowledge of community resources. Knowledge of agency procedures. Ability to write clear, concise, informative reports.
8. Teaches patients and families nursing procedures and good health practices. Interprets to patient and family the implications of the diagnosis—includes the patient and family in goal setting and plan of care according to their ability.	Knows teaching/learning principles. Ability to adapt to patient and family level of understanding and ability.
9. Plans for the use of ancillary agency personnel and supervises their performance.	Knowledge of the legal functions of the RN, LPN, H-HHA. Knowledge of the legal functions of the RN, LPN, H-HHA in the agency.
10. Organizes and manages caseload efficiently.	Good organizational skills.
a. Plans travel routes for optimum economy and efficiency.	Knowledge of area and travel routes Ability to use maps.

TABLE 22-3   Milwaukee Visiting Nurse Association's job and personnel specifications for a public nurse II—cont'd

Duties and responsibilities	*Basic requirements*
b. Establishes priorities within own caseload.	
c. Plans frequency of visits.	
d. Completes necessary records and reports as required within set time limits.	
11. May be assigned additional responsibilities. (Committees, research, etc.)	
Professional conduct:	
1. Accepts agency philosophy, purpose, and objectives	Knowledge of.
2. Follows agency policies and procedures.	Knowledge of.
3. Demonstrates good inter-personal relationships.	Recognizes how behavior affects others.
4. Uses proper resources to deal with stress.	
Professional growth:	
1. Participates in performance evaluation.	Motivated towards self-improvement.
2. Takes responsibility for own professional growth.	

Section B—personnel specifications

1. Wisconsin professional nurse registration.

2. Graduate of baccalaureate program accredited by the National League of Nursing and American Public Health Association.

3. Two years current experience in community health nursing.

Reproduced by permission of the Visiting Nurse Association of Milwaukee, Wis, undated.

to standards established for care. Direct mechanisms must also be used to ensure that each client serviced by the agency receives care equal to or better than established standards. Ongoing evaluation of one's professional performance is important, because it can provide a safeguard for quality client care, promote professional development, and facilitate the identification of professional strengths as well as professional needs.

All nursing personnel must be evaluated on the basis of specified criteria; these criteria should reflect all aspects of nursing performance expected in a given setting. Careful attention must be given to the development of criteria that identify how well a nurse utilizes the nursing process. Often there is a greater emphasis on personal appearance, quantitative counts of visits, and adherence to time policies than to nursing care given. These factors should not be ignored when reviewing staff performance, but they should not be the only focus of the staff evaluation process.

Developing job and personnel specifications that focus on the critical components of nursing practice is the first step in developing appropriate evaluation criteria which reflect all aspects of nursing performance. An example of such specifications developed by one Visiting Nurse Association for a Public Health Nurse II position is presented in Table 22-3. Note particularly in these specifications that the nurse's duties and responsibilities emphasize nursing functions and specifically identify what the community health nurse needs to accomplish in relation to client care. This type of delineation aids in the identification of relevant evaluation categories when nurses are developing evaluation tools.

Community health nurses at all levels, from administrators to staff, have a responsibility to become involved in the evaluation process. Nurses who actively participate in the development of tools for measurement of care and the evaluation process will be more satisfied with the results.

Take the initiative to become involved. It will be a learning experience which will have long-lasting effects on the delivery of your nursing care.

Implementation of Evaluation Measurements

Developing measurement tools and procedures to facilitate use of these tools takes time and a commitment to the value of professional accountability. It took the nursing staff at the Oakland County Health Department, for example, approximately one and one-half years to develop an acceptable audit tool, and then several more years to refine the audit procedures. This agency was successful in achieving its goal because adequate time was allocated for the development of a quality assurance program. Responsibilities were adjusted so that nurses could focus attention on quality assurance without feeling the pressures of caseload demands.

Administrative support during the development and implementation phases of a quality assurance program is essential. Without administrative support, it is highly unlikely that staff will be allowed sufficient time to prepare adequate measurement tools and evaluation procedures. Administrators can also help to reduce the resistance to change and to obtain funds for staff development activities. Many agencies have found that nurses feel threatened when new evaluation measurements are instituted; staff development programs can reduce this threat.

When implementing a quality assurance program, nurses should be oriented to the use of the tools as well as the *process* procedures. They should be allowed to verbalize their anxieties and lack of understanding in a supportive atmosphere. At times, committee members who have had the chief responsibility for developing the measurement tools become frustrated when all staff members do not seem to accept the tools as readily as they have. This especially occurs when committee members forget how long it took them to accomplish their task and to understand the process involved. Members of evaluation committees must recognize that all personnel need time to air their concerns, just as they had time during the development phase. It should not be expected that staff

will grasp the concepts of quality assurance without thought, debate, and resistance.

Make Interpretations

Data from all evaluation procedures should be examined to make interpretations about the quality of nursing care being provided in a particular setting. One tool alone, such as the nursing audit, cannot provide a sufficient data base to determine if quality is present or lacking. In addition, data from multiple sources are often needed to identify the real cause for inadequate care.

The purpose of evaluation is to identify discrepancies between established standards and criteria and actual nursing practice. Evaluation assessments should be specific enough to identify both strengths and needs in the current level of nursing care. In general, most agencies have found that both strengths and needs do exist. If either is found lacking when analyzing evaluation data, the measurement tools and the process for using these tools should be reevaluated. The tools may be too general and broad to discriminate between safe and unsafe care. On the other hand, the tools may be appropriate, but staff may need additional orientation to use them effectively. When they are using the nursing audit for the first time, it is not uncommon to find nurses assuming that certain care was given, even if it was not documented in the family service record. This may be an inappropriate assumption that covers up deficiencies in nursing care.

In order to make interpretations about discrepancies between standards and actual practice, measurement data must be organized and grouped so that a composite picture is clearly visualized. Summary reports should be developed so that the combined results of multiple efforts can be examined and patterns of care identified. Interpretations about overall agency quality must be based on *patterns* occurring over time, rather than on selected record reviews at a given time. Individual staff performance should be evaluated on the basis of *patterns* as well, rather than on one or two select incidents.

After individual audit committee members at the Oakland County Health Department finish

Monthly summary report

Nursing audit report _____
              (Month) (Day) (Year)

_____
/s/ Chairman, Nursing Audit Committee

Number of family folders reviewed ☐

Overall evaluation by number of family folders	Outstanding	Satisfactory	Incomplete	Unsatisfactory
	☐	☐	☐	☐

Category name	Outstanding	Satisfactory	Incomplete	Unsatisfactory	Total
I. Observation of situation					
II. Evaluate total situation and draw up plans for nursing plans					
III. Implementation of nursing plans					
IV. Coordination of other services—intra- and interagency					
V. Recording format					

Function	Outstanding	Satisfactory	Incomplete	Unsatisfactory
I	49–64	33–48	17–32	0–16
II	49–64	33–48	17–32	0–16
III	28–36	19–27	10–18	0–9
IV	15–20	10–14	5–9	0–4
V	12–14	8–11	4–7	0–3

Record score range

149–198 = Outstanding
100–148 = Satisfactory
 51– 99 = Incomplete
  0– 50 = Unsatisfactory

Summary of comments:

Figure 22-5   Oakland County Division of Health, Public Health Nurse Family Record Audit: monthly summary report. (Reproduced by permission of the Nursing Division, Oakland County Division of Health, Pontiac, Mi.)

their audit reviews, they complete a summary report, like the one presented in Figure 22-5. It is then shared with administration and staff. This summary report helps agency personnel to quickly identify strengths and deficiencies in nursing care. It also allows for comparisons from one audit review to another, because change is depicted numerically.

Identify Course of Action

Once strengths and weaknesses in the delivery of nursing practice have been delineated, alternative interventions should be identified to correct deficiencies in care. In addition, nurses should receive positive feedback about their strengths. Staff members who receive only negative feedback can become discouraged with nursing and may be less motivated to make necessary changes.

To identify alternative courses of action for correcting deficiencies, nurses must first analyze why certain problems are occurring. For example, perhaps the recording of the nursing staff demonstrates very little follow-up and evaluation of nursing interventions. There are several reasons why this may be happening, including lack of knowledge, insufficient time allocated for recording, inadequate caseload management skills, unshared values, limited resources, and poor staff morale. Discourse among nurses to find the reasons for the problems should occur before change actions are identified. If the problem is due to inadequate resources to meet client needs rather than lack of knowledge, planning for continuing education programs would be inappropriate. Time allocated for continuing education in this situation would probably only increase the probability that all client needs were not being met. Administrative action to secure further resources or to reevaluate job expectations would be more appropriate.

Input from the nursing staff is essential for determining the best course of action to correct deficiencies in the delivery of nursing care. An administrative mandate which specifies that changes must occur immediately will frustrate staff members if they have not been allowed to voice their opinions about the help they need to alter their actions. Most nurses are interested in providing quality care. They will resist change, however, if they are not actively involved in selecting the appropriate course for change.

Choose Action

Two major activities should occur when choosing change actions: (1) discussion about the advantages and disadvantages of suggested remedial actions and (2) development of a plan for implementing the selected change strategy. Refer again to the situation in which record audits reflect inadequate follow-up and evaluation of nursing in-

terventions. If the major problem identified in this situation is poor documentation due to lack of skill, remedial actions might include conducting a total staff continuing education program which focuses on recording skills, weekly individual supervisory and staff conferences to discuss strengths and needs relative to recording, or self-study by individual staff members. If the majority of the nurses are having difficulty with recording, it probably would be most advantageous to initiate a staff development program. If, on the other hand, only a few nurses are having problems, a staff development program might be very costly to the agency in time and money. If it is determined that a staff continuing education activity is needed, a plan should be developed to ensure that this selected action is implemented.

When discussing the pros and cons of alternate change strategies, agency and community resources should be examined. Often, existing resources are not utilized because it is felt that an "outside expert" or a consultant can do a better job. Frequently this is not the case. Nurses are more motivated to make necessary changes when their talents and skills are recognized and supported. They also become committed to helping others during the change process when they are actively involved, because they believe they have something to contribute. The outside expert frequently does not become actively involved in the change process. This person often shares knowledge and then agency personnel are left to decide how to make changes based on newly gained information. There are times when outside resources should be used; however, such help should be used with discretion because it can be costly and may not help an agency to accomplish what it hopes to achieve.

Planning for change increases the probability that change will occur. It also increases the likelihood that activities will be orderly and predictable and less stressful to staff. Although the entire staff should be involved in developing action plans, one person must be delegated the responsibility and authority to see changes implemented. Group decision making spreads responsibility and often results in no one coordinating and taking responsibility for implementing alternatives.

Take Action

Improvement of nursing care is the primary objective of any quality assurance program. Action must be taken if this is to occur; merely defining problems is not enough. Decisions about various alternative approaches must be made and correction measures implemented, because merely having a discussion about change produces few results.

Taking action to alter practice is one of the most significant components of a quality assurance program. It demonstrates that nurses really do assume accountability for the care provided by members of their profession. It supports the belief that quality assurance should be the responsibility of a profession rather than the responsibility of legal authorities.

Corrective action must be carefully documented and evaluated to determine whether or not it has altered practice. Other actions may be needed if the selected one does not result in desired change. If, for instance, a staff development program does not improve the documentation on client service records, supervisors may have to increase their conference time with individual staff members to help them with their recording skills. The quality assurance cycle should continue even if change does occur. Ongoing monitoring is essential in order to maintain quality standards for practice over time.

PARTNERS IN QUALITY ASSURANCE

The quality assurance model (Figure 22-1) presented at the beginning of this chapter illustrates that individual nurses, the nursing profession, and clients all share responsibility for maintaining high professional standards of nursing practice (Model shows, 1976, p. 23). Input from the client is essential for determining values important to recipients of care. Client feedback is also crucial for the identification of deficiencies in practice on an ongoing basis. It is important that clients have an effect on all components of a quality assurance program because nursing is responsible for ensuring quality of care with clients.

Agencies are utilizing a variety of methods to obtain client input about quality care. Telephone or face-to-face interviews, client satisfaction tools, and client representation on advisory boards are a few examples of ways in which community agencies involve clients in quality assurance. It is important to recognize that the term *client* is not limited to the actual recipient of care: community health agencies have multiple clients such as physicians, hospital discharge planners, community groups, third-party payors, and consumers of care. Methods should be established to obtain input and feedback from all client groups.

Nursing practice, education, and research (Figure 22-1) provide knowledge and experience which aid in the development of a sound quality assurance program. Nurses involved in any of these activities must be willing to share their findings so that others can benefit from their experiences. Practitioners, educators, and researchers must be committed to quality assurance and must work toward refining tools and processes which will facilitate nurses' quality assurance efforts.

In the community health setting, research is needed to validate the effectiveness of the preventive health approach to nursing practice. Further data are also needed to determine if community health nurses are actually meeting the needs of the population as a whole. The tools discussed previously in this chapter were designed to evaluate nursing care with individual clients. Structure, process, and outcome criteria must be developed to identify discrepancies in care to the community. This is crucial if community health nurses are going to continue to subscribe to the belief that their client is the community.

ESTABLISHING A QUALITY ASSURANCE PROGRAM

Professional accrediting bodies, such as the National League for Nursing (NLN) and the Joint Commission on Accreditation of Healthcare Organizations (JCAHO), and third-party payors are recommending that community health agencies have a planned and systematic quality assurance program which focuses on the actual delivery of client care (Gottlieb, 1988; Harris, 1988; McCann and Rooney, 1988). The American Nurses' Association (ANA, 1986, Standards of Home

Health, p. 5) recommends that home health agencies have a quality assurance program which addresses both clinical and administrative aspects of the organization. Most agencies with a well-developed quality assurance program focus on both the actual delivery of client care and the administrative components of quality.

Like other programs, one which concentrates on quality assurance should include a set of objectives; specified services, activities, and time parameters for achieving these objectives; and essential resources needed to develop, implement, and evaluate the overall program (refer to Chapter 12). A manager or administrator in the organization should be assigned the responsibility for developing a written quality assurance plan, ensuring that program objectives are met, and implementing program services and activities in a timely manner. Aspects of a program can easily be neglected if responsibility for quality assurance is not clearly identified. A written plan assists all personnel in the agency to identify essential elements of quality assurance and helps agency staff to articulate its quality assurance efforts to others.

There are various approaches and models for developing a quality assurance program (Daniels, 1987; Gottlieb, 1988; Gould, DiPasquale Ruane, 1988; Martin and Scheet, 1988; McCann and Rooney, 1988). However, common elements found in most of these approaches are similar to the components in the ANA model previously discussed in this chapter. Values in relation to quality are identified, quality assessment standards and criteria are developed, clinical performance is measured in terms of these standards and criteria, action is taken to eliminate deficiencies, and corrective action is assessed to determine the effectiveness of these actions.

A quality assurance program being developed to evaluate actual care delivered to clients should be designed to monitor the quality and appropriateness of client care and to resolve identified problems (Joint Commission on Accreditation of Hospitals, 1983). The minimum activities to evaluate quality and appropriateness should include "supervisory and technical review of clinical records, peer review which includes shared home visits, utilization review, incident reporting, contin-

uing and in-service education, multidisciplinary reviews of patient care where appropriate, and patient opinion surveys" (Gottlieb, 1988, p. 11). Data obtained from these activities should be systematically organized and evaluated against performance standards and criteria.

Administrative aspects of an agency greatly influence the level of care provided to consumers. In order for an organization to deliver quality care, it must have an organizational structure which facilitates effective and efficient service delivery, sufficient and appropriate resources to adequately meet service demands, and established processes to address changes in health care delivery. Administrative aspects of a quality assurance program include such components as written clinical and personnel policies and procedures, the hiring of qualified staff, educational processes which expand clinical competency, and personnel and fiscal management activities.

Ensuring quality of care is a professional responsibility which protects clients and advances practice in an organization. An organization needs to establish a quality assurance program which best meets its needs. This involves identifying the level of care acceptable to the agency and evaluating agency standards against established practice norms. It also involves examining carefully specified requirements of legal bodies such as licensure boards, third-party payors, and other organizations that influence agency practice. Detailing the requirements of all organizations involved in the delivery of community health nursing services is beyond the scope of this text.

INTEGRATION OF UTILIZATION REVIEW, RISK MANAGEMENT, AND QUALITY ASSURANCE ACTIVITIES

Escalating health care costs and complex changes in health care delivery have resulted in increased concern over cost containment and legal issues affecting community-based health care agencies. This has led to an emphasis being placed on utilization review and risk management activities.

Utilization review is a process designed to evaluate "the appropriateness of client admissions and discharges; the appropriate and adequate use of personnel; and over- and underutilization of services" (NLN, 1985, p. 48). This process focuses on the delivery of services in a cost-effective and efficient manner and utilizes a client record review to identify if the amount and type of services provided were appropriate to the needs of the clients and appropriate for the agency to provide. Patient classification systems assist agencies in predicting the kind and amount of service needed by client groups with specific characteristics. Although patient classification systems have been more widely used in acute care settings, there are several available community-oriented classification systems designed to predict service needs (Ballard and McNamara, 1983; Churness, Kleffel, Onodera and Jacobson, 1988; Daubert, 1979; Hardy, 1984; Harris, Santoferraro and Silva, 1985).

Risk management is a process designed to identify, evaluate, address, and prevent potential and actual risks which increase the chances of legal liability (Tehan and Colegrove, 1987). Tehan and Colegrove (1987, p. 71) believe that home care agencies face significant risk in relation to the delivery of patient care services, assessment of caregiver competency, and employee health and safety. Nonprofit and public community agencies face similar risks (Knapp, 1989). Community-based agencies are currently placed in a position of assuring quality care with limited resources, while delivering increasingly complex client services and containing costs. This has exposed agencies to increased risks and has provided a stimulus for agencies to develop risk management programs. A risk management program focuses on such matters as the monitoring of staff selection, orientation, and on-going educational processes; the development of policies to ensure client and employee safety; the evaluation of unsafe client and employee incidents; and the development of educational materials to enhance caregiver/client competency.

While risk management, utilization review, and quality assurance are separate programs with distinctive and separate foci, they are related and have some overlap (Harris, 1988, p. 400). Selected aspects of utilization review and risk management focus on the provision of optimal or quality care as defined by professional standards (Spratt, 1984). For example, judgments about appropriateness of care during the utilization review process are based on established criteria or norms. Inappropriate services do not promote optimal or quality care. To ensure quality care, risk management, utilization review, and quality assurance activities should be integrated and coordinated to achieve a balance among the goals of the three programs. If this coordination is lacking, an agency may neglect aspects of each of these programs (Harris, 1988, p. 400).

SUMMARY

Members of a profession are responsible for developing and upholding standards of professional practice. They must ensure that care provided by all members is equal or better than the standards established to assure a satisfactory level of quality. Monitoring of practice on an ongoing basis is essential in order to protect society from incompetent and unqualified practitioners. Changing societal demands make it even more critical that nurses evaluate the delivery of nursing care, because there is a trend toward emphasizing control of professional practice. There is no question that if nursing does not assume accountability for its actions, others will govern nurses' actions for them. Professionals are functioning in an era of quality assurance.

Quality assurance is a dynamic process involving a series of actions designed to evaluate nursing care. It also includes the implementation of measures designed to improve deficiencies found during evaluation efforts. It is a systematic, ongoing evaluation for the purpose of determining what type of nursing care is being provided, how this care is provided, and the outcome of nursing services to the client. Three partners—individual nurses, the nursing profession, and clients—all share responsibility for maintaining high-quality standards of professional practice. Nurses in service, education, and research must work together to refine evaluation measurements and processes that can facilitate quality assurance efforts.

APPENDIX 22-1

Oakland County Division of Health: Public Health Nurse Family Record Audit

Definitions of criterion measurements for audit committee

I. Observation of situation:

A. *Physical environment:*
   Definition: Description and location of where visit occurs, and noted changes.
   1. Physical structure—apartment, condo, colonial house, etc.
   2. Interior and exterior environmental conditions.
   3. Location—rural, urban, suburban, next to highway, etc.
   4. Specific visit data (includes visit in park, corner drugstore, television blaring, children demanding attention, neighbor visiting; other disruptive factors).
   5. Safety factors (throw rugs in home where elderly reside, fenced yard for preschool children, etc.).
   Location: In data base.
   Frequency: Physical environment described at least once in total record.
   Scoring: Yes   At least three (3) of the factors in definition.
          Partial Minimum of two factors in definition.
          No   None or one factor in definition.

B. *Social environment:*
   Definition: Description of:
   1. Family constellation.
   2. Patterns of interactions with the family, e.g., who relates to whom?
   3. Quality of relationships within family, e.g., hostile, supportive, positive, etc.
   4. Religious or ethnic influences, e.g., supportive or non-supportive.
   Location: Data base (Numbers 2, 3, and 4 under definition). Family data sheet (Number 1 under definition).
   Frequency: Social environment described at least once in total record.
   Scoring: Yes   At least three (3) of the definition factors.
          Partial Two (2) of the definition factors.
          No   One (1) or none of the definition factors.

C. *Economic environment:*
   Definition: Identified source of income (may include how it is used).
   Location: Family data sheet.
   Frequency: Economic environment identified at least once in record.
   Scoring: Yes   Source of income identified on family data sheet.
          Partial Identified in data base, but not found on family data sheet.
          No   Source of income not identified in total record.

D. *Educational environment:*
   Definition: Description of formally or informally acquired knowledge of adult family members who are served.
   Location: Family data sheet or data base.
   Frequency: Educational environment of each adult family member described once in total record.
   Scoring: Yes   Educational environment of all adult family members who receive service. May be inferred from professional occupation, e.g., lawyer, architect, etc., but not from non-professional.
          Partial Educational environment of some but not all, adult members described.
          No   No reference to educational environment mentioned in total record.

E. *Emotional environment:*
   Definition: Description of demonstrated feelings, verbal and/or nonverbal, such as hostility, joy, sorrow, apathy, hate, love, reverence.
   Location: Data base.
   Frequency: Emotional environment described at least once in total record.
   Scoring: Yes   Emotional environment described in relation to at least two family members or to family as a unit. If only one member is family, score as yes.
          Partial Description of demonstrated feelings on less than two family members.
          No   Emotional environment not recorded.

F. *Problems and needs as seen by family:*
   Definition: Viewpoint of problems/needs identified by each family member with whom PHN interacts.

APPENDIX 22-1

Oakland County Division of Health: Public Health Nurse Family Record Audit—cont'd

Location: Data base, plans, or nursing diagnosis.

Frequency: At least once in record.

Scoring: Yes   Viewpoint of each family member with whom PHN interacts.

         Partial   Recorded viewpoint of at least one family member with whom PHN has interacted.

         No   Viewpoint of no family member present in total record.

G. *Problems and needs as seen by the PHN:*

Definition: PHN evaluates problems and needs of entire family.

Location: In data base, plans, or nursing diagnosis.

Frequency: Recorded at least one time for each family member.

Scoring: Yes   If each family member mentioned at least one time in record.

         Partial   If some members are not mentioned in record.

         No   NA

H. *Resources:*

Definition: Description of existing or previous sources of support and assistance.

1. Medical resources.
2. Dental resources.
3. Other agencies (social, counseling, etc.)
4. Friends, relatives, neighbors.

Location: Family data sheet.

Frequency: Described at least one time in record.

Scoring: Yes   Applicable medical and/or professional resources listed on family data sheet and significant other resources.

         Partial   Not all medical or professional resources listed in data sheet although other resources are listed.

         No   No resources listed.

II. Evaluate total situation and draw up plans for nursing action:

A. *Available information is reviewed:*

Definition: Information is gathered and reviewed from such sources as referral source, other family records, other PHNs, physicians, school records, dentists, and other agencies servicing the family. The key words are *available and applicable.*

Location: On family data continuation sheet and family data sheet.

Frequency: NA

Scoring: Yes   A notation on family data sheet or family data continuation sheet that all available or applicable information was reviewed.

         Partial   Need for additional information is indicated but no statement on family data sheet or family data continuation sheet.

         No   Referral information missing from family data sheet.

B. *Assessment of needs:*

Definition: PHN evaluates all patient/family members who have needs and identifies problems.

Location: Assessed needs as found in data base and nursing diagnosis, or data base and plans.

Frequency: PHN updates needs as expected outcomes (EO) are met.

Scoring: Yes   If written in data base and plans or data base and nursing diagnosis.

         Partial   (1) Written in data base but not in nursing diagnosis or plans.

                  (2) No evidence of reassessment as indicated by EO dates, or resolution column is not completed.

         No   Needs/problems not found in data base.

C. *Family and patient coping abilities:*

Definition: Statement of how family deals with situations, or meets difficulties.

Location: Statement in data base.

Frequency: Minimum of one such statement in family folder.

Scoring: Yes   If statement found in data base.

         Partial   NA

         No   Statement missing.

D. *Acceptability of nursing service:*

Definition: Statement of family response to PHN service.

Continued.

APPENDIX 22-1

Oakland County Division of Health: Public Health Nurse Family Record Audit—cont'd

***

Location: Statement found in data base.

Frequency: Minimum of one (1) statement in family folder.

Scoring: Yes   If statement in data base.

         Partial   NA

         No   No such statement in data base.

E. *Barriers to action:*

Definition: Identification of restraints to family movement restricting and obstructing PHN intervention. (These may be as diverse as mental or physical handicaps, individual PHN limitations, social or economic factors, language barriers, or improper timing of PHN action.) Absence of barriers to action is implied unless barriers are specified in dictation.

Location: In data base and/or summary.

Frequency: NA

Scoring: Yes   All unmet expected outcomes are explained in data base and/or summary.

         Partial   Some unmet expected outcomes not explained in data base and/or summary.

         No   If no reasons given in data base and/or summary for not meeting expected outcomes.

F. *Nursing diagnosis:*

Definition: Statement on nursing diagnosis and expected outcomes flowsheet (Form N634).

1. Nursing diagnosis based on information stated in data base and nursing action.

2. Contributing factor(s) must include implication for PHN intervention.

3. Nursing diagnosis must be written by end of second visit and as PHN/family work on additionally identified problems.

Location: From N634 Form under nursing diagnosis column.

Frequency: A minimum of one (1) nursing diagnosis, and additions when PHN/family work on other identifiable problems.

Scoring: Yes   Each nursing diagnosis contains all factors in definition.

         Partial   One of the definition factors missing in one or more nursing diagnosis.

         No   Contains none of the definition factors.

G. *Written expected outcomes (EO's)*

Definition: A statement of intended or realistically anticipated client/family behavioral change by a certain time.

1. Measurable.

2. Client/family oriented.

3. Re-evaluation date.

Location: On N634 Form under expected outcome column.

Frequency: A minimum of one (1) expected outcome per nursing diagnosis.

Scoring: Yes   All expected outcomes comply with expected outcome definition factors.

         Partial   One or more expected outcomes missing at least one factor.

         No   No expected outcomes; or all expected outcomes missing at least one factor.

H. *Written nursing plans:*

Definition: Written activities to continue on-going assessment and reach expected outcomes. The activities may be performed by PHN, client, family, or other agencies/resources.

1. Each specific plan numbered.

2. As plan completed, PHN has written in parenthesis after item (met and date) in ink and initialed.

3. Purpose and timing of next visit recorded.

4. *If appropriate,* plans should include:

     a. Feedback to referring agency/resource.

     b. When contracting with family, PHN to indicate what the PHN and client/family will do.

     c. A list of potential or suspected problems identified by PHN or family for future assessment; identified problems deferred until future visits also to be identified.

Location: Stated (listed) after nursing action category as *plans.*

Frequency: Minimum—plan or plans stated one time per visit.

Scoring: Yes   Plan(s) conforms to definition.

         Partial   Plans as listed non-specific and vague; plans consistently do not conform to definition.

         No   No plans listed after each visit.

APPENDIX 22-1

Oakland County Division of Health: Public Health Nurse Family Record Audit—cont'd

III. Implementation of Nursing Plans:
    A. *Evidence of planning with family:*
        Definition: PHN and client/family establish activities or tasks to achieve a mutually agreed upon outcome.
        1. Statement that PHN had discussed plan.
        2. Statement that family agreed to plan.
        Location: Data base and nursing action and plans.
        Frequency: NA
        Scoring: Yes   Statement that PHN discussed the plan; statement that family agreed to plan.
                 Partial Either factor in definition missing.
                 No   Both factors in definition missing.
    B. *Evidence of PHN action:*
        Definition: Written evidence of teaching, counseling, supervision, demonstration, direct care, referral, evaluation, teaching tools, completion of forms, referrals given, PHN role and/or Oakland County Health Division service, or telephone calls made on home visit.
        Location: Under nursing action based on information in data base.
        Frequency: Each visit
        Scoring: Yes   All nursing actions based on information in data base.
                 Partial Not all nursing action based on information in data base.
                 No   No nursing action is based on information in data base.
    C. *Evidence of PHN follow-up:*
        Definition: Evidence of PHN follow-up to carry out or attempt to carry out each plan.
        Location: Found in nursing action or data base.
        Frequency: Evidence of follow-up for each plan.
        Scoring: Yes   Evidence of follow-up is for each plan as defined.
                 Partial Evidence of follow-up is missing one or more times.
                 No   No evidence of follow-up found in record.
    D. *Evidence of PHN flexibility:*
        Definition: PHN actions are restated in response to changing family situation and needs.
        Location: Nursing diagnosis, expected outcomes, resolution, nursing action, or nursing plans.
        Frequency: When indicated.
        Scoring: Yes   Indication of response based on changes indicated in data base as defined above or no indication of changing family situation or needs.
                 Partial NA
                 No   There is evidence of changing situation and needs in data base but not reflected in either nursing diagnosis, expected outcomes, resolution, nursing action, or nursing plans.
    E. *Assessment of expected outcomes* (EO's)
        Definition: Ongoing evaluation of expected outcomes as service is provided.
        Location: Under resolution column and expected outcomes.
        Frequency: When indicated.
        Scoring: Yes   All expected outcomes are indicated as met or unmet with date in resolution column, and dates of EO's are revised. If indicated in data base, new EO's should be added.
                 Partial One or more EO's do not meet "yes" criteria.
                 No   No data in resolution column.
    F. *Legal practice:*
        Definition: Recording indicates PHN's adherence to mandated law (Nursing Practice and State Communicable Disease Laws, etc.).
        Location: Throughout record.
        Frequency: Throughout record.
        Scoring: Yes   There is no evidence of illegal practice.
                 Partial No partial possible.
                 No   Evidence of illegal practice.

Continued.

APPENDIX 22-1

Oakland County Division of Health: Public Health Nurse Family Record Audit—cont'd

IV. Coordination of Other Services—Intra- and Inter-Agency:
    A. *Referral to other services:*
        Definition: If need is identified by family or PHN for referral to other services, PHN directs family towards a specific agency or community resource. May include communication with other services before family is seen by other resources.
        Location:
        1. In data base.
        2. Nursing actions.
        3. Plans.
        4. If utilized should be listed on family data sheet.
        Frequency: NA
        Scoring: Yes   If no need indicated; or if need identified in data base and resources discussed or referral made under nursing action.
                Partial Referral in nursing action with no need identified in data base.
                No   Need indicated in data base, not found or discussed in nursing action or plans.
    B. *Follow-up of referrals made by PHN:*
        Definition: Evidence that PHN obtained information about if/how the family acted upon the referral (either from family or service agency).
        Location: In subsequent data base, or plans, or expected outcomes.
        Frequency: NA
        Scoring: Yes   No need indicated, or status of referral is indicated in the data base or date of referral is written after the plan for the referral, or resolution column completed reflects referral was completed and date of completion.
                Partial Statement in data base that family acted on referral in resolution column or in plans.
                No   No written or oral feedback as defined can be found.
    C. *Feedback to source of referral:*
        Definition: Feedback is written or verbal communication to the source of referral after some action has been taken by PHN.
        Location: Written feedback is found at the back of family folder in the form of a copy of the letter, a continuing patient care form (CPC), or another type of referral form. A statement should appear under plans on the family data continuation sheet with the date it was returned. Verbal feedback is indicated as an entry on the family data continuation sheet.
        Frequency: Each written referral should have a carbon copy of feedback at the back of the family folder.
        Scoring: Yes   1. Feedback if returned to all professional referral sources found under "Referral Source" on the family data sheet in written or oral form.
                        2. The absence of feedback to a non-professional source is accepted as the PHN's decision "it would be unwise or unnecessary."
                        3. Self-referrals are scored *yes.*
                Partial A response to each professional referral source cannot be found.
                No   No written or oral feedback as defined can be found.
    D. *Clarification of agency roles:*
        Definition: PHN explained applicable Health Division services and PHN role (i.e., community and school service as well as Child Health Conference, Communication Clinic, Family Planning).
        Location: Nursing action.
        Frequency: Minimum of one time.
        Scoring: Yes   A statement that PHN explained role and agency services.
                Partial A statement that PHN explained only role or services, not both.
                No   No statement that agency role and services were explained.
    E. *Conferences on behalf of family:*
        Definition: A communication to facilitate provision of health services to individual and family as need indicated. This includes PHN's supervisor, other professionals or non-professionals.
        Location: Family data continuation sheet.

APPENDIX 22-1

Oakland County Division of Health: Public Health Nurse Family Record Audit—cont'd

---

Frequency: When indicated.

Scoring: Yes   1. If no need indicated and no conference is recorded.

2. Conference recorded including content and conclusions.

Partial   Conference recorded but content or conclusions not included.

No   Conference recorded as having been held but content and conclusions both missing.

V. Record Format:

A. *Family record forms complete:*

Definition: Family data sheet (N644) must be completed on all lines or columns with at least one entry under address, referral information, and significant notes. All family members must be listed.

1. Identifying information complete (District/Census Tract; family name; address and phone and changes; referrals received information; roster with sex, marital status, relation to head, and birth date).

2. Admission dates complete for all roster names and current for the year in which the last coded contact occurred *(in pencil).*

3. Immunization information for each family member including dates complete enough for assessment for each immunization listed, or a notation if dates unknown to the family (in pencil).

4. Significant notes to include notations pertinent to the household member(s): diagnosis, "deceased," "out of household," etc., if applicable.

5. Occupation/source of income/education must have at least one entry and include information found in the data base.

6. Agency, medical, dental, or other resources must have at least one entry and include information found in data base.

7. Date coded closed must be completed.

Scoring: Yes   All of the above information included in the record.

Partial   One or more of "2" through "7" missing unless "optional" or NA.

No   None.

B. *Agency dictation format used:*

Definition:

1. Continuation sheet (N662) to include the areas of data base, nursing action, and plans in each coded visit.

2. Nursing diagnosis and EO sheet (N634) with at least one nursing diagnosis and EO, with resolution column complete.

3. Summary sheet (N667) with at least one summary statement or transfer or closing summary.

Scoring: Yes   All criteria in above definitions are met.

Partial   One or more of the above missing.

No   None of above factors.

C. *Summaries are recorded:*

Definition:

1. Every 12 home visits or 18 months, whichever comes first.

2. At the time of record transfer or closure.

3. As a summary statement at the time of transfer or closure if two or less home visits and/or other contacts have been made.

4. A summary to be written within three (3) months after closure of service to family.

Location: On summary sheet (N667).

Frequency: As defined.

Scoring: Yes   All applicable criteria in definition are met.

Partial   Summaries are done but not on required schedule.

No   No criteria in definition are met.

D. *Order of closed family record:*

Definition: (Sequence:)

1. Family data sheet—N664.

2. Continuation sheets—N662.

3. Nursing diagnosis and EO—N634 (may go before or after summary sheet).

4. Summary sheets (green)—N667.

5. Reports and letters, etc: grouped and placed in reverse chronological order (most current on top).

Scoring: Yes   Sequence of record followed as in definition.

Partial   Sequence of record not followed.

No   Any part of the record missing.

Continued.

APPENDIX 22-1

Oakland County Division of Health: Public Health Nurse Family Record Audit—cont'd

E. *Evidence of supervisory review:*
   Definition:
   1. Signature with initial and last name and title at least once in the body of the record, and a minimum of one time a year when record is open longer than a year.
   2. Signature with initial and last name and title after the closing or transfer entry.
   3. Initials on summary sheets.
   Scoring: Yes   Conditions met.
            Partial   Any one of the conditions missing.
            No   Conditions not met.

F. *Evidence of PHN review:*
   Definition:
   1. Each dictation and summary is signed in ink with first initial, last name, and title (PHN).
   2. Corrections that change the meaning of the sentence are made in ink and initialed with a date.
   3. Signature and date after last entry on Expected Outcome sheet.
   Scoring: Yes   Each entry signed and corrections made as defined.
            Partial   Each entry signed and corrected but not as defined.
            No   Not all entries are signed and/or obvious errors are not corrected.

Reproduced by permission of the Nursing Division, Oakland County Division of Health, Pontiac, MI, undated.

REFERENCES

American Nurses' Association (ANA): A plan for implementation of the standards of nursing practice, Kansas City, Mo, 1975, The Association.

American Nurses' Association: Standards of home health nursing practice, Kansas City, Mo, 1986, The Association.

American Nurses' Association, Council of Community Health Nurses: Standards of community health nursing practice, Kansas City, Mo, 1986, The Association.

Ballard S and McNamara R: Quantifying nursing needs in home health care, Nurs Res 32(4):236-241, 1983.

Bappert KG and Blom LR: Supervisory needs of community health nurses, unpublished master's thesis, University of Michigan, Ann Arbor, Mi, 1983.

Buck JN: Measuring the success of home health care, Home Health Nurse 6(3):17-23, 1988.

Burnside IM: Nursing and the aged, New York, 1976, McGraw-Hill.

Christy TE: The first 50 years, Am J Nurs 71:1778-1784, 1971.

Churness UH, Kleffel D, Onodera ML, and Jacobson J: Reliability and validity testing of a home health patient classification system, Public Health Nurs 5:135-139, 1988.

Daniels K: Planning for quality in the home care system. In Fisher K and Gardner K, eds: Quality and home health care: redefining the tradition, Chicago, Il, 1987, Joint Commission on Accreditation of Healthcare Organizations, pp 38-42.

Daubert EA: Patient classification system and outcome criteria, Nurs Outlook 27:450-454, 1979.

Donabedian A: Evaluating the quality of medical care, Milbank Q 44:166-206, 1966.

Donabedian A: Some issues in evaluating the quality of nursing care, Am J Public Health 59:1833-1836, 1969.

Duffy SA and Fairchild N: Educational needs of community health nursing supervisors, Public Health Nurs 6:16-22, 1989.

Ervin NE, Chen SPC, and Upshaw H: Development of a public health nursing quality assessment measure, Quality Rev Bull 15(5):138-143, 1989.

Gordon M: Manual of nursing diagnosis 1988-1989, St Louis, 1989, CV Mosby Co.

Gottlieb HJ: Quality assurance: a blueprint for improved patient care and service, Home Health Nurse 6(3):11-12, 1988.

Gould EJ and DiPasquale Ruane N: Quality assurance in home health. In Harris MD, ed: Home health administration, Owings Mills, Md, 1988, National Health, pp 393-439.

Hardy JA: A patient classification system for home health patients, Caring 3(9):26-27, 1984.

Harris MD: Home health administration, Owings Mills, Md, 1988, National Health.

Harris MD, Santoferraro C, and Silva S: A patient classification system in home health care, Nurs Economics 3:276-282, 1985.

Health Care Financing Administration: Conditions of participation: home health agencies, 42CFR, Part 484, Sections 484.1-484.52, Washington, DC, 1989, US Department of Health and Human Services.

Joint Commission on Accreditation of Hospitals: Hospice self-assessment and survey guide, Chicago, 1983, The Commission.

Keller (Beach) ES: The continuing education needs of community health nurses in Michigan and factors influencing these needs as perceived by these nurses and their supervisors, Ann Arbor, 1978, University of Michigan (unpublished doctoral dissertation).

Kensky AD: Cultural influences on the Jewish patient. In Clemen S and Will M, eds: Family and community health nursing: a workbook. Ann Arbor, 1977, University of Michigan.

Knapp MB: Legal concerns affecting nonprofit community agencies that serve the elderly, Quality Rev Bull 15(3):86-91, 1989.

Knollmueller RN: Educational needs of home health care agency supervisors. In Fisher K and Gardner K, eds: Quality and home health care: redefining the tradition, Chicago, 1987, Joint Commission on Accreditation of Healthcare Organizations, pp 38-42.

Lalonde B: Assuring the quality of home care via the assessment of client outcomes, Caring 7(1):20-24, 1988.

Lesnik MJ and Anderson BE: Nursing practice and the law, ed 2, Philadelphia, 1955, Lippincott.

Libey T and Storfjell J: Standards of care for the aging, a course paper submitted in partial fulfillment of course requirements for N515, Advanced Study of the Nursing Process, University of Michigan, Community Health Nursing Graduate Program, Ann Arbor, November 1978.

Lysaught JP: An abstract for action, New York, 1970, McGraw-Hill.

Martin KS and Scheet NJ: The Omaha System: providing a framework for assuring quality of home care, Home Health Nurse 6(3):24-28, 1988.

McCann BA and Rooney AL: Striving for excellence in home care: a quality assurance approach, Caring 7(10):15-19, 1988.

Minnesota Department of Health, Office of Community Health Services, Section of Community Nursing: Outcome criteria: public health nursing services and home health care services, Minneapolis, 1979, Minnesota Department of Health.

Model shows dynamic concept of quality assurance, Am Nurse, p 23, February 28, 1976.

More V and Masterson AS: Hospice care systems, structures, process, costs, and outcomes, New York, 1987, Springer.

National League for Nurses, Council of Home Health Agencies and Community Health Services: Administrator's handbook for the structure, operation and expansion of home health agencies, New York, 1985, The League.

Papers on the national health guidelines: baselines for setting health goals and standards, DHEW Pub No HRA 77-640, Washington, DC, 1977, Health Resources Administration.

Phaneuf MC: The nursing audit: self-regulation in nursing practice, New York, 1976, Appleton-Century-Crofts.

Public Law 92-603: Section 246E, Title XI, General Provisions and (B) Professional Standards Review, Social Security Amendments of 1972, Ninety-Second Congress HRI, October 30, 1972.

Ramey JG: Setting nursing standards and evaluating care, J Nurs Adm 3:17-25, 1973.

Rinke LT and Wilson AA: Outcome measures in home care; vol II Service, New York, 1988, National League for Nursing.

Rinke LT and Wilson AA: Client-oriented project objectives, Caring 7(1):25-29, 1988.

Sabatino CP: The "Black Box" of home care quality: a report of the American Bar Association, Presented by Chairman, Select Committee, US House of Representatives, Pub No 99-537, Washington, DC, August 1986, US Government Printing Office.

Schmadl JC: Quality assurance: examination of the concept, Nurs Outlook 27:462-465, 1979.

Sienkiewicz JI: Patient classification in community health nursing, Nurs Outlook 32:319-321, 1984.

Simmons DA, Martin KS, Crews CC, and Scheet NJ: Client management information system for community health nursing agencies, NTIS Accession No HRP-0907023, Springfield, Va, 1986, National Technical Information Service.

Spratt CE: How one hospital copes with the demands of quality assurance. In Tobias RB, ed: A study guide in quality assurance and utilization review, Camp Hill, Pa, 1984, American College of Utilization Review Physicians.

Tehan J and Colegrove SL: Risk management and home health care: the time is now. In Fisher K and Gardner K, eds: Quality and home health care: redefining the tradition, Chicago, 1987, Joint Commission on Accreditation of Healthcare Organizations.

Wandelt MA and Ager JW: Quality patient care scale, New York, 1974, Appleton-Century-Crofts.

Wandelt MA and Stewart DS: Slater nursing competencies rating scale, New York, 1974, Appleton-Century-Crofts.

Weed LL: Medical records, medical education and patient care, Chicago, 1970, Year Book.

SELECTED BIBLIOGRAPHY

Accreditation Division for Home Care and Community Health, National League for Nursing: Accreditation criteria, standards, and substantiating evidences, New York, 1987, The League.

Bernal H: Levels of practice in a community health agency, Nurs Outlook 23:364-369, 1978.

Ceglarek JE and Rife JK: Developing a public health nursing audit, J Nurs Adm 10:37-43, 1977.

Flynn BC and Ray DW: Current perspectives in quality assurance and community health nursing, J Community Health Nurs 4:187-197, 1987.

Hand JS, Bruno P, Feffer DA, and Plath SL: Home health audit tool—at last, Home Health Rev 4:15-22, 1981.

Harrington C: Quality, access, and costs: public policy and home health care, Nurs Outlook 36:164-166, 1988.

Jackson MM and Lynch P: Applying an epidemiological structure to risk management and quality assurance activities, Quality Rev Bull 11(10):306-312, 1985.

Lang NM and Clinton JF: Assessment of quality of nursing care. In Werley HH and Fitzpatrick JJ, eds: Annual review of nursing research, vol 2, New York, 1984, Springer.

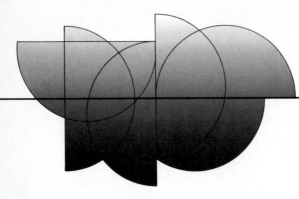

23

Challenges for the Future

If you do not think about the future, you cannot have one.

JOHN GALSWORTHY
SWAN SONG, 1928

OBJECTIVES

Upon completion of this chapter, the reader will be able to:

1. *Describe how technology will change the health care delivery system.*
2. *Relate changes in the acute care delivery system to service provision in the home setting.*
3. *Discuss significant nursing challenges in the next decade.*
4. *Identify ethical issues encountered by community health nurses and the role of an ethics committee in addressing these issues.*
5. *Explain how political involvement can shape the health care system.*
6. *Discuss the concept "health care for all."*

What is the future for community health nursing? As Chapter 1 demonstrated, political and social events helped to shape the development of community health nursing leaders like Florence Nightingale and Lillian Wald, and in turn shaped the nursing profession. Such events continue to shape nursing and will do so in the future.

Nursing needs to plan for the future. This planning will allow us to contribute to change instead of only being reactive to it. Nurses need to be instrumental in shaping the health care of tomorrow, as well as meeting the challenges that tomorrow will bring. The revolution that is occurring in health care is putting increased emphasis on disease prevention and health promotion, the realization that there are limitations to what health science can do, and the need to control the astronomical increases in health care costs (Wilson, 1988, p. 402).

It remains to be seen how community health nursing will meet growing challenges, such as health care delivery and accessibility issues, consumer accountability, nursing liberation, reimbursement and role changes, the nursing shortage, changing demands in nursing education, expanding need for nursing research, ethical issues, and politics and nursing. There is a certain amount of risk taking in predicting and planning the future. However, community health nursing will be viable and relevant only as we are willing to take these risks.

HEALTH CARE DELIVERY AND ACCESSIBILITY

Technology has driven changes in the health care delivery system and will continue to do so (Christman, 1987, p. 217). Twenty years ago VCRs, PCs, and CDs were unknown to the general public and now are commonplace. Today corresponding types of complex and sophisticated technology are being introduced into the health care system. New medicines and vaccines are being developed, complicated operating room equipment is being utilized, genetic engineering is being explored, and in vitro fertilization is being done. It is difficult for health care workers to keep up with the rapid pace of technology, but staying proficient is

crucial to the provision of safe and quality health care. As the year 2000 approaches, technologic advances will increase sharply, and every reader of this text will be affected by them in some way. More diagnostic and treatment services will continue to be delivered outside the hospital in settings such as the home, clinics, outpatient centers, and long-term care facilities. The inpatient setting will become more technically sophisticated, and increasingly specialized in providing only the most critical and intensive care (McMannis Associates, 1989).

Futurists predict the following health care delivery system (McMannis Associates, 1989): *Super tertiary advanced technology centers* of 200 or 300 beds, located regionally, that provide care for the most seriously ill who require 24-hour intensive care; *Community care centers* of 50 to 75 beds located in suburban areas that are less sophisticated and less expensive than the technology centers; *Comprehensive ambulatory care centers* that provide mainstream medicine and surgery on an outpatient basis; *Diagnostic and therapeutic treatment centers* which will handle rehabilitative and restorative care for the aging population; and *extended care facilities* that are multilevel and provide care for people with chronic and long-term care needs. The incidence and prevalence of chronic and long-term conditions are significant and rising (refer to Chapters 11 and 17). People with these conditions have created an ongoing demand for nursing care. It will be a challenge to nursing to stay in the forefront of care to this population group and to provide quality comprehensive services.

Service provision in the home care setting has become a reality and is growing rapidly. Home care agencies and services are found in both the public and private sectors, and the private, for-profit sector is evidencing amazing growth. This has been due largely to the incentive under prospective payment to discharge patients as early as possible. Health care is shifting to the home and community, and the demand for nursing services is increasing dramatically. Nursing faces a major challenge in meeting these demands.

Lack of accessibility to health care services often results from the service not existing in the first place, lack of knowledge about the service, inability to pay for the service, or inability/difficulty in accessing the services (e.g., transportation). The cost of health care is a critical obstacle to accessibility, and we have reached a point in the United States at which the average person cannot afford to be sick (Maraldo, 1989, p. 302). Accessibility of health care for many at-risk and underserved populations, such as inner city and rural residents, the aged, people who are handicapped, and the medically indigent, is an urgent need that must be addressed.

CONSUMER INVOLVEMENT

Consumers of health care as well as professionals are recognizing the importance of finding ways to meet the needs of underserved populations in our society. Sophisticated consumers are having more to say about the type of care they receive and are increasingly being seen as key members of the health care team. Consumer groups, such as the American Association of Retired Persons (AARP), are advocating needed services for their members. This has prompted providers of care to be more responsive to consumer demands and needs.

Effectiveness and efficiency in the delivery of quality health care services are prime foci for improvement in all health care settings. In this era of limited resources, these foci are essential. Evidence of unmet health care need is prevalent among many segments of the American population and will continue to exist until more appropriate health care delivery patterns are developed. This challenge for the future cannot be ignored. Involving consumers in addressing this challenge can strengthen the position of health care professionals who are advocating needed changes.

NURSING LIBERATION: REIMBURSEMENT AND EXPANDED ROLES

Nurses have recognized that changes must occur in traditional nursing roles in order to address the current challenges in the health care delivery system. The role of the nurse is expanding and greater opportunities for nurses are available. Nurses are providing many preventive health ser-

vices for the "healthy" population, and cost-effective fee-for-service activities. Research on the cost effectiveness of the nurse provider reflects that nurses can reduce health care costs, while at the same time improve access to health care and quality of care (Ten trends, 1986, p. 19). More states are enacting legislation that allows reimbursement for nursing services. The nursing profession can expect resistance from organized medicine in relation to this "competition," and nursing's expanded role, especially as the medical profession faces a personpower surplus with the potential of lost revenue (Ten trends, 1986, p. 18).

A recent and interesting nursing role predicted for the 1990s and beyond is that of the *traveling nurse*. The idea originated with TravCorps, Inc. of Massachusetts in 1978. In 1981, Humana Corporation established its Mobile Nurse Corps to enable its numerous hospitals in 20 states to have adequate nursing staff during periods of high admission and emergencies; there are now more than 70 mobile nurse agencies in the United States (Baumann JR, 1990, p. 8D). Traveling nurses go from one assignment to another around the country and are being used in community-based as well as institutional settings. *Working Woman* listed the traveling nurse as one of the 25 "hottest" careers of the 1990s (Baumann JR, 1990, p. 8D). Nursing roles and job opportunities in *occupational health, gerontology, preventive health, health education, and long-term care* are expanding, many nurses are needed in these areas, and many academic programs are increasingly addressing the need to prepare nurses for such roles.

It will be a challenge to nursing to adapt to the roles necessary to meet increasingly complex and diverse health care needs. As interesting and exciting new roles emerge and traditional roles change, continuing education will be an integral part of role fulfillment.

THE NURSING SHORTAGE

Today's nurse is better educated and better paid, and has more opportunities than ever before (Lass, 1990, p. 5D). Nurses—not doctors or other health care professionals—provide more than 80 percent of all direct patient care (Hawken, 1990, p. 5D). At the same time, across the nation there is a shortage of nurses that is putting the quality of patient care in jeopardy.

By the year 2000, the USDHHS predicts a shortage of almost 600,000 baccalaureate-prepared nurses, and this shortage is expected to reach more than 1 million by the year 2020 (Joel, 1990, p. 7D). By the year 2000 there will be a need for twice as many nurses with masters and doctoral degrees as will be available (Lass, 1990, p. 5D). One has only to peruse the classified ads in the local newspaper to appreciate that many hospitals and community health nursing agencies are desperate for nurses and are making tempting recruitment offers.

One outcome of the nursing shortage is that international nurses are being recruited to the United States to help fill the gap (Baumann LA, 1990, p. 8D). However, international nurses may not be familiar with the American health care system, health care resources, culture or language, all of which raise additional quality of care issues. The nursing shortage, and its effect on the quality of care, will be a major issue in the 21st century. Ways to prepare all nurses to successfully function in our health care system must be addressed.

NURSING EDUCATION

Educators will need to rise to the challenges and prepare nurses to function in the new health care delivery system. All nurses will also have to stand firm as training programs for physician assistants and technicians are suggested as a solution to resolving the personpower shortage. These types of personnel are not prepared to provide nursing care, and thus cannot alleviate the nursing shortage.

Addressing the nursing shortage challenge will undoubtedly result in a number of nontraditional educational settings being developed and implemented. Career ladders in nursing will need to be reassessed and facilitated. Options, such as masters programs that provide both basic and advanced preparation for professionals with college degrees in other areas will need to be expanded.

There is a growing need for graduate education for nurses (Moccia, 1989, p. 16; Ten trends, 1986, p. 19). There is also a need for continuing education to help nursing faculty and other nurses keep up to date on advances and technology. Issues such as level of entry into practice, funding of nursing education, and continuing education must be addressed in the 21st century.

NURSING RESEARCH

Nursing research reached new heights with the establishment of the National Center for Nursing Research (NCNR) within the National Institutes of Health. Research is an essential part of nursing as well as a career opportunity (Hinshaw, 1988, p. 54). Approximately 45 to 50 schools of nursing now offer doctoral degrees for nurses interested in doing research (Hinshaw, 1990, p. 8D). The emphasis on nursing research has been impressively supported by the major nursing organizations, has broadened nursing's theoretical base, and has added to the prestige of the profession.

In 1981, the American Nurses' Association put forth priority areas for nursing research that remain applicable. These are as follows:

1. Promoting health, well-being, and competency for personal care among all age groups
2. Preventing health problems throughout the life-span that have the potential to reduce productivity and satisfaction
3. Decreasing the negative impact of health problems on coping abilities, productivity, and satisfaction
4. Ensuring that the care needs of particularly vulnerable groups are met through appropriate strategies
5. Designing and developing health care systems that are cost effective in meeting the nursing needs of the population
6. Promoting health, well-being, and competency for personal health in all age groups

In 1989, the National Center for Nursing Research reaffirmed the need to focus research activities on health promotion across the life-span, nursing care needs of vulnerable groups, and the development of health care delivery systems to meet the nursing needs of at-risk aggregates. The priority research areas NCNR has under consideration address these areas. Research is an exciting area of nursing that should show great strides during the next decade.

Community health nursing, by definition, deals with populations across all age groups and focuses on prevention and health planning for vulnerable groups. Thus, nurses in this practice area are in a unique position to identify significant, researchable questions relative to the ANA's and NCNR's priorities. Participating in research activities is one way for the practitioner to begin to address the challenges of the future. Becoming involved in political activities and ethical decision making are other ways to ensure that cost-effective, quality health care is available to people in need.

ETHICS IN COMMUNITY HEALTH NURSING PRACTICE

Rapid changes in the health care delivery system have made life more complex and have provoked dilemmas never before faced by consumers or health care providers. It is becoming increasingly difficult for professionals in many situations to discern what should or should not be done. Appendix 9-1 (pp. 328–330) is a scenario of some of the questions raised by the participants in sophisticated health care of a child: Should a child have to live her or his life in a hospital? Is such a life of enough quality to make it meaningful? Is the terrible expense for the care of one such child possible, and what will happen when increasing numbers of children need the same care? How justly are the rest of the children in the family being treated when one family member consumes so much time?

The ability to preserve lives that once could not be saved and governmental cutbacks in health care spending have forced community health nurses to examine the concept of human rights and choices. Cost containment has produced many ethical questions in health care and is forcing us into a two-tiered system of health care—

one for those who can pay and one for those who cannot (Ten trends, 1986, p. 18).

Community health nurses must make decisions about whose rights prevail and which client they should serve when resources are not sufficient for meeting the needs of *all* client groups. They must also examine how their choices about the delivery of health care services have impacted on various consumers and consumer groups. Gaining an understanding of ethics can assist nurses to better deal with these complex and often confusing practice issues.

Ethics is the study of choices made by individuals and groups in their relationships to one another. The development of a code of ethics is basic to a profession because it provides a means for that profession to regulate its practice. It also helps its members to make choices relative to clinical practice concerns.

A code indicates a profession's acceptance of the responsibility and trust with which it has been invested by society. Upon entering the profession of nursing, each person inherits a measure of the responsibility and trust that has accrued to nursing over the years and the corresponding obligation to adhere to the profession's code of conduct and relationships for ethical practice (American Nurses' Association, 1985).

The American Nurses' Association adopted its code in 1950; it is revised periodically (ANA, 1985). The most recent revision was published in 1985.

Professional codes of ethics are statements encompassing rules that apply to persons in professional roles and that are *voluntarily* adopted by the group themselves (Beauchamp, 1982). Many national organizations involved in promoting quality health and health-related services are increasingly developing a code of ethics for their membership. These codes are designed to preserve the basic rights of clients in an honest and ethical manner. For example, the National Association for Home Care (NAHC) adopted its Code of Ethics in 1982 to demonstrate to the general public that NAHC and its individual members stand for integrity and the highest ethical standards. NAHC's Code of Ethics elaborates on patient rights and responsibilities; relationships to other provider agencies; responsibility to NAHC; fiscal responsibilities; marketing and public relations; responsibilities to employees; and processes for handing code violations (NAHC, 1982).

In a *perfect* world, everyone's rights and choices are respected. However, in the *real* world, some people are more respected than others (lawyers receive more respect than sanitation workers), and some people are often not respected at all (the poor and the disabled). Human choices are affected by one's attitude and environment. For example, some nurses believe that selective abortion should be the right of all women. Others believe, due to cultural influences or to personal or religious beliefs, that abortion is categorically wrong. Changes in our society are making choices such as these much more difficult. Naisbitt (1984) describes one of the megatrends in the United States as a move from an either/or option to a multiple-options situation: There is no longer any objectively "right" answer to many questions, which presents ethical dilemmas for professionals in all health care settings. These dilemmas include multiple-option situations such as how to deal with conflicting needs of patients and caregivers; when to hospitalize a terminally ill client; resolving conflicts between what is ordered and what is needed; allowing "death with dignity"; maintaining agency standards of productivity while competently meeting increasingly complex care needs of clients; giving pain medication even if early death might be an unavoidable consequence of pain control; and provision of service based on payor regulations (Lund, 1989; Michigan Home Health Assembly, 1990; Pignatello, Moulton, and Eng, 1988).

Ethics attempts to identify, examine, and justify human acts by applying certain principles to determine the right thing to do in specific situations (Wellman, 1975, p. 317). Curtain and Flaherty (1982) write that there are two ethical approaches which influence decision making: normative and nonnormative. Individuals using normative approaches work within definite interpretations of right and wrong. In contrast, individuals who support nonnormative approaches deny that universal rules for making decisions exist. They use basically subjective internal processes such as emotivism, skepticism, and relativism. Rightness and wrongness are determined within situations and not by them. Utilizing the nonnormative approach, a decision to abort a fetus might be considered unethical for a woman at one point in time, and completely ethical for this *same woman* at another point in time. Those who use the normative approach state that there are universal principles of right and wrong that should not be broken and would not consider abortion wrong at one time and right at another. However, this view also holds that general principles are interpreted differently by different people. Each approach has its strengths and weaknesses and neither one is completely adequate for all ethical decision making.

To discuss complex ethical issues, some writers are advocating the development of ethics committees that can deal with complex questions of client care as well as policy making and budget and personnel decisions (Aroskar, 1984). Roles and functions of such a committee could include the following (Lynn, 1983):

1. Identifying the types of cases that should be reviewed
2. Assuring correct determination of decision-making competence
3. Providing a responsive mechanism that assures that the interests of all parties, especially those of the patient, have been adequately represented in decision making (thus protecting the competent patient)
4. Reviewing surrogate applicants for patients who cannot make their own decisions
5. Protecting the incompetent patient's interests
6. Reviewing and revising institutional decision-making policies related to ethical concerns
7. Educating the committee and others in the institution
8. Determining which cases need attention from outside the institution, such as the courts

9. Considering how economic costs will be considered in making patient care decisions and in the development of related policies

Ethics committees are most often found in inpatient settings. This, however, should not be the norm. Community health nurses regularly encounter ethical dilemmas that are difficult to resolve, such as when to allow adolescents the right to make choices about health care which differ from their parents' choices and when to ask for legal intervention when parents are neglecting their children. Assistance from an ethics committee can help nurses in the community to more effectively handle these and other complex issues. At times, nurses leave a practice field, because they have not been successful in resolving the ethical dilemmas which they encounter in that field. Support from colleagues might prevent this.

An in-depth discussion about ethics and ethical issues in community health nursing practice is far beyond the scope of this text. A pamphlet issued by the American Nurses' Association (1982), *Ethics References for Nurses,* provides a valuable guide for identifying resources available in the field of ethics. Use of these resources is encouraged; ethical dilemmas cannot be avoided in the community health setting.

POLITICAL INVOLVEMENT

The most powerful approach that nurses can take to shape the future is the political approach. It is vital that nurses understand, actively participate in, and provide leadership in politics and the political process (Wilson, 1988, p. 403). Nurses comprise the largest group of health care providers in the country, and numbers alone give them a powerful majority. Today's nurses are becoming more politically active, visible, and powerful and are providing leadership in health care delivery. They must continue to grow in their sophistication and use of politics and expand their involvement in political activities.

Nurses sit on local and state boards of health, in policy positions for local, state, national and international governments and organizations, and in the executive offices of many private corporations (Hawken, 1990, p. 5D). National nursing groups have organized for political action, and are becoming increasingly effective. The establishment of the National Center for Nursing Research is an example of their political "savvy" and expertise. Nursing has the opportunity to shape a national health plan (Maraldo, 1989, p. 304), and exert influence nationally on health policies.

Politics can be defined as the art of influencing the actions of others for the purposes of promoting specified goals and protecting one's interests (Kalisch and Kalisch, 1976). Political action usually involves activities directed toward influencing the behavior of governmental officials and other individuals in powerful positions. Politics and nursing are inseparable and, in fact, politics *is* an integral part of nursing. The relationship between federal legislation and health care (costs, programs, education and services) cannot be denied. The federal government is heavily involved in health care and has a great influence on it through legislation and funding.

The political arena is where health care decisions are made, decisions that will bear on health care for all of us. More than 2500 health-related bills and resolutions are introduced into every 2-year federal congressional session (Davis, Oakley, and Sochalski, 1982). Not all of these are major pieces of legislation, and only a few will be enacted into law, but it is evident that the federal government is involved in health care. Nurses need to have an impact on this legislation! Thus, they need to keep abreast of what is happening and disseminate this information to others, and they must be persistent in their efforts to influence decisions about health care policy.

Politics involve people: Nurses have highly developed people-oriented skills that present a real political advantage. Use these skills when working with legislators and officials. Getting to know people in politically influential positions can help one to achieve community health goals.

Politicians are open to the opinions of their constituents, even if they do not agree with them. They know they may not be reelected if their constituency is ignored or does not like what they are doing. Many members of Congress are more impressed with a constituent's story than they are with the sophisticated analyses or extensive reports that pass before them (Donley, 1979, p. 1948).

There are many levels of political involvement for nurses. Kalisch and Kalisch (1981) have described levels ranging from spectator to gladiator. The spectators have gone one level above political apathy and are in the process of exposing themselves to political stimuli and collecting political information. From spectator, one moves into transitional activities such as writing letters, sending telegrams, making phone calls, arranging meetings with officials and legislators, making political contributions, and attending political meetings. This is usually done on an individual basis. Once the nurse moves into group or collective activities, he or she is moving into the gladiator role. Gladiator activities can include political campaign work such as helping a candidate to be elected or working against the election of an unresponsive candidate, running for political office, taking an active role in the political aspects of professional organizations, lobbying, and seeking to get legislation passed or changed.

Nurses need political organization: the potential of an organized, informed group is unlimited. Nurses need to support the organized political activities that already exist through their professional organizations. The American Nurses' Association and the National League for Nursing are very active politically. The ANA has established congressional district coordinators in each of the nation's 435 congressional districts to ensure that all nurses in each district are registered to vote, that they have all the necessary information about candidates and issues, and mainly that they *vote.*

Perhaps one of our priorities should be to have nurses elected to Congress so they can explain firsthand to fellow representatives or fellow senators what this country's health care problems are and what nurses could do to alleviate them. Nurses have the knowledge and skills needed to make significant changes in our health care system.

HEALTH CARE FOR ALL: A MAJOR CHALLENGE FOR THE 1990s

The American Public Health Association (APHA) has openly and aggressively championed the right to "health care for all" in the United States. This is a noble goal, and one that will take much time and effort to achieve. In 1963, President Lyndon Johnson shared with the American public that "Yesterday is not ours to recover but tomorrow is ours to win or lose." This statement is wholly applicable to the state of health care. We must move ahead to a better health care delivery system. We must focus on the future rather than lament about the past, and we must learn from our mistakes. Although data suggest that there are significant difficulties in our health care system that presently prevent the nation from providing comprehensive health care, these obstacles can be overcome. The United States has had a long list of accomplishments in health care delivery and has a strong potential for achieving major public health accomplishments.

The 1990s will bring many challenges as well as opportunities. "Health for all" will be a major battle to win in the next decade. This will involve *taking action* to address emerging threats to the health of the public while containing continuing long-existing threats. These threats include *immediate crises,* such as the AIDS epidemic and inadequate health care for disadvantaged aggregates; *enduring problems,* such as injuries, chronic illness, and infant mortality; and *impending crises,* such as long-term care needs of populations across the life-span and control of toxic wastes (Institute of Medicine, 1988, p. 1).

The "health for all" challenge emphasizes access to health care which will enable all people to lead productive and satisfying lives. It involves addressing the inequities in society and within the health care system which prevent people from achieving health, and it focuses on the shared responsibility of people for their own health. This battle requires implementing strategies that promote broad-based planning for health and development rather than for health services only. It demands a strong emphasis on political action, policy formulation, multidisciplinary practice, sound managerial functioning, and constituency building (Maglacas, 1988; Institute of Medicine, 1988). Constituency building is a "must." Current and future threats to our nation's public health will require collective action if they are to be resolved.

Let us as community health nurses think about the future so that we have the very best one possible! Let us follow Lillian Wald and lead the way.

SUMMARY

Community health professionals face many challenges. They are being asked to assume responsibility for care of unprecedented complexity and to plan services for multiple, diverse population groups. They must make some difficult decisions about the best means of allocating scarce resources, which often presents ethical dilemmas not easily solved. Competition has increased the number of selected types of community-based services, especially reimbursable home health care, but has not necessarily strengthened services for those most in need. There is, for example, a limited supply of appropriate long-term care resources, even though the demand for these resources is dramatically increasing.

Sophisticated technology, spiraling health care costs, demographic changes, and political decisions are dramatically influencing future directions in the health care delivery system. Community-based care is emphasized, preventive health services are promoted, self-care is stressed, and competition among health care providers is fostered. These trends present both challenges and opportunities for health care providers and consumers alike. To shape the future, health professionals must be risk takers. They must handle ethical dilemmas and engage in research activities to document the need for and the effectiveness of preventive health services, and they must be politically *active*.

REFERENCES

American Nurses' Association (ANA): Code for nurses with interpretive statements, ANA Pub Code No G-58, Kansas City, Mo, 1985, The Association.

ANA: Research priorities for the 1980s: generating a scientific basis for nursing practice, ANA Pub Code No D-68, Kansas City, Mo, 1981, The Association.

ANA: Ethics references for nurses, ANA Pub Code No G-159, 3M, Kansas City, Mo, 1982, The Association.

Aroskar M: Institutional ethics committees and nursing administration, Nurs Economics 2:132-136, 1984.

Baumann JR: Nursing opportunities in America. Traveling nurses: trend of the 90s, USA Today, p 8D, January 25, 1990.

Baumann LA: Nursing opportunities in America: international nurses, USA Today, p 8D, January 25, 1990.

Beauchamp TL: Philosophical ethics, New York, 1982, McGraw-Hill.

Christman L: A view to the future, Nurs Outlook 35(6):216-218, 1987.

Curtain L and Flaherty J: Nursing ethics: theories and pragmatics, Bowie, Md, 1982, Brady.

Davis CK, Oakley D, and Sochalski JA: Leadership for expanding nursing influence on health policy, J Nurs Adm 12:15-21, 1982.

Donley R: An inside view of the Washington health scene, Am J Nurs 79:1946-1952, 1979.

Donley R: Health policy and nursing practice—a vision of the 21st century, Paper presented at conference. New Directions for Nursing: The Future is Now, University of Tennessee (Knoxville) College of Nursing, June 16, 1984.

Hawken PI: Nursing opportunities in America: nursing education for the 21st century, USA Today, p 5D, January 25, 1990.

Hinshaw AS: The national center for nursing research: challenges and initiatives, Nurs Outlook 36(2):54, 56, 1988.

Hinshaw AS: Nursing opportunities in America. Research: a career opportunity for nurses, USA Today, p 8D, January 25, 1990.

Institute of Medicine: The future of public health, Washington, DC, 1988, National Academy Press.

Joel LA: Nursing opportunities in America: growing demand for BSN-prepared nurses, USA Today, p 7D, January 25, 1990.

Kalisch BJ and Kalisch PA: A discourse on the politics of nursing, J Nurs Adm 6:29-34, 1976.

Kalisch BJ and Kalisch PA: Politics of nursing, Philadelphia, 1981, Lippincott.

Lass LY: Nursing opportunities in America. Today's nurses: better education, better paid, more opportunities, USA Today, p 5D, January 25, 1990.

Lund M: Nursing home dilemmas, Geriat Nurs 10:298-300, 1989.

Lynn J: The role and functions of institutional ethics committees: the President's commission view, Paper presented at the Conference on Institutional Ethics Committees: Their Role in Medical Decision Making, Washington, DC, April 21, 1983.

Maglacas AM: Health for all: nursing's role, Nurs Outlook 36:66-71, 1988.

Mahler H: What is health for all? World Health, pp 3-5, November 1979.

Mallison MB: Gender gap in politics, Am J Nurs 83:175, 1984.

Maraldo PJ: Home care should be the heart of a nursing-sponsored national health plan, Nurs Health Care 10(6):301-304, 1989.

McMannis Associates, Health Care Strategy Group: Technology 2000: a window to the future, Washington, DC, 1989, The Associates.

Michigan Home Health Assembly, Ethics Committee: Ethical dilemmas experienced by professionals in home health care, unpublished research project, East Lansing, Mi, 1990, The Assembly.

Moccia P: 1989: shaping a human agenda for the nineties. Trends that demand our attention as managed care prevails, Nurs Health Care 10(1):15-17, 1989.

Naisbitt J: Megatrends. Ten new directions transforming our lives, New York, 1984, Warner.

National Association for Home Care (NAHC): Code of ethics, Washington, DC, 1982, The Association.

Office of Information and Legislative Affairs: National Center for Nursing Research: facts about funding, Bethesda, Md, 1989, National Center for Nursing Research.

Pignatello CH, Moulton P, and Eng MA: Ethical concerns of home health administration: the day-to-day issues. In Harris MD, ed: Home health administration, Owings Mills, Md, 1988, National Health.

Ten trends to watch, Nurs Health Care 7(1):17-19, 1986.

Wellman C: Morals and ethics, Glenview, Il, 1975, Scott, Foresman.

Wilson LM: The American health care revolution, Am Assoc Occupat Health Nurs J 36(10):402-407, 1988.

SELECTED BIBLIOGRAPHY

Fry S: Dilemma in community health ethics, Nurs Outlook 31:176-179, 1983.

Fry S: Rationing health care, Nurs Econ 1:165-169, 1983.

Maraldo PJ: Politics, a very human matter, Am J Nurs 82:1104-1105, 1982.

Maraldo PJ: Nursing as a political force—making our own destiny, Paper presented at conference New Directions for Nursing. The Future Is Now, University of Tennessee (Knoxville) College of Nursing, June 16, 1984.

Milio N: The realities of policymaking: can nurses have an impact? J Nurs Adm 14:18-23, 1984.

Puetz B: Networking for nurses, Rockville, Md, 1983, Aspen.

Rosner D: Health care for the "truly needy": nineteenth-century origins of the concept, Milbank Q 60:355-385, 1982.

Silva M: Ethics, scarce resources, and the nurse executive, Nurs Economics 2:11-18, 1984.

Stewart MJ: From provider to partner: a conceptual framework for nursing education based on primary health care premises, Adv Nurs Sci 12:9-23, 1990.

Ward P: Public health nursing and the future of public health, Public Health Nurs 6:163-168, 1989.

INDEX

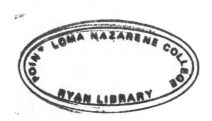

Ingredients for Success.

NEW!
POCKET GUIDE TO FAMILY ASSESSMENT
AND INTERVENTION
Karen Mischke Berkey, RN, PhD; Shirley M.H. Hanson, RN, PMHNP, PhD, FAAN
(0-8016-5886-1) December 1990. Approx. 250 pages.
This handy spiral-bound reference provides a framework for assessing families and implementing effective intervention strategies. Employing a holistic approach to family care, it includes theory as well as valuable assessment, intervention, and evaluation techniques.

NEW!
PERSPECTIVES IN FAMILY AND COMMUNITY HEALTH
Karen Saucier, RN, PhD
(0-8016-4338-4) March 1991. Approx. 512 pages.
This collection of state-of-the-art articles reflects the contemporary practice of community health nursing. The text provides a wide variety of valuable perspectives on issues, trends, research, and the application of community health nursing techniques. A few "classic" articles which provide timeless or historical perspectives are interwoven with the contemporary views.

HEALTH PROMOTION THROUGHOUT THE LIFE SPAN
2nd Edition
Carole Edelman, RN, MS; Carole Lynn Mandle, RN, PhD
(0-8016-3260-9) 1990. 616 pages.
This popular text addresses the important role of the nurse in the promotion of health and prevention of illness. The updated second edition develops related theory and presents essential skills nurses need in the effective provision of nursing care to the healthy person.

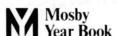

**Mosby
Year Book**

To order ask your bookstore manager or call toll-free 800-426-4545. We look forward to hearing from you soon.